ELSEVIER
SAUNDERS

3251 Riverport Lane
St. Louis, MO 63043

EQUINE EMERGENCIES: TREATMENT AND PROCEDURES,
FOURTH EDITION

ISBN: 978-1-4557-0892-5

ISBN: 978-1-4557-0892-5

Vice President and Publisher: Linda Duncan
Content Strategy Director: Penny Rudolph
Content Manager: Shelly Stringer
Publishing Services Manager: Catherine Jackson
Project Manager: Carol O'Connell
Design Direction: Karen Pauls

Working together
to grow libraries in
developing countries

www.elsevier.com • www.bookaid.org

Printed in India

Last digit is the print number: 9   8   7

Equine
EMERGENCIES
Treatment and Procedures

Fourth Edition

EDITORS

James A. Orsini, DVM, DACVS
Associate Professor of Surgery
New Bolton Center
School of Veterinary Medicine
University of Pennsylvania
Kennett Square, Pennsylvania

Thomas J. Divers, DVM, DACVIM, DACVECC
Professor
Large Animal Medicine
Cornell University College of Veterinary Medicine
Cornell University Hospital for Animals
Cornell University
Ithaca, New York

Contributors

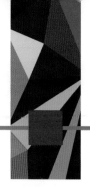

Helen Aceto, PhD, VMD
Assistant Professor of Veterinary Epidemiology, Director of
   Biosecurity
Department of Clinical Studies—New Bolton Center
School of Veterinary Medicine
University of Pennsylvania
Kennett Square, Pennsylvania
Contagious and Zoonotic Diseases
Standard Precautions and Infectious Disease Management

Robert Agne, DVM
Associate
Podiatry
Rood and Riddle Equine Hospital
Lexington, Kentucky
Foot Injuries

Ellison Aldrich, VMD
Large Animal Surgery Resident
Department of Clinical Sciences
College of Veterinary Medicine and Biomedical Sciences
Colorado State University
Fort Collins, Colorado
Emergency Diagnostic Endoscopy

Fairfield T. Bain, DVM, MBA, DACVIM, ACVP, DACVECC
Clinical Professor of Equine Internal Medicine
Department of Veterinary Clinical Sciences
College of Veterinary Medicine
Washington State University
Pullman, Washington
Hyperbaric Oxygen Therapy
Respiratory System—Respiratory Tract Emergencies
Respiratory System—Strangles: Diagnostic Approach and
   Management

Alexandre Secorun Borges, DVM, MS, PhD
Professor, Large Animal Internal Medicine
Department of Clinical Sciences
Sao Paulo State University–UNESP
Botucatu, SP, Brazil
Emergency Diseases Unique to Countries Outside the Continental
   United States: South America

Benjamin R. Buchanan, DVM, DACVIM, DACVECC
Brazos Valley Equine Hospital
Navasota, Texas
Snake Envenomation

Alexandra J. Burton, BSc, BVSc, DACVIM
Large Animal Medicine
College of Veterinary Medicine
The University of Georgia
Athens, Georgia
Emergency Treatment of Mules and Donkeys

Stuart C. Clark-Price, DVM, MS, DACVIM, DACVA
Assistant Professor of Anesthesia and Pain Management
Department of Veterinary Clinical Medicine
University of Illinois
Urbana, Illinois
Anesthesia for Out of Hospital Emergencies

Kevin T. Corley, BVM&S, PhD, DACVIM, DACVECC, DECEIM, MRCVS
Specialist, Equine Medicine and Critical Care
Anglesey Lodge Equine Hospital
The Curragh, Co
Kildare, Ireland
Director
Veterinary Advances Ltd
The Curragh, Co
Kildare, Ireland
Foal Resuscitation

J. Barry David, DVM, DACVIM
Hagyard Equine Medical Institute
Lexington, Kentucky
Gastrointestinal System—Acute Infectious and Toxic Diarrheal
   Diseases in the Adult Horse

Elizabeth J. Davidson, DVM, DACVS, DACVSMR
Associate Professor in Sports Medicine
Department of Clinical Studies—New Bolton Center
School of Veterinary Medicine
University of Pennsylvania
Kennett Square, Pennsylvania
Musculoskeletal System—Diagnostic and Therapeutic Procedures
Musculoskeletal System—Arthrocentesis and Synovial Fluid Analysis
Musculoskeletal System—Temporomandibular Arthrocentesis
Musculoskeletal System—Cervical Vertebral Articular Process
   Injections
Musculoskeletal System—Sacroiliac Injections

Stephen G. Dill, DVM, DACVIM
Certified by the International Veterinary Acupuncture Society
Certified by the American Veterinary Chiropractic Association
Remington, Virginia
Complementary Therapies in Emergencies: Acupuncture

Thomas J. Divers, DVM, DACVIM, DACVECC
Professor
Large Animal Medicine
Cornell University Hospital for Animals
Department of Clinical Sciences
Cornell University College of Veterinary Medicine
Cornell University
Ithaca, New York
Emergency and Critical Care Monitoring
Emergency Laboratory Tests and Point-of-Care Diagnostics
Gastrointestinal System—Acute Salivation (Ptyalism)
Gastrointestinal System—Stomach and Duodenum: Gastric Ulcers
Gastrointestinal System—Diarrhea in Weanlings and Yearlings
Gastrointestinal System—Acute Infectious and Toxic Diarrheal
  Diseases in the Adult Horse
Liver Failure, Anemia and Blood Transfusion
Nervous System—Neurologic Emergencies
Respiratory System—Respiratory Tract Emergencies
Urinary System—Urinary Tract Emergencies
Shock and Systemic Inflammatory Response Syndrome
Temperature Related Problems: Hypothermia and Hyperthermia
Euthanasia/Humane Destruction
Adverse Drug Reactions, Air Emboli, and Lightning Strike
Specific Acute Drug Reactions and Recommended Treatments
Equine Emergency Drugs: Approximate Dosages and Adverse Drug
  Reactions

Tamara Dobbie, DVM, DACT
Staff Veterinarian in Reproduction
Department of Clinical Studies—New Bolton Center
George D. Widener Hospital for Large Animals
School of Veterinary Medicine
University of Pennsylvania
Kennett Square, Pennsylvania
Reproduction System—Stallion Reproductive Emergencies
Reproduction System—Mare Reproductive Emergencies
Monitoring the Pregnant Mare
Emergency Foaling

Bernd Driessen, DVM, PhD, DACVA, DECVPT
Professor of Anesthesiology
Department of Clinical Studies—New Bolton Center
School of Veterinary Medicine
University of Pennsylvania
Kennett Square, Pennsylvania
Pain Management

Edward T. Earley, DVM, FAVD/Eq
AP Residency
Dentistry
Cornell University Hospital for Animals
Cornell University
Ithaca, New York
Partner
Laurel Highland Veterinary Clinic, LLC
Williamsport, Pennsylvania
Gastrointestinal System—Dental Radiology Ambulatory Techniques
Gastrointestinal System—Upper Gastrointestinal Emergencies: Teeth

David L. Foster, VMD, DAVDC
Adjunct Associate Professor
Large Animal Surgery—Equine Dentistry
George D. Widener Hospital for Large Animals
New Bolton Center
School of Veterinary Medicine
University of Pennsylvania
Kennett Square, Pennsylvania
Owner/Veterinarian
Equine Dental Services of New Jersey
Morganville, New Jersey
Gastrointestinal System—Aging Guidelines
Gastrointestinal System—Upper Gastrointestinal Emergencies: Teeth

José García-López, VMD, DACVS
Associate Professor
Large Animal Surgery
Clinical Sciences
Cummings School of Veterinary Medicine
Tufts University
North Grafton, Massachusetts
Musculoskeletal System—Adult Orthopedic Emergencies

Rachel Gardner, DVM, DACVIM
BW Furlong and Associates
Oldwick, New Jersey
Caring for the Down Horse

Janik C. Gasiorowski, VMD, DACVS
Department of Surgery
Mid-Atlantic Equine Medical Center
Ringoes, New Jersey
Biopsy Techniques
Burns, Acute Soft Tissue Swellings, Pigeon Fever, and Fasciotomy
Respiratory System—Temporary Tracheostomy

Earl M. Gaughan, DVM, DACVS
Clinical Professor
Virginia-Maryland Regional College of Veterinary Medicine
Duck Pond Drive, Phase II
Virginia Tech
Blacksburg, Virginia
Burns, Acute Soft Tissue Swellings, Pigeon Fever, and Fasciotomy

Raymond J. Geor, BVSc, MVSc, PhD, DACVIM, DACVSMR,
  DACVN (Honorary)
Professor and Chairperson
Large Animal Clinical Sciences
College of Veterinary Medicine
Michigan State University
East Lansing, Michigan
Nutritional Guidelines for the Injured, Hospitalized and Postsurgical
  Patient

Rebecca M. Gimenez, PhD
President
Technical Large Animal Emergency Rescue, Inc.
Macon, Georgia
Disaster Medicine and Technical Emergency Rescue

Nora S. Grenager, VMD, DACVIM
Fredericksburg, Virginia
Burns, Acute Soft Tissue Swellings, Pigeon Fever, and Fasciotomy

Eileen S. Hackett, DVM, PhD, DACVS, DACVECC
Assistant Professor of Equine Surgery and Critical Care
Department of Clinical Sciences
College of Veterinary Medicine and Biomedical Sciences
Colorado State University
Fort Collins, Colorado
Emergency and Critical Care Monitoring
Emergency Laboratory Tests and Point-of-Care Diagnostics
Quick Reference Protocols for Emergency and Clinical Conditions
Equine Emergency Drugs: Approximate Dosages and Adverse Drug Reactions

R. Reid Hanson, DVM, DACVS, DACVECC
Professor Equine Surgery
J.T. Vaughan Hospital
Department of Clinical Sciences
College of Veterinary Medicine
Auburn University
Auburn, Alabama
Burns, Acute Soft Tissue Swellings, Pigeon Fever, and Fasciotomy

Joanne Hardy, DVM, PhD, DACVS, DACVECC
Clinical Associate Professor
Veterinary Large Animal Clinical Sciences
College of Veterinary Medicine
Texas A&M University
College Station, Texas
Musculoskeletal System—Pediatric Orthopedic Emergencies

Patricia M. Hogan, VMD, DACVS
Hogan Equine LLC
Cream Ridge, New Jersey
Emergencies of the Racing Athlete

Samuel D. A. Hurcombe, BSc, BVMS, MS, DACVIM, DACVECC
Assistant Professor of Equine Emergency & Critical Care
Veterinary Clinical Sciences
College of Veterinary Medicine
The Ohio State University
Columbus, Ohio
Emergency Problems Unique to Draft Horses

Nita L. Irby, DVM, DACVO
Lecturer, Clinical Sciences
Cornell University College of Veterinary Medicine
Cornell University
Ithaca, New York
Ophthalmology

Sophy A. Jesty, DVM, DACVIM (LAIM and Cardiology)
Assistant Professor of Cardiology
Clinical Sciences
College of Veterinary Medicine
University of Tennessee
Knoxville, Tennessee
Cardiovascular System

Amy L. Johnson, DVM, DACVIM (LAIM and Neurology)
Assistant Professor of Large Animal Medicine and Neurology
Department of Clinical Studies—New Bolton Center
School of Veterinary Medicine
University of Pennsylvania
Kennett Square, Pennsylvania
Nervous System—Diagnostic and Therapeutic Procedures
Nervous System—Neurologic Emergencies

Jean-Pierre Lavoíe, DMV, DACVIM
Professor
Department of Clinical Sciences
Faculty of Veterinary Medicine
Université de Montréal
Montreal, Canada
Respiratory System—Respiratory Tract Emergencies

David G. Levine, DVM, DACVS
Staff Surgeon
George D. Widener Hospital for Large Animals
New Bolton Center
School of Veterinary Medicine
University of Pennsylvania
Kennett Square, Pennsylvania
Regional Perfusion, Intraosseous and Resuscitation Infusion Techniques

Olivia Lorello, VMD
Intern
B.W. Furlong & Associates
Equine Veterinarians
Oldwick, New Jersey
Blood Collection
Medication Administration and Alternative Methods of Drug Administration
Intravenous Catheter Placement

K. Gary Magdesian, DVM, DACVIM, DACVECC, DACVCP
Professor and Henry Endowed Chair in Emergency Medicine and Critical Care
Veterinary Medicine: Medicine & Epidemiology
School of Veterinary Medicine
University of California—Davis
Davis, California
Neonatology

Tim Mair, BVSc, PhD, DECEIM
Director
Bell Equine Veterinary Clinic
United Kingdom
Emergency Diseases Unique to Countries Outside the Continental United States: Europe

Rebecca S. McConnico, DVM, PhD, DACVIM
Professor of Veterinary Medicine—Equine Internal Medicine
Department of Veterinary Clinical Sciences
Veterinary Teaching Hospital
School of Veterinary Medicine
Louisiana State University;
Equine Branch Director
Louisiana State Animal Response Team (LSART)
Affiliate of the Dr. WJE Jr. Foundation/Louisiana Veterinary Medical Association
Baton Rouge, Louisiana
Flood Injury in Horses

Jay Merriam, DVM, MS
Adjunct Clinical Instructor of Equine Sports Medicine
Large Animal Medicine
Cummings School of Veterinary Medicine
Tufts University;
Sports Medicine
Massachusetts Equine Clinic
Uxbridge, Massachusetts
Emergency Treatment of Mules and Donkeys

Linda D. Mittel, MSPH, DVM
Senior Extension Associate
Department of Population and Diagnostic Sciences
Animal Health Diagnostic Center
Cornell University College of Veterinary Medicine
Cornell University
Ithaca, New York
Emergency Treatment of Mules and Donkeys

James N. Moore, DVM, PhD, DACVS
Distinguished Research Professor and Josiah Meigs Distinguished
   Teaching Professor
Large Animal Medicine
College of Veterinary Medicine
The University of Georgia
Athens, Georgia
Gastrointestinal System—Acute Gastric Dilation
Gastrointestinal System—Acute Abdomen: Colic

P.O. Eric Mueller, DVM, PhD, DACVS
Associate Professor of Surgery
Chief of Staff
Large Animal Hospital
Department of Large Animal Medicine
College of Veterinary Medicine
The University of Georgia
Athens, Georgia
Gastrointestinal System—Acute Gastric Dilation
Gastrointestinal System—Acute Abdomen: Colic

SallyAnne L. Ness, DVM, DACVIM
Large Animal Internal Medicine
Department of Clinical Sciences
Cornell University College of Veterinary Medicine
Cornell University
Ithaca, New York
Blood Coagulation Disorders

Joan Norton, VMD, DACVIM
Norton Veterinary Consulting and Education Resources
Noblesville, Indiana
*Laboratory Diagnosis of Bacterial, Fungal and Viral, and Parasitic
   Pathogens*
Gene Testing
Shock and Systemic Inflammatory Response Syndrome

James A. Orsini, DVM, DACVS
Associate Professor of Surgery
Director, Laminitis Institute—PennVet
Director, *Equi-Assist*
Department of Clinical Studies—New Bolton Center
School of Veterinary Medicine
University of Pennsylvania
Kennett Square, Pennsylvania
Blood Collection
*Medication Administration and Alternative Methods of Drug
   Administration*
Intravenous Catheter Placement
Venous Access via Cutdown
Biopsy Techniques
Emergency Diagnostic Endoscopy
Gastrointestinal System—Diagnostic and Therapeutic Procedures
Gastrointestinal System—Upper Gastrointestinal Emergencies: Teeth
Gastrointestinal System—Stomach and Duodenum: Gastric Ulcers
Musculoskeletal System—Diagnostic and Therapeutic Procedures
Musculoskeletal System—Arthrocentesis and Synovial Fluid Analysis
Musculoskeletal System—Temporomandibular Arthrocentesis
Musculoskeletal System—Endoscopy of the Navicular Bursa
Respiratory System—Diagnostic and Therapeutic Procedures
Respiratory System—Temporary Tracheostomy
Urinary System—Diagnostic and Therapeutic Procedures
Laminitis
Emergencies of the Racing Athlete
*Equine Emergency Drugs: Approximate Dosages and Adverse Drug
   Reactions*

Israel Pasval, DVM
Haklait Mutual Society for Veterinary Services in Israel
*Emergency Diseases Unique to Countries Outside the Continental
   United States: The Middle East*

John F. Peroni, DVM, MS, DACVS
Associate Professor
Large Animal Medicine
College of Veterinary Medicine
The University of Georgia
Athens, Georgia
Gastrointestinal System—Acute Gastric Dilation
Gastrointestinal System—Acute Abdomen: Colic

Robert H. Poppenga, DVM, PhD, DABVT
Professor of Diagnostic Veterinary Toxicology
California Animal Health & Reed Safety Laboratory
School of Veterinary Medicine
University of California—Davis
Davis, California
Toxicology

Birgit Puschner, DVM, PhD, DABVT
Professor
Department of Molecular Biosciences and The California Animal
   Health and Food Safety Laboratory System
School of Veterinary Medicine
University of California—Davis
Davis, California
Toxicology

Rolfe M. Radcliffe, DVM, DACVS, DACVECC
Lecturer, Large Animal Surgery and Emergency Critical Care
Department of Clinical Sciences
Cornell University College of Veterinary Medicine
Cornell University
Ithaca, New York
Thoracic Trauma

Michael W. Ross, DVM, DACVS
Professor of Surgery (CE)
Department of Clinical Studies—New Bolton Center
School of Veterinary Medicine
University of Pennsylvania
Kennett Square, Pennsylvania
*Imaging Techniques and Indications for the Emergency Patient—
    Scintigraphic Imaging*

Amy Rucker, DVM
MidWest Equine
Columbia, Missouri
Laminitis

Christopher Ryan, VMD, DABVP
Resident in Radiology
Department of Clinical Studies—Philadelphia
School of Veterinary Medicine
University of Pennsylvania
Philadelphia, Pennsylvania
*Imaging Techniques and Indications for the Emergency Patient—
    Digital Radiographic Examination*

Montague N. Saulez, BVSc, MS, DACVIM-LA, DECEIM, PhD
Equine Internist
Western Cape
South Africa
*Emergency Diseases Unique to Countries Outside the Continental
    United States: South Africa*

Barbara Dallap Schaer, VMD, DACVS, DACVECC
Associate Professor (CE)
Department of Clinical Studies—New Bolton Center
School of Veterinary Medicine
University of Pennsylvania
Kennett Square, Pennsylvania
*Medication Administration and Alternative Methods of Drug
    Administration*
Emergency Diagnostic Endoscopy
Gastrointestinal System—Diagnostic and Therapeutic Procedures
Respiratory System—Diagnostic and Therapeutic Procedures
Urinary System—Diagnostic and Therapeutic Procedures
Contagious and Zoonotic Diseases
Standard Precautions and Infectious Disease Management

Peter V. Scrivani, DVM, DACVR
Assistant Professor
Department of Clinical Sciences
Cornell University College of Veterinary Medicine
Cornell University
Ithaca, New York
*Imaging Techniques and Indications for the Emergency Patient—
    Computed Tomography (CT) and Magnetic Resonance Imaging
    (MRI)*

JoAnn Slack, DVM, MS, DACVIM
Assistant Professor
Large Animal Cardiology and Ultrasound
Department of Clinical Studies—New Bolton Center
School of Veterinary Medicine
University of Pennsylvania
Kennett Square, Pennsylvania
*Imaging Techniques and Indications for the Emergency Patient—
    Ultrasonography: General Principles and System and Organ
    Examination*

Nathan Slovis, DVM, DACVIM, CHT
Director
McGee Medical Center
Hagyard Equine Medical Institute
Paris, Kentucky
Gastrointestinal System—Acute Diarrhea: Diarrhea in Nursing Foals

Dominic Dawson Soto, DVM, DACVIM
Associate
Loomis Basin Equine Medical Center, Inc.
Penryn, California
Medical Management of the Starved Horse

Ted S. Stashak, DVM, MS, DACVS
Professor Emeritus Surgery
Department of Clinical Sciences
College of Veterinary Medicine and Biomedical Sciences
Colorado State University
Fort Collins, Colorado
*Integumentary System: Wound Healing, Management, and
    Reconstruction*

Tracy Stokol, BVSc, PhD, DACVP (Clinical Pathology)
Associate Professor
Population Medicine and Diagnostic Sciences
Cornell University College of Veterinary Medicine
Cornell University
Ithaca, New York
Cytology

Brett S. Tennent-Brown, BVSc, MS, DACVIM, DACVECC
School of Veterinary Science
The University of Queensland
Gatton, Queensland, Australia
*Emergency Diseases Unique to Countries Outside the Continental
    United States: Australia and New Zealand*

Christine L. Theoret, DMV, PhD, DACVS
Professor
Department de Biomédecine Vétérinaire
Faculté de Médecine Vétérinaire
Université de Montréal
Quebec, Canada
*Integumentary System: Wound Healing, Management, and
    Reconstruction*

Regina M. Turner, DVM, PhD, DACT
Associate Professor
Department of Clinical Studies—New Bolton Center
School of Veterinary Medicine
University of Pennsylvania
Kennett Square, Pennsylvania
Reproductive System—Stallion Reproductive Emergencies
Reproductive System—Mare Reproductive Emergencies
Emergency Foaling

Dirk K. Vanderwall, DVM, PhD, DACT
Associate Professor
Department of Animal, Dairy, and Veterinary Sciences
School of Veterinary Medicine
Utah State University
Logan, Utah
Reproduction System—Stallion Reproductive Emergencies
Reproduction System—Mare Reproductive Emergencies

Andrew William van Eps, BVSc, PhD, DACVIM
Senior Lecturer in Equine Medicine
School of Veterinary Science
The University of Queensland
Gatton, Queensland, Australia
Emergency Diseases Unique to Countries Outside the Continental United States: Australia and New Zealand

Pamela A. Wilkins, DVM, MS, PhD, DACVIM, DACVECC
Professor of Equine Internal Medicine and Emergency and Critical Care
Veterinary Clinical Medicine
College of Veterinary Medicine
University of Illinois
Champaign-Urbana, Illinois
Perinatology and the High-Risk Pregnant Mare

Jennifer A. Wrigley, CVT
Director of Nursing—*Equi*-Assist
Department of Clinical Studies—New Bolton Center
School of Veterinary Medicine
University of Pennsylvania
Kennett Square, Pennsylvania
Emergencies of the Racing Athlete

Jean C. Young, LVT, VTS
Medicine Technician
Large Animal Medicine
Cornell University Hospital for Animals
Equine/Farm Animal Clinic
Cornell University College of Veterinary Medicine
Ithaca, New York
Emergency Laboratory Tests and Point-of-Care Diagnostics

DEDICATION

Two great legends of Large Animal Medicine, Surgery and Reproduction:
FRANCIS H. FOX, DVM, Cornell '45, and ROBERT B. HILLMAN, DVM, Cornell '55

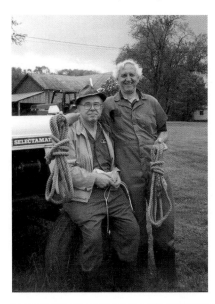

Drs. Fox and Hillman touched the lives of many veterinary students, residents, and faculty during their combined 120 years of devotion to veterinary medicine at Cornell University. We, with thousands of others, are fortunate to have learned the art and science of veterinary medicine from their wisdom. Dr. Fox retired his stethoscope in 2010 and Dr. Hillman remains an active clinician in the Department of Theriogenology at Cornell today. Good friends, mentors, and colleagues, they embody the highest level of professionalism, enjoyment in teaching, and advancing clinical science, combined with a "few" pranks along the way.

With the greatest of pleasure and distinction, this edition is dedicated in their honor.

Thomas J. Divers and James A. Orsini

There are other incredible individuals who guide our lives with awe-inspiring leadership, wisdom, creativeness, and generosity. To these devoted friends, advocates, and idealists, this book is likewise dedicated.

James A. Orsini

JOHN K. & MARIANNE S. CASTLE

MARGARET HAMILTON DUPREY

MARY ALICE MALONE

ELIZABETH R. MORAN

MICHAEL J. & DENISE (POSTH) ROTKO

2013

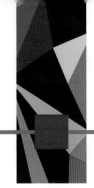

Preface

The fourth edition of *Equine Emergencies: Treatment and Procedures* continues to build on the foundation started in 1998 with the publication of the first edition. This edition is an expanded and thoroughly updated volume that provides our colleagues with a comprehensive and detailed resource for the most "common" and "not so common" procedures and treatments needed to manage any equine emergency. The information is the most detailed of any of the previous editions, while offering a point-by-point checklist of "what to do" and "what not to do" when caring for the horse emergency. Our goal is to continue to provide the most current, in-depth information for essentially every equine emergency, and this edition has been reviewed to include every step in most procedures, as well as recommendations and selection of medications. The format is similar to the third edition, but is more precise in illustrations, protocols, procedures, and treatments, clearly differentiating it from other equine emergency texts currently available.

We recognize that there is more than one way to diagnose and treat an equine emergency patient or to perform a procedure, and to that extent this text is not a maxim but the compilation of experienced clinicians from both academia and private practice writing about emergency procedures and treatments in their own specialty areas. There are 18 new chapters, with every part updated and comprised of feedback from our colleagues, friends, and mentors who regularly treat equine emergencies.

Here are some of the highlights of the fourth edition:

- Every page was planned, reviewed, and reorganized in an easy-to-understand format.
- Many new figures have been added to this edition, and the existing figures have been redrawn for clarity and usability to aid in illustrating key points.
- 18 new chapters include topics covering hyperbaric oxygen therapy, venous cut-down, critical care monitoring, quick reference treatment protocols for the most common emergency conditions, newer imaging techniques, emergency foaling, problems unique to the draft horse, caring for the down horse, flood injuries, racing athlete emergencies, snake envenomation, managing the starved horse, and alternative therapies.
- Appendices have been expanded with access to essential information in a format that reduces the risk of error. Two good examples are the "equine emergency drugs" and "quick reference protocols for emergency conditions" for any clinical crisis.
- The number of equine emergency diseases, diagnostic procedures, and treatments has grown considerably since the first edition of the book was published, which has necessitated an increased number of pages for each edition. In order to keep the fourth edition of the book "manageable" as your emergency companion, references for each chapter have been placed on the companion website at www.equine-emergencies.com. The website also provides us with the ability to add updates.
- This edition is also available as an e-book publication. This should prove invaluable as the book will now be available in a searchable format, "anywhere and anytime."

The ability to find information easily and by clinical complaint has been enhanced by Elsevier's superb publishing team, addressing the concerns that you shared with us from previous editions. We believe we have succeeded in meeting your expectations with a dependable and durable resource for all your equine emergencies. We know that all reference books have limitations and that "best practices" come from past and repeated experiences; we hope that this textbook provides you with the information you need on a daily basis. After you have had a chance to become "comfortable" with this edition and see and read the revisions and new changes, please share with us your comments. Thanks to everybody who has spoken, written, or e-mailed us and to all who have contributed in a large or small way to the fourth edition.

James A. Orsini
Thomas J. Divers

Acknowledgments

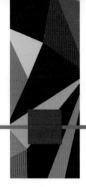

The fourth edition of *Equine Emergencies: Treatment and Procedures* is here today because of the commitment and contribution of more than 60 authors, colleagues, friends, and family. Elsevier's unparalleled publishing team was supportive of all our new ideas, beginning with the decision to make this edition an e-book: leading the group, Shelly Stringer, Content Manager; Carol O'Connell, Project Manager; Penny Rudolph, Content Strategy Director; Catherine Jackson, Publishing Services Manager; and Jeanne Robertson, Medical Illustrator. Writing a book never seems to get easier and, in truth, this edition was more than two years in the making. The skills and knowledge, based on a lifetime of experiences, provided to us by mentors, colleagues, and students, has made it possible for us to provide you this book to meet virtually all your emergency needs.

Our contributing authors exceeded all our expectations not only in the quality of their information but in their professionalism and desire to produce the highest quality reference book.

We also want to thank the many authors who wrote for the previous editions; their pearls of wisdom continue to serve us well. We want to also acknowledge our professional and personal "advisers" for their steadfast support. Thank you (JAO) John K. and Marianne Castle, Dr. Willard Daniels, Dr. William Donawick, Bob and Margaret H. Duprey, William S. Farish, Dr. John Garafalo, Robert Huffman, Roy & Gretchen Jackson, Dr. William Kay, Dr. John Lee, Mary Alice Malone, Marian and Gib McIlvain, Elizabeth R. Moran, Ellen & Herb Moelis, Dr. Roy Pollock, Dr. Charles Ramberg, Michael Rotko, Dr. Wayne Schwark, Vonnie & Larry Steinbaum, and Carol & Mark Zebrowski; and remember those recently lost much too early in life: Robert Davies, Dr. Teresa Garafalo, and Denise Rotko. Thank you (TJD) Drs. Jill Beech, Dilmus Blackmon, Doug Byars, Sandy deLahunta, Lisle George, Jack Lowe, Brad Smith, Bud Tennant, Robert Whitlock, and the late John Cummings and Bill Rebuhn, all of whom helped guide my career, and to the absolutely wonderful 45 equine medicine residents and innumerable practicing veterinarians who have all taught me so much more than I have taught them. I especially thank Dr. Jim Orsini for his personal friendship and his leadership in editing this fourth edition of *Equine Emergencies*.

We also want to recognize Sue Branch, Molly Higgins, Tia Jones, Kate Shanaghan, Cindy Stafford, Patty Welch, and Jennifer Wrigley, who, in many different ways, made sure that we reached this level of eminence, met our deadlines, and that all the pieces of the book fit as designed. Their support with the "big and not so big" details was always handled with professionalism, patience, and humor. Lastly, a very special thank you goes to Dr. Nora Grenager, who was instrumental in editing all the proofs, checking and rechecking, and adding a level of expertise and skill that was so much more than we could have hoped for. Nora, you are simply astounding!

Dr. Tom Divers is not only co-editor but an honored colleague and close friend. Without his experience, patience, and depth of knowledge, the fourth edition could not have been completed. We want to recognize our loving families (JAO), Toni, Colin, and Angela, and (TJD) Nita, Shannon, Bob, and Reuben for their unending patience, and finally our parents, Anne and Sal and Robert and Hattie, for teaching us the importance of integrity, patience, and persistence.

James A. Orsini
Thomas J. Divers

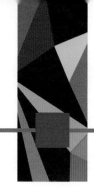

Contents

PART I

Emergency Procedures and Diagnostics

SECTION I Important Diagnostic and Therapeutic Procedures for Emergency Care

CHAPTER 1

Blood Collection

Olivia Lorello and James A. Orsini

Blood collection from a vein is a routine procedure commonly performed during patient evaluation. Many diagnostic tests require whole blood or serum. Often, specific additives are necessary in blood collection tubes to prevent coagulation (Table 1-1).

Venipuncture of the External Jugular Vein

The external jugular vein is most accessible and is found easily within the jugular groove along the ventral aspect of the neck. The vein can be safely accessed in the cranial half of the neck where muscle (omohyoideus muscle) interposes between the vein and the underlying carotid sheath containing the carotid artery. The vein fills most rapidly if distended by digital pressure just below the intended venipuncture site. Stroking the vein distally causes motion waves higher up, which is helpful if the distended vein is not readily visible.

Equipment
- 18- to 20-gauge, 1- to 1½-inch (2.54- to 3.75-cm) Vacutainer[1] needle (or a 10-mL syringe and 20-gauge needle for fractious patients)
- Vacutainer cuff
- Appropriate Vacutainer tube or tubes

Procedure
- Screw the protected, short end of the needle into the Vacutainer cuff.
- Distend the vein, and swab the venipuncture site with alcohol.
- Align the needle parallel with the vein, opposite the direction of the blood flow.
- Insert the needle through the skin at a 45-degree angle, and then redirect it in a parallel direction once the vein lumen has been entered.
- Attach the Vacutainer tube by pushing the cover of the tube onto the short, protected needle in the Vacutainer cuff. The vacuum draws blood into the tube to the appropriate level. If additional tubes are needed, switch tubes while leaving the needle and cuff in place.

---

[1]Vacutainer needles, cuffs, and blood tubes (Becton-Dickinson Vacutainer Systems, Rutherford, New Jersey).

Venipuncture of the Transverse Facial Vein

The transverse facial vein in the head is commonly used in adults or nonfractious patients to sample small volumes of blood for a packed cell volume or total solids determination. *Practice Tip: Up to 35 mL can be taken from this site at one time. The vein runs ventral to the facial crest and parallel to the transverse facial artery (Fig. 1-1, A).*

Equipment
- 22- to 25-gauge, 1- to 1½-inch (2.5- to 3.75-cm) needle
- 3-mL syringe
- Appropriate Vacutainer or hematocrit tube or tubes

Procedure
- Swab the area beneath the facial crest with alcohol.
- Align the needle perpendicular to the skin beneath the facial crest, at the level of or just rostral to the medial canthus, and push the needle through the skin until bone is encountered. Attach the syringe, if not already attached, and withdraw the needle while aspirating until the needle is in the vein lumen.
- A Vacutainer needle and tube may be used to collect blood.

Alternate Sites for Venipuncture

Fig. 1-1, *B*, illustrates other venipuncture sites:
- The superficial thoracic vein in the cranial and ventral third of the thorax caudal to the point of the elbow
- The cephalic vein on the medial aspect of the forelimb
- The medial saphenous vein on the medial aspect of the hind limb

If the sample is collected in a syringe, immediately transfer the sample to a Vacutainer tube because the sample begins to clot as soon as it is drawn. Push the needle through the cover of the Vacutainer tube and let the vacuum draw the blood from the syringe. *Practice Tip: Actively pushing blood into the tube damages the blood cells.* Mix the anticoagulant into the sample by gently rotating the tube upside down several times. The sample should last for several hours if properly mixed and kept cool (4° C/39.2° F). To prevent hemolysis, serum should be separated from whole blood by means of centrifugation if the sample is to sit for longer than several hours.

Table 1-1	Blood Tubes for Diagnostic Procedures	
Color of Top of Vacutainer Tube	**Additive**	**Analysis Possible**
Red or red/black	None	Chemistry studies; viral antibody studies; crossmatch*; hormones; bile acids
Purple	Na EDTA	Hematologic studies: CBC and platelet counts; bone marrow analysis; immunohematology; Coombs test; fluid cytology; crossmatch,* PCR
Green	Na heparin	Chemistry studies (i-STAT); blood gases; therapeutic drugs; lymphocyte typing
Yellow	Acid citrate	Crossmatch*; blood typing, dextrose, PRP
Blue	Na citrate	Coagulation studies: fibrinogen, PT, PTT, AT; bone marrow supernatant
Gray	Na fluoride/ K oxylate†	Glucose measurement when submission to lab will be delayed

AT, Antithrombin; *CBC,* complete blood cell count; *EDTA,* ethylenediaminetetraacetic acid; *K,* potassium; *Na,* sodium; *PCR,* polymerase chain reaction; *PRP,* platelet rich plasma; *PT,* prothrombin time; *PTT,* partial thromboplastin time; *SDH,* sorbitol dehydrogenase.
*Both red or red/black and purple are required.
†May cause some hemolysis.

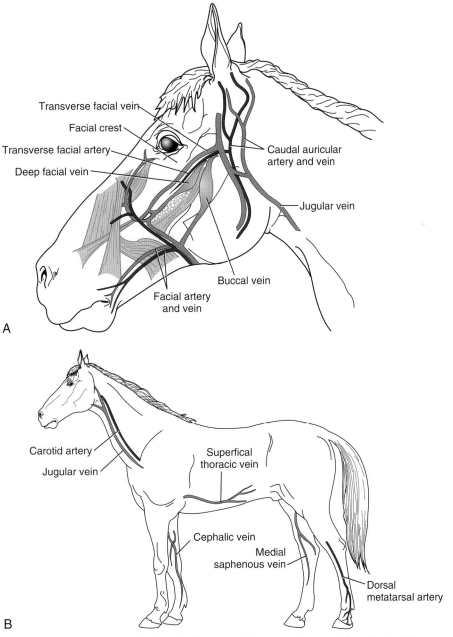

Figure 1-1   Veins and arteries used for blood collection. **A,** Veins and arteries accessible in the head; **B,** alternate sites for vein and artery sampling.

Practice Tip: *Hemolysis has a significant effect on many values, such as: calcium (increased), sodium (decreased), chloride (decreased), creatinine (increased), alkaline phosphatase (increased), potassium (increased), magnesium (increased), alanine aminotransferase (increased), and lactate dehydrogenase (increased). Glucose is artifactually low after 60 minutes because of red cell glycolysis. Slides for a differential are best made soon after the sample is obtained.*

Complications

A hematoma often forms if a large-gauge needle is used or if the vein is excessively traumatized and blood continues to escape from the venipuncture site. Hematoma formation or excessive bleeding from a venipuncture site may indicate a coagulopathy in a critically ill patient. Keeping the head elevated and applying direct pressure to the puncture site may minimize this complication. If a hematoma occurs, warm compresses, topical anti-inflammatories (diclofenac sodium) and a compression bandage may expedite healing.

Thrombosis of the vein is an uncommon complication that can occur if the vascular endothelium is damaged from repeated venipuncture. Septic thrombophlebitis can occur if the site becomes infected.

Arterial Puncture

Arterial puncture is most commonly performed for arterial blood gas analysis, which is an excellent indicator of respiratory and metabolic conditions. Several arteries are suitable for sampling (see Fig. 1-1). In the adult horse, arterial blood samples can be taken from the transverse facial artery, facial artery, caudal auricular artery, and in tractable patients, from the dorsal metatarsal artery. The carotid artery may be used in the adult horse, but this artery is often associated with significant hematoma formation, and contamination with venous blood is possible. In foals, arterial blood gas samples are usually taken from the dorsal metatarsal artery, located along the plantar lateral aspect of the third metatarsus, or the brachial artery, accessible on the medial aspect of the humerus.

Equipment
• 20- or 25-gauge, 1- to 1½-inch (2.54- to 3.75-cm) needle
• Heparinized plastic syringe or prepared arterial blood gas syringe[2]
• Gauze sponges soaked in alcohol

Procedure

The transverse facial artery can be palpated caudal to the lateral canthus of the eye, running roughly parallel to the zygomatic arch (see Fig. 1-1, *A*). The facial artery can also be palpated as it courses from that location to the mandible and can be accessed at any palpable point along this path. Carefully palpate the pulse before arterial puncture. When using a commercially prepared syringe designed for arterial sampling, withdraw the plunger of the syringe to the volume of blood needed for arterial sample. The procedure is as follows:
• Clean the area thoroughly with alcohol gauze sponges. While palpating the pulse, puncture the artery with the needle. If the artery has been punctured, provided the patient has appropriate arterial blood pressure, bright red blood flows into the syringe, filling the syringe until the plunger is reached. If a conventional syringe is used, withdraw the syringe plunger to allow arterial blood to fill the heparinized syringe.
• Remove any air from the syringe immediately. ***Important:*** Blood gas analysis should be performed within minutes of sampling to obtain the most accurate results. If values other than blood gases are to be analyzed, the sample can be placed into a heparinized tube (green top tube) and cooled.
• As soon as the needle is withdrawn, apply digital pressure over the puncture site with a gauze sponge for several minutes.

Complications
• As with venipuncture, the most common complication is hematoma formation. Use the smallest-gauge needle possible to minimize vessel trauma, and apply pressure to the artery until bleeding stops.
• Local skin infiltration of 2% local anesthetic directly over the site for needle puncture improves patient compliance and may decrease injury to the vessel wall.

[2]MICRO A.B.G., Arterial Blood Sampler (Marquest Medical Products, Inc., Englewood, Colorado).

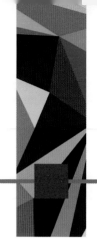

CHAPTER 2

Medication Administration and Alternative Methods of Drug Administration

Olivia Lorello, Barbara Dallap Schaer, and James A. Orsini

Multiple routes of administration exist for equine pharmaceuticals. Route of administration profoundly affects the pharmacokinetics of a drug. The pharmaceutical package insert describes the acceptable routes of administration and is a valuable source of information. Before administering any medication, it is appropriate to consult the package insert regarding any risks that might be associated with the actual handling of the drug. Directions for medication handling should be followed strictly. Table 2-1 gives an overview of the most common routes of medication administration.

Oral Drug Administration

The oral route is the most convenient route of administration and is associated with the fewest complications. This route is ideal for client/owner drug administration. Drugs designed for oral administration are prepared as tablets, granules, powders, suspensions, and pastes.

Many horses eat powders, granules, and crushed tablets mixed with a palatable food (sweet feed, pellets, chopped apples, and applesauce).

For difficult or anorectic patients, medications can be mixed or dissolved in water and administered using a dose syringe.[1] Adding molasses, corn syrup, apple sauce, gelatin such as Jell-O, or other palatable substances encourages acceptance by the patient. Medications in paste or suspension form should be administered as follows:
- Properly restrain the head.
- Make sure the mouth is cleared of food.
- Place a hand over the bridge of the nose, and place a thumb at the corner of the mouth in the interdental space to facilitate dose syringe placement. Carefully place the dose syringe between the buccal mucosa and the molars, and angle it over the tongue.
- Spread the medicine evenly over the back of the tongue and dispense slowly to encourage swallowing.

Administration of medication through a nasogastric tube is useful for individuals who refuse oral dosing or who need a large volume of medication delivered. Nasogastric tubing also ensures that the entire dose is delivered:

- See Nasogastric Tube Placement (Chapter 18, p. 157).
- Medication is delivered easily with a large, 400-mL dose syringe[2] that fits on the end of most nasogastric tubes.
- After administering the medication, deliver a dose syringeful of water and then air to ensure that all of the drug has cleared the tube.
- Leave the syringe attached or kink the tube when removing it to reduce the risk of aspiration.

Complications

The complete dose often is not delivered unless it is administered through a nasogastric tube.

Practice Tip: *Some drugs are inactivated in the stomach of herbivores, so check to be sure that the drug is intended for oral use in horses. Modifying the drug formulation by crushing and combining with other medicines and vehicles can adversely affect the pharmacokinetics of the prescribed drug(s).*

Use of the oral route may result in high drug levels/ concentrations in the gastrointestinal tract, which can cause gastrointestinal irritation and inflammation and potentially alter normal bacterial flora, resulting in diarrhea and colic.

Intramuscular Administration

Intramuscular administration typically results in slower absorption and comparably lower peak blood levels than the intravenous route. Because of this, frequency of administration of medications intramuscularly is usually lower. As with oral administration, many owners are comfortable administering drugs intramuscularly. Several large muscle masses are suitable for drug administration (Fig. 2-1). Consider the following:
- Small volumes (10 mL or less) may be administered in the neck in the indented triangular space that lies above the cervical vertebrae, below the nuchal ligament, and a handbreadth in front of the cranial border of the scapula.
- The lower halves of the semitendinosus and semimembranosus muscles are suitable for large volumes. Proper restraint of the horse is needed, and the person dispensing the drug should stand as close to the horse's side as possible to avoid personal injury.

---

[1]Dose syringe with catheter tip (35 or 60 mL), Monoject (Sherwood Medical, St. Louis, Missouri).

[2]A 400-mL nylon dose syringe (J.A. Webster, Inc., Sterling, Massachusetts).

- Large volumes also may be administered in the pectoral muscles (pectoralis descendens) between the front limbs.

Procedure

- Clean the site with an alcohol- or chlorhexidine-soaked swab until the gross dirt is removed.
- Use a 1½-inch, 22-, 20-, 19-, or 18-gauge needle, depending on the viscosity of the medicine to be delivered.
- Quickly stick the needle through the skin up to the hub.
- Attach the drug-filled syringe to the needle and aspirate to ensure that the needle is not in a vessel.
- Ideally, inject no more than 5 to 10 mL in any one site. For large volumes, the needle may be redirected without pulling out of the skin after injecting each 5- to 10-mL aliquot.

Table 2-1	Medication Administration Methods	
Route	**Advantages**	**Disadvantages**
Oral	Less technical	Incomplete dose, drug bioavailability
Intramuscular	Less technical	Muscle soreness
Intravenous	Immediate and predictable blood concentration of drug; controlled infusion rate	Need venous access
Topical (intrauterine, intramammary, intracystic, ophthalmic)	Local drug delivery	Varied technicality
Inhaled	Fewer systemic side effects	Requires equipment

- When dosing must be repeated, rotate between muscle groups to avoid repeated injury to any one muscle.

Complications

Abscess formation is an occasional complication. Clean the skin thoroughly before injecting, and choose a site that is easily drained if this complication occurs.

Clostridial myositis has been associated with the intramuscular administration of flunixin meglumine and should be avoided (see p. 618).

Muscle soreness, specifically neck soreness, is fairly common and is related to drug irritation and associated inflammation, the volume administered, and the site of administration. Injection sites in high-motion areas should be avoided. Avoid repeated intramuscular injection in foals.

Severe drug reactions can occur if certain drugs (e.g., procaine penicillin G) are inadvertently injected in a vessel (see Chapter 22, p. 374).

Intravenous Administration

Use of the intravenous route provides immediate blood levels of the drug but typically requires more frequent administration. Medication must be administered slowly (at a rate of approximately 1 mL per 5 seconds) or diluted in sterile water or saline solution, especially if the particular drug is known to cause any type of adverse reaction.

The external jugular vein is most commonly used for medication delivery. Venipuncture should be only in the cranial third of the neck. See Fig. 1-1 for the location of venipuncture sites.

Equipment

- Alcohol-soaked gauze
- 18-, 19-, or 20-gauge 1½-inch (3.75-cm) needle
- Syringe with medication

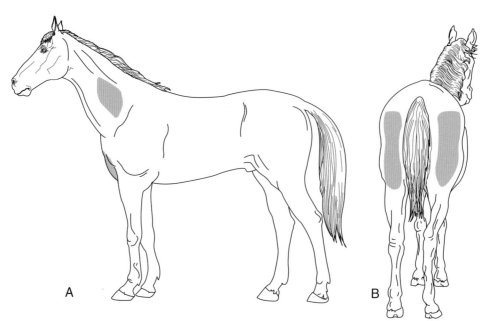

Figure 2-1   Sites for intramuscular drug delivery *(shaded areas)*. **A,** Lateral view. **B,** Posterior view.

Procedure
- Clean site with an alcohol wipe until gross dirt is removed.
- Ideally, detach the syringe from the needle. While holding off the vein below the venipuncture site, align the needle directly over the vein, opposite the blood flow. Experienced clinicians may prefer to leave the syringe attached to the needle.
- Push the needle through the skin and enter the vein; blood fills the hub of the needle if the needle is in the vein. If blood is pulsing from the hub of the needle, an artery may have been entered accidentally, and the needle must be redirected. Venipuncture is commonly performed with the syringe and needle attached; however, experience is needed to ensure that medication is not administered accidentally into an artery.
- Once the needle has been properly placed, advance the needle to the hub, confirm correct placement, and attach the syringe to the needle without changing the needle position. Always check correct placement of the needle by drawing back on the syringe and confirming a flashback of blood in the syringe before injecting the solution. Recheck the position of the needle between injections of each 5 mL.
- Frequent and long-term administration of intravenous drugs requires an indwelling catheter to reduce injury to the vein and improve patient cooperation. See intravenous catheter placement (Chapter 3, pp. 9-11).

Complications
Caution: Accidental intraarterial injection is life-threatening with most substances and may result in rapid seizure activity (see Chapter 22, p. 374). Using a large-bore needle and entering the vein with the needle detached increase the likelihood of detecting arterial puncture.

Accidental delivery of a caustic substance (e.g., phenylbutazone) outside the vein (perivascular) can result in necrosis and sloughing of the surrounding skin.

Thrombosis and infection of the vein are uncommon. The risk increases with frequent venipuncture, especially if the medication is known to be irritating to the vessel lumen.

Topical Administration
Medication may be administered topically using the skin, eyes, and mucous membranes and within body cavities (intravaginal, intrauterine, intracystic, intramammary, and intrarectal) for a direct local effect. Drugs approved for topical use are special preparations in ointments, creams, pastes, sprays, and powders. Possible whole-body effects should be considered because in many cases, the drugs are absorbed systemically. Certain oral medications (e.g., metronidazole/aspirin) may be made into solution and delivered per rectum in patients who are not able to receive medications by mouth.

Rectal Administration
Rectal administration of drugs is used to produce local or systemic effects. Absorption is inconsistent but can be useful in patients unable to take medications, intended for systemic use, by mouth (e.g., postoperatively).

Drugs can be suspended in 1 to 2 oz (30 to 60 mL) of water and introduced rectally through a soft feeding tube and 60-mL syringe. Caution must be taken during rectal administration of any drug. The patient should be restrained appropriately and adequate lubrication should be used.

Inhalation/Nebulization
Local delivery methods of aerosolized medications to the respiratory tract of horses include:
- Nebulizers
- Metered-dose inhalers (MDIS)
- Dry powder inhalers

These types of drug delivery methods allow a higher concentration of drug to reach the target site while minimizing side effects.

These methods are used primarily to treat recurrent airway obstruction (RAO) and inflammatory airway disease (IAD) through bronchodilation and by reducing inflammation and can also be used in treating respiratory distress. Drugs commonly administered this way include:
- β_2-adrenergic agonists
- Glucocorticoids

Transdermal/Cutaneous Administration
Use of the transdermal or cutaneous dosage form, in which the drug is incorporated in a stick-on patch and is applied to an area of thin, clipped or shaved skin, is increasingly more common in clinical practice. As opposed to topical delivery, in which rate of delivery is controlled by absorption through the skin, the rate of drug absorption is also controlled by the delivery system (patch). Drugs administered by this route include:
- Fentanyl[3]
- Nitroglycerin[3]
- Scopolamine
- Estrogen

Note: Absorption may be erratic!

Intrasynovial Administration
The decision to administer drugs intraarticularly should be made after considering the potential complications of altering the intraarticular environment. Direct intrasynovial administration naturally produces much higher drug levels in a joint than does use of the systemic route and is commonly used to treat degenerative joint disease and infectious arthritis. Medications to be injected intraarticularly should be considered carefully for their potential to cause irritation or inflammation. Use of drugs specifically labeled for intraarticular use is the safest. Certain acid or basic drugs may be modified by the addition of a buffering solution before intrasynovial injection. Sites for intraarticular injection and the relevant anatomic features are described in Chapter 21.

---

[3]Drugs with pharmacologic transdermal absorption studies in horses.

Table 2-2	Alternative Routes of Medication in Emergent Situations		
Route	**Drug**	**Indication**	**Dose**
Tracheal Mucosa	Epinephrine	Anaphylaxis, asystole	0.1-0.2 mg/kg (anaphylaxis) 0.3-0.5 mg/kg (asystole)
Sublingual	Detomidine hydrochloride	Sedation*	40 µg/kg
Intraosseous	Fluids	Lack of venous access†	20 mL/kg crystalloid then reassess
Intranasal	Phenylephrine hydrochloride	Nasal/pharyngeal edema	10 mg diluted to 10 mL
Intracardiac	Potassium chloride	Ventricular fibrillation‡	225 mL
Nebulization	Aminophylline	Respiratory distress, pulmonary edema	5 mg/kg
Inhaler	Albuterol	Bronchospasm	720 µg

*When IV access is not available. Larger dose may be needed in excited horses. Do not get medication in administrator's eye or mouth!
†Foals only.
‡If electrical defibrillation is not available.

Intrathecal Administration

The intrathecal route of drug administration is used only to achieve direct spinal analgesia, perform myelography, or treat meningoencephalitis. Medication is administered directly into the subarachnoid space. See Chapter 22, p. 339; medication must be nontoxic, of normal pH, and preservative free.

Epidural Administration

Epidural drug administration is used for anesthesia for urogenital surgery and pain management (see Chapter 49, p. 760). Medications injected into the epidural space include:

- Local anesthetics (lidocaine, mepivacaine, and bupivacaine)
- α_2-adrenergic agonists (xylazine, detomidine)
- Narcotics (morphine)

The sacrococcygeal interspace or the first and second coccygeal interspaces (more common) are sites for epidural injection.

Equipment

- Stocks for restraint
- Twitch, sedation, or both (detomidine/xylazine and butorphanol tartrate)
- Clippers
- Material for sterile scrub
- Sterile gloves
- 2% local anesthetic; 5-mL syringe; 22-gauge, 1-inch needle
- 18-gauge, 10.2-cm, thick-walled Tuohy needle; 18-gauge Teflon epidural catheter with stylet or 18-gauge, 1½-inch (3.75-cm) needle
- 12-mL syringe (sterile)

Procedure

- Restrain the patient in stocks. Sedate using xylazine, 0.2 to 1.1 mg/kg IV, and butorphanol, 0.01 to 0.1 mg/kg IV to effect.
- Clip and aseptically prepare an area over the first coccygeal interspace. The first coccygeal interspace (Co_1-Co_2) is the first palpable depression on the midline caudal to the sacrum.
- Subcutaneously inject 1 to 2 mL of 2% mepivacaine (Carbocaine[4]) to desensitize the skin.
- Make a stab incision through the skin to facilitate passage of the epidural needle. An 18-gauge (Periflex[5]) Tuohy needle is inserted on the midline into the interspace and is directed cranially and ventrally at a 45-degree angle to the rump. Entrance into the epidural space is confirmed by a loss of resistance to passage of the needle; correct placement of the needle is confirmed by the ability to inject 5 to 10 mL of air without resistance.
- Thread an 18-gauge, polyethylene epidural catheter (Accu-Bloc Periflex) through the Tuohy needle into the epidural space, and secure it to the skin for repeated drug administration.
- If an 18-gauge, 1½-inch (3.75-cm) hypodermic needle is used for the procedure, a stab incision is not required.

Complications

Incomplete block can be caused by the presence of congenital membranes, adhesions from previous epidural procedures, location of the epidural catheter or needle in the ventral epidural space, or escape of the epidural catheter tip through the intervertebral foramen.

Alternative Routes of Drug Administration

Some of the less common routes of drug administration may be useful in emergent situations where intravenous access is difficult, intramuscular administration is dangerous, oral drug administration is too slow acting, or alternative and less common methods have higher efficacy. Table 2-2 describes unique routes of administration and common indications.

---

[4]Carbocaine-V (Pharmacia-Upjohn Co., Division of Pfizer, Inc., New York).
[5]Burrow Accu-Bloc Periflex, 18-gauge polyethylene epidural catheter (Burrow Medical, Inc., Bethlehem, Pennsylvania).

CHAPTER 3

Intravenous Catheter Placement

Olivia Lorello and James A. Orsini

Placement of Intravenous Catheter

- Intravenous catheters are used for:
  - Administration of large volumes of fluids
  - Maintenance of continuous fluid therapy
  - Intravenous medications
  - Parenteral nutrition
  - Blood sampling
- The size and catheter type needed depend on the intended use (Table 3-1).
- Large-gauge, 5-inch (12.5-cm) catheters (14-, 12-, or 10-gauge) are used to administer intravenous fluids rapidly to adult patients in need of shock fluid volume boluses.
- *Practice Tip: Bilateral jugular venous catheters may be used for rapid, large-volume fluid replacement in the treatment of severely dehydrated patients.* **Important:** Large-bore catheters are more likely to cause thrombophlebitis, cellulitis, or both.
- A 16-gauge, 5-inch catheter is recommended if frequent intravenous access is required for administration of medications only or in foals. Such a catheter is NOT typically suitable for intravenous fluid administration in an adult horse.
- Catheters are available for short-term[1] and long-term[2] use. In patients that are critically ill, long-term catheters made of polyurethane are commonly used. Short-term catheters, often made of fluorinated ethylene propylene polymer, are typically only left in for a maximum of 3 days, whereas long-term catheters can be maintained for several weeks. The jugular vein is most accessible for catheter placement.
- *Practice Tip: If the jugular vein cannot be used, the cephalic and superficial (lateral) thoracic veins are suitable alternatives for catheters (see Fig. 1-1).*
  Note: Most veterinarians refer to this vein as the lateral thoracic, but as in Fig. 1-1, its proper name is superficial thoracic vein.
- *Note:* The following technique applies to simple over-the-needle catheter placement. Guidewire catheters[3] are available in longer lengths and for long-term use. Instructions for placement accompany each catheter, but similar preparation and techniques should be followed.

Equipment

- Material for aseptic preparation of catheter site
- Clippers
- Sterile gloves
- Appropriate over-the-needle catheter
- Heparin saline flush (2000 units of heparin in 500 mL of saline solution)
- 2-0 nonabsorbable suture
- Rapid-acting glue (cyanoacrylate) optional
- 20- or 35-mL syringe
- Extension set[4] filled with heparinized saline solution
- Intermittent injection cap[5]
- Elasticon roll[6] (optional)

Procedure

- Choose an area in the cranial third of the jugular groove for catheter placement. Superficial (lateral) thoracic catheters should enter the vein at the yellow circle in Fig. 4-1.
- Clip the area for aseptic preparation, making sure that the area is large enough to facilitate aseptic placement of the catheter.
- Aseptically prepare the entire clipped area for catheter placement. Don sterile gloves to minimize contamination of the catheter and site.
- Remove the protective sleeve on the catheter, and loosen the cap on the stylet. The catheter should be handled *only* at the hub.
- Distend the jugular vein by placing three fingers (or knuckles) in the jugular groove on the cardiac side to the proposed catheter site.
- Position the catheter so that it is parallel to the jugular groove and directed with the flow of blood in the vein.
- Enter percutaneously at a 45-degree angle, and advance the catheter and stylet until blood appears at the catheter hub.

---

[1]BD Angiocath (Becton, Dickinson and Company, Franklin Lakes, New Jersey).

[2]Milacath polyurethane catheter-over-needle (Mila International, Inc., Florence, Kentucky).

[3]Guidewire catheters (14- or 16-gauge, 8-inch; Mila International, Inc.). Single- and double-lumen styles are available. Central venous catheter (14- or 16-gauge, 8-inch; Arrow International, Inc., Reading, Pennsylvania).

[4]Extension set (7-inch or 30-inch; Abbott Laboratories Inc., Abbott Park, Illinois). Large animal extension set (large-bore, 7-inch; International Win, Ltd., Kennett Square, Pennsylvania).

[5]Injection cap (along with Luer-Lok; Baxter Healthcare Corp., Deerfield, Illinois).

[6]Elasticon (Johnson and Johnson Medical, Inc., Arlington, Texas).

Table 3-1	**Commonly Used Catheters and Their Clinical Indications***				
Brand/Material	**Length**	**Design**	**Gauge**	**Indications**	
Angiocath[†]/ FEP polymer	5-inch (12.5 cm)	Over-the-needle	14, 12, 10	Short-term use (up to 3 days) Fluid resuscitation	
			16	Short-term use (up to 3 days)	
Milacath[‡]/ Polyurethane[§]	5.25-inch (13 cm)	Over-the-needle	14, 12	Long-term use (3-4 weeks) Fluid resuscitation, septic/critically ill	
			16	Long-term use (3-4 weeks) Foals, septic/critically ill	
Milacath[‡]/ Polyurethane	8-inch (20 cm)	Over-the-wire, available with multiple lumens	14 or 16	Long-term use (3-4 weeks) Lateral thoracic catheterization, foals, parenteral nutrition, septic/critically ill	
Arrow[‖]/ Polyurethane	28-inch (70 cm)	Over-the-wire	16	Central venous pressure measurements	

FEP, Fluorinated ethylene propylene.
*NOTE: This table references common examples, but numerous appropriate products are available.
[†]BD Angiocath (Becton, Dickinson and Company, Franklin Lakes, New Jersey).
[‡]Milacath polyurethane catheter-over-needle (Mila International, Inc., Florence, Kentucky).
[§]Polyurethane is less thrombogenic than FEP—the first choice for septic and critically ill patients.
[‖]Guidewire catheters (14- or 16-gauge, 8-inch; Mila International, Inc.). Single- and double-lumen styles are available. Central venous catheter (14- or 16-gauge, 8-inch; Arrow International, Inc., Reading, Pennsylvania).

- When the catheter is within the vein lumen, angle the catheter parallel to the jugular groove and advance the catheter and stylet slightly, confirming that the catheter is still appropriately placed.
- Stabilizing the stylet, slide the catheter down the vein lumen. The catheter should advance without resistance. Remove the stylet.
- Attach the extension set tubing and injection cap.
- Confirm catheter placement in the vein by aspirating blood into the extension set. Blood should flash back easily. Flush the catheter with heparinized saline solution.
- Use cyanoacrylate adhesive to anchor the catheter hub to the skin (optional).
- Secure the catheter hub to the skin using suture, taking care not to kink the catheter or puncture the jugular vein. Additionally secure the extension set to the skin in several places.
- The extension set is usually left exposed for ease of inspection for catheter-associated problems, or it can be covered by a sterile dressing and an Elasticon bandage placed around the neck.
- Bandages should be used to protect the catheter and insertion site in down patients such as foals to minimize catheter disruption and contamination.
- To deliver fluids, remove the injection cap and attach the extension set to an intravenous administration set.[7]

Catheter Use and Maintenance

- Injection caps should be replaced daily or as needed.
- The injection port should be wiped with an alcohol swab before each needle insertion.

- All catheters need to be flushed with 5 to 7 mL of heparinized saline solution every 4 to 6 hours to maintain patency.
- Patency should be checked each time the catheter is flushed and before administration of any medications.
- Check patency by attaching a syringe filled with heparinized saline solution and aspirating to achieve a flashback of blood; slowly inject in 5 to 7 mL of heparinized saline solution.
- Failure to achieve a flashback may be due to the following:
  - Clotted blood in the catheter
  - Kinking of the catheter or extension set
  - Loose attachment of the injection cap or extension set
  - Positional effect of the patient's head or neck
- If no flashback is seen, gently inject 5 to 7 mL of heparinized saline solution into the catheter and draw back. The catheter may need to be replaced if a flashback is not confirmed.
- When administering medication through a catheter, choose an injection port close to the catheter; clamp off any fluids that are flowing through the catheter, and check for a flashback, followed by injecting 5 mL of heparinized saline solution before the first drug, between each drug, and after the last drug is administered.
- ***Important:*** Certain drugs precipitate when mixed. Flushing sufficient heparinized saline solution to clear the extension set and catheter between each drug administered minimizes this complication. If any precipitation is seen, immediately stop medication administration and attempt to retrieve precipitate from the catheter by directly attaching a syringe to the catheter and withdrawing the injected contents.
- Drugs should be administered slowly. Medications known to cause adverse systemic reactions should be administered even more slowly and should be diluted.

[7]Stat large animal IV set (large-bore, 10 feet long; International Win, Ltd.).

- When replacing a catheter, use an alternate vein to minimize phlebitis.
- If possible, do not catheterize the same venipuncture site until the venipuncture site is healed.
- Use a long-term over the wire catheter if venous access is required for more than 6 days to avoid injury to the vein.
- ***Practice Tip:*** *If inserted and maintained properly, long-term catheters can, in many cases, be left in place for weeks.*

Complications

- Thrombophlebitis, phlebitis, or local cellulitis is a complication of long-term and, on rare occasion, short-term venous access (catheterization).
- Examine the catheter site twice daily for swelling, heat, and pain.
- A small circle of reactive skin at the site of skin puncture is not unusual, but thickening—induration—at this site and any associated heat or pain are abnormal and require immediate removal of the catheter.
- Careful palpation of the entire vein, paying particular attention to the location of the tip of the catheter within the vein, should also be performed twice daily.
- ***Important:*** Phlebitis can be a cause of fever and an increase or decrease in nucleated cell count.

- Phlebitis usually is responsive to local therapy (hot packing, topical dimethyl sulfoxide with or without antimicrobial agent, and/or topical 1% diclofenac sodium) but must be monitored closely because continued progression of serious complications such as septic thrombus or abscess would necessitate more aggressive treatment.
- ***Important:*** Antimicrobial treatment should be directed against *Staphylococcus* spp. pending culture and susceptibility results.
- If an ultrasound examination demonstrates fibrin strands in the vein and when infection is suspected in the perivascular area, systemic antibiotics should be used.
- Embolization of the catheter can occur if the catheter is severed accidentally or breaks off. This is an uncommon occurrence if the catheter is examined frequently and is replaced as needed.
- Thoracic radiography, sonography, or fluoroscopy can be used to locate the catheter. Interventional radiographic techniques are sometimes successful for catheter retrieval and may be more likely to be tried if the catheter is located in the heart and is imaged easily.
- ***Note:*** An embolized catheter that "travels" to the lung and is left there generally does not cause any long-term problems.

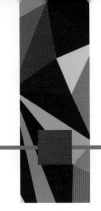

CHAPTER 4

Venous Access via Cutdown

James A. Orsini

Venous access via cutdown ("venous cutdown") involves making a small skin incision over a vein to facilitate intravenous (IV) catheterization. This simple surgical procedure is used in the medical management of the seriously ill foal or adult horse when routine catheterization is not possible. It is especially useful in the severely hypotensive patient when entry into a peripheral vein is made difficult because of poor vascular filling or when large-bore catheter placement is needed for resuscitation purposes.

The cutdown technique is an excellent method of obtaining venous access in a number of emergency situations. However, caution is needed; although complications are rare, they are potentially serious. They can be prevented by using good surgical technique and removing the catheter as soon as possible after completion of the resuscitative/supportive therapy.

Although the cutdown procedure is simple to perform, it needs to be completed rapidly and effectively in an emergency situation. Therefore, a thorough understanding of the anatomy associated with the target vessel, the surgical procedure, and its potential complications are important to know well.

Indications

Venous cutdown is indicated in the critically ill patient when vascular access is essential, but a less invasive option is unsuccessful or not feasible. Examples include:
- Very small patients (e.g., a premature foal)
- Any patient in profound shock
- Patients with phlebitis, thrombosis, or fibrosis/sclerosis that renders the most favored vein or access site unusable

Contraindications

Venous cutdown is contraindicated in the following situations:
- When a less invasive alternative is available
- When performing the procedure would cause excessive delay in resuscitation of the patient (In such cases, intraosseous infusion may be the better option; see Chapter 5, p. 17.)
- When infection is present in the region of the cutdown site
- When edema or other swelling is present over the target vein
- In the presence of injury proximal to (limb vein), caudal to (facial or jugular vein), or cranial to (lateral thoracic vein) the cutdown site (i.e., between the cutdown site and the heart)

- In the presence of a coagulation disorder
- When healing is impaired or host defense mechanisms are compromised

In every case in which venous cutdown may be indicated, the need to perform the procedure should be weighed carefully against the potential risks.

Anatomical Sites

Although venous cutdown may be used to gain access to any superficial vein, the most commonly used are the following (Fig. 4-1):
- External jugular vein
- Superficial thoracic vein
- Facial vein
- Cephalic vein
- Saphenous vein (and, less often, the lateral saphenous vein)

Patient selection is important when using any vein other than the jugular vein. Vessel size, access, and patency; restraint for the procedure; and catheter maintenance after the procedure must each be considered. For example, although the recumbent neonate's cephalic or saphenous vein may present an attractive option, maintaining a patent catheter in these vessels once the foal is mobile can be challenging.

Equipment

Because venous cutdown is performed primarily for the purpose of IV catheter placement, the items needed for catheterization must be assembled and ready for use. Taking the time to gather all needed equipment, supplies, and the fluids or medications that are to be given intravenously before starting the procedure is particularly important in the critically ill patient.

The items needed include the following:
- Materials and supplies for large-bore IV catheter placement (see Chapter 3, p. 9)
- Sterile local anesthetic solution (e.g., mepivacaine, 2%), 2 to 3 mL, with a 25-gauge, ½- to 1-inch needle
- Sterile surgical drapes (optional but recommended)
- Tourniquet (optional and only for use on a limb)
- Sterile minor surgery instrument pack, or at least a scalpel handle, curved hemostats, iris scissors, and needle holders
- Sterile scalpel blade, ideally #10, #11, or #15 (i.e., a small blade)
- Sterile surgical sponges (e.g., 4- × 4-inch gauze pads)

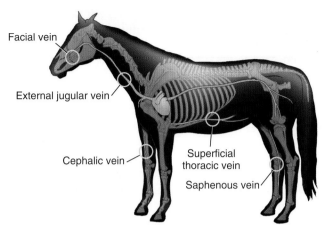

Figure 4-1 The most commonly used anatomical sites for venous cutdown are the external jugular vein, superficial thoracic vein, facial vein, cephalic vein, and saphenous vein.

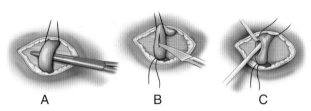

Figure 4-2 The surgical procedure for the venous cutdown is fundamentally the same for all appropriate sites in the equine patient. **A,** Isolating and elevating the vein; **B,** venotomy; **C,** threading the catheter into the vein.

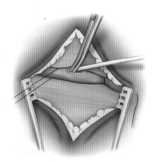

Figure 4-3 The use of ligatures and a curved mosquito hemostatic forceps to facilitate access to the venous lumen for catheter insertion.

- Sterile monofilament suture material, such as 3-0 or 2-0 polyglactin 910 (Vicryl)[1] or equivalent, if not included with the catheter equipment and appropriate skill suture
- Plastic venous dilator (optional)
- Sterile wound dressing and routine bandaging material as appropriate for the chosen site

Procedure

Regardless of the vein to be catheterized, the cutdown procedure is essentially the same, so the following instructions generally apply to all suitable sites in the equine patient (Figs. 4-2 and 4-3). However, although the surgical approach to the vein is uniform, there are two options for seating the catheter in the vein:

- Standard cutdown
- Mini-cutdown

Most of the time, the mini-cutdown can be used. It is simpler and faster than the standard procedure, and when successful, it carries no greater risk for complications. However, when catheterization via the mini-cutdown is taking too long or is likely to damage the vein, the standard cutdown must be used without delay. It is wise to begin every venous cutdown procedure prepared to perform the standard cutdown if necessary.

Standard Cutdown

The standard cutdown procedure is performed as follows:

- Restrain the patient as appropriate for the chosen site and the patient's temperament, position, and medical condition.
- Prepare the site as directed for IV catheter placement (see Chapter 3, p. 9); if necessary, enlarge the clipped area to ensure an aseptic surgical field and catheter placement.
- Occlude the vein on the cardiac side beyond the prepped area, as for IV injection or catheter placement. If possible, apply a tourniquet proximal to the site when using the cephalic or saphenous vein, and if necessary, tuck a folded surgical swab under the tourniquet directly over the path of the vein to ensure complete occlusion. A similar approach may be used to keep the jugular vein occluded for the procedure: a thick wad of gauze or a roll of bandage is strapped tightly into the jugular groove at the base of the neck and held in place by a couple of layers of Elastikon[2] wrapped snugly around the horse's neck. *However, if occluding the vessel in this way takes more than about 30 seconds to perform, then simply have an assistant apply digital pressure to occlude the vein.*
- Inject 2 to 3 mL of local anesthetic subcutaneously over the vein and either side of the vessel at the cutdown site, taking care to avoid injecting into the vein. (If the patient is unconscious or obtunded, skip this step.)
- Repeat the surgical prep if necessary. Don sterile gloves.
- Cover the surgical site with sterile drapes, leaving a small window (approximately 3 × 3 inches [7.5 × 7.5 cm] or as appropriate for the site) directly over the vein.
- Carefully make a small skin incision over the vein, perpendicular (at right angles) to the vein. An incision 1 to 2 inches (3 to 5 cm) in length usually is adequate. (A longitudinal incision made parallel to the vein reduces the risk of damaging the vessel and associated neurovascular structures, but it may not provide sufficient exposure.) Incise through the full thickness of the skin so that the subcutaneous tissues may be identified within the incision.
- Bluntly dissect the subcutaneous tissues from the vein by spreading them gently with a curved hemostat parallel to the course of the vein, with the tips of the hemostat pointed downward, toward the vein. Gently blot any blood as

[1]Vicryl (Ethicon Inc., Johnson and Johnson Company, Somerville, New Jersey).

[2]Elastikon (Johnson and Johnson Medical, Inc., Arlington, Texas).

needed with a sterile surgical sponge. Bleeding is usually minimal unless the vein is inadvertently cut.

At this point, either insert the catheter into the vein (see Mini-Cutdown, later) or proceed with the standard technique.

- Isolate the vein from the adjacent tissues and mobilize it for a length of approximately ½ to 1 inch (1 to 3 cm). If necessary, use a tissue spreader or other self-retaining retractor for a wider field of view.
- Following mobilization of the vein, use a hemostat to pass a pair of sutures under the vein, proximal and distal to the catheterization site, for stabilization.
- Tie the distal ligature and leave the ends long enough to allow manipulation of the vein (Fig. 4-2). Leave the proximal ligature untied so that the vein can be moved or occluded as needed for catheter insertion and to control backflow of blood (which is achieved by simply lifting up on the suture and vein) (see Fig. 4-2, A).
- Using a hemostat placed between the two sutures, elevate the vein to flatten it. Doing so provides good visualization, immobilizes the vessel, and limits bleeding when the vessel is incised. Alternatively, place gentle traction on the proximal suture to control oozing at the venous puncture site.
- Using the tip of the scalpel blade or iris scissors, carefully make a small incision in the near wall of the vein, at a 45-degree angle to the vein and extending only one third to one half of the vessel's diameter (see Fig. 4-2, B). ***Practice Tip:*** *If the venotomy is too small, the catheter may pass into the adventitia of the vein rather than into the lumen. However, if the incision is too large, the vein may tear completely. A longitudinal incision may be made in the vein instead, but it is more difficult to identify the vessel lumen using this approach; hence, the recommendation for an oblique venotomy incision.*
- Carefully thread the catheter into the lumen of the vein through the venotomy incision (see Fig. 4-2, C). Threading the catheter into the vein often is the most difficult and time-consuming part of the procedure. Care is needed to correctly identify the vessel lumen and to avoid dissection of the vessel wall with the catheter tip, penetration of the far wall of the vessel (i.e., going all the way through the vein with the catheter), and lodging of the catheter tip into a venous valve. It is also important to use a catheter that is not too large for the chosen vein.
- A plastic venous dilator may be used to identify and expand the vessel lumen to facilitate catheter placement. (The dilator has a small pointed tip that opens the lumen before the catheter tip is advanced.) ***Practice Tip:*** *As an alternative, a sterile 20-gauge needle, bent at a 90-degree angle, or curved mosquito hemostatic forceps (see Fig. 4-3) can serve as a dilator by elevating the near, proximal wall of the vein at the venotomy site. In most cases, a venous dilator is not needed in the adult horse.*
- Once the catheter is advanced into the vessel lumen, use a syringe to remove any air from the catheter, and connect the catheter to the extension set or IV tubing.

- Secure the proximal ligature around both the vessel and the catheter to prevent the catheter from dislodging. Remove the distal ligature.
- Remove the tourniquet or other occlusive device/pressure; suture the skin incision closed, taking care not to kink or crush the catheter, and secure the catheter to the skin as for routine IV catheter placement.
- Apply a topical antimicrobial ointment and sterile dressing over the site and cover or bandage in place as appropriate for the location.

Mini-cutdown

The mini-cutdown technique is a variation on the standard approach that is designed to preserve the integrity of the vein and avoid the time-consuming steps of mobilizing and placing sutures around the vein. It is the preferred method and in most cases is easy to do in both foals and adults.

- Follow the instructions for the standard approach, up to the point at which the vein is bluntly dissected from the subcutaneous tissues.
- Carefully insert the catheter tip through the near wall of the vessel and advance it as described in Chapter 3 for routine IV catheterization. Take particular care to seat the catheter tip within the vessel lumen before advancing it; avoid dissecting the near wall or penetrating the far wall if the vein is undistended or only partially distended because of circulatory collapse. Begin at the distal-most extent of the exposed vein, in case the first attempt at catheter placement is unsuccessful.
- If the catheter cannot be easily seated within the vessel on the first or second attempt, consider proceeding with the standard approach to avoid further vessel damage and delay.
- Once the catheter is properly placed in the vein, aspirate any air from the catheter, attach the extension set or IV tubing, release the tourniquet, suture the skin incision, and otherwise complete the catheter placement as described earlier for the standard approach.

Aftercare

- Follow the instructions given in Chapter 3 for IV catheter care. In addition, inspect the cutdown site at least once a day, and follow routine wound care for surgical incisions. Remove the skin sutures 10 to 14 days after placement.

Risks and Complications

Although the risk is slight with careful patient selection and surgical technique, the following complications are possible:

- Hemorrhage or hematoma may occur from inadvertent "nicking" of the vein during cutdown. If the damage to the vein is slight and the vein is catheterized anyway, then perivascular leakage of fluid or medication may be an added complication.
- Infection, either perivascular (as with any surgical procedure) or intravascular (septic thrombophlebitis, bacterial endocarditis, or systemic sepsis as with any IV catheterization) may develop.

- Failure to achieve central access and resuscitation in a timely manner may result in the death of the patient.
- Phlebitis, thrombosis, or embolism may occur as with any IV catheterization.
- Damage to surrounding anatomical structures, such as an adjacent artery or nerve, may be incurred during the cutdown procedure.
- Wound dehiscence may occur as with any surgical procedure.
- To avoid injury to adjacent structures, it is important to select a site for cutdown in which the vein is well isolated and use the *mini-cutdown technique* whenever possible.

Incisional infection is a potential complication, as with any surgical procedure. With due care, the risk is minimal, although the patients typically requiring venous cutdown are profoundly compromised, so they may be inherently at greater risk for incisional infection and for septic thrombophlebitis than are healthier patients. Therefore, broad-spectrum systemic antimicrobial coverage may be a prudent precaution in patients requiring venous cutdown.

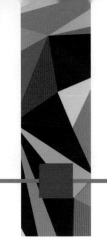

CHAPTER 5

Regional Perfusion, Intraosseous, and Resuscitation Infusion Techniques

David G. Levine

Regional Perfusion

Intravenous antimicrobial regional limb perfusion (RLP) has been described as an effective method of treating distal limb infections in horses. This is true for septic arthritis, osteomyelitis, cellulitis, and other soft tissue infections. Various techniques have been described, all with the goal of achieving high concentrations of an antimicrobial in the synovial, osseous, and soft tissue structures of the distal limb while limiting systemic side effects and cost. Aminoglycosides, specifically amikacin, are most commonly used both for their concentration-dependent mechanism of action and for their effectiveness against common equine orthopedic pathogens. Ideally, antimicrobials should be selected based on culture and susceptibility results if possible before treatment is initiated. This is not always practical because RLP is frequently used in high-risk musculoskeletal cases where culture results are not known. Examples of antimicrobials that have been used in the perfusate include aminoglycosides (gentamicin and amikacin), beta-lactams (penicillins, cephalosporins, carbapenems), enrofloxacin, and vancomycin. The majority of reports on RLP have evaluated the technique in horses under general anesthesia, which obviates their usefulness as a field technique. More recent reports on RLP performed in standing horses have shown lower concentrations of antimicrobials in the target tissues and a wider variation in data. Modifications in technique to include wider tourniquets and discouraging movement with proper sedation have shown more positive results. Although RLP can be used for septic arthritis, direct injection of the joint obtains higher concentrations of antimicrobials for longer periods of time and should be considered if there is no other soft tissue damage in the region. Intraosseous routes also can be used (see p. 17). In cases of intravenous regional limb perfusion, the procedure is most commonly performed using a tourniquet with the patient appropriately sedated. A tourniquet is applied to the limb proximal to the vascular access point and the site of suspected or confirmed infection. Either arterial or venous sites can be used with no difference in tissue concentration between the arterial and venous routes. Wide rubber tourniquets or pneumatic tourniquets should be used and the patient kept quiet and immobile to limit movement of the limb resulting in leakage of the perfusate proximal to the tourniquet and dislodging of the intravenous catheter. A long-term catheter can be placed in the perfusion vessel, although this may cause tissue irritation, phlebitis, and thrombosis of the catheterized vessel as sequelae. A butterfly catheter can be used for each treatment and works well for single or repeated perfusions.

Equipment

- Material for aseptic preparation
- Clippers
  - Clipping the perfusion site is clinician dependent.
  - The site is best clipped if the vessel is difficult to appreciate.
- Sterile gloves
- Appropriate over-the-needle catheter—20 to 23 gauge if being left in place for more than one perfusion—or a butterfly catheter[1]—size 21 to 27 gauge for daily use
- Heparinized saline flush (2000 units of heparin in 500 mL of saline solution) for catheters that are left in place for additional perfusions
- Elasticon tape
- Tourniquet—wide rubber or pneumatic[2]
- ***Practice Tip:*** *Use 40 to 60 mL of balanced electrolyte solution containing the equivalent of one third of the calculated systemic dose of the parenteral antimicrobial agent dose chosen for infusion. Twenty milliliters of perfusate can be used if the tourniquet is placed below the carpus/tarsus and the digital vessels are being used.*

Procedure

- Appropriately sedate the patient.
  - Alpha$_2$-agonist mixed with butorphanol is commonly used. The suggested dose is 0.01 mg/kg of detomidine mixed with 0.01 mg/kg butorphanol, IV or IM.
- Place the tourniquet.
- Aseptically prepare the skin overlying the catheter insertion site.
- Introduce the catheter into the selected vessel.

  Often the cephalic or saphenous vein is used and the tourniquet is placed above the site of perfusion. For distal limb

---

[1]Surflo Winged Infusion Set, 25 gauge, 19 mm (Terumo Medical Co., Somerset, New Jersey).
[2]ATS 1000 (Aspen Labs, Zimmer, Inc., Warsaw, Indiana).

perfusions, the tourniquet can be placed on the metacarpus/metatarsus and the digital vessels used.

- Perfuse the limb with 40 to 60 mL of a balanced electrolyte solution containing one third to the full systemic dose of the selected antimicrobial agent.
- Inject the perfusate over 1 to 3 minutes, checking frequently to ensure proper catheter placement within the vessel.
- Remove the tourniquet 20 to 30 minutes after injection of the perfusate.
- Place a secure bandage over the perfusion site.

Complications

- Improper placement of the tourniquet results in diffusion of the drug above the tourniquet. Using a narrow tourniquet results in low concentrations of the antimicrobials in target tissues. ***Practice Tip:*** *Rule-of-thumb: the width of the tourniquet used for the procedure should approximate the diameter of the limb above the site being perfused.*
- Movement of the patient during perfusion results in leakage of the perfusate proximal to the tourniquet and lower concentrations of perfusate to target tissues. Local perineural analgesia or additional sedation may be required to achieve a full 20 to 30 minutes of perfusion without movement. However, leaving the tourniquet on longer than 30 minutes may result in vessel and nerve injury.
- Repeated perfusions can cause local inflammation and thrombosis of the vessel. Application of topical diclofenac sodium cream[3] followed by a support bandage helps decrease the inflammation.

Intraosseous and Fluid Resuscitation Infusion Technique

Intraosseous infusion technique (IIT) can be used for a rapid delivery of medication and/or fluid when intravenous access is limited or *not* possible. This is most often used in neonatal foals where severe dehydration causes collapse of peripheral vessels. Uptake of medication or fluid is similar to that of intravenous injection; the cortex of the long bones prevents collapse during periods of hypovolemia. IIT is also used for regional delivery of medication such as regional/local antimicrobial perfusion of the lower limb with a tourniquet applied above the bone being perfused. Although regional intravenous perfusions are shown to have similar or better antimicrobial levels at the target tissue, some clinicians prefer the IIT route for cases in which multiple repeated infusions are required. This preference is attributed to regional intravenous perfusions becoming progressively more challenging because of local vessel irritation over time.

Equipment

- Sedation—depending on age and type of perfusion:
  - Adults—alpha$_2$-agonist (xylazine, detomidine) +/- butorphanol (see p. 315)
  - Foals may not need sedation if hypovolemic

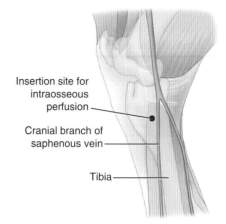

Figure 5-1   Cross-sectional anatomy of the intraosseous infusion site.

- Material for aseptic preparation
- Clippers
- Sterile gloves
- Local anesthesia: 2% mepivacaine (Carbocaine)
- #15 or #10 scalpel blade or disposal scalpel
- 12- or 15-gauge intraosseous needles/Sur-fast Cook[4] intraosseous needle/cannulated screws
- Heparin saline solution
- Crystalloid solution, lactated Ringer solution
- Perfusate for regional perfusion of antimicrobials (see Chapter 21, p. 303)
- Sterile bandage material

Practice Tip: *In newborn foals, alternatively, an 18- or 16-gauge needle can be used. In these cases, the needle is not left in place and should be replaced with an intraosseous needle, or intravenous access should be secured.*

Procedure

- Place the equine patient in a safe, clean, and warm environment.
- Position the foal in lateral recumbency for fluid resuscitation procedure.

Infiltrate the intraosseous site with mepivacaine superficially and deep to the bone.

- If performing an antimicrobial perfusion, place a tourniquet above the bone being perfused *after* the intraosseous needle or cannulated screw is secured in the medullary cavity.
  - Leave the tourniquet on for 20 to 30 minutes.
- Aseptically prepare the intraosseous site:
  - Most often the third metacarpus/metatarsus is used.
  - The proximal medial one third of the tibia 3 cm distal to the tendinous—a flat area devoid of vessels—band of the semitendinosus muscle is an alternate site (Fig. 5-1).
- ***Practice Tip:*** *A branch of the saphenous vein crosses the tibia 2 cm distal to the infusion site. The nutrient foramen*

---

[3]SURPASS, Boeringer Ingelheim (St. Joseph, Missouri).

[4]Sur-fast Intraosseous Infusion Needle Set, #C-DINH-12-2.3-PA (12 gauge, 2.3 cm) or #C-DINH-15-1.8-pa (15 gauge, 1.8 cm) (Cook Critical Care, Inc., Bloomington, Indiana).

is 2 to 3 cm distal to the infusion site near the popliteal line in the center of the tibial shaft.

- Using the scalpel blade or a disposal scalpel, incise the skin and subcutaneous tissues until contacting bone.
- Using the intraosseous needle—designed with placement stylet—or a large-gauge needle, apply a downward pressing and twisting motion against the bone until a loss of resistance is felt. If using a cannulated screw, drill a thread hole equal to the core diameter of the screw being used and then tap creating screw threads.
- Entrance into the medullary cavity is confirmed by aspirating blood or marrow contents.
- Flush the needle with 5 to 10 mL of heparinized saline solution.
- The intraosseous needle can be removed after infusion of a maximum of 1 L of crystalloid solution or it is secured in place. The needle should be flushed with heparinized saline every 4 to 6 hours to maintain patency. For long-term use, a cannulated screw may be more effective than a needle.
- Place a sterile wrap over the intraosseous site to maintain sterility.

Complications

- Subperiosteal or subcutaneous leakage of fluids or malposition of the intraosseous needle can result in partial occlusion of the needle. The leakage can cause a local tissue reaction but is usually only a temporary problem.
- Fractures can be caused by poor needle placement or creation of a large bony defect proportionally to the size of the patient.
- Occlusion of the needle or screw by a clot is the major limiting factor with this procedure. Although effective for quick resuscitation, long-term use is often *not* possible.

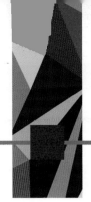

CHAPTER 6

Biopsy Techniques*

Janik C. Gasiorowski and James A. Orsini

Tissue biopsy often is helpful in antemortem diagnosis of disease and generally is not considered an emergency procedure. Depending on disease location, biopsy procedures can be associated with a certain degree of risk. In these cases, these procedures are often used for treatment or prognosis purposes only. In this chapter, biopsy techniques for different types of tissues are discussed, but the following practice tips apply to all tissue types.

Practice Tips:
- *Samples should be sent to a veterinary pathologist or specialist with the appropriate anamnestic and descriptive information.*
- *Biopsy specimens should be less than 1 × 1 cm for proper formalin fixation.*
- *The formalin-to-tissue volume ratio is 10:1.*
- *Samples should not be allowed to freeze during transport.*

Specialized Equipment

Biopsy of the skin and fine-needle aspiration of cysts and lymph nodes can be done with basic equipment as described later. Specialized instrumentation can make deeper, more complex biopsy procedures less invasive and improve histologic sample architecture. The operator must be familiar with the selected instrument before attempting to collect a sample. Practice before clinical use is highly recommended.

Most manual and automated biopsy needles have centimeter demarcations. Newer needles are etched for enhanced sonographic visibility.

Manual Biopsy: Soft Tissue[1]

The notched stylet is deployed from the cannula and the instrument is inserted into the target tissue (Fig. 6-1). The sharp cannula is then manually pushed back down while the stylet is held firmly in place. The sharp cannula cuts the tissue capturing a specimen in the notch of the stylet.

Manual Biopsy: Endoscopic[2]

Tissue samples may be obtained through the biopsy channel of flexible endoscopes. The biopsy forceps are long flexible cables with articulating jaws at the end controlled by thumb loops on the operator's end. The instrument is passed through the endoscope with the jaws closed. Once the target tissue is endoscopically located, the biopsy instrument is advanced and a tissue sample grasped. Frequently, the sample is too large to be retracted through the biopsy channel, so the entire endoscope/forceps/tissue combination is removed together to retrieve the biopsy sample.

Manual Biopsy: Bone[3]

These instruments consist of a trocar-tipped stylet and a strong cannula with a serrated end. The large T-shaped handle is held firmly in the palm while the instrument is advanced through the cortical bone in a drilling/rotational manner.

Automatic Biopsy: Soft Tissue[4]

Spring-loaded biopsy needles function similarly to the manual soft tissue biopsy needle previously described. A spring mechanism is loaded and the needle is placed into the target tissue. Activating the trigger deploys the notched stylet and then the cannula in the same process depicted in Fig. 6-1.

Automatic Biopsy: Bone[5]

This instrument is much like the manual Jamshidi needle but is powered by a battery-powered drill. It can be used to obtain bone marrow core or aspirate samples and has been associated with less pain and better sample histologic architecture.

Skin Biopsy

Skin biopsy is used in cases of undiagnosed skin disease, usually in cases of treatment failure or persistent clinical signs. Biopsy should be performed early in the disease process, preferably within 3 weeks, because the histopathologic findings are difficult to interpret in chronic cases. Punch biopsy or wedge biopsy (elliptical incision) usually is performed. Punch biopsy is preferred, except for sampling of vesicular, bullous, or ulcerative lesions, for which a wedge biopsy is more useful.

---

*We recognize and appreciate the contribution of Barbara Dallap Schaer, in the third edition, on which this chapter is based.
[1]Tru-Cut biopsy needle (Cardinal Health, McGaw Park, Illinois).
[2]EndoJaw biopsy forceps (Olympus, Inc., Center Valley, Pennsylvania).
[3]Jamshidi disposable bone marrow biopsy/aspiration needle (Baxter Healthcare Corporation, Deerfield, Illinois).
[4]TZ Spring-loaded biopsy needle (Gallini Medical Devices, Grand Rapids, Michigan).
[5]OnControl Bone Marrow Biopsy System (Vidacare Corporation, San Antonio, Texas).

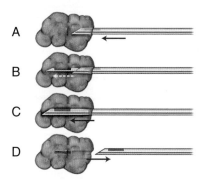

Figure 6-1   A, The biopsy needle is placed into the target tissue. **B,** The notched stylet is deployed. **C,** The cutting cannula is pushed back down over the notched stylet, capturing the sample. **D,** The entire instrument, with the biopsy inside, is removed.

Equipment

- 6- or 8-mm cutaneous biopsy punch[6] or a #15 scalpel blade for wedge biopsy
- 2% mepivacaine (Carbocaine) for local anesthesia, 25-gauge needle, and 3- to 10-mL syringe
- Rat-toothed forceps
- Metzenbaum scissors
- Needle holders
- Sterile gauze sponges
- 2-0 nonabsorbable suture
- 10% buffered formalin

Procedure

- Select areas representative of disease. A biopsy should include the lesion, point of transition, and normal skin.
- *Do not* wash or scrub the intended sample site or remove lesion crusts. This may result in disruption of the tissue architecture or removal of informative sample portions.
- Local anesthetic is infiltrated in the subcutaneous tissue beneath the area to be sampled. Do not inject directly through the intended sample to minimize histologic artifacts. Mark the anesthetized area.
- Punch biopsy: Select the site and rotate the biopsy punch while applying firm pressure until the instrument cuts through the dermis. Because the biopsy specimen is adherent to subcutaneous fat, grasp it with a forceps and separate it from the fat with Metzenbaum scissors.
- Wedge biopsy: Use a scalpel blade to make an elliptical skin incision; sharply incise the subcutaneous fat with scissors to free the sample.
- Be careful not to create a tissue artifact.
- Place the sample on a tongue depressor, subcutaneous fat side down, and immerse the tongue depressor in formalin. The tongue depressor preserves sample architecture during transport. Michel medium is typically used for immuno-fluorescence tests and is not a good preservative for histo-pathologic testing.

---

[6]Baker's biopsy punch (Baker Cummins Dermatologicals, Inc., Miami, Florida).

- Close the wound with a simple interrupted or cruciate suture pattern. Deep or large wedge biopsies may require two-layer closure.

Complications

Although infection is a rare complication, exercise extreme caution with biopsies performed near synovial structures or in contaminated areas. If dehiscence occurs, clean daily and allow healing by second intention. If a large wedge biopsy is in a high-motion area, restrict exercise for 1 week to decrease the risk of dehiscence.

Biopsy of Mass, Nodule, and Cyst

Cutaneous masses, nodules, and cysts are sampled by means of aspiration or excisional biopsy. Fine-needle aspiration yields a cellular sample and is differentiated cytologically as infectious, allergic, parasitic, or neoplastic. *Excisional* biopsy describes complete removal of a mass for treatment versus *incisional* biopsy, which refers to removal of a piece of tissue representative of the lesion. In both cases, histopathologic examination is used to confirm a diagnosis.

Equipment
Fine-Needle Aspiration

- 20-gauge, 1- to 1½-inch (2.5- to 3.75-cm) needle and 20-mL syringe
- Microscope slides

Excisional Biopsy

- Material for aseptic preparation
- 2% mepivacaine (Carbocaine) for local anesthetic
- #10 or #15 blade and handle
- Rat-toothed forceps
- Metzenbaum scissors
- Needle holder and suture scissors
- Sterile 4 × 4-inch gauze sponges
- Container with 10% buffered formalin
- 1-0/2-0 nonabsorbable suture

Procedure
Fine-Needle Aspiration

- Insert the needle with attached syringe into the center of the mass.
- Aspirate sample material into the needle and *not* into the syringe barrel.
- Redirect the needle several times without leaving the mass or contaminating the aspirate with normal tissue. If blood contaminates the sample, repeat the procedure with a new needle and syringe in a new location if possible. Release the negative pressure before withdrawing.
- Make a slide for cytologic examination by disconnecting the needle, filling the syringe with air, reattaching the needle, and expelling the needle contents onto a slide. Smear the aspirate for blood, or compress it between two slides and pull them apart. Allow the slides to air-dry.
- Aspirate a fluid-filled mass or cyst in a similar manner, sampling 1 to 2 mL of fluid to make a smear.

- Stain the slides with Wright or Diff-Quik stain. Send stained and unstained slides to a pathologist for interpretation.

Excisional Biopsy

- Aseptically prepare the area of the mass to be excised. *Do not* scrub if the surface is important for histologic interpretation.
- Inject a local anesthetic into the subcutaneous tissue or create a ring block.
- Make an elliptical incision around the mass and undermine the subcutaneous tissue with scissors.
- Place the tissue in formalin. If the mass is larger than 1 cm in diameter, section it longitudinally into 1-cm-wide samples.
- Close the subcutaneous and skin layers. Tension-relieving suture patterns such as a vertical mattress pattern or near-far-far-near suture pattern can be used if necessary.
- Restrict exercise to handwalking for 7 to 10 days.

Complications

See Skin Biopsy, Complications, p. 20.

Lymph Node Aspiration

Fine-needle aspiration of enlarged or abnormal lymph nodes is adequate for cytologic examination and can be helpful in differentiating infectious and neoplastic causes of lymphadenopathy. Complications are unusual.

Equipment

- 22-gauge, 1½-inch (3.75-cm) needle
- 10-mL syringe
- Microscope slides

Procedure

- Stabilize the lymph node with one hand, and insert the needle with attached syringe into the center of the lymph node.
- Please see technique description for Fine-Needle Aspiration (see p. 20).
- Allow the slides to air-dry. Stain slides with Diff-Quik. Send stained and unstained slides to a pathologist experienced in reading equine cytologic samples because the cytologic diagnosis of lymphosarcoma is difficult in the horse.

Renal Biopsy

Biopsy of the kidney is unusual because renal disease is well characterized with serum biochemical and renal function tests. Indications include renal masses and undiagnosed causes of renal failure. Percutaneous renal biopsy entails some risk and is performed only when the information is likely to affect treatment or outcome. Because perirenal hemorrhage is the primary complication associated with this procedure, prior clotting profile evaluation is recommended; clotting problems associated with renal failure in horses are uncommon. The right kidney is easily viewed with ultrasound, and biopsy should be performed with sonographic guidance to obtain an accurate sample and reduce the risk of complications. Biopsy of the left kidney is also performed under sonographic guidance.

Equipment

- Sedative (xylazine hydrochloride and butorphanol tartrate)
- 14-gauge, 6-inch (15-cm) soft tissue biopsy needle; manual or automatic
- #15 scalpel blade
- Clippers
- Material for aseptic preparation
- Sterile gloves
- 2% mepivacaine (Carbocaine) or other suitable local anesthetic, 25-gauge needle, and 3-mL syringe
- Sterile sleeve and sterile lubricant for ultrasound-guided biopsy of the right kidney
- 10% buffered formalin

Procedure

- Sedate patient to minimize motion during the procedure.

Right Kidney Ultrasound-Guided Biopsy

- The right kidney is located between the 15th and 17th intercostal spaces ventral to the lumbar processes.
- Clip the hair over the area, and perform an aseptic scrub.
- Place the ultrasound transducer in a sterile sleeve, and identify a site to sample away from the renal vessels. Alternatively, the biopsy location is determined by ultrasound examination followed by a "nonguided" Tru-Cut biopsy.
- Inject a local anesthetic subcutaneously at the biopsy site; repeat the sterile scrub.
- With sterile, gloved hands, make a stab incision and advance the biopsy needle through the stab incision to the kidney. The needle is directed obliquely in an attempt to sample cortical tissue only and avoid the renal medulla, renal pelvis, and hilar and renal vessels.
- If needed, a second assistant can perform sonographic guidance during the procedure. The needle appears as a hyperechoic line on the ultrasound screen and may be directed obliquely to avoid the renal vessels, pelvis, and medulla. *Note:* Be familiar with operation of the selected biopsy unit.
- Place the biopsy specimen in 10% formalin.

Left Kidney Biopsy

- The left kidney is more loosely attached to the abdominal wall and may require stabilization per rectum during the biopsy procedure. The kidney must remain motionless during needle placement. Successful biopsy of the left kidney requires sonographic guidance.
- Skin preparation and biopsy techniques are identical to those of ultrasound-guided biopsy of the right kidney.

Complications

Infection and peritonitis occur if sterile technique is not maintained or if the rectum is perforated. If rectal tissue or feed material is found, begin systemic antimicrobial therapy. Do not perform a biopsy on a suspected renal abscess because of the risk of infection.

Bleeding is a potential complication if the needle penetrates the renal artery or vein or one of the accessory arteries entering the caudal pole of the kidney. Central venous pressure and lactate levels should be monitored in patients with acute, significant blood loss. Packed cell volume and total protein should be monitored for several days on a renal biopsy patient. A clotting profile should be considered before the renal biopsy.

Hematuria is not uncommon and generally resolves spontaneously in 12 to 24 hours.

Liver Biopsy

Percutaneous biopsy of the liver is a simple procedure indicated in the treatment of patients with undiagnosed liver disease. Histopathologic findings often can define the liver disease as infectious, toxic, or obstructive/congestive.

Note: Sonographic guidance should be used to ensure that the biopsy specimen is obtained from an affected section of liver.

Equipment
- Sedative (xylazine hydrochloride and butorphanol tartrate)
- 14-gauge, 6-inch (15-cm) soft-tissue biopsy needle; manual or automatic
- #15 scalpel blade
- Clippers
- Sterile scrub
- 2% local anesthetic, 25-gauge needle, and 3-mL syringe
- Sterile gloves
- 10% buffered formalin

Procedure
- Perform clotting times (prothrombin time [PT] and partial thromboplastin time [PTT]) and platelet count before biopsy of the liver. PT and PTT are often abnormal in horses with liver failure; however, if the platelet count is normal and the biopsy is important for treatment planning, proceed with the biopsy.
- Using ultrasound guidance, locate a portion of the liver between the 6th and 15th intercostal spaces of the right lower to upper abdomen, respectively. Clip the hair and select an affected area of liver for biopsy.
- A liver biopsy can be performed "blindly" (without ultrasound) from the right 14th intercostal space in a line drawn from the point of the shoulder to the tuber coxae. Occasionally the liver cannot be seen on the right, and it is necessary to perform a biopsy of the liver, under ultrasound guidance, on the left at the level of the elbow, just caudal to the diaphragm.
- Sedate the patient for the procedure.
- Aseptically prepare the selected site.
- Inject a local anesthetic subcutaneously; perform a second aseptic preparation.

- With sterile, gloved hands, make a stab incision, insert the biopsy needle into the incision, and advance it in a cranial and ventral direction.
  Practice Tip: *Know the correct operation of the biopsy needle before using it.*
- Place the biopsy specimen in 10% formalin and another sample in an aerobic/anaerobic transport tube if a bacterial culture is indicated.

Complications

Although rare, excessive bleeding can occur, especially with existing coagulopathy secondary to liver disease. A coagulation profile is usually performed before liver biopsy. Monitor all patients for signs of bleeding for 48 hours after the procedure. If the platelet count is normal, bleeding is uncommon even in the face of a prolonged PT and PTT.

Infection (cellulitis, peritonitis) is unlikely if sterile technique is maintained. *Do not* perform a biopsy on liver abscesses. Accidental biopsy of the colon mandates systemic antibiotic therapy. If the liver is small on the right side of the horse, it may be necessary to approach the liver via the caudal thorax. Pneumothorax is a possible complication with this approach because of the track of the biopsy instrument through the diaphragm to the liver.

Lung Biopsy

Percutaneous biopsy of the lung is used in the evaluation of patients with diffuse lung disease or nonbacterial causes of focal pulmonary disease, if radiography, ultrasonography, and bronchoalveolar lavage do not provide a diagnosis.

Although deaths have been reported to occur, generally speaking, lung biopsy is safe and easy to perform.

Biopsy may be performed in a percutaneous, thoracoscopic, or an open manner. Manual or automated biopsy needles (previously described) are most commonly used for percutaneous biopsy. Endoscopic staplers,[7] bipolar cautery devices,[8] and ligating loops[9] have been used for thoracoscopic and open biopsy procedures. Open biopsy is usually performed only during procedures in which the thorax is already open. Percutaneous biopsy is most commonly performed and is described in the following.

Equipment
- Sedative (xylazine hydrochloride)
- Material for aseptic preparation
- Clippers
- Sterile gloves
- 2% local anesthetic, 22-gauge, 1½-inch (3.75-cm) needle, and 3-mL syringe
- #15 scalpel blade
- 14-gauge, 15-cm Tru-Cut biopsy needle
- 2-0 nonabsorbable suture on a straight or curved needle
- 10% buffered formalin

---

[7]Endo GIA (Covidien-AutoSuture, Boulder, Colorado).
[8]LigaSure Vessel Sealing System (Covidien, Boulder, Colorado).
[9]SURGITIE (Tyco Healthcare, Pointe Claire, Quebec, Canada).

Procedure

- Sedation is determined by the temperament of the patient.
- The most common site for biopsy, when lung disease is diffuse, is the right seventh or eighth intercostal space. Place the needle approximately 8 cm above the level of the olecranon and at the cranial aspect of the rib to avoid the intercostal vessels.
- Clip the hair, and perform a gross scrub.
- Infiltrate a local anesthetic into the subcutaneous tissues and parietal pleura.
- Perform a final aseptic scrub at the site of needle puncture.
- With sterile, gloved hands, make a stab incision through the skin.
- Advance the biopsy needle through the skin, muscle layer, and parietal pleura in a cranial and medial direction and continue during end inspiration for an additional 2 cm into lung parenchyma.
  Note: You must be familiar with the operation of the biopsy unit so that the biopsy can be performed quickly and successfully for sample collection.
- Place the tissue in 10% formalin.
- Close the skin incision using a simple cruciate pattern.

Complications

A small volume of air may leak into the thorax before the skin is closed and should not cause a problem. Hemoptysis may occur and is rarely a problem. Fatal tension pneumothorax rarely occurs after lung biopsy (see Chapter 25, p. 470, and Chapter 46, p. 729).

Bone Marrow Biopsy

Bone marrow biopsy or aspirate is a useful procedure to determine causes for changes in peripheral blood cell count or cell morphology. The finding of possible neoplastic or abnormal cells in the circulating blood is an indication for bone marrow biopsy. This procedure is used to differentiate primary hematopoietic disease (lymphosarcoma, multiple myeloma, myeloproliferative disease), compensatory marrow changes (iron deficiency anemia, anemia of chronic disease), and red cell hypoplasia due to administration of erythropoietin. Bone marrow is analyzed by means of aspiration or core biopsy. A sample for complete blood cell count drawn at the time of biopsy should be submitted with the biopsy sample.

Equipment

- Sedative (xylazine hydrochloride and butorphanol tartrate)
- Material for aseptic preparation
- Clippers
- Sterile gloves
- 2% local anesthetic, 25-gauge needle, and 3-mL syringe
- #15 scalpel blade
- For aspiration: 15-gauge, 2-inch (5-cm) bone marrow needle (Jamshidi[3])
- For core biopsy: 11-gauge, 4-inch (10-cm) bone marrow needle

- 12-mL Luer-Lok syringe with anticoagulant (10% disodium EDTA), Petri dish, and microscope slides if aspiration is performed (more commonly used of the two procedures)
- 10% buffered formalin if a biopsy specimen is submitted

Procedure

- The fourth, fifth, or sixth sternebrae are the most common sites; the marrow cavity lies just below the periosteum. The tuber coxae can be used for biopsy in individuals less than 4 years of age. The tibial crest can serve as yet another site.
- *Practice Tip: When obtaining samples from sternebrae, it is very important not to breach the far cortex because the apex of the heart lies directly above the biopsy site.*
- Sedation is recommended.
- Infiltrate a local anesthetic into the subcutaneous tissues and periosteum.
- Clip the hair, and perform aseptic preparation.
- With sterile, gloved hands, make a small stab incision.

Bone Marrow Aspiration

- Insert the needle and stylet through the skin and advance it to the periosteum. A rotational motion is needed to advance the needle through the cortex and into the marrow cavity. Once in the marrow cavity, the needle is firmly seated.
- Remove the stylet and attach the syringe. Aspirate the bone marrow with negative pressure on the plunger; aspirations should be short and gentle. Excessive negative pressure results in blood contamination of the sample.
- Place the sample in a Petri dish. Remove the marrow spicules and place them on a microscope slide. Prepare a squash smear by positioning one slide on top of the other and gently pulling them apart. Send both stained (Diff-Quik) and unstained slides to the laboratory.
- The concentration of acid-citrate-dextrose (ACD) solution used to collect bone marrow for stem cell culture ranges from 7% to 20%.
- *Practice Tip: Use 5 mL ACD solution in a 35-mL syringe, 14% concentration.*
- Other variables involved in the collection of bone marrow weigh far more heavily on outcome than does the ACD concentration. Many use heparin as the alternative; however, ACD solution is preferred because it preserves the platelets better than heparin.
- *Note:* Always check with the laboratory that is going to process the stem cells for their specific recommendations.

Bone Marrow Biopsy

- Insert the biopsy needle through the skin and advance it to the cortex.
- Remove the stylet. Continue to advance the cannula for another 2 cm using a forceful rotational movement.
- A rotational thrust of the needle should detach the specimen; withdraw the needle.
- The stylet is used to push the biopsy specimen out of the needle and into a formalin container.

Complications

Hemorrhage can occur and rarely is clinically significant unless the patient has thrombocytopenia or another clotting deficiency. Osteomyelitis is rare.

Muscle Biopsy

Histopathologic examination of muscle samples is useful whenever disease of muscle fibers, neuromuscular junctions, or peripheral nerves is suspected. This is a minor surgical procedure performed on a standing horse. Samples of diseased and normal muscle should be collected. If polysaccharide storage myopathy (PSSM) is suspected, biopsy of the semimembranosus muscle is preferred. For motor neuron disease, the biopsy is performed on the muscle at the tail head (sacrocaudalis dorsalis medialis).

Practice Tip: Formalin may not be the preservative of choice, depending on the specific analysis. Place a 1-inch biopsy sample between saline dampened 4×4s and ship overnight in a hard container in ice packs is preferred method for diagnosing PSSM by the University of Minnesota laboratory. A moist gauze sponge with excess saline removed and the sample not "floating" or frozen is recommended. Contact the pathology laboratory before performing a muscle biopsy for specific preservative recommendations.

Equipment

- Material for aseptic scrub
- Clippers
- Sterile gloves
- 2% local anesthetic, 25-gauge needle, and 5-mL syringe
- #10 scalpel blade and handle
- Metzenbaum scissors
- Tongue depressor
- 0 or 2-0 absorbable and nonabsorbable suture
- Appropriate fixative or saline

Procedure

- Sedation is determined by the temperament and state of debilitation of the patient.
- The sample should be approximately 5 mm wide, 20 mm long, and 5 mm thick and should be parallel to the direction of the diseased muscle fibers.
- Clip the hair, and perform a gross scrub at the biopsy site.
- Infiltrate a local anesthetic into the subcutaneous tissues. *Do not* inject anesthetic into the muscle; this affects the histopathologic findings.
- Perform an aseptic scrub.
- With sterile, gloved hands, incise the skin over the muscle belly. Use blunt dissection to separate the skin from the muscle belly. Remove a muscle sample using sharp dissection.
- Secure the sample to a tongue depressor or muscle biopsy clamp[10] with stay sutures to prevent sample shrinkage. The

sample should be minimally handled to prevent crush artifacts.
- Close the incision in two layers to minimize dead space.
- If a biopsy of atrophied gluteal or back muscle is needed, a Tru-Cut biopsy or similar instrument is used for sampling.

Complications

Infection is uncommon, but dehiscence of semimembranosus muscle can occur.

Endometrial Biopsy

Endometrial biopsy is a useful procedure to evaluate infertility.

Important: Rule out pregnancy before biopsy to avoid iatrogenic abortion. The procedure is best performed during estrus.

Equipment

- Sedative (xylazine hydrochloride and butorphanol tartrate)
- Scrub material
- Sterile sleeve (shoulder length)
- Sterile lubricant[11]
- 70-cm alligator punch[12] (sterile)
- Bouin fixative

Procedure

- Sedation is recommended. Ideally the mare is restrained with a twitch, in stocks.
- Tie the mare's tail to the side.
- Scrub the perineum with a dilute antiseptic solution (povidone-iodine or chlorhexidine) and rinse with water.
- With a sterile, gloved arm, digitally dilate the cervix, and gently guide the biopsy instrument through the cervix.
- Advance the biopsy instrument into the uterus and with the gloved arm in the rectum, confirm instrument placement.
- Via rectal palpation, depress a portion of the uterine mucosa between the jaws of the tissue and close the instrument to obtain the sample. Take endometrium only; full-thickness biopsy is contraindicated.
- Place the sample in the appropriate fixative and process within 24 hours.

Complications

Abortion can occur if the mare is pregnant at the time of biopsy. Perform a complete reproductive examination before biopsy. The cervix should be closed if the mare is pregnant.

Endometritis can occur if bacterial pathogens are introduced into the uterus.

References

References can be found on the companion website at www.equine-emergencies.com.

[10]Rayport muscle biopsy clamp (Allegiance Health Care, Edison, New Jersey).

[11]Priority Care Sterile Lubricating Jelly (First Priority, Inc., Elgin, Illinois).
[12]Jackson uterine biopsy forceps (Jorgensen Laboratories, Inc., Loveland, Colorado).

CHAPTER 7

Hyperbaric Oxygen Therapy

Fairfield T. Bain

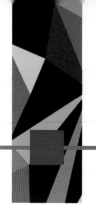

Although hyperbaric oxygen therapy (HBOT) is not new to the human medical field, it has only recently become available as a treatment option for equine patients. In human medicine, HBOT is most widely known for the treatment of decompression sickness (aka "the bends") for divers and more recently for a variety of medical conditions. Hyperbaric oxygen therapy is an FDA-approved medical therapy for certain conditions in human medicine.

Indications for HBOT for humans from the Undersea and Hyperbaric Medical Society are:
- Air or gas embolism
- Carbon monoxide poisoning
- Clostridial myositis and myonecrosis (gas gangrene)
- Crush injury, compartment syndrome, and other traumatic ischemia
- Decompression sickness
- Arterial insufficiencies:
  - Central retinal artery occlusion
  - Enhancement of healing in selected problem wounds
- Severe anemia
- Intracranial abscess
- Necrotizing soft tissue infections
- Osteomyelitis (refractory)
- Delayed radiation injury (soft tissue and bony necrosis)
- Compromised grafts and flaps
- Acute thermal burn injury

Equine patients have many conditions similar to those indications listed for human HBOT. This technology may be applicable to several emergency conditions or trauma, especially wounds associated with:
- Poorly vascular traumatized tissue and flaps
- Burn injury
- Soft tissue infections (e.g., tendon sheath infections)
- Clostridial myositis
- Bone infections (osteomyelitis)
- As in human medicine, HBOT is often used as an adjunctive treatment along with other medical therapies, such as anti-inflammatory medications and antimicrobial agents.
- There is increasing clinical experience with HBOT for the equine patient with certain traumatic injuries, infections, or potentially necrotizing processes.
- The rational application of hyperbaric oxygen as an adjunct to current medical management should be considered for certain emergent conditions in the equine patient.

Physiology of Hyperbaric Oxygen Therapy

- *Practice Tip: HBOT works using the principles of gas under pressure.*
- It is a mode of therapy in which the patient breathes 100% oxygen at pressures greater than normal atmospheric pressure.
- In the hyperbaric chamber, the horse is exposed to almost 100% oxygen under increasing pressure.
- Some principles of physics of gases are useful to understanding the effects of hyperbaric oxygen.
  - At sea level, breathing air, we are exposed to a pressure of 14.7 pounds per square inch (psi) or 760 millimeters of mercury (mm Hg).
  - Air is comprised of 79% nitrogen and 21% oxygen, containing a partial pressure of approximately 160 mm Hg of oxygen (21% × 760 mm Hg).
  - In hyperbaric medicine, a common unit of pressure used is Atmospheres Absolute (ATA); sea level = 1 ATA ("normal atmospheric pressure").
  - In diving, each 33 feet (or 10 meters) of seawater, the pressure increases 1 ATA.
  - Therefore, at 33 feet of seawater (fsw), the absolute pressure is 2 ATA.
  - At 66 feet of seawater, the absolute pressure is 3 ATA. The comparisons to depths in seawater are important because they are the relative pressures that a patient is exposed to for clinical hyperbaric oxygen treatments.
  - The critical feature of oxygen under pressure is that the partial pressure of inspired oxygen (FiO_2) increases exponentially.
  - Using 100% oxygen at 2 ATA, the horse is breathing in 2 atmospheres of 100% oxygen—or 760 mm Hg × 2 = 1520 mm Hg.
  - At 3 ATA, the horse is breathing in 3 atmospheres worth of 100% oxygen or 760 mm Hg × 3 = 2280 mm Hg equaling 14 times the amount one would breathe in room air at sea level.
  - Most clinical applications for the equine patient involve treatment between 2.0 to 2.5 ATA resulting in dramatic increases in the partial pressure of oxygen

(PaO$_2$) within arterial blood. Treatment protocols for the equine patient are based on experience with human patients and animal models. ***Practice Tip:*** *The goal is to use the lowest pressure possible to accomplish the clinical end point, such as tissue salvage or resolution of infection.*

- In normal physiology, most of the arterial oxygen content (CaO$_2$) is comprised of oxyhemoglobin.
- During HBOT, there is a progressive increase in the concentration of oxygen dissolved in plasma.
- It is the dissolved oxygen that results in the physiological effects of hyperbaric oxygen.
- ***Important:*** With medical applications of HBOT, 3 ATA is the maximum pressure used for patient treatment (because of the increased risk of oxygen seizures at higher concentrations of oxygen), with most treatments being between 2.0 to 2.5 ATA.

- The mechanisms of action of HBOT are mediated by the increased concentration of dissolved oxygen in the plasma.
- These can include:
  - Improved oxygenation of hypoxic tissues within complicated or hypoxic wounds
  - Vasoconstriction resulting in decrease in edema
  - Improved antimicrobial activity and increased bacterial killing by neutrophils
  - Modulation of neutrophil adhesion to endothelial cells in ischemia-reperfusion injury
- The ability to save hypoxic tissue within complicated wounds may reduce time for repair and return to function.
- Although there are no controlled clinical trials in the horse, there appears to be an application for hyperbaric oxygen to treat tissue in such wounds in the equine trauma patient.

●〉 WHAT TO DO

HBOT for the Equine Patient
Clostridial Myositis
- Horses with rapidly progressing clostridial myositis represent a unique challenge, with current clinical management aimed at reducing the amount of tissue lost by necrosis from vascular injury.
- Often, the overlying skin is already necrotic by the time of detection and examination by a veterinarian.
- There is evidence that HBOT may impair clostridial toxin function and help salvage skin and muscle within the affected regions.
- Early treatment with hyperbaric oxygen has been performed in an effort to save as much tissue as possible.

Burn Injury
- Burn injuries occur less frequently in the horse; the challenge is with severe skin injury, when necrosis, pain, and the additional insult of smoke inhalation injury are part of the clinical findings. HBOT is in common use for treatment of human burn patients for both clinical conditions.
- Mechanisms shown to benefit the burn patient include:
  - Improvement of oxygenation in hypoxic patients
  - Injured skin
    - Reduction of edema
    - Improved microcirculation
    - Reduced inflammatory responses
    - Faster epithelialization
    - Improved wound healing
- ***Practice Tip:*** *HBOT is considered a primary treatment for smoke inhalation injury.*

Soft Tissue Infections
- Soft tissue infections, especially of the lower limb, can be difficult to manage with routine therapy including antimicrobial agents, anti-inflammatory medications, and surgical drainage or lavage.
- The addition of HBOT may be useful in bacterial killing by leukocytes and improving antimicrobial function in inflamed, hypoxic tissue.
- A similar effect can be expected in cases of bone infections in which necrotic bone may be preventing adequate penetration and function of antimicrobial agents.

Ischemia-Reperfusion Injury
- There is research and clinical experience in animals and humans supporting a benefit of hyperbaric oxygen in ischemia-reperfusion injury.
- In the equine patient, gastrointestinal and smoke inhalation injury involve similar mechanisms of neutrophil adhesion to capillary endothelial cells.
- HBOT is used in some equine hospitals postoperatively for patients with strangulating intestinal lesions to decrease injury associated with ischemia-reperfusion. ***Practice Tip:*** *Large colon torsion represents the most common example of ischemia-reperfusion injury in the equine patient.*
- Ultrasound monitoring of colon thickness and serum protein concentrations as a marker of intestinal mucosal protein loss are useful as objective measures of colon wall health and viability. Both can be used to assess and monitor the clinical response when using HBOT in the postoperative period for these patients.

Neurologic Injury
- New information supports the potential benefits of HBOT for traumatic brain injury and possibly spinal injury.
- There is also evidence suggesting HBOT may be useful in repair of peripheral nerve injury by increasing growth factors and other mechanisms of stimulating axonal budding.
- ***Practice Tip:*** *Peripheral nerve injury in the horse, brachial plexus or radial nerve injury, are examples of injuries that could benefit from hyperbaric oxygen in the early post-trauma period—the first 24 to 48 hours.*

Complicated Wounds and Skin Flaps
- While not every wound needs hyperbaric oxygen treatment, some large wounds with hypoxic injury to the skin, underlying tissues, and large skin flaps may benefit from HBOT.
- The goal is to minimize tissue necrosis and loss from hypoxia in order to reduce the time for wound healing.

◉〉 WHAT NOT TO DO

HBOT Contraindications

- The most common clinical condition for which there may be a contraindication in the horse is when the potential for pneumothorax exists.
- This might include thoracic trauma in the adult and birth trauma in the neonate where rib fracture with secondary pulmonary injury and pneumothorax can occur.
- At-risk equine patients should be examined for the presence of pneumothorax before being treated with hyperbaric oxygen.

- Changes in atmospheric pressure can result in pain and injury to the tympanic membrane in human patients. The pain from pressure changes appears unusual in the horse, possibly because of the ability to accommodate for pressure changes by the guttural pouch.
- ***Practice Tip:*** *Horses with sinus or guttural pouch disorders should be monitored closely during HBOT for signs of increasing discomfort or irritability that may indicate gas trapping and pain associated with pressure changes.*

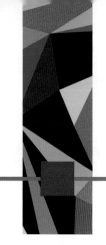

CHAPTER 8

Complementary Therapies in Emergencies: Acupuncture

Stephen G. Dill

Acupuncture can serve as an adjunctive modality for equine emergencies. This chapter addresses when acupuncture may prove valuable for specific emergency conditions and provides basic guidelines for what to do with acupuncture. Although a discussion of specific acupuncture diagnostic and therapeutic techniques is beyond the scope of this chapter, veterinarians seeking training in acupuncture can find approved programs listed later in the chapter.

Background Information on Acupuncture

Acupuncture is reported to have local and systemic physiologic effects, making it useful in the treatment of emergencies. Acupuncture helps the body achieve "homeostasis and balance." If a biologic system is functioning in an abnormal way—hyperactively or hypoactively—acupuncture restores normal balance. For example, if there is a hyperimmune response (e.g., allergies or autoimmune disease), acupuncture modulates the hyperactive immune system. Conversely, if the immune system is hypoactive, as occurs in stress or an immunodeficient state, acupuncture may be useful in improving immune function.

Many studies have been reported on how acupuncture works. The effects of acupuncture occur primarily through the nervous system, with endorphins, enkephalins, serotonin, and other neurotransmitters playing important functions.

Blood flow is vital to health and healing; acupuncture can regulate blood flow to tissues and therefore is useful as part of the treatment plan for many conditions, including laminitis, thromboembolic colic, intermittent claudication, and cerebrovascular accidents (CVAs), for example. Early in the treatment of CVAs in people, neurologists recommend caution in performing acupuncture for this condition because of the risk of increasing blood flow to the region of bleeding and aggravating the clinical condition.

In addition to affecting blood flow, acupuncture is also reported to affect gastrointestinal (GI) motility and provide analgesia. As such, it is particularly useful in postoperative ileus. It is also indicated in many types of colic because of its ability to normalize both hypo- and hyperactive GI motility. A theoretical concern with the use of acupuncture in colic is that it reduces the horse's response to pain; therefore, an accurate assessment of pain is less reliable as a clinical marker in differentiating a medical from a surgical patient. Generally, in surgical cases of colic, the period of analgesia with acupuncture is relatively short in duration.

Acupuncture has several other effects on a biological system, making it a useful adjunct for the treatment of emergency conditions affecting the motility of the bile duct, bladder, and uterus. It not only acts as an antiemetic and thermoregulator but also affects endocrine imbalances and hormone levels, general cardiovascular status, cardiac rhythm, spinal cord function after trauma, airway constriction, apnea, and other functions. Emergency conditions that may benefit from acupuncture treatment are listed in Box 8-1.

Clinical response may occur within minutes to hours following acupuncture treatment. Treatment intervals for emergencies may vary from twice a day to every few days, depending on the specific circumstances.

●〉 WHAT TO DO

Acupuncture for Emergency Cases

- Know the specific clinical problems where acupuncture can be a valuable adjunct in care.
- Identify a certified veterinary acupuncture specialist to call for consultation.
- Take a veterinary acupuncture training course to become familiar with the technique and indications for its use.
- Treat early—the likelihood of a favorable outcome increases with early treatment.
- Repeat treatments are often indicated for best results.
- Treatment intervals vary depending on specific circumstances.
- Acupuncture is considered a safe method of treatment; understand the limitations and precautions when using acupuncture in clinical practice.

●〉 WHAT NOT TO DO

Acupuncture

- Acupuncture needles should not be inserted through a contaminated or infected area.
- Acupuncture may be used to treat pregnant mares and even to prevent abortion; however, certain acupuncture points and techniques should be avoided because they can cause an abortion.

Other Features of Clinical Acupuncture

Approximately 1 in 10 equine patients treated for a variety of gait abnormalities is "stiff gaited" for 1 to several days after treatment. The stiffness is minor in severity and of no clinical consequence; it is best to alert owners of this adverse side effect to avoid unnecessary concern. This uncommon side effect is less likely to occur in treating equine emergencies.

Box 8-1 Emergency Conditions That May Benefit from Treatment with Properly Performed Acupuncture

Disease/Condition
Colic—a wide variety of etiologies
Anterior enteritis
Colitis/diarrhea
Rectal prolapse
Choke/megaesophagus
Cholelithiasis
Liver disease
Shock
Hemorrhage, generalized or localized
Septicemia
Laminitis
Congestive heart failure
Cardiac arrhythmias
Syncope
Cardiopulmonary resuscitation
Respiratory arrest
Burns
Heat stroke
Pyrexia
Allergies/anaphylaxis
Immune-mediated diseases
COPD/RAO
Pneumonia
Renal disease
Urolithiasis
Bladder paralysis
Seizures
Cerebrospinal trauma/inflammation
Peripheral nerve trauma
Musculoskeletal trauma/injury
Tendon/ligament trauma/sprain/bowed tendon
Neck/thoracolumbar pain
Gait abnormalities
Exertional rhabdomyolysis
Uveitis, keratitis, corneal ulcers
Prevention of abortion
Retained placenta
Metritis
Uterine prolapse
As an aid in fetal malposition
Insufficient lactation
Mastitis

COPD, Chronic obstructive pulmonary disease; *RAO,* recurrent airway obstruction.

Acupuncture treatment can provide pain relief in the terminally ill equine patient. Although these patients often appear more alert and comfortable and have more energy for a short period of time after treatment, they may die shortly after this phase of apparent improvement. The clinical response often benefits the equine patient and owner; however, owners should be advised of the likely course of events so that they are not surprised by the sudden deterioration after an apparent clinical improvement.

The extremely weak patient can be treated with acupuncture, but it is recommended to use a minimal number of needles with mild needle stimulation during the treatment.

Acupuncture is effective in and of itself, but in some instances, results are improved using Chinese herbs. Yunnan Paiyao,[1] also spelled Baiyao, has been used for many years in China with reportedly good results in treating abnormal bleeding. A suggested dose for a 500-kg horse is 15 mg/kg PO q12h. Other Chinese herbal combinations useful for bleeding that may be more tailored to the individual condition of the patient also are available.

Developing an Expertise in Clinical Acupuncture

Veterinarians not trained in the use of acupuncture but who want to use acupuncture in clinical practice should seek advanced training or refer cases to a certified veterinary acupuncturist. Training programs in veterinary acupuncture are found on the following websites: www.ivas.org, www.tcvm.com, and www.colovma.org.

Contact information for several organizations follows:
International Veterinary Acupuncture Society
www.ivas.org
1730 South College Ave.
Suite 301
Fort Collins, CO 80525
Chi Institute
www.tcvm.com
9700 West Hwy 318
Reddick, FL 32686
CVMA Medical Acupuncture for Veterinarians
www.colovma.org
191 Yuma St
Denver, CO 80223

These groups list contact information for certified veterinarians on their websites for ease of referral. Unless you have firsthand experience with a referring veterinarian for acupuncture treatment, it is best to refer a clinical case to a certified veterinarian. Certification assures you and your client that the clinician has a specified level of knowledge about veterinary acupuncture. One other group providing contact information for certified veterinarians in acupuncture as well as continuing education (but no certification course) includes:
American Academy of Veterinary Acupuncture
www.aava.org
PO Box 1058
Glastonbury, CT 06033

This chapter provides basic information to guide veterinarians in the treatment of equine emergencies using acupuncture as an adjunct modality. The training opportunities coupled with the bibliographic references (reference list is available on the companion website) can assist the veterinarian in better caring and advising horse owners on the benefits of acupuncture.

References

References can be found on the companion website at www.equine-emergencies.com.

[1]Yunnan Paiyao (Baiyao), Kan Herbs, www.Kanherb.com, 831-438-9450.

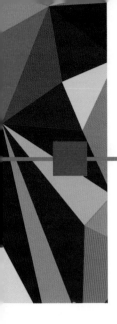

Emergency Imaging, Endoscopy, Laboratory Diagnostics, and Monitoring

CHAPTER 9

Laboratory Diagnosis of Bacterial, Fungal, Viral, and Parasitic Pathogens

Joan Norton

- It is frequently difficult to differentiate bacterial, viral, parasitic, or fungal diseases based on clinical signs alone.
- To appropriately treat an infectious disease, the causative agent must be identified.
- ***Practice Tip:*** *Proper sample collection, transport containers, shipping conditions, and transport media are critical to the laboratory confirmation of an infectious agent. Most samples can be shipped chilled using an ice pack. Do* not *use ice packs for anaerobic samples.*

- Interpreting laboratory results must take into account:
  - Signalment and case information
  - History
  - Clinical signs
  - Other laboratory data
- Knowledge of potential agents is important when requesting testing and interpreting the results.

●〉 **WHAT TO DO**

Bacterial Samples and Testing

- Selection of collection swabs, transport media, transport container, shipping and handling, and temperature requirements depends on the suspected pathogen—aerobic versus anaerobic.
- Collect sample using aseptic technique before debridement or exploration of the affected site.
- If possible, discontinue antimicrobial therapy for a minimum of 24 hours before sample collection.
- For an unopened abscess, the capsule should be aseptically prepared before aspiration or incision for collection of fluid or abscess samples from the deepest part of the area of interest. Liquids should be placed in a sterile container and culture swabs in bacterial transport media.
- Samples also may be collected via aspiration with a sterile needle and syringe. Transfer the sample to an appropriate transport media or container for testing.
- Immediately place the sample in the appropriate transport medium, keeping in mind that anaerobic samples are sensitive to room air.
- ***Practice Tip:*** *Anaerobic samples must be placed in anaerobic transport media and not chilled. Grossly purulent material (i.e., Strangles) can sometimes be culture negative even with proper technique used in sampling and handling. Swabbing the depths of the abscess can improve culture results.*
- Samples for blood culture are placed in blood culture bottles. Anaerobic and aerobic blood culture bottles should be inoculated as per manufacturer's instructions. Hair overlying the vein is clipped and the skin aseptically prepared and allowed to dry before venipuncture. Change needles, and wipe bottle tops with alcohol, and allow to air-dry before injecting the sample into the blood culture bottle.

- ***Practice Tip:*** *Do* not *chill blood culture samples.*
- Urine samples degrade rapidly and should be refrigerated quickly and transported to the laboratory within 48 hours. Colony counts should be requested.
- Fecal samples, for aerobic bacterial culture, are placed in a clean container. Because a large number of organisms are normally present, request *only* the pathogens you suspect.
- ***Practice Tip:*** *Fecal cultures for anaerobic organisms (e.g., Clostridia sp.) are placed in anaerobic transport media. Toxins for C. difficile and C. perfringens are thermal labile. Fecal samples for toxin testing are stored in a plastic (not Styrofoam) container at 2° C to 8° C immediately after collection and processed within 48 hours. Longer storage is possible at −20° C.*
- Fecal swabs are *not* appropriate for toxin testing.
- Samples should arrive at the testing laboratory within 24 hours of collection.
- Uterine cultures are performed using a guarded sterile swab:
  - Prepare the perineum using an antiseptic wash.
  - A sterile, lubricated, gloved hand is inserted into the vagina; gently dilate the cervix with one finger.
  - Guide the swab through the cervix before pushing the tip out of the protective covering. **Important:** Be sure to retract the swab into the sleeve before removing it from the uterus and vagina.
  - The end of the swab is broken off and placed in an appropriate culture transport system.
- Solid tissue samples for culture are transported in a leak proof container and are kept moist with a small amount of sterile saline and refrigerated. Do *not* submerge the sample in saline. Necropsy samples should be taken within 4 hours of death and placed

●〉 WHAT TO DO—cont'd

in individually labeled containers with the specimens clearly identified.

- Bacterial morphology characteristics and Gram stain of samples can be performed if an air-dried glass slide sample is submitted. Smears of the samples should be air dried and heat fixed for Gram stain and microscopic examination. These slides are shipped so that they remain dry during transport! Do *not* place in a container with ice packs!

- Cytology samples are prepared and examined in house or referred.
- Thin smears should be prepared, dried, and stained with a Diff-Quik type stain and Gram stain to assist in determining the infectious agent.

●〉 WHAT NOT TO DO

Bacterial Samples and Testing

- *Do not* send syringes and/or needles containing samples to the laboratory for testing.
- Anaerobic samples *do not* survive at room air for more than 20 minutes.
- Repeated freezing and thawing of samples is to be avoided.
- *Do not* submit fecal swabs for toxin testing!
- *Do not* submerge tissue samples in saline solution submitted for bacterial culture.
- Do *not* chill blood culture bottles for shipping.
- Do *not* open tops of blood culture bottles.
- Do *not* allow air-dried microscope slide samples to become wet.

●〉 WHAT TO DO

Fungal Samples and Testing

- Testing for fungal infections is rarely an emergency unless mycosis is suspected in cases of progressive ocular, intestinal, skin, vascular, or pulmonary disease.
- Most fungal samples are cultured using the same transport media for bacteria culture.
- For skin samples, hair is plucked and deeper skin scrapings prepared with a #10 scalpel blade.
- Placing mineral oil on the skin before scraping prevents loss of the sample.
- The samples are placed in a sterile vial for transport.
- Hair removed for fungal culture should be placed in a dry container and shipped at room temperature to prevent overgrowth of bacterial and fungal contaminants.
- *Practice Tip: Fungal cultures typically take much longer than bacterial cultures and therefore results can be delayed up to 2 to 3 weeks. Contact the laboratory for fungal sensitivity testing.*
- Fungal spores, hyphae, or filamentous cells may be identified on Gram stain prepared as previously described for microscopic slide evaluation for bacteria.
- Gram stain and cytologic examination of corneal scrapings are recommended if fungal keratitis is suspected (see Chapters 11 and 23, pp. 41 and 406).
- *Note:* Fungal hyphae are commonly seen on the transtracheal wash of horses with recurrent airway obstruction (RAO; heaves) that are housed in barns. In these individuals, the fungal contamination does *not* require treatment.

●〉 WHAT TO DO

Viral Samples and Testing

- The chances of isolating a virus from a sample are highest in the early stages of infection.
- Sampling areas vary with causative agent.
- Respiratory viruses are best recovered from nasal swabs or EDTA whole blood samples in the case of EHV-1.
- Neurologic viruses are often recovered from CSF, fresh brain tissue, and EDTA samples.
- Enteric viruses (rotavirus and coronavirus) are recovered/tested from feces.
- *Practice Tip: If unsure of correct sample procedure, always contact the testing laboratory or take multiple samples and request the laboratory to use the appropriate sample.*
- Viral transport media is a good transport media for viral isolation and viral PCR.
- EDTA blood, transtracheal wash (TTW), and tissues also can be used.
- If possible, consult with testing laboratory before collecting samples!
- *Practice Tip: Chilled samples (use refrigeration or ice packs for overnight shipping) increase the chance for viral recovery.*
- If viral transport media is *not* available, place swab into a plain sterile red-top tube with 1 to 2 drops of sterile saline.
- Fluid samples obtained from affected areas—vesicles, tracheal aspirates, or feces—should be collected with a moistened swab and placed in viral transport media and refrigerated or frozen before shipping.
- Blood samples for viral isolation and serology should be collected into plain red-top and EDTA tubes and shipped chilled, but *not* frozen.
- Positive virus isolation may be observed as early as 5 to 7 days for certain viruses; definitive identification may take longer.
- Negative samples are held and final analysis determined at 30 days after culture.
- Paired serum antibody titers are helpful for diagnosis.
- *Practice Tip: Serum samples are taken 2 to 4 weeks apart; a fourfold increase in titer between samples confirms exposure.*
- *Important for Rabies:*
  - All neurologic cases with rabies in the differential diagnosis should be submitted for fluorescent antibody (FAB) testing and for histopathology changes characteristic of the disease. Consider rabies regardless of vaccination history.
  - Chilled brain tissue, including the cerebellum and brain stem, is submitted.
    - Samples can be collected from a suspect animal that died a few days earlier but this is not ideal.

● WHAT TO DO—cont'd

- **Contact the County Department of Health for assistance and the testing laboratory for specific sampling and shipping details.**
  - Do *not* submit the entire head.
  - Wear latex gloves, surgical mask, and glasses during sample collection.
  - *Do not* use power saws (including Stryker saws), which can aerosolize the virus. Remove the cerebellum and some brainstem using a large spoon.
  - Refrigerate specimens before shipment. Do *not* fix tissues with chemical preservatives.
  - Place specimens in at least two separately sealed plastic bags with gel-type cold packs in a Styrofoam-insulated cardboard box.
  - Disinfect all instruments and surfaces with a 10% solution of household bleach mixed in water.

● WHAT NOT TO DO

Viral Sample and Testing
- *Do not* use bacterial transport media for viral samples.

● WHAT TO DO

Parasite Samples and Testing
- Blood parasites: Piroplasmosis
  - EDTA blood and serum are required for testing.
  - This is a foreign animal disease (FAD); confirming the disease or suspicion of the disease requires that appropriate authorities are notified.
  - Validation testing is required by a national and/or veterinary state laboratory.
- Respiratory: Fluid obtained from TTW may show migrating parasites or lung worms. Fluid is placed in an EDTA tube and shipped chilled.
- Fecal parasites: Feces should be placed in a sealed leak proof container for fecal flotation. **Sample should be kept chilled or ova may hatch!**
  - ***Practice Tip:*** *Often with clinical cyathostomiasis, fecal examinations are negative.*
  - Clinical history and signs often assist in confirming parasites.
- Neurologic parasites:
  - EPM antemortem samples ideally include CSF in both an EDTA (for cytology) and clot tube along with serum for serum:CSF antibody ratio.
  - Postmortem samples include neurologic tissue.
  - *Parelaphostrongylus tenuis* and *Halicephalobus* sp.—Post mortem samples include histology of the spinal cord for *P. tenuis* or brain/brainstem for *Halicephalobus* and PCR testing of the affected tissue. Samples are placed in formalin and frozen at necropsy.

● WHAT TO DO

Molecular Testing
Polymerase Chain Reaction (PCR)
- Polymerase chain reaction (PCR) testing is available to identify the presence of DNA in a variety of bacterial, viral, and parasitic pathogens.
- Samples for respiratory disease—EHV-1, -4, -5, EIV, rhinitis virus A and B, *Rhodococcus equi,* and *Streptococcus equi subspecies equi*—can be obtained from nasal swabs, pharyngeal or guttural pouch washes *(Strep. equi),* tracheal aspirates, or bronchoalveolar lavage (BAL) (EHV-5).
- EDTA whole blood is submitted for EHV-1 in the viremic stage—Potomac horse fever, *Anaplasma phagocytophilum,* and other agents causing bacteremia or viremia.
- PCR can be performed on feces to identify DNA from *Salmonella* spp, beta-coronavirus, *Neorickettsia ehrlichia,* and *Lawsonia intracellularis.*
- Contact laboratory for additional fecal PCR tests.

● WHAT TO DO

Summary of Laboratory Testing for Pathogens
- Laboratory diagnostics are critical to obtain a definitive diagnosis.
- Veterinary laboratories often have specific requirements for testing.
- Before testing, contact the laboratory to obtain important information on sample collection, testing, shipping, and handling of samples.
- If contacting the testing laboratory before sample collection is *not* possible, multiple samples should be taken, and the laboratory should be instructed/contacted for best samples and testing use.
- Submit samples to an American Associated Veterinary Laboratory Diagnosticians (AAVLD) certified laboratory whenever possible for best practices and sample recovery.

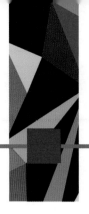

CHAPTER 10

Emergency and Critical Care Monitoring

Thomas J. Divers and Eileen S. Hackett

- Monitoring procedures for the emergency or critically ill horse vary depending on the equipment available and financial limitations.
- Monitoring can be
  - Basic
  - Advanced
  - Goal directed
- Basic monitoring depends on repeated clinical examination in addition to some basic observations (e.g., urine production).
- Advanced monitoring requires diagnostic equipment (e.g., I-STAT, ultrasound, electrocardiogram [ECG]).
- Goal-directed monitoring is a combination of basic and advanced, while numeric goals are set for specific clinical variables, such as heart rate and physiologic data—Pao_2 and glucose. Point of care laboratory monitoring is discussed in Chapter 15.
- Monitoring the emergency and critical care patient is intended to provide information on:
  - Global and local perfusion
  - Oxygenation
  - Organ function
  - Sepsis
  - Electrolyte and acid-base status
  - Metabolism
  - Complications
- ***Practice Tip:*** *The goal of monitoring is to allow early and appropriate changes in treatments and guide prognosis.*
- Global tissue perfusion is determined by monitoring:
  - Heart rate
  - Hydration status
  - Mucous membrane color
  - Pulse pressure
  - Temperature of extremities
  - Urine production (basic monitoring)
- The color of mucous membranes and capillary refill are determined by:
  - Cardiac output
  - Vasomotor tone
  - Hemoglobin concentrations
  - Bilirubin concentrations
- Advanced monitoring of tissue perfusion includes measuring:
  - Blood pressure
  - PvO_2

- Pulse oximetry—SpO_2 (***Note:*** SpO_2 is generally 3% less than actual SaO_2.)
- Blood and fluid lactate concentration
- Echocardiography—estimate cardiac output and access chamber dimensions and function
- Oncotic pressure—estimated by plasma protein concentration
- Cardiac troponin-I (cTnI) concentration
- Blood pressure measurements are generally performed by direct and indirect methods (see p. 34, for details).
- Inadequate cardiac preload to the heart is most commonly a result of intravascular dehydration in adult horses; in septic foals, vasomotor tone dysfunction may be a more common cause and should be closely monitored in the critical care equine patient.
- Basic monitoring of cardiac preload is observed by clinical evidence of dehydration—skin turgor, wetness of mucous membranes, and speed of jugular filling after manual obstruction.
- Measurement of central venous pressure (CVP) is ideal for monitoring cardiac preload, but the technique is *not* always easy to perform and is *not* needed in most cases. Please see pp. 35-36, for details.
- Measurement of urine specific gravity is an easy and often underutilized means of monitoring hydration status; fluid therapy needs; and in some cases, renal function.
- Oxygenation of tissues is monitored by clinical and laboratory perfusion markers as discussed earlier in addition to monitoring:
  - Hemoglobin (Hgb) values
  - PaO_2
  - End-tidal CO_2—nasal or endotracheal capnograph—can be used to determine proper placement of endotracheal tube (a near zero recording could indicate the endotracheal tube is in the esophagus or patient expired) or as an estimate of cardiac output in shock patients ($ETCO_2$ is low in shock unless $PaCO_2$ is elevated) or as a guide to effective resuscitation. Endotracheal measurement is more reliable than intranasal measurement.
  - Other pulmonary function (e.g., auscultation, endoscopy, ultrasound)
  - Other oxygen supply/delivery monitoring—mucous membrane color, lactate, PvO_2
- Monitoring of plasma electrolytes, complete blood count (CBC) (including plasma color), and organ function/

disease tests are very important in the emergency and/or critical adult or foal and are used as a supplement to the clinical monitoring.

- Abnormalities found in the CBC and blood chemistry results may provide information not detected by the other monitoring methods.
- Monitoring blood glucose is particularly important in sick foals, as is serum creatinine in all ages of critically ill horses, while electrolyte monitoring is important in horses and foals with diarrhea and renal disease.
- Monitoring the CBC, especially the presence or absence of toxic changes in neutrophils, band neutrophils, and platelet count, is necessary along with information on the primary disease. Clinical findings, combined with laboratory results, determine the severity of the disease and the need for and duration of hoof cryotherapy to prevent laminitis.
- Drug monitoring is an advanced part of monitoring the critical care equine patient.
- Measuring aminoglycoside plasma concentrations is important to determine efficacy and early toxicity.
  - *Practice Tips:*
  - *Peak levels—30 min after IV administration is associated with efficacy.*
  - *Toxicity—associated with trough levels*
  - *In life-threatening sepsis, gentamicin peak levels are 8 to 10 µg/mL and amikacin 25 to 30 µg/mL, corresponding to 10× the minimum inhibitory concentration (MIC) of the susceptible pathogen.*
  - *Trough levels should be <1 µg/mL gentamicin or <3 µg/mL amikacin.*
  - *Peak levels are determined by plasma collection 30 min after IV administration and 60 min after IM administration.*
  - *Trough levels are determined on plasma taken just before the next scheduled dose is given. Adjusting the dose of potentially toxic drugs is discussed in Appendix 4, p. 815.*
- Other monitoring procedures are discussed in the chapters identified below:
  - ECG[1] and Doppler monitoring in the cardiovascular system and treatment of systemic inflammatory response syndrome (SIRS) (see Chapter 32)
  - Blood gases,[2] pulse oximetry, lactate, cTnI, and end tidal CO_2 (ETCO$_2$) in the respiratory, perinatology, neonatology, and treatment of SIRS (see Chapter 15)
  - Abdominal distention, colic, gastric reflux, abdominal ultrasound, peritoneal fluid changes in gastrointestinal and ultrasound (see Chapters 14 and 18)
  - Urine production and CVP (see p. 35 and Chapter 26, p. 489) and treatment of SIRS (see Chapter 32, p. 567)

- Changes in neurologic status (see Chapter 22, p. 341)
- Monitoring the pregnant mare (see Chapter 27, p. 497)
- Monitoring of the feet for early evidence of laminitis (see Chapter 43)
- Monitoring of incisions or wounds for infection (see Chapter 19, p. 243)
- Using the clinical examination and laboratory testing prevents or detects early complications in the critically ill horse and prevents serious and life-threatening complications such as renal dysfunction and electrolyte abnormalities as previously discussed.
  - Laminitis, drug toxicity, and thrombophlebitis
  - Proper biosecurity protocols and monitoring reduces nosocomial infections.
  - Monitoring the nutritional status of the critically ill horse and providing appropriate nutritional intervention is often overlooked and is discussed in Chapter 51, p. 768.

Blood Pressure Monitoring

- Arterial blood pressure (BP) measurement is used to detect alterations in circulatory function and response to therapy.
- Low arterial pressure is seen in multiple disease states including:
  - Heart failure
  - Blood loss
  - Massive fluid loss
  - Acute trauma
  - Sepsis
- *Practice Tip: Systemic pressure support, ideally using fluid therapy, improves organ function and ameliorates deleterious effects of circulation disturbances.*

Indirect Blood Pressure

- Blood pressure monitoring is performed using oscillometric pressure cuffs.
- Although less accurate than direct pressure measurement, this indirect method is noninvasive and generally well tolerated in horses and foals (Box 10-1).
- An occlusive cuff is placed over an easily accessible artery, usually on the tail or limb. The base of the tail is used in adults and the metatarsal artery in foals. Cuffs should be the appropriate size.
  - Cuff width should be 40% of the limb circumference or 25% to 35% of the tail circumference, and bladder length should be 80% of the tail circumference.
  - *Practice Tip: Narrow cuffs overestimate pressure and wide cuffs underestimate pressure.*
  - Purchasing multiple sizes of cuffs allows blood pressure measurement, regardless of variations in age and size.

---

[1]A new ECG recording device is now available for the iPhone—AliveCor Veterinary Heart Monitor for iPhone 4/4S per Dr. Marc Kraus, Cornell University.

[2]As a rule, arterial blood gas analysis is used when monitoring pulmonary function, whereas venous blood gases are helpful when monitoring other organ dysfunction and shock.

Box 10-1	Indirect BP Reference Values	
Adult:		Foal:
99-125 mm Hg (systolic)		80-125 mm Hg (systolic)
54-91 mm Hg (diastolic)		60-80 mm Hg (diastolic)

- ***Practice Tip:*** *Indirect measurements often underestimate actual blood pressure by 10 to 20 mm Hg. If the heart rate displayed on the blood pressure monitor does not correlate with the auscultable heart rate, then blood pressure value is likely incorrect!*
- The cuff is attached to a commercially available pressure recording device, which reports systolic and diastolic pressure readings and heart rate.
- *Note:* The reported heart rate should be consistent with the actual heart rate to ensure the most accurate measurement.
- Quiet restraint, maintenance of the head at a neutral level, and obtaining multiple readings improve accuracy.

Direct Blood Pressure

- Blood pressure is evaluated directly through the use of an arterial catheter. This method is invasive and likely to have improved accuracy over indirect methods, especially in the severely ill (Box 10-2).
- Convenient catheterization sites are:
  - Transverse facial artery in adults (20-gauge catheter)
  - Lateral metatarsal artery in foals (18- or 20-gauge catheter)
- Aseptic preparation of arterial catheterization sites is recommended.
- Local anesthetic infiltration is helpful in conscious horses before percutaneous catheterization.
- Blood pressure can be continuously measured by connection of the catheter and fluid-filled extension sets to an electronic pressure monitor.
- Arterial pressure wave tracings are visible; systolic, diastolic, and mean arterial pressures are measured.
- ***Practice Tip:*** *Extension set tubing length should be limited and air bubbles flushed from the line to improve pressure measurement.*
- Clean catheter insertion technique and application of direct pressure on catheter removal minimizes hematoma formation.

Central Venous Pressure Monitoring

- CVP estimates the volume of venous blood pumped through the heart and is measured within the cranial vena cava by insertion of a long catheter into this region using the jugular vein for access.
- CVP is an approximation of right atrial pressure.
- CVP is measured using a CVP catheter kit or a 24-inch intravenous catheter.[3-5]
  - The tip of the catheter must be in the anterior vena cava or right atrium, approximately 50 cm from the jugular insertion in the midcervical area of the average-size adult horse. Jugular vein pressures are lower than CVP.
  - In foals, the catheter position can be determined by radiographs; in adult horses it is best determined by observing consistent but minor changes (0.5 cm H_2O) in the measurement associated with breathing and changes in intrapleural pressure.

Box 10-2	Direct BP Reference Values	
Adult:	Foal:	
126-168 mm Hg (systolic)	129-168 mm Hg (systolic)	
85-116 mm Hg (diastolic)	65-83 mm Hg (diastolic)	
110-133 mm Hg (mean)	82-108 mm Hg (mean)	

Box 10-3	CVP Reference Value Measurements	
Adult:	Foal:	
6-18 cm H_2O	3-12 cm H_2O	
8-12 mm Hg	2-9 mm Hg	

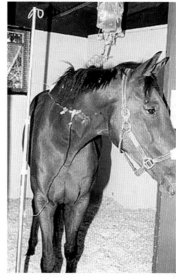

Figure 10-1 CVP monitoring in a horse using a water manometer. The manometer is taped to an IV pole so that it remains in the same position in relation to the base of the heart for each measurement.

- Normal values for adult horses and foals are in Box 10-3.
- ***Practice Tip:*** *Changes over time are likely more important than the actual values, which can overestimate the actual CVP.*
- The zero position on the manometer must remain at the exact same level (estimated at base of the heart or point of the shoulder) on the horse for each measurement (Fig. 10-1).
- The head position of the horse should be nearly the same for each measurement. Head height decreases CVP.
- Electronic monitors[6] generally measure approximately 2 cm lower than a water manometer.
- ***Practice Tip:*** *To convert cm water CVP to mm Hg, multiply by 0.73554.*

---

[3]Intracath (Deseret Medical, Inc., Franklin Lakes, New Jersey).
[4]Equine 19-G, 90-cm long line catheter (Mila International, Inc., Erlanger, Kentucky).
[5]Central Catheter Set (Arrow International, Reading, Pennsylvania).
[6]Medtronic Lifepak 12 (Medtronic Physio-Control, Inc., Redmond, Washington).

| Box 10-4 | **CVP Based End Points of Fluid Resuscitation** |

Adult: 15-24 cm H$_2$O—*Stop* fluid therapy

| Box 10-5 | **Conditions Associated with Low CVP Values** |

- Vasodilation
- Hypovolemia
- Inappropriate reference point
- Inadequate insertion distance

| Box 10-6 | **Conditions Associated with High CVP Values** |

- Volume overload
- Right heart dysfunction
- Vasoconstriction
- Pericardial and pleural effusion
- Pneumothorax
- Positive-pressure ventilation
- Ventricular catheterization
- Catheter occlusion
- Inappropriate reference point

- Pressure can be measured by connecting the catheter and fluid-filled extension set(s) to a manometer or pressure transducer device.
  - *Practice Tip:* Small oscillations in the fluid meniscus with breathing indicate catheter tip location.
  - Large fluctuations in fluid meniscus indicate overinsertion of the catheter tip within the heart.
  - A consistent reference point should be used.
  - *Practice Tip:* In the standing horse, the reference point is the point of the shoulder. In the recumbent horse, the reference point is the sternum.
- Quiet restraint is used and multiple readings are recorded.
- More important than single CVP measurements are trends recorded over time or in response to treatment (Boxes 10-4 to 10-6).

References

References can be found on the companion website at www.equine-emergencies.com.

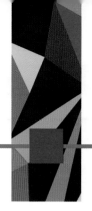

Cytology

Tracy Stokol

Cytologic Evaluation

Cytologic evaluation is a useful technique for the equine practitioner.

- Minimal equipment is required: glass slides, syringes, needles.
- Smears can be prepared in the field for later staining and examination.
- Solid tissue lesions and body fluids can be aspirated and imprints can be prepared from biopsy specimens for rapid assessment and a potential diagnosis.

The ability to obtain a cytologic diagnosis depends on smear quality and cellularity and the proficiency of the cytologist.

- Slides of poor cellularity or quality (slowly dried, smudged cells) are rarely diagnostic.
- Some smears (even if cellular) are not diagnostic. Biopsy and histopathologic examination may be required.

- Proficiency requires extensive training and practice.
- To enhance skills, duplicate slides can be kept and results compared with that of a clinical pathologist. Cytologic smears can be compared with histopathologic diagnosis from biopsies.

There are inherent limitations in the diagnostic accuracy of cytologic evaluation:

- Smears only represent the aspirated site. Focal or multifocal lesions may be missed.
- Aspirates do *not* evaluate tissue architecture, which can be crucial for diagnosing certain tumors and differentiating inflammation from neoplasia in some circumstances.
- Connective or fibrous tissue (e.g., sarcoids) exfoliates poorly on aspiration or imprints.
- Cystic or fluid-filled lesions are often nondiagnostic. Aspirate cyst walls or solid tissue where possible.

●❯ WHAT TO DO

Preparation of Cytologic Specimens

Interpretation is optimized by preparing high-quality slides for examination. Smear quality is influenced by specimen collection, slide preparation, slide staining, and sample storage and handling.

Collecting the Specimen

Tissue Aspirates

Aspirate solid organs or mass lesions with a 21- to 22-gauge needle and 5- to 12-mL syringe, applying a gentle suction force when the needle is located within the tissue to dislodge cells. Redirect the needle and re-aspirate several times (without exiting the tissue) to maximize the sampled region. When finished aspirating, remove the needle from the syringe, fill the syringe with air, and then replace the needle. Place the bevel of the needle close to the slide surface, and then use the air-filled syringe to gently expel the aspirated tissue onto *several* slides. Gently spread the tissue on the slide using the squash technique (see the following and Figs. 11-1 and 11-2) and rapidly air-dry the smears (for more, see below).

- Larger-bore needles yield thick tissue chunks (which do not smear well) and increase blood contamination.
- Smaller-bore needles may rupture cells, leading to nondiagnostic specimens.
- Smaller-volume syringes do not provide enough vacuum pressure to disrupt tissues.
- Vigorous suction or expulsion onto slides causes blood contamination and may rupture cells.
- A good aspirate looks "dry." Vigorous suction and exiting the tissue during aspiration collects cells into the needle hub or syringe barrel, from where they cannot be retrieved.

- Multiple slides permit additional staining procedures, such as a Gram stain.

Fluid Specimens

Techniques for obtaining samples of pulmonary secretions (tracheal wash and bronchoalveolar lavage [BAL]) and body cavity fluids (peritoneal [PTF], pleural [PLF], cerebrospinal [CSF], and synovial [SF]) are discussed elsewhere (see specific organ system chapters).

- Purple-top tubes containing ethylenediaminetetraacetic acid (EDTA) are preferred because EDTA preserves cell morphology, inhibits (but does not prevent) bacterial growth, and blocks clot formation.
- Collection of bloody fluids into a non-anticoagulant (red-top) tube is worthwhile to determine if the sample clots (helps differentiate hemorrhage from blood contamination).
- If bacterial culture or measurement of biochemical analytes (e.g., glucose or enzymes) is desired, submit a portion of the fluid in a sterile non-anticoagulant (red-top) tube. If prolonged shipping is likely, use a microbiologic transport system for culture.
- Always make smears from freshly collected fluid to optimize cytologic results (for more, see below).

Surgical Biopsies/Necropsy Tissues

Because result turnaround time is quicker for cytology than histopathology, examination of cytologic slides from these samples can potentially yield a rapid diagnosis. Also, correlating cytologic to histopathologic results is useful for improving diagnostic cytologic skills. Cytologic smears (imprints and scrapings) can be prepared from surgical biopsies or necropsy specimens (see the following).

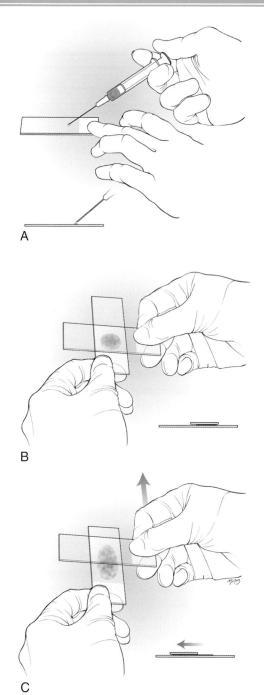

A

B

C

Figure 11-1 *Preparation of a squash smear from an aspirate.* **A,** After aspirating the lesion, place the tip of the needle, bevel side down, onto the surface of a clean glass slide just in front of the frosted end. Depress the plunger and gently expel a small amount of the aspirate onto the slide; multiple slides can be prepared simultaneously. A drop that is 4 to 5 mm in diameter is ideal. **B,** Place a second slide (spreader slide) directly on top of the first slide with the drop. This squashes the drop. The spreader slide can be placed perpendicular (as shown) or parallel to the bottom slide. Allow the drop to spread between the two surfaces; just allow the two slide surfaces to be in contact, do not place any additional pressure on either slide. **C,** Gently, using a smooth steady but swift motion, move the spreader slide forward; this spreads the drop of fluid along the length of the slide, creating a thin smear. Then rapidly air-dry the slide. The spreader slide can be reused to squash one or two additional slides, and then it is discarded. Note that if too large a drop of the aspirate is placed on the slide, the slides may not separate easily and a feathered edge is not obtained.

- Cells deteriorate rapidly after death, so collect samples ASAP after euthanasia. Little diagnostic information is yielded from autolyzed tissues and body cavity fluids obtained at necropsy.
- Avoid exposure of slides and fluid samples to formalin (liquid or fumes), which introduces a staining artifact (Fig. 11-3).

Preparation of Glass Slides

General Principles

Prepare slides as soon as practical after collection. This is particularly important for fluid samples for the following reasons:

- Cells in fluid samples remain alive and functional after collection.
  - Bacteria are phagocytized by neutrophils, simulating sepsis. This can occur quite rapidly after sample collection (within an hour).
  - Red blood cells are phagocytized by macrophages, simulating previous hemorrhage. This can occur within a few hours of sample collection.
- With time, cells become pyknotic or begin to lyse in vitro and become unrecognizable.
- With time, bacterial overgrowth may occur, affecting cell counts (bacteria are counted as cells) and obscuring or lysing cells, yielding nondiagnostic specimens.

Use new, precleaned glass slides, preferably with frosted ends: Do not wash slides and reuse. Label slides (specimen, site, patient identification) on frosted end in *pencil*. Ink from marker pens (including permanent markers) dissolves during staining.

Always rapidly air-dry slides, preferably with a hair dryer (on the high setting and holding the back or noncellular side of the slide near the nozzle of the hair dryer during drying). Heat fixing is not required. Cells do not spread in slowly dried smears, obscuring detail and hindering evaluation.

- Neutrophils can be misidentified as lymphocytes.
- Bacteria are difficult to detect intracellularly when cells are "balled up."
- Cells are difficult to distinguish by size; for example, lymphoblasts resemble lymphocytes.

Smear Preparation Technique

For all specimens, avoid placing the sample near or at the slide edges. These areas are missed with most automated stainers and are difficult to examine with higher-power objectives. General smear types for fluids and aspirates are wedge and squash smears (see Figs. 11-1 and 11-2) and for surgical biopsy/necropsy, tissue samples are imprints and scrapings.

- WEDGE: Blood, fluids of low viscosity (peritoneal, pleural, nonmucoid cyst fluid)
- SQUASH: Aspirates, viscid fluids (tracheal wash, synovial fluid, mucus or mucoid fluids), tissue scrapings
- IMPRINTS: Surgical biopsy or necropsy tissues
- SCRAPINGS: Surgical biopsy or necropsy tissues—best technique if firm or fibrous

Aspirates

Gently make squash smears as soon as the sample is expelled onto the slide and then rapidly air-dry. If the aspirate yields nonmucoid fluid, wedge smears also can be made.

- Heavy-handedness ruptures cells, producing strands of nuclear debris (which may mimic fungal hyphae or bacterial chains), and prevents cell identification, yielding nondiagnostic samples.

Body Cavity Fluids

Smears are prepared using a wedge or squash technique (see Figs. 11-1 and 11-2) from unconcentrated (direct) or concentrated (sediment)

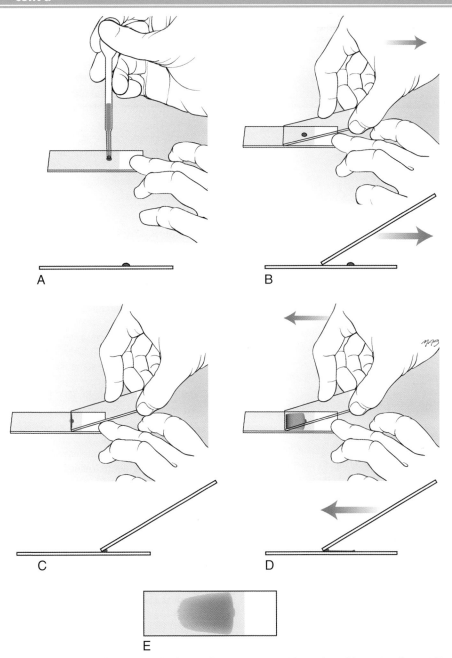

A

B

C

D

E

Figure 11-2 *Preparation of a wedge (or blood) smear from an aspirate.* **A,** Place a drop of the aspirated material just in front of the frosted edge of a slide; ideally, this should be 4 to 5 mm in diameter. For body fluid specimens, a plastic Pasteur pipette or microhematocrit tube can be used to dispense the drop. It is difficult to control the size of the drop with a Pasteur pipette; to obtain a small drop, touch the tip of the pipette gently to the slide surface (do not squeeze the bulb). A microhematocrit tube can be gently tapped to yield a small drop on the slide surface. **B,** Place the spreader slide directly onto the bottom slide, in front of the drop, and then slide it backward such that the edge of the spreader slide contacts the entire drop. **C,** The drop then spreads along the edge of the spreader slide. **D,** Using a swift, smooth motion and maintaining *even* contact between the slides (this is essential), gently push the spreader slide and the drop of fluid along the full length of the slide. Rapidly air-dry the slide. Do not place any pressure on the spreader slide and avoid lifting up the spreader slide as you reach the end of the smear. The angle between the spreader and bottom slide is important: it should be approximately 40 degrees as shown in the side view. If the angle is too low or too high, the resulting smear is too long or too short, respectively. It is important to maintain this angle along the entire length of the smear. If making multiple smears, use a clean edge (fresh spreader slide) for each new smear. **E,** The ideal final smear does not extend more than three fourths along the length of the slide and has a feathered edge.

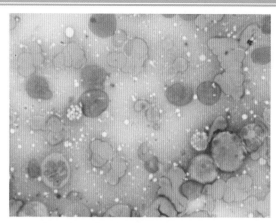

Figure 11-3 *Formalin artifact.* Formalin imparts a bluish green hue to the smear and prevents adequate staining. Formalin vapors can leak from lids of closed containers, so lids should be sealed with parafilm if shipping with cytologic slides (Wright stain, 1000× magnification).

fluid. Fluid can be concentrated to optimize cell yield. The need for concentration is determined by cell counts in laboratories but can be subjectively judged from fluid opacity and turbidity.

- Opaque/turbid/flocculent fluids are usually highly cellular: Make direct smears.
- Clear/transparent fluids are poorly cellular: Make sediment smears.

Concentration/sedimentation can be achieved by low-speed centrifugation (e.g., urine centrifuge). After centrifugation, most of the supernatant is removed (with a pipette or by rapidly inverting the centrifuge tube), leaving a small volume (about 0.25 mL) for resuspending the pellet (which may not be visible in samples of low cellularity). A small drop of the resuspended pellet is then placed on a slide for making smears. The pellet cannot be used for cell counts, so only concentrate a portion of the sample, leaving the balance for counts and for the laboratory to make their own smears from unadulterated fluid. Diagnostic laboratories prepare sediment smears with the foregoing technique but also have cytocentrifuges, which are used for maximally concentrating poorly cellular specimens (e.g., CSF).

Surgical Biopsies/Necropsy Specimens

To obtain the best imprints, do the following:

- Always use a freshly cut surface and gently blot with gauze or tissue to remove excess tissue fluid or blood from the surface to be imprinted.
- Gently touch or roll the tissue surface onto several glass slides, making several (three to four) imprints per slide. It is preferable to make fewer imprints on several slides than multiple imprints on one or two slides.

Firm fibrous tissue may not exfoliate and often requires a more vigorous scraping technique:

- If the sample is large enough, take a scalpel blade (e.g., size #10) and use the edge of the blade perpendicular to the cut surface to gently scrape off cells.
- Touch, tap, or wipe off the accumulated tissue on the blade edge onto a slide and make squash smears (using firmer pressure than usual because these are thick specimens).

Keys to Preparing Top-Quality Smears

- Prepare ASAP after collection; use clean, high-quality glass slides (preferably with frosted ends for ease of labeling).
- Concentrate a portion of fluid specimens if poorly cellular (transparent or clear).
- Use a fresh-cut, blotted surface for imprints or scrapings.
- Be gentle when making smears—use even contact, no-to-little pressure.
- Rapidly air-dry the smear.
- Label with patient identification or owner name and site/fluid type.
- Make several slides so that additional staining procedures can be performed as needed and duplicates can be kept for comparing results, if desired.

Staining

Romanowsky-Type or Polychromatic Stains

The Romanowsky-type or polychromatic stains are the standard cytologic stains and are based on combinations of azure (blue, basic) and eosin (red, acidic) dyes. Basic dyes bind to acidic structures (DNA, RNA), staining them various shades of blue and purple, whereas the acidic dye stains alkaline structures in the cytoplasm different shades of red. Examples of these stains are Wright (used by most veterinary laboratories), May-Grünwald, Giemsa, and "quick" polychromatic stains (e.g., Diff-Quik, Dip Stat, STAT III). These latter stains are widely used in veterinary practice but have some disadvantages to the aforementioned stains:

- Understaining is common (Fig. 11-4); hence it is good practice to examine slides before adding oil or coverslips to determine whether staining is adequate (i.e., nuclei should be blue, and red blood cells [RBCs] should be red).
  - Thick, cellular or proteinaceous samples require longer staining time. Thin, lightly cellular samples with normal protein stain adequately with the routine procedure.
  - Slides can be restained if staining is inadequate. (**Note:** Omit the fixation step and add to the appropriate staining jar.)
- Granules within mast cells and some lymphocytes (cytotoxic T cells or natural killer cells) stain poorly or not at all. This can lead to misidentification of these cells.
- Nucleoli are more prominent and may lead to a suspicion of neoplasia in nonneoplastic lesions.
- Nuclear chromatin is more homogeneous. Clinical pathologists often use chromatin patterns to help identify cell maturity (e.g., lightly stippled chromatin = immaturity), particularly in lymphoid cells; these subtle features are lost with quick stains.
- Color is more "black and white," lacking the complexity of shades with Wright's stain that is helpful.
- Bacteria and fungi can multiply in the stain and adhere to the slides (Fig. 11-5). These can be readily mistaken for true pathogens.
- Methodologic issues are the following:
  - The alcohol in the first fixation step evaporates rapidly.
  - ***Practice Tip:*** *To prolong shelf life, store in a sealed container and place in staining jars only when needed.*
  - Deterioration in staining quality occurs with time and repeated use. If this occurs, refresh the stain.
  - Stain precipitates develop in older stains and can mimic bacteria (Fig. 11-6). If this becomes problematic, discard the old stain, clean the staining jars (with ethanol or methanol), and replenish with fresh stain. Heavily stained jars may need to be replaced.

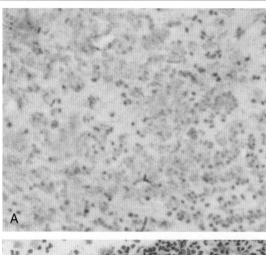

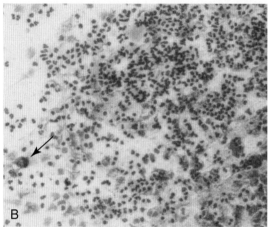

Figure 11-4 Understained direct smears of a tracheal wash. **A,** In this inadequately stained smear, individual cells cannot be distinguished from background mucus. **B,** After restaining, numerous neutrophils and a single macrophage *(arrow)* are readily identified in a streaky mucoid background (Diff-quik, 200× magnification). Restaining of previously stained slides is possible if the smears have not been already oiled or coverslipped.

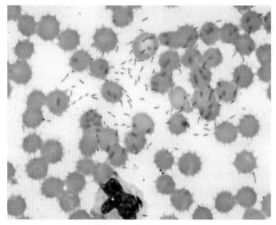

Figure 11-5 Contaminant bacteria. Contaminant bacteria in quick polychromatic stains are large bacilli, found throughout the smear. They overlie cells and are slightly out of the plane of focus (Diff-quik, 1000× magnification).

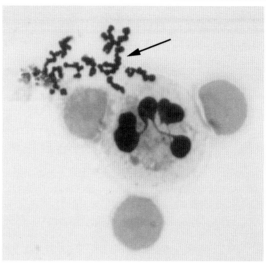

Figure 11-6 Stain precipitate. Stain precipitate *(arrow)* can be difficult to distinguish from bacterial cocci. Bacteria are more uniform in size, shape, and appearance than precipitate and stain blue rather than purple with a Wright stain (Wright stain, 1000× magnification).

Keys to Staining with Quick Polychromatic Stains
- Follow staining protocols recommended by the manufacturer, but increase staining times in the red and blue dyes or "double" stain if smears are thick.
- Allow slides to air-dry and do not touch when drying.
- Examine smears before adding oil or coverslips. If staining is inadequate, restain.
- Take good care of the stains; replace them often and do not top up, to minimize stain precipitate and bacterial growth.

Other Stains
Gram Stain
All bacteria (except Mycobacterium sp.) stain blue with the polychromatic stains, but the Gram stain is needed to classify them as gram-positive or gram-negative. Adequate decolorization (which can be challenging in thick specimens) is essential.
- If cell nuclei are stained red, the smear has been adequately decolorized.
- **Practice Tip:** *Gram stains should not be interpreted if cell nuclei are blue or black (gram-negative bacteria may not decolorize sufficiently and appear gram-positive).*

Prussian Blue Stain
Hemosiderin (a storage form of iron derived from breakdown of hemoglobin within mononuclear phagocytes) stains greenish-brown to gray-black in Romanowsky-type stains but can be difficult to distinguish from phagocytized cell debris or other pigments. Prussian blue stains ferric iron (in the form of hemosiderin) blue and is a useful stain to confirm whether an intracellular pigment is hemosiderin (which is definitive evidence of prior hemorrhage when observed in macrophages from most cytologic specimens).

Fungal Stains
Fungi or yeast are usually readily observed in Romanowsky-stained cytologic specimens, because they stain blue. However, degrading fungal hyphae can be difficult to identify, particularly when they are present in the center of necrotic cellular debris, which frequently

accompanies these infections. Fungal hyphae are readily identified in cytologic specimens with a silver stain (Fig. 11-7).

Cytochemistry/Immunocytochemistry

Cytochemistry and immunocytochemistry are used to determine cell lineage in cytologic smears (only unstained smears). The main use for

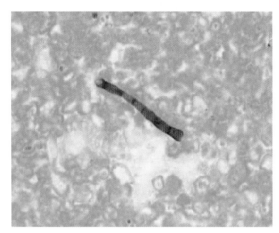

Figure 11-7 Fungal hyphae. Fungal hyphae can be difficult to detect in a Romanowsky-stained cytologic smear, particularly when the hyphal walls are degrading and surrounded by necrotic cellular debris. A Gomori-Grocott methenamine silver (GMS) stain clearly demonstrates fungal hyphae, which stain black in a green background (GMS stain, 1000× magnification).

these techniques is classification of hematopoietic neoplasms (leukemia, lymphoma) but they can also be applied to solid tumors. Immunocytochemistry usually requires an acetone- or formalin-fixation step (depending on the antigen).

- Cytochemistry detects cytoplasmic enzymes by their ability to cleave specific substrates. Granulocytes and monocytes are usually rich in these enzymes (e.g., myeloperoxidase), so these stains are frequently employed for classification of acute leukemia in horses. Some of these enzymes are also expressed in solid tumors and their presence can help confirm a specific tumor diagnosis (e.g., osteosarcomas express high concentrations of alkaline phosphatase). This technique is restricted to blood or cytologic specimens because formalin-fixation destroys enzyme activity.
- Immunocytochemistry detects surface or intracellular antigens with antibodies and is mostly used for identifying lymphocyte subtypes, such as helper T cells (express CD3 and CD4), cytotoxic T cells (express CD3 and CD8), and B cells (express surface IgM or CD19-like molecules) in blood or cytologic specimens. Antigens expressed in certain types of solid tumors can also be detected, thus helping to confirm a specific diagnosis (e.g., von Willebrand factor in hemangiosarcoma, cytokeratin for differentiating a carcinoma from a sarcoma). More antibodies can be applied to cytologic than histologic specimens because some antigens are destroyed by formalin-fixation (e.g., CD4 and CD8). When this technique is used to classify or type hematopoietic cells, it is called immunophenotyping.

Cytologic Assessment

Evaluation of smears made from aspirates or imprints consists of microscopic examination only. Complete assessment of fluid specimens from body cavities (peritoneal, pleural, cerebrospinal, synovial) entails, in addition to microscopic examination, the following:

- **Nucleated cell and RBC counts:** Veterinary laboratories use automated counters, but counts can be done in practice using a hemocytometer and a diluting delivery device (e.g., Leuco-Tic[1]). *Point-of-care analyzers (e.g., LaserCyte,[2] HemaTrue,[3] VetScan,[4] Forcyte[5]) can be of variable accuracy for performing cell counts of fluids. The Forcyte is advertised as being approved for joint and peritoneal fluid cell counts. Most of the machines are used in practice to measure cell counts on fluids, they may be insufficiently sensitive to detect low counts and fibrin, small clots, or viscous samples can plug the tubing. Counts can also be estimated from well-prepared direct smears of fluids; however, this requires substantial experience.*
  - Analyzer counts include all nucleated cells, including mesothelial cells; that is, counts do not equal a white blood cell count.

- Analyzers "see" bacterial clumps, protozoa, and debris as nucleated cells, yielding erroneous cell counts.
- TOTAL PROTEIN: Value is measured by refractometer and used interchangeably with specific gravity. For cellular or bloody fluids, total protein is measured using the supernatant of a centrifuged aliquot. *Note:* Total protein by refractometer values may be falsely increased in lipemic samples or in underfilled EDTA tubes (<0.2 mL fluid in a 3- or 5-mL EDTA tube) because EDTA contributes to the refractive index. The latter artifact is more common in aspirates from body cavities that yield low volume (e.g., SF).
- **Microscopic examination of smears:** The type of smear made from fluid specimens differs between laboratories but is usually based on cell counts:
  - Poorly cellular (nucleated cell counts <3000 cells/µL): Cytospin
  - Moderately cellular (nucleated cell counts between 3000 and 30,000 cells/µL): Sediment
  - Highly cellular (nucleated cell counts >30,000 cells/µL): Direct (unconcentrated)
  - Very bloody fluids (red blood cell count >1,000,000 cells/µL): Direct and buffy coat
- If only a small volume of fluid is obtained from a body cavity of the horse, preparation of smears for microscopic examination should be the top priority. Specific diagnostic information (e.g., degenerate neutrophils and intracellular bacteria) typically is gained only from smear examination.

---

[1]Bioanalytic GmbH, Umkirch/Freburg, Germany.
[2]IDEXX Laboratories, Inc., Westbrook, Maine.
[3]Heska, Loveland, Colorado.
[4]Abaxis Veterinary Diagnostics, Union City, California.
[5]Oxford Science, Inc., Oxford, Connecticut.

●› WHAT TO DO

Storage and Handling

Most veterinarians refer cytologic specimens to a veterinary diagnostic laboratory for examination.

- Contact the laboratory ahead of time to obtain recommended procedures for sample handling and submission.
- Provide a complete history, including pertinent clinical signs, a detailed description of the lesion, and results of imaging studies (if available). This is essential information, allowing the clinical pathologist to provide the best possible interpretation and suggest additional diagnostic testing, as appropriate.
- Label all slides/tubes correctly (see Smear Preparation Technique, p. 38). **Note:** Tape or adhesive labels become unreadable after staining, adhere to the stainer, or detach during staining.
- Submit all smears, preferably unstained.
  - Clinical pathologists can use their preferred stain and perform other stains, as needed.
  - Smear quality/content cannot be judged from gross appearance before staining. A smear may "look" cellular, but on staining it may consist of debris or blood, with no intact cells.
  - Diagnostic tissue may only be present on one of several smears. Many clinicians will stain a slide to ensure adequate cellularity. Also submit this slide (it may be the only diagnostic sample).
- Ship slides in secure, break-proof containers.
  - Use plastic slide holders. Cardboard slide boxes are inadequate; slides often break and shatter within them.
  - Use protective packaging for added security (bubble wrap, peanuts).
  - **Practice Tip:** Do not refrigerate slides. Moisture forms and lyses cells when the slides warm up.
- With fluids, consider the following:
  - Store fluids refrigerated, then ship on cool packs to the laboratory ASAP. Avoid direct contact with a frozen cold pack (wrap the tubes in paper towels); freezing lyses cells.
  - Submit with smears prepared immediately after collection to overcome storage artifacts (phagocytic activity, bacterial overgrowth, cell lysis). Specify smear type (direct or sediment).
  - Protect from temperature extremes (heat or cold); for example, do not leave in the sun in the heat of summer.
- Protect all specimens (slides, fluids) from formalin fumes/liquid. Ship cytologic preparations separately from jars of formalinized tissue, if needed.

Keys to Specimen Storage and Handling

- Provide a complete and detailed history.
- Label slides/tubes appropriately.
- Submit all smears, even if prestained.
- Keep fluid specimens cold at all times.
- Avoid temperature extremes, formalin fumes, and moisture on slides.
- Ship ASAP after collection.

- Measurement of protein content and nucleated cell counts provides supportive information only and the latter can be estimated from direct smears.

Microscopic Examination

The most important aspect of slide examination is consistency; develop a consistent technique and avoid shortcuts. This ensures thoroughness and minimizes errors. A definitive diagnosis may not always be obtained; however, the general disease process (inflammation or neoplasia) can often be recognized quickly if a logical, systematic approach is used. A definitive diagnosis is not always necessary for immediate case management; preliminary findings may modify the diagnostic plan or dictate initial treatment. When in doubt as to the interpretation or diagnostic or pathologic relevance of any cytologic finding, always submit specimens to a clinical pathologist for evaluation.

- Scan the smear with a 4× to 10× objective to evaluate staining quality, identify areas of cellularity, and locate the optimal area for examination (thin, adequately spread and cells intact).
- During scanning, look for large objects such as cell clusters, crystals, foreign bodies, parasites, and fungal hyphae.
- Once an optimal area or unique feature has been located, perform a detailed examination ideally with an oil-immersion objective (50× to 100×). A 40× objective must be used with a glass coverslip (place a drop of oil on the slide and then apply the coverslip).
  - Identify the cells: Normal tissue residents (e.g., ciliated columnar epithelial cells in a tracheal wash), reactive (e.g., fibroblasts), inflammatory, or neoplastic.
  - Look for infectious agents (100× is required to identify bacteria).
- Recognize artifacts/incidental findings that commonly lead to misdiagnosis:
  - Smudged cells have been disrupted during smear preparation (Fig. 11-8). Do not examine these cells; nuclear and cell outlines and cytoplasmic features should be clearly identifiable. Nuclear streaming from smudged cells can resemble fungal hyphae or chains of bacteria. Some cells are inherently fragile and rupture more easily:
    ○ Lymphocytes, particularly if neoplastic (lymphoma)
    ○ Degenerate neutrophils in septic conditions
    ○ Endocrine neoplasms
  - Stain precipitate can be difficult to distinguish from bacterial cocci (see Fig. 11-6).

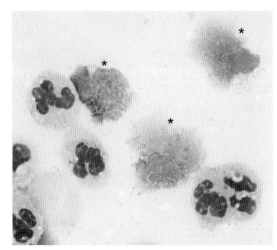

Figure 11-8 Smudged or "basket" cells. Smudged cells (*) have been ruptured during smear preparation and are ignored during cytologic evaluation (Wright stain, 1000× magnification).

- Starch granules from glove powder (Fig. 11-9) can be mistaken for a foreign body.

◉〉 WHAT TO DO

Keys to Effective Microscopic Evaluation

Develop a consistent, thorough technique.
- Only examine adequately stained smears; restain if needed.
- Scan at 4× to 10× and identify areas of interest. Avoid thick areas with poorly spread cells.
- Examine in detail at 40× to 100×.
- When uncertain of a diagnosis or relevance of an observation finding, refer the specimen to a clinical pathologist.

General Disease Processes

Hemorrhage

Erythrocytes (RBCs) are an inevitable component of most cytologic specimens. The key is to distinguish between blood contamination and true hemorrhage.
- **Practice Tip:** *For specimens collected from body cavities, observe the fluid as it enters the syringe/tube. A fluid that starts off clear and then becomes red (or vice versa) is blood contaminated.*

- An aliquot of bloody fluids can be placed in a red-top tube to evaluate for clot formation. Clotting indicates blood contamination, peracute pathologic hemorrhage, or a splenic tap (for abdominocentesis).
- **Practice Tip:** *Blood that has been lost into body cavities defibrinates rapidly; hence, most true hemorrhagic effusions do not clot.*
- A red or reddish brown supernatant suggests prior hemorrhage (RBCs lyse with time). RBCs may lyse in vitro if the specimen is handled inappropriately (vigorously shaken, exposed to extreme heat or cold, stored for prolonged times).
- Platelets indicate blood contamination or peracute hemorrhage.
- Erythrophages and hemosiderophages (Fig. 11-10) indicate prior hemorrhage.
- Erythrophagia occurs within a few hours in vitro in bloody fluids, so these cells can be artifacts if smears are not prepared promptly after collection.
- **Note:** Hemosiderophages do not develop in vitro (cells cannot survive long enough to produce hemosiderin), so they always indicate prior hemorrhage.

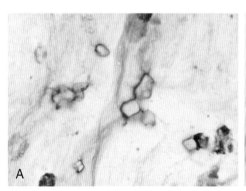
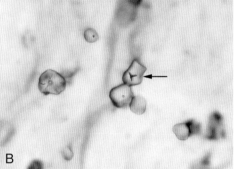

Figure 11-9   Starch granules in a tracheal wash. **A,** Starch granules are large, irregular, square to hexagonal, colorless to greenish blue refractile crystals from latex glove powder. **B,** They have a characteristic central cross *(arrow)* or depression that can be identified by adjusting the focus.

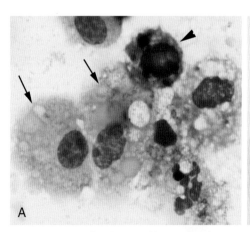
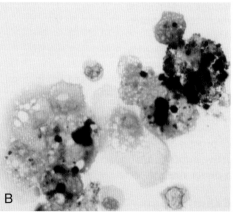

Figure 11-10   Erythrophages and hemosiderophages in a tracheal wash from a horse with exercise-induced pulmonary hemorrhage. **A,** Macrophages containing phagocytized red blood cells (erythrophages; *arrows*) and variable amounts of dusky light brown to black pigment (hemosiderophages; *arrowhead*) are seen (Wright stain). **B,** The cytoplasmic pigment stains blue to black (depending on amount) with Prussian blue, confirming that it is hemosiderin (Prussian blue stain, 1000× magnification).

- Hematoidin crystals (Fig. 11-11): These bright yellow rhomboidal crystals are a form of bilirubin produced from hemoglobin in tissues under hypoxic conditions and indicate prior hemorrhage.
- ***Practice Tip:*** *It is impossible to differentiate between peracute hemorrhage (too early for erythrophagocytosis) and blood contamination by cytologic examination alone. In both instances, platelets may be seen and there are no erythrophages or hemosiderophages. Observation of the fluid during collection for evidence of blood contamination may be key in these cases, along with ultrasonographic examination of the body cavity (hemorrhage is more echoic than transudate or exudate fluid) and clinical signs. With hemorrhage the fluid is generally uniform in color but with blood contamination there may be streaks of blood mixed with the body cavity fluid.*

Keys to Recognizing Hemorrhage

- Changes in red coloration during sample collection indicate blood contamination.

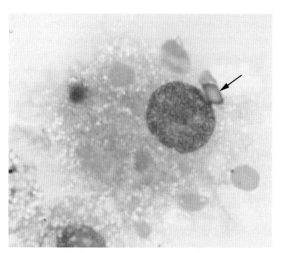

Figure 11-11 Hematoidin crystals. These bright yellow refractile crystals (seen within an erythrophage, *arrow*) are a form of bilirubin produced from hemoglobin under conditions of low oxygen tension and indicate prior hemorrhage (Wright stain, 1000× magnification).

- RBCs with platelets mean blood contamination or peracute hemorrhage.
- Erythrophages, hemosiderophages, and hematoidin crystals mean prior hemorrhage.
- Erythrophages, hemosiderophages, hematoidin, RBCs, and platelets mean recent and prior hemorrhage or blood contamination with prior hemorrhage.
- Erythrophages, with no hemosiderophages or hematoidin, in stored fluid samples may be an in vitro artifact.

Inflammation

Because neoplasia is relatively rare in horses, the goal of emergency cytologic evaluations is to detect or rule out an inflammatory process and potential causative microorganism. Inflammation is identified by increased numbers of inflammatory cells and is classified by the types of cells, specifically neutrophils, eosinophils, lymphocytes, and macrophages (also called histiocytes). Mast cells and basophils are rarely seen as part of the inflammatory response in horses. The type of inflammatory cells can also imply duration.

- *Suppurative:* Neutrophils composing >85% to 90% of inflammatory cells implies that inflammation is acute or of short duration. This is often, but not always, due to bacterial infection. Neutrophils can be further described by their appearance (Fig. 11-12):
  - Nondegenerate: Neutrophils resemble their counterparts in blood; that is, nuclei are intact with condensed chromatin.
  - Degenerate: Neutrophils have swollen, distended, and vacuolated cytoplasm and are undergoing karyolysis (pale, swollen, disrupted nuclei). These changes are often, but not always, seen with inflammation of infectious (bacterial) cause. ***Note:*** Neutrophils swell in vitro with storage of fluid samples, mimicking degenerative change. Thus, assessment for degenerate neutrophils should be done only in smears of fresh fluid.
  - Pyknosis and karyorrhexis: Nuclei condense and fragment. This indicates apoptosis (programmed cell death) or necrosis and is usually not due to infectious causes.

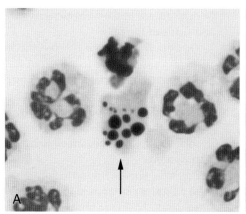 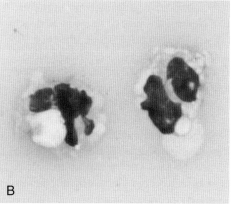

Figure 11-12 Neutrophil appearances in cytologic specimens. **A,** Nondegenerate neutrophils have segmented nuclei, mature condensed nuclear chromatin, and pink cytoplasmic granules. A single neutrophil, displaying nuclear condensation and fragmentation (karyorrhexis) is undergoing programmed cell death (apoptosis; *arrow*). **B,** Degenerate neutrophils have swollen nuclei with lighter chromatin (karyolysis) and increased amounts of vacuolated cytoplasm that lacks pink granules (Wright stain, 1000× magnification).

- *Lymphocytic:* Mostly lymphocytes are found, particularly small cells with some large or reactive forms. Some plasma cells may be seen. This implies a more chronic process or an antigenic stimulus.
- *Histiocytic:* Macrophages dominate. These can be vacuolated or nonvacuolated and may display phagocytic activity (leukocytes, RBCs, secretory products, nonspecific debris). Some may be multinucleated. Typically, this implies long-standing inflammation or inflammation resulting from persistent antigens, for example, foreign bodies, fungi, or mycobacteria. Histiocytic inflammation is frequently used synonymously with *granulomatous* inflammation, although the latter is a term best reserved for histologic specimens (which have architectural features of granulomas).
- *Eosinophilic:* Many eosinophils are found, perhaps with a few mast cells and/or basophils. This implies a hypersensitivity response to allergens or parasites.
- *Mixed:* Samples consist of a mixture of inflammatory cells. This is further classified by the cells present, for example, lymphoplasmacytic, neutrophilic, and histiocytic.
  - Nonsuppurative: Mixture of lymphocytes and macrophages with few neutrophils. This implies that inflammation is chronic or of longer duration.
  - *Neutrophilic histiocytic (pyogranulomatous):* Mixture of nondegenerate neutrophils (60% to 70%) and macrophages (30% to 40%), with low numbers of plasma cells and lymphocytes. Multinucleated macrophages are common, with some foreign body giant cells (nuclei arranged irregularly in the cell). This is usually caused by foreign bodies and fungal or higher bacterial (e.g., mycobacteria) infections. ***Note:*** The term *pyogranulomatous* is best reserved for histologic lesions with characteristic architectural features (circular lesions consisting of a central core of neutrophils, surrounded by histiocytes with some multinucleated giant cells). The term *mixed neutrophilic histiocytic inflammation* is preferred for cytologic specimens.
- *Septic inflammation: Septic* is a modifying term used when intracellular bacteria are observed. The inflammatory response is usually suppurative but can be mixed (neutrophilic histiocytic). Neutrophils may or may not be degenerate, depending on the causative agent. ***Practice Tip:*** *Bacteria can be rapidly engulfed by phagocytes in vitro, so this diagnosis is most clearly made from smears prepared from fresh specimens.*

Keys to Cytologic Examination of Inflammation
- Classification is by the predominant type(s) of cells.
- Cell type implies duration; that is, acute = neutrophilic, and chronic = mixed, lymphocytic, or histiocytic.
- Cell type implies cause; for example, degenerate neutrophils = bacterial infection, and eosinophils = allergens or parasites.
- Septic inflammation is indicated by intracellular bacteria and degenerate neutrophils.
- Intracellular bacteria in stored fluid samples may not be pathogenic; they could be an artifact of delayed sample submission. Similarly, neutrophils may take on a degenerate appearance with storage.

Neoplasia
Neoplasia is infrequent in horses. Neoplasms may incite inflammation (through necrosis or secretion of cytokines), induce paraneoplastic responses (e.g., hypercalcemia with some squamous cell carcinomas or lymphomas), or cause body cavity effusions.
- Cytologically, malignant neoplasia is recognized by abnormalities in cell size, shape, and nuclear features; that is, cells display cytologic criteria of malignancy. Reliable recognition of these features can be difficult and generally should be confirmed by a clinical pathologist.
- Malignancy also can be diagnosed when certain cell types are found in atypical locations; for example, keratinized squamous cells are an abnormal finding in PTF or a deep aspirate of a mass and suggest an underlying squamous cell carcinoma.
- It is difficult to distinguish benign neoplasms from hyperplastic lesions because the cells have similar cytologic features and do not demonstrate malignant features. Histologic examination of tissue architecture is required.
- Some malignant neoplasms are difficult to diagnose because the cells resemble their normal counterparts and lack abnormal features, for example, endocrine tumors and equine lymphoma. Histopathologic examination is required for a definitive diagnosis in these settings.
- Neoplasia may be misdiagnosed in inflammatory states. Inflammatory conditions, especially when chronic, can cause morphologic changes (dysplasia, metaplasia) in local tissue cells (epithelial, mesothelial, or mesenchymal) that can mimic malignancy. It may not be possible to rule out the presence of neoplasia without histologic examination or until the inflammation is treated or controlled with appropriate antimicrobial therapy.
- Many tumors are secondarily inflamed, which can be due to necrosis or an immune response to the neoplasm, making the diagnosis of neoplasia difficult in some cases.
- Neoplasms are initially characterized by the arrangement and shape of the cells:
  - *Discrete cell or round cell tumors:* Individual (or discrete) cells that are usually round. Examples include lymphoma, mast cell tumor, and histiocytic tumors.
  - *Mesenchymal tumors:* Individual cells with spindled or tapering shapes. Loose aggregates, sometimes associated with extracellular matrix, may be found. Examples include sarcoid, fibrosarcoma, hemangiosarcoma, and melanoma.
  - *Epithelial tumors:* Round to polygonal cells that exfoliate in adhesive clusters and individually. Examples include squamous cell carcinoma, tumor of cutaneous basilar epithelium (basal cell tumor), and mesothelioma.
  - *Endocrine tumors:* Small uniform cuboidal to round cells that exfoliate in packets or dense clusters and rupture easily. Examples include thyroid adenomas and C-cell tumors.

Keys to Cytologic Examination of Neoplasia

- Neoplasia is identified by cytologic criteria of malignancy.
- Inflammation alone may cause changes in cells that mimic neoplasia.
- Many tumors may be secondarily inflamed and/or necrotic.
- Classification is by cell shape and arrangement: discrete, mesenchymal, epithelial, endocrine.

Peritoneal Fluid

PTF analysis is a valuable tool most commonly used as part of the diagnostic repertoire in horses with colic. Results provide evidence of inflammation, sepsis, hemorrhage, intestinal ischemia, and gastrointestinal rupture, although they are not always specific as to the nature of the underlying lesion. PTF analysis might also be diagnostic in horses with ruptures of the urinary tract and occasionally neoplasia involving abdominal organs.

Normal Peritoneal Fluid

PTF can be readily aspirated from many normal horses (approximately 100 to 300 mL is available for sampling; see Chapter 18, p. 158 for procedures). PTF is a dialysate of plasma with low nucleated cell counts and protein and is classified as a transudate.

- *Clarity and color:* Fluid is clear to slightly turbid, colorless to light yellow (can usually read lines on a paper through the fluid-filled tube).
- *Protein:* <2.5 g/dL. Normal PTF has little fibrinogen and does not clot.
- *RBC count:* <1000 cells/μL, unless the sample is blood-contaminated. PTF contains no erythrophages.
- *Nucleated cell count:* <5000 cells/μL in adult horses.
  - Some healthy horses can have counts as high as 10,000 cells/μL; however, counts between 5000 and 10,000 cells/μL are considered suspect in an ill horse. Normal postpartum mares should have normal nucleated cell counts and protein.
  - Counts are lower in foals: <1500 cells/μL.

- *Smear examination:*
  - Nucleated cells are a mixture of neutrophils (50% to 70%) and macrophages (30% to 50%), with low numbers of lymphocytes, mast cells, and mesothelial cells (Figs. 11-13 and 11-14). Eosinophils are rare.
  - Neutrophils are nondegenerate. Some may be pyknotic (indicating senescence).
  - Macrophages are often vacuolated. A few may contain phagocytized neutrophils (leukophages) or phagocytic debris. Erythrophages should not be seen in smears made from fresh samples.
  - Mesothelial cells are seen as single cells or small, round clusters. They have a central round nucleus, abundant light purple cytoplasm, and peripheral "corona." Occasionally, mesothelial cells detach mechanically in flat sheets and are more polygonal (see Fig. 11-14).
  - Nonpathogenic findings include starch granules (see Fig. 11-9), rolled-up dark blue keratinized squamous epithelial cells from the skin (also called keratin "bars"), microfilariae (from a free-living nonpathogenic

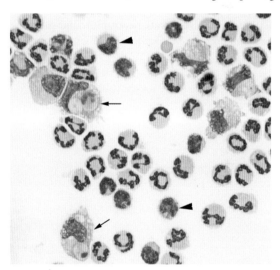

Figure 11-13 Normal peritoneal fluid. Nondegenerate neutrophils and macrophages dominate, with low numbers of small lymphocytes *(arrowheads)* and mesothelial cells (not pictured). A few leukophages *(arrows)* are seen (Wright stain, 500× magnification).

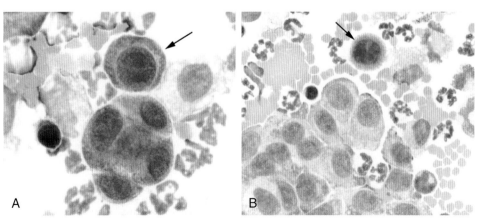

Figure 11-14 Mesothelial cells in pleural fluid. **A,** Mesothelial cells are large, round cells with central nuclei and abundant purple cytoplasm. They exfoliate into fluids as individual cells *(arrow)* or small clusters (1000× magnification). **B,** Mechanically desquamated mesothelial cells are more elongate and detach in flat sheets (an individual mesothelial cell is shown alongside for comparison, *arrow;* Wright stain, 500× magnification).

nematode *Setaria*), and carboxymethylcellulose (bright purple to magenta granules in macrophages and free in the background after intraperitoneal administration of "belly jelly" to prevent postoperative adhesions).

- *Biochemical analytes:*
  - Levels of low-molecular-weight/water-soluble substances (e.g., glucose and urea) are similar to those in blood. These diffuse readily across the mesothelium and equilibrate quickly. Lactate is similar in blood and peritoneal fluid in normal horses.
  - Levels of high-molecular-weight substances (e.g., most enzymes, creatinine, and most proteins) are lower than in blood. These are less diffusible and take longer to equilibrate.

Key Features of Normal Peritoneal Fluid
- Clear to slightly turbid and colorless to light yellow
- Nucleated cell count: <5000 cells/μL in adults and <1500 cells/μL in foals
- Low RBC count
- Total protein: <2.5 g/dL
- Mixture of nondegenerate neutrophils and macrophages; few lymphocytes, mesothelial cells, mast cells, and eosinophils; some leukophages and apoptotic cells; no bacteria or erythrophages

Enterocentesis

Practice Tip: *Accidental puncture of the intestine is a potential complication of abdominocentesis that produces a transient, usually asymptomatic, peritonitis. Enterocentesis rarely can cause deleterious sequelae in adult horses, such as intestinal lacerations, cellulitis (always check site for 2 to 4 days following an enterocentesis, especially if the horse is not on antibiotics), or abscessation.*

- Sample is turbid, flocculent, and greenish brown, with a fetid odor.
- Results vary, depending on whether PTF was simultaneously sampled:
  - *Enterocentesis alone:* Many bacteria of various sizes and shapes (bacilli and cocci). Protozoa (from the cecum or colon) and plant debris may also be seen.
  - *Enterocentesis and abdominocentesis:* Mixture of the aforementioned organisms/structures with normal PTF cells. Neutrophils are nondegenerate and bacteria are not phagocytized (assuming promptly made smears of freshly collected fluid; Fig. 11-15).

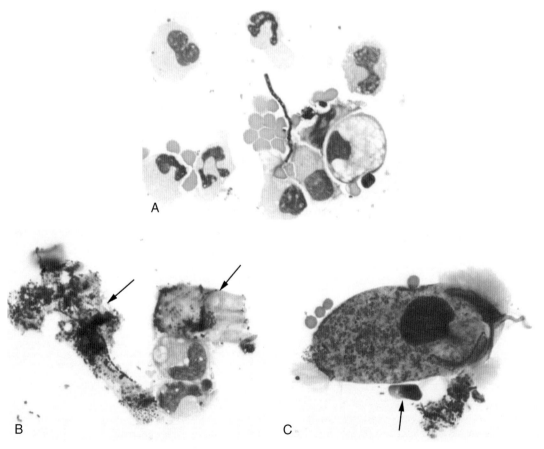

Figure 11-15 Enterocentesis with partial abdominocentesis. **A,** A long filament of bacterial rods is seen extracellularly, together with nondegenerate neutrophils from peritoneal fluid. Bacteria were not phagocytized. **B,** Plant debris *(arrows)* with a mixed population of bacterial rods and cocci (some adhered to the debris) are seen alongside peritoneal macrophages (1000× magnification). **C,** A large protozoan from a different area of the same sample, with a small lymphocyte *(arrow)* and plant debris, is shown. The protozoan indicates that the site of enterocentesis was the large colon or cecum (Wright stain, 500× magnification).

- Enterocentesis can be impossible to differentiate from a peracute gastrointestinal (GI) rupture on cytologic examination alone but should be suspected in a horse that is not displaying clinical signs of a GI rupture (e.g., severe or absence of pain, endotoxemia, and hypovolemic shock).

Colic

Assessment of PTF, interpreted along with clinical signs, can be useful indicators of GI compromise and the need for surgical intervention in horses with colic caused by strangulating obstructions (e.g., volvulus, torsion, or incarceration).

- In early stages of colic, PTF may be normal.
- The first changes that occur with intestinal ischemia are an increased RBC count and erythrophagia, often accompanied by increased protein. This is most often due to venous congestion and results in a red-tinged, slightly turbid fluid. At this stage, the nucleated cell count is normal. Lactate in peritoneal fluid begins to increase above blood values.
- As ischemia worsens, inflammatory cells infiltrate the intestinal wall and peritoneal cavity. At this stage, the nucleated cell count (mostly neutrophils) and protein are increased, with a variable RBC count. The fluid is grossly turbid and may be flocculent. PTF lactate is increased. Dark red-brown fluid has been associated with intestinal necrosis. Bacteria may not be seen until the intestinal wall is devitalized sufficiently to leak or rupture. Once the latter occurs, plant debris and mixed bacteria are seen (intracellularly and extracellularly) along with an increased nucleated cell count (predominantly degenerate neutrophils).
- In some GI conditions causing colic—for example, enteric foreign bodies and impactions—PTF may remain normal throughout. Erythrophagia alone (with normal protein) may be seen in some impactions causing serosal vascular congestion.
- Horses suffering from acute GI rupture typically present with colic and shock. The site of rupture can affect the character of PTF. Varying amounts of plant material may be seen, regardless of site.
  - *Gastric:* A large amount of fluid is released into the abdomen, diluting PTF. The fluid is turbid, brown, and grainy. Smears have a granular background and can be acellular or contain low numbers of large, flattened light blue keratinized squamous cells (not keratin bars) from the squamous portion of the stomach.
  - *Intestinal (small or large):* Mixed bacterial population of rods and cocci along with low numbers of degenerate neutrophils with phagocytized bacteria (Fig. 11-16). In peracute cases, the fluid may mimic an enterocentesis.
  - *Cecal/colonic:* Protozoa, together with phagocytized bacteria in degenerate neutrophils, indicates a rupture at these sites. If large volumes of ingesta are released into the abdomen, this can mimic an enterocentesis.
- Nucleated cell counts and protein are often normal in acute ruptures; however, bacteria and debris can result in erroneous counts. Therefore, clinical signs and cytologic

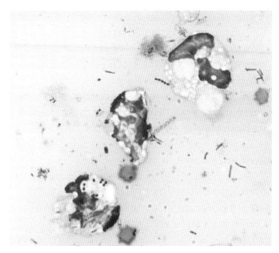

Figure 11-16 Peritoneal fluid from a horse with colic resulting from an intestinal rupture. Degenerate neutrophils have phagocytized a mixed flora of bacteria in this cytospin preparation. The peritoneal fluid nucleated cell count was normal (1000 cells/µL), despite cytologic evidence of sepsis (Wright stain, 1000× magnification).

examination of the fluid are essential for a definitive diagnosis.

Exudates

Exudative effusions indicate an inflammatory stimulus in the peritoneal cavity. This can be due to septic (e.g., *Actinobacillus* infection) or nonseptic causes. Nonseptic causes include: devitalization and necrosis of the GI wall following ischemic injury or neoplasia, chemical injury (e.g., urine peritonitis, seminoperitoneum, or hemoperitoneum commonly following castration), and abdominal surgery.

- Fluid is turbid (from increased cells) and discolored. Flecks of fibrin may impart a flocculent appearance. A visible pellet is seen in centrifuged samples with high nucleated cell counts.
- Nucleated cell counts are >5000 cells/µL and usually much higher.
- Total protein is elevated (>2.5 g/dL) and the sample may clot because of a high fibrinogen content.
- Inflammation is typically suppurative (>85% to 90% neutrophils). In sepsis, neutrophils are usually degenerate but can be nondegenerate. Nondegenerate neutrophils with high neutrophil counts (>20,000 cells/µL) are typical of a primary peritonitis caused by *Actinobacillus equuli*.
- Intracellular bacteria may be identified. The absence of bacteria or degenerate neutrophils does not rule out sepsis and these fluids should be cultured regardless.
  - A mixed bacterial population suggests an intestinal origin.
  - A single bacterial species suggests a primary peritonitis or abscessation, rather than intestinal leakage/rupture.
- PTF pH and glucose are decreased in septic peritonitis; however, some horses with nonseptic peritonitis have similar results. These tests should not be used in isolation for diagnosis of sepsis. Both tests need to be performed immediately after collection because anaerobic glycolysis

and glucose consumption occur in vitro, producing arti-factual changes that resemble sepsis.

- *Practice Tip: Identification of phagocytized bacteria in a freshly prepared sample and a positive bacterial culture remain the gold standards for sepsis.*
- Abdominal surgery alone can induce a sterile, asymptomatic peritonitis. Nucleated cell counts (mostly neutrophils) can remain high (>30,000 cells/μL) for longer than a week after surgery. Neutrophils are usually nondegenerate, and bacteria are absent.

Hemorrhagic Effusions

RBCs are typically seen in low numbers in PTF. An increased number of RBCs can be seen with the following conditions:

- *Blood contamination:* Platelets are usually observed, but there is no erythrophagia. Contamination may be observed by changes in red coloration during sample collection.
  - *Practice Tip: Hemorrhage or diapedesis into the abdominal cavity: The tap is uniformly bloody and does not clot in a red-top tube. This is commonly observed in association with a devitalized GI tract. Cytologic indicators of prior hemorrhage/diapedesis include erythrophages, hemosiderophages, absence of platelets (if hemorrhage is not ongoing), and hematoidin crystals. An increased RBC count and erythrophagia (often accompanied by an elevated protein) may be the first indicators of intestinal ischemia or serosal vascular congestion.*
- *Hemorrhagic effusion/hemoperitoneum:* The fluid resembles frank blood and does not clot. The RBC count is >1,000,000 cells/μL, with a measurable packed cell volume (PCV). There is cytologic evidence of prior hemorrhage. Causes include trauma (splenic tears, hematomas), ruptured abdominal vessels (e.g., uterine artery during foaling), neoplasia (hemangiosarcoma, ovarian tumors), and coagulopathies (e.g., hemophilia A).
  - *Practice Tip: Splenic tap: The fluid resembles a hemoperitoneum; however, the fluid clots if placed in a noncoagulated tube. The fluid PCV is similar to or greater than blood and there is no cytologic evidence of hemorrhage. Splenic elements (lymphocytes, hematopoietic precursors) may be seen but are not a consistent or reliable finding.*

Neoplasia

Neoplasia usually manifests with chronic symptoms (weight loss, weakness, and intermittent colic) in horses. Tumors involving the GI tract can cause acute abdominal pain, particularly if they result in hemoperitoneum, peritonitis (from necrosis), GI ischemia (e.g., strangulating lipomas), or rupture.

- Tumors can cause any type of abdominal effusion including transudates, exudates, hemoperitoneum, chyle, and GI ruptures.
- Neoplastic cells may be observed in PTF, permitting a definitive diagnosis, for example, lymphoma, gastric squamous cell carcinoma (Fig. 11-17), mesothelioma, adenocarcinoma, and malignant melanoma (Fig. 11-18).

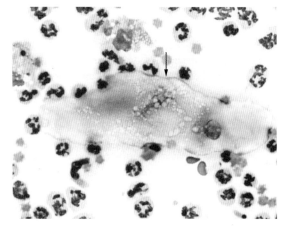

Figure 11-17 Squamous cells in the peritoneal fluid of a horse with a squamous cell carcinoma. A cluster of two large, elongate, fully keratinized squamous epithelial cells with retained nuclei permit a diagnosis of squamous cell carcinoma from a direct smear of peritoneal fluid in a horse with a concurrent exudative peritonitis (Wright stain, 500× magnification). Note that nucleated keratinized squamous cells (with no neoplastic features) may be seen in PTF of foals and adult horses with gastric rupture.

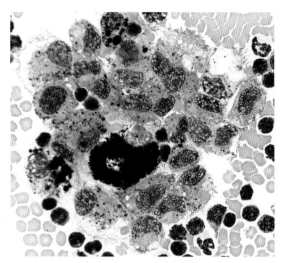

Figure 11-18 Melanophages in the peritoneal fluid of a horse with malignant melanoma. Numerous macrophages with variable amounts of black melanin pigment in their cytoplasm (melanophages) were seen in this peritoneal fluid sample from a gray horse. The melanin originated from a metastatic melanoma, which was confirmed on necropsy examination (Wright stain, 500× magnification).

- Absence of neoplastic cells does not exclude neoplasia because most equine abdominal tumors do not exfoliate cells into PTF.
- Mesothelial cells can become reactive in effusions and may be mistaken for neoplastic cells. They exhibit increased cytoplasmic basophilia, increased nuclear-to-cytoplasmic ratios, multinucleation, and large prominent nucleoli. In these settings, it can be difficult, even for an experienced cytopathologist, to discriminate between a reactive or inflammatory process and neoplasia.

Other Conditions

- *Seminoperitoneum:* Perforation of the female reproductive tract during breeding may introduce sperm into the abdominal cavity, inciting a sterile peritonitis. Free sperm and phagocytes (neutrophils and macrophages) containing sperm heads are diagnostic findings.

- *Uroperitoneum:* Urinary bladder ruptures are not uncommon in neonatal foals and also can occur in adult male horses with urolithiasis or in postpartum mares. Nucleated cell counts are initially normal, but a sterile suppurative peritonitis develops with time.
  - ***Practice Tip:*** *Uroperitoneum can be definitively diagnosed by higher creatinine levels in PTF than peripheral blood (creatinine equilibrates slowly across the peritoneal lining). In adult horse cases, and rarely in foals, calcium carbonate crystals can be seen in PTF and are similarly diagnostic.*

- *Lipid-rich effusions:* Lipid-rich effusions are usually seen as a consequence of leakage of chylomicron-rich GI lymph due to lymphangiectasia, lymphatic hypertension, or lymphatic blockage. These are true chylous effusions and are rare in horses. In neonatal foals these effusions are slightly more common and lipid-rich effusions have been attributed to congenital lymphatic defects, or less commonly, pancreatitis, whereas in adult horses they occur with lymphatic obstruction, presumably caused by colonic torsions or mesenteric abscesses. In foals the lipid-rich effusions may resolve without known cause. In chylous effusions, the fluid is grossly white or pink/red (if bloody) and opaque and may develop a "cream" layer on refrigeration (indicating the high triglyceride content). A visible sediment does not usually form on centrifugation or standing. Measurement of PTF triglyceride concentrations is helpful for diagnosis; values are higher than serum. Nucleated cell counts are variable and consist mostly of small lymphocytes. Macrophages containing phagocytized clear fat globules may be seen. With long-standing effusions, neutrophilic inflammation may develop from the irritating effects of chyle (such fluids may form a visible sediment). PTF with similar gross features (chylous-like) may be seen in suckling foals with acute gastric rupture or horses with pancreatitis. Gastric rupture can occur in foals as a consequence of perforating ulcers, which results in leakage of milk into the peritoneal cavity and a concurrent suppurative peritonitis. This is a clear emergency that is usually fatal unless surgical intervention is immediate. One foal at our hospital with an acute gastric rupture and visible milk in peritoneal fluid had a remarkably quick recovery after surgical repair. Clinical signs and imaging findings should help differentiate a gastric rupture (e.g., pneumoperitoneum with a fluid line) from other causes of lipid-rich effusions in foals. ***Practice Tip:*** *Acute pancreatitis has recently been recognized in 2- to 5-day-old foals. Foals typically present with anorexia, depression, neurologic signs, and hypovolemic shock. Consistent clinical chemistry findings are hypoglycemia, increased lipase and amylase concentrations, and gross lipemia due to hypertriglyceridemia. PTF is grossly turbid (from fat) and red/orange (from concurrent hemorrhage) (Fig. 11-19). PTF lipase and amylase concentrations are higher than blood, which may facilitate*

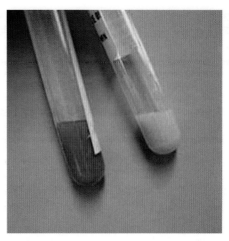

Figure 11-19   Peritoneal fluid and serum from a foal with pancreatitis. Gross lipemia and hemorrhage is evident in the uncentrifuged PTF sample *(left tube)*. The serum sample is also lipemic *(right tube)*. Both samples had high triglyceride content. The lipid-rich nature of the PTF may be due to a true chylous effusion (leakage of lymph) or potential liberation of fat from abdominal adipose tissue by pancreatic enzymes.

diagnosis. Protein is also increased, although this may be an artifact (lipid contributes to the refractive index). Some foals may have concurrent inflammation (peritonitis), but high nucleated cell counts in PTF are not a consistent feature of this condition. Prompt recognition and aggressive treatment are important because the prognosis is generally poor.

● WHAT TO DO

Keys to Interpretation of Abnormal Peritoneal Fluid Cytologic Findings

- *Do not* interpret cytologic results in isolation; clinical signs are crucial.
- *Do not* exclude an underlying pathologic condition based on normal nucleated cell counts and/or protein. Both may be normal in acute GI ruptures, neoplastic effusions, uroperitoneum, and pancreatitis.
- *Enterocentesis:* Suspect enterocentesis if there are mixed bacteria, plant debris or protozoa, and "normal" PTF cells in partial taps, particularly if the horse does not exhibit signs typical of GI ruptures.
- *Colic:* Progressive changes from normal to increased RBC count, erythrophagia and increased protein, to suppurative inflammation, to GI rupture/leakage.
- *GI rupture:* Plant material and large numbers of a mixed bacterial population phagocytized within degenerate neutrophils. Sample may contain keratinized squamous cells only or acellular grainy fluid in acute gastric rupture. In foals, acute gastric rupture can grossly resemble a chylous effusion.
- *Exudates:* Septic or nonseptic suppurative inflammation of variable cause is evident.
- *Hemorrhagic effusion:* Greater than 1 million RBCs per microliter, measurable PCV, nonclotting fluid, erythrophages, hemosiderophages, hematoidin crystals, and platelets (if acute or recent) are found.
- *Seminoperitoneum:* Suppurative to mixed inflammation is present and free sperm and phagocytized sperm heads may be seen.
- *Uroperitoneum:* Normal results or a mild exudate, creatinine in PTF is greater than blood, and calcium carbonate crystals in adults and, rarely, foals may be seen.

SECTION II Emergency Imaging, Endoscopy, Laboratory Diagnostics, and Monitoring

- *Pancreatitis:* Grossly turbid and red/orange (from fat and hemorrhage), amylase and lipase in PTF are greater than blood, high protein (may be a false increase from fat), normal or mildly increased nucleated cell count.
- *Neoplasia:* Various types of effusions can occur; neoplastic cells may not be visible; differentiate from reactive mesothelial cells.

Pleural Fluid

Thoracentesis is performed when there is evidence of pleural effusion based on clinical examination (auscultation, percussion) and imaging studies (radiography, ultrasonography; see Chapter 25, p. 459, for procedures). Like PTF, normal pleural fluid (PLF) is a dialysate of plasma, and interpretation of cytologic results is identical to that described for PTF. Conditions causing PLF accumulation are the following:

- *Inflammation:* Pleuropneumonia with its sequelae (lung abscesses, infarction) is the most common cause of pleural effusion in horses. This is infectious in origin and can be precipitated by stress (transport, racing). The fluid is cloudy to flocculent and yellow or red. Nucleated cell counts are high, and bacteria are usually phagocytized within degenerate neutrophils. **Note:** *A fetid smell to the fluid suggests infarction and a guarded prognosis!*
- *Neoplasia:* These neoplasms can be primary intrathoracic (e.g., lymphoma, which is the most common tumor causing pleural effusion, or mesothelioma) or metastatic (e.g., melanoma or squamous cell carcinoma) tumors (Fig. 11-20). Neoplastic cells may not exfoliate into the fluid with some tumors but are fairly common with lymphoma, especially if the fluid is red. With mesothelioma, PLF is commonly yellow and flocculent in appearance.
- *Chylothorax:* The condition has been reported in foals with presumed congenital lymphatic defects or diaphragmatic hernias and in adults with obstruction or destruction of pleural lymphatic vessels by a primary intrathoracic hemangiosarcoma.

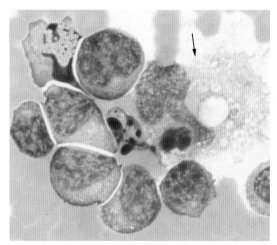

Figure 11-20 Lymphoblasts in the pleural fluid of a horse with lymphoma. Many large lymphoblasts (some apoptotic) are seen alongside a leukophagocytic macrophage *(arrow)* in a sediment smear of pleural fluid from a horse. These were diagnostic for lymphoma (Wright stain, 1000× magnification).

- *Miscellaneous:* Exudative pleural effusions have been reported following pericarditis and *Anoplocephala* metacestode infection.

Key Features of Normal Pleural Fluid
- Clear to slightly turbid and colorless to light yellow
- Nucleated cell count: <5000 cells/μL
- Low RBC count
- Total protein: <2.5 g/dL
- Normal PLF is a mixture of nondegenerate neutrophils and macrophages; few lymphocytes, mesothelial cells, mast cells, and eosinophils; some leukophages and apoptotic cells; and no bacteria or erythrophages.

Pericardial Fluid
- Pericardial fluid is rarely submitted for laboratory examination, but the following conditions can be diagnosed by pericardial fluid analysis:
  - *Septic pericarditis:* Usually yellow turbid or flocculent fluid, neutrophilic inflammation with or without bacteria. *Actinobacillus* sp. is the most common isolate.
  - *Nonseptic pericarditis:* Associated with fever and presumed viral infection. Fluid is often red with a mixture of lymphocytes, plasma cells, and neutrophils.
  - *Neoplasia:* May see neoplastic cells such as lymphoma (fluid is frequently red).

Synovial Fluid

As for other body cavity fluids, synovial fluid (SF) is a dialysate of plasma. However, SF is modified by secretion of large amounts of glycosaminoglycans, particularly hyaluronic acid, by synovial membrane cells. SF bathes joints and tendons, providing lubrication and growth factors and preventing concussive injury. SF analysis is indicated in horses with lameness, evidence of joint effusion, or skin lacerations in proximity to a joint (to assess for possible joint penetration). Some SF (at least 0.5 mL) can be aspirated from most joints. Tendon sheath fluid can also be aspirated; interpretation is similar to joint fluid.

The two main disease processes affecting equine joints are traumatic/degenerative and inflammatory disease, which are distinguished based on nucleated cell counts and cell types:
- Traumatic/degenerative = low numbers of mononuclear cells.
- Inflammation = high numbers of neutrophils. Because immune-mediated arthropathies are not common in horses, sepsis is the usual cause of inflammatory joint disease.

Normal Synovial Fluid
- *Color and clarity:* Clear, colorless to slightly yellow
- *Texture:* Highly viscous because of hyaluronic acid. Use squash preparation method to prepare thin smears.
  - Viscosity is assessed subjectively by fluid "stringiness." If a drop of SF is placed on a slide using a needle/syringe or pipette, a strand of fluid (at least 1 to 2 cm long) should form as the needle/pipette tip is drawn away.

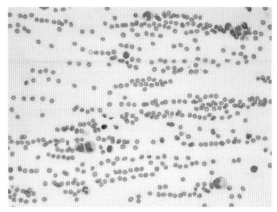

Figure 11-21   Normal joint fluid. Erythrocytes and synovial fluid cells (macrophages, lymphocytes) line up in rows ("windrowing") in this blood-contaminated joint fluid aspirate, indicating normal viscosity (Wright stain, 200× magnification).

- Fluid dries slowly; rapidly air-dry smears.
- Viscosity imparts a pink granular background and causes "windrowing" of cells (arranged in lines in the direction of smearing (Fig. 11-21). Windrowing may not be seen in poorly cellular fluids with normal viscosity.
- Viscosity may affect accuracy of cell counts (difficult to attain repeatable counts) and microscopic examination (slow drying).
- Some normal SF can gel (thixotropism), making it impossible to count cells, measure protein, or prepare smears. Hyaluronidase can be added to liquify the sample.
- *Cell counts:* Nucleated counts are <1000 cells/μL, with few RBCs.
- *Total protein by refractometer:* <2.5 g/dL
  - ***Practice Tip:*** *A low yield (<0.25 mL) may falsely increase protein of samples collected into EDTA. EDTA contributes to the refractive index (pure EDTA has a "total protein" of 9.0 g/dL by refractometry), mimicking degenerative joint disease.*
- *Smear examination:*
  - Nonvacuolated macrophages and small lymphocytes dominate (also termed *large* and *small mononuclear cells,* respectively).
  - Neutrophils are <10% and nondegenerate. This percentage may be higher in poorly cellular (but normal) or blood-contaminated fluids.
  - Low numbers of synovial lining cells (synoviocytes) can be seen. These can be difficult to distinguish from macrophages.

Key Features of Normal Synovial Fluid

- Clear, colorless, and viscous
- Nucleated cell count: <1000 cells/μL
- Low RBC count
- Total protein: <2.5 g/dL
- Mixture of nonvacuolated macrophages, small lymphocytes, and synoviocytes, with <10% neutrophils

Traumatic or Degenerative Joint Disease

- No gross abnormalities may be detected (normal color, clarity, viscosity). Viscosity may be reduced if there is joint effusion (dilutional effect).
- In some cases, the only indication of an arthropathy is an increased volume of cytologically normal fluid.
- Nucleated cell counts are normal to slightly increased (usually <5000 cells/μL).
- Total protein is normal to slightly increased.
- Distribution of cell types is normal. Macrophages might be vacuolated.
- Cartilage fragments and osteoclasts may be seen, representing cartilage damage and cartilage erosion to subchondral bone, respectively. Cartilage fragments may also be mechanically dislodged during aspiration in joints with small synovial spaces or little fluid.
- Traumatic injury may cause joint hemorrhage. In acute cases, this can resemble blood contamination, but there should be some evidence of hemorrhage (erythrophages, hemosiderophages) on microscopic examination if long-standing.
- Acute joint trauma can mimic inflammatory joint disease. Trauma induces a transient neutrophilic inflammatory response (nucleated cell counts can be as high as 12,000 cells/μL with >50% neutrophils). This should resolve over a few days to a more typical degenerative profile.
- Degenerative joint disease may be the final outcome of traumatic injury.

Inflammatory Joint Disease

Inflammatory joint disease is due to acute trauma (see previous discussion) or sepsis; however, the latter is far more common. ***Note:*** There are reports of presumptive immune-mediated arthropathy (secondary to bacterial infections such as *Rhodococcus equi* in foals and presumed idiopathic in older equines).

- Fluid is yellow to creamy, hazy, with decreased viscosity and may be flocculent. Fibrin clumps may enmesh cells, which decreases the nucleated cell count.
- Nucleated cell counts are high, usually >5000 cells/μL and up to several hundred thousand per microliter.
- Neutrophils dominate and are usually nondegenerate, even with sepsis.
- Total protein is increased (>2.5 g/dL).
- Bacteria are rarely identified in septic arthropathies but may be seen in joint fluids from septic foals. The absence of bacteria in septic fluids has been attributed to bacterial colonization of the synovium; however, cultures of synovial membrane biopsies have not proved to be more sensitive than SF cultures.
- It can be difficult, if not impossible, to identify joint inflammation (or joint involvement in lacerated skin wounds) if the fluid is moderately to severely blood contaminated. The latter increases nucleated cell counts, neutrophil percentages, and total protein.

Other Conditions

There have been isolated reports of eosinophilic synovitis, lymphocytic synovitis (due to *Borrelia burgdorferi* or villonodular synovitis), fungal arthritis (due to *Candida* sp.), and chemical synovitis (e.g., intraarticular antibiotic or silicone injections). Chronic bleeding may induce a mild neutrophilic synovitis.

Practice Tip: *A marked neutrophilic inflammatory response (mean of 50,000 nucleated cells/μL) with increased total protein (mean of 5 g/dL) is induced within 6 hours of intraarticular injection of autologous or allogeneic mesenchymal stem cells. The nucleated cell count returns to normal by 72 hours; however, the total protein remains increased.*

Keys to Interpretation of Abnormal Synovial Fluid Cytologic Specimens

- Normal results do *not* rule out degenerative joint disease.
- Sepsis is the primary differential diagnosis for an inflammatory (neutrophilic) arthropathy.
- Acute trauma can mimic a septic arthritis by inducing a neutrophilic synovitis. This is usually transient, and the nucleated cell count is usually <12,000 cells/μL.
- *Degenerative and traumatic joint disease* shows normal to decreased viscosity; nucleated cell count usually <5000 cells/μL, consisting of mononuclear (large and small) cells with <10% neutrophils; and normal to mildly increased protein. SF results may be completely normal.
- *Inflammatory disease:* Decreased viscosity, high nucleated cell count (>5000 cells/μL), and protein (>2.5 g/dL), mostly nondegenerate neutrophils are evident. Bacteria may not be seen even in cases of septic arthritis.

Tracheal Wash and Bronchoalveolar Lavage

Techniques for collection of transtracheal wash (TTW) or BAL samples are described elsewhere (see Chapter 25, p. 451, for procedures). These techniques are performed in horses with clinical signs referable to the respiratory tract (cough, nasal discharge, respiratory distress), as part of the diagnostic evaluation for poor performance in athletic horses, or to detect exercise-induced pulmonary hemorrhage (EIPH). Tracheal washes can be performed through an endoscope or transtracheally. Collection technique affects interpretation (see the following); thus it is important to identify how tracheal wash specimens are collected. ***Note:*** Unlike other body fluids, total protein concentrations are not measured.

Tracheal Wash Versus Bronchoalveolar Lavage

Tracheal wash samples most directly reflect pathologic processes that involve bacterial infection of the lung, focal noninfectious diseases, such as pulmonary hemorrhage, or larger airway disorders, whereas BALs *usually* represent diffuse lower airway disease.

- **Practice Tip:** *Tracheal wash samples are preferred for evaluation of infectious respiratory disease (except for EHV-5), whereas BALs are often preferred for diffuse chronic lower airway inflammatory disease. Cytologic results of these two*

specimens are different and do not always correlate with each other.

- *Sample site:* Tracheal wash samples are less sensitive than BALs for detecting diseases affecting the lower airways (bronchioles and alveoli). BALs only detect abnormalities affecting the sample site and may miss nondiffuse lesions (e.g., BALs may be normal in pneumonia if a non-affected area of lung is lavaged and do not demonstrate the mucus or cellularity observed on tracheal washes in racehorses with inflammatory airway disease or mucopus syndrome).
- *Mucus:* Mucus is a normal component of tracheal washes but should be lacking in BALs. In BALs, mucus indicates contamination with upper airway constituents, which clouds interpretation. Indeed, BALs submitted to diagnostic laboratories are usually filtered to remove any contaminating mucus.
- *Cell counts:* Cell counts are not performed on tracheal washes but are done on BALs with a hemocytometer (counts are usually below the detection limit of automated analyzers).
- *Cell types:* Differential counts are routinely performed on BALs but not tracheal washes. Alveolar macrophages and upper airway epithelial cells (ciliated columnar and goblet) dominate in tracheal washes, whereas macrophages and lymphocytes are the most abundant cells in BALs. Few upper airway epithelial cells should be seen in BALs.
- **Practice Tip:** *A higher number of neutrophils (usually <10%, with up to 25% being observed in stabled horses without inflammatory airway disease) are seen in tracheal washes than in BALs (up to 5%).*
- *Bacteria:* Cultures are more likely to be positive in tracheal washes than BALs in horses with sepsis and in healthy horses (normal flora reside in the lower trachea).
- *Incidental findings:* ***Note:*** Tracheal washes are more likely to contain environmental contaminants, such as pigmented fungal elements, than BALs.

Normal Tracheal Wash Cytologic Findings

- Sample should contain visible mucous flecks or strands.
  - Samples lacking mucus are unlikely to be representative (cells are caught up within mucus).
  - Mucus is thick and dries slowly. It is important to prepare squash preps of the mucus and to rapidly air-dry the slides.
  - Mucus forms purple to pink strands or variably sized granules in smears. Mucin granules could be mistaken for bacteria, but are lighter stained and more variable in shape (Fig. 11-22).
  - Mucus or Curshmann's spirals are dark, tightly wound spirals of mucus (see Fig. 11-22). They usually indicate increased mucous production from airway irritation but may be seen in healthy horses.
- Alveolar macrophages dominate, with <10% neutrophils. Stabled horses can normally have up to 25% neutrophils. Lymphocytes, eosinophils, and mast cells may be seen in low numbers. Some macrophages may be multinucleated.

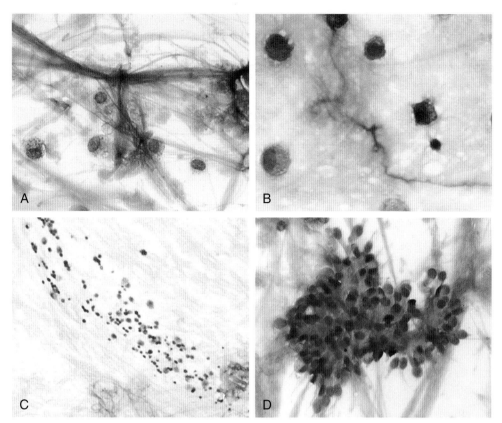

Figure 11-22 Normal tracheal wash. **A,** Thick strands of mucus and alveolar macrophages. **B,** Alveolar macrophages surround a mucus spiral. **C,** A stream of light purple mucin granules. **D,** Cluster of ciliated columnar epithelial cells (Wright stain, 500× magnification).

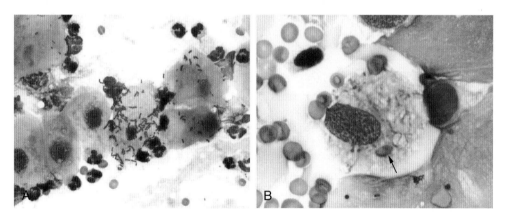

Figure 11-23 Incidental findings in a tracheal wash. **A,** Oropharyngeal contamination from an endoscopic wash: Large squamous cells with adherent bacteria, together with nondegenerate neutrophils (indicating concurrent inflammation), are seen. Bacteria are not phagocytized. Red blood cells suggest concurrent hemorrhage (500× magnification). **B,** A green-blue dematiaceous fungal spore *(arrow)* is adhered to an alveolar macrophage and is an environmental contaminant (Wright stain, 1000× magnification).

- Ciliated columnar epithelial cells and goblet cells occur individually or in clusters (see Fig. 11-22).
- Extracellular bacteria (mixed population) may be present, particularly if there is oropharyngeal contamination (see the following).
- *Transtracheal collection:* RBCs may be seen from collection-induced hemorrhage. Rarely, fully keratinized squamous cells from the skin can contaminate these washes. If the catheter folds and extends into the pharynx, the wash may contain oropharyngeal cells and/or commensal bacteria.

- *Endoscopic collection:* RBCs are rare in nontraumatic collections, and their presence usually indicates recent airway hemorrhage. Some degree of oropharyngeal contamination is present; hence, bacterial cultures are more likely to be positive. This can be reduced by using guarded endoscopes.
- *Incidental findings:*
  - Oropharyngeal contamination: The wash contains nonkeratinized squamous epithelial cells from the oropharynx, with or without adherent bacteria (Fig. 11-23).

Mixed bacteria are also found extracellularly; however, none should be phagocytized.

- Dematiaceous (pigmented) fungal hyphae and/or spores may be seen in the background or adhered to macrophages (see Fig. 11-23). These are environmental contaminants and are more frequently observed in washes from stabled horses (especially horses with recurrent airway obstruction [RAO]) or those fed hay in close confinement (e.g., round bales). These fungi can exacerbate/initiate RAO but can be seen in horses without this disease.

Normal Bronchoalveolar Lavage Cytologic Findings

- No mucus
- Nucleated cell count: 200 to 400 cells/µL
- Mixture of macrophages (30% to 75%) and lymphocytes (20% to 50%) with <5% neutrophils. Some mast cells (1% to 2%), with rare eosinophils (<1%). Macrophages may be multinucleated. Ciliated columnar epithelial and goblet cells are absent, unless there is upper airway contamination (these are excluded from differential counts).
- Rarely see dematiaceous fungal elements; may see extracellular bacteria from the oropharynx
- No to few RBCs
- The site of sampling (left or right lung) and volume of infusate may affect cell proportions.

Keys to Normal Tracheal Wash and Bronchoalveolar Fluid Cytologic Examination

- *Tracheal wash:* Contains mucus, macrophages, respiratory epithelial cells, <10% neutrophils (<25% neutrophils in stabled horses)
  - RBCs can be normal in a TTW; oropharyngeal contamination is expected if collected via endoscopy (minimized by a guarded endoscope).
- *BAL:* Little or no mucus, 200 to 400 nucleated cells/µL, mixture of macrophages and lymphocytes, <5% neutrophils, 1% to 2% mast cells, <1% eosinophils
- *Incidental findings:* Oropharyngeal contamination (squamous cells with adherent bacteria, extracellular mixed bacteria), environmental inhabitants (dematiaceous fungal elements), glove powder

Inflammation

Inflammation can result from infectious (bacterial, fungal, viral) and noninfectious causes. Common noninfectious diseases include RAO (also known as heaves or chronic obstructive pulmonary disease) and the syndrome of inflammatory airway disease (IAD) of younger performance horses.

- *Suppurative inflammation:* >85% to 90% neutrophils. This can be due to pneumonia, RAO, or IAD. Degenerate neutrophils usually indicate sepsis. Mucus is thin and mucous spirals are usually absent with sepsis or severe suppurative inflammation.
- *Mixed inflammation:* Increased numbers of nondegenerate neutrophils, with macrophages (often multinucleated) and

fewer lymphocytes; also called "chronic-active" inflammation. Mucus is frequently observed in strands, with some mucous spirals. These features are typical, but not specific, for RAO; similar results are seen with interstitial pneumonia, resolving infections, and pulmonary multinodular fibrosis (associated with equine herpes virus type-5 [EHV-5] infection).

- *Eosinophilic inflammation:* Caused by parasitic infections (e.g., *Dictyocaulus arnfieldi* in horses housed with donkeys and *Parascaris equorum* in foals or yearlings) or fungal infections (e.g., *Cryptococcus*). Eosinophilia is an uncommon cytologic finding in RAO.

●❯ WHAT TO DO

Pneumonia

- Tracheal washes are usually diagnostic, and BALs are not generally indicated.
- Washes contain large amounts of thin mucus that does not form strands or spirals.
- Inflammation is typically suppurative but may be mixed and resemble RAO. Neutrophils are often degenerate.
- Hemorrhage (hemosiderophages, erythrophages, hematoidin) may occur as a sequela.
- One may identify a causative agent:
  - *Bacteria:* Rhodococcus equi is a common pathogen in foals <5 months of age and causes pneumonia and pulmonary abscessation. The bacterium is a small, pleomorphic, gram-positive rod often forming "Chinese letter" shapes (Fig. 11-24). Infection usually incites a mixed neutrophilic histiocytic inflammatory response, and neutrophils may not be degenerate.
  - *Fungi:* Pneumocystis carinii can accompany *Rhodococcus* pneumonia in young foals (<3 months). Cyst and ameboid ("trophozoite") forms are easily overlooked or mistaken for necrotic cellular debris (Fig. 11-25). BALs may be more sensitive than tracheal washes for detecting this fungus. A Gomori-Grocott methenamine silver (GMS) stain also highlights the organism.
  - *Aspiration:* **Note:** Oropharyngeal cells and commensal bacteria accompany a suppurative inflammatory response. Neutrophils are degenerate and phagocytizing bacteria, which distinguishes this from oropharyngeal contamination.

Nonseptic Inflammatory Airway Disease

Nonseptic inflammatory airway disease encompasses two conditions associated with inflammation (usually neutrophilic), airway obstruction, and hypersensitivity to inhaled environmental allergens or molds (e.g., *Alternaria* sp.): RAO and the syndrome of IAD.

- RAO: RAO is synonymous with heaves or chronic obstructive pulmonary disease, and typically affects older (>10 years) stabled horses. A summer pasture-associated RAO has been identified in several areas.
  - Diagnosis can be readily obtained by history, clinical examination, and tracheal wash or BAL findings.
  - Increased amounts of thick, tenacious mucus with numerous mucous spirals are evident.
  - Tracheal wash samples show a suppurative to mixed (neutrophils and macrophages) inflammatory response.

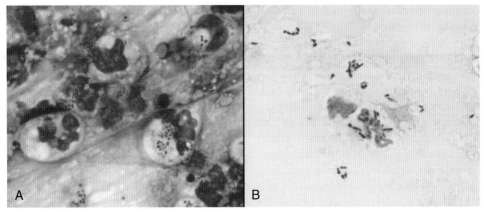

Figure 11-24 *Rhodococcus equi* pneumonia in a tracheal wash from a foal. **A,** There is a suppurative inflammatory response consisting of degenerate neutrophils. Small pleomorphic bacilli are phagocytized and free in the background (Wright stain). **B,** Bacilli are gram-positive and form "Chinese letters," compatible with *R. equi* (Gram stain, 1000× magnification).

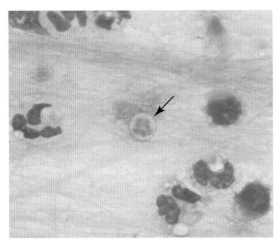

Figure 11-25 *Pneumocystis carinii* in a tracheal wash from a 2-month-old foal. A single cyst with 8 spores is observed in the center of the field *(arrow).* Surrounding cells are mostly nondegenerate neutrophils. Note that this organism is now considered a fungus, even though outdated protozoal terminology for the different stages of the organism is still applied (Wright stain, 1000× magnification).

Neutrophils are nondegenerate, and multinucleated macrophages are frequent. Eosinophils are uncommon.
- May see clusters of hyperplastic columnar epithelial cells (darker blue and more cuboidal than normal) with increased numbers of goblet cells.
- Extracellular bacteria may be present, usually a mixed flora, although there may be a uniform population of diplococci *(Streptococcus zooepidemicus).* The pathogenic significance of extracellular bacteria is uncertain, but culture is indicated in these settings. Bacteria are more likely to be pathogenic if they are phagocytized, and cultures yield moderate to heavy growth.
- Dematiaceous fungal elements may be numerous.
- BALs are characterized by increased total nucleated cell counts, comprising >20% neutrophils (higher neutrophil percentage than that seen with IAD). Increased proportions of mast cells and eosinophils are uncommon.

- IAD: This is a common entity in young racing horses. Many consider BAL to be the diagnostic technique of choice although large airway disease may still play a significant role in the disorder!
  - IAD is associated with poor performance in young athletic horses (<5 years).
  - Mucous production is variable but often appears increased if the horse is scoped following exercise. The amount of mucus seen on endoscopy may be more diagnostic for the condition than the cellular inflammation noted on microscopic exam of the TTW.
  - Tracheal wash findings are similar to RAO: neutrophilic to mixed inflammation, extracellular bacteria, and dematiaceous fungi.
  - BALs: Total nucleated cell counts may be increased and consist of mixed cells (neutrophils, lymphocytes, and macrophages). In rare cases, there is only histiocytic inflammation (mostly macrophages with many multinucleated forms). Counts are frequently within normal limits, but the distribution of cell types is abnormal although variable. There may be increased proportions of neutrophils (10% to 13%, usually <20%), lymphocytes (>50%), mast cells (4%), and eosinophils (4% to 10%). Some horses may only have increased eosinophil and/or mast cell percentages.

Hemorrhage

Hemorrhage can be due to exercise (EIPH) or can result from lung injury of various causes (e.g., inflammation, smoke inhalation, or neoplasia).
- Hemorrhage is suspected when RBCs are observed in tracheal washes collected via an endoscope. RBCs are an expected finding in a TTW.
- Hemorrhage is confirmed by erythrophagia (fresh samples only) and identification of hemosiderin pigment within macrophages or hematoidin crystals.
- Small amounts of hemosiderin may not be detected on Wright-stained smears. Also, other pigments (carbon, phagocytic debris) may be mistaken for hemosiderin.

- It is useful to confirm the presence or absence of hemosiderin with a Prussian blue stain (see Fig. 11-10).
- Hemosiderophages can persist in pulmonary secretions for 1 to 3 months after a bout of hemorrhage; that is, they do not reflect recent hemorrhage.

Other Conditions

- *Neoplasia:* Pulmonary neoplasia is rare in horses and includes primary (pulmonary adenocarcinoma, granular cell tumor) and metastatic (e.g., hemangiosarcoma, squamous cell carcinoma, or malignant melanoma) neoplasms. Tracheal washes and BALs are insensitive diagnostic procedures because neoplastic cells may not invade the airways.
- *Multinodular pulmonary fibrosis:* This form of interstitial pneumonia has been associated with equine herpes virus type-5 infection and should be suspected in an adult presenting with weight loss, fever, tachypnea or respiratory distress and having a severe nodular interstitial pulmonary pattern on radiographic examination. Cytologic findings are not specific and include neutrophilic inflammation with thick mucus in tracheal washes and mixed, mostly neutrophilic inflammation, with vacuolated and multinucleated macrophages, and increased proportions of granular lymphocytes and mast cells in BALs. Viral inclusions are rare and difficult to conclusively identify in cytologic specimens. The disease is best confirmed on lung biopsy, which demonstrates characteristic fibrosis and neutrophilic histiocytic inflammation in alveoli. PCR can be used to identify EHV-5 in the BAL fluid or lung biopsy.

⊙⟩ WHAT TO DO

Keys to Interpretation of Abnormal Tracheal Wash and Bronchoalveolar Lavage Cytologic Findings

- *Oropharyngeal contamination:* Nonkeratinized squamous epithelial cells with adherent bacteria; mixed bacterial population, none phagocytized
- *Suppurative inflammation:* With nondegenerate neutrophils, suspect IAD (e.g., RAO in older horses and IAD in young athletic horses), primary bacterial infections, and interstitial pneumonia. With degenerate neutrophils, look for a bacterial cause and suspect pneumonia or primary bacterial infections (e.g., shipping pleuropneumonia). Culture is indicated.
- *Rhodococcus equi pneumonia:* Young foals with suppurative inflammation, nondegenerate or degenerate neutrophils, and pleomorphic small bacterial rods forming "Chinese letters." Consider underlying *P. carinii* infection.
- *Mixed inflammation:* Caused by RAO, IAD, interstitial pneumonia (including multinodular pulmonary fibrosis), and resolving infections
- *Eosinophilic inflammation:* Parasitic or fungal cause; may not see causative organism
- *RAO:* Increased amounts of thick mucus, neutrophilic to mixed inflammation, nondegenerate neutrophils, and multinucleated macrophages; affects older horses (>10 years)

- *IAD:* BALs are preferred. Nucleated cell counts may be increased but are usually normal; however, there are increased proportions of neutrophils (<20%), lymphocytes, eosinophils, or mast cells. IAD affects young horses (<5 years). Endoscopy after exercise is recommended.
- *Hemorrhage:* RBCs (endoscopic wash), hemosiderin (confirm with Prussian blue stain), hematoidin, erythrophages. Hemosiderophages do not necessarily indicate recent hemorrhage.

Cerebrospinal Fluid

CSF is secreted by cells in the choroid plexus and brain and is of low cellularity and low-protein. CSF can be collected from atlanto-occipital and lumbosacral sites (see Chapter 22, p. 340, for procedures) and should be submitted in EDTA (unless a need for culture is anticipated). Because of extremely low protein, cells rapidly lyse in vitro, affecting counts and cell evaluation. Specimens must be kept cool and submitted for analysis within 24 hours of collection. Specific, highly sensitive techniques are required to measure protein, although urine dipsticks can provide a reasonable approximation of protein values. Because of low cellularity, cell counts are performed manually with a hemocytometer, and cytospin smears are essential for microscopic examination. CSF results can provide evidence of inflammation and trauma. However, CSF abnormalities are not specific for any particular disease, and many horses with clinical signs referable to the central nervous system have normal CSF results (e.g., equine protozoal myelitis).

Normal Cerebrospinal Fluid Results

- *Clarity and color:* Transparent and colorless. Any turbidity or color is abnormal.
  - Normal neonatal foals may have slightly yellow CSF.
- *Nucleated cell count:* 0 to 5 cells/µL
- *RBC count:* Negligible, unless the sample is blood-contaminated; no erythrophages.
- *Protein:* 60 to 120 mg/dL (most normal horses are <80 mg/dl)
- *Smear examination:*
  - Differential cell counts are often done, particularly if the nucleated cell count is increased.
  - Nucleated cells are mononuclear cells (lymphocytes and macrophages). Neutrophils are infrequent, unless there is blood contamination.
  - Incidental findings include clusters of ependymal lining cells, extracellular whorls of granular pink myelin, squamous epithelial cells from the skin, and glove powder.
- *Biochemical analytes:*
  - Glucose, potassium, calcium, and enzymes are lower in CSF than plasma.
  - Glucose in the CSF is further lowered with CNS bacterial sepsis.
  - Sodium, chloride, and magnesium are higher in CSF than plasma.

Key Features of Normal Cerebrospinal Fluid

- Samples should be kept cool and submitted ASAP to the laboratory.
- Clear and colorless
- Nucleated cell count: 0 to 5 cells/μL
- Macrophages and lymphocytes: rare neutrophils
- Protein: 60 to 120 mg/dL

Abnormal Cerebrospinal Fluid Results

CSF results are categorized by the type of inflammation; however, none of the inflammatory profiles are specific for individual diseases. Therefore, CSF analysis is only one diagnostic tool and not definitive in itself (see Chapter 22, p. 342).

Grossly Identifiable Abnormalities of Cerebrospinal Fluid

- Turbidity can be due to increased cells, bacteria, epidural fat, or radiographic contrast media.
- Red-tinged or red fluid indicates blood contamination or subarachnoid hemorrhage.
- Yellow fluid (xanthochromia) indicates prior hemorrhage or icterus (conjugated or direct bilirubin can cross an intact blood-brain barrier, whereas this barrier must be compromised to permit passage of unconjugated or indirect bilirubin).
- Creamy, white fluid indicates greatly increased nucleated cell counts (pleocytosis).

General Categories of Abnormal Cerebrospinal Fluid

- *Suppurative inflammation:* Fluid is turbid and may be opaque, depending on counts. Protein concentration is usually increased. Neutrophils dominate and may be nondegenerate, even if there is a bacterial infection (similar to SF). Causes include bacterial sepsis, variable immunodeficiency syndrome in adults, eastern equine encephalitis, abscesses, and trauma (e.g., subdural hemorrhage or previous CSF tap).
- *Lymphocytic inflammation:* Small lymphocytes dominate, with rare large or reactive forms. Plasma cells may be seen. Inflammation is typical of viral infections (nucleated cell counts are normal or only mildly increased in most cases), including West Nile virus, but can also be seen in horses with primary spinal lymphoma, neuroborreliosis, or compressive lesions. ***Note:*** Increased proportions of granular lymphocytes (cytotoxic T or natural killer cells) may be seen in necrotizing or viral conditions (e.g., equine herpes myeloencephalopathy, which normally has a normal cell count), but are not specific for these disorders.
- *Eosinophilic inflammation:* Inflammation results from protozoal, parasitic (e.g., migrating nematodes), and fungal infections. This is rare in the horse except for *Parelaphostrongylus tenuis*.
- *Mixed inflammation:* Mixture of cells; neutrophils or mononuclear cells can dominate. Causes include fungal infections (e.g., *Cryptococcus,* Fig. 11-26), prior myelography (radiographic contrast media induce a

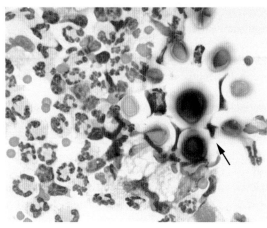

Figure 11-26 *Cryptococcus neoformans* in cerebrospinal fluid. An aggregate of large blue yeasts with thick nonstaining capsules *(arrow)* are surrounded by a mixed inflammatory infiltrate (neutrophils, lymphocytes, macrophages) in a horse with *Cryptococcus* meningitis (Wright stain, 1000× magnification).

mild meningitis), viral infections, and verminous (e.g., *Halicephalobus*) encephalomyelitis.
- *Blood contamination:* Fluid is red-tinged. RBCs settle after sedimentation, leaving a clear, colorless supernatant. Blood contamination (depending on degree) affects interpretation, particularly the ability to detect underlying inflammation (blood adds leukocytes, increasing nucleated cell counts and neutrophil percentages, and protein). Published formulas to correct nucleated cell counts and protein for the degree of blood contamination are of dubious accuracy (1 WBC for every 500 to 1000 RBCs). Platelets and RBCs, but no erythrophages or hemosiderophages, are visible.
- *Hemorrhage:* Fluid may be red-tinged with a RBC-rich sediment after centrifugation if hemorrhage is acute. Erythrophages, hemosiderophages, and hematoidin crystals may be observed. With time, RBCs disintegrate within the arachnoid space, causing xanthochromia.

Specific Conditions

Trauma/Compressive Lesions

- CSF is usually normal with compressive disorders, such as cervical spondylomyelopathy.
- Acute trauma may result in hemorrhage (see previous discussion). Sample may be red (recent hemorrhage) to yellow (from past hemorrhage).
- The nucleated cell count and protein may be mildly increased.

Septic Bacterial Meningitis

- ***Practice Tip:*** *Infection mostly occurs in neonatal foals and adults with variable immunodeficiency syndrome.*
- Fluid is turbid, yellow, creamy, or white.
- Infection produces the highest cell counts, which are due to a neutrophilic pleocytosis. Neutrophils are typically nondegenerate.
- Increased protein is typical.
- Bacteria may not be observed.

Viral Encephalitis
- Results are variable and may be normal.
- Classic findings are a mild lymphocytic pleocytosis and/or increased protein (including West Nile virus encephalomyelitis and Eastern encephalomyelitis virus infections). Some samples may be xanthochromic. Western encephalomyelitis tends to be more neutrophilic.
- A neutrophilic pleocytosis can be seen with acute infections (e.g., eastern equine encephalomyelitis [EEE]).
- Equine herpes virus type-1 (EHV-1) causes a vasculitis with resulting neurologic signs (equine herpes myeloencephalopathy). CSF may be normal or can display xanthochromia and increased protein. Total nucleated cell counts are often normal or may be increased with a lymphocytic pleocytosis. Increased proportions of granular lymphocytes may be seen (but are not specific).

Equine Protozoal Myelitis *(Sarcocystis Neurona)*
- CSF findings are usually normal.
- May see a mild mixed (neutrophils, macrophages, lymphocytes) pleocytosis and mildly increased protein.
- Increased creatine kinase is not a reliable finding. Creatine kinase can be falsely high from contamination of CSF with dural or epidural fat.

- Comparing SAG 2,3,4 ELISA antibody in serum and CSF can provide valuable information on intrathecal antibody production and the likelihood of disease.

●› WHAT TO DO

Keys to Interpretation of Abnormal Cerebrospinal Fluid Cytologic Findings
- Normal results do not rule out an underlying pathologic condition. Results are often normal in degenerative, compressive, infectious (e.g., protozoal and viral), and neoplastic diseases.
- Neutrophils are nondegenerate, and bacteria are rarely observed in sepsis.
- Hemorrhage is usually due to trauma.
- *Suppurative inflammation:* Consider bacterial, acute viral infections, abscesses, and trauma.
- *Lymphocytic inflammation:* Consider viral infections, lymphoma, and compressive lesions.
- *Mixed inflammation:* Consider various causes.

References
References can be found on the companion website at www.equine-emergencies.com.

CHAPTER 12

Emergency Diagnostic Endoscopy

Barbara Dallap Schaer, Ellison Aldrich, and James A. Orsini

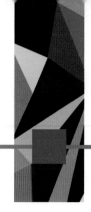

Endoscopy is a valuable diagnostic tool routinely performed in equine practice. Endoscopy allows direct visualization of the upper and lower airway, esophagus, stomach, duodenum, urethra, and bladder. This procedure can be used to further characterize abnormalities identified with other imaging modalities, such as digital radiography and ultrasonography, and to identify lesions that are undetectable with other methods. Samples (biopsy specimens and aspirates) can be obtained transendoscopically for culture, cytology, and histologic examination. Regardless of the system examined, endoscopy should be performed systematically. A thorough knowledge of applied anatomy is necessary to "drive" the endoscope and to differentiate normal from abnormal.

Types of Endoscopes

Many of the flexible endoscopes used in equine practice have been designed for use in humans. The most commonly used flexible endoscopes are either fiber-optic endoscopes or videoendoscopes. Both are adapted easily for procedures on horses. A fiber-optic endoscope is portable and considerably less expensive than a videoendoscope but produces inferior image quality. Often, the light source is of lower wattage on a fiber-optic endoscope than on the videoendoscope. The image is viewed through an eyepiece on the endoscope, so only one person can view the examination unless the endoscope is adapted for a teaching head. A videoendoscope has excellent image quality that is projected onto a monitor. The examination can be seen by all and can be recorded. The unit is generally not suited for field use because it is not easily portable. Recently, a dynamic respiratory endoscope was developed to assess laryngeal function in the horse exercising in its natural setting, as opposed to on a treadmill. Endoscopes should have a biopsy channel and a system for air and water delivery. The size of the endoscope required depends on the anatomic site examined and the size of the patient (see later).

Equipment

- Appropriately sized flexible fiber-optic endoscope,[1] or videoendoscope[2]
- Saline bowl with warm water

- Biopsy forceps, grasping forceps, polypectomy snares, and polyethylene tubing, which are accessories available with each unit
- 30-mL syringe for transendoscopic aspirates

Procedure

- Two to three persons are needed to perform endoscopic examinations.
- Sedation, a twitch, or both may be needed depending on the patient and the system examined. The patient is best restrained in stocks or in a stall.
- The endoscope should be arranged to minimize injury to the operators, patient, and equipment.
- Familiarity with the mechanics of the endoscope is necessary, as is manipulation of the endoscope tip in all directions. The air and water controls are operated from the handpiece; typically, the red button delivers air, and the blue button delivers water.
- Lubricate the endoscope with warm water or a small amount of sterile lubricating jelly[3] (avoid lubricating the tip of the endoscope).
- Passage of the endoscope is described separately for each system.
- Water delivered to the tip of the endoscope cleans the lens; air is delivered to dilate the cavity and improve the examination.
- *Biopsy* is performed by means of advancing the biopsy instrument through the biopsy channel until it protrudes 2 to 3 cm beyond the tip of the endoscope. Manipulate the instrument to obtain a sample and withdraw. Place the specimen in an appropriate fixative.
- Transendoscopic *aspiration* is performed by means of passing sterile polyethylene tubing through the biopsy channel until it extends 2 to 3 cm past the tip of the endoscope. Aspirate a sample using a 30- to 60-mL syringe. Administering sterile saline solution frequently facilitates the aspiration. Place the sample directly onto slides or into an EDTA Vacutainer tube.

[1]Flexible fiber-optic endoscopes: 11-mm outer diameter, 100 cm long; 12-mm outer diameter, 160 cm long; and 8-mm outer diameter, 150 cm long (Karl Storz Veterinary Endoscopy-America, Inc., Goleta, California).

[2]Flexible videoendoscopes: GIF Type Q140 Gastrointestinal Videoscope (9.8-mm outer diameter, 200 to 250 cm long), SIF 100 (11.2-mm outer diameter, 300 cm long), and CF 100 TL (12.9-mm outer diameter, 200 or 300 cm long). (Available by special order from Olympus America, Inc., Center Valley, Pennsylvania).

[3]K-Y lubricating jelly (Johnson and Johnson Medical, Inc., Arlington, Texas); H-R lubricating jelly (Carter Products, Division of Carter-Wallace, Inc., New York, New York).

- The endoscope should be cleaned with antiseptic solution and rinsed after each use.

Gastrointestinal System: Esophagus, Stomach, Duodenum, Rectum and Small Colon Endoscopy

Endoscopy allows examination of the esophagus, stomach, duodenum, rectum, and distal small colon. Endoscopy is the method of choice for confirming the presence of gastric and duodenal ulceration and can aid in the diagnosis of rectal tears.

Procedure

The procedure is as follows:

- The endoscope must be 225 to 300 cm long for complete examination of the stomach and duodenum in adults. A 200-cm endoscope is the minimal length for cursory examination of the stomach in an adult.
- Adults should be fasted for 8 to 12 hours before gastroscopy, and weanling foals should be fasted for 6 to 8 hours. If the duodenum is being examined, longer fasting periods may be required—24 hours for adults. Do *not* fast nursing foals.
- Sedation is generally required.
- See Nasogastric Tube Placement (see Chapter 18, p. 157) for passage of the endoscope into the esophagus. Confirm entrance into the esophagus to prevent damage to the endoscope.
  Practice Tip: Retroflexion of the long endoscopes in the pharynx and entering the oral cavity can be avoided if the view is clear and unobstructed at all times. To prevent damage to the endoscope, a short nasogastric tube may be passed into the proximal esophagus and used as a cannula.
- Insufflation assists passage and examination of the esophagus, cardiac sphincter, and stomach.
- Both the lesser curvature of the stomach and opening of the duodenum are best seen after retroflexion of the scope within the air-filled stomach. Once the scope passes into the duodenum, the duodenal papillae and bile secretion may be noted. On rare occasions an obstructing biliary stone may be seen. Biopsy of the stomach or duodenum can be easily performed with a biopsy instrument passed through the open channel of the scope.

Laparoscopy

Laparoscopy is a valuable diagnostic and surgical tool, which is performed under standing sedation or general anesthesia. In the colic patient, laparoscopy can be used to confirm suspected lesions if rectal palpation and other diagnostic modalities do *not* offer a definitive diagnosis. Laparoscopic evaluation is also useful for evaluating adhesions of the gastrointestinal or reproductive tracts, obtaining biopsies (e.g., hepatic, renal, intestinal), or as part of a chronic colic workup. As a surgical application, laparoscopy provides a minimally invasive alternative to laparotomy, smaller incisions, and decreased postoperative pain. In addition, the right and left flank approaches, which are performed standing, offer better access to several structures in the caudodorsal abdomen *not* readily visualized during ventral midline laparotomy.

Indications

Laparoscopic surgery can be used to:

- Address rectal tears
- Repair mesenteric rents
- Perform ovariectomies and cryptorchidectomies
- Break down adhesions
- Repair bladder ruptures
- Perform nephrosplenic ablation or colopexy

Laparoscopy requires specialized equipment, expertise, and a thorough knowledge of the laparoscopic anatomy.

Laparoscopes

Videolaparoscopes are in widespread use in human medicine and have gained popularity in equine practice over the last decade. Conventional telescopes utilize the Hopkins system, with a rod-shaped quartz lens, which is connected to a light source and camera head. Laparoscopic images are relayed to a monitor for the surgeon to view and still images and video footage can be recorded. More recently, direct videolaparoscopes link the charge-coupled devices directly to the end of the scope, eliminating the rod-lens system. Standard laparoscopes are 10 mm in diameter and range from 30 to 60 cm in length, depending on the manufacturer. The scope is straightforward—0° angle, allowing maximal illumination—or oblique—25° or 30° angle—which is preferred by some surgeons because it minimizes interference with instruments and provides a superior panoramic view.

Equipment

- Laparoscopic telescope[4]
- Camera to process and transmit images for viewing and recording
- Light source (xenon or halogen) attached to a fiber-optic cable
- Color monitor to display video images
- Cannulas, with pyramidal trocars and/or blunt obturators, through which instruments are introduced and removed minimizing trauma to tissue
- Insufflator and compressed CO_2 tanks to create a pneumoperitoneum, allowing visualization and operating space for instruments
- Laparoscopic hand instruments (with handles typically 30 to 45 cm) such as grasping forceps, scissors, Babcock forceps, injection needles, plus any procedure-specific instruments
- Electrosurgery unit
- Suction unit

---

[4]Ten-millimeter scopes (preferred); 5-mm scopes (foals), Stryker offers 5-mm and 10-mm IDEAL EYES Laparoscopes in 30-cm and 45-cm lengths.

Procedure

If a peritoneal fluid sample is desired, abdominocentesis should be performed before laparoscopy because CO_2 insufflation can lead to erroneous results. Laparoscopic surgery requires a surgeon, one assistant, anesthetist, and an operating room (OR) technician. The principle of *"triangulation"* is used when choosing the locations of instrument portals to provide the best view of the surgical field, with instrument and scope converging on the surgical site.

Flank Approaches

Both the right and left flank approaches, performed with the patient standing, offer excellent imaging of most abdominal structures, particularly those located dorsally in the abdomen. Partial evaluation of the opposite side of the abdomen is possible by transrectally moving the terminal descending colon and advancing the scope under the rectum to the opposite side of the abdomen. Feed is typically withheld for 24 hours before surgery. Although fasting improves visualization in general, some structures (i.e., the pelvic flexure and portions of the dorsal and ventral colons) may be obscured by loops of small intestine and small colon in the fasted patient.

- The patient is restrained in stocks and sedated with intravenous xylazine or detomidine and butorphanol. The horse's head can be rested on a stand or suspended from the stocks.
- The tail is wrapped and tied to the stocks to prevent contamination of the surgical field.
- Rectal palpation is performed to ensure that no viscera are present directly beneath the paralumbar fossae before trocar introduction.
- The surgical field is clipped, aseptically prepared, and draped.
- Local anesthesia of the skin and underlying musculature is achieved with 10 to 30 mL of 2% lidocaine or mepivacaine infiltrating the surgery portal sites.
- A 1- to 2-cm incision is made for the laparoscope portal between the tuber coxae and the last rib, through the crus of the internal abdominal oblique muscle.
- Insufflation with CO_2 is performed to distend the abdomen to 10 to 15 mm Hg of pressure. Insufflation is performed before introducing the scope, but this increases the risk of insufflating the retroperitoneal space.
- Instrument portals are created at appropriate locations, depending on the intended procedure, under direct visualization to avoid trauma to viscera.
- Typically, the abdominal viscera are examined systematically from cranial to caudal. The scope is initially in a sublumbar position and then oriented into the pelvic canal to evaluate structures within the caudal abdomen.
- Portals less than 10 mm are closed in a single layer, while larger portals require multiple-layer closure.

Right Flank

The following structures are visualized via a *right* flank approach:

Cranial Abdomen
- Diaphragm
- Right, quadrate and caudate lobes of the liver
- Hepatoduodenal ligament
- Omental bursa
- Cranial duodenal flexure, descending duodenum, and mesoduodenum
- Caudal vena cava
- Portal vein
- Epiploic foramen
- Portion of the stomach
- Right dorsal colon
- Right perirenal fascia

Caudal Abdomen
- Base of cecum, lateral and ventral cecal bands
- Duodenum and mesoduodenum
- Jejunum
- Small colon and mesocolon
- Rectum and mesorectum
- Bladder and associated ligaments
- Males:
  - Right spermatic cord, ductus deferens, mesorchium and vaginal ring
- Females:
  - Right ovary, mesovarium, oviduct, broad ligament and uterine horn

Left Flank

The following structures are visualized via a *left* flank approach:

Cranial Abdomen
- Diaphragm
- Esophageal notch
- Stomach and gastrosplenic ligament
- Left liver lobe and triangular ligament
- Lateral and dorsocranial aspects of the spleen
- Jejunum
- Left perirenal fascia, kidney, nephrosplenic ligament and space

Caudal Abdomen
- Jejunum
- Small colon and mesocolon
- Rectum and mesorectum
- Bladder and associated ligaments
- Males:
  - Left spermatic cord, ductus deferens, mesorchium, and vaginal ring
- Females:
  - Left ovary, mesovarium, oviduct, broad ligament, and uterine horn

Ventral Midline Approach

The ventral midline approach is performed with the patient under general anesthesia and placed in dorsal recumbency. Depending on the structure(s) of interest, positioning (i.e., Trendelenburg, head lower, or reverse Trendelenburg, head higher) may be helpful to allow examination of structures in the most caudal and cranial aspects of the abdomen. Ventral midline laparoscopy offers the best access to ventral abdominal structures and allows visualization of right and left urogenital structures.

- The surgical field is clipped, aseptically prepared, and draped.
- Three laparoscope portals are created on the midline:
  - Retroxiphoid portal 10 cm caudal to the xiphoid cartilage
  - Preumbilical portal 15 cm cranial to the umbilicus
  - Umbilical portal
- Insufflation with CO_2 is performed to distend the abdomen to 10 to 15 mm Hg of pressure.
- Instrument portals are created under direct visualization as described for the flank approach.
- Portals are closed similar to the flank approach.
  The following structures are seen via the *ventral midline* approach:
- Diaphragm
- Falciform and round ligaments
- Right, left, and quadrate liver lobes
- Stomach
- Spleen
- Sternal and pelvic flexures of the large colon
- Right and left ventral colon
- Cecal apex
- Cecocolic fold
- Jejunum
- Small colon
- Rectum and mesorectum
- Pre-pubic tendon
- Right and left urogenital structures[5]

Complications

The most common complications associated with laparoscopic surgery are:

- Inadvertent trauma or penetration of abdominal viscera
- Laceration of the caudal epigastric and circumflex iliac vessels
- Insufflation of the retroperitoneum, especially in fat horses

Other complications associated with sedation, anesthesia, and dorsal recumbency should also be considered. Proper training and thorough knowledge of anatomy reduces these risks. *Practice Tip: It is recommended to have a plan to convert the minimally invasive procedure to an open procedure if necessary.*

Respiratory System: Upper and Lower Airway Endoscopy

Endoscopy of the airway is indicated in the evaluation of patients with nasal discharge, epistaxis, coughing, dyspnea, dysphagia, facial asymmetry, respiratory noise, or exercise intolerance. This is the method of choice for diagnosing

[5]Trendelenburg positioning is usually required to access the bladder, ovaries, and vaginal ring.

ethmoid hematoma, laryngeal hemiplegia, epiglottitis, epiglottic entrapment, dorsal displacement of the soft palate, guttural pouch empyema and mycosis, exercise-induced pulmonary hemorrhage, tracheal trauma or stricture, temporohyoid osteoarthropathy, and congenital abnormalities of the upper airway (e.g., cleft palate). This procedure also assists in the diagnosis of paranasal sinusitis and pulmonary infection or abscess.

Procedure

The procedure is as follows:

- The endoscope should be 150 to 200 cm long and 9 mm in outside diameter for examination of the entire airway; a 9-mm-diameter endoscope is the largest size that can be passed safely in a foal.
- Do *not* sedate the patient, if possible, because sedation can affect the function of the pharynx and the larynx. Sedation is recommended for examination of the lower airway to reduce coughing.
- Pass the endoscope into either nostril and systematically evaluate the upper airway structures, taking care not to injure the ethmoid turbinates. Maintain a clear line of sight during the entire examination.
- The larynx and pharynx can be evaluated first to observe laryngeal function; degree of lymphoid hyperplasia; epiglottic positioning; and the arytenoids' appearance, positioning, and movement. Often evaluation of the nasal passages is performed upon withdrawal of the endoscope.
- The trachea can be entered by passing the scope between the arytenoid cartilages. Tracheal rings are seen if the scope has been properly introduced. Note any abnormal discharge, mucosal inflammation, cysts, or masses. *Caution:* The scope can retroflex in the pharynx and enter the oral cavity, damaging the instrument. Ensure an unobstructed view to prevent this problem.
- Entering the guttural pouch is aided with a biopsy instrument or endoscopic brush as a guide, or it can be performed by means of passing a Chambers catheter up the opposite nostril and "flipping" open the opposite pouch opening.
- *Practice Tip: Spray the trachea with 4 to 6 mL of sterile 2% lidocaine or Cetacaine (benzocaine, butyl aminobenzoate, and tetracaine hydrochloride) spray through the biopsy channel to decrease coughing if the lower respiratory tract is examined.*
- 20 to 30 mL of 2% lidocaine can be infused on the epiglottis to lift the epiglottis.
- The nasomaxillary opening is located in the caudal middle meatus and can be reached with a 9-mm-diameter scope. Drainage from the paranasal sinuses into the middle meatus may be seen in cases of sinusitis.

Sinoscopy

Endoscopic examination of the paranasal sinuses—sinoscopy—involves making a small incision through the skin and periosteum over the sinus of interest, creating a portal for the endoscope using a trephine, and then inserting the endoscope into the sinus cavity. Fluid or tissue samples may also be collected and local treatment of the sinus instituted during the procedure. An intranasal approach has been described, involving the creation of a portal through the dorsal turbinates into the conchofrontal sinus using a laser, but presented here is the standard transcutaneous approach.

Indications

Sinoscopy provides direct access to the interior of the paranasal sinuses, so it is used when the disease process has been localized to the sinuses. Its indications and benefits include:

- Direct visual assessment for space-occupying lesions (e.g., cysts and tumors), hemorrhagic lesions (e.g., progressive ethmoid hematoma, fungal plaques, or erosions), alveolar (tooth root) abscesses, other changes to the mucosa, and skull fractures involving the sinuses
- Collection of fluid and/or tissue samples for microbial culture and antimicrobial sensitivity testing, cytology, and/or histopathology
- Initiation of local therapy, such as lavage, with or without antimicrobials; cautery; and laser ablation

Anatomy

When performing sinoscopy, the portal site of choice depends on the sinus of primary interest. Of the six paranasal sinuses, three are routinely accessed directly using a transcutaneous approach:

- Frontal—conchofrontal—sinus
- Caudal maxillary sinus
- Rostral maxillary sinus

Although there is communication among the various paranasal sinuses, there is normally *no* communication between the corresponding sinuses on the left and right sides of the head.

Frontal Sinus

The most useful approach to the paranasal sinuses is one in which the portal is made into the frontal sinus directly over the frontomaxillary foramen. This natural communication between the frontal and caudal maxillary sinuses allows easy passage of an endoscope. It is also the approach least likely to inadvertently damage "structures" within the sinus or contaminate the surgical site with purulent exudate should a sinus contain free fluid.

The position for trephination is determined thus:

- A horizontal line is imagined at the level of the medial canthus of the eyes, and the portal is made 5 mm (¼ inch) above this line, 5 cm (2 inches) lateral to the midline of the face. Fig. 12-1, *A*, describes a slight variation in the anatomical landmarks used for frontal sinoscopy.
- The distances, and all others, describe the position in the average 450-kg (1000-lb) horse; appropriate adjustments should be made for the significantly larger or smaller patient.

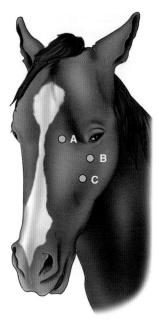

Figure 12-1 Sites for paranasal sinus trephination in an adult. **A,** Draw a horizontal line from the midline to the medial canthus and trephine at a location 1 cm axial to the midpoint of this line, or approximately 2/3 of the distance from the midline to the medial canthus. **B,** Caudal maxillary sinus. Trephine at a location 3 cm rostral from the medial canthus and 3 cm dorsal from the facial crest. **C,** Rostral maxillary sinus. Trephine at a location half the distance along a line drawn from the medial canthus to the rostral end of the facial crest.

Caudal Maxillary Sinus

- The caudal maxillary sinus is readily accessed for sinoscopy via the frontal approach.
- If direct access to the maxillary sinus is required, or if the sphenopalatine sinus is the area of primary interest, then the portal should be located on the dorsolateral side of the face, 2 cm rostral and 2 cm ventral to the medial canthus of the eye (Fig. 12-1, *B*).
- This location usually places the portal just dorsal to the caudal cheek teeth and avoids the infraorbital canal.
- ***Practice Tip:*** *Both structures are vulnerable with this approach, particularly the tooth roots in a young horse, so care must be taken when creating the portal and inserting the endoscope.*

Rostral Maxillary Sinus

- In almost all horses, the rostral maxillary sinus is completely separated from the caudal maxillary sinus by a bony septum.
- The septum is *not* in a consistent location relative to any external landmarks, so the most reliable approach to this sinus, and the least likely to cause damage to the tooth roots, is one guided by radiographs.
- Alternatively, the endoscope is passed into the caudal maxillary sinus via the frontal approach and advanced until it reaches the septum. With the septum illuminated and the light faintly visible through the clipped skin overlying it, the portal can be accurately placed over the rostral maxillary sinus (i.e., just rostral to the lighted area).
- Typically, this portal will be 3 to 4 cm (about 1½ inches) caudal to the infraorbital foramen, and 1 cm ventral to a

line imagined between the infraorbital foramen and the medial canthus of the eye (Fig. 12-1, *C*).

- The age of the horse must be taken into consideration when entering the maxillary sinuses via these dorsolateral approaches.
- *Note:* There may be little or no room for the endoscope in a young horse <6 years of age, because of the space-occupying effect of reserve crown on the maxillary cheek teeth.
- Radiography of the skull is a very useful screening procedure and guide before embarking on sinoscopy of the maxillary sinuses in a horse 10 years of age or younger.

Equipment

The following items are needed:

- Sedation: detomidine—10 µg/kg IV, with or without butorphanol—0.025 mg/kg IV; having xylazine—0.3 to 0.5 mg/kg IV—on hand is useful in case additional sedation is required during the procedure.
- Clippers
- Chlorhexidine or povidone-iodine surgical scrub, isopropyl alcohol, and roll cotton for sterile skin preparation
- Sterile local anesthetic solution (e.g., mepivacaine, 2%, 1 to 3 mL, with 25-gauge, ½- to 1-inch needle); having an additional 5 to 10 mL drawn up in a syringe is useful in case the horse reacts to movement of the endoscope within the sinuses.
- Sterile minor-surgery instrument pack, or at least sterile scalpel handle, hemostat, tissue forceps, and needle holders
- Sterile self-retaining tissue retractors—optional, but recommended
- Sterile scalpel blade
- Sterile surgical sponges (e.g., 4- × 4-inch gauze pads)
- Sterile 15-mm diameter trephine, or as appropriate for the size of the endoscope
- Sterile flexible endoscope
- Any items needed for sterile fluid or tissue sampling as appropriate for the particular case
- Sterile saline or polyionic solution for sinus lavage, 1 liter, warmed to body temperature
- Sterile Foley catheter or other tubing if needed for repeated sinus lavage following sinoscopy
- Sterile 2-0 monofilament suture material

  Practice Tip: The trephine opening should be at least 5 mm larger in diameter than the endoscope so that the endoscope can be inserted into the sinus with ease and manipulated without damaging the surrounding tissue. If using a pediatric endoscope or a rigid arthroscope, a Steinmann pin of suitable diameter may be used in place of the trephine. If a Foley catheter is to be placed and left in situ for repeated lavage after sinoscopy, then matching the diameter of the catheter to that of the trephine helps keep the catheter in place.

Procedure

The basic procedure is the same for all three approaches described earlier:

- Sedate the horse.
- Clip an area at least 3 × 3 inches over the trephination site.
- If desired, place a mark on the skin where the portal is to be created using a felt-tip pen or other permanent marker.
- Aseptically prepare the skin for sterile surgery.
- Anesthetize the skin over the trephination site with local anesthetic.
- Make a skin incision 2.5 to 3 cm (1 to 1¼ inch) in length, parallel to the long axis of the head.
- Continue the incision through the subcutaneous tissue and periosteum; with the rostral maxillary sinus approach, gently elevate the levator nasolabialis muscle dorsally before proceeding.
- Retract the skin and periosteum with a self-retaining retractor or a hemostat to expose the bone; undermine the periosteum as needed.
- Place the cutting edge of the trephine flat against the bone and, with light but steady pressure, rotate the trephine repeatedly in an oscillating fashion to cut a circular hole through the bone.
- Remove the bone plug; when using a large trephine, the bone plug may be saved in a sterile container and kept moist with sterile saline for later replacement if it is intact.
- If there is free fluid in the sinus, aseptically collect a sample for laboratory analysis; aspirate any remaining fluid if it is sufficient to impede visibility within the sinus.
- Insert the endoscope into the portal and advance/direct the tip as needed for thorough visualization of the sinus cavity or cavities.
- If necessary, provide additional sedation or infuse a small amount of local anesthetic onto the mucosa if the patient reacts to manipulation of the endoscope within the sinus.
- Take samples of affected tissue using the biopsy instrument and perform treatments as indicated (e.g., cautery, excision, laser ablation).
- Liberally lavage the sinus with warm sterile saline/ polyionic solution via the endoscope, or remove the endoscope and lavage using a sterile catheter, to avoid dislodging a clot; this step may be skipped or modified for hemorrhagic lesions.
- If leaving an indwelling catheter in situ for repeated lavage, suture the skin closed around the catheter and secure the catheter to the skin.
- If not leaving a catheter in place, either replace the bone plug and suture the wound closed or allow the open portal and wound to close by second intention.

  If bleeding occurs during the procedure, the options depend on the severity of the bleeding:
- If the bleeding is relatively minor, wait a couple of minutes and then reassess; carefully resume the procedure once the bleeding has stopped.
- If the bleeding is moderate and electrocautery or laser cautery of the site is not possible, remove the endoscope

and leave the horse standing quietly in a bedded stall; if sinoscopy is still necessary, carefully resume the procedure the following day (provided that epistaxis has stopped), protecting the surgical site with a sterile dressing in the interim.
- If the bleeding is severe, uncontrollable, and potentially life-threatening, consider sinusotomy via frontonasal bone flap under general anesthesia to gain better access and provide hemostasis within the sinus cavity using sterile gauze packing.

Aftercare
- Administer antibiotics and anti-inflammatory therapy as appropriate for the case.
- Remove the skin sutures 10 to 14 days after the procedure.
- If the portal is left to close by second intention, clean around the site at least twice a day until the wound closes.
- If a catheter is left in the sinus, lavage at least once a day with warm sterile saline or polyionic solution and an anti-microbial drug or antiseptic solution (e.g., povidone-iodine) as appropriate for the case. Remove the catheter and allow the wound to close by second intention once lavage is no longer needed.

Complications
With careful technique and site selection, complications are uncommon, although they can be mild to serious:
- Bleeding from the damaged sinus mucosa, and especially from the ethmoid turbinates
- Damage to the thin bone plate overlying the tooth roots, exposing the tooth roots to infection from respiratory commensals or pathogens
- Damage to the thin bone plate of the infraorbital canal, potentially resulting in chronic obstruction
- Infection of the bone, subcutaneous tissues, or skin if purulent material from the sinus spills from the portal
- Subcutaneous emphysema around the portal site—generally mild and self-limiting.
- Cosmetic defect—bony depression or swelling—at the portal site
  These complications are largely avoided by:
- Attention to the anatomy of the paranasal sinuses
- Performing the trephination slowly and carefully
- Guiding the tip of the endoscope through the labyrinth of the sinuses using direct visualization
- Taking a lateral radiograph of the skull before proceeding is also worthwhile, particularly when it reveals fluid in the sinus of interest. Using the external landmarks of the skull as a guide, a trephination site can be chosen that is above the fluid line yet still within the boundaries of the sinus.

Thoracoscopy
Thoracoscopy provides a minimally invasive technique to examine several intrathoracic structures for diagnostic and therapeutic purposes. The procedure is performed in the standing sedated horse or under general anesthesia allowing direct visualization of the lungs, pleura, portions of the esophagus, diaphragm, and intrathoracic vessels.

Indications
- Obtaining lung or lymph node biopsies
- Evaluating pleuropneumonia, abscesses, and drain placement
- Pneumonectomy
- Pericardectomy
- Evaluating and debriding intrathoracic adhesions
- Repair of diaphragmatic hernias
- Diagnosing esophageal neoplasia

Equipment
- Laparoscopic telescope[6]
- Camera to process and transmit images for viewing and recording
- Light source (xenon or halogen) attached to a fiber-optic cable
- Color monitor to display video images
- Stainless steel teat cannula
- Cannulas/trocars with stopcock adaptors for attaching suction
- Hand instruments such as grasping forceps, scissors, blunt probes, injection needles, plus any procedure-specific instruments
- Electrosurgery unit
- Suction unit

Procedure
- The procedure is typically well tolerated, despite the creation of a unilateral pneumothorax. Administration of intranasal oxygen is recommended during the procedure.
- ***Practice Tip:*** *Although uncommon, some mature horses lack an intact mediastinum and can develop bilateral pneumothorax. Therefore, it is important to have cannulas with stopcocks for rapid attachment of suction if it becomes necessary to reverse the pneumothorax.*
- It is important that portal incisions include only the skin and subcutaneous tissue
- Penetration of the intercostal musculature and thoracic cavity should be with a cannula and sharp trocar to create a good seal around the cannula to prevent air from escaping during surgery and subcutaneous emphysema developing postoperatively. ***Practice Tip:*** *When introducing the cannula and trocar, it is important to angle the instruments caudally to avoid lacerating the intercostal vessels and nerves, which follow the caudal face of each rib.*
- The placement of the scope portal depends on the intrathoracic structures of interest and knowing the anatomy of the thorax. Portals made in the cranial intercostal spaces

---

[6]Ten-millimeter scopes (preferred); Stryker offers 5-mm and 10-mm IDEAL EYES Laparoscopes in 30-cm and 45-cm lengths.

require additional blunt dissection of subcutaneous fat and muscle; manipulation of the scope is more difficult and frequently causes discomfort to the patient because the cranial ribs are less compliant.

- The patient is restrained in stocks and sedated with intravenous xylazine or detomidine and butorphanol. The horse's head can be rested on a headstand or suspended overhead from the stocks.
- The tail should be wrapped and secured to prevent contamination of the surgical field.
- The surgical field should be clipped, aseptically prepared, and draped.
- Local anesthesia is achieved with 8 to 15 mL of 2% lidocaine or mepivacaine, either by local infiltration of subcutaneous, muscular, and pleural tissue at the surgery portal sites or by depositing the anesthetic along the caudal border of the designated rib space and the ribs immediately cranial and caudal to the entrance site for the scope.
- A 1- to 2-cm incision is made ventral to the serratus dorsalis muscle through the skin and subcutaneous tissue in the designated intercostal space.
- Blunt dissection of the subcutaneous tissue and fascia may be necessary, particularly in the more cranial rib spaces.
- A teat cannula is used to penetrate the intercostal muscles and parietal pleura allowing air into the thorax for several breaths, creating a unilateral pneumothorax. Alternatively, active insufflation with CO_2 can be used to collapse the lung.
- A cannula and sharp trocar combination is introduced through the skin incision, angled caudally, and into the thoracic cavity using a gently twisting motion.
- If pleural fluid is present, it should be removed with suction before beginning the thoracic examination.
- Instrument portals are created in a similar fashion at appropriate locations, depending on the intended procedure.
- When the procedure is completed, suction is used to reverse the pneumothorax with the scope still in place, visualizing reinflation of the lung. Portals can be closed in a single layer with nonabsorbable suture material, or in multiple layers, using an absorbable material to close the intercostal muscles.

Anatomy

- The following anatomic structures are visualized during thoracoscopy from either the right or left hemithorax:
  - Pleural surface of ribs and intercostal muscles
  - Dorsal, lateral, diaphragmatic, and mediastinal lung surfaces; caudal lung lobe
  - Pulmonary ligament
  - Costal and hiatal diaphragm
  - Dorsal mediastinum
  - Thoracic portion of the esophagus
  - Aorta
  - Esophageal artery and vein

- Bronchoesophageal artery and vein
- Dorsal intercostal arteries and veins
- Sympathetic trunk
- Dorsal and ventral branches of the vagus nerve
- Caudal mediastinal lymph nodes
- Tracheobronchial lymph node
- ***Practice Tips:*** *In the right hemithorax only, the azygos vein, pulmonary veins, and thoracic duct can also be seen. The heart base and main stem bronchi can only be seen from the left hemithorax.*

Complications

- Although rare in the adult horse, the lack of an intact mediastinum leads to a bilateral pneumothorax, which must be reversed ASAP!
- Horses with pulmonary compromise (i.e., severe pleuropneumonia) may *not* tolerate unilateral pneumothorax well. These individuals become hypoxemic and require immediate reversal of the pneumothorax. Administration of 100% oxygen may also be beneficial.
- Lung lacerations and subcutaneous emphysema have also been reported (see Chapter 46, p. 734).

Urinary System—Urethra and Bladder Endoscopy
Indications

- Hematuria, pollakiuria (frequent urination), dysuria, and tenesmus are common reasons for endoscopy of the lower urinary tract. (see Chapter 26, p. 492.)

Anatomy

- The urethra in the female is approximately 6 to 8 cm (2 to 3 inches) in length and is easily dilated for access to the bladder.
- The external urethral orifice of the mare is at the cranial/anterior portion of the vestibule at the junction of the vaginovestibular fold.
- The urethra in the male is approximately 75 to 90 cm (30 to 35 inches) in length. The colliculus seminalis is located a few centimeters caudal to the most proximal part of the urethra and is the opening for the ducts of the ductus deferens and seminal vesicles. The prostatic ducts are on either side of colliculus seminalis.
- The bulbourethral glands open dorsally several centimeters caudal to the colliculus seminalis.
- The urethra ends at the glans penis and extends 1 to 2 cm as an urethral process.
- The bladder is relatively distensible with a capacity of >4 L of urine in an average size horse.
- The ureters open in the dorsal bladder neck or trigone, near the urethra.

Equipment

- The endoscope should be at least 100 cm long and 9 mm or less in diameter for examination of the urethra and bladder. Longer endoscopes are often required for examining male horses.

Procedure

- Perform the procedure using aseptic technique.
- Cold-sterilize the endoscope in Cidex OPA[7] disinfectant for 30 minutes. Rinse the endoscope with sterile saline before use. Flush the biopsy channel.
- Sedation is recommended for stallions and geldings. Administer 0.4 to 0.6 mg/kg xylazine, 0.01 mg/kg butorphanol, and 0.02 mg/kg acepromazine—geldings *only*—IV for restraint and relaxation.
- Perform a sterile scrub of the distal penis and external urethral process; if applicable, catheterize the bladder and evacuate the urine. See Urinary Tract Catheterization on Chapter 26, p. 485.

---

[7]Cidex OPA, ortho-phthalaldehyde solution (Advanced Sterilization Products, Ethicon, Inc., Irvine California).

- Using sterile gloves, lubricate the length of the endoscope with sterile lube, avoiding the tip.
- Advance the endoscope using the same technique as described for catheterization of the bladder.
- Systematically evaluate the urethra and the bladder, using insufflation to improve the examination. Insufflation normally causes the urethral vessels to appear engorged.
- ***Practice Tip:*** *Ureteral openings are best seen by retroflexion of the scope in the bladder.*

Complications

- With prolonged air insufflation of the urethra, arterial air embolism and death can occur.

References

References can be found on the companion website at www.equine-emergencies.com.

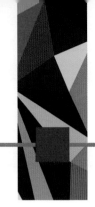

CHAPTER 13

Gene Testing

Joan Norton

- Sequencing of the horse genome has opened the door for a multitude of genetic tests with applications that include:
  - Predicting hair coat
  - Diagnosing disease
  - Identifying carrier horses
  - Preventing disease through responsible breeding
- In order to maximize the value of this information, clinicians must understand the diseases and conditions where genetic testing exists and how to properly collect the appropriate samples for evaluation.

Coat Color

- Coat color genetic testing, generally, does *not* have medical implications but is important for clients who are breeding for specific hair coats.
- Genetic testing is available to determine the base coat color (Red/Black Factor) or the distribution of black pigment controlled by the Agouti gene.
  - Dilutions are genetic mutations that alter the base coat color.
  - Testing is available for Champagne, Cream, Pearl, and Silver dilutions.
  - Age-related total hair depigmentation
  - The Gray modifier also can be identified.
- Several genes have been linked to coat pattern and testing is available for the:
  - Appaloosa
  - Sabino
  - Splashed White
  - Tobiano
  - Dominant White
  - Roan and Dun zygosity

Lethal White Overo Syndrome (LWOS)

- Lethal white overo syndrome (LWOS) occurs when an American Paint Horse is born homozygous for the overo pattern.
- *Practice Tip: Phenotypically these foals have all or nearly all white coats and blue eyes.*
- These foals have ileocolonic aganglionosis, leading to dysmotility of the colon, colic, and death.
- Horses that are heterozygous for the overo gene have a spotted coat color pattern commonly known as "frame" or "frame overo"; however, coat pattern alone does *not* always correlate with LWO heterozygosity. The

overo pattern may be obscured by other spotting patterns.
- *Laboratory Testing:* Twenty mane or tail hairs with roots attached can be submitted to the University of California at Davis Veterinary Genetics Laboratory (www.vgl.ucdavis.edu/services/horse.php), Animal Genetics, Inc. (www.horsetesting.com/CA.htm).

Lavender Foal Syndrome (LFS)

- Lavender foal syndrome (LFS) is an autosomal recessive disorder seen in Arabian foals.
- These foals are born with a coat color dilution that lightens the tips of the coat hairs, or sometimes the entire hair shaft, and display a variety of neurologic deficits including:
  - Inability to sit sternal or stand
  - Strabismus or nystagmus
  - Seizure-like activity
- No other biochemical or hematologic abnormalities are seen in these cases, and they fail to respond to treatments.
- No typical histopathologic lesions are seen on postmortem examination.
- *Laboratory Testing:* Twenty mane or tail hairs with roots attached can be submitted to Animal Health Diagnostic Center, College of Veterinary Medicine, Cornell University (http://ahdc.vet.cornell.edu/sects/Molec/), the University of California at Davis Veterinary Genetics Laboratory (www.vgl.ucdavis.edu/services/horse.php), Animal Genetics, Inc. (www.horsetesting.com/CA.htm). Rooted hairs, whole blood in EDTA, or a bristled style cheek swab can be submitted to Veterinary Genetics Services (www.vetgen.com/equine-CA-service.html).
- An assay to detect the deletion associated with LFS has been developed and is now available through the Animal Health Diagnostic Center at Cornell University. Testing of breeding horses is recommended to avoid breeding carriers to each other. *Sampling:* The assay generally requires the submission of hair roots pulled from the mane or tail. Pulled hair samples should be trimmed to a 4-inch (10-cm) length and taped to a hair sample sheet. Samples from each horse should be placed in individual envelopes, sealed, and attached to a LFS submission form. Other samples may be tested, including whole blood samples collected in lavender-top blood tubes containing ethylenediaminetetraacetic acid (EDTA).

Dermatologic Genetic Conditions
Hereditary Equine Regional Dermal Asthenia (HERDA)

- Hereditary equine regional dermal asthenia (HERDA), also known as hyperelastosis cutis (HC), is a recessive genetic skin disease predominately found in the American Quarter Horse.
- This disorder is characterized by a lack of adhesion within the layers of skin because of a defect in the genes coding for collagen.
- Clinically, the superficial layers of the epidermis are easily pulled from the deeper connective tissue.
- *Practice Tip: Areas under saddle seem to be most prone to these lesions and it is often not until the horse is broken to the saddle that this problem is identified.*
- *Laboratory Testing:* Twenty mane or tail hairs with roots attached can be submitted to the University of California at Davis Veterinary Genetics Laboratory (www.vgl.ucdavis.edu/services/horse.php), Animal Genetics, Inc. (www.horsetesting.com/CA.htm).

Junctional Epidermolysis Bullosa (JEB)

- Junctional epidermolysis bullosa (JEB) is an autosomal recessive disease also known as red foot disease or hairless foal syndrome.
- Two separate genetic mutations have been identified:
  - JEB1, occurring in Belgian Draft horses and related Draft breeds
  - JEB2, which is seen in American Saddlebred horses
- This disorder is caused by a mutation of the γ2 subunit of the laminin 5 gene inhibiting the production of laminin γ2 polypeptide that anchors the epidermis to the dermis and is involved in hoof attachment.
- *Practice Tip: Lesions in the affected horses typically arise at the pressure points at 4 to 5 days of age.*
- These lesions quickly grow larger, creating patches all over the foal's body and possible detachment of the hoof wall. Other clinical signs include oral ulcers and premature eruption of the incisors.
- *Laboratory Testing:* Twenty mane or tail hairs with roots attached can be submitted to the University of California at Davis Veterinary Genetics Laboratory (www.vgl.ucdavis.edu/services/horse.php), Animal Genetics, Inc. (www.horsetesting.com/CA.htm).

Muscular Genetic Disorders
Hyperkalemic Periodic Paralysis (HYPP)

- Hyperkalemic periodic paralysis (HYPP) is an autosomal dominant point mutation in the α-subunit of the voltage gated sodium channels in the myocytes passed down from the Quarter Horse stallion "Impressive."
- HYPP is characterized by:
  - Sporadic episodes of muscle tremors, shaking, or trembling
  - Weakness and collapse
  - Concurrent hyperkalemia during an episode
  - Respiratory obstruction

- Homozygote horses are more severely affected than heterozygotes, and even foals, if homozygous, may be severely affected.
- *Laboratory Testing:* Twenty mane or tail hairs, with roots attached, can be submitted to the University of California at Davis Veterinary Genetics Laboratory (www.vgl.ucdavis.edu/services/horse.php), Animal Genetics, Inc. (www.horsetesting.com/CA.htm) or whole blood in an EDTA tube. Or, 20 mane or tail hairs with roots attached can be submitted to the University of Minnesota Neuromuscular Diagnostic Laboratory (www.vdl.umn.edu/guidelines/equineneuro/home.html).
- Treatment and prevention of these episodes are discussed in Chapter 22, p. 357.

Polysaccharide Storage Myopathy (PSSM)

- Polysaccharide storage myopathy (PSSM) is a glycogen storage disease that causes a variety of signs ranging from rhabdomyolysis to poor performance.
- PSSM type 1 is a mutation in the GSY1 gene found in over 20 breeds and most commonly affects Percherons, Belgium, Paint, and Quarter Horses. In Quarter Horses the prevalence in halter horses is >25%, but low in racing Quarter Horses. The prevalence in Warmbloods is variable depending upon origin of the breed but is generally much higher for type 2 PSSM than for type 1 PSSM. The prevalence of PSSM is low in breeds such as Shires, Clydesdales, Throughbreds, Standardbreds, and many others.
- PSSM type 2 genetic mutation is yet to be identified.
- *Practice Tip: A majority of Quarter Horses have type 1 PSSM, but the majority of Warmblood and Draft horses have type 2 PSSM.*
- *Laboratory Testing:* Whole blood in an EDTA tube or 20 mane or tail hairs with root attached can be submitted to the University of Minnesota Neuromuscular Diagnostic Laboratory (www.vdl.umn.edu/guidelines/equineneuro/home.html), the University of California at Davis Veterinary Genetics Laboratory (www.vgl.ucdavis.edu/services/horse.php), or Animal Genetics, Inc. (www.horsetesting.com/CA.htm).

Malignant Hyperthermia

- Malignant hyperthermia is a mutation in the ryanodine receptor 1 (RyR1) gene that causes a dysfunction in the sarcoplasmic receptors of skeletal muscles resulting in excessive release of calcium into the myoplasm.
- Clinical signs include:
  - Hyperthermia
  - Tachycardia
  - Tachypnea
  - Hyperhidrosis
  - Muscle rigidity
  - Death
- Episodes can be triggered by anesthesia, stress, exercise, or concurrent myopathies.

- Homozygote horses are more severely affected than heterozygotes.
- *Laboratory Testing:* Whole blood in an EDTA tube or 20 mane or tail hairs with roots attached can be submitted to the University of Minnesota Neuromuscular Diagnostic Laboratory (www.vdl.umn.edu/guidelines/equineneuro/home.html) or Animal Genetics, Inc. (www.horsetesting.com/MH.htm).

Glycogen Branching Enzyme Deficiency (GBED)

- Glycogen branching enzyme deficiency (GBED) is a fatal disease seen primarily in Quarter Horses. Foals lack the glycogen branching enzyme needed to store glycogen in its branched form.
- This mutation results in late-term abortion and still-births and is responsible for 3% of all Quarter Horse abortions.
- *Practice Tip: Affected foals are weak, unable to stand and maintain adequate body temperature, may develop seizures, or die peracutely.*
- *Laboratory Testing:* Twenty mane or tail hairs with roots attached can be submitted to the University of California at Davis Veterinary Genetics Laboratory (www.vgl.ucdavis.edu/services/horse.php), Animal Genetics, Inc. (www.horsetesting.com/CA.htm) and rooted hairs, whole blood in EDTA, or a bristled style cheek swab can be submitted to Veterinary Genetics Services (www.vetgen.com/equine-CA-service.html).

Other Genetic Disorders
Cerebellar Abiotrophy

- Cerebellar abiotrophy is a neurologic autosomal recessive genetic condition found almost exclusively in Arabian horses.
- The mutation leads to degeneration of the Purkinje cells in the cerebellum leading to intention tremors and ataxia.
- *Practice Tip: Clinical signs do not manifest until 6 weeks to 4 months of age.*
- *Laboratory Testing:* Twenty mane or tail hairs with roots attached can be submitted to the University of California at Davis Veterinary Genetics Laboratory (www.vgl.ucdavis.edu/services/horse.php), Animal Genetics, Inc. (www.horsetesting.com/CA.htm), and rooted hairs, whole blood in EDTA, or a bristle style cheek swab can be submitted to Veterinary Genetics Services (www.vetgen.com/equine-CA-service.html).

Congenital Stationary Night Blindness

- Congenital stationary night blindness (CSNB) is a condition seen in Appaloosa and Miniature Horses, with a Leopard patterned (LP) hair coat and linked with the LP gene that leads to a defect in neural transmission through the rod pathway involving the inner nuclear layer.
- Clinical signs include diminished or absent night vision.
- *Laboratory Testing:* Twenty mane or tail hairs with roots attached can be submitted to Animal Genetics, Inc. (www.horsetesting.com/CA.htm).

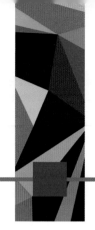

CHAPTER 14

Imaging Techniques and Indications for the Emergency Patient

DIGITAL RADIOGRAPHIC EXAMINATION

Christopher Ryan

- Digital radiography (DR) provides a rapid and noninvasive technique to obtain diagnostic information in the equine emergency setting.
- The wide exposure latitude of digital radiographic systems compared with screen-film radiography equals a broader range of exposures, which are still likely to result in a diagnostic image.
- It is important to remember that image quality in DR also depends on hardware and software, which can be extremely variable among manufacturers.
- Poor image processing algorithms can lead to disappointing images compared with carefully taken, high quality screen-film radiographs.
- Digital radiographic systems provide a tentative diagnosis and therapeutic plan to be implemented at the initial exam without the need to wait for film processing (especially in emergency situations); field evaluation of radiographs should never serve as the final diagnostic assessment.
- Radiographic displays on portable units are typically of low resolution and the field emergency setting tends to be filled with interruptions and distractions.
- It is always recommended that a final evaluation be performed in a quiet and controlled environment, preferably using medical grade diagnostic grayscale monitors.
- Indications for radiographic evaluation of the equine patient in emergency situations include:
  - Acute onset of severe lameness
  - Wounds and lacerations
  - Penetrating foreign body
  - Laminitis
  - Trauma and suspected fracture
  - Head trauma with neurologic signs, epistaxis, or palpable skull fractures/depressions

Patient Preparation

- In many emergency situations diagnostic anesthesia is often *not* needed to localize the site of lameness.
- A comprehensive physical examination including the use of hoof testers should provide reasonable localization and selection of the area of interest to be examined radiographically.
- Following physical examination and assessment, sedation may be necessary to obtain good quality radiographs.
  - Commonly used sedatives are:
    - Xylazine HCl (0.2-1.1 mg/kg IV)
    - Detomidine HCl (0.01-0.02 mg/kg IV)
    - Butorphanol tartrate (0.02-0.04 mg/kg IV) for added duration and analgesic effects
  - Sedatives should be used *cautiously,* especially in the orthopedic emergency situation, to avoid excessive ataxia.
- The area of interest should be cleaned to prevent superimposition of dirt and debris on the radiographs.
  - *Feet*—a hoof pick and wire brush are useful to remove dirt from sole and sulci. The sulci can then be packed with a moldable modeling compound[1] to eliminate gas superimposition shadows on the radiographs due to air trapped in the sulcus.
  - *Limbs*—use a grooming brush to remove dust and dirt.

General Technique

- ***Practice Tip:*** *A minimum of two orthogonal projections is recommended for any radiographic study. Evaluation of joints, long bones, and feet may require multiple oblique views to provide a better understanding of the three-dimensional conformation of the region of interest and any pathology.*
- Proper radiographic technique including kVp, mAs, and source-to-detector distance, should be chosen to allow adequate visualization of bony and soft tissue structures.
- Many portable x-ray generators are limited in both kVp and mAs, which can lead to increased exposure times and motion artifact, especially on thicker body parts.
- A generator stand can help eliminate operator motion.
- With digital radiograph systems, the algorithms used to process raw image data are important in the final radiograph.
- Overexposure of the imaged study may result in loss of soft tissue detail, missing important lesions.

---

[1]Play-dough (Hasbro, Inc., Pawtucket, Rhode Island).

- Underexposure can lead to increased noise in the image creating a grainy appearance.
- Proper protective gear including lead gowns, gloves, and thyroid shields should be worn by those taking the radiographs; a cassette holder is useful for positioning of the digital detector. Set up the radiographic equipment and enter patient demographic information into the system before working with a patient; this eliminates time wasted once a horse is sedated. A lead marker identifying the limb and taped to the digital detector serves as a backup for limb identification and directionality (e.g., medial vs. lateral) in cases of mislabeling.

Distal Limb and Foot

- Specific emergency situations that warrant radiography of the foot or distal limb include:
  - Penetrating wounds to the sole
  - Fractures
  - Lacerations
  - Laminitis
  - Subsolar abscesses

Penetrating Foot Injuries

- Puncture wounds to the sole or frog may be superficial or deep and risk injury to:
  - Solar germinal epithelium
  - Digital cushion
  - Deep digital flexor tendon
  - Distal sesamoidean impar ligament
  - Coffin bone
  - Navicular bone
  - Synovial structures including:
    - Digital flexor tendon sheath
    - Navicular bursa
    - Distal interphalangeal joint
- The anatomic structure involved is determined by the depth and direction of the penetrating injury.

Acute Puncture Wound

- If the penetrating object remains in place, survey radiographs of the foot help in assessment of the anatomic structures involved.
- If the foreign object is no longer present and a puncture wound is suspected, a sterile metallic malleable probe may be inserted into an identified tract before radiographic examination, to better define depth and direction of the tract (Fig. 14-1).
- The foot, and especially the sole, should be thoroughly cleaned before exploring any tracts with a sterile probe.

Chronic Puncture Wound

- Radiographs are indicated to help rule out:
  - Septic osteitis of the coffin bone
  - Septic arthritis
  - Fractures
  - Sequestrum formation

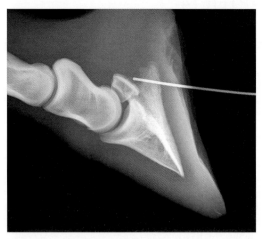

Figure 14-1   Lateromedial radiograph of the foot with malleable probe placed in a solar puncture wound. Note the probe contact with the navicular bone.

- Special procedures, such as positive contrast arthrography/bursography or fistulography, can be helpful in determining the extent of injury and possible affected structures.

Arthrography/Bursography/Tenography
Equipment

- Clippers
- Material for aseptic preparation
- Sterile gloves
- 5- to 20-mL syringe containing iodinated positive contrast media, Iohexol,[2] 240 mg/mL, and 20- to 22-gauge needle. A 20- to 22-gauge spinal needle is required for navicular bursography.
- Blood collection tubes (ethylenediaminetetraacetic acid [EDTA] tube and red-top tube) and sterile 5- to 10-mL syringe for collection of synovial fluid

Procedure

- An approach to the joint, bursa, or tendon sheath is chosen separate from the wound site and any significant soft tissue swelling (Fig. 14-2).
- Clip the hair and thoroughly clean skin in the area of the synovial structure to be evaluated, including an aseptic preparation.
- A needle is placed using aseptic technique and a sample of synovial fluid for cytology, culture, and sensitivity is taken, if indicated, and can be obtained either by free flow or aspiration with a syringe.
- Contrast media is injected. Use a sufficient volume to distend the synovial compartment.
- Radiographs are obtained immediately after contrast medium injection.
- Passive flexion of the limb is performed to distribute the contrast throughout the synovial cavity.
- Orthogonal radiographic views of the area of interest are generally recommended; under certain circumstances, a single view may be sufficient.

---

[2]Omnipaque (GE Healthcare, Princeton, New Jersey).

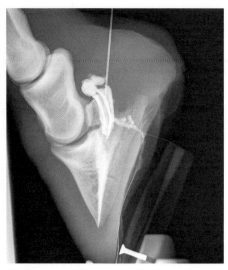

Figure 14-2   Lateromedial radiograph of same foot shown in Fig. 14-1. Contrast media has been injected into the navicular bursa, providing evidence that the wound tract extends into the solar surface.

- Multiple oblique views may be needed to best define a communication between a synovial structure and a wound.
- An appropriately chosen kVp helps enhance image contrast by maximizing the photoelectric effect of the x-ray beam with the limb. ***Practice Tip:*** *The kVp should be greater than twice the 33.2 keV k-edge of the iodine in the contrast media (i.e., a kVp value ≥67) to maximize photoelectric effect.*

Contrast Fistulography

- Wound communication with a synovial compartment is typically easier to identify with positive contrast arthrography, bursography, or tenography.
- Contrast media also may be directly instilled into a wound tract to determine possible communication with a synovial structure (Fig. 14-3).

Equipment

- Material for aseptic preparation
- Sterile gloves
- 5- to 20-mL syringe containing iodinated positive contrast media (e.g., Iohexol) and 18- to 22-gauge over-the-needle catheter or sterile teat cannula.

Procedure

See procedure for arthrography/bursography/tenography (see p. 74).

Wounds and Lacerations

- Radiographs are recommended for limb wounds to rule out injury to underlying bony structures including:
  - Nondisplaced fractures
  - Hairline fractures of long bones (Fig. 14-4)
  - Avulsions of tendon and ligament origins and insertions (Fig. 14-5)

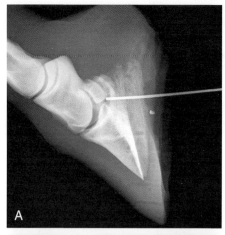
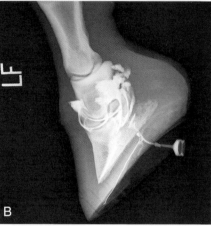

Figure 14-3   **A,** Lateromedial radiograph of the foot with malleable probe placed in a solar puncture wound. Note that the probe extends to the impar ligament distal to the navicular bone and likely into the coffin joint. **B,** Same foot as shown in Fig. 14-3, *A*, with contrast injected into the solar wound tract. Contrast is visible throughout the distal interphalangeal (coffin) joint.

- Radiopaque foreign bodies also may be seen, which are *not* evident on physical examination or wound exploration (Fig. 14-6).
- In chronic cases, especially in the presence of a draining tract, radiographs may help rule out a bone sequestrum (Fig. 14-7).
- Positive contrast studies may be used to determine a communication of a wound with a joint or other synovial structure (bursae, tendon sheaths) and are often better in identifying a synovial communication than positive contrast fistulography.
- Positive contrast fistulography may be used in wounds to the limb, especially in puncture wounds with deep pocket formation.
- The procedure is similar to that described for penetrating wounds of the sole.

Laminitis

See Chapter 43, p. 697.

Equipment—Digital Radiographs

- Wooden blocks are needed on which to place the feet. The height of the blocks depends on the size of the x-ray

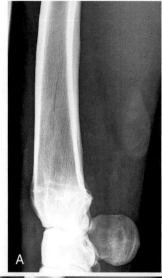

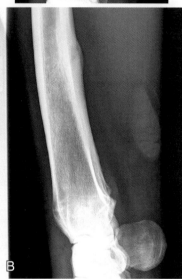

Figure 14-4   A, Lateromedial view of the distal radius in which a radiolucent hairline fracture is evident in the mid- to distal diaphysis. **B,** Same horse as Fig. 14-4, *A,* after 4 weeks of stall rest. Smooth periosteal and endosteal callus is present along the mid-diaphyseal caudal cortex.

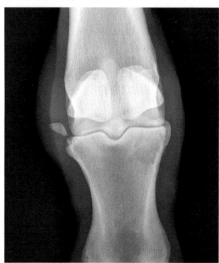

Figure 14-5   Dorsoplantar view of the left hind fetlock in which there is an avulsion fracture at the insertion of the lateral collateral ligament with marked fragment displacement and associated soft tissue swelling.

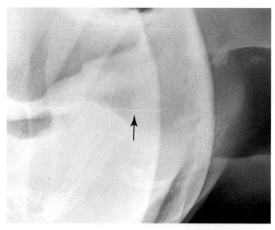

Figure 14-6   Lateral view centered on the pharynx. A metallic wire foreign body is present just cranial to the larynx *(black arrow).*

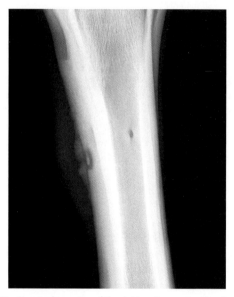

Figure 14-7   Dorsopalmar view of the right metacarpus with a focal radiolucent cortical defect containing a central bony opacity and surrounding periosteal reaction and soft tissue swelling consistent with a sequestrum.

generator; measure from floor to center of collimator and subtract ¾ inch (1.9 cm). The blocks should ideally have two wires at 90° to each other embedded in the top surface.
- Markers using a short malleable wire or barium paste are useful for identifying the coronary band and dorsal hoof wall. ***Practice Tip:*** *The dorsal hoof wall marker should extend from the coronary band nearly to the weight-bearing surface.*

Procedure
- Clean feet as previously described.
- The left and right feet are positioned on the blocks for even weight bearing. Place the feet as close to the medial and palmar/plantar edge of the block as possible to minimize the object-detector distance (the distance between the DR plate and the foot); blurring of the anatomy results when this distance is increased. Metacarpi/metatarsi (cannon) bones should be positioned vertically.

- Lateromedial and dorsopalmar views are generally sufficient for evaluation of the laminitic foot, though palmar margin views are sometimes indicated. Additionally, small metallic markers are useful to identify the point of the frog.
- When radiographing the foot for laminitis, the x-ray beam should be centered ¾ inch (1.9 cm) above the weight-bearing surface of the foot and parallel with the ground.

Venograms

See Chapter 43, p. 701.

- Positive contrast digital venography (venograms) is a useful imaging technique in evaluating the foot, especially in cases of laminitis.
- Deficits in perfusion of the foot and reperfusion of injured area(s) can be assessed and followed with serial venograms.
- Venograms have proven useful in establishing a more accurate prognosis and developing treatment plans.
- Lack of improvement of the vascular pattern on serial venograms is a strong indicator that current treatment is *not* working, or the foot pathology is so severe that the chance of tissue repair is poor.

Venogram Technique

See Chapter 43, p. 701.

Equipment

- Material for aseptic preparation
- 3- to 5-mL syringe per foot of local anesthetic agent (e.g., mepivacaine hydrochloride [Carbocaine])
- Tourniquet—simple surgical tubing, Esmarch bandage, or pneumatic tourniquet
- Over-the-needle catheter (20 to 22 gauge, 1.25 inch [3.0 cm]) or butterfly catheter (21 to 23 gauge). A 7- or 30-inch (18- or 76-cm) intravenous extension set attached to the catheter reduces the risk of the catheter dislodging while injecting.
- 20 to 30 mL iodinated contrast media (Iohexol). Use 10- to 12-mL syringes to reduce back pressure when injecting.
- Sterile gauze and elastic bandage (Vet-Wrap)

Procedure

See Chapter 43, pp. 701-704.

- The digital radiograph equipment should be set up with patient demographic information entered before beginning the procedure. For sedation, use an alpha-2 agonist such as xylazine or detomidine.
- Perform a palmar nerve block at the level of the proximal sesamoid bones (abaxial sesamoid nerve block). Clean the soles of the feet after perineural analgesia.
- Survey lateromedial and dorsopalmar radiographs are taken before tourniquet application or contrast administration. Aseptically prepare the skin overlying the catheter site (lateral or medial palmar digital vein).

- Apply the tourniquet at the level of the fetlock.
- The distended lateral palmar digital vein is catheterized distal to the proximal sesamoid bone. Connect the extension set to the catheter and infuse 20 to 30 mL of positive contrast media. ***Practice Tip:*** *A typical Thoroughbred foot usually requires approximately 20 mL; a large Warmblood or Draft horse foot may need up to 30 mL of contrast. Partially flex the carpus to unload the deep digital flexor tendon without removing the foot from the block while injecting the second-half of the contrast volume.* When the injection is completed, the syringe and extension set can be taped to the tourniquet.
  Practice Tip: *Use hemostats to occlude the extension set after completing the injection or else the back pressure will cause the syringe to fill from the vein.*
- Lateromedial and dorsopalmar radiographs are immediately repeated as described above.
- The tourniquet is removed before the catheter and a pressure bandage is applied after the procedure, compressing the venipuncture site.

Technical Errors

- Filling defects are due to inadequate contrast volume from poor tourniquet application or insufficient volume of contrast agent (Fig. 14-8).
- Perivascular injection from the catheter dislodging or leaking of contrast around the catheter
- Excessive time between contrast injection and radiographs leads to "blurring" due to diffusion of contrast into the extracellular space.
- Areas of interest for critical evaluation on the digital venogram include:
  - Coronary plexus
  - Coronary papillae
  - Sublamellar plexus
  - Circumflex vessels
  - Sole papillae
  - Terminal arch
    Practice Tip: *Until you have performed many venograms, have a colleague who is familiar with venograms analyze the images to gain the most information from the procedure.*

Fractures/Acute Non–Weight-Bearing Lameness

- In cases of an acute non–weight-bearing lameness, a fracture may be the etiology (see Chapter 21, p. 315) based on physical examination.
- If radiographs can be safely and efficiently obtained in a field emergency setting, they may provide accurate assessment of the injury and prognosis.
- Fractures within the hoof capsule (e.g., distal sesamoid bone [navicular bone] or distal phalanx [coffin bone] fractures) have few changes on physical examination other than severe lameness.
- The foot should be prepared for radiographs as described on p. 73.

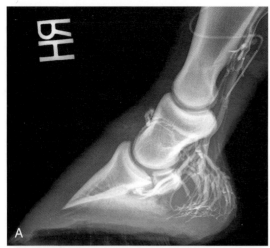

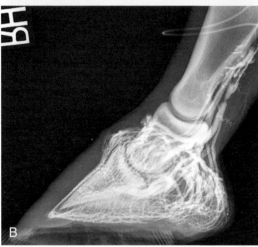

Figure 14-8   A, Lateromedial digital venogram in which the tourniquet provided inadequate venous occlusion, leading to inadequate contrast volume within the digital vasculature. **B,** Reapplication of tourniquet and injection of an additional volume of contrast media, leading to adequate digital vasculature distention.

- Articular fractures are best seen on dorsoproximal-palmarodistal views.
- Nonarticular fractures of the palmar processes may require dorsal 45° lateral (or medial) palmarodistal oblique views to visualize.
- *Practice Tip: Care must be taken not to confuse separate centers of ossification of the palmar processes of the coffin bone or bipartite distal sesamoid bones with fractures.*
- Palmaroproximal-palmarodistal oblique (skyline) views are best at demonstrating fractures of the navicular bone.

Skull Radiography

- Skull radiographs are indicated when evaluating:
  - Dental disease
  - Disorders of the paranasal sinuses/nasal cavities
  - Traumatic injuries

Dental Radiography

- Field radiographs of the dental arcades are typically performed with a smaller detector panel (9 × 11 inch/23 ×

28 cm) compared with a referral hospital, which uses a 14- × 17-inch/36- × 43-cm panel (see Chapter 18, p. 164).
- Wide collimation, providing a larger field of view, is useful, especially with the smaller panels for easier identification of anatomic structures.
- Radiographic technique may need to be increased compared to the lower technique needed for evaluation of air-filled paranasal sinuses, guttural pouches, or pharyngeal/laryngeal regions.

Fractures

- Fractures of the skull occur as one of three types:
  - Fractures of the mandible
  - Depression fractures of the skull
  - Separation along suture lines
- Fractures of the mandible may be unilateral or bilateral, and superimposition on lateral radiographic views makes interpretation difficult. Thirty-five degree to 45° ventrolateral to ventrodorsal oblique views (Fig. 14-9) of each mandible can eliminate superimposition (Fig. 14-10).
- Fractures of the incisors are best seen with intraoral views, directing the x-ray beam orthogonal to a plane tangential to the incisor tooth surface at the gingival margin.
- Depression fractures of the bones overlying the paranasal sinuses or nasal passages typically involve the frontal, nasal, lacrimal, or maxillary bones. The zygomatic arch also may be involved in fractures of the orbit.
  - Oblique views at various angles better demonstrate the presence and types of fractures. Horses that flip over backwards are prone to fractures of the base of the skull. The suture between the basisphenoid and basioccipital bone is particularly at risk for fracture. *Practice Tip: Do not mistake the normal suture line, which may be seen until between 2 and 5 years of age, for a fracture* (Fig. 14-11).
  - Radiographic signs of trauma may reveal an increase in soft tissue opacity in the region of the normally air-filled guttural pouches secondary to injury to the longus capitis muscles and bleeding (Fig. 14-12).

Procedure

- Appropriately sedate the patient.
- Use a rope halter to eliminate superimposition of metallic buckles and clasps.
- Radiopaque markers can be placed on external swellings to aid in determining significance of radiographic abnormalities.

Digital Radiography Artifacts

- Although errors in exposure technique are reduced with the wide exposure latitude of digital radiographic systems, technique errors such as poor positioning and failure to adequately center the x-ray beam on the region of interest are similar to screen-film radiographs.

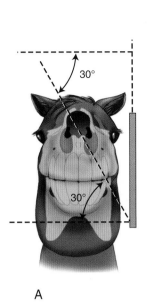

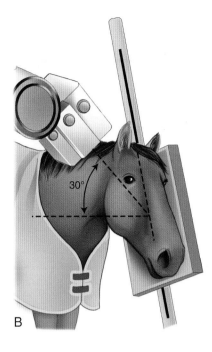

Figure 14-9 Schematic demonstrating positioning for oblique views of the mandible. (Adapted from Obrien. Handbook of Equine Radiography. Saunders-Elsevier 2010.)

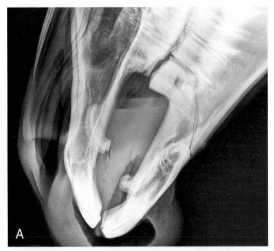

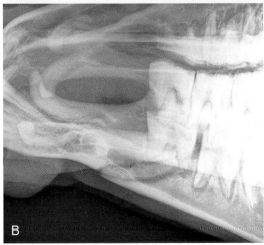

Figure 14-10   A, Lateral view of the rostral mandible in which the side of the fracture *cannot* be determined. **B,** Oblique view of the rostral mandible clearly shows the fracture involving the left rostral mandible. The right rostral mandible was normal in the opposite oblique view (not shown).

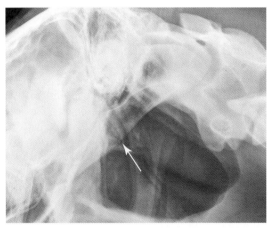

Figure 14-11 Lateral radiograph of a 7-month-old weanling showing a normal spheno-occipital suture *(white arrow).*

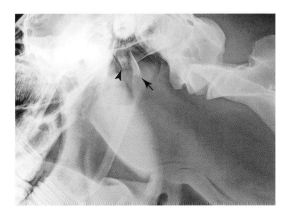

Figure 14-12 Basisphenoid-basioccipital fracture. Notice how the suture is wider and more distinct than in Fig. 14-11 *(arrowhead).* There is also a large displaced ventral bone fragment *(arrow)* and obliteration of the gas-filled guttural pouches, with soft tissue opacity representing hemorrhage from the longus capitis muscles.

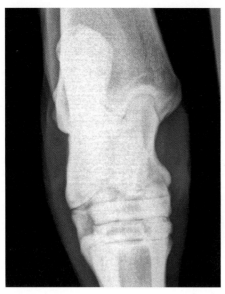

Figure 14-13   Dorsoplantar view of the tarsus with a marked grainy appearance due to underexposure. Increasing the exposure technique remedies the artifact.

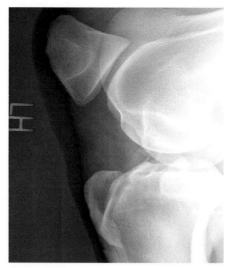

Figure 14-14   Overexposed lateral view of the stifle in which the cranial soft tissues are no longer visible because of saturation of the detector elements. "Planking" artifact is also visible to the left of the stifle.

- Digital systems add a new set of artifacts to recognize and to correct. These are divided into the categories of:
  - Exposure artifacts
  - Image processing artifacts

Exposure Artifacts

- Image processing of an underexposed radiograph causes the image to appear of diagnostic quality. Zooming in demonstrates a grainy, noisy, mottled, or pixilated image because of a decrease in the signal-to-noise ratio (Fig. 14-13).
- Overexposure causes detector elements in a flat panel to become saturated and saturated pixels are set to the same maximal gray-scale value.
  - If a calibration mask is used to correct for nonuniformity in the detector panel, the mask may become visible as "planking" or wide bars/rectangles in the final image (Fig. 14-14).
  - *Correction* is simply repeating the radiograph at a lower exposure.
- A calibration "mask" is used to correct irregularities in a detector panel and is created by making full exposures of a panel.
  - Anything between the x-ray source and panel when the exposure is made for the mask can become incorporated into the digital mask including:
    - Anything on the collimator window (e.g., splashed contrast media)
    - Debris on the panel
  - Panels used in equine practice are generally held in various positions; the mask artifacts may *not* appear in the same location and appear as a single or pair of light and dark "ghostlike" artifacts.
- Radiofrequency interference occurs if a detector is placed close to a radiofrequency source or there is a break in the

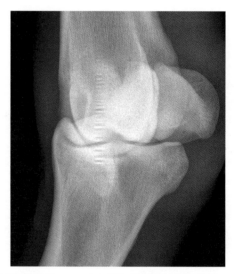

Figure 14-15   Radiofrequency interference artifact. Note the narrow vertical band of thin, parallel horizontally stacked lines dorsal to the proximal sesamoid bones.

shielding of the detector or its cable. These artifacts appear as narrow bands of thin, parallel stacked lines and are variable in length (Fig. 14-15). Consider replacing cables with worn, frayed, or broken shielding.

- "Ghosting" occurs in systems that utilize photodiodes in the detector panel (most equine systems) and are seen if an exposure is taken too quickly because of differences in retained charge in the photodiodes. A faint "ghost" image of the prior exposure appears superimposed on the subsequent exposure.

Image Processing Artifacts

- Excessive edge-enhancement can lead to dark halo formation known as "Uberschwinger" or "rebound" effect.

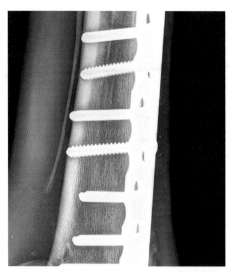

Figure 14-16 Rebound artifact due to edge enhancement algorithms (typically unsharp masking). Notice the radiolucent halos within the cortical bone surrounding the screw ends.

- The halos typically occur around very dense or radiopaque structures such as metallic implants or dense cortical bone and can mimic disease processes such as osteolysis associated with orthopedic implant loosening (Fig. 14-16) or pneumothorax.
- Clipping occurs when an inappropriate look-up table (LUT) is applied in the preprocessing step of image processing. Appearance is similar to Fig. 14-14.
- Information about soft tissues can be lost, and despite changing brightness and contrast during viewing, no information is present in thinner soft tissue regions.
- Overexposure can also lead to a clippinglike artifact.

ULTRASONOGRAPHY: GENERAL PRINCIPLES AND SYSTEM AND ORGAN EXAMINATION

*JoAnn Slack**

Ultrasound Examination

The ultrasound examination is a noninvasive method of obtaining rapid diagnostic information in the emergency setting. Ultrasonography is particularly useful in the rapid assessment of the horse for the following:
- Trauma
- An acute condition of the abdomen
- Respiratory distress and pneumonia
- Evaluation of fetal well-being in high-risk pregnant mares
- Ocular emergencies

Echocardiography is useful for assessing the horse with cardiovascular emergencies and is discussed beginning on Chapter 17, p. 150.

*We recognize and appreciate the contribution and original work of Virginia B. Reef, DVM, DACVIM, in the previous editions of *Equine Emergencies*.

●》 WHAT TO DO

Ultrasound Examination
Patient Preparation
The best images are obtained by clipping the hair from the skin over the area to be examined using a #40 surgical clipper blade.
- Shaving the skin is usually not necessary.
- If clipping is not an option, wetting the hair and skin thoroughly with warm water along the lay of the hair or spraying the area with alcohol may be sufficient for a diagnostic quality image.
- The skin should be scrubbed clean with surgical soap and water.
- Ultrasound coupling gel should be applied to the skin.
- If there is an acute laceration or puncture wound, the examination should be performed aseptically, using sterile ultrasound gel or sterile K-Y jelly and a sterile ultrasound "condom" or surgical glove to cover the transducer.

Ocular ultrasound can be performed by placing the transducer directly on the eye or on the eyelid. The transcorneal approach requires instillation of topical anesthetic and placement of an auriculopalpebral nerve block. Although this method provides the best images of the cornea, it is not tolerated by all horses. The transpalpebral approach is well tolerated by most horses and may be the only option in cases of severe eyelid swelling or large periocular masses. Sterile ultrasound gel or K-Y jelly is indicated in either approach. A standoff allows for better near-field visualization.

Emergency Musculoskeletal Examinations

Ultrasonographic assessment of horses with a recent history of trauma, severe lameness, or a penetrating wound or laceration helps the clinician differentiate areas of muscle injury from injury to bone, tendons, ligaments, joints, tendon sheaths, or the surrounding soft tissue structures. Fractures can be diagnosed in horses in which routine radiographs are *not* diagnostic or in patients with fractures in areas that are *not* amenable to routine radiography. In a horse with a laceration or a penetrating wound, the extent of damage to the synovial and tendinous or ligamentous structures in the area can be evaluated, and the presence and location of foreign material can be determined.

Normal Ultrasonographic Findings in the Equine Musculoskeletal System

Each tendon and ligament should be evaluated in two mutually perpendicular planes. The normal size, shape, and sonographic characteristics should be similar between the same anatomic tissues in opposing limbs. The unaffected limb can be used as a control, if necessary.
- Most tendons and ligaments have a homogeneous echoic appearance with a parallel fiber pattern.
  - The proximal suspensory ligament has a more heteroechoic appearance caused by varying amounts of muscle fibers, connective tissue, and fat at the origin and in the proximal suspensory body.
  - The biceps tendon also contains connective tissue and fat and therefore has a slightly more heterogeneous ultrasonographic appearance.

- The tendon sheath appears as a thin echoic structure with a thinner hypoechoic lining. Normally, anechoic intrathecal fluid is minimal.
  - A small collection of anechoic fluid is normally imaged in the carpal sheath between the deep digital flexor tendon and inferior check ligament and within the tarsal sheath between the deep digital flexor tendon and inferior check ligament remnant.
- A bursa is a potential space that normally contains little or no discernible fluid. The normal ultrasonographic appearance of muscle and bone is unique to each and should be compared with that in the contralateral limb, if abnormalities are suspected.
- Normal muscle has a unique speckled pattern when imaged in its short axis and a unique striated pattern when imaged in its long axis.
- The normal bony surface echo is a thin echoic line of uniform thickness, which is smooth, except in the region of normal bony protuberances.
  - Articular cartilage is anechoic and varies in thickness, depending on its location.
  - A soft tissue layer immediately adjacent to the bone is present in all nonarticular areas.
    Practice Tip: *Each joint has a characteristic ultrasonographic appearance with varying thickness of the joint capsule and synovium but this should be similar in both limbs.*
- The joint capsule is a slightly thicker, echoic, usually curvilinear structure with a thin layer of hypoechoic synovium within.
  Note: Joint fluid is anechoic.

Abnormal Ultrasonographic Findings in the Musculoskeletal System

Indications for an emergency musculoskeletal ultrasonographic examination include:
- Considerable swelling with associated heat and sensitivity
- Severe lameness
- Laceration
- Penetrating wound
- Suspected fracture that is *not* seen radiographically
- An area in which radiographic images cannot be obtained

Severe Tendinitis or Desmitis

Significant enlargement of a tendon or ligament with complete disruption of its fiber pattern is consistent with rupture of the tendon or ligament. The injured tendon may appear anechoic, hypoechoic, or echoic depending on how much time has elapsed since the injury and whether an organized clot is contained within the lesion (Fig. 14-17). Significant peritendinous or periligamentous soft tissue swelling is usually present.

Practice Tips:
- *Fetlock drop is found with severe suspensory desmitis and superficial digital flexor tendinitis.*
- *The toe flipping up with weight bearing is consistent with rupture of the deep digital flexor tendon.*
- *Subluxation of the proximal interphalangeal joint occurs with severe oblique distal sesamoidean desmitis and rupture of the superficial digital flexor tendon in the pastern.*
- *Flexion of the stifle with extension of the hock is consistent with a ruptured peroneus tertius tendon.*

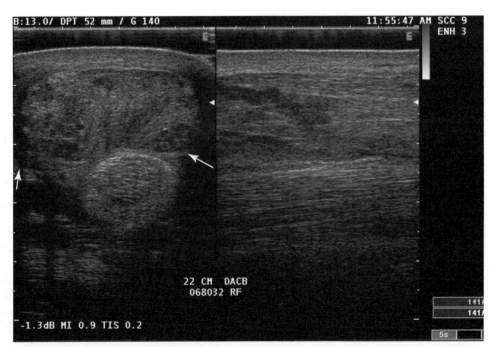

Figure 14-17 Sonogram of the metacarpal region obtained from a horse with a ruptured superficial digital flexor tendon and dropped fetlock. Note the significant enlargement, complete fiber disruption, and hematoma formation within the superficial digital flexor tendon *(arrows)*.

Severe Tenosynovitis or Bursitis

Significant distention of the tendon sheath or bursa with fluid and fibrin is most consistent with a septic tenosynovitis or bursitis. It can occur in horses with recent intrathecal or intrabursal hemorrhage or active, nonseptic inflammation within the tendon sheath or bursa.

- Fibrin appears as filmy, hypoechoic strands or clumps within the synovial fluid (Fig. 14-18).
- Fluid in an infected tendon sheath or bursa can appear anechoic, hypoechoic, or echoic depending on the protein content and cellularity of the synovial fluid.
- Acute bleeding into a synovial structure usually has a swirling echoic appearance. Anechoic fluid with hypoechoic loculations and echoic masses is consistent with recent hemorrhage.

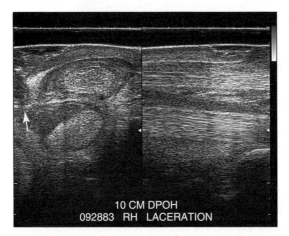

Figure 14-18   Sonogram of the tarsal sheath from a horse with a penetrating wound/laceration of the proximomedial metatarsal region. Note the hypoechoic fibrin within the tarsal sheath *(arrow),* surrounding the superficial and deep digital flexor tendons.

- Disruptions of the tendon sheath or bursa resulting in the formation of a synovial fistula are identified by the discontinuity in the tendon sheath or bursa and the adjacent, usually anechoic, periarticular fluid accumulation.

Myositis and Muscle Rupture

Enlargement of the affected muscle belly occurs with myositis. The ultrasound changes in muscle echogenicity and the presence or absence of muscle striations are indicative of the type of pathologic muscle condition present.

- Muscle edema results in the muscle appearing less echoic than normal but retaining its normal striations.
- Increased muscle echogenicity with loss of the normal striations is consistent with a postanesthetic myopathy.
- A more heterogeneous sonographic appearance with loss of the normal muscle fiber pattern is consistent with a necrotizing myositis.
  - The detection of pinpoint hyperechoic echoes consistent with free gas in the muscle or muscle fascia, and in the absence of a tract lined with gas associated with a penetrating wound, is consistent with a clostridial myositis.
- Cavitation of the most severely affected muscle often is seen associated with liquefaction necrosis.

Areas of muscle fiber disruption are the most common muscle injuries detected by ultrasonography. Muscle tears in horses are most frequently seen in the hind limb and shoulder muscles. The affected muscles can be diagnosed by carefully tracing the involved muscles from their origin to insertion.

- Anechoic fluid-filled areas with hypoechoic loculations are imaged within the muscle belly (Fig. 14-19).
- Large anechoic loculated fluid-filled areas are usually imaged between the adjacent muscle fascia and in the adjacent subcutaneous tissues.

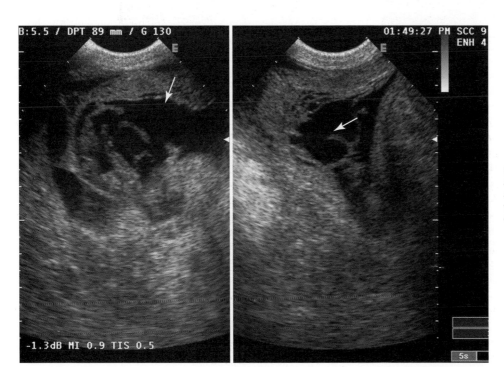

Figure 14-19   Sonogram of a horse with a semimembranosus muscle tear. An anechoic serum fluid pocket *(arrows)* with hypoechoic fibrin strands are present within the muscle belly.

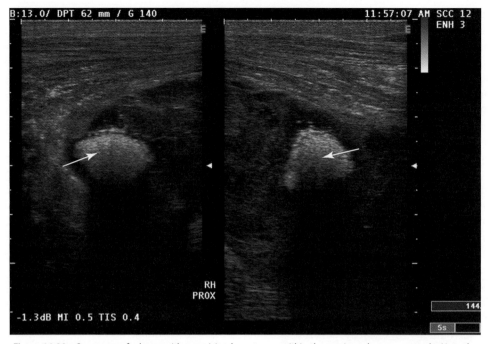

Figure 14-20   Sonogram of a horse with organizing hematomas within the semimembranosus muscle. Note the discrete echogenic masses *(arrows)* surrounded by hypoechoic fluid. The masses cast acoustic shadows from their far surfaces consistent with aging clots.

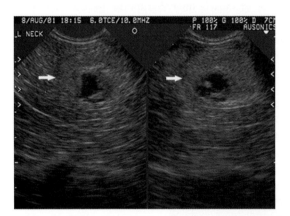

Figure 14-21   Sonogram of the left side of the neck obtained from a horse with disseminated skeletal muscle hemangiosarcoma. Note the echoic round to oval mass in the superficial musculature *(arrows)* with the anechoic area of cavitation (necrosis and hemorrhage).

- The free edge of a completely disrupted muscle may be imaged floating in the anechoic loculated fluid.
- Echoic masses consistent with clot are often imaged within the intramuscular, interfascial, or subcutaneous hematoma.
  - Acoustic shadows may be cast from the far side of these clots as they become more organized (Fig. 14-20).

Muscle neoplasms, particularly hemangiosarcomas, should always be considered in the differential diagnosis of horses with acute severe muscle disruption, especially when multiple sites are involved.

- Individuals with skeletal muscle hemangiosarcoma often have discrete echoic masses in the muscle; however, anechoic loculated heterogeneous masses may be imaged in areas of tumor necrosis (Fig. 14-21).

Fractures

The ultrasonographic diagnosis of a fracture depends on imaging the fracture line or fracture fragment in two mutually perpendicular ultrasound planes.

- A nondisplaced fracture is diagnosed when there is a break in the normal hyperechoic bony surface echo in an area where there is not a normal vascular channel.
- A hyperechoic bony structure casting an acoustic shadow that is distracted from the underlying parent portion of the bone in two mutually perpendicular ultrasound planes is consistent with a displaced fracture fragment. Anechoic loculated fluid is usually present in the adjacent soft tissues.
  Practice Tip: *Disruption of the surrounding musculature is commonly imaged with comminution or displacement of the fracture fragment.*
- Echoic masses are frequently detected within the anechoic loculated fluid that is consistent with a clot.
  Practice Tip: *Ultrasound is the best method for diagnosing fractured ribs (Fig. 14-22).*

Severe Synovitis

Considerable distention of the joint with fluid and fibrin is indicative of a severe synovitis.

- Flocculent, hypoechoic to echoic synovial fluid may be imaged in septic arthritis.
- A hemarthrosis is suggested by the presence of large quantities of uniformly echoic synovial fluid, particularly in individuals with periarticular hematomas.
- Thickening of the joint capsule and synovium is also frequently imaged in patients with severe synovitis, regardless of its cause.

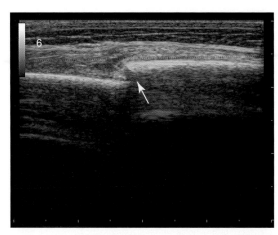

Figure 14-22   Sonogram of a right sixth rib fracture from a neonatal foal. The image is a long axis view, with dorsal to the right of the image. The distal rib fragment is displaced toward the thoracic cavity *(arrow)*. Note the fluid pocketing in the overlying soft tissues consistent with hematoma/seroma formation.

- Significant periarticular hypoechoic soft tissue swelling is usually present surrounding the joint capsule in individuals with severe synovitis.
  - Anechoic loculated fluid surrounding the joint is most consistent with a traumatic synovitis.
- Disruptions of the joint capsule resulting in the formation of a synovial fistula are identified by the discontinuity in the joint capsule and the adjacent periarticular fluid accumulation.
- Joint instability or radiographic findings of avulsion fractures associated with the origin or insertions of the collateral ligaments should prompt sonographic evaluations of the collateral ligaments associated with that joint, looking for disruption of the fibers of the collateral ligament.
  - Enlargement of the collateral ligament, with disruption of its fiber pattern and a decrease in its echogenicity, is consistent with collateral desmitis. The ligament may be difficult or impossible to identify in areas of complete rupture. Comparison with the contralateral limb is helpful in deciding on the degree of injury sustained.

Lacerations and Puncture Wounds

Ultrasonographic examination of puncture wounds and lacerations should be done after aseptic preparation of the area. Puncture wounds should be examined by ultrasonography before a contrast study is performed because the air injected with the contrast media impairs visualization of the underlying structures, limiting the usefulness of the ultrasonographic examination. The sonographic examination should begin superficially and gradually progress deeper until the full extent of the tract is determined.

- The tracts usually appear as hypoechoic linear or tubular paths containing various amounts of anechoic fluid and hyperechoic gas.
- Hyperechoic free gas echoes are usually seen at the skin surface of the puncture wound or laceration and decrease

in number as the tract or laceration extends deeper. These gas echoes are usually pinpoint and cast small gray acoustic shadows.

- A foreign body appears as an echoic to hyperechoic structure within the tract of the puncture wound or laceration.
  - ***Practice Tip:*** *Wood, the most common foreign body detected in horses, is hyperechoic and casts a strong black acoustic shadow from its near surface. Glass is also hyperechoic and casts a strong acoustic shadow.*
  - Needles, nails, wires, and BB gun pellets produce the typical metallic reverberation artifact.
  - Tubular hyperechoic structures that cast weak acoustic shadows may represent a piece of hoof.
- Always look for more than one foreign body.
- The type of foreign body and the position of the ultrasound beam relative to the foreign body determine the type of acoustic shadow cast by the foreign body.

Emergency Abdominal Examinations

- Diagnostic ultrasound is helpful in the assessment of the foal or adult with an acute condition of the abdomen.
- The findings on ultrasonographic examination help differentiate surgical from medical causes of colic.
- Diagnostic ultrasonography provides a window for noninvasive evaluation of the gastrointestinal viscera and abdominal organs and can guide other diagnostic procedures such as abdominocentesis.
- Transrectal ultrasonographic examination of abnormalities detected on rectal palpation can also be performed to clarify the rectal findings further.

Normal Ultrasonographic Findings in the Equine Gastrointestinal Tract

Large and small intestinal echoes are imaged from the ventral abdomen in the foal, whereas in the adult, only large intestinal echoes are usually imaged from this window. A few loops of jejunum may be imaged in the midventral abdomen in some adults. Only large intestinal echoes are usually imaged in the intercostal spaces (ICSs) and the flank.

- Large intestinal echoes are recognized by their large semicircular, sacculated appearance.
- The large intestinal wall is hypoechoic to echoic with a hyperechoic gas echo from the mucosal surface that normally measures 3 mm or less in thickness.
- Peristaltic waves are normally visible.
- The right dorsal colon is imaged ventral to the liver in the tenth to fourteenth ICSs.
- The cecum is imaged in the right paralumbar fossa.
- The gastric fundic echo is imaged as a large semicircular structure medial to the spleen at the level of the splenic vein in the left ninth to twelfth ICSs ventral to the diaphragm and ventral lung.
  - The wall of the stomach is hypoechoic to echoic with a hyperechoic gas echo from the mucosal surface and can measure up to 7.5 mm in thickness.
- The duodenum is imaged medial to the right lobe of the liver, adjacent to the right dorsal colon, beginning at

approximately the tenth ICS and can be followed caudally around the caudal pole of the right kidney.

- The duodenum appears as a small oval or circular structure (when sliced in its short axis) with a hypoechoic to echoic wall ≤3 mm thick.
- The duodenum usually appears partially collapsed with regular waves of fluid ingesta imaged during real-time scanning.
- The jejunum is rarely visualized in the adult except adjacent to the stomach and occasionally in the midventral to caudal left side of the abdomen, whereas in the foal the jejunum is readily seen along the floor of the ventral abdomen.
  - The small intestinal echoes are recognized by their small tubular and circular appearance.
  - The wall of the jejunum is hypoechoic to echoic with a hyperechoic echo from the mucosal surface and is usually ≤3 mm thick.
  - Some anechoic fluid ingesta and hyperechoic "gassy" ingesta are often imaged in the lumen of the jejunum.
  - Peristaltic waves are normally visible.
- The ileum is rarely imaged transcutaneously but may be imaged transrectally in the adult as a slightly thicker (4 to 5 mm), more muscular segment of small intestine in the dorsal caudal abdomen with visible peristaltic activity.
- Only a small amount of anechoic peritoneal fluid is usually imaged within the peritoneal cavity cranioventrally.

Abnormal Ultrasonographic Findings in the Equine Gastrointestinal Tract

Practice Tip: Significant increases in the thickness of the intestinal wall, coupled with considerable distention of the lumen and a lack of visible peristaltic activity, are ultrasonographic indications of significant intestinal compromise. Considerable fluid distention of the stomach should prompt nasogastric decompression.

Herniation

Surgical colic is caused by herniation of the abdominal viscera into the thoracic cavity, scrotum, umbilicus, or through the body wall.

Umbilical

- Gastrointestinal viscera, peritoneal fluid, or omentum is imaged in the external umbilicus.
- Measure the size of the hernia.
- Determine the viability of entrapped or incarcerated intestine.
  - Measure wall thickness, intestinal distention, and evaluate peristalsis.
- If the hernia is more involved, look for internal umbilical remnant infection, subcutaneous abscess, and/or enterocutaneous fistula.

Inguinal

- Gastrointestinal viscera or omentum is imaged in the enlarged scrotal sac.
- Determine the viability of the entrapped or incarcerated intestine.

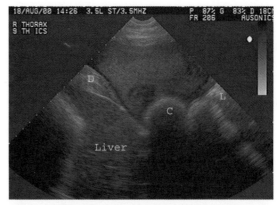

Figure 14-23 Sonogram of the right side of the thorax obtained in the ninth intercostal space from a horse with a diaphragmatic hernia. The right side of the image is dorsal, and the left side is ventral. Notice the echoic swirling fluid consistent with a hemothorax *(top)*, the white hyperechoic circular sacculated colon *(C)* in the thoracic cavity adjacent to the lung *(L)*, and the muscular part of the diaphragm *(D)* dorsal to the liver.

  - Measure wall thickness, intestinal distention, and evaluate peristalsis.
- Perform a rectal examination in the stallion, and evaluate the small intestine to determine the degree of distention proximal to the obstruction.

Diaphragmatic

- Gastrointestinal viscera, omentum, or abdominal organs imaged in the thoracic cavity (Fig. 14-23)
- The herniated viscera entrapped in the rent in the diaphragm displaces the lung dorsally.
- The approximate size of the hernia can be estimated by the number of ICSs affected and whether it is imaged on one or both sides of the thorax.
- Determine the viability of entrapped or incarcerated intestine.
  - Measure wall thickness, intestinal distention, and evaluate peristalsis.
- A diaphragmatic hernia could be missed by ultrasonography if located in the center of the diaphragm or if the herniated viscera are *not* in contact with the thoracic wall.

Abdominal Wall Hernias and Rupture of the Prepubic Tendon

- Determine the viability of the entrapped or incarcerated intestine.
  - Measure wall thickness and intestinal distention, and evaluate peristalsis.
- Identify the intestine involved and the presence and locations of adhesions.
- Evaluate the muscles and/or tendon of the abdominal wall.
  - Measure the size of the defect, and evaluate the edges of the hernial ring.

Nephrosplenic Ligament Entrapment/ Left Dorsal Displacement

Ultrasonographic findings consistent with a nephrosplenic ligament entrapment (NSE) include the following:

- The presence of large colon between the spleen and body wall in the left caudal abdomen

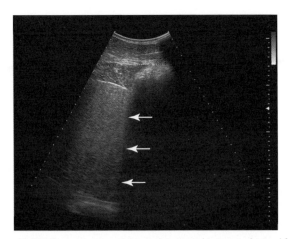

Figure 14-24   Transcutaneous abdominal sonographic image obtained from the left fifteenth intercostal space showing horizontal dorsal border of spleen *(arrows)* due to gas shadowing of large colon within nephrosplenic space. Dorsal is to the right of the image.

- The dorsal splenic border appearing horizontal and displaced ventrally to the middle of the abdomen (Fig. 14-24)
- An inability to see the tail of the spleen or left kidney transcutaneously. This should *not* be used as the sole sonographic criteria for the diagnosis of NSE because these structures may occasionally be obscured from view by gas in the large or small colon in horses without NSE.
- The stomach may be ventrally displaced and visible from the ventral abdomen.
- *Practice Tip: The sonogram can be used to determine whether treatment with phenylephrine, followed by lunging or rolling the horse, has corrected the nephrosplenic ligament entrapment successfully.*
  - In horses with either acute or chronic intermittent colic, the large colon may be seen between the spleen and body wall, but the left kidney is still visible. This may represent a variation of NSE or left dorsal displacement.

Right Dorsal Displacement of Large Colon
The diagnosis of right dorsal displacement is based on:
- Identification of a mesocolonic vein adjacent to the right body wall in the mid-right abdomen, in approximately the eleventh to thirteenth intercostal spaces (Fig. 14-25).
- If the mesocolonic vein *cannot* be visualized running horizontally against the abdominal wall this does *not* rule out a right displacement. A displacement can occur without rotation, in which case, the vessel is *not* against the peritoneum.
- Other sonographic findings include:
  - Inability to see the right liver lobe
  - Small intestine dorsal to the right liver lobe
  - Inability to see the duodenum
  - Concurrent colon impaction

Sand Colic
- Small, pinpoint granular hyperechoic echoes, casting multiple acoustic shadows, are imaged in the ventralmost portion of the affected intestine.

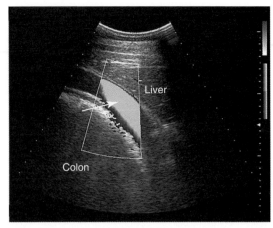

Figure 14-25   Transcutaneous abdominal sonographic image obtained from the right thirteenth intercostal space showing distended colonic mesenteric vessel adjacent to right body wall and medial margin of right liver lobe. Doppler interrogation demonstrates blood flow within the vessel *(arrow)*. Right dorsal displacement of the large colon was confirmed at surgery. Dorsal is to the right of the image.

- There is loss of normal sacculations in the affected portion of large intestine as it is flattened by the weight of the intraluminal sand.
- There are greatly decreased or absent peristaltic movements of the sand-containing ventral portion of the colon.

Enterolithiasis
- Rarely does this condition show up in images because the affected colon is *not* usually seen from a transcutaneous or rectal "window."
- A large, hyperechoic mass, casting a strong acoustic shadow, might be within the lumen of the intestine if the affected portion of intestine is adjacent to the ventral body wall and there is *not* gas between the mucosa and the stone.
- Wall thickness may be increased.
- Decreased to absent peristalsis occurs in the affected segment of intestine.
- Enteroliths may be hard to visualize on ultrasound examination because of the large amount of gas in the large intestine.

Intussusception
- Characteristic ultrasonographic findings associated with the invagination of one loop of intestine (intussusceptum) into another loop of intestine (intussuscipiens) are the following:
  - Target or "bull's eye" sign appears in the affected portion of intestine (Fig. 14-26).
  - The strangulated intestine usually has thickened, edematous, hypoechoic walls.
  - Little or no peristaltic activity is imaged in the affected portion of intestine.
  - Often fibrin is imaged between the intussusceptum and intussuscipiens.
  - Distended, fluid-filled intestine is imaged proximal to a strangulated portion of intestine.

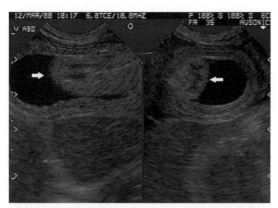

Figure 14-26   Sonograms of a jejunal-jejunal intussusception obtained from a foal. Notice the target or "bull's eye" appearance of the short axis section *(right image)* of the jejunum at one end of the intussusception. The *arrow* points to the intussusceptum.

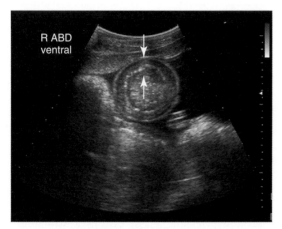

Figure 14-27   Transcutaneous abdominal sonographic image of thick-walled loop of small intestine from horse with strangulating lipoma. Note the increased echogenicity of the wall of the small intestine *(arrows)*.

- Jejunal intussusception is usually imaged from the ventral-most portion of the abdomen and is most common in foals.
- Ileal intussusception is usually imaged rectally or transcutaneously in the caudodorsal abdomen and is most common in yearlings and young horses.
- Large bowel intussusception usually involves the ileum and large bowel and is imaged most frequently from the right side of the abdomen because the cecum or right ventral colon is involved. This condition is most common in adult horses.

Strangulating Small Intestinal Disorders and Small Intestinal Volvulus

- Characteristic ultrasonographic findings are the following:
  - The strangulated small intestine usually has thickened, edematous, hypoechoic walls with little or no peristaltic activity (Fig. 14-27).
  - Small intestinal loops are turgid and fluid filled.
  - Luminal contents are anechoic or layered with echoic ventral particulate ingesta.
  - Distended, fluid-filled small intestine is imaged proximal to the strangulated small intestine.

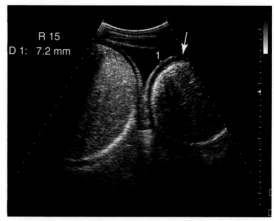

Figure 14-28   Transcutaneous abdominal sonographic image of a loop of dilated small intestine with muscular hypertrophy. Note prominent hypoechoic muscular layer of the small intestinal wall *(arrow)*.

- Distended, thick-walled small intestine most frequently is detected in the ventral portion of the abdomen because of its increased weight.
- ***Practice Tip:*** *There may be overlap in the sonographic appearance of strangulating and nonstrangulating lesions. The ultrasound findings should always be interpreted in light of the clinical picture.*
- Diagnosis of the specific cause of strangulation is often not possible.

Intestinal Masses

- Ultrasonographic findings with intraluminal, intramural, or mesenteric masses obstructing the passage of ingesta are as follows:
  - Focal, mural anechoic to echoic masses within the intestinal wall often make up the lumen of the affected portion of intestine.
  - Echoic areas of narrowed irregular bowel wall have been imaged in horses with mural stricture.
  - Thickening of the muscular layer of the wall of the small intestine is indicative of idiopathic muscular hypertrophy, detectable transrectally and transcutaneously (Fig. 14-28).
  - Intraluminal hemorrhage appears as echogenic clots or echoic swirling fluid.
- Mural masses in the adult may be the following:
  - Abscesses
  - Intestinal carcinoids
  - Leiomyomas
  - Granulomas
  - Hematomas
  - Fibrosis
- Mural masses in foals or young horses may be abscesses.
- Diffuse thickening of the bowel is seen with hypoxic injury to the bowel, enterocolitis, or infection with *Lawsonia intracellularis*.

Impaction

Characteristic ultrasonographic findings of impaction include the following:

- A round or oval echoic distended viscus, lacking sacculations, often measuring 20 to 30 cm or more in the adult.
- Meconium appears as hypoechoic, echoic, or hyperechoic masses in the lumen of the large colon, small colon, or rectum.
- The bladder can be used as an "acoustic window" to evaluate the rectum and small colon immediately dorsal to it.
  Practice Tip: Ascarids appear as hyperechoic to echoic tubular structures that are often knotted into a mass in the lumen of the intestine. (See Chapter 18, p. 199.)
- Isolated ascarid worms are often imaged in fluid-distended colon.
- Intestinal wall thickness may be normal or increased.
  Note: Foals that are anorectic for one or more days normally have a corrugated-appearing cecal wall.
- A large acoustic shadow is cast from the impacted ingesta adjacent to the colonic mucosa.
- Distention of the colon proximal to the impaction is usually present, making ultrasonographic evaluation of the impaction easier.
- Little or no peristaltic activity of the affected intestine occurs.
- Impactions can be imaged only transcutaneously when the impacted large colon or cecum is adjacent to the body wall or fluid is interposed between the affected portion of the intestine and the body wall.
- Impactions usually can be imaged from the flank or side of the abdomen in horses with cecal or right dorsal colon impactions.
- Small colon impactions have been imaged from the flank in miniature horses.
- In adults, small or large colon impactions can be imaged transrectally if palpable.

Large Colon Torsion

Characteristic ultrasound findings include the following:
- Colon wall thickness is ≥9 mm when measured along the ventral abdomen in adult horses with historical and physical examination findings consistent with a surgical lesion of the large colon (Fig. 14-29).

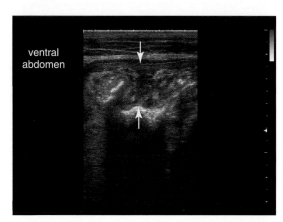

Figure 14-29 Sonographic image obtained from transcutaneous ventral abdominal window. The large colon wall is markedly thickened and heteroechoic *(arrows)*. In a horse with appropriate clinical signs, this finding is diagnostic for a large colon volvulus.

- *Practice Tip: Colon wall thickness is highly specific and moderately sensitive when measured in this patient population. A similar sonographic appearance of the large colon may occur with colitis.*

Medical Colic
Proximal Duodenitis-Jejunitis
Characteristic ultrasonographic findings of proximal duodenitis-jejunitis include the following:
- Fluid distention of the stomach and duodenum
- Usually decreased or absent duodenal motility consistent with an ileus; this can be variable!
- Intestinal wall that may be thickened with variable echogenicity
- Presence or absence of duodenal stricture

Enterocolitis
Characteristic ultrasonographic findings of enterocolitis include the following:
- Fluid distention of the intestinal tract is apparent, especially the cecum and colon. (See Fig. 18-76, p. 233.)
- The intestinal wall may be thickened more than normal, particularly with severe inflammatory bowel disease.
- "Shreds" of intestinal mucosa may be imaged in the intestinal lumen.
- Significant fluid distention of the stomach should prompt nasogastric decompression.
- Neonatal foals with necrotizing enteritis may have sonographically detectable gas in the intestinal wall called "pneumatosis intestinalis." This finding indicates a guarded to poor prognosis.

Cholangiohepatitis and Elevated Biliary Enzymes
Characteristic ultrasonographic findings include the following:
- Hepatomegaly
- Increased echogenicity of the hepatic parenchyma
- Biliary distention and echoic bile within biliary tree
- Presence of thickening of the bile ducts
- Presence of hepatoliths

Gastric Distention and Delayed Gastric Emptying
Ultrasonographic findings include the following:
- Circular to oval gastric echo distended with anechoic to hypoechoic fluid or echoic to hyperechoic ingesta is seen on the left side of the abdomen.
  - *Practice Tip: Echoic fluid or hypoechoic fluid containing echoic lumps in foals is milk.*
  - Layering of the dorsal gas, ventral fluid, and if present, even more ventral ingesta is often imaged.
- Imaging the gastric echo over five or more ICSs on the left side of the abdomen is consistent with significant gastric distention.
- Imaging the gastric echo on the right side of the abdomen is rare and is consistent with severe gastric distention.
- A greatly enlarged gastric echo filled with hyperechoic material casting an acoustic shadow extending over five or more ICSs on the left side of the abdomen is detected with gastric impaction.

- A mass with a complex pattern of echogenicity in the wall of the stomach, often with invasion into the adjacent spleen or liver parenchyma, is consistent with a gastric squamous cell carcinoma. This pattern is most common in older horses.
- Gastric emptying problems are identified when large amounts of ingesta persist unchanged in the stomach in a fasted, anorectic, or "refluxing" individual on repeat examinations. Always consider in Friesian horses with colic.

Right Dorsal Colitis

Ultrasonographic findings include the following:
- The right dorsal colon can be imaged most consistently in the right eleventh, twelfth, and thirteenth ICSs axial to the liver and below the ventral margin of the lung. The wall thickness of the right dorsal colon of normal horses measures up to 0.36 cm in these ICSs.
- Horses with right dorsal colitis have wall thicknesses that measure from 0.60 cm to greater than 1.0 cm. The wall may appear hypoechoic secondary to edema or have echogenic infiltrate, and mucosal irregularities may be present. Comparison of the wall thickness of the right dorsal colon to the right ventral colon may aid in identifying cases with less significant thickening (Fig. 14-30).
- Decreased thickness of the colon wall may be associated with successful treatment or rarely thinning before rupture.

Abdominal Abscess

Characteristic ultrasonographic findings include the following:
- Abdominal abscesses are anechoic, hypoechoic, or filled with echoic material and are often multiloculated, especially in the foal with *Rhodococcus equi* infections.
- Hyperechoic echoes representing free gas may be detected, suggesting concurrent anaerobic infection.
- Large or small intestine may be adhered to the wall of the abscess and thus its movement restricted.

- Abdominal abscesses in foals are detected in the ventral abdomen associated with *Rhodococcus equi* abscesses involving the mesenteric lymph nodes.
- In the adult, abdominal abscesses may be detected in the ventral abdomen but are also frequently found dorsally associated with the root of the mesentery, cecum, and large colon.
- Abdominal abscesses are infrequently reported in the adult associated with the liver.

Peritonitis

Characteristic ultrasonographic appearance is as follows:
- Anechoic, hypoechoic, or echoic fluid
- Presence of flocculent, composite fluid
- Presence of fibrin and/or adhesions between the serosal surfaces of the intestine and the abdominal wall
- Free gas echoes and particulate echogenic debris, which are consistent with a ruptured viscus (Fig. 14-31).

The abdomen, gastrointestinal, and abdominal viscera should be examined thoroughly for the source of the peritonitis, such as an abdominal abscess or devitalized area of bowel.

Hemoperitoneum

- Homogeneous, hypoechoic to echoic swirling cellular fluid is consistent with hemoperitoneum (Fig. 14-32).
- The spleen, liver, and kidneys should be carefully examined to be sure that a rupture of one of these organs is not the cause of the hemoperitoneum.
  - Anechoic, loculated fluid within the spleen, liver, or kidney or in the subcapsular space is indicative of organ trauma.
- A very small spleen supports splenic contraction associated with significant blood loss.
- Rupture of the middle uterine artery often results in a large volume of blood in the broad ligament with a smaller quantity of blood free in the peritoneal cavity.

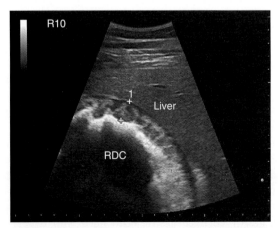

Figure 14-30 Transcutaneous abdominal sonogram obtained from the right tenth intercostal space. Note the markedly thickened and heterechoic wall of the right dorsal colon. The remainder of the large colon was of normal thickness and echogenicity (between cursors). Dorsal is to the right of the image.

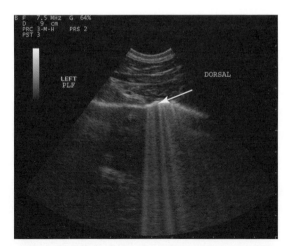

Figure 14-31 Sonogram of a weanling with a ruptured stomach. Note the hyperechoic free gas echoes *(arrow)* along the dorsal aspect of the abdomen diagnostic for rupture of a gastrointestinal viscus. The definitive site of the rupture could not be determined by sonography.

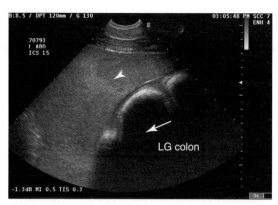

Figure 14-32   Sonogram of a horse with hemoperitoneum. Note the echoic cellular fluid *(arrowhead)* adjacent to the hyperechoic gas echo of the large colon *(arrow)*. In real time the fluid takes on a characteristic swirling appearance diagnostic of active hemorrhage.

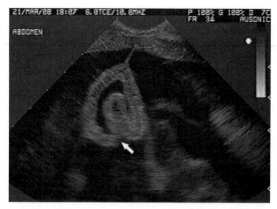

Figure 14-33   Transverse sonogram of the urinary bladder obtained from a foal with uroperitoneum and a ruptured bladder. Notice the collapsed and folded appearance of the bladder. Although it appears as if the rupture may be located on the dorsal surface of the bladder *(arrow)*, the defect is not readily visible. Surrounding the bladder is a large volume of anechoic fluid within the peritoneal cavity; the gastrointestinal viscera are floating in this fluid.

Emergency Urinary System Examinations

Normal Ultrasonographic Findings in the Equine Urinary Bladder

The equine urinary bladder is a round to oval fluid-filled structure with a hypoechoic to echoic bladder wall. *Practice Tip: The urine in the foal urinary bladder should be anechoic, whereas the urine contained in the adult urinary bladder has a composite echoic appearance caused by the mucus and crystalluria.*

Abnormal Ultrasonographic Findings in the Equine Urinary Bladder

Uroperitoneum

Definition: Uroperitoneum is a large accumulation of the urine within the peritoneal cavity associated with a defect in the urinary tract that allows urine to flow into the peritoneal cavity.

• Uroperitoneum occurs most frequently in the equine neonate in the immediate postpartum period.
• In the adult, uroperitoneum is most common in the postpartum mare.
• The location of the urinary tract defect can be determined by the sonographic appearance of the urinary bladder, ureters, urachus, and retroperitoneal space.
• A large quantity of fluid in the peritoneal cavity is consistent with uroperitoneum.
• The fluid is usually anechoic but becomes more echoic as the uroperitoneum becomes more long-standing and a chemical peritonitis develops.
• The gastrointestinal viscera normally float in the peritoneal fluid and urine contained within the peritoneal cavity.
• A folded, collapsed urinary bladder is consistent with a rupture of the urinary bladder (Fig. 14-33).
• Fluid around the urachus and in the retroperitoneal space along the ventral abdomen with an intact urinary bladder is indicative of a defect in the urachus.
• Retroperitoneal fluid around the kidney(s) with an intact urinary bladder is consistent with a ureteral defect(s).

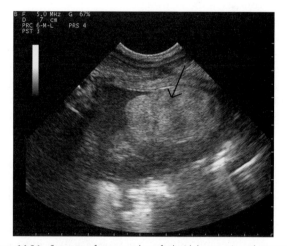

Figure 14-34   Sonogram from a newborn foal with hematuria and stranguria resulting from a cystic hematoma. A hypoechoic homogeneous clot is present within the urinary bladder *(arrow)*. The urine is hypoechoic with a swirling cellular pattern consistent with ongoing hemorrhage.

Cystic Hematomas in Foals

• Hemorrhage into the urinary bladder may be seen in the early postpartum period associated with trauma to the umbilicus.
• Active hemorrhage into the bladder appears as echogenic swirling fluid with or without the presence of clots. As a hematoma forms and organizes, a heteroechoic mass becomes visible surrounded by anechoic urine (Fig. 14-34).
• The urachus and umbilical arteries also may contain large echogenic masses consistent with blood clots. In the normal foal, the urachus is only a potential space and should *not* contain fluid or clots. The umbilical arteries normally have sludging blood and may be seen to pulsate for the first 24 hours after birth.

Ultrasonography in High-Risk Pregnancies

Fetal Well-Being in High-Risk Pregnancies

Ultrasonographic evaluation of the fetus and its intrauterine environment from a transcutaneous and transrectal approach provide the clinician with important information when evaluating the high-risk pregnant mare (see Chapter 30, p. 520). Severe illness of the mare, premature udder development, premature lactation, or an abnormal vaginal discharge should prompt a complete transcutaneous and transrectal ultrasonographic evaluation of the fetus to determine its well-being. Prompt intervention may improve the outcome for foals born to high-risk mares. The normal late-gestation mare has a single fetus in anterior presentation, dorsopubic position. The nonfetal horn is usually evident from the ventral abdominal window in late gestation.

Biophysical Profile

The equine biophysical profile (see Chapter 30, p. 526) consists of seven parameters that, if normal, support the delivery of a normal fetus (Table 14-1). Each of these parameters is assigned a score of 2 if it is normal and 0 if it is abnormal for a "perfect" biophysical profile of 14. The equine biophysical profile consists of the following:

- Breathing movements: Regular breathing movements should be present in the late gestation fetus.
- Cardiac rate and rhythm: The mean resting fetal heart rate in the late gestation equine fetus is 75 beats/min with a heart rate range detected by ultrasonography of ±15 beats/min and a regular rhythm. If the gestation is prolonged, the fetal heart rate continues to slow to as low as 57 beats/min if the gestation length is <344 days. The heart rate can slow to 50 beats/min if the gestation length is 320 to 360 days and to as low as 41 beats/min if the gestation length is >360 days.
- Fetal aortic diameter: The fetus in late gestation should have an aortic diameter that is approximately 23 mm.
- Fetal movement and tone: The normal fetus is active during the examination with periods of activity imaged for more than 50% of the scanning time. The normal fetus has muscular tone and should *not* appear flaccid.
- Fetal fluids: Ample quantities of amniotic and allantoic fluid should surround the normal late-term fetus. Between 0.8 and 14.9 cm of amniotic fluid and 4.7 to 22.1 cm of allantoic fluid should surround the normal fetus.
- Uteroplacental thickness: The normal mean thickness of the uterus and the chorioallantois combined should be 11.5 mm (see Chapter 27, p. 498).
- Uteroplacental separation: The uterus and chorioallantois should be associated closely with one another with no imaged areas of separation or only small focal areas imaged.

Abnormal Fetal and Maternal Findings in the High-Risk Pregnant Mare

- *Practice Tip: The inability to image the nonfetal horn in late gestation is a good ultrasonographic indication of a twin pregnancy.*
- The detection of two contiguous chorioallantoic membranes, usually perpendicular to the uterus, also signals the presence of a twin pregnancy.

Table 14-1	Equine Biophysical Profile*		
Fetal or Maternal Measurement		**Patient**	**Abnormal**
Fetal Heart Rate (HR) and Rhythm			
Rhythm		—	Irregular or absent
Low HR <320 days' gestation (beats/min)		—	<57
Low HR 320-360 days' gestation (beats/min)		—	<50
Low HR >360 days' gestation		—	<41
High (postactivity) HR (beats/min)		—	>126
HR range (beats/min)		—	> 50 or <5
Fetal Breathing			
Rhythm		—	Irregular or absent
Fetal Aortic Diameter (mm)			
$Y = 0.00912 \times X + 12.46$		$Y \pm 4 \times$ S.E. (5.038)	> or < $Y \pm X \times$ S.E. (5.038)
Fetal Activity and Tone			
Fetal activity		—	Absent
Fetal tone		—	Absent
Fetal Fluid Depths			
Maximal allantoic fluid depth (cm)		—	<4.7 or >22.1
Maximal amniotic fluid depth (cm)		—	<0.8 or >18.5
Uteroplacental Thickness			
Uterus and chorioallantois (mm)		—	<3.9 or >21
Uteroplacental contact			
Areas of discontinuity		—	Large
Biophysical profile score		—	≤10 = negative outcome; 12 = high risk for negative outcome

SE, Standard error; *X*, pregnant mare's weight in pounds; *Y*, Predicted aortic diameter.
*Calculation of biophysical profile: Assign 2 points to each category if all evaluations are normal; assign 0 points to each category if one of the evaluations is abnormal.

- The imaging of two separate thoraxes confirms the presence of twin fetuses; two different fetal heart rates are usually detected if both fetuses are alive.
- The fetal aortic diameters and thoracic diameters generally differ in size, with one of the twins smaller than the other.
- The twin fetuses may have different presentations, with the posterior presentation abnormal.
- *Practice Tip: If the head of the fetus is imaged in late gestation from the ventral abdominal window, the mare is likely to need assistance at the time of delivery.*

- Torsion of the umbilical cord with significant distention of the urinary bladder has been identified in fetuses in utero and has resulted in the abortion or death of the fetus.
- Other fetal abnormalities also may be identified that may affect fetal health.
- Thickening of the amnion is also abnormal and may be detected in mares with a severe placentitis.
- Increased echogenicity of the fetal fluids may be seen in mares with placentitis or meconium-stained fetus.
- Increased echogenicity of the fetal fluids has not been correlated with an adverse outcome in the late gestation fetus, only when these findings are detected earlier in gestation.

Abnormal Biophysical Profile

Practice Tip: *If two or more of the seven parameters are abnormal—a score of 10 or less—the foal delivered is likely to be compromised.*

- Breathing movements: Irregular or absent fetal breathing movements are abnormal in the late gestation fetus. This abnormality may be associated with acute intrauterine hypoxia.
- Cardiac rate and rhythm:
  - A heart rate of <57 beats/min is abnormal for calculation of the biophysical profile if the gestation length is <320 days.
  - A heart rate of <50 beats/min is abnormal if the gestation length is 320 to 360 days.
  - A heart rate of <41 beats/min is abnormal if the gestation length is >360 days.
  - An irregular heart rhythm, a heart rate in excess of 126 beats/min, or a heart rate range in excess of 50 beats/min or <5 beats/min is also abnormal in the late gestation fetus.
  - These abnormalities may be associated with acute intrauterine hypoxia.
- Fetal aortic diameter: An aortic diameter of <18 mm or >27 mm is abnormal in the late gestation fetus. A smaller-than-normal aortic diameter is indicative of intrauterine growth retardation or the presence of twins.
- Fetal movement and tone: Absent fetal activity or a flaccid appearance to the fetus is abnormal. These abnormalities may be associated with acute intrauterine hypoxia.
- Fetal fluids: Hydrops should be considered when >14.9 cm of amniotic fluid (hydrops amnii) or >22.1 cm of allantoic fluid (hydrops allantois) surrounds the fetus. A fetus that is *not* surrounded by adequate amounts of fetal fluids (<0.8 cm amniotic or <4.7 cm allantoic) is distressed.
  - Intrauterine hypoxia and premature rupture of the fetal membranes may be responsible for the decreased quantities of fetal fluid.
- Umbilical cord: Torsion of the umbilical cord can result in considerable distention of the fetal urinary bladder and abortion (Fig. 14-35).
- Uteroplacental thickness: A combined uteroplacental thickness of <3.9 mm or >21 mm is abnormal for the calculation of the biophysical profile. Treatment of the mare for suspected placentitis often is initiated when

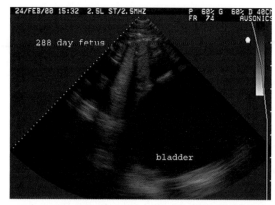

Figure 14-35 Sonogram of a 288-day fetus with significant distention of the urinary bladder. The foal was aborted shortly after the sonogram was performed. Marked twisting of the umbilical cord was present at birth.

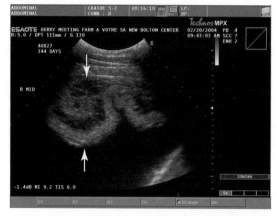

Figure 14-36 Sonogram from a horse with placentitis. Note the considerable thickening and loculations present within the uteroplacental unit (between *arrows*).

the combined uteroplacental thickness is 15 mm or greater (Fig. 14-36).
- Uteroplacental separation: Premature placental separation is supported when there is a large and/or progressive area of separation between the uterus and chorioallantois.

Emergency Thoracic Examinations

Thoracic ultrasonography is helpful in assessing the foal or adult with severe lower respiratory tract problems. Almost the entire thorax can be evaluated by ultrasonography, including the cranial mediastinal region. The affected side or sides of the thorax, and "pinpointing" the location of lesions, can be determined in most individuals because the involved lung segment is usually pleural based. The character of pleural fluid can be determined by ultrasonography.

The type and severity of underlying pulmonary parenchymal disease can be diagnosed and differentiated:
- Consolidation
- Pleuropneumonia
- Abscesses
- Pneumothorax
- Granulomas
- Tumors in the lung or pleural cavity

- Penetrating thoracic wounds
- Diaphragmatic hernias

The thoracic ultrasound examination findings can be used to formulate a more accurate prognosis for survival and to select appropriate treatment and monitoring response to therapy. Survival of horses with pleuropneumonia is more likely if pleural fluid, fibrin, loculations, free gas echoes, or parenchymal necrosis are *not* detected on the initial ultrasonographic examination.

Normal Ultrasonographic Appearance of the Lung and Pleural Cavity

- The lung is seen on both sides of the thorax from the sixteenth to seventeenth ICSs cranially to the fourth ICS.
- The cranial mediastinum is pictured only from the right third ICS in normal horses.
- The lung covers the cranial and caudal mediastinum in most individuals, although a hypoechoic soft tissue mass (thymus) may be imaged in youngsters ventral and medial to the right apical lung lobe and cranial to the heart.
- Fatty tissue also may be seen in this area and around the heart, most commonly detected in ponies and fat horses. Fat is usually slightly more heterogeneous and echogenic than thymus and continues caudally around the heart into the caudal mediastinum.
- The normal visceral pleural edge of the lung is a straight hyperechoic line with characteristic equidistant reverberation—air artifacts—indicating normal aeration of the pulmonary periphery.
- In real time, the visceral pleural edge of the lung glides ventrally across the diaphragm with inhalation and dorsally with exhalation, "the gliding sign."
- *No* pleural fluid or a small accumulation (up to 3.5 cm) of anechoic pleural fluid in the most ventral portions of the thorax may be detected.
- The curvilinear diaphragm is thick and muscular ventrally and thin and tendinous caudodorsally.

Abnormal Ultrasonographic Appearance of the Lung and Pleural Cavity: Pleural Disease

Pleural Effusion

Characteristic ultrasonographic findings include the following:

- Anechoic, hypoechoic, or echoic space is visible between the lung (visceral pleura), thoracic wall (parietal pleura), diaphragm, heart, and on either side of the mediastinal septum.
- Composite fluids are complex and more echogenic than normal, containing fibrin, cellular debris, a higher cell count and total protein concentration, and/or gas.
- Sonographic patterns of pleural fluid include anechoic, complex nonseptated, and complex septated fluid.
  - Anechoic fluid represents a transudate or modified transudate.
  - Increased echogenicity of the fluid indicates an increased cell count or total protein concentration.

- Blood within the pleural cavity—hemothorax—has a hypoechoic to echogenic swirling pattern and may be septated.
  Practice Tip: *Hemangiosarcoma should always be considered in the differential diagnosis of hemothorax.*
- Clotting in pleural fluid appears as soft, echoic masses.
- The cells and cellular debris in pyothorax are more echogenic, heavier, and in the most ventral location, whereas the less cellular fluid or gas cap is detected dorsally.
- Fibrin appears hypoechoic with a filmy to filamentous or frondlike appearance.
- Fibrous adhesions are rigid and echoic, often distorting the structures to which they are attached during one phase of respiration and restricting pulmonary mechanics.
- Free gas within the fluid (polymicrobullous fluid) is imaged as small, very bright, pinpoint, hyperechoic echoes within pleural fluid.
  - More free gas echoes are imaged dorsally in the pleural fluid.
  - The microbubble echoes move in various directions depending on respiratory motion, cardiac motion, and the patient's movements.
  - The free gas echoes adhere to the fibrinous pleural surfaces and initially may be detected only adjacent to fibrin.
  - Free gas echoes may be compartmentalized in only one portion of the thorax.
  - Free gas echoes are usually caused by an anaerobic infection within the pleural cavity (Fig. 14-37).
- The largest accumulation is ventral.
- Compression of normal lung (compression atelectasis), retraction of the lung toward the pulmonary hilus, and a ventral lung tip that floats in the surrounding fluid are apparent if there is no ventral consolidation of the lung.
- The pericardial-diaphragmatic ligament, a normal pleural reflection of the parietal pleura over the diaphragm and heart, is pictured as a thick membrane floating in pleural fluid.

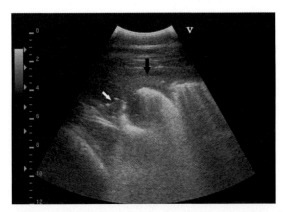

Figure 14-37 Sonogram of the right side of the thorax obtained from a horse with anaerobic pleuropneumonia. Note the hypoechoic consolidated lung *(black arrow)* and the sonographic air bronchogram visible as a tubular hyperechoic structure within the consolidated lung. The hyperechoic free air in the pleural space *(white arrow)* is associated with the fibrin strands present on the axial surface of the lung. These sonographic findings are consistent with an anaerobic fibrinous pleuropneumonia.

- The thoracocentesis should be performed several centimeters above the normal ventral margin of the thorax caudal to the heart where nonloculated pleural fluid or the largest pocket of loculated fluid is imaged (usually the seventh ICS).
- Care should be used so that the thoracocentesis does *not* occur immediately adjacent to the heart or too ventrally in the thorax in a patient with a large pleural effusion, below the ventral attachment of the diaphragm to the chest wall.
- Loculations between the parietal and visceral pleural surfaces of the lung, diaphragm, pericardium, and inner thoracic wall limit pleural fluid drainage.
- The fluid level and the extent of pulmonary parenchymal consolidation or abscessation present generally correspond to the volume of pleural fluid recovered by thoracocentesis.
  - Less than 1 L of fluid may be recovered with pleural fluid only around the cranioventral lung tip.
  - A pleural fluid line level with the point of the shoulder corresponds to the recovery of 1 to 5 L of pleural fluid per side.
  - A pleural fluid line to midthorax corresponds to 5 to 10 L of pleural fluid per side.
  - A pleural fluid line to the top of the thorax corresponds to 20 to 30 L of pleural fluid per side.
- The detection of fibrinous pleuropneumonia, with or without loculations, warrants a guarded prognosis initially and the initiation of broad-spectrum antimicrobial therapy, after obtaining a transtracheal fluid aspirate and pleural fluid aspirate for culture and susceptibility testing.
- If free gas echoes are detected in pleural fluid, a guarded to grave prognosis should be given, and broad-spectrum antimicrobial therapy, including appropriate coverage for anaerobic microorganisms (e.g., metronidazole) should be initiated immediately before results of culture and susceptibility testing are available.
- The cost-effectiveness of treatment must be considered because horses with anaerobic pleuropneumonia are likely to require a longer period of antimicrobial treatment and are unlikely to return to their prior performance level, if they survive.

Pneumothorax

Characteristic ultrasonographic findings with free air dorsally in the thoracic cavity include the following:
- A soft tissue density echo is detected between the dorsal free gas echo and the ventral aerated lung echo in the area of pulmonary atelectasis.
- A gas-fluid interface occurs with hydropneumothorax (pleural effusion and pneumothorax).
- The gas-fluid interface moves simultaneously in a dorsal to ventral direction with respiration, the "curtain sign," reproducing the movements of the diaphragm.
  - This finding is best seen with pleural effusion, parenchymal consolidation, or atelectasis.

- ***Practice Tip:*** *A bronchial-pleural fistula is the most common cause for hydropneumothorax.*
- A pneumothorax without pleural effusion is more difficult to detect by ultrasonography because gas free in the pleural cavity and air within the lung have the characteristic hyperechoic reflection and reverberation artifacts with periodicity. Sliding of gas echo is absent with pneumothorax.
  - Small hypoechoic irregularities with comet tail artifacts are absent dorsally in the area of the pneumothorax.
- To detect pneumothorax in patients without pleural effusion, the scan should begin at the most dorsal aspect of the thorax and continue ventrally, looking for a break in the characteristic reverberation air artifact.

Noneffusive Pleuritis
- Fibrin without fluid between the pleural surfaces is more difficult to detect because there is *no* fluid separating parietal and visceral pleural surfaces.
- Examine the parietal and visceral pleural interface carefully during inspiration and expiration, evaluating lung movement relative to the parietal pleura.
- Characteristic ultrasonographic findings include the following:
  - Rough or erratic movement of the visceral pleural lung surface occurs across the parietal pleura.
  - Absence of any movement between these surfaces during respiration is consistent with dry pleuritis or adhesions.
  - Ensure that the patient is taking deep breaths because shallow respiration may mimic a dry pleuritis.

Abnormal Ultrasonographic Appearance of the Lung and Pleural Cavity: Pulmonary Disease
Compression Atelectasis
Compression atelectasis occurs whenever the lung parenchyma is collapsed by fluid, air, or viscera (e.g., individuals with diaphragmatic hernia) occupy space in the thorax that normally contains lung.

Characteristic ultrasonographic findings include the following:
- The lung is collapsed and without air, leaving this portion of lung hypoechoic—echogenicity of soft tissue.
- The atelectic lung is retracted toward the hilus.
- Linear air echoes may be imaged in larger airways and squeeze together as they converge toward the root of the lung.
- The atelectic lung floats on top of and within the pleural fluid.

Consolidation
Characteristic ultrasonographic findings are as follows:
- An irregular visceral pleura with radiating comet tail artifacts is a nonspecific finding seen in individuals with acute or mild pneumonia.
- Irregular anechoic to hypoechoic areas are surrounded by normally aerated lung.

- Sonographic air bronchograms may or may not be present, pictured as distinctive hyperechoic linear air echoes in anechoic or hypoechoic lung.
- Sonographic fluid bronchograms may or may not be present, pictured as nonpulsatile, anechoic tubular structures in anechoic or hypoechoic lung.
- Fluid bronchiectasis may or may not be present, represented as an enlarging diameter of the fluid bronchogram toward the periphery.
- Air and fluid bronchograms become larger as they converge toward the root of the lung.
- The consolidation is usually cranioventral with the right lung being more commonly and more severely affected.
  Practice Tip: *Often, if the ultrasound examination is performed very early in the course of the disease and the pneumonia is severe, the pneumonia appears less extensive and later tends to coalesce into larger areas of consolidation.*
- The small hypoechoic areas of early consolidation may be seen only during exhalation.
- A large area of consolidated lung is usually wedge-shaped, poorly defined, and hypoechoic.
- Hepatization of lung parenchyma occurs with severe consolidation, resulting in an ultrasonographic appearance similar to that of the liver.
- Multiple small hyperechoic gas echoes in a severely consolidated or hepatized lung are suggestive of an anaerobic pneumonia.
- A rounded or bulging anechoic area suggests severe consolidation, often progressing to pulmonary necrosis or abscess formation.
- A gelatinous-appearing lung occurs with parenchymal necrosis. These necrotic areas either cavitate and form an abscess or rupture into the pleural space, creating a bronchial-pleural fistula.
- The detection of parenchymal necrosis also warrants a grave to guarded prognosis initially. Individuals with parenchymal necrosis also should be treated aggressively with broad-spectrum antimicrobials targeted for anaerobes.
- The cost-effectiveness of treatment should be considered because horses with parenchymal necrosis are likely to require a long period of antimicrobial treatment and are unlikely to return to their prior performance level, if they survive.
- The number of treatment days is also likely to be longer for horses with pleuropneumonia when fibrin, loculations, pulmonary parenchymal necrosis, or abscesses are detected by ultrasonography.

Pulmonary Edema

- Interstitial and alveolar pulmonary edema can be seen by sonography in cases of left ventricular failure and acute respiratory distress syndrome.
- Characteristic ultrasound findings include the following:
  - Marked, diffuse, coalescing "comet tail" artifacts emanating from nonaerated areas of the visceral pleural surface (Fig. 14-38).

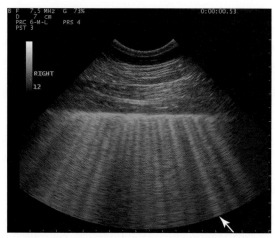

Figure 14-38   Sonogram from a horse with heart failure and severe pulmonary edema resulting from acute rupture of a mitral valve chordae tendineae. Numerous coalescing comet tail artifacts *(arrow)* are present emanating from the visceral pleural surface.

- This is in contrast to rare or occasional comet tail artifacts that can be seen resulting from a variety of conditions that interrupt the normal aeration at the visceral pleural surface.
- A small anechoic pleural effusion also may be present in cases of heart failure.

Bronchial-Pleural Fistula or Abscess

Definition: A bronchial-pleural fistula is a communication between a bronchus and the pleural cavity that results in a pneumothorax. The fistula is usually the result of a necrotizing pneumonia that becomes a walled-off bronchial-pleural abscess.

Characteristic ultrasonographic findings include the following:

- A cavitation involving the visceral edge of the lung with hyperechoic air echoes and sonolucent fluid echoes imaged in real time and moving from the gelatinous area of pulmonary necrosis into the pleural space
- Presence or absence of pleural effusion

Pulmonary Abscess

A pulmonary abscess is a cavitary area in the lung parenchyma lacking bronchi or vessels and filled with purulent fluid.

Characteristic ultrasonographic findings include the following:

- An anechoic or hypoechoic area lacking air or fluid bronchograms is apparent with acoustic enhancement of lung deep to the sonolucent area.
- The material contained may vary from anechoic to hyperechoic, depending on the type of exudate present.
- Loculations or compartmentalization of the abscess may occur.
- Encapsulation (uncommon) may occur.
- Hyperechoic free gas echoes may be mixed with the exudate, suggesting anaerobic infection.

- A dorsal gas cap may be present, indicative of a bronchial communication and probable anaerobic infection.
- In foals with multiple *Rhodococcus equi* abscesses, many abscesses involve the pulmonary periphery and therefore are detectable by ultrasonography. Foals with abscesses >2 cm may require antibiotic treatment and close monitoring.

Pulmonary Fibrosis or Diffuse Granulomatous Disease, Metastatic Neoplasia

Characteristic ultrasonographic findings include the following:

- Small hypoechoic to echoic soft tissue masses scattered throughout the lung periphery (Figs. 14-39 and 14-40).
- Usually homogeneous, rarely heterogeneous
- Lack of bronchial and normal vascular structures within the masses

Cranial Mediastinal Abscess

Characteristic ultrasonographic findings include the following:

- Walled-off, usually encapsulated mass of hypoechoic to echoic fluid and fibrin is present cranial to the heart.

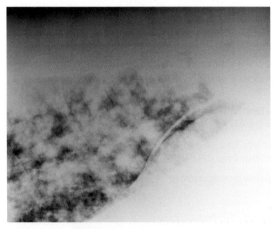

Figure 14-39   Radiographic image of a horse with equine multinodular pulmonary fibrosis.

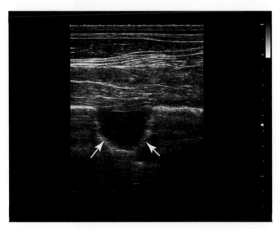

Figure 14-40   Ultrasonographic images of a horse with equine multinodular pulmonary fibrosis. *Arrows* point to the typical sonographic appearance of pulmonary fibrosis. At the periphery of the lung, the normal aeration is interrupted by hypoechoic homogenous nodules.

- Caudal displacement of the heart occurs, and signs of cranial vena cava obstruction develop in patients with large cranial mediastinal abscesses.

Cranial Mediastinal Neoplasia

Neoplastic infiltration of the lymphoid tissue in the cranial mediastinal, caudal cervical, or bronchial lymph nodes results in a large space-occupying mass in the cranial mediastinum.

Characteristic ultrasonographic appearance includes the following:

- Homogeneous or heterogeneous hypoechoic to echoic soft tissue mass displaces the lung dorsally and the heart caudally.
- Mass usually is associated with a large anechoic pleural effusion.
- Caudal displacement of the heart occurs.
- The mass is usually lymphosarcoma, although it may be seen in individuals with mesothelioma or hemangiosarcoma.
- The mass can usually be imaged from the third ICS and may extend dorsally and cranially toward the thoracic inlet and up the ventral neck with cervical lymph node involvement.

Emergency Ocular Examinations

Practice Tip: *Ocular ultrasonography is indicated when conditions exist that preclude a complete standard ophthalmologic examination or when retrobulbar injury or disease is suspected.*

- Sonographic evaluation may be the only diagnostic tool available in cases in which severe palpebral or third eyelid swelling is present.
- Ultrasonography of the posterior segment is useful when anterior segment or vitreous abnormalities such as corneal edema, hyphema, or vitreous hemorrhage prevent visualization of the fundus.
- Sonographic findings can aid in formulating a prognosis for vision and can guide clinical decision making regarding medical or surgical interventions.
- Ocular ultrasound should be performed with extreme care in horses with severe corneal injury and risk of perforation or globe rupture.

Normal Ultrasonographic Findings in the Equine Eye

The globe and the periorbital and retrobulbar soft tissues and bone can be evaluated easily using high-frequency transducers (5.0 to 14.0 MHz) available to most equine practitioners. Linear "transrectal" transducers used for reproductive studies give good images of the globe and superficial periorbital tissues, although the retrobulbar space may be inadequately visualized in some horses. Axial sections of the eye are the most common obtained. The lens surfaces and optic nerve are placed in the center of the scan, and different axial sections are obtained by rotating the probe marker from the 12 o'clock position (axial vertical or transverse section) to the 3 o'clock or 9 o'clock positions (horizontal axial or sagittal section).

Practice Tip: Comparisons should always be made with the normal contralateral eye when possible. Ultrasound biomicroscopic imaging with a 50-MHz or higher transducer is the optimal sonographic method for evaluating the cornea and anterior segment. This equipment is *not* routinely available to most equine emergency clinicians and therefore is not described.

- The axial globe length should be measured from the cornea to the retina and compared with the normal eye. Mean axial globe length has been reported for extirpated adult equine eyes (38.4 ± 2.22 mm male, 40.45 ± 2.4 mm female), adult miniature horses (33.7 ± 0.07 mm, A-mode ultrasound), and adult horses of various non–draft breeds (39.23 ± 1.26 mm, B-mode ultrasound).
- The cornea appears as a smooth, convexly curved echogenic line along the most anterior aspect of the globe.
- The anterior chamber is anechoic but may contain reverberation artifacts that can extend through the lens and posterior segment. Anterior chamber depth is measured from the corneal surface to the central anterior lens capsule. Mean anterior chamber depth has been reported to be 5.63 ± 0.86 mm in adult horses and a similar 5.6 ± 0.03 mm in adult miniature horses.
- The posterior chamber normally is *not* seen.
- The iris appears as an echoic irregular band extending from the pupillary margin to the margins of the globe. The ciliary body is immediately posterior to and continuous with the iris. The corpora nigra (granula iridica) appears as an echogenic mass on the anterior aspect of the iris at the dorsal and sometimes ventral pupillary margins. Iris cysts can be incidental findings and can appear as anechoic spherical structures within the corpora nigra (Fig. 14-41).

- The lens is anechoic with the anterior and posterior margins of the lens capsule seen as echogenic lines. Mean lens thickness has been reported to be 11.75 ± 0.80 mm in adult horses and 10.3 ± 0.006 mm in adult miniature horses.
- The vitreous should be uniformly anechoic. The gain should be increased when examining the vitreous in order to avoid missing fine vitreous opacities caused by scatter and sound attenuation by the lens.
- The retina, choroid, and sclera appear in combination as a concave echoic band along the posterior aspect of the globe. These structures cannot be distinguished from each other in the normal eye.
- The retrobulbar muscle, fat, and optic nerve appear as varying echogenicities posterior to the globe. The optic nerve is cone shaped and homogeneous in appearance. Homogeneous, hypoechoic fat may be seen surrounding the optic nerve in many horses. The extraocular muscles are also hypoechoic but mottled in appearance. The normal bony orbit is deep to the extraocular muscles, appears smooth and hyperechoic, and casts a strong acoustic shadow.

Abnormal Ultrasonographic Findings in the Equine Eye

- Sonography can aid in the evaluation of numerous emergency ocular conditions.
- Ocular pathologic conditions such as:
  - Retinal detachments
  - Vitreous and retrobulbar hemorrhages
  - Lens dislocation
  - Scleral rupture

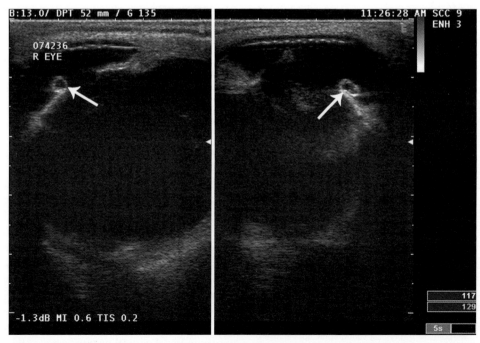

Figure 14-41   Sonogram from a horse with iris cysts. Note the anechoic circular structures present on the ventral medial aspect of the iris *(arrows).*

- Globe rupture
- Foreign body retention
- Orbital fractures—can be identified by sonography in the traumatized eye
- Ultrasound can be used to detect corneal abnormalities when severe eyelid swelling prevents direct examination.
- Ultrasound can be used to differentiate buphthalmos from exophthalmos and to identify underlying causes for each.

Cornea and Anterior Chamber
- Corneal ulcers cause a thickened, irregular, or pitted appearance to the cornea.
- Corneal edema appears as a diffusely thickened and hypoechoic cornea.
- Corneal stromal abscesses appear as focal areas of corneal thickening and increased echogenicity. Stromal abscesses should be evaluated closely for the presence of a foreign body.
- Synechiae appear as hypoechoic strands between the cornea and iris—anterior synechiae (Fig. 14-42)—or between the iris and anterior lens capsule—posterior synechiae.
- Hyphema, hypopyon, and inflammatory exudates cause increased echogenicity of the anterior chamber. Differentiation between these infiltrates is usually *not* possible.
- The anterior chamber depth can be increased in cases of uveitis or glaucoma.
- Iris prolapse is diagnosed any time the iris is imaged away from its normal position.

Lens Displacement and Rupture
- With lens luxation, the echogenic lens capsule is imaged in an abnormal position anterior or posterior to its normal location or may appear to move freely between the anterior chamber and vitreous (Fig. 14-43). Lateral luxations at the level of the iris also can be imaged. Acute lens luxation may be seen together with vitreous hemorrhage.
- Lens rupture is characterized by discontinuity of the lens capsule with echogenic lens material in the surrounding aqueous or vitreous.

Vitreous Opacities and Detachment
- Vitreous opacities can occur with hemorrhage, inflammation, vitreous degeneration, asteroid hyalosis, and detachment of the vitreous.
- Vitreous opacities are imaged as areas of increased echogenicity within a normally anechoic vitreous. Increasing the far field gain is often necessary to visualize these opacities.
- Severe acute hemorrhage into the vitreous appears as a diffuse increase in echogenicity that can fill the entire cavity. As the hemorrhage organizes, discrete echogenic masses and strands become visible. Vitreous inflammation can be difficult to distinguish from organizing hemorrhage but is typically characterized by multifocal strands of varying echogenicities. Discrete abscesses may be seen within the vitreous and appear as homogeneous echogenic masses (Fig. 14-44).
- The vitreous body is gelatinous and may separate from the retina—vitreous detachment—producing a space that may fill with hypoechoic effusion or hemorrhage. The interface between the vitreous and hemorrhage or effusion is seen as a moderately weak echogenic line that may mimic a retinal detachment if a persistent adhesion of the vitreous exists at the optic nerve head.

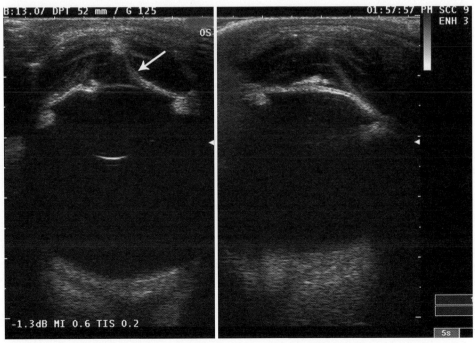

Figure 14-42   Sonogram from a horse with anterior synechiae and corneal ulceration. Hypoechoic strands of fibrin *(arrow)* can be seen extending from the anterior surface of the iris to the cornea.

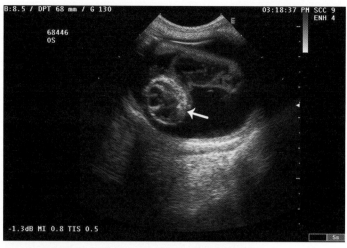

Figure 14-43 Sonogram from a horse with luxation of the lens. The lens is displaced ventrally into the vitreous *(arrow)*. The lens is rounder than normal with a thick hyperechoic capsule and striated hyperechoic and hypoechoic lines consistent with cataractous changes. Hypoechoic strands and hypoechoic loculated areas within the vitreous are most consistent with fibrin.

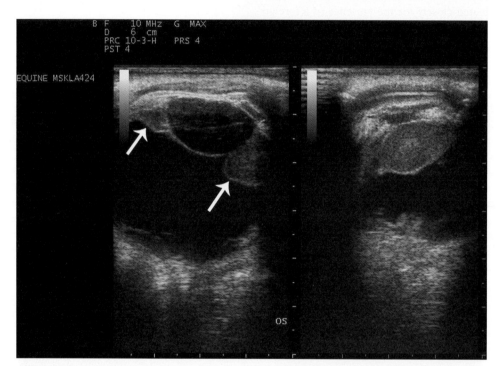

Figure 14-44 Sonogram from a horse with a mass within the vitreous. The hypoechoic homogeneous mass *(arrows)* just behind the dorsal and ventral aspects of the ciliary body and lens is most consistent with an abscess.

Retinal Detachment

- Complete retinal detachment is seen as an echogenic "V-shaped" structure with the apex of the "V" at the optic disk and the tips of the "V" just behind the ciliary body—seagull sign (Fig. 14-45). This appearance is created because connective tissue attachments of the retina to the optic disk and ora ciliaris usually remain even with complete detachment, although disinsertion from the ora ciliaris has been reported.

- With recent-onset retinal detachment the retina is very thin and somewhat mobile within the vitreous. The mobility is less than that of vitreous fibrin strands. Vitreous hemorrhage may be seen concurrently.

- With chronicity, the detached retina becomes thickened and less mobile, and adhesions may form between the

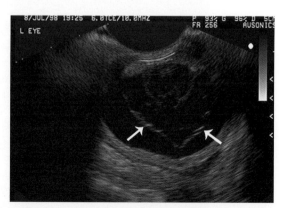

Figure 14-45 Sonogram from a horse with a complete retinal detachment. The retina *(arrows)* is lifted from the choroid but still attached at the optic disk and ora ciliaris forming a V-shaped structure within the vitreous.

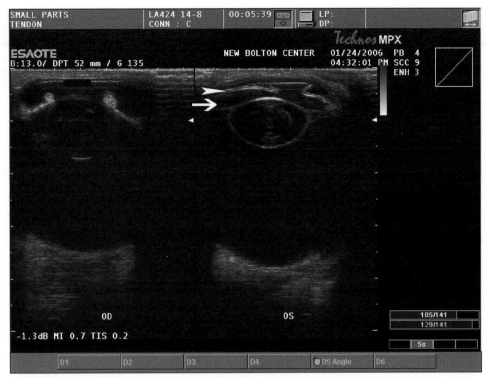

Figure 14-46   Sonogram from a horse with glaucoma of the left eye. The left globe is enlarged compared with the right. Iris bombe is evidenced by anterior displacement of the iris *(arrowhead)* and anechoic fluid within the posterior chamber *(arrow)*. Cortical cataracts are present in both eyes.

retina and posterior lens capsule. Dystrophic mineralization also may occur and appears as hyperechoic areas that cast acoustic shadows.

- Combined retinal and choroidal detachment has been reported in the horse and should be considered as a differential diagnosis when significant thickening of a detached retina is detected.
- Partial or focal retinal detachment appears as an elevated, immobile, thin line at the periphery of the globe.

Scleral Rupture

- With scleral rupture, the scleral margins are ill-defined or indistinguishable from surrounding tissues. Localization of discrete scleral tears with ultrasound has *not* been reported.
- Because blunt trauma is the most likely reason for scleral rupture, hemorrhage into the vitreous, anterior chamber, and/or retrobulbar space is commonly seen. Combined choroidal and retinal detachments are reported in horses with scleral rupture, but the sonographic appearance has *not* been described.

Foreign Bodies

- Intraocular foreign bodies usually appear as echogenic or hyperechoic structures. They can be found anywhere within the orbital or periorbital tissues or within corneal stromal abscesses.
- Wood and glass are echogenic and cast acoustic shadows. Metal has a characteristic reverberation artifact. Fracture

fragments also cast strong acoustic shadows and should be considered as a possible differential diagnosis, prompting careful evaluation of the bony orbit.

Glaucoma

- Glaucoma is recognized by sonography as an increased axial globe length compared with the normal contralateral eye or published normals.
- Corneal edema is seen with primary, secondary, and congenital glaucoma. Secondary glaucoma also has signs of intraocular inflammation such as posterior synechiae and cataract formation. Lens luxation and iris bombe also may occur.
- Iris bombe appears as a thickened iris that bulges toward the cornea. The anterior displacement of the iris causes the posterior chamber to become visible (Fig. 14-46).
- The iris and ciliary bodies should be closely evaluated for masses that may be blocking the iridocorneal angle. Melanomas of the uveal tract may have a homogeneous, hypoechoic, or echoic sonographic appearance or may have a more heterogeneous appearance. Hyperechoic areas that cast acoustic shadows consistent with areas of calcification also can be seen within melanomas.

Ruptured Globe

- A ruptured globe appears smaller than normal and the intraocular structures are difficult to recognize. It can be difficult to distinguish the borders of an acutely ruptured globe from surrounding periocular hemorrhage.

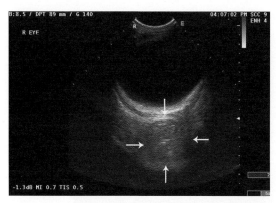

Figure 14-47 Sonogram from a horse with a retrobulbar mass. The well-circumscribed, circular retrobulbar mass *(arrows)* is homogeneous and hypoechoic. Doppler ultrasound interrogation of the mass revealed it to be highly vascular.

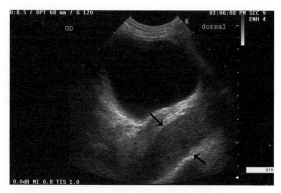

Figure 14-48 Sonogram from a horse with a periorbital abscess. Note the hypoechoic fluid pocket *(arrows)* dissecting along the dorsal and posterior aspect of the orbit.

Retrobulbar Masses

- Retrobulbar masses are a cause of exophthalmos in horses because of the enclosed bony orbit. Abscesses, hemorrhage, cysts, neoplasia, and cellulitis can cause exophthalmos.
- Comparison with the normal contralateral eye is critical for identifying small or indistinct retrobulbar masses.
- Retrobulbar masses can sometimes be appreciated by scanning over the supraorbital fossa.
- Retrobulbar hemorrhage may appear anechoic or hypoechoic depending on the "age" of the hematoma. Acute hemorrhage appears diffusely hypoechoic. As a hematoma organizes, echogenic clots are surrounded by anechoic fluid. Mature blood clots can be echogenic and may cast acoustic shadows from their distal borders. This is in contrast to calcified tissue and most foreign material, for these cast shadows from their near surfaces.
- Numerous retrobulbar neoplasms have been reported in the horse, and ultrasound cannot provide a histopathologic diagnosis. Discrete homogeneous masses are most characteristic of lymphosarcoma, although carcinomas and neuroendocrine tumors have been reported with similar sonographic appearances. Aggressive tumors are more typically diffuse and heteroechoic and may invade the bony orbit (Fig. 14-47).
- Retrobulbar abscesses contain hypoechoic to echogenic material that is sometimes layered. The fluid is usually contained within a well-defined echogenic capsule (Fig. 14-48). The area should be scanned carefully for an associated foreign body.

Orbital Fractures

- Orbital fractures are seen as disruptions in the normally smooth, hyperechoic cortical bone surface.
- Fracture fragments are hyperechoic linear structures that are distracted from the underlying parent bone. Impingement of the globe by these fracture fragments is an indication for surgical repair.
- An orbital fracture involving the wall of the paranasal sinuses occurs with periorbital emphysema. Periorbital emphysema is characterized by hyperechoic gas echoes that cast gray acoustic shadows and interfere with visualization of the deeper tissues.

Summary

Ultrasonography is valuable in the emergency setting because it is a noninvasive imaging modality that can be used in a wide variety of areas, helping the clinician to determine the cause of the emergency and providing useful diagnostic information that can help one formulate a prognosis and treatment plan.

SCINTIGRAPHIC IMAGING

Michael W. Ross

A comprehensive review of nuclear medicine is beyond the scope of this chapter and readers are referred to the bibliography for additional information. Clinical nuclear medicine involves *in vivo* use of radioisotopes in the diagnosis and management of clinical disease. Several terms are used synonymously with nuclear medicine, including: *nuclear scintigraphy, bone scintigraphy,* and *gamma scintigraphy,* and although these terms differ slightly, for horses, most clinicians refer to bone scintigraphy, the technique most commonly performed. Bone scintigraphy is highly sensitive compared with digital radiography and can detect as little as 10^{-13} g of radiopharmaceutical in bone compared with grams before a lesion is detected using radiography. Many factors limit sensitivity, specificity, and accuracy of bone scintigraphy including:

- Time from radiopharmaceutical administration to image acquisition
- Body part to camera distance
- Shielding
- Motion
- Time from injury to image acquisition—an important consideration in the utility of nuclear medicine in emergency management.
- Ambient temperature and peripheral perfusion
- Amount of background radiation

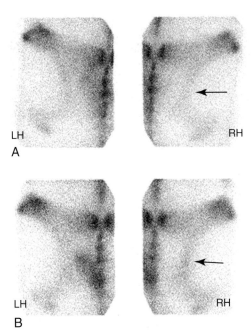

LH

RH

A

LH

RH

B

Figure 14-49 **A,** Initial (2 days after injury) and 7-day follow-up. **B,** Uncorrected delayed (bone) phase dorsal pelvic scintigraphic images of a 3-year-old Thoroughbred colt that slipped and fell on the right hind limb. At 2 days after injury, the scintigraphic study failed to identify a fracture in the ilial body, seen as a focal area of increased radiopharmaceutical uptake 7 days later *(arrows)*. False-negative scans occur during pelvic imaging early after injury because factors such as motion, background radiation, distance, and shielding can interfere with scan acquisition and interpretation.

Example: A horse is found to be acutely, non–weight-bearing lame, and a pelvic fracture is suspected. A combination of negative factors including high background radiation, motion, endogenous shielding, and distance reduce sensitivity of pelvic and other axial skeletal scintigraphic imaging and that of upper limb imaging would warrant delaying immediate pelvic scintigraphy (Fig. 14-49). False-negative scans can occur early after traumatic injury, and scintigraphic examination is best delayed until maximum sensitivity can be achieved—7 to 10 days after injury—see later. High sensitivity—94.4%— in horses with extremity fractures is reported, but a lack of sensitivity (true positives) in pelvic imaging is suggested. Specificity—true negatives—is low compared with other modalities because disparate diseases can similarly alter blood flow and binding sites in bone.

- Scintigraphic lesions that are difficult to differentiate are:
  - Direct trauma (osteitis) and fracture
  - Stress-related bone injury, including fracture and osteoarthritis
  - Infection (infectious osteitis and, less frequently, osteomyelitis)
  - Osteochondrosis
  - Enostosis-like lesions
  - Neoplasia

Accuracy is improved by acquiring several images from different angles, minimizing factors affecting sensitivity, and knowing the history. ***Example:*** A focal area of increased

radiopharmaceutical uptake (IRU) in the caudolateral tibial cortex of a 2-year-old Thoroughbred (TB) filly would undoubtedly represent stress-related bone injury rather than a rare bone tumor.

General Considerations

- Radiographs depict activity in bone that occurred in the past several days to years.
- Scintigraphy is a *functional* evaluation of bone at the time of imaging.
- ***Practice Tip:*** *Scintigraphic evidence of bone activity means active bone formation—bone modeling—is occurring that might take weeks to be seen radiologically. Therefore, a major advantage of scintigraphy is early detection of bone injury.*
- ***Important:*** Scintigraphy is unlikely to accurately reflect changes in bone that occurred longer than 3 to 4 months before imaging. Horses given substantial rest before examination are *not* good candidates unless the examination is a follow-up to assess healing.
- The most common and useful radioisotope is technetium-99m (^{99m}Tc). ^{99m}Tc, a short-lived (metastable) radioisotope with a half-life of 6 hours, is ideal for radiation safety and tissue retention.
- ^{99m}Tc is excreted almost entirely through the kidneys, so containing and monitoring urine is extremely important.
- ^{99m}Tc is produced when ^{99}Mo decays to ^{99}Tc and the metastable (^{99m}Tc) radioisotope gives off a gamma ray (140 keV) that is used for imaging.
- Commercially, ^{99}Mo/^{99m}Tc generators can be purchased for use in large hospitals, but an alternative, cost-effective method is the daily purchase of individual doses without the need to house generators. This service is generally available Monday through Saturday and if located close to a nuclear pharmacy.
- Studies can be performed on an emergency basis during daytime hours—the only limitation is availability of radioisotope—or anytime, if a generator is available; having a generator available means radioisotope is always available.
- Directly from the generator, ^{99m}Tc is in the ionic form of sodium ^{99m}Tc pertechnetate (Na^{99m}TcO$_4$) that can be injected or mixed with a bone-seeking agent or pharmaceutical.
- Radiation is measured in curies (Ci) or millicuries (mCi); becquerels (Bq), megabecquerels (MBq), and gigabecquerels (GBq) are also used. One mCi is equal to 37MBq.
- ***Practice Tip:*** *The recommended dose of ^{99m}Tc is 0.4 to 0.5 mCi (14.8 to 18.5 MBq)/kg, totaling 150 to 2 Na^{99m}TcO$_4$ is injected intravenously, but only flow and pool-phase studies can be performed.*
- For most equine studies, Na^{99m}TcO$_4$ is mixed with a pharmaceutical.
- For bone, ^{99m}Tc is bound to methylene diphosphonate (MDP), or hydroxymethane/hydroxymethylene diphosphonate (HDP).

When Can a Bone Scan Be Done in an Emergency Situation?

- *Practice Tip: Binding of radiopharmaceutical has a direct effect on decisions such as timing of the nuclear medicine study and interpretation. This is clinically important when considering if a horse is a candidate for a scintigraphic examination in an emergency situation.*
- The exact mechanism of binding of ^{99m}Tc-HDP to bone is unclear. ^{99m}Tc-HDP is believed to bind to exposed sites on the inorganic hydroxyapatite crystal.
- Binding sites are exposed under normal and pathologic conditions in areas of actively remodeling bone or in soft tissues undergoing mineralization.
- ^{99m}Tc-MDP uptake occurs by the processes of chemical adsorption onto, and by direct integration into, the crystalline structure.
- Other possible mechanisms for increased uptake include incorporation into the organic matrix or local hypervascularity.
- Radiopharmaceutical may dissociate with incorporation of ^{99m}Tc and MDP individually into the organic and inorganic phases, respectively.
- ^{99m}Tc-MDP adsorption might depend on pH and the presence of phosphates, calcium compounds, and other cations.
- *Practice Tip: There is a common misconception that blood flow is most important in determining the amount of radiopharmaceutical delivered to an area of injury. Radiopharmaceutical uptake is not simply the result from changes in local blood flow; blood flow is likely increased in sites of actively remodeling bone.*
- Although increased blood flow does *not* significantly affect a bone scan, adequate blood flow is necessary to deliver radiopharmaceutical to available binding sites in bone.
- Rather than measuring blood flow, delayed (bone phase) images reflect changes in bone metabolism.
- *Important:* A 3-phase bone scan—flow (vascular), pool (soft-tissue), and delayed (bone) phases—can detect increased perfusion and soft-tissue inflammation if present, but it is metabolic activity of bone that influences the amount of radiopharmaceutical uptake.
- Decreased blood flow, caused by infarction or ischemia, can greatly affect a bone scan but is an unusual clinical problem (see photopenia later). An equine patient with severe lameness and extremities cool to the touch, where avascular necrosis is suspected, and in cases in which severe wounds or breakdown injuries have damaged arterial supply, a 3-phase bone scan can be diagnostic. Catheterization of peripheral vessels and positive contrast radiographic studies are *not* necessary if scintigraphic examination can be performed.
- *Practice Tip: The most important aspects of ^{99m}Tc-MDP binding relate to timing of the scan and the stage of modeling (formation). In actively remodeling bone, osteoclastic activity predominates during bone resorption, whereas osteoblastic activity dominates during bone modeling.*
- Modeling occurs independently or in conjunction with remodeling in cancellous and cortical bone.
- *Practice Tip: The high sensitivity of bone scintigraphy is attributed to increased osteoblast activity that precedes morphologic changes visible radiologically.*
- Site and stage of binding are important from a clinical perspective.
- *Practice Tip: Binding sites for ^{99m}Tc-MDP are created by osteoblast activity during bone modeling, and maximal IRU occurs 8 or 12 days after bone injury.*
- *Note:* An acute fracture caused by direct trauma may *not* be scintigraphically evident for several days. Acute, traumatic injury differs from stress-related bone injury, because the latter, particularly common in racehorses, results from a continuum of bone changes that might lead to stress or catastrophic fractures and osteoarthritis.
- Microfracture, periosteal callus, and subchondral bone damage precede the development of stress or complete fracture in the dorsal cortex and distal articular surface of the third metacarpal bone (McIII), the third metatarsal bone (MtIII), humerus, tibia, and pelvis.
- In horses with acute lameness from stress-related bone injury, bone scan findings usually are immediately positive because bone modeling is ongoing.
- *Practice Tip: In horses with stress-related bone injury, a bone scan result is likely to be positive long before catastrophic fracture occurs, an important advantage of scintigraphy compared with radiography.*
- *Practice Tip: In horses with traumatic injury, such as an acute pelvic or other upper limb fracture, a false-negative scan during the acute phase may result from lack of modeling.*
- Other factors resulting in false-negative results include:
  - Distance
  - Shielding
  - High background activity
  - Motion
- *Example 1:* A horse developed acute hind limb lameness during hospitalization and suspecting a pelvic fracture involving the acetabulum, clinicians performed scintigraphic examination on day 2, but the scan result was negative. Seven days later faint IRU appeared consistent with fracture.
- *Example 2:* A horse being shipped for scintigraphic examination 24 hours later was caught underneath a bar in the trailer while attempting to back out, injuring the lumbar region. Scintigraphic examination in this horse revealed a positive result demonstrating lag phase in some horses is short (Fig. 14-50). In this example, it was *not* necessary to wait for days after injury to see acute bone trauma.
- *Practice Tip: In the distal limbs, lag phase is variable but early detection of bone injury can be valuable in clinical decision making (Figs. 14-51 and 14-52).*
- *Photopenia* is an unusual scintigraphic finding. Theoretically, if blood supply is *not* adequate during flow and pool-phases, radiopharmaceutical concentrations

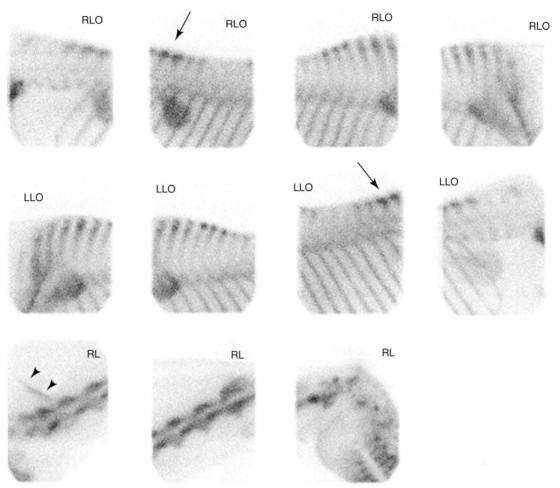

Figure 14-50   Left and right lateral delayed phase scintigraphic images of the axial skeleton of an aged Warmblood that sustained a trailer accident approximately 24 hours before imaging. Focal intense increased radiopharmaceutical uptake can be seen *(arrows)* involving the dorsal spinous processes of the lumbar vertebrae. Active bone modeling is attributed to acute injury based on history and presence of soft tissue swelling that developed immediately after injury. Increased radiopharmaceutical uptake can be seen in skeletal muscle or the laminar portion of the ligamentum nuchae *(arrowheads);* skeletal muscle behaves like bone, and damage can be seen in delayed phase images.

sufficient to differentiate normal from abnormal bone are *not* achieved.
- Causes of *photopenia* include:
  - Bone infarct
  - Abscess, intense resorption
  - Sequestrum
- *No* known equine disease involves only bone resorption without modeling.
- *Photopenia* is seen rarely when portions of bone are surgically removed or displaced out of view.
- In flow phase images of horses with lameness abolished with regional analgesia (palmar digital/nerve block), there is often reduction of blood flow in the affected limb, seen as a *photopenic* region between the coronary band and distal aspect of the foot on dorsal images.
- A relative reduction in blood flow when compared with the contralateral limb may reflect chronic reduction in weight bearing; this finding does *not* persist in pool-phase or delayed images.
- *Photopenia* seen in clinical cases:

- Subperiosteal abscess of the olecranon process with photopenia in pool-phase images believed caused by fluid accumulation and compression of nearby vessels
- Proximal tibia in delayed phase images caused by severe effusion of the overlying lateral femorotibial joint compartment
- Delayed phase images caused by infectious osteitis, bone sequestration, and distal limb ischemia
  Practice Tip: *Damaged skeletal muscles behave like damaged bone, and in general, injury to skeletal muscle is seen in delayed phase scintigraphic images soon after injury or onset of clinical signs. A lag phase of 24 to 48 hours may be necessary, but usually injury can be detected immediately.*

●》 **WHAT TO DO**

Nuclear Scintigraphy Emergency
- Rarely would scintigraphy be required to evaluate a horse during off-hours or on a weekend.

- Scintigraphic examinations can be scheduled during working hours for most horses even if a clinical decision must be made based on the results of a bone scan.
- Scintigraphy can be extremely valuable and help with clinical decisions if these guidelines are followed:
  - Injury to the distal extremities, including the elbow and stifle and continuing to the distal aspect of the forelimbs/hind limbs: To avoid *false-negative* scintigraphic findings, a bone scan should be delayed for 48 to 72 hours after a traumatic incident or the onset of acute, severe lameness (scan may be positive earlier).
  - Injury to the upper limbs and axial skeleton, except pelvis: To avoid *false-negative* scintigraphic findings, a bone scan should be delayed 72 to 96 hours after a traumatic incident (though scan may be positive earlier).
  - Injury to the pelvis: Given the inherent problems with pelvic imaging, to avoid *false-negative* scintigraphic findings, a bone scan should be delayed for 10 days (scan may be positive earlier).
  - To evaluate vascular integrity of the distal extremities, 3-phase scintigraphic imaging is employed immediately after onset of injury or acute, severe lameness.
  - To image damaged skeletal muscle, scintigraphic imaging is employed immediately after injury or onset of acute, severe lameness, but waiting 24 to 48 hours may be reasonable.

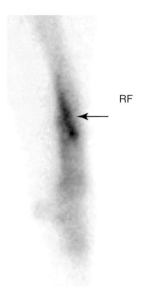

Figure 14-51 Lateral delayed phase scintigraphic image of a stallion sustaining a breeding accident 7 days earlier (dorsal is to the right and proximal is uppermost). The horse was "fracture lame" in the right forelimb (RF), and although clinical signs incriminated bone trauma of the radius, radiologic findings were normal. A proposed surgical procedure being done under general anesthesia was canceled when linear, focal intense increased radiopharmaceutical uptake indicating the presence of an oblique fracture was identified *(arrow)*. Early and accurate diagnosis was valuable in clinical decision making.

Figure 14-52   A, Craniocaudal digital radiographic image of the left cubital (elbow) joint of a horse sustaining a wound over the lateral aspect 5 days before admission. **B** and **C,** Flexed lateral and dorsal delayed phase scintigraphic images taken the same day showing focal intense increased radiopharmaceutical uptake (IRU) *(arrows)* of the distal, lateral aspect of the left radius (*S,* sternum). While radiologically normal, focal IRU indicated the presence of substantial bone injury in this horse, explaining persistent lameness and lack of clinical improvement. **D,** Craniocaudal digital radiographic image taken 12 days later clearly identifies bony injury *(arrow)*. Early diagnosis using scintigraphy in horses after traumatic injury can give answers and reinforce clinical decisions.

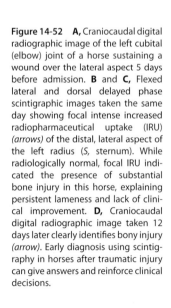

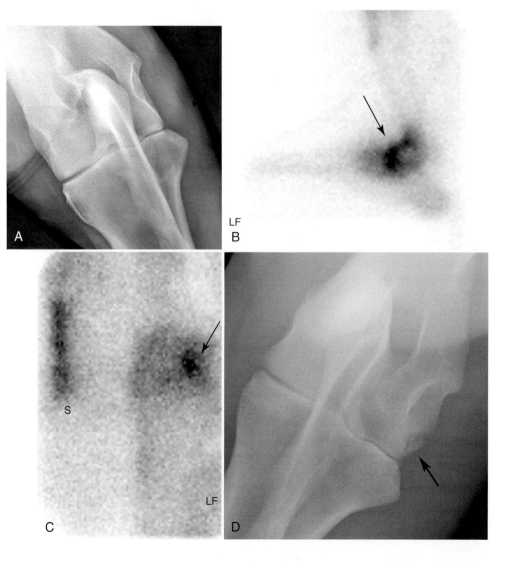

COMPUTED TOMOGRAPHY (CT) AND MAGNETIC RESONANCE IMAGING (MRI)

Peter V. Scrivani

Computed tomography (CT) and magnetic resonance imaging (MRI) are techniques that allow for noninvasive depiction of patient morphology and function that is unsurpassed using other diagnostic methods. When used appropriately, these imaging methods provide useful information that contributes to improved patient care by superior diagnostic accuracy, better determination of lesion extent for treatment planning, improved prognostication, and enhanced ability to monitor disease progression and response to treatment. Without thoughtful selection of the examinations, patient care may be affected by an increase in cost to the owner, increased patient risk because of general anesthesia and recovery from anesthesia, and case mismanagement because of incorrect or incomplete acquiring of information. Therefore, it is important to understand the competitive advantages and disadvantages of these two modalities, in addition to their clinical indications, to optimize the care of the equine emergency patient.

Practice Tip: *CT is good for a rapid examination and when spatial resolution is important: MRI is best suited for contrast resolution.*

CT uses X-rays to determine the density of body structures, and a computer to reconstruct images of the patient in any anatomic plane or three dimensions. CT is good for a rapid examination and when spatial resolution is important. Quick examinations are important when patient motion (e.g., respiratory or heart motion) is a concern. Spatial resolution refers to the ability of the scanner to discriminate that two adjacent high-contrast objects are separate structures. The high spatial resolution of CT makes this modality good for depicting bone detail (Fig. 14-53). CT, nevertheless, is also good for certain types of soft-tissue imaging (e.g., thoracic and abdominal imaging). MRI measures the response of protons within the body to high-frequency radio waves when placed in a strong magnetic field. MRI is best when contrast resolution is important. Contrast resolution is the ability to

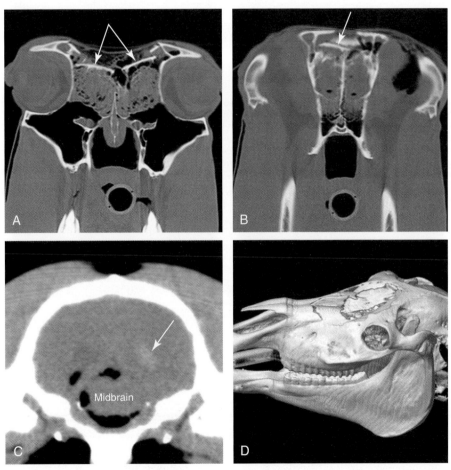

Figure 14-53   CT scans of an 8-year-old, Quarter horse mare that was kicked in the face. **A,** Transverse CT scan (bone algorithm) at the level of the eyes. **B,** Transverse CT scan (bone algorithm) through the frontal sinuses and olfactory bulbs. **C,** Transverse CT scan (soft-tissue algorithm) of the brain. **D,** Three-dimensional surface volume CT reconstruction (bone algorithm) of the head. Note the compression fracture that predominantly involves both frontal bones (**A, B,** and **D**). The fracture fragments are ventrally displaced into the nasal cavity and frontal sinuses *(arrows)* but not into the cranial cavity. The fracture lines, however, communicate with the cranial cavity allowing gas to surround the midbrain (**C**). Additionally, a small focus of bleeding is visible *(arrow).*

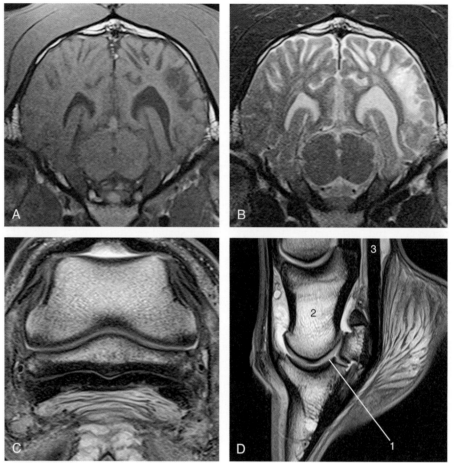

Figure 14-54   MRI scans of a 1.5-year-old, Thoroughbred colt with an area of chronic necrosis in the left cerebral hemisphere (**A** and **B**), and a normal 6-year-old, Quarter gelding (**C** and **D**). **A,** Transverse T1-weighted MRI scan of the brain at the level of the midbrain. **B,** Transverse T2-weighted MRI scan of the brain at the level of the midbrain. **C,** Transverse, proton density (PD) MRI scan through the middle phalanx, navicular bone, and deep digital flexor tendon. **D,** Sagittal PD MRI scan of the digit. Note the excellent contrast resolution that allows differentiation of numerous tissue types such as articular cartilage *(1)*, bone *(2)*, and tendons *(3)*. Also, compare the brain images to the CT scan of the brain in Fig. 14-53, *C.*

distinguish between differences in tissue intensity in an image. For example, the differences in intensity of gray matter, white matter, and cerebrospinal fluid are much greater on MRI than CT, making it easier to differentiate these tissues using MRI. Similarly, MRI is excellent for musculoskeletal imaging because of its ability to differentiate cartilage, tendons, ligaments, cortical bone, and marrow (Fig. 14-54).

Practice Tip: *The types of CT or MRI examinations that may be performed are limited by the configuration of the scanner and the size and shape of the horse.*

In the adult, typically either modality may be used to examine the head and distal limbs. CT usually can also examine at least the cranial half of the neck. MRI is more variable in what parts may be examined because of the different scanner configurations (e.g., open versus closed magnet). In foals and miniature horses, CT is also used to examine the thorax and abdomen.

- This chapter does not discuss the technical issues surrounding patient preparation and image acquisition, which typically require a technician with specialized training.

- The time it takes to acquire and properly interpret CT and MRI images should be factored into any plan for patient management.

- In most cases, CT or MRI should be considered as an elective procedure that is performed in stabilized patients. There are few indications for CT and MRI that are *truly* emergencies.

- Whereas each imaging modality is ideally suited for examining particular conditions, most modalities can provide diagnostic information on a wide range of conditions, and the selection of the imaging method frequently is based on equipment availability.

Emergency CT/MRI Examinations
Head

- For acute trauma without neurologic deficit, radiography generally is sufficient for the initial evaluation. CT or MRI may be performed to identify additional injuries or document the extent of known injuries.

- For acute trauma associated with neurologic deficits, CT or MRI may be performed to document the extent of injury and guide a plan for emergency treatment (e.g., for compression fractures, subdural hematomas).

- For acute neurologic deficits without trauma, CT or MRI may be performed to determine the cause of clinical signs and determine if emergency treatment is justified.

Spine

- For acute trauma, radiography generally is sufficient for the initial evaluation. CT or MRI may be performed to identify additional injuries or document the extent of known injuries and guide a plan for treatment.
- When acute extraaxial spinal-cord compression is suspected (e.g., epidural hematoma, trauma), myelography, CT, or MRI may be performed to formulate a plan for emergency treatment.

Musculoskeletal

- For musculoskeletal infections, ultrasonography typically is usually adequate to identify fluid pockets for draining. Radiography typically is useful in identifying osteomyelitis, although MRI is more sensitive and not specific. MRI may be helpful for differentiating necrotizing infectious fasciitis that requires aggressive surgical management for decompression (see Chapter 35, p. 622).
- For acute bone trauma, radiography generally is sufficient for the initial evaluation. If the results of radiography are negative and an occult fracture is suspected, then bone nuclear scintigraphy (see p. 102) or MRI may be performed.

- For an acute fracture, CT or MRI may be performed to determine the extent of the fracture immediately before repair (e.g., medial condylar fracture). Three-dimensional CT reconstructions are helpful in planning surgical repair of complex fractures.
- For acute soft-tissue trauma, ultrasonography generally is sufficient for the initial evaluation. MRI may be performed, especially for penetrating wounds to identify the anatomic structures involved.

Thorax/Abdomen

- For acute respiratory distress, radiography and/or ultrasonography generally are the best guides for treatment planning. CT may be performed, although the need for general anesthesia limits its usefulness.
- For a suspected abscess, radiography and/or ultrasonography generally are sufficient for the initial evaluation. If the results are negative, then CT should be considered.
- For colic, the diagnosis often is made without imaging or with ultrasonography. CT or radiography (most practical) may be performed, especially to detect enteroliths.

References

References can be found on the companion website at www.equine-emergencies.com.

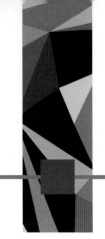

CHAPTER 15

Emergency Laboratory Tests and Point-of-Care Diagnostics

Eileen S. Hackett, Thomas J. Divers, and Jean C. Young

Point-of-Care Diagnostics

Definition: "Point-of-care testing" is diagnostic testing performed at or near the patient. These analyses are important and, in many cases, essential in evaluating the emergency or critical care equine patient. Point-of-care devices are oftentimes portable and are used patient-side in a hospital setting or on the farm. ***Practice Tip:*** *The primary advantage of point-of-care testing is the ability to obtain immediate results, allowing adjustments in patient treatment and minimizing the need to send and await sample results from a clinical pathology laboratory.* Other benefits include:

- Convenience
- Lower cost compared with purchase of bench equipment
- Less maintenance of laboratory-based diagnostic equipment

This allows more frequent monitoring of critically ill patients and provides trends on the changing clinical picture. Sample volumes are generally tiny, which is important in the monitoring of smaller patients. Information gained from point-of-care testing devices is best used when the operator has a complete understanding of the:

- Methodology of the device
- Use instructions
- Species-specific precision
- Accuracy

Advantages of Point-of-Care Testing

- Immediate access, if cartridges are at room temperature[1]
  - Store boxes of cartridges in the refrigerator, where the shelf life is 1 to 2 years.
  - Most cartridges must be kept at room temperature for 4 hours before use.
  - Therefore, keep one or two of each test set at room temperature if the shelf life is only 2 weeks.
- User-friendly equipment—both point-of-care and small benchtop equipment
- Small amounts of blood needed (often only 1 to 3 drops) for point-of-care testing
- Results within 30 seconds to 10 minutes

Disadvantages of Point-of-care Testing

- Quality control can be an issue if storage, testing temperature, and cartridge expiration date are *not* adhered to. Some values are consistently incorrect. With the i-STAT 1[2] portable clinical analyzers, there is an inconsistent underestimation of hematocrit (Hct).
- Tests must be conducted at temperatures of approximately 18° to 30° C (64° to 86° F). Although this temperature range is recommended, samples tested at temperatures as low as 50° did *not* result in noticeable erroneous values.

Laboratory Tests
Blood Gases and Blood Chemistries

- For in-hospital use, portable blood gas or chemistry analyzers are useful for providing rapid information on oxygenation, ventilation, acid-base status, ionized calcium, and creatinine, among other analytes.
- ***Practice Tip:*** *Convenient sites for arterial sampling include the transverse facial artery, facial artery, and lateral metatarsal artery.* (See Chapter 1, p. 4.) To sample, palpate the arterial pulse, insert syringe and needle at a 45-degree angle where the pulse is the strongest, expel air, mix well, and either evaluate immediately or place in ice bath. Arterial oxygen values can change significantly in 15 minutes and acid-base after 30 minutes at room temperature. Samples can be stored in ice for 4 to 6 hours with little change in values. Air bubbles will increase PO_2 and decrease PCO_2 within 2 minutes.
- The i-STAT[3] and IRMA,[4] are point-of-care analyzers commonly employed for these uses.
- Blood is collected in heparinized syringes for measurement of blood gases and in a heparinized syringe or heparin tube for chemistry analysis.
- Results are displayed on the handheld machine within 1 to 3 minutes with printing and/or storage capability.
- Because critically ill equine patients with marked changes in the respiratory and other parameters may need immediate corrective treatment, point-of-care technology is a natural choice to provide immediate therapeutic direction.

---

[1]Store test cartridges in the refrigerator to increase the shelf life to 1 to 2 years. Most cartridges must be kept at room temperature for 4 hours before use. Therefore, keep one or two of each test set at room temperature if the shelf life is only 2 weeks.

[2]Abaxis Vet Scan (Abaxis, Union City, California).

[3]VetScan i-STAT 1 (AbbottPointOfCare.com, Princeton, New Jersey, www.AbbottPointOfCare.com).

[4]International Technidyne Corporation, Edison (New Jersey, www.itcmed.com/products/irma-trupoint-blood-analysis-system).

- The i-STAT 1 is marketed by Abaxis and measures the same analytes as the previous i-STAT, with the addition of cardiac troponin I (cTn-I), an expanded Chem 8, and activated clotting time (ACT) and prothrombin time.
- This system has been extensively used during the past several years with accurate and uniform results, except for Hct, which is sometimes falsely low. Hemoglobin (Hgb) is also measured.
- Hct and plasma protein, actually total solids, are best measured with a microhematocrit centrifuge and a refractometer. A variety of cartridges are available for the i-STAT (approximate cost, $7 to $16 USD each except for cTn-I which is $27 USD).
- The most useful test kits are the following:
  - i-STAT CG8+—Na^+, K^+, glucose, P_{O_2}, S_{O_2} (oxygen saturation), P_{CO_2}, T_{CO_2} (total carbon dioxide), HCO_3^-, pH, ionized Ca^+, base excess (BE)*
  - i-STAT EC8+—K^+, Na^+, Cl^-, pH, P_{CO_2}, P_{O_2}, T_{CO_2}, HCO_3^-, BE, glucose, anion gap, blood urea nitrogen (BUN)*
  - i-STAT 6+—K^+, Na^+, Cl^-, blood urea nitrogen (BUN), glucose*
  - i-STAT 4+—pH, P_{CO_2}, P_{O_2}, lactate, HCO_3^-, T_{CO_2}, SaO_2, BE
  - i-STAT 3+—Na^+, K^+, Cl^{-*}
  - i-STAT Crea—creatinine—*be careful comparing with automated methods because the value is often different by 0.1 to 0.3 mg/dL in healthy horses and foals.*
  - i-STAT cTn-I—Cardiac troponin I is available on the new i-STAT 1 analyzer; elevations in cTn-I are specific for myocardial injury. The initial value has some prognostic importance, but the change in value over time is most important!
  - i-STAT CHEM 8+—BUN, creatinine, ionized Ca^+, glucose, Na^+, K^+, Cl^- available on new i-STAT 1 analyzer
  - i-STAT G—glucose
  - ACT—activated clotting time—normal range needs to be validated for the horse
- The portable clinical analyzer performed similarly to the benchtop blood gas analyzer for evaluation of lactate and glucose concentrations, but not pH, in synovial fluid.
- The older i-STAT equipment has been phased out and replaced by the i-STAT 1; service for the older machines may not be available after 2012.
  Practice Tip: A basic interpretation of blood gas results is provided in Table 15-1.

Glucose

- Changes in glucose regulation are well documented in equine critical care.
- *Practice Tip: Direction and degree of alteration is associated with illness severity and prognosis.*
- Point-of-care glucometry is historically inaccurate relative to reference chemistry values in horses and foals.
- A major limitation of glucometry is the predominance of human glucometer use in veterinary medicine.

Table 15-1	Primary Classification of Acid-Base Disorders and Expected Alterations in Blood Gas Parameters	
Acid-Base Disorder	**Primary Change**	**Compensatory Change**
Respiratory acidosis, $P_{CO_2} > 46$ mm Hg	$\uparrow P_{CO_2}$	$\uparrow HCO_3^-$
Respiratory alkalosis, $P_{CO_2} < 36$ mm Hg	$\downarrow P_{CO_2}$	$\downarrow HCO_3^-$
Metabolic acidosis, $HCO_3^- < 22$ mEq/L	$\downarrow HCO_3^-$	$\downarrow P_{CO_2}$
Metabolic alkalosis, $HCO_3^- > 28$ mEq/L	$\uparrow HCO_3^-$	$\uparrow P_{CO_2}$

- Human glucometers contain algorithms that improve measurement accuracy of whole blood glucose in this species-specific population.
- A major species difference, affecting accuracy of whole blood glucose measurement with a glucometer designed for humans, is the intracellular to plasma glucose ratio.
- Veterinary-specific glucometers allow accurate whole blood glucose measurement in a variety of species.
- A veterinary glucometer, AlphaTRAK,[5] is validated for healthy and critically ill horses and foals. This glucometer uses 0.3 μL of whole blood with results in 25 seconds. Assure Chronimed, Inc.[6] and Accu-Chem[7] are two other instruments used to measure blood glucose. These test instruments appear to be accurate at predicting severity of hypoglycemia but may *not* have the same accuracy in reporting the level of hyperglycemia. Glucose also can be measured with the i-STAT.

Lactate

- Increases in blood lactate are used in equine critical care as a marker of disease severity and prognosis.
- Reports document blood lactate derangements in critically ill adults and foals with:
  - Sepsis
  - Gastrointestinal accidents
  - Other disease etiologies
- Lactate measurement can be performed with a point-of-care device—Accutrend—validated in critically ill horses. This lactate meter uses less than 20 μL of whole blood or plasma and provides results within 60 seconds.
- Lactate can also be measured quickly (1 minute), accurately, and inexpensively using the Lactate Pro.[8]
- Whole blood or cellular samples (i.e., peritoneal fluid) should be measured within 30 minutes, or the lactate may increase from sample storage.

[5]AlphaTRAK1 (Abbott Laboratories, Abbott Park, Illinois, www.alphatrakmeter.com).
[6]Assure Chronimed, Inc., Minnetonka, Minnesota, www.pointofcare.net.
[7]Accu-Chem Boehringer Ingelheim Corp., Ingelheim, Germany, www.boehringeringelheim.com.
[8]Lactate Pro (Veterinary Supply, Inc. 800-330-1522).

- *Practice Tip:* *When peritoneal fluid lactate is increased and above the value found in blood, this is an indicator of intestinal strangulation.*
- It is recommended that plasma lactate be used more reliably to evaluate trends in serial lactate measurements.
- Transient elevations in lactate are commonly seen in early life in neonatal foals; however, decreases to adult levels are expected by 24 to 72 hours.
- *Practice Tip:* *Elevations in lactate are present in most critically ill horses; the initial value* and *the change in lactate concentration following appropriate treatment/resuscitation can both indicate prognosis!*

Cardiac Troponin

- *Practice Tip:* *Elevation of cardiac-specific troponin I (cTn-I) is an indicator of myocardial injury, and changes in the protein provide diagnostic and prognostic information.*
- Cardiac injury in horses can be secondary to:
  - Myocarditis
  - Sepsis
  - Rattlesnake envenomation
  - Cantharidin intoxication
  - Other causes—primary or secondary to multiple organ dysfunction syndrome (MODS)
- A point-of-care analyzer capable of measuring cTn-I is validated in horses, both in horses with normal values and in those with experimental monensin intoxication resulting in cardiac disease.
- The ELISA analyzer (VetScan i-STAT 1) uses 17 μL of plasma or plasma fraction of whole blood with results in 10 minutes. This point-of-care analyzer is commonly used in equine hospitals. The cTn-I measurement cartridge increases its utility and is equivalent to a benchtop immunoassay for cTn-I. Normal range of cTn-I for this analyzer is 0.0 to 0.06 ng/mL in horses. This analyzer has a reportable range of up to 50 ng/mL; however, performance has *not* been evaluated at levels above 35 ng/mL.

Bench Chemistry Analyzers

A number of small, easy-to-use bench chemistry analyzers are available for equine practice and use heparinized whole blood, serum, or plasma. All analyzers provide results within minutes.

- IDEXX Vet Test Chemistry Analyzer[9] has an equine health profile—albumin, aspartate aminotransferase (AST), BUN, Ca^{2+}, creatine kinase (CK), creatinine, gamma-glutamyltransferase (GGT), glucose, lactate dehydrogenase, total bilirubin, total protein—and additional single slide test for some additional analytes that can be useful in equine practice (Mg^{2+}, NH_3, P, lactate, and triglyceride). One advantage of this machine is the ability to measure blood ammonia; however, it must be performed within 10 to 15 minutes after collection.

- IDEXX VetStat Electrolyte and Blood Gas Analyzer[10] can provide results of single use *cassettes*.
- Heska SpotChem EZ[11] has panels and individual tests. This instrument can be used to measure albumin, AST, BUN, total Ca^{2+}, CK, creatinine, GGT, glucose, Mg^{2+}, P^+, K^+, total bilirubin, total protein, and triglycerides.
- Abaxis VetScan[12] has an equine profile plus with albumin, AST, BUN, Ca^{2+}, CK, creatinine, GGT, globulin, glucose, K^+, Na^+, total bilirubin, Tco_2, and total protein.

Complete Blood Cell Count (CBC)

- There are automated systems for determining equine total white blood cell count and differential counts, red cell count and indexes, and platelet count.
- One instrument is the Vet ABC-Diff Hematology Analyzer,[13] previously marketed by Heska or their newer HemaTrue Hematology Analyzer.[14]
- IDEXX has the LaserCyte or ProCyte[15] and Abaxis the VetScan HM5 Hematology System,[16] which also uses small volumes of blood combined with ethylenediaminetetraacetic acid (EDTA) with results in minutes.
- The hemogram machines have special cards that are inserted to improve accuracy in testing equine CBCs.
- Mean corpuscular volume (MCV), red blood cell distribution width (RDW), and mean platelet volumes (MPVs) are reported with at least the ProCyte and VetScan, which can be helpful in determining if an anemia or thrombocytopenia is regenerative.
- Platelet counts on the machines may be underreported; however, the ProCyte does report if there is clumping. One can detect platelet clumps by examining the feathered edge of the blood film. If platelet clumping is causing a pseudothrombocytopenia, which is *not* uncommon in equine EDTA samples, clumps of platelets are seen along with any other large components of the blood at the feathered edge.
- The ability of machines to accurately perform differential counts and total counts on synovial or peritoneal and pleural fluid must be confirmed.[17]
- Identification of immature neutrophils, toxic neutrophils, *Anaplasma phagocytophilum* (Figs. 15-1 and 15-2), or neoplastic cells must be identified by microscopic examination. The Diff-Quik stain is the best method of staining cells for this type of examination.
- Fibrinogen can be measured by an automated system using the VetScan VSpro[18] in less than 15 minutes and is

---

[9]IDEXX Vet Test Chemistry Analyzer (IDEXX Laboratories, Westbrook, Maine).

[10]IDEXX VetStat Electrolyte and Blood Gas Analyzer (IDEXX Laboratories, Westbrook, Maine).

[11]Heska SpotChem EZ (Heska, Loveland, Colorado).

[12]Abaxis VetScan (Abaxis, Union City, California).

[13]Vet ABC-Diff Hematology Analyzer (Heska, Loveland, Colorado).

[14]HemaTrue Hematology Analyzer (Heska, Loveland, Colorado).

[15]LaserCyte or ProCyte (IDEXX Laboratories, Westbrook, Maine).

[16]VetScan HM5 Hematology System (Abaxis, Union City, California).

[17]The Forcythe hematology analyzer (generation III) has been evaluated for measuring WBC counts in peritoneal and joint fluids. (Oxford Science Inc., Oxford, Connecticut.)

[18]VetScan VSpro (Abaxis, Union City, California).

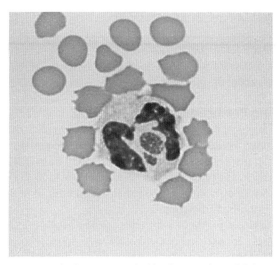

Figure 15-1 Wright-Giemsa stain of a blood smear of an adult horse from northern Virginia with fever and leg edema. The light blue bodies in the neutrophil are *Anaplasma phagocytophilum* morulae.

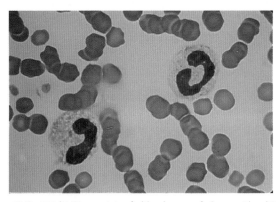

Figure 15-2 Wright-Giemsa stain of a blood smear of a horse with colitis. The lower neutrophil is curved and nonsegmented (a band neutrophil), and the cytoplasm of both neutrophils has foamy vacuolation and purplish-staining granules (toxic granulation), suggesting severe toxemia.

portable for out of the hospital use. It can also measure prothrombin time (PT) and partial thromboplastin time (PTT).

- Another method for measuring fibrinogen is using microhematocrit tubes and a refractometer. Two tubes of the same blood sample are tested: one after spinning; and the other after spinning, heating for 2 minutes at 58° C, and spinning again. *The difference between the two is the fibrinogen.* Example: If the first tube reads 7.2 g/dL and the heated tube reads 7.0 g/dL, this equates to 200 mg/dL of fibrinogen.
- Serum amyloid A (SAA): An acute phase hepatic-derived protein can be measured at the acute phase protein laboratory University of Miami (800-596-7390) in the United States or using a convenient on-site benchtop testing in Europe (Equinostic[19]).
- The advantages of SAA are:
  - Very low values in normal horses/foals (0 to 30 mg/L)

- Dramatic elevations (often 100×) within 6 hours, peaking at 24 to 36 hours after acute local or systemic inflammation
- Samples are very stable at room temperature or when refrigerated for several days.
- SAA increases with tissue trauma (e.g., postsurgery), but SAA is *not* supposed to increase with recurrent airway obstruction (RAO).
  Practice Tip: One possible disadvantage in measuring SAA is its sensitivity to inflammation; elevations may not *be clinically significant in some horses.*

Urinalysis

- Multiple commercially available urinary test strips, such as Multistix[20] and Chemstrip,[21] may be used to identify leukocytes, protein (may be falsely elevated in some horses), pH, blood (hemoglobin or myoglobin), bilirubin, and glucose.
- A refractometer may be used to determine specific gravity.

Osmometer

- An osmometer can be used to accurately determine osmotic pressure, which is the principal force opposing the exit of fluid from the vascular space.
- A small benchtop Colloid Osmometer[22] is commonly used for determining osmotic pressure in equine patients. The machine must be calibrated before every test and should be flushed just before using. This can be useful if colloids are being administered because their administration does *not* allow accurate measurement of osmotic pressure by refractometer determination of total solids (TS).
- *Practice Tip: Normal osmotic pressure in the adult horse is 20 to 22 mm Hg and slightly less in the foal—18 to 20 mm Hg. If colloids have* not *been used, a TS measurement of 7.0 is comparable to an osmotic pressure of 21 mm Hg; this can vary depending on the albumin/globulin ratio, which also affects the osmotic pressure.*
- Discolored plasma, high glucose, and high urea increase TS values, resulting in a falsely elevated protein measurement.
- *Practice Tip: The TS of 6% hetastarch is 3.2, and osmotic pressure is 30 mm Hg; the osmotic pressure of 25% albumin is 70 mm Hg.*

Coagulation Analyzer

- An easy-to-use machine, SCA2000,[23] has been used for rapid determination of PT.
- *Practice Tip: Normal values on fresh whole blood: PT = 12 to 18 seconds and PTT = 97 to 137 seconds. Citrated whole blood: PT = 14 to 22 seconds; PTT = 131 to 199 seconds.*

---

[19]Equinostic (Copenhagen, Denmark).

[20]Multistix (Bayer Corporation, Pittsburgh, Pennsylvania, www.bayerus.com).

[21]Chemstrip (Roche Diagnostics Corporation, Indianapolis, Indiana, www.poc.roche.com).

[22]Colloid Osmometer (Wescor, Logan, Utah).

[23]SCA2000 by Synbiotics (Lyon Cedex, France, and IDEXX).

- Activated clotting time can be measured on the i-STAT 1 but is *only* prolonged with severe (95%) factor deficiencies. Prothrombin time cartridges have recently been introduced and validation in horses is needed.
- Platelet aggregometry (PF-100) can be performed in horses, but reference ranges are wide; 60.5 to 115.9 seconds with collagen-ADP cartridges.

Foal Immunoglobulin

- Semiquantitative measures of foal IgG are commonly in use in hospitals and on farms to determine success of passive transfer.
- The SNAP test foal IgG ELISA[24] is used with serum or whole blood, obtaining results in <10 minutes. The interpretation of the test depends on color change and provides a 400 mg/dL and 800 mg/dL calibration spot in addition to a color change for unknown sample. This device is more accurate in the measurement of IgG concentrations <400 mg/dL or >800 mg/dL; intermediate concentrations are less accurate than those measured by radial immunodiffusion assay.
- A quantitative IgG assay[25] for use in foals allows a more precise prediction of passive transfer and does *not* rely on color change interpretation. This system uses a turbidimetric immunoassay and is highly correlated with the radial immunodiffusion assay—the gold standard of measurement. The test requires separation of plasma from whole blood and measures a small volume of plasma (25 μL), with results in 15 minutes, including preparation time.
- *Practice Tip: There are faster methods of analysis, allowing quicker foal treatment compared with the radial immunodiffusion assay, which requires approximately 24 hours for results under laboratory conditions.*

Colostrometer

- *Practice Tip: Colostrometers are useful in equine medicine within 24 hours of foaling and are used to both evaluate individual mares in preventing inadequate passive transfer and for colostrum harvest and storage.*
- The JorVet Equine Colostrometer[26] uses 15 mL of colostrum and compares its weight to that of distilled water in a column to determine specific gravity.
- A considerably smaller quantity of colostrum is needed to evaluate specific gravity using an equine colostrum refractometer.[27] The equine colostrum refractometer is highly portable and uses only a few drops of colostrum. This colostrometer reports specific gravity (Brix%) and gives a colostrum quality assessment of very good, good, fair, or poor, relative to the inferred colostral IgG concentration. The refractometer also allows adjustments for temperature compensation within an operational range of 10° to 30° C (50° to 86° F).

Foaling Prediction

- A foaling predictor test is used to help predict time of foaling, based on changes in colostral electrolytes that occur just before foaling. Several products are available for this test. The FoalWatch kit[28] uses 1.5 mL of milk and 9 mL of distilled water mixed together with a drop of indicator solution in a titret ampule.
- *Practice Tip: Mares with milk calcium >200 to 250 ppm (mg/L) are likely to foal within 24 to 72 hours.*
- Another foaling predictor test is the Predict-A-Foal kit,[29] using 3 to 4 drops of milk and a water hardness color change strip to predict foaling within 12 hours.
- Foal prediction tests do *not* use sufficient quantities of milk to raise concerns of colostrum deprivation of foals.
- These are not good predictors of time for delivery in mares with placentitis.

IDEXX 3-4 DX

- The IDEXX 3DX or 4DX[30] can be used to detect antibody against *Borrelia burgdorferi*; results should be read at 8 minutes after initiating the SNAP test. Any light blue color should be considered a positive test result.
- A 4DX is now available and includes antibody testing for *Anaplasma phagocytophilum*. This test may not be highly sensitive in the early clinical disease in horses because 7 or more days may be required after infection in order for IgM antibodies to develop.

Tox A/B Quik Chek

- The Tox A/B Quik Chek[31] can be used for rapid (25 minutes) detection of *Clostridium difficile* toxins A or B in feces.
- Gram stains can be used to determine type of organism present in samples such as tracheal wash and pleural fluid.

Fecal Occult Blood Test

- Equine feces can be tested quickly for blood using kits called SUCCEED.[32]
- Results are available in 5 minutes.
- There can be some false results for either hemoglobin or albumin.
- Many other test tablets are available for use in detecting occult blood in feces.

[24]SNAP test foal IgG ELISA (IDEXX Laboratories, Westbrook, Maine, www.idexx.com/view/xhtml/en_us/equine/in-house-diagnostics/snap-tests/foal-igg.jsf?SSOTOKEN=0).

[25]IgG assay (Animal Reproduction Systems, Chino, California, http://arssales.com/equine).

[26]JorVet Equine Colostrometer (Jorgensen Laboratories, Loveland, Colorado, www.jorvet.com).

[27]Equine colostrum refractometer (Animal Reproduction Systems, Chino, California, http://arssales.com/equine).

[28]FoalWatch kit (CHEMetrics, Calverton, Virginia, www.chemetrics.com/instructions/i1700.pdf).

[29]Predict-A-Foal kit (Animal Reproduction Systems, Chino, California, http://arssales.com/equine).

[30]IDEXX 3DX or 4DX (IDEXX Laboratories, Westbrook, Maine).

[31]Tox A/B Quik Chek (Inverness Medical, Princeton, New Jersey).

[32]SUCCEED (Freedom Health, LLC, Aurora, Ohio).

Blood Gas Interpretation
See Table 15-1 for the classification of acid-base disorders and the expected alterations in blood gas parameters.

Respiratory Compensation for Metabolic Acid-Base Disturbances
- Prompt
- Often dramatic changes in P_{CO_2}

Metabolic Compensation for Respiratory Acid-Base Disorders
- Hours to days
- Dramatic changes in HCO_3^- are *not* likely.

- A primary disorder (look at pH) with proper compensation has HCO_3^- and P_{CO_2} changing in the same direction. The pH does *not* fully return to normal and may or may not be restored to a normal range.
- HCO_3^- and P_{CO_2} values moving in opposite directions is suggestive of a primary metabolic and respiratory disturbance.

References
References can be found on the companion website at www.equine-emergencies.com.

PART II

Emergency Examination and Management of Organ Systems

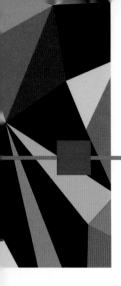

SECTION I   Body and Organ Systems

CHAPTER 16

Blood Coagulation Disorders

SallyAnne L. Ness

- As the complex interactions between the cellular and vascular contributions to coagulation become increasingly recognized, the traditional coagulation cascade should be considered one of several components of coagulation, rather than the precise order by which clotting is achieved.
- The perennial historical perspective of coagulation provided by Dr. Rudolf Virchow in 1845 views the general rules of coagulation as being:
  - A disruption of the vascular integrity
  - Changes in the hemodynamics or stasis of blood flow
  - Changes in the concentration of substances that promote and/or inhibit coagulation
- Recognition of components such as antithrombin III; proteins C and S; and homeostasis between tissue and platelet activators and inhibitors is pivotal to understanding the myriad of coagulation participants that respond to the activation process, subsequent coagulation, fibrinolysis, and anticoagulation.
- Coagulation disorders are represented by the following:
  - Hypercoagulation (thrombosis)
  - Hypocoagulation (bleeding diathesis)
- A normal coagulation system can be present in the presence of a hemorrhagic crisis because of physical disruption of the vascular integrity, as in external trauma or spontaneous internal vascular rupture—aortic root rupture, uterine artery hemorrhage, or guttural pouch mycosis.
- Initial assessment of the bleeding patient should aim to differentiate between *vessel injury* or *vascular disease* and *systemic coagulopathy* leading to bleeding diathesis.
- *Practice Tip: In horses, thrombotic disorders are more common than hemorrhagic diatheses.*
- Inflammation and sepsis are known initiators of systemic coagulation pathways via activation of the intrinsic coagulation cascade by circulating proinflammatory mediators such as:
  - Endotoxin
  - Tumor necrosis factor–alpha (TNF-α)
  - Lipoproteins
  - Growth factors
- Activation of endothelial cells and circulating monocytes stimulates the expression of tissue factor, an important

initiator of thrombin formation in both health and disease.
- In the septic patient, systemic hypercoagulability is potentiated by an overall reduction in endogenous anticoagulant factors including:
  - Antithrombin III (AT-III)
  - Tissue factor pathway inhibitor (TFPI)
  - Activated protein C (aPC)

Hypercoagulation: Thrombophilia and Thrombosis

- Hypercoagulation is common in horses and is associated with:
  - Abnormally elevated platelet counts (thrombocytosis)
  - Arteritis (cranial mesenteric arteritis)
  - Vasculitis (purpura hemorrhagica)
  - Idiopathic iliac thrombosis
  - Spontaneous or sepsis-associated limb arterial thrombosis in foals
  - Laminitis
  - Pulmonary infarction
  - Deficiencies of antithrombin III and protein C or protein S cofactors
  - Inhibition of fibrinolysis
  - Consumptive coagulopathies (disseminated intravascular coagulation [DIC]).
- DIC can exhibit laboratory evidence of hypocoagulation (prolonged clotting times and thrombocytopenia) while the individual has clinical evidence of hypercoagulation, thrombophilia, and no overt signs of bleeding.
- Thrombophlebitis in horses frequently occurs as a sequela to systemic inflammation and loss of antithrombin III following:
  - Endotoxemia
  - *Salmonella* and other causes of infectious colitis
  - Nonsteroidal anti-inflammatory drug (NSAID) toxicity
  - Pleuritis
  - Toxic metritis
  - Large colon volvulus
  - Following intravenous administration of irritating or hypertonic solutions (phenylbutazone, enrofloxacin).

Hypocoagulation: Bleeding Disorder and Diathesis Tendencies

- Hypocoagulation in the horse can be associated with:
  - Thrombocytopenia (immune mediated or acquired)
  - Thrombasthenia (abnormal platelet function)
  - Toxicosis (warfarin/anticoagulant rodenticides toxicity, moxalactam and related antibiotics)
  - Inherited disorders (hemophilia A, von Willebrand disease)
  - Primary fibrinolysis (hyperplasminemia)
- It also occurs in advanced DIC as a consumptive coagulopathy with secondary fibrinolysis.
- Rapid volume replacement with hetastarch and/or crystalloid fluids following severe blood loss can result in dilution of coagulation factors and loss of normal hemostatic ability.
- Bleeding disorders can be acute or chronic.

Clinical Signs of Hemorrhage and Thrombosis

- Obvious clinical signs of thrombosis or hemorrhage can be *inapparent* because of skin pigmentation and hair coat.
- Clinical signs suggestive of primary hemostatic defects (platelet and von Willebrand factor disorders) include petechial or ecchymotic hemorrhage of the mucous membranes and conjunctiva. Epistaxis also may occur.
- Clinical signs suggestive of secondary hemostatic defects (coagulopathies) include:
  - Hematoma formation
  - Hemarthrosis
  - Intracavitary hemorrhage
- Vascular thrombosis may result in partial or complete ischemia of tissues supplied by the affected vessels (e.g., limb arterial thrombosis in septicemic foals).
- The full extent of thrombotic lesions may be inapparent until identified at surgery or postmortem examination.
- Antemortem diagnosis can be established with ultrasound identification of intravascular clot formation or with Doppler ultrasound detection of decreased blood flow.
- Thrombophilia manifests clinically as:
  - Jugular thrombosis
  - Asymmetric cold limbs (saddle thrombus)
  - Hypothermic lameness during increased exercise
  - The presence of regional edema in conjunction with petechial or ecchymotic hemorrhage (purpura, vasculitis)
- Thrombophilia may be associated with acute hemolytic anemias.

◆◆ WHAT TO DO

Coagulopathy with Blood Loss

- Treatments are principally aimed at the following:
  - Volume replacement with crystalloids including hypertonic saline
  - Colloids such as whole blood, plasma, and hetastarch. **Note:** Hetastarch is contraindicated in patients with evidence of hypocoagulability.

- An acute bleed is commonly accompanied by changes in vital signs—tachycardia, tachypnea, and hypothermia—and pale mucous membranes.
- Peracute aortic root rupture with collapse and death usually occurs in stallions during or after breeding.
- Uterine-ovarian artery rupture is most often acute and can occur before or after parturition.
- A subcutaneous hematoma may follow trauma or spontaneous hemorrhage.
- Ultrasound evaluation of body cavities or acute subcutaneous swellings may show the presence of extraneous "swirling smoke" fluid indicative of free blood within a space (Fig. 16-1).
- Epistaxis, genitourinary hemorrhage, melena, and petechial or ecchymotic lesions may be present.
- Overt epistaxis can be caused by exercise-induced pulmonary hemorrhage (EIPH), guttural pouch mycosis, ethmoidal hematoma, sinusitis, trauma, and coagulation deficiencies, including thrombocytopenia.

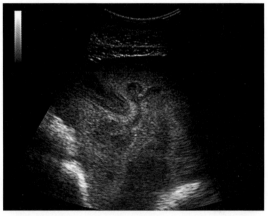

Figure 16-1 Ultrasound image of a hemoabdomen in a horse with warfarin toxicity demonstrating characteristic "swirling smoke" appearance of blood within a body cavity.

Laboratory Assessment of Coagulation

- The following laboratory tests are available for evaluation of hemostasis in the equine patient. Screening tests are categorized into:
  - Tests of primary hemostasis (platelet plug formation)
  - Tests of secondary hemostasis
    - Tests of fibrin clot formation and breakdown (fibrinolysis)
- The following specialized tests may necessitate referral of samples to a research laboratory following consultation:
  - Coagulation factors
  - von Willebrand disease
  - Antibody-coated platelet
  - Protein assays
- *Note:* If known laboratory values are not available, a normal control sample is recommended to aid in the interpretation of individual results.
- Platelet counts:
  - False platelet aggregation can occur in ethylenediaminetetraacetic acid (EDTA) and therefore may necessitate sample collection in sodium citrate for quantitative counts.

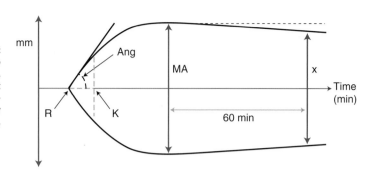

Figure 16-2 Typical thromboelastogram with measured parameters: R = time to the initiation of clot formation, K = time for the tracing to achieve a set clot strength, Ang = Angle, the rate of clot formation, MA = maximum amplitude, the greatest clot strength, χ = clot strength at 60 minutes after MA, CL60 = 100× (χ/MA). (From Epstein, KL et al: Thromboelastography in 26 healthy horses with and without activation by recombinant human tissue factor, *J Vet Emerg Crit Care* 19(1): 96-101, 2009.)

- A scan of a hematologic slide for adequate platelet numbers by a laboratory technician is accurate in detecting inadequate numbers. ***Practice Tip:*** *At least 10 platelets per high-powered field (magnification: ×1000) is considered adequate if clumping of platelets is* not *observed.*
- Template bleeding time:
  - In vivo evaluation of primary hemostasis and platelet plug formation following vascular injury.
  - The hair distolateral to the accessory carpal bone is clipped and a template bleeding device is used to produce a small incision.
  - Filter paper is used to absorb blood 1 to 2 mm below the incision site.
  - Timing starts when the incision is made and ends when bleeding stops; reported normal bleeding time for healthy horses ranges from 2 to 6 minutes, and may be prolonged with both quantitative—thrombocytopenia—and qualitative—von Willebrand disease, Glanzmann thrombasthenia—disorders.
- Platelet function analysis (PFA-100[1]):
  - A point-of-care assay validated in horses for evaluation of primary hemostasis. Cartridges coated in collagen and ADP activate platelets and simulate platelet adhesion and aggregation after vascular injury.
  - The PFA-100 is able to identify inherited, acquired, and drug-induced thrombocytopathies, including functional disorders in which platelet counts may be normal—von Willebrand disease, Glanzmann thrombasthenia—and can be used to monitor response to aspirin therapy.
- Activated clotting time (ACT):
  - Point-of-care evaluation of secondary hemostasis, specifically the intrinsic and common pathways
  - Deficiencies in factors V, VIII, IX, X, XI, XII, prothrombin (factor II), or fibrinogen result in prolonged ACT.
- Activated partial thromboplastin time (aPTT):
  - Point-of-care evaluation of secondary hemostasis, specifically the intrinsic and common pathways
  - Similar to evaluation by ACT but with higher sensitivity
  - Deficiencies in factors V, VIII, IX, X, XI, XII, prothrombin (factor II) or fibrinogen result in prolonged aPTT.

- Can be used to monitor heparin therapy with the goal to prolong the aPTT to 1.5 times pretreatment baseline levels.
- Prothrombin time (PT):
  - Aids in the evaluation of the extrinsic coagulation system, specifically the extrinsic and common pathways and their ability to convert fibrinogen to fibrin
  - Deficiencies in tissue factor (factor III), factors V, VII, X, prothrombin, or fibrinogen result in prolonged PT.
  - Often used to detect or monitor vitamin K antagonist anticoagulants (e.g., warfarin, [Coumadin])
- Fibrinogen:
  - Quantification of fibrinogen can be performed by means of heat precipitation, fibrometer, or point-of-care automated analyzer (VetScan VSpro[2]).
  - Decreased fibrinogen levels may be observed with DIC, but this is a less sensitive test in horses compared with other species.
- Fibrin degradation products (FDPs):
  - Evaluation of primary (fibrinogenolysis without clot formation) or secondary (clot dissolution) fibrinolysis.
  - Elevated FDP concentrations suggest increased fibrinogenolysis or fibrinolysis activity, and may be observed with DIC, severe inflammatory processes, and hemorrhagic disorders.
- D-dimers:
  - End product of fibrinolysis
  - D-dimers are released following cleavage of fibrin bonds by plasmin.
  - Differs from FDPs in that it is specific for fibrinolysis (i.e., dissolution of fibrin generated from active thrombin production).
  - Elevated D-dimers are common in foals <1 week of age, presumably due to resolution of umbilical vessel clots.
- Thromboelastography (TEG):
  - A point-of-care hemostatic assay that records changes in the viscoelastic properties of whole blood from initiation of clot formation through fibrinolysis (Fig. 16-2).
  - It can detect both hypocoagulopathies and hypercoagulopathies and may be a more accurate representation of

[1]PFA-100 (Dade-Behring, Newark, Delaware).

[2]VetScan VSpro (Abaxis, Union City, California).

global in vivo hemostasis than traditional coagulation assays, which only evaluate isolated components of the coagulation cascade and do not incorporate contributing cellular elements.

- Specific activators such as tissue factor or kaolin may be added to expedite coagulation.
- Hemoscopic TEG PlateletMapping is a modified TEG assay designed specifically to assess platelet function.
- Polycythemia has been shown to induce hypocoagulabilty on TEG without concurrent changes in other coagulation parameters, and dilution of plasma coagulation factors by increased red cell mass may be an important confounder when interpreting TEG in horses with elevated hematocrits.
- TEG reference intervals vary significantly among different laboratories and personnel.

Blood Clotting Disorders

Thrombocytopenia

- Thrombocytopenia is not an uncommon clinical finding in equine practice and is usually associated with a severe systemic inflammatory response or as a result of immune-mediated platelet removal by the spleen.
- Infectious diseases such as infection with *Anaplasma* (formerly *Ehrlichia equi*) and equine infectious anemia (EIA) are commonly associated with thrombocytopenia.
- The autoimmune phenomena can result from:
  - Viral infection
  - Abscessation
  - Neoplasia (especially hemangiosarcoma)
  - Colostral antibodies
  - Drug-associated causes
    ○ Trimethoprim-sulfa products are the most common offender
  - Idiopathic causes
- If thrombocytopenia occurs in conjunction with autoimmune hemolytic anemia (a positive result on Coombs test), the disorder is known as Evans syndrome and is more commonly associated with a primary neoplasia or abscess.
- An unusual thrombocytopenia (often severe) with oral vesicles and skin lesions has been reported in foals and appears to be an immune reaction to colostral antibodies.
- A low platelet count can be evident on a blood smear or by absolute count.
- *Practice Tip:* Petechiation typically is observable with platelet counts in the 40,000 to 60,000 per microliter range. A more serious bleed (epistaxis) can occur in the 10,000 to 20,000 per microliter range, and life-threatening hemorrhage can develop at less than 10,000 per microliter.
- Blood samples can be tested at specialized laboratories such as Kansas State University (www.vet.ksu.edu/depts/dmp/service/immunology/index.htm) for antibody-coated platelets and/or a regenerative platelet response, reticulated (messenger RNA) platelets.

  ○ Increased mean platelet volume (MPV) reported on some hematology analyzers is another indication of regenerative platelet response
- The platelet count can be normal during clinical evidence of bleeding if the underlying disorder is related to platelet function rather than quantity (e.g., Glanzmann thrombasthenia, von Willebrand disease, drug-induced thrombocytopathy [aspirin-induced bleeding has not been reported among horses]).

●〉 WHAT TO DO

Thrombocytopenia

- Most foals with colostral-associated thrombocytopenia recover with or without steroid therapy. Stall confinement until platelet counts are above 40,000 per microliter is recommended.
- Management of platelet autoimmune deficiencies consists primarily of administration of corticosteroids. Dexamethasone is considered the most effective drug as long as caution is practiced regarding an associated laminitis. Doses may vary from a low of 10 mg to a high of 80 mg per adult, preferably administered intravenously with a 20-gauge needle or per os (PO) every 12 or 24 hours as divided doses.
- Azathioprine, 3 mg/kg PO q24h, can be used for refractory cases or when steroids are contraindicated. Alternatively, azathioprine can be used in addition to dexamethasone when platelet counts are extremely low (<10,000 per microliter).
- *Practice Tip: For severe thrombocytopenia believed to be immune mediated, both drugs can be used simultaneously!*
- Platelet counts should be measured every 3 to 6 days until numbers reach levels consistent with near-normal values, and then steroid administration can be tapered. In suspected cases of immune-mediated platelet destruction (e.g., those with splenomegaly), the use of vincristine, 0.004 mg/kg (2 mg/450 kg horse) IV weekly, can be combined with the steroid, q24h for 3 to 5 days, twice a week for 1 to 2 weeks, and finally once a week until the platelet counts are stable, to increase platelet release from the bone marrow.
- A plasma transfusion has been beneficial in some horses, allegedly as a source of blocking antibody. Plasma or whole blood collected in plastic bags provides a source of platelets that may inhibit bleeding. If the thrombocytopenia is a result of increased consumption, there is little benefit from the transfusion.
- Fresh frozen plasma may have hemostatically functional platelet microparticles.

Clinical Presentation

- Horses and foals with severe sepsis or systemic inflammatory syndrome frequently have moderately low platelet counts (50,000 to 80,000).
- Although an unfavorable prognostic finding, abnormal bleeding rarely occurs unless other coagulation parameters—PT, PTT, DIC—are abnormal.

Clotting Factor Deficiencies

- Clotting factor deficiencies are relatively uncommon among horses.
- Hemophilia A is the most common inherited disorder.
  - Foals with hemophilia A are usually colts (X-linked trait) that present with hemarthrosis of many joints or bleed excessively from minor wounds.

- The aPTT (intrinsic system) is prolonged, and factor VIII is deficient.
- Factor VIII–associated deficiency occurs with von Willebrand disease and is linked with qualitative deficiencies in platelet function that cause an increase in the in vivo bleeding time test results.
- Warfarin or warfarin-derivative anticoagulant toxicity in horses overdosed with Coumadin or with inadvertent access to rodenticide compounds produces clinical signs of bleeding related to antagonism of vitamin K–dependent factors (II, VII, IX, X). Prolonged therapy with exogenous vitamin K may be required, depending on the inciting compound. Generally both PT and PTT are prolonged with warfarin toxicity; however, only PT may be prolonged in the early stages of toxicity.
- Protein C is also vitamin K dependent. Some lactam and beta-lactam antibiotics, most notably moxalactam and carbenicillin, are capable of causing hypoprothrombinemia. Advanced liver disease often results in intrinsic and extrinsic factor deficiencies (see liver disease, Chapter 20, p. 268).

▶ WHAT TO DO

Coagulopathy
- Fresh frozen plasma is the preferred treatment.
- Vitamin K_1, 500 mg subcutaneously (SQ) q12-24h for an adult horse, is the required treatment for warfarin toxicity. *Do not administer intravenously.*

Disseminated Intravascular Coagulation (DIC)
- DIC is an acquired hypercoagulable syndrome characterized by the deposition of fibrin throughout the microvascular.
- DIC always occurs secondary to a primary disease process capable of inducing systemic activation of coagulation; including but not limited to:
  - Sepsis
  - Systemic inflammatory response syndrome
  - Endotoxemia
  - Trauma
  - Immune reaction
  - Multiple organ dysfunction (MODS) or failure
- DIC is a true consumptive coagulopathy and is associated with a poor prognosis.
- DIC can be acute or chronic and can be local or systemic.
- The full gamut of coagulation (activation, coagulation, fibrinolysis, and anticoagulation) may be present but is rarely proportional in horses, *with multisystemic thrombosis being the most prevalent clinical sign.*
- The diagnosis of DIC can be made by clinical evidence of hypercoagulation or hypocoagulation (or both) and some or all of the following laboratory abnormalities:
  - Prolonged activated coagulation time, PT, aPTT
  - Decreased platelet count and fibrinogen levels
  - Elevated levels of fibrin degradation products and/or D-dimers

- The level of antithrombin III (heparin cofactor) often is less than 60% to 70% of normal.
  - Deficiency of anticoagulant proteins C and S may also occur
- Microscopic examination of blood smears may show increased sheared red cells (schistocytes) consistent with a microangiopathic hemolytic anemia (MAHA).
- Occasionally in end-stage DIC, platelet and coagulation factor depletion produces clinical signs of bleeding; however, most cases of equine DIC are characterized by hypercoagulability and thrombophilia, and observed morbidity and mortality are generally the result of microvascular thrombosis and subsequent organ failure.

▶ WHAT TO DO

Disseminated Intravascular Coagulation
- Treat for the primary disorder, if known, and direct treatments that slow the consumptive process.
- Crystalloids and colloids are the mainstay of treatment. If there is evidence of bleeding (less common than thrombosis in the horse), high doses of hetastarch should *not* be used.
- Heparin in conjunction with normalizing plasma antithrombin III levels has traditionally been recommended at dosages of 40 to 80 IU/kg SQ or IV q6-8h. Subcutaneous dosing can result in local swelling, and unfractionated heparin has been associated with secondary anemia and thrombocytopenia. *Adverse heparin reactions are* not *known to occur with the use of low-molecular-weight heparins (dalteparin, 50 to 100 IU/kg SQ q24h; enoxaparin, 0.5 to 1 mg/kg [40 to 80 IU/kg] SQ q24h).*
- Blood and plasma transfusions are controversial in regard to adding "fuel to the fire" by providing additional components for the continuation of the consumptive process and infarctive thrombosis. However, absolute contraindications also are rare. If supported based on clinical or laboratory results, plasma transfusion is indicated whenever low antithrombin III levels are present or suspected.
- Treatment of DIC often is difficult and must be individualized to include the primary disorder. The prognosis is usually poor with systemic DIC.
- ***Note:*** The key word is *individualized treatment.*

Therapeutic Intervention of Hemostasis and Anticoagulation
- Medical therapies that affect the coagulation system are becoming increasingly available to practitioners. The choice of therapy will depend on the clinical diagnosis and the nature of the presenting coagulopathy. The following are potential therapies for various coagulation abnormalities in the equine patient:
  - Administer plasma products at 10 to 15 mL/kg IV.
  - Administer vitamin K_1 at 500 mg SQ q12-24h for warfarin toxicity. *Do not administer intravenously.*
  - Administer heparin at 40 to 80 IU/kg SQ or IV q6-8h. Subcutaneous dosing can result in local swelling, and unfractionated heparin has been associated with secondary anemia and thrombocytopenia. *Adverse heparin reactions are* not *known to occur with the use of low-molecular-weight heparins (dalteparin, 50 to 100 IU/kg*

SQ q24h; enoxaparin, 0.5 to 1 mg/kg [40 to 80 IU/kg] SQ q24h).

- Administer aspirin at 10 to 20 mg/kg PO or per rectum every other day (EOD). Aspirin is still one of the most common platelet inhibitors used in both human and equine medicine. Its effect is through inhibition of platelet arachidonic acid and thromboxane, which may stimulate platelet activation/aggregation. Although aspirin inhibits thromboxane in healthy horses, it may have an inconsistent effect on platelet aggregation in normal horses and a minimal effect in horses with inflammatory diseases.

- Administer platelet aggregation antagonist clopidogrel (Plavix), 2 mg/kg PO q24h, following a 4-mg/kg loading dose. Clopidogrel effectively decreases ADP-induced platelet aggregation in horses, and its therapeutic application for equine diseases associated with platelet activation (laminitis, thrombosis) is currently being evaluated.

- ***Practice Tip:*** *There are many activators of platelets in horses with inflammatory disease, and aspirin may inhibit collagen activation but not ADP and vice versa for clopidogrel. Therefore, both drugs could be used concurrently. When given orally, antiplatelet effects can be seen in less than 6* hours and persist for 2 or more days. Administer fibrinolysins—thrombolytics such as streptokinase, urokinase, and tissue plasminogen activator (TPA).

- Administer antifibrinolytic agents—plasminogen inhibitors such as epsilon-aminocaproic acid (Amicar), 5 to 20 g diluted IV q6-8h.

- Administer conjugated estrogen (Premarin), 25 to 50 mg slowly IV in saline/adult horse for uterine bleeding. Conjugated estrogens have occasionally been reported to be of value in decreasing chronic bleeding from sites other than the uterus. Mechanism of activity is unproven and is believed to increase factor VIII activity.

- Administer Yunnan Baiyao, 2 bottles (8 g) PO q12h. This is a traditional Chinese herbal medicine that has been used as a hemostatic drug for over 100 years. It has recently been shown in human patients to reduce postoperative hemorrhage; however, its efficacy in horses is unknown.

References

References can be found on the companion website at www.equine-emergencies.com.

Drs. Ness, Orsini, and Divers would like to acknowledge and thank Dr. Doug Byars for his contributions to this chapter in all previous editions of this book and to his generous sharing of knowledge in this and many other areas of equine medicine.

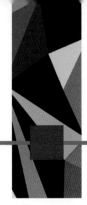

CHAPTER 17

Cardiovascular System

*Sophy A. Jesty** *

Physical Examination

- A complete cardiovascular examination of a horse includes:
  - Auscultation of the heart
  - Auscultation of both lung fields
  - Palpation of the precordium
  - Palpation of the arterial pulses
  - Evaluation of the venous system, mucous membranes, and capillary refill time
  - Overall assessment of the patient's health
- In the emergency setting, the horse usually is distressed, and only a resting examination is indicated. The patient's clinical condition should be assessed as quickly as possible so that the appropriate lifesaving treatment, if needed, can be instituted.

Auscultation of the Heart

- Auscultation of the heart is performed from both sides of the thorax.
  - Heart rate, rhythm
  - Intensity of heart sounds
  - Characterize murmurs or transient sounds associated with the cardiac cycle.
- Normal heart rate is 28 to 44 beats/min in an adult at rest and may be as high as 80 beats/min in a foal; the average for an equine neonate is 70 beats/min.
- *Practice Tip: The most common physiologic rhythm in horses is normal sinus rhythm.*
- *Practice Tip: Second-degree atrioventricular (AV) block is the most common vagally mediated arrhythmia detected in normal horses.*
- Sinus arrhythmia, sinus bradycardia, and sinoatrial (SA) block also occur in normal individuals with high resting vagal tone.
- Identify heart sounds, and characterize their timing and intensity. Up to four heart sounds can be auscultated in normal horses (Table 17-1).
- Auscult the heart over all four valve areas (Fig. 17-1).
- Characterize murmurs by their intensity, timing, duration, quality, point of maximal intensity, and radiation (Table 17-2).

Other Aspects of the Physical Examination

- Palpate the precordium over both sides of the chest to detect precordial thrills or abnormal apex beats—accentuated, faint, or displaced.
- Evaluate the arterial pulses simultaneously with cardiac auscultation to determine that they are synchronous with every heartbeat.
- Assess the quality of the arterial pulses in the facial or transverse facial artery and in the extremities.
- Evaluate the jugular vein, saphenous vein, and other peripheral veins for distention and pulsations.
- Perform auscultation of both lung fields at rest and, if possible, with the patient breathing into a rebreathing bag. The rebreathing bag should *not* be used if the horse is in severe respiratory distress.

Electrocardiogram

Diagnosis of rhythm disturbances is made with an electrocardiogram (ECG).

- Obtain a complete 6-lead or 12-lead ECG whenever possible (Table 17-3; Fig. 17-2). In an emergency, the base-apex lead may be all that is needed to accurately diagnose the rhythm disturbance present in the equine patient.
- The base-apex lead gives the clinician large, easy-to-analyze complexes, and the electrodes usually can be properly applied with minimal resistance from the horse.
- The base-apex lead can be easily obtained in a recumbent horse when obtaining a full 12-lead ECG may be difficult. The electrodes can be applied at the heart apex and the jugular groove on the same side of the patient if necessary.
- The base-apex lead is the best monitoring lead for radio-telemetry ECG systems, for continuous 24-hour Holter ECG monitoring, and for monitoring cardiac rhythms in critically ill patients, during antiarrhythmic therapy, or during pericardiocentesis.
- Transtelephonic ECG systems should be avoided if possible during an emergency. The clinician transmitting the ECG usually is not able to evaluate the ECG as it is being obtained because he or she does *not* see the ECG tracing. Instead, the clinician has to wait for the assessment of the person receiving the ECG to select an appropriate treatment.
- ECGs can be performed onsite using the i-Phone and the AliveCor heart monitor.[1] The ECG can be visualized immediately and emailed for consultation if needed.

*Acknowledging and thanking Virginia B. Reef for her contributions in previous editions of *Equine Emergencies*.

[1]Alivecor, Inc., Woodside, CA 94062.

Echocardiogram

- Diagnosis and assessment of the severity of valvular, pericardial, myocardial, or great vessel disease are made with an echocardiogram.
- If the horse is too distressed to stand for an echocardiogram, this diagnostic test can often be delayed until the horse is more stable. Signalment, history, and clinical examination are often enough to allow for the initiation of appropriate therapy without the immediate need for an echocardiogram.
- An echocardiogram reveals structural or functional changes to the heart.

Arrhythmias

Arrhythmias can be classified as bradyarrhythmias or tachyarrhythmias.

- Cardiac arrhythmias occur commonly in horses and rarely necessitate antiarrhythmic therapy.
- Certain cardiac arrhythmias, however, can be life threatening and necessitate emergency treatment.
- *Practice Tip: Rapid tachyarrhythmias and profound bradyarrhythmias are most likely to necessitate immediate*

CARDIO

Table 17-1	Equine Heart Sounds		
Sound	**Genesis**	**PMI**	**Quality**
S$_1$	Early ventricular contraction, abrupt deceleration of blood associated with tensing of the AV valve leaflets and AV valve closure, opening of the semilunar valves, and vibrations associated with ejection of blood into the great vessels	L apex	Loud, high frequency Longer, louder, lower pitch than S$_2$
S$_2$	Closure of the semilunar valves, abrupt deceleration of blood in the great vessels, opening of the AV	L base	Loud, high frequency Sharper, short, higher valves pitch than S$_1$
S$_3$	Rapid deceleration of blood in the ventricles at the end of the rapid ventricular filling phase	L apex	Soft, low frequency Lower pitch than S$_2$
S$_4$	Vibrations associated with blood flow from atria to ventricles during atrial contraction	L base	Soft, low frequency Lower pitch than S$_1$

AV, Atrioventricular; *L,* left; *PMI,* point of maximal intensity.

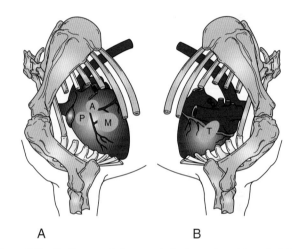

Figure 17-1 Cardiac auscultation areas in the horse viewed from the left **(A)** and the right **(B)** side of the thorax. *Shaded areas* represent the respective valve areas. *P,* Pulmonic valve; *A,* aortic valve; *M,* mitral valve; *T,* tricuspid valve.

Table 17-2	Characterization of the Common Equine Cardiac Murmurs					
Murmur	**Intensity (Grade)**	**Timing**	**Duration**	**Quality/Shape**	**PMI**	**Radiation**
Physiologic	1-2	S	E, M, L, HS	Low frequency	A, P, Mi, T	
(flow)	1-3	D	E, M, L	Decrescendo	A, P, Mi, T	
MR	1-6	S	HS, PS	Mixed, plateau	Mi A	DCa DCr
MVP	1-6	S	M-L	Crescendo	Mi	DCa
TR	1-6	S	HS, PS	Mixed, plateau	T	DCr, DCa
TVP	1-6	S	M-L	Crescendo	T	
AR	1-6	D	HD	Low frequency, decrescendo musical, decrescendo	A	DCr Apex (left)
PR	1-6	D	HD	Low frequency, musical, decrescendo	P	Apex (right)
VSD	3-6	S	HS, PS	Mixed, plateau	T	P

A, Aortic valve; *AR,* aortic regurgitation; *D,* diastolic; *DCa,* dorsocaudal; *DCr,* dorsocranial; *E,* early; *HD,* holodiastolic; *HS,* holosystolic; *L,* late; *M,* mid; *Mi,* mitral valve; *MR,* mitral regurgitation; *MVP,* mitral valve prolapse; *P,* pulmonic valve; *PMI,* point of maximal intensity; *PR,* pulmonic regurgitation; *PS,* pansystolic; *S,* systolic; *T,* tricuspid valve; *TR,* tricuspid regurgitation; *TVP,* tricuspid valve prolapse; *VSD,* ventricular septal defect.

CARDIO

Table 17-3	Electrode Placement for Complete 12-Lead Electrocardiogram
Lead	**Placement**
Lead I: LA-RA	Left foreleg (left arm) electrode placed just below the point of the elbow on the back of the left forearm. Right foreleg (right arm) electrode placed just below the point of the elbow on the back of the right forearm.
Lead II: LL-RA	Left hind leg (left leg) electrode placed on the loose skin at the left stifle in the region of the patella. Right foreleg (right arm) electrode placed just below the point of the elbow on the back of the right forearm.
Lead III: LL-LA	Left hind leg (left leg) electrode placed on the loose skin at the left stifle in the region of the patella. Left foreleg (left arm) electrode placed just below the point of the elbow on the back of the left forearm.
aV_R: RA-CT	Right foreleg (right arm) electrode placed just below the point of the elbow on the back of the right forearm. The electrical center of the heart or central terminal × 3/2.
aV_L: LA-CT	Left foreleg (left arm) electrode placed just below the point of the elbow on the back of the left forearm. The electrical center of the heart or central terminal × 3/2.
aV_F: LL-CT	Left hind leg (left leg) electrode placed on the loose skin at the left stifle in the region of the patella. The electrical center of the heart or central terminal × 3/2.
CV_6LL: V_1-CT	V_1 electrode placed in the sixth intercostal space on the left side of the thorax along a line parallel to the level of the point of the elbow. The electrical center of the heart (central terminal).
CV_6LU: V_2-CT	V_2 electrode placed in the sixth intercostal space on the left side of the thorax along a line parallel to the level of the point of the shoulder. The electrical center of the heart (central terminal).
V_{10}: V_3-CT	V_3 electrode placed over the dorsal thoracic spine of T7 at the withers. Electrical center of the heart. The dorsal spine of T7 is located on a line encircling the chest in the sixth intercostal space (central terminal).
CV_6RL: V_4-CT	V_4 electrode placed in the sixth intercostal space on the right side of the thorax along a line parallel to the level of the point of the elbow. The electrical center of the heart (central terminal).
CV_6RU: V_5-CT	V_5 electrode placed in the sixth intercostal space on the right side of the thorax along a line parallel to the level of the point of the shoulder. The electrical center of the heart (central terminal).
Base-apex: LA-RA	Left foreleg (left arm) electrode placed in the sixth intercostal space on the left side of the thorax along a line parallel to the level of the point of the elbow. Right foreleg (right arm) electrode placed on the top of the right scapular spine.

treatment to control the arrhythmia and relieve the signs of cardiovascular collapse.

- An ECG is necessary to confirm the diagnosis of the rhythm disturbance auscultated and to choose the appropriate treatment.
- Perform continuous ECG monitoring on all horses with potentially life-threatening arrhythmias to monitor cardiac rhythm and response to treatment.
- ***Practice Tip:*** *Supraventricular and bradyarrhythmias are common in horses recovering from general anesthesia, and supraventricular arrhythmias are frequent in horses after high-intensity exercise. In both situations the arrhythmias are generally benign.*
- ***Practice Tip:*** *Ventricular arrhythmias are less common and should be considered more serious. These arrhythmias commonly occur in Standardbred racehorses immediately after racing throughout the rapid deceleration phase. All of the Standardbred horses in a clinical study rapidly converted to normal rhythm after finishing the race.*

Bradyarrhythmias

Complete (Third-Degree) Atrioventricular Block

- Rare
- Usually associated with inflammatory or degenerative changes in the AV node

- Severe exercise intolerance and frequent syncope are common
- Resting heart rate (ventricular rate) usually <20 beats/min, with a more rapid, independent atrial rate.

Auscultation

- Loud, regular S_1 and S_2
- Slow ventricular rate (<20 beats/min)
- Rapid, regular independent S_4, usually 60 beats/min; occasional bruit de canon sounds caused by the summation of S_4 with another heart sound—S_1, S_2, or S_3

Electrocardiogram

- Atrial rate is rapid—more P waves than QRS-T complexes.
- P-P interval is regular.
- *No* evidence exists of AV conduction, and *no* consistent relationship is found between P waves and QRS-T complexes; PR intervals are variable.
- Abnormal QRS-T configuration, usually wide and bizarre, is unassociated with the preceding P waves (Fig. 17-3).
- The escape pacemaker is junctional or ventricular.
- The R-R interval is usually regular but is irregular when more than one QRS-T configuration is present in association with complexes arising from different areas in the ventricle (Fig. 17-4).

CARDIO

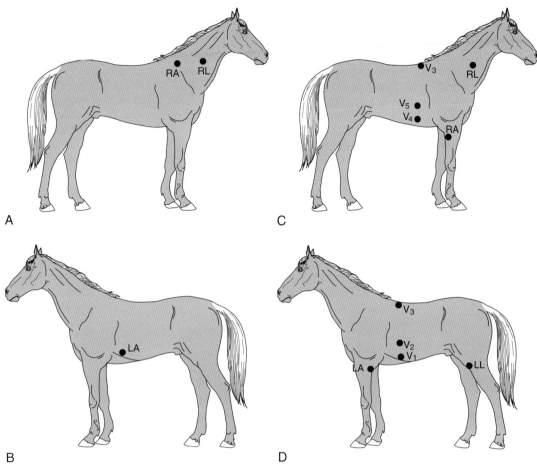

Figure 17-2 Sites for lead placement for obtaining a base-apex electrocardiogram (**A** and **B**) and a complete electrocardiogram (**C** and **D**) in a horse. The *black circles* represent the sites of attachment for the electrodes. **A,** Position of the electrode on the right side of the patient for recording a base-apex electrocardiogram with the electrodes from lead I. *RA,* right foreleg (right arm); *RL,* right hind leg (right leg). **B,** Position of the electrode on the left side of the patient for recording a base-apex electrocardiogram with the electrodes from lead I. *LA,* Left foreleg (left arm). **C,** Position of the electrode on the right side of the patient for recording a complete electrocardiogram. *RA,* Right foreleg (right arm); *RL,* right hind leg (right leg); V_3, third chest lead (V_{10}); V_4, fourth chest lead (CV_6RL); V_5, fifth chest lead (CV_6RU). **D,** Position of the electrode on the left side of the patient for recording a complete electrocardiogram. *LA,* Left foreleg (left arm); *LL,* left hind leg (left leg); V_1, first chest lead (CV_6LL); V_2, second chest lead (CV_6LU); V_3, third chest lead (V_{10}).

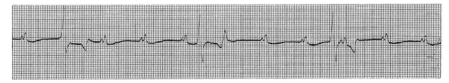

Figure 17-3 Base-apex electrocardiogram of a horse with complete heart block. Large, wide QRS complexes are evident and are not associated with the preceding P waves. There is complete atrioventricular dissociation with a rapid, regular atrial rate of 70 beats/min and a slow, regular ventricular rate of 20 beats/min. The P-P interval is regular, and the R-R interval is regular. This electrocardiogram was recorded at a paper speed of 25 mm/s with a sensitivity of 10 mm/mV.

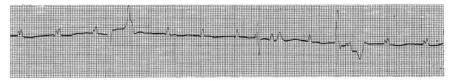

Figure 17-4 Lead II electrocardiogram of a horse with third-degree AV block. Wide and bizarre QRS complexes of differing morphologies are evident and are not associated with the preceding P waves. There is complete atrioventricular dissociation with a rapid regular atrial rate of 70 beats/min and a slow, irregular ventricular rate of 30 beats/min. The P-P interval is regular, and the R-R interval is irregular. This electrocardiogram was recorded at a paper speed of 25 mm/s with a sensitivity of 10 mm/mV.

Complete (Third-Degree) Atrioventricular Block

- Treatment should be aggressive when arrhythmia is diagnosed.
- *Vagolytic drugs:* Atropine or glycopyrrolate should be administered intravenously at a dose of 0.005 to 0.01 mg/kg as a bolus. ***Note:*** Vagolytic drugs usually are unsuccessful in restoring sinus rhythm; side effects include tachycardia, arrhythmias, decreased gastrointestinal motility, and mydriasis.
- *Sympathomimetic drugs* speed idioventricular rhythm. These drugs should be used with care, or *not* at all, if other ventricular ectopy is present because they may exacerbate ventricular arrhythmias.
- Isoproterenol, 0.05 to 0.2 mg/kg/min, is indicated when syncope is present and if *no* ventricular ectopy is detected. Rapid tachyarrhythmias are an undesirable side effect. If tachyarrhythmias occur, stop isoproterenol infusion and manage ventricular arrhythmias with lidocaine or propranolol.
- Corticosteroids: Dexamethasone is indicated in high doses (0.05 to 0.22 mg/kg) administered IV (preferably), IM, or PO, in the hope that reversible inflammatory disease is present in the region of the AV node.
- Laminitis, immune suppression, and iatrogenic renal insufficiency are undesirable side effects of corticosteroid use in the care of horses. These side effects occur most frequently after prolonged use of large doses of corticosteroids or in horses with metabolic disease treated with even modest doses.
- Implantation of a cardiac pacemaker: Pacemakers provide definitive management of third-degree AV block if no response is seen with medical therapy. Permanent transvenous pacemakers have been implanted successfully in horses with third-degree AV block (Figs. 17-5 and 17-6). Temporary transvenous pacemakers can be tried in the treatment of horses with advanced second-degree or complete AV block until a permanent transvenous pacemaker can be inserted.
- Temporary transvenous pacemakers are less successful in capturing the cardiac rhythm because these pacing wires are *not* embedded in the myocardium, but instead are just placed against the endocardial surface.

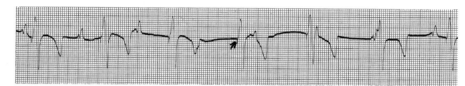

Figure 17-5   Base-apex electrocardiogram of a horse with third-degree AV block treated with a pacemaker with a single pacing electrode in the right ventricle. The pacing spike *(arrow)* initiates the ventricular depolarization at a rate of 50 beats/min. There is a completely independent, slightly faster atrial rate of 60 beats/min and complete atrioventricular dissociation. The QRS complexes appear wide and bizarre. The P-P interval is regular, and the R-R interval is regular. This electrocardiogram was recorded at a paper speed of 25 mm/s with a sensitivity of 10 mm/mV.

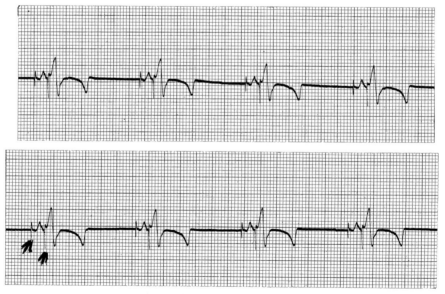

Figure 17-6   Continuous base-apex electrocardiogram of a horse with third-degree AV block with a pacemaker with an atrial pacing electrode in the right atrium and a ventricular pacing electrode in the right ventricle (dual chamber, dual sensing, dual action [DDD] pacemaker). The earlier pacing spike causes atrial depolarization *(first arrow),* and the later pacing spike causes ventricular depolarization *(second arrow).* The atrial and the ventricular rates are 50 beats/min and are associated with one another. The P-P and R-R intervals are regular. The atrial electrode has the ability to sense inherent electrical depolarization of the atria and does not pace the atria if the sinus rate increases, thus allowing the patient to exercise. The ventricular lead can be programmed to pace with either an inherent or a paced atrial depolarization. This electrocardiogram was recorded at a paper speed of 25 mm/s with a sensitivity of 5 mm/mV.

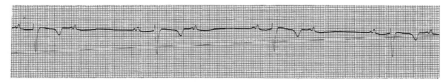

Figure 17-7   Base-apex electrocardiogram of a horse with advanced second-degree AV block with 2:1 conduction. Every other P wave is not followed by a QRS complex, but every QRS complex present is preceded by a P wave at a normal PR interval (440 ms). The P-P interval is regular, and the R-R interval is regular. The atrial rate is slightly increased at 50 beats/min with a slow ventricular rate of 25 beats/min. This electrocardiogram was recorded at a paper speed of 25 mm/s with a sensitivity of 5 mm/mV.

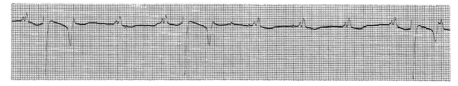

Figure 17-8   Base-apex electrocardiogram of a horse with advanced second-degree AV block with variable conduction. Every P wave is not followed by a QRS complex, but every QRS complex present is preceded by a P wave at a normal PR interval (480 ms). The P-P interval is regular, and the R-R interval is irregular. The atrial rate is slightly increased at 60 beats/min with a slower than normal ventricular rate of 20 beats/min. This electrocardiogram was recorded at a paper speed of 25 mm/s with a sensitivity of 5 mm/mV.

Advanced (Second-Degree) Atrioventricular Block

- May also be associated with severe exercise intolerance and collapse
- Can be seen with electrolyte imbalances (e.g., hypercalcemia), digitalis toxicity, and AV nodal disease
- Should be investigated thoroughly and managed aggressively (see p. 143) in the hope of preventing progression of the dysfunction to third-degree AV block

Auscultation

- Regular S_1 and S_2
- Slow to low-normal heart rate, usually 8 to 24 beats/min
- S_4 preceding each S_1 and regular S_4 in pauses for each period of second-degree AV block

Electrocardiogram

- Rapid atrial rate
- Regular P-P interval
- Evidence of AV conduction (consistent PR intervals) for some P-QRST complexes
- Some P waves do *not* have associated QRS-T complexes..
- Normal QRS-T configuration is associated with the preceding P waves (Figs. 17-7 and 17-8)
- R-R interval is usually regular but may be irregular in some horses (see Fig. 17-8).

Sinus Bradycardia, Sinus Arrhythmia, and Sinoatrial Block

- Sinus bradycardia, sinus arrhythmia, and SA block occur in fit horses but are less common than second-degree AV block.

Auscultation

- Regular S_1 and S_2 with a pause in rhythm (SA block) or rhythmic variation of diastolic intervals (sinus bradycardia and sinus arrhythmia)
- Pause in rhythm equal to one diastolic pause or a multiple of the shortest diastolic pause (SA block)
- Slow to low-normal heart rate, usually 20 to 30 beats/min

- S_4 preceding each S_1 that can be auscultated
- *No* S_4 in pauses for each period of SA block

Electrocardiogram

- Slow to low-normal atrial rate
- Irregular P-P interval
- Evidence of AV conduction (consistent PR interval)
- Normal QRS-T complex associated with the preceding P waves
- R-R interval rhythmically irregular (sinus bradycardia and sinus arrhythmia) or regularly irregular (SA block), with a diastolic pause equal to the number of beats blocked at the SA node

●❯ WHAT TO DO

Sinus Bradycardia, Sinus Arrhythmia, Sinoatrial Block

- Usually manifestations of high vagal tone disappear with exercise or the administration of vagolytic (atropine or glycopyrrolate, 0.005 to 0.01 mg/kg IV) or sympathomimetic (isoproterenol, 0.05 to 0.2 µg/kg/min) drugs. Although *not* evaluated for this use, N-butylscopolammonium bromide (Buscopan) at 0.3 mg/kg IV is an alternative treatment.

Sinoatrial Arrest

- An uncommon arrhythmia in horses, which could be a manifestation of extreme vagal tone or sinus node dysfunction

Auscultation

- Regular S_1 and S_2 with a prolonged pause in the rhythm—more than two diastolic intervals
- Slow to low-normal heart rate, usually 20 to 30 beats/min but may be lower if pathologic
- S_4 preceding each S_1 and usually can be auscultated
- *No* S_4 in pauses for period of SA arrest

Electrocardiogram

- Slow to low-normal atrial rate
- Regularly irregular P-P interval

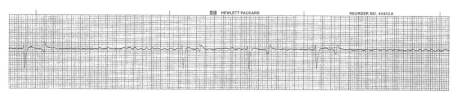

Figure 17-9   Base-apex electrocardiogram of a horse with atrial fibrillation. Irregularly irregular R-R intervals, absence of P waves, and presence of baseline f waves are evident. The QRS morphology is normal, as is the ventricular rate (30 beats/min). This electrocardiogram was recorded at a paper speed of 25 mm/s with a sensitivity of 5 mm/mV.

- Evidence of AV conduction (consistent PR interval)
- Normal QRS-T complex associated with the preceding P waves
- R-R interval regularly irregular, with a diastolic pause equal to more than two diastolic intervals; should disappear with exercise or the administration of a vagolytic or sympathomimetic drug
- ***Practice Tip:*** *Prolonged periods of SA arrest, profound sinus bradycardia, or high-grade SA block may indicate sinus node dysfunction. These horses should be evaluated carefully with an exercising ECG and the response of the horse to vagolytic and sympathomimetic drugs determined. Sinus node disease is rare in horses, but inflammatory and degenerative changes must be considered as possible etiologic factors.*

⦿ WHAT TO DO

Sinoatrial Arrest

- A course of high-dose corticosteroids (dexamethasone, 0.05 to 0.22 mg/kg IV) should be initiated for patients with life-threatening abnormalities of sinus rhythm in the hopes of addressing any inflammatory component.
- As with other extreme bradyarrhythmias, pacemaker implantation is the treatment of choice if sinus arrest is persistent, causing clinical signs, or is life threatening.

Sick Sinus Syndrome

- Periods of profound sinus bradycardia and tachycardia have *not* been reported in horses.
- Definitive treatment would be pacemaker implantation.

Tachyarrhythmias

Atrial Fibrillation

- Occurs frequently in patients and rarely necessitates emergency therapy.
- Often *not* a tachycardia unless concurrent with heart failure
- Many horses have little or no underlying cardiac disease and come to medical attention because of exercise intolerance. Other presenting problems include tachypnea,

dyspnea, exercise-induced pulmonary hemorrhage, myopathy, colic, and congestive heart failure. Atrial fibrillation can be an incidental finding during a routine examination.
- Resting heart rate usually is normal, although the rhythm is irregularly irregular and S$_4$ *cannot* be auscultated.
- Intensity of peripheral pulses is variable depending on the preceding RR interval.
- Cardiac output in patients with atrial fibrillation and no underlying cardiac disease is normal at rest.

Auscultation

- Heart rate usually is normal—28 to 44 beats/min—although atrial fibrillation can occur at any heart rate.
- Irregularly irregular diastolic periods occur.
- ***Practice Tip:*** *Detecting atrial fibrillation can be challenging because the heart rate is usually normal, and the irregularly irregular rhythm is easily missed if the examination is brief. If there is a suspicion of atrial fibrillation, slight excitement of the horse increases the heart rate and makes the rhythm easier to detect.*
- S$_4$ is absent.

Electrocardiogram

- Irregularly irregular R-R intervals (Fig. 17-9)
- *No* P waves
- Rapid baseline fibrillation (f) waves
- Normal QRS-T complexes

⦿ WHAT TO DO

Atrial Fibrillation

- Cardioversion—pharmacologic or electrical—from atrial fibrillation to normal sinus rhythm is generally required for the horse to perform successfully, but cardioversion should *not* be considered an emergency procedure.

  Practice Tip: *Quinidine sulfate is usually administered orally at a dose of 20 mg/kg q2h to the fasted horse. If >3 doses are required and quinidine serum measurements are not available, it is common practice to increase the dosage interval to q6h. Intravenous quinidine gluconate is more expensive and not as reliable in conversion but is safer and does not require fasting. It is routine to administer 1 to 2 mg/kg IV every 10 minutes, and an accepted practice is not to exceed 12 mg/kg total dose. Although the IV quinidine treatment may appear to have no effect on heart rate or ECG during treatment, the horse may convert within the next 24 hours after treatment.*

▶ WHAT TO DO

Quinidine Toxicity

- Horses may present as emergency cases with quinidine toxicity from attempts to convert atrial fibrillation to normal sinus rhythm. Adverse cardiac and intestinal events are most common.
- Therapeutic level of quinidine: 2 to 5 µg/mL
- Toxic level of quinidine: >5 µg/mL
- The detection of any significant adverse reactions or signs of quinidine toxicity (Box 17-1) should prompt discontinuation of quinidine administration and may require additional treatment if the induced problem is serious (Box 17-2 and Fig. 17-10).
- Obtain a plasma sample for determination of plasma quinidine concentration. Plasma electrolyte concentrations and a creatinine concentration also should be determined if the adverse or toxic effects are cardiovascular.
- **_Important:_** Administration of digoxin and quinidine together results in rapid elevations of serum digoxin concentration and the possible development of digoxin toxicity. Plasma digoxin concentrations nearly double with concurrent administration of quinidine sulfate.
- Therapeutic range of digoxin: 0.5 to 1.5 ng/mL
- Digoxin toxicity manifests as anorexia, depression, colic, or the development of other cardiac arrhythmias (Fig. 17-11).

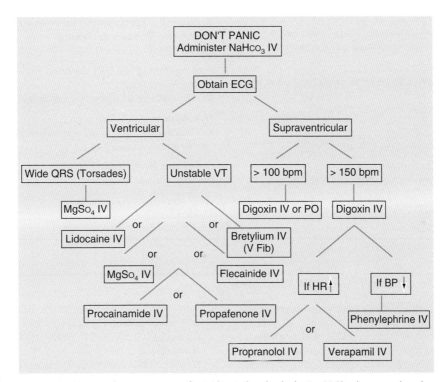

Figure 17-10 Decision tree for management of quinidine-induced arrhythmias. *BP,* Blood pressure; *bpm,* beats per minute; *ECG,* electrocardiogram; *HR,* heart rate; *IV,* Intravenously; *PO,* per os (by mouth); *V Fib,* ventricular fibrillation; *VT,* ventricular tachycardia.

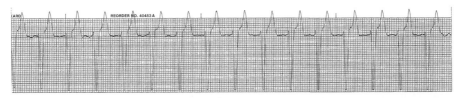

Figure 17-11 Base-apex electrocardiogram of the horse in Fig. 17-9 after treatment with quinidine sulfate and digoxin. This patient has atrial fibrillation with monomorphic ventricular tachycardia and digoxin toxicity. Large, wide QRS complexes are ventricular in origin, P waves are absent, and baseline f waves are evident. This electrocardiogram was recorded at a paper speed of 25 mm/s with a sensitivity of 5 mm/mV.

Box 17-1   Adverse Reactions and Toxic Side Effects of Quinidine Sulfate and Quinidine Gluconate Treatment

1. Depression
Rx: Occurs in all treated horses, no treatment needed

2. Paraphimosis
Rx: Occurs in all treated stallions or geldings, no treatment indicated unless persistent after discontinuation of treatment

3. Urticaria, Wheals
Rx: Discontinue quinidine; if severe, administer corticosteroids, antihistamines, or both

4. Nasal Mucosal Swelling
Snoring
Rx: Monitor degree of airflow; discontinue quinidine if there is a significant decrease in nares airflow

Upper Respiratory Tract Obstruction
Rx: Discontinue quinidine; sign of quinidine toxicity; if severe, administer corticosteroids, antihistamines, or both; insert nasotracheal tube, preferably, or perform emergency tracheostomy

5. Laminitis
Rx: Discontinue quinidine; administer analgesics and other treatment as indicated

6. Neurologic
Ataxia
Rx: Discontinue quinidine; sign of quinidine toxicity

Bizarre Behavior: Hallucinations?
Rx: Discontinue quinidine; sign of quinidine toxicity

Convulsions
Rx: Discontinue quinidine; sign of quinidine toxicity; administer anticonvulsants as indicated

7. Gastrointestinal
Flatulence
Rx: Occurs in many treated horses; treatment not needed

Diarrhea
Rx: Usually resolves with discontinuation of drug; discontinue drug administration if diarrhea is severe

Colic
Colic may occur because of intestinal distention associated with the vagolytic properties of quinidine or immediately after receiving the first oral dose, believed caused by the irritating effect of quinidine on gastric ulcers.
Rx: Usually resolves with administration of flunixin meglumine; use other analgesics as needed; sign of quinidine toxicity

8. Cardiovascular
Tachycardia: Supraventricular or Ventricular—Uniform, Multiform, Torsades de Pointes
Rx: See Box 17-2, Table 17-4

Prolongation of the QRS duration (>25% of pretreatment value)
Rx: Discontinue quinidine; sign of quinidine toxicity

Hypotension
Rx: Discontinue quinidine; administer phenylephrine if needed (see Box 17-2, Table 17-4)

Congestive Heart Failure
Rx: Discontinue quinidine; administer digoxin if not already administered

Sudden Death
Rx: Cardiopulmonary resuscitation

Box 17-2   Management of Quinidine-Induced Arrhythmias

Determine whether arrhythmia is supraventricular or ventricular (see Figs. 17-13, 17-14, 17-16, and 17-17):
- Obtain another electrocardiogram (ECG) lead if unable to determine whether rhythm is supraventricular or ventricular. Look for change in QRS configuration from normal or preceding QRS configuration. Record ECG during entire treatment with radiotelemetry, if possible.
- Measure/monitor blood pressure if possible.
- Don't panic!

If arrhythmia is supraventricular:
- If rate is sustained at >100 beats/min, administer diltiazem, 0.125 mg/kg IV slow bolus or digoxin, 0.0022 mg/kg IV (1 mg/1000 lb or 450 kg) or 0.011 mg/kg PO (5 mg/1000 lb or 450 kg).
- If rate is sustained at >150 beats/min or pressures are poor, administer diltiazem, 0.125 mg/kg IV slow bolus or digoxin, 0.0022 mg/kg IV (1 mg/1000 lb/450 kg). Can repeat the dose of either diltiazem or digoxin IV in relatively short period if necessary. Administer NaHCO$_3$, 1 mEq/kg IV (450 mEq/1000 lb or 450 kg).

If rate remains elevated or pressures are poor:
- Administer propranolol: 0.03 mg/kg IV (13.5 mg/1000 lb or 450 kg), to slow heart rate.
- Administer phenylephrine: 1 µg/kg/min IV to effect, up to 0.01 mg/kg total dose to improve blood pressure. Phenylephrine also slows the heart rate.

- Administer verapamil: 0.025 to 0.05 mg/kg IV (11.25 to 22.5 mg/1000 lb or 450 kg) every 30 minutes. Can repeat up to 0.2 mg/kg (90 mg/1000 lb or 450 kg) total dose.

If arrhythmia is ventricular:
- If wide QRS tachycardia (torsades de pointes) is present, administer MgSO$_4$, 1 to 2.5 g/450 kg per minute IV to effect up to 25 g/1000 lb or 450 kg. Administer in rapid IV drip over 10 minutes or in bolus if necessary.

If ventricular tachycardia is unstable:
- Administer lidocaine hydrochloride: 20 to 50 µg/kg/min or 0.25 to 0.5 mg/kg very slowly IV (225 mg/1000 lb or 450 kg). Can repeat in 5 to 10 minutes.
- Administer MgSO$_4$: 1 to 2.5 g/450 kg/min IV to effect up to 25 g/1000 lb or 450 kg. Administer in rapid IV drip over 10 minutes or in bolus if necessary.
- Administer procainamide: 1 mg/kg/min IV (450 mg/min/1000 lb or 450 kg) to a maximum of 20 mg/kg (9 g/1000 lb or 450 kg).
- Administer propafenone: 0.5 to 1 mg/kg IV (225 to 450 mg) in 5% dextrose slow IV over 5 to 8 minutes.
- Administer bretylium: 3 to 5 mg/kg IV (1.35 to 2.25 g/1000 lb or 450 kg). Can repeat up to 10 mg/kg total dose.

Electrocardiographic Changes Associated with Quinidine Toxicity

- Prolongation of QRS complex
  - Prolongation of the QRS complex duration to greater than 25% of the pretreatment QRS complex duration is an indication of quinidine toxicity (Fig. 17-12).
  - Prolongation of the QT interval also occurs.
- Rapid supraventricular tachycardia
  - Supraventricular tachycardia occurs in patients being treated for atrial fibrillation with quinidine; it is associated with a sudden release of vagal tone at the AV node, an idiosyncratic reaction not associated with quinidine toxicity.
- Heart rates of 200 beats/min occasionally occur and are potentially life threatening (Fig. 17-13). Immediate therapy (see Box 17-2) is needed to slow the ventricular response rate and prevent deterioration of the patient's cardiovascular status.

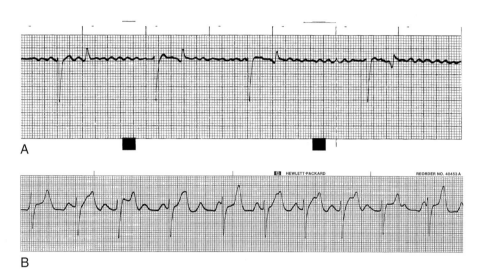

Figure 17-12   Base-apex electrocardiograms of a horse with atrial fibrillation, before **(A)** and after **(B)** treatment with quinidine sulfate, causing prolongation of the QRS complex. Irregularly irregular R-R intervals, no P waves, and baseline f waves are evident in the pretreatment electrocardiogram **(A)** with a QRS complex duration of 100 ms. After treatment with four doses of quinidine sulfate, the QRS complexes increased to 140 ms **(B),** and the ventricular rate increased to 60 beats/min. Large P waves are occurring regularly, buried in many of the QRS and T complexes associated with an atrial tachycardia (atrial rate of 150 beats/min) with block. A quinidine plasma concentration measured at this time was elevated. These electrocardiograms were recorded at a paper speed of 25 mm/s with a sensitivity of 5 mm/mV.

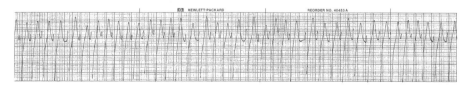

Figure 17-13   Base-apex electrocardiogram of a horse with atrial fibrillation that developed a rapid supraventricular tachycardia with a heart rate of 210 beats/min after the second dose of quinidine sulfate. R-R intervals are slightly irregular, P waves are absent, and the morphology of the QRS complex for the base-apex lead is normal. The f waves are not visible because of the rapid ventricular response rate. This electrocardiogram was recorded at a paper speed of 25 mm/s with a sensitivity of 5 mm/mV.

●› WHAT TO DO

Quinidine-Induced Arrhythmias

- Administer one or more of the following until desired clinical response:
  - Diltiazem: 0.125 mg/kg IV.
  - Digoxin: 0.0022 mg/kg IV.
  - NaHCO₃: 1 mEq/kg IV.
- If pressures are poor, administer phenylephrine: 1 to 2 µg/kg/min.
- If heart rate remains elevated, administer propranolol (0.03 mg/kg IV) although *not* before diltiazem, if used, has been metabolized.

- Supraventricular tachycardia is associated with decreased cardiac output at rest and may deteriorate into other, more life-threatening ventricular arrhythmias (Fig. 17-14).
- Sustained ventricular response rates of >100 beats/min (Fig. 17-15) in patients being treated for atrial fibrillation with quinidine should be controlled before quinidine administration is continued to prevent further deterioration of the cardiac rhythm.

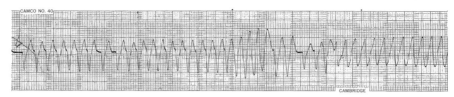

Figure 17-14 Base-apex electrocardiogram of a horse with atrial fibrillation and rapid supraventricular tachycardia that developed after two doses of quinidine sulfate and then deteriorated into paroxysms of ventricular tachycardia. R-R intervals are irregular, P waves are absent, and the morphology of the QRS complex is normal for a base-apex lead on the left side of the strip. These findings are consistent with rapid atrial fibrillation (i.e., supraventricular tachycardia) at a heart rate of 240 beats/min. This rhythm then deteriorates into a paroxysm of ventricular tachycardia followed by two supraventricular complexes and then a period of more sustained ventricular tachycardia with a heart rate of 270 beats/min. The f waves are not visible because of the rapid ventricular rate. This electrocardiogram was recorded at a paper speed of 25 mm/s with a sensitivity of 2 mm/mV.

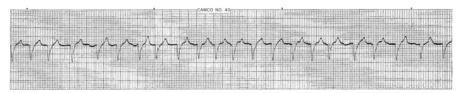

Figure 17-15 Base-apex electrocardiogram of a horse with rapid atrial fibrillation and a heart rate of 130 beats/min. R-R intervals are irregular, P waves are absent, and the baseline f waves are small. This electrocardiogram was recorded at a paper speed of 25 mm/s with a sensitivity of 2 mm/mV.

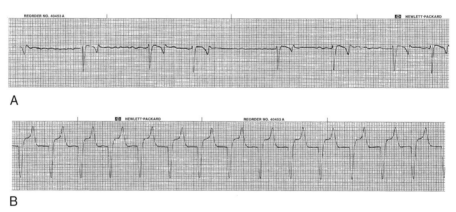

Figure 17-16 Base-apex electrocardiogram of a horse with atrial fibrillation **(A)** that developed uniform ventricular tachycardia **(B)** 15 minutes after the first dose of quinidine sulfate was administered. **A,** R-R intervals are irregular, P waves are absent, and baseline f waves are present. These findings are characteristic of atrial fibrillation. The resting heart rate is 40 beats/min. **B,** Wide and bizarre QRS complexes with the T wave oriented in the opposite direction to the QRS complex are consistent with complexes that are ventricular in origin. The ventricular complexes are monomorphic, and the heart rate is 90 beats/min. The baseline f waves are barely visible on the electrocardiogram, and no P waves are present. These electrocardiograms were recorded at a paper speed of 25 mm/s with a sensitivity of 5 mm/mV.

Ventricular Arrhythmias Associated with Quinidine

- If a large number of ventricular premature depolarizations, ventricular tachycardia (Fig. 17-16), or multiform ventricular complexes are detected, quinidine administration should be stopped.
- If the ventricular arrhythmias do *not* disappear, intravenous administration of antiarrhythmic drugs should be instituted, usually beginning with lidocaine, 20 to 50 μg/kg/min slowly IV (Tables 17-4 and 17-5).

- Ventricular arrhythmias induced by quinidine administration usually are idiosyncratic. These arrhythmias are associated with the proarrhythmic effect of antiarrhythmic drugs and are *not* associated with quinidine toxicity (Fig. 17-16).
- Quinidine-induced torsades de pointes, a wide ventricular tachycardia (Fig. 17-17), is more likely to occur in hypokalemic patients (Fig. 17-18).

Table 17-4 Antiarrhythmic Therapy

Drug	Indication	Dosage
Amiodarone	VT, SVT	5 mg/kg IV loading, then infusion of 0.83 mg/kg/h
Atropine or glycopyrrolate	Sinus bradycardia, vagally induced arrhythmias	0.005-0.01 mg/kg IV
Bretylium tosylate	Life-threatening VT, ventricular fibrillation	3-5 mg/kg IV, can repeat up to 10 mg/kg total dose
Dexamethasone	VT, complete atrioventricular block	0.05-0.22 mg/kg IV or IM
Diltiazem	SVT, ventricular rate control	0.125 mg/kg IV over 2 min, repeated every 5-12 min, up to 5 doses
Flecainide	Acute AF, ventricular and atrial arrhythmias	1-2 mg/kg infused at the rate of 0.2 mg/kg per minute
Lidocaine*	VT, ventricular arrhythmias	0.25 mg/kg (bolus), then 0.5 mg/kg very slowly IV to effect, can repeat in 5-10 minutes; repeat up to 3 times
$MgSO_4$	VT	1-2.5 g/450 kg/min IV to effect, not to exceed 25 g total dose
Phenylephrine HCl	Quinidine toxicosis, arterial hypotension	1 to 2 μg/kg/min; hypotension, 1 to 2 μg/kg/min
Phenytoin	Digoxin toxicity, atrial arrhythmias	5-10 mg/kg IV first 12 hours, then 1-5 mg/kg IV q12h or 20 mg/kg PO q12h for 3 or 4 doses, followed by 10-15 mg/kg PO q12h; plasma levels should be monitored and should be between 5-10 mg/mL; abnormally high concentrations may cause drowsiness or recumbency
Procainamide	VT, AF, ventricular and atrial arrhythmias	1 mg/kg/min IV, not to exceed 20 mg/kg IV 25-35 mg/kg q8h PO
Propafenone†	Refractory VT, AF, ventricular and atrial arrhythmias	0.5-1 mg/kg in 5% dextrose slowly IV to effect over 5-8 min 2 mg/kg PO q8h
Propranolol	Unresponsive VT and SVT	0.03 mg/kg IV 0.38-0.78 mg/kg PO q8h
Quinidine gluconate	VT, AF	0.5-2.2 mg/kg (bolus) q10min to effect; not to exceed 12 mg/kg‡ IV total dose
Quinidine sulfate	AF, VT, atrial and ventricular arrhythmias	22 mg/kg via nasogastric tube q2h until converted, toxic, or plasma (quinidine) level is 3-5 mg/mL; continue quinidine sulfate q6h until converted or toxic§
$NaHCO_3$	Quinidine toxicosis, atrial standstill, hyperkalemia	1 mEq/kg IV; can be repeated; decreases free quinidine
Verapamil	SVT	0.025-0.05 mg/kg IV q30min; can repeat to 0.2 mg/kg total dose

AF, Atrial fibrillation; *SVT*, supraventricular tachycardia; *VT*, ventricular tachycardia.
*Lidocaine without epinephrine for intravenous injection.
†Not available for intravenous injection in North America.
‡Most horses can tolerate only 12 mg/kg IV total dose if given at 1 to 2.2 mg/kg q10min.
§Not to exceed 6 doses q2h (most horses can tolerate only 4 doses q2h).

Table 17-5 Adverse Effects of Antiarrhythmic Drugs

Drug	Adverse Effect	Cardiovascular Effect
Amiodarone	Diarrhea, colic	Prolongation of QRS, proarrhythmic
Atropine	Ileus, mydriasis	Tachycardia, arrhythmias
Bretylium tosylate	GI disorder	Hypotension, tachycardia, arrhythmias
Digoxin	Depression, anorexia, colic	SVPD, VPD, SVT, VT
Flecainide	Agitation, neurologic	Prolonged QRS and QT intervals, proarrhythmic effect, negative inotrope
Lidocaine	Excitement, seizures	VT, sudden death
$MgSO_4$		Hypotension
Quinidine	Depression, paraphimosis, urticaria, wheals, nasal mucosal swelling, laminitis, neurologic disorders, GI	Hypotension, SVT, VT, prolonged QRS and QT intervals, CHF, sudden death, negative inotrope
Phenytoin	Sedation, drowsiness, lip and facial twitching, gait deficits, recumbency, seizures	Arrhythmias
Procainamide	GI, neurologic disorders, similar to effects of quinidine	Hypotension, SVT, VT, prolonged QRS and QT intervals, sudden death, negative inotrope
Propafenone	GI, neurologic disorders, similar to effects of quinidine, bronchospasm	CHF, AV block, arrhythmias, negative inotrope
Propranolol	Lethargy, worsening of COPD	Bradycardia, third-degree AV block, arrhythmias, CHF, negative inotrope
Verapamil		Hypotension, bradycardia, AV block, asystole, arrhythmias, negative inotrope

AV, Atrioventricular; *CHF*, congestive heart failure; *COPD*, chronic obstructive pulmonary disease; *GI*, gastrointestinal; *SVPD*, supraventricular premature depolarizations; *SVT*, supraventricular tachycardia; *VPD*, ventricular premature depolarizations; *VT*, ventricular tachycardia.

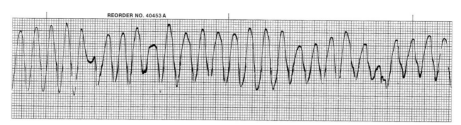

Figure 17-17   Base-apex electrocardiogram of a horse with atrial fibrillation that had received two doses of quinidine sulfate and developed a "sine wave" ventricular tachycardia (torsades de pointes). The QRS complexes and T waves twist around the baseline and are difficult to differentiate from one another. The plasma potassium level was normal at this time. This electrocardiogram was recorded at a paper speed of 25 mm/s with a sensitivity of 2 mm/mV.

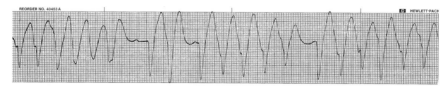

Figure 17-18   Base-apex electrocardiogram of a horse with atrial fibrillation that had received six doses of quinidine sulfate and developed torsades de pointes, which was managed immediately with an intravenous infusion of $MgSO_4$. Widened QRS complexes and T waves are evident, as is twisting of the QRS complexes and T waves around the baseline. This sign is present although the torsades de pointes is resolving. This horse was hypokalemic (2.4 mEq/L) and was receiving an intravenous infusion of $MgSO_4$ at the time of this electrocardiogram. The ventricular rate is 110 beats/min. An occasional f wave is present. The wide QRS complex tachycardia resolved with magnesium and potassium replacement fluids. This electrocardiogram was recorded at a paper speed of 25 mm/s with a sensitivity of 5 mm/mV.

●〉 WHAT TO DO

Quinidine-Induced Torsades De Pointes

• Intravenous infusion of $MgSO_4$ at a rate of 1 to 2.5 g/450 kg/min should be instituted immediately for quinidine-induced torsades de pointes.

●〉 WHAT TO DO

Quinidine-Associated Adverse Effects

See Box 17-1 for a summary of quinidine adverse effects.

Gastrointestinal Signs

• Flatulence is common: Quinidine administration does *not* need to be discontinued.
• Oral ulcerations: They are associated with oral administration of quinidine; therefore, oral administration of quinidine sulfate is contraindicated—use nasogastric intubation.
• Diarrhea usually occurs with higher doses of quinidine and usually resolves after discontinuing quinidine treatment.
• Only one case of quinidine-induced diarrhea culturing positive for *Salmonella* organisms is reported.
• Colic associated with quinidine toxicity: Discontinue quinidine administration; administer analgesics as needed.

• Colic occurring *immediately* after administration of the first quinidine dose suggests gastric ulcer pain. Discontinue oral quinidine and use IV quinidine gluconate, if available and appropriate; use transvenous electrical cardioversion or treat gastric ulcers first before beginning oral quinidine.

Sudden Death

• Believed to be associated with deterioration of rapid supraventricular or ventricular tachycardia to ventricular fibrillation or cardiac arrest
• Sudden death underscores the importance of continuous ECG monitoring (Fig. 17-19) and rapid management of any arrhythmias that occur.

Hypotension

• Monitor pulse pressure or blood pressure for quinidine-induced hypotension.
• Discontinue quinidine administration; if hypotension is severe, administer phenylephrine: 0.1 to 0.2 mg/kg/min to effect.

Congestive Heart Failure

• Occurs in individuals with severe underlying myocardial dysfunction or compensated congestive heart failure (inappropriate patients for cardioversion with quinidine).
• Negative inotropic effects of quinidine manifest only at higher drug doses.

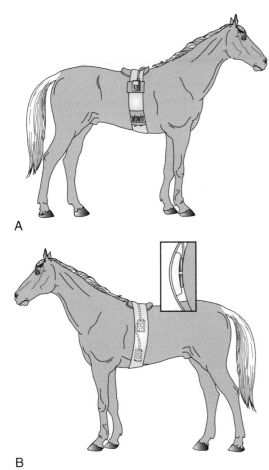

A

B

Figure 17-19 Contact electrodes in place under a surcingle for obtaining an electrocardiogram by means of radiotelemetry. **A,** Withers pad and the surcingle are in place in the girth area, and the telemetry box is taped to the upper rings of the surcingle just below the withers. **B,** Placement of the grounded electrodes on the left side of the patient under the moistened sponges are held in place by the surcingle. Care must be taken to ensure close contact between the patient's skin and the contact electrodes in the area near the withers and in the girth area. The upper grounded electrode (negative electrode) should be placed on the flat portion of the dorsal thorax. The lower grounded electrode (positive electrode) should be placed in the flat portion of the girth area or on the sternum, whichever area ensures better contact.

- Discontinue quinidine administration; treat with digoxin, 0.0022 mg/kg IV, and furosemide, 1 to 2 mg/kg IV, if needed.

Upper Respiratory Tract Obstruction

- Monitor nasal airflow for quinidine-induced upper respiratory tract obstruction resulting from nasal mucosal swelling.
- If airflow through the external nares decreases, discontinue quinidine administration.
- ***Practice Tip:*** *Decreased airflow is indicative of quinidine toxicity.*
- Insert a nasotracheal tube if airflow through the external nares continues to decrease.
- If obstruction is severe, administer corticosteroids, antihistamines, or both.
- Emergency tracheostomy may be necessary for some patients if a nasotracheal tube is *not* inserted when a significant decrease in airflow is first detected (see Chapter 25, p. 456).

Urticaria, Wheals

- Discontinue quinidine administration.
- If severe, administer antihistamines and corticosteroids.

Paraphimosis

- Transient in all geldings and stallions
- Disappears with discontinuance of treatment and return of plasma quinidine concentrations to negligible levels. It is *not* necessary to stop quinidine treatment.

Laminitis

- Rare
- If digital pulses are increased, discontinue quinidine administration.
- If patient is uncomfortable, administer analgesics.

Neurologic Signs

- Ataxia, bizarre behavior, seizures
- Indicative of quinidine toxicity
- Discontinue quinidine administration; anticonvulsants may be indicated if seizures occur.

⦿〉 WHAT TO DO

Horses with Congestive Heart Failure and Atrial Fibrillation

- From 10% to 15% of horses with atrial fibrillation have severe underlying cardiac disease and congestive heart failure.
- The resting heart rates of these individuals are elevated (>60 beats/min) and may exceed 100 beats/min (Fig. 17-20).
- Clinical signs of left-sided heart failure or right-sided heart failure may be present.
- Murmurs of tricuspid or mitral regurgitation usually are present; however, patients with severe aortic regurgitation also may have congestive heart failure.
- ***Practice Tip:*** *These patients are* not *candidates for cardioversion to sinus rhythm.*
- Treatment of these horses is directed at slowing the ventricular response rate (heart rate) and supporting the failing myocardium.

- Digoxin: 0.0022 mg/kg IV q12h or 0.011 mg/kg PO q12h, is the drug of choice because of its vagal and positive inotropic effects (see Table 17-6).
- If heart rate is *not* controlled adequately with digoxin alone, propranolol, diltiazem, or verapamil is used in the same way as for other supraventricular tachycardias (see p. 138, Other Supraventricular Tachycardias). Beta-blockers and calcium channel blockers should *not* be used concurrently to avoid an excessive decrease in inotropy and chronotropy.
- Furosemide therapy is used in the treatment of patients with ventral or pulmonary edema (see p. 146, Congestive Heart Failure).
- Afterload reducers (vasodilators), such as hydralazine or benazepril are added in the treatment of patients with severe mitral or aortic regurgitation (see section on Congestive Heart Failure, p. 148).

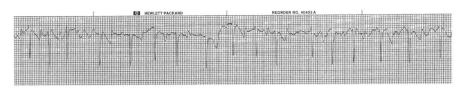

Figure 17-20   Base-apex electrocardiogram of a horse with atrial fibrillation and congestive heart failure. Heart rate is rapid (110 beats/min), R-R interval is irregular, P waves are absent, and baseline f waves are present. These findings are consistent with atrial fibrillation. This electrocardiogram was recorded at a paper speed of 25 mm/s with a sensitivity of 5 mm/mV.

Table 17-6	Drug Therapy for Horses with Myocardial Disease, Valvular Heart Disease, and Congestive Heart Failure	
Drug	**Indication**	**Dosage**
Aspirin	Thrombophlebitis, endocarditis	10-20 mg/kg PO or per rectum
Dexamethasone	Myocarditis, arrhythmias	0.05-0.22 mg/kg IV or IM
Digoxin	Congestive heart failure, atrial tachyarrhythmias, control of rapid ventricular response in atrial fibrillation or flutter	0.0022 mg/kg IV q12h (maintenance dose); 0.0044-0.0075 mg/kg IV q12h (loading dose administered for only 2 doses, rarely used); 0.0022-0.00375 mg/kg IV q12h to control ventricular response rate in atrial fibrillation; 0.011-0.0175 mg/kg PO q12h
Dobutamine	Cardiogenic shock, hypotension, complete atrioventricular block (emergency therapy)	1-5 mg/kg per minute IV
Enalapril or Benazepril	Mitral and aortic regurgitation	Enalapril, 0.5 mg/kg PO q12h; Benazepril, 0.5 mg/kg PO q24h
Furosemide	Edema	1-2 mg/kg subcutaneous, IM, or IV as needed or followed by 0.12 mg/kg/h as a CRI; 1-2 mg/kg PO q12h (maintenance); PO has poor bioavailability and not recommended
Hydralazine	Mitral regurgitation	0.5-1.5 mg/kg PO q12h or 0.5 mg/kg IV (decreases peripheral resistance for at least 4 hr)
Milrinone	Congestive heart failure, low cardiac output	10 µg/kg/min IV; 0.5-1 mg/kg PO q12h

Other Supraventricular Tachycardias

- Atrial tachycardia and other supraventricular tachycardias other than atrial fibrillation are uncommon in horses.
- Signs of cardiovascular collapse can occur when heart rate is high (>150 beats/min)

Auscultation
- Rapid regular rhythm

Electrocardiogram
- Atrial and ventricular rates are elevated; AV association is maintained
- P-P and R-R intervals are regular, and PR intervals are consistent.
- Sometimes, depending on the heart rate, the P waves can be "buried" in the preceding QRS-T complex and are impossible to appreciate. It is helpful to acquire the ECG at a paper speed of 50 mm/s rather than the conventional 25 mm/s.
- QRS-T morphology is similar to a normal sinus beat morphology.
- P waves may appear dissimilar to P waves of normal sinus beats.

Echocardiogram
- Often the only abnormality is that associated with significant tachycardia (i.e., ventricular dyssynchrony).
- If the atrial tachycardia is due to underlying myocarditis or cardiomyopathy, chamber dilation or a decrease in systolic function may be seen.

- ***Practice Tip:*** *If atrial tachycardia is due to myocarditis, cardiac troponin I (cTn-I) is increased.*
- Occasionally, supraventricular rhythms result from atrial dilation, so enlarged atria may be seen.

⏺ WHAT TO DO

Other Supraventricular Tachycardias
- The goal of therapy is to slow the ventricular rate. This can be accomplished by slowing the ventricular response to the atrial depolarizations (i.e., by slowing conduction through the AV node) or by breaking the underlying rhythm.
- Calcium channel blockers, beta-blockers, and digoxin work to slow AV nodal conduction.
- ***Practice Tip:*** *Calcium channel blockers and beta-blockers should* not *be used concurrently, for their combined negative chronotropic and inotropic effects are dangerous.*
- Administer one or more of the following until desired clinical response:
  - Diltiazem: 0.125 mg/kg IV over 2 minutes and up to 5 doses
  - Verapamil: 0.025 to 0.05 mg/kg IV q30min up to 0.2 mg/kg
  - Propranolol: 0.05 mg/kg IV up to 0.1 mg/kg
  - Digoxin: 0.0022 mg/kg IV q12h or 0.011 mg/kg PO q12h
  - Sodium channel blockers are used in an attempt to break the underlying rhythm.
  - Procainamide: up to 1.0 mg/kg/min IV up to 20 mg/kg

Ventricular Tachycardia

- The clinical signs of congestive heart failure become more severe the longer ventricular tachycardia is present and the higher the heart rate.
- ***Practice Tip:*** *Clinical signs of congestive heart failure develop more rapidly in horses with higher heart rates.*
- Clinical signs of low-output heart failure also develop more rapidly when the rhythm is multiform rather than uniform.
- Generalized venous distention, jugular pulsations, ventral edema, and pleural effusion develop in patients with sustained uniform ventricular tachycardia at a rate of 120 beats/min.
- Some patients also have pericardial effusion, pulmonary edema, and ascites.
- Syncope has been detected in horses with uniform ventricular tachycardia and a heart rate of 150 beats/min.

Auscultation

- Rapid, regular rhythm if monomorphic; rapid, irregular rhythm if polymorphic
- Heart sounds often loud and varying in intensity

Electrocardiogram

- Ventricular rate is elevated, usually >60 beats/min, with slower independent atrial rate.
- P-P interval is regular.
- P waves are "buried" in QRS-T complexes with AV dissociation.
- ECG shows regular R-R interval (monomorphic) or irregular R-R interval (polymorphic) ventricular tachycardia.

- Abnormal QRS-T complexes are unrelated to the preceding P wave. All abnormal QRS-T waves have same configuration (monomorphic), or several different QRS-T wave configurations are detected (polymorphic).
- Monomorphic ventricular tachycardia occurs when the ectopic focus originates from one place in the ventricle and produces only one abnormal QRS-T configuration (Fig. 17-21).
- Polymorphic ventricular tachycardia occurs when the ectopic ventricular complexes originate from more than one focus in the ventricle or when electrical propagation from a single site is variable. Abnormal QRS-T complexes of different morphologies are seen (Fig. 17-22). Polymorphic ventricular complexes are associated with increased electrical heterogeneity, which carries with it an increased risk of development of a fatal ventricular rhythm.
- R on T, a QRS complex occurring within the preceding T wave (Fig. 17-23), indicates significant electrical heterogeneity and increases the risk of development of ventricular fibrillation.
- Torsades de pointes, in which the QRS and T complexes twist around the baseline (Fig. 17-24), is another ventricular rhythm that can deteriorate rapidly into ventricular fibrillation and cause sudden death. These cases are observed briefly in horses after racing and rapidly convert to normal rhythm in most cases.

Echocardiogram

- In most horses the only abnormality is that associated with the rhythm disturbance (i.e., ventricular dyssynchrony)

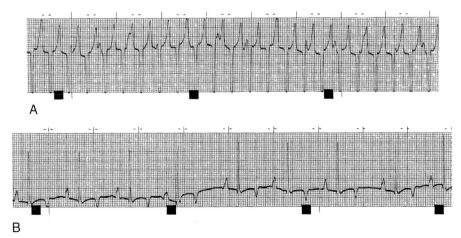

Figure 17-21   Lead II electrocardiogram of a horse with uniform ventricular tachycardia before **(A)** and after **(B)** cardioversion. **A,** Wide and bizarre negative QRS complexes with the T wave oriented in the opposite direction, which is an abnormal QRS morphology for lead II in the horse. A rapid, regular ventricular rate of 150 beats/min and slower regular atrial rate of 90 beats/min are evident. The R-R interval and P-P interval are regular. The P waves are buried in the QRS and T complexes and are disassociated with the QRS complexes. This electrocardiogram was recorded at a paper speed of 25 mm/s with a sensitivity of 5 mm/mV. **B,** Tall positive QRS complex with a negative T wave deflection after each P wave. The P wave morphology changes from beat to beat, and the P-P and R-R intervals are not perfectly regular. This electrocardiogram shows slight sinus arrhythmia with a wandering pacemaker at a heart rate of 50 beats/min immediately after cardioversion from sustained monomorphic ventricular tachycardia. This electrocardiogram was recorded at a paper speed of 25 mm/s with a sensitivity of 10 mm/mV.

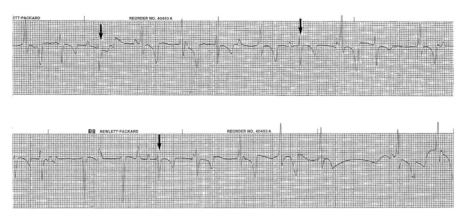

Figure 17-22   Continuous base-apex electrocardiogram of a horse with polymorphic ventricular tachycardia. Multiple morphologies of the QRS and T complexes appear wide and bizarre compared with the few normal QRS and T complexes *(arrows)*. The R-R intervals are irregular, but the P-P intervals are regular. The underlying atrial rate is 60 beats/min, with a heart rate of 70 beats/min. This electrocardiogram was recorded at a paper speed of 25 mm/s with a sensitivity of 5 mm/mV.

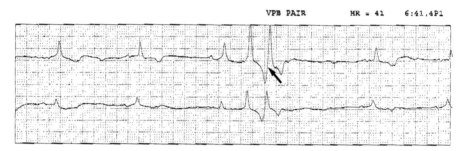

Figure 17-23   Base-apex electrocardiogram obtained with a 24-hour Holter recorder for a horse with multiple ventricular premature depolarizations, pairs of ventricular premature depolarizations, and paroxysms of ventricular tachycardia. The R on T occurs with the pair of ventricular premature depolarizations *(arrow)*. The heart rate is 41 beats/min. This electrocardiogram was recorded at a paper speed of 25 mm/s with a sensitivity of 10 mm/mV.

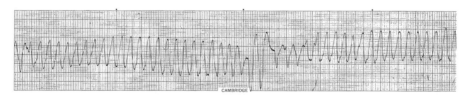

Figure 17-24   Base-apex electrocardiogram of a horse with torsades de pointes ventricular tachycardia with a heart rate of 280 to 300 beats/min. Wide QRS complex tachycardia and slurring of the distinction between the QRS complex and the T wave are evident, and the electrocardiogram appears to oscillate around the baseline. This electrocardiogram was recorded at a paper speed of 25 mm/s with a sensitivity of 2 mm/mV.

- Severe concurrent myocardial dysfunction may be detected in horses with multiform ventricular tachycardia and indicates probable widespread myocardial necrosis (Fig. 17-25).
- ***Practice Tip:*** *Treatment is indicated if the equine patient is showing clinical signs at rest attributable to the arrhythmia:*
  - Rate is excessively high
  - Rhythm is polymorphic
  - R on T complexes are detected (Box 17-3)
- The selection of an appropriate antiarrhythmic agent for a patient with ventricular tachycardia depends on:

Box 17-3	Indications for Immediate Management of Ventricular Tachycardia

Clinical signs of cardiovascular collapse
    Rapid heart rate (>120 beats/min)
    Polymorphic ventricular tachycardia
    Detection of R on T complex

- Severity of the arrhythmia
- Associated clinical signs
- Suspected causative factor
- Availability of appropriate antiarrhythmic drugs (see Table 17-4)

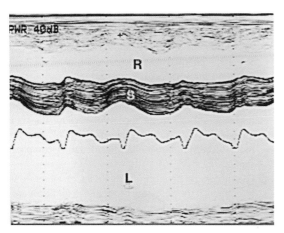

Figure 17-25 M-mode echocardiogram of a horse with polymorphic ventricular tachycardia, severe left ventricular dysfunction, and left-sided congestive heart failure. Systolic dysfunction of the left ventricular free wall is evident. This echocardiogram was obtained from the right parasternal window in the left ventricular position with a 2.5-MHz sector scanner transducer. An electrocardiogram is superimposed for timing. *L,* Left ventricle; *R,* right ventricle; *S,* interventricular septum.

●❯ WHAT TO DO

Ventricular Tachycardia
- *Practice Tip: Lidocaine—without epinephrine—is readily available and is the most rapidly acting drug.*
- **Lidocaine** must be administered carefully and in small doses (0.25 to 0.5 mg/kg, slow IV bolus) because of the central nervous system excitement and seizures associated with larger doses. Diazepam, 0.05 mg/kg IV, is used to control the excitability or seizures that may result from lidocaine.
  - Therapeutic plasma concentration is 1.5 to 5 mg/mL.
- Other sodium channel blockers (see Table 17-4):
  - Quinidine gluconate: 1 to 2.2 mg/kg IV as a bolus
  - Procainamide: 1 mg/kg/min IV
  - Phenytoin: 8 mg/kg IV followed by 10 to 15 mg/kg q12h
  - Flecainide: 1 to 2 mg/kg infused at the rate of 0.2 mg/kg/min
  - All are administered more slowly or in graded doses
- All these drugs have negative inotropic effects when administered at high doses but often are effective in converting ventricular tachycardia in horses.

- Propranolol, 0.03 mg/kg IV, also has negative inotropic effects and is rarely successful in converting horses with ventricular tachycardia.
- Propranolol should be tried, however, in the treatment of patients that do *not* respond to other antiarrhythmics. Therapeutic plasma concentrations of propranolol range from 20 to 80 ng/mL in horses.
- **MgSO$_4$:** 1 to 2.5 g/450 kg/min IV, for 10 to 20 minutes often is effective in the management of refractory ventricular tachycardia in horses. MgSO$_4$ is the drug of choice for quinidine-induced torsades de pointes and has *no* negative inotropic effects. MgSO$_4$ does cause hypotension.
- MgSO$_4$ is effective in the treatment of horses that have a normal or low magnesium level and usually is administered slowly.
- Amiodarone, 5 mg/kg IV, can be used to treat ventricular arrhythmias.
  - In human beings, an initial intravenous bolus is followed by oral dosing for maintenance therapy. In horses, oral dosing is *not* recommended because it yields low and inconsistent blood levels. The therapeutic level in humans is 1 to 2.5 mg/L.
- Bretylium tosylate, 3 to 5 mg/kg IV repeated up to a 10 mg/kg total dose, is reserved for patients with severe, life-threatening ventricular tachycardia or ventricular fibrillation.
- Intravenous propafenone should be reserved for patients with refractory ventricular tachycardia. Propafenone is currently *not* available in the United States. Therapeutic plasma concentrations are between 0.2 and 3.0 mg/mL in horses.
- All antiarrhythmic drugs may have adverse effects and can be proarrhythmic (see Table 17-5).

Cardiopulmonary Resuscitation

Cardiopulmonary resuscitation (CPR) of an adult horse (for foal CPR, see (Chapter 29, p. 513) should be approached according to the same systematic principles applied to CPR of humans and small animals. The major difference is the size of the patient with cardiac arrest. The **ABCD** of CPR reminds the clinician of the order in which cardiopulmonary resuscitation is approached.
- *A* stands for establishing an airway
- *B* for breathing for the patient
- *C* for establishing circulation
- *D* for drugs that should be administered

●❯ WHAT TO DO

Cardiopulmonary Resuscitation (CPR)
Establish an Airway if Obstruction Is Present
- An airway is easily established with the nasotracheal placement of a smaller endotracheal tube or the orotracheal placement of a larger endotracheal tube.
- If orotracheal or nasotracheal intubation is *not* possible, emergency tracheostomy can be performed, and the endotracheal tube can be inserted into the trachea through the tracheostomy site (see Chapter 25, p. 456).
- The cuff should be inflated, and the endotracheal tube should be attached to a demand valve or anesthetic machine.
- If an endotracheal tube is *not* available, a 10-foot length of Tygon tubing with a ½-inch (1.25-cm) internal diameter should be inserted nasotracheally and attached to the flow regulator of an E-size oxygen cylinder.

Breathe for the Patient
- This is the immediate priority for newborn foals and horses with apnea that maintain a heartbeat.
- Four to six breaths per minute are reportedly adequate to maintain normal Pao$_2$ for a horse.
- With a demand valve or large-animal anesthesia machine, the rebreathing bag can be compressed to between 20 and 40 cm H$_2$O.
- The oxygen flow rate—100% O$_2$—should be adjusted so that there is moderate expansion of the thorax in 2 to 3 seconds.
- When Tygon tubing and intranasal oxygen are used, the horse's nose and mouth must be occluded and released alternately.

Establish *Circulation in Cardiac Arrest*

- This is the first priority if the airway is patent.
- The peripheral arterial pulses should be checked, and the heart should be auscultated to verify cardiac arrest.
- An ECG must be obtained to determine the type of cardiac arrhythmia present in the patient with cardiac arrest (e.g., pulseless electrical activity, asystole, or ventricular fibrillation).
- ***Important:*** An airway must be established for the horse before reestablishment of circulation. Chest compressions are the next priority and should be started even before attempting mechanical ventilation!
- The horse should be in lateral recumbency, ideally in right lateral recumbency, with the head level or lowered.
- An ECG is obtained with external or internal cardiac massage to determine the rhythm being generated or initiated during CPR.
- *External cardiac massage*
  - Forceful and rapid compressions of the horse's chest right behind the horse's elbow with the resuscitator's knee or hands (if the patient is small) are performed.
  - Begin at the rate of 60 to 80 compressions per minute.
  - This is difficult to perform on adults and is rarely successful.
  - Monitor the peripheral pulse to determine whether cardiac compressions are adequate.
- Internal cardiac massage
- Attempt this *only* if external cardiac compression is unsuccessful.
- Internal cardiac massage is associated with a large number of postoperative complications in the horse—pneumothorax, pleuropneumonia, and severe lameness
- Successful intracardiac compression requires an incision in the fifth intercostal space with retraction of the fifth and sixth ribs or a fifth rib resection and manual compression of the left ventricle.
- Compress the heart 40 to 60 times per minute.
- Compressions can be performed through an incision in the diaphragm if the patient is undergoing exploratory celiotomy.

Drugs Administered for Cardiac Arrest

- Determine the type of cardiac arrest that is being experienced by the equine patient. Further therapeutic intervention depends on whether asystole or ventricular fibrillation is present (Box 17-4).
- Administer drugs into a central vein, the cranial vena cava, if possible, or otherwise into the jugular vein as close to the central vein as possible.
- *Asystole (Fig. 17-26)*
  - Epinephrine should be administered intravenously: 0.1 mg/kg IV bolus followed by 0.01 to 0.02 mg/kg/min, or intratracheally—10× dose; intracardiac administration is used as a last resort.
  - Periods of asystole must be recognized and intervention begun immediately for treatment of horses to be successful.
- *Ventricular fibrillation (Fig. 17-27)*
  - Epinephrine is unlikely to be successful.
  - Administer antiarrhythmic drugs with efficacy against ventricular fibrillation (preferable) or refractory sustained ventricular tachycardia.

- Administer bretylium tosylate: 3 to 5 mg/kg IV; can repeat this up to 10 mg/kg total dose.
- Administer amiodarone: 5 mg/kg IV.
- Successful pharmacologic defibrillation of an adult with antiarrhythmic drugs has *not* been performed.
- Successful electrical defibrillation of one 350-kg horse and several foals have been reported. External defibrillation in larger horses is unlikely to be successful because the transthoracic impedance is too high. Internal defibrillation should be more successful, but the postresuscitation complications are significant.
- Pharmacologic or electrical defibrillation or both should be attempted, if the necessary drugs and defibrillator are available and the pre-existing condition of the patient is *not* terminal.
- Intravenous fluid administration is given at the rate of 20 mL/kg/h during resuscitation of a horse to maintain normal or elevated mean circulatory pressures. ***Practice Tip:*** *Maintaining normal or elevated mean circulatory pressure during CPR increases the probability of a favorable outcome for the canine patient and is likely for an equine patient. An exception to this rule is a patient with end-stage congestive heart failure, in which fluids exacerbate the underlying problem.*

Box 17-4   Cardiopulmonary Resuscitation and Treatment of the Horse

Establish an Airway
- Nasotracheal placement of an endotracheal tube
- Orotracheal placement of an endotracheal tube

Asystole
- Initiate external cardiac massage.
- ***Practice Tip:*** *If no heartbeat, inject epinephrine, 0.01 mg/kg IV followed by 0.01 to 0.02 mg/kg/min, or 0.1 to 0.2 mg/kg intratracheally and ventilate vigorously for 4 to 5 breaths.*
- Epinephrine is given by means of intracardiac administration as a last resort and is injected into the left ventricle.
- Continue CPR, checking the peripheral pulse for effectiveness.
- Establish an IV line and administer lactated Ringer's solution rapidly.
- Reevaluate CPR and ECG findings. If unable to establish a pulse within 2 minutes, open the chest at the sixth intercostal space and begin cardiac massage.

Ventricular Fibrillation
- Initiate or continue CPR.
- Defibrillate.
  - Administer 5 mg/kg bretylium tosylate intracardiac (IC).
  - Use an electrical defibrillator (direct current) at appropriate W-s/kg. Use adequate amounts of electrode paste on the skin and no alcohol, which is flammable.
  - ***Practice Tip:*** *Mix potassium chloride, 1 mEq/kg with acetylcholine, 6 mg/kg, and inject IC.*

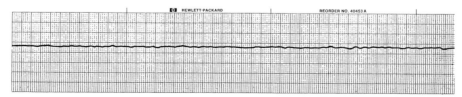

Figure 17-26   Base-apex electrocardiogram of a horse with asystole. The electrocardiogram recorded line is flat with some baseline undulations and no evidence of atrial or ventricular electrical activity. This electrocardiogram was recorded at a paper speed of 25 mm/s with a sensitivity of 5 mm/mV.

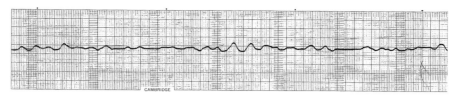

Figure 17-27 Base-apex electrocardiogram of a horse with ventricular fibrillation. Baseline fibrillation waves are fine, and there is no evidence of coordinated atrial or ventricular depolarization. This electrocardiogram was recorded at a paper speed of 25 mm/s with a sensitivity of 5 mm/mV.

CARDIO

●❯ WHAT TO DO

Postresuscitation Treatment
- Calcium in the form of calcium chloride or calcium gluconate (0.1 to 0.2 mEq/kg, slowly IV over 5 to 10 minutes), although highly controversial, may be indicated to increase the force of myocardial contraction and counteract the effects of hypocalcemia and hyperkalemia.
- Once a normal sinus rhythm has been restored, dobutamine (1 to 5 μg/kg/min IV) is the drug of choice for maintaining cardiac output and arterial blood pressure.
- The use of $NaHCO_3$ is controversial and is *not* indicated if circulation is restored rapidly, because large volumes of $NaHCO_3$ can cause:
  - Hyperosmolality
  - Hypernatremia
  - Hypocalcemia
  - Hypokalemia
  - Decreased affinity of hemoglobin for oxygen
- Small doses of $NaHCO_3$ may be indicated to manage metabolic acidosis and hyperkalemia in horses that have experienced a prolonged period of cardiac arrest.

Electrolyte Disturbances Causing Cardiac Arrhythmias

Hyperkalemia
- Potassium is the major intracellular cation (150 meq/L) and sodium is the major extracellular cation (140 mg/L). This pattern is the result of the sodium-potassium exchange pump (Na^+-K^+-ATPase) on cell membranes sequestering potassium in the cell and extruding sodium.
- Only 2% of the total body potassium stores are found outside of cells, limiting the value of plasma potassium measurements as an index of total body potassium.
- ***Practice Tip:*** *Elevated potassium concentrations can cause cardiac arrhythmias. Increases in total body potassium to plasma potassium concentration is "often" reflected by a <5% increase in total body potassium for every 1 mEq/L increase in plasma concentration.*
- Hyperkalemia is most frequently recognized in foals with uroperitoneum but is occasionally seen in adults with acute renal failure.
- Hyperkalemia is also seen in Quarter Horses with hyperkalemic periodic paralysis.
- Clinical signs include:
  - Stiffness
  - Muscle weakness
  - Muscle fasciculations
  - Muscle spasm
  - Respiratory stridor
  - Recumbency
  - Death
- Death is caused by paralysis of the pharyngeal and laryngeal muscles or by cardiac arrhythmias associated with hyperkalemia.
- Cardiac arrhythmias may or may not be detected, but an ECG should be obtained for adults or foals with a plasma potassium concentration >6 mEq/L.

Electrocardiogram
- Tall, peaked T waves are detected when plasma potassium concentration reaches 6.2 mEq/L (Fig. 17-28).
- Progressive slowing of conduction and decreased excitability result in cardiac arrest or ventricular fibrillation.
- Broadening and flattening of the P waves, prolonged PR intervals, and bradycardia develop, conduction slows, and excitability decreases. Atrial arrest or atrial standstill develops.
- Atrial and ventricular premature depolarizations and ventricular tachycardia have been reported.
- Widened QRS complexes are further indications of severe (near lethal) hyperkalemia.
- The QT interval is *not* a reliable indicator of hyperkalemia.

●❯ WHAT TO DO

Hyperkalemia
- Uroperitoneum must be managed aggressively as soon as it is diagnosed because these foals are at high risk of developing cardiac arrhythmias, particularly when they are under general anesthesia during surgical repair of the ruptured bladder, urachus, or ureter.
- Ventricular premature complexes, ventricular tachycardia, third-degree AV block, and atrial standstill have been reported in foals with uroperitoneum.
- Sodium deficit should be replaced slowly at the rate of 0.5 mEq/h.
- Administer 0.45% to 0.9% NaCl, IV.
- $NaHCO_3$, 1 mEq/kg IV, helps drive potassium intracellularly.
- Between 5% and 50% dextrose IV also may be needed to help drive the potassium intracellularly.
- Administer 5% dextrose, 0.5 mL/kg, and 0.9% saline solution IV.
- If the foregoing measures are unsuccessful, administer regular insulin, 0.1 IU/kg IV with 0.5 to 1 g/kg dextrose IV to drive potassium

CARDIO

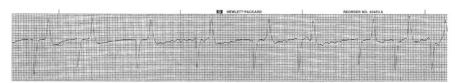

Figure 17-28   Base-apex electrocardiogram of a horse with hyperkalemia (plasma K⁺ concentration 6.6 mEq/L) and a creatinine level of 24 mg/dl. Tall, tented T waves (2.5 mV) are typical of hyperkalemia. This horse also had atrial fibrillation. R-R intervals are irregular, P waves are absent, and baseline f waves are present with a heart rate of 50 beats/min. This electrocardiogram was recorded at a paper speed of 25 mm/s with a sensitivity of 5 mm/mV.

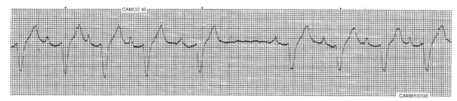

Figure 17-29   Base-apex electrocardiogram of a horse with hypokalemia (plasma K⁺ concentration, 1.4 mEq/L), sinus arrhythmia, and a heart rate of 50 beats/min. Greatly widened QRS and T complexes reflect delayed conduction and abnormal ventricular repolarization. This electrocardiogram was recorded at a paper speed of 25 mm/s with a sensitivity of 5 mm/mV.

into the cell. ***Practice Tip:*** *Add 5 mL of the foal's blood to the fluid to prevent the insulin from adhering to the fluid administration bag.*

- If severe cardiac arrhythmias or atrial standstill are detected, calcium gluconate, 4 mg/kg, can be administered slowly (over a 10-minute period) to effect.
- Calcium gluconate should be discontinued if bradycardia occurs after calcium administration.
- Gradual drainage of the uroperitoneum should be performed in conjunction with intravenous fluid replacement therapy, as indicated previously.
- Surgical correction of the uroperitoneum should be performed after medical stabilization of the foal.

Hyperkalemic Periodic Paralysis

- Adult horses experiencing an acute episode of hyperkalemic periodic paralysis experience signs such as recumbency, respiratory stridor, or trembling.
- Serum potassium concentration often is >6 mEq/L; draw blood to measure serum potassium concentration.

◉〉 WHAT TO DO

Hyperkalemic Periodic Paralysis

- Administer 0.2 to 0.4 mL/kg of 23% calcium borogluconate solution IV.
- Administer 6 mL/kg 5% dextrose solution IV or 1 mL/kg 50% dextrose IV.
- Administer NaHCO₃, 1 to 2 mEq/kg IV.
- Insulin may be used as recommended previously, but regular monitoring of blood glucose concentration is required for the following 24 hours.

Hypokalemia

- ***Practice Tip:*** *Total body potassium equals approximately 50 mEq/kg of body weight. A decrease in total body potassium to plasma potassium often reflects a 10% deficit in total*

body potassium for every 1 mEq/L decrease in potassium plasma concentration.

- Common among horses with heat exhaustion with concurrent hypochloremia, hypocalcemia, and metabolic alkalosis
- Also occurs in equine patients, both horses and foals, with severe diarrhea

Electrocardiogram

- Prolongation of the QT interval is an indication of hypokalemia.
- Supraventricular and ventricular arrhythmias occur.
- Atrial tachycardia with block (Fig. 17-29) and junctional tachycardia are common supraventricular arrhythmias among patients with hypokalemia.
- Ventricular tachycardia, torsades de pointes, and ventricular fibrillation can occur with severe hypokalemia.

◉〉 WHAT TO DO

Hypokalemia

- Replace calculated potassium deficit slowly intravenously, adding potassium chloride (KCl), 20 to 40 mEq/L or more to fluids; do *not* exceed a rate of 0.5 mEq/kg/h. Serum potassium concentration should be monitored during treatment. Intravenous fluids given at a rapid rate may cause significant kaliuresis and can impede the correction of hypokalemia.
- Administer KCl: 0.1 to 0.2 g/kg PO, if the gastrointestinal tract is patent. This is the right way to correct hypokalemia if time permits and the gastrointestinal (GI) tract is normal.
- Correct other electrolyte abnormalities, if present, and do *not* cause diuresis with excessive intravenous fluid administration unless the patient has volume contraction.

Hypomagnesemia

- Magnesium deficiency is usually associated with hypokalemia or hypocalcemia.

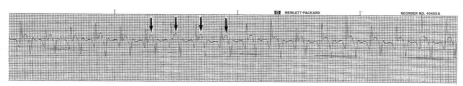

Figure 17-30   Lead II electrocardiogram of a horse with severe hypomagnesemia (Mg^{2+} concentration 0.7 mg/dL), hyperkalemia (K^+ concentration 6.2 mEq/L), and azotemia (creatinine concentration 6.0 mg/dL). Rapid, regular rhythm with a ventricular rate of 100 beats/min. The QRS complexes are normal for lead II, but the P waves are buried in the QT complex *(arrows),* suggesting junctional tachycardia. The T waves are large (1 mV and spiked). This electrocardiogram was recorded at a paper speed of 25 mm/s with a sensitivity of 10 mm/mV.

Electrocardiogram

- Serious ventricular arrhythmias are most likely in patients with significant hypomagnesemia, but supraventricular tachycardia (Fig. 17-30) and atrial fibrillation also occur in patients with severe hypomagnesemia.
- PR interval is prolonged, QRS complex is widened, ST segment is depressed, and T wave is peaked.

●〉 WHAT TO DO

Hypomagnesemia

- Administer $MgSO_4$, 1 to 2.5 g/450 kg/min IV at a rate *not* to exceed 25 g/450 kg, and follow it with oral $MgSO_4$ supplementation, 0.2 to 1 g/kg.

Hypocalcemia

- Hypocalcemic tetany, lactation tetany, transport tetany, and eclampsia are *uncommon* in horses.
- When associated with lactation, hypocalcemia often occurs after peak lactation, approximately 60 to 100 days postpartum.
- *Practice Tip: Occasionally, hypocalcemia occurs after prolonged or strenuous exercise, especially in hot weather, during prolonged transport, or in horses with diarrhea.*
- Hypocalcemia occurs among horses fed a diet low or deficient in calcium. Magnesium also may be deficient in the diet, which can lead to multiple cases of hypocalcemia on a farm.
- Hypocalcemia occurs among horses with cantharidin (blister beetle) toxicosis.
- Hypocalcemic tetany caused by hypoparathyroidism may occur in young foals.
- Hypoalbuminemia reduces the total serum concentration of calcium and of protein-bound calcium but *not* of ionized calcium.
- To measure serum calcium more accurately in patients with hypoalbuminemia and if ionized calcium cannot be measured, do the following:
  - Corrected calcium = Measured calcium (mg/dL) − albumin (g/dL) + 3.5
  - Ionized calcium is measured on the i-STAT (see Chapter 15, p. 111).
- Alkalosis reduces the concentration of ionized calcium in the blood. Two different clinical syndromes occur among horses with moderate to severe hypocalcemia:
  - Horses with a low serum calcium level, 5 to 8 mg/dL, and low serum magnesium concentration have tetany with:

  - Tachycardia
  - Synchronous diaphragmatic flutter
  - Laryngospasm with loud, labored breathing
  - Trismus
  - Protrusion of the nictitans
  - Dysphagia
  - Abdominal pain
  - Goose-stepping
  - Stiff hind limb gait
  - Ataxia may be present
  - Rhabdomyolysis, convulsions, coma, and death may follow.
- Horses with an even lower serum calcium concentration (<5 mg/dL) and normal serum magnesium concentration may have:
  - Flaccid paralysis
  - Mydriasis
  - Stupor
  - Recumbency

Electrocardiogram

- ECG abnormalities other than tachycardia are rare.
- Atrial or ventricular premature complexes or ventricular tachycardia is occasionally detected.
- Cardiac arrest or ventricular standstill may occur.
- *Practice Tip: QT interval is inversely correlated with ionized plasma calcium concentration.*

●〉 WHAT TO DO

Hypocalcemia

- Administer intravenous infusion of calcium gluconate: 4 mg/kg slowly (over a 10-minute period) to effect.
- Analyze the horse's ration and ensure an adequate calcium-to-phosphorus ratio (1.3 to 2:1) and adequate magnesium in the diet.

Hypercalcemia

- Hypercalcemia occurs among horses with:
  - Chronic renal failure
  - Lymphosarcoma
  - Paraneoplastic syndromes
  - Hypervitaminosis D and
  - After ingestion of *Cestrum diurnum; Cestrum diurnum* contains 1,25-dihydroxycholecalciferol and may induce hypervitaminosis D.
- Hyperphosphatemia occurs and is an early and reliable indicator of vitamin D intoxication or idiopathic calcinosis.

- Hypercalcemia, with normal or high phosphorus, results in soft tissue mineralization and mineralization of the heart and blood vessels, especially aorta, pulmonary artery, coronary arteries, and endocardium.

Electrocardiogram
- Initially heart rate slows, and sinus arrhythmia and partial AV block are detected.
- Tachycardia and extrasystoles are common findings.
- Atrial and ventricular tachycardia may occur.
- QT interval inversely correlates with ionized plasma calcium concentration.
- Cardiac arrest, ventricular fibrillation, or ventricular standstill is a lethal event.

●❯ WHAT TO DO

Hypercalcemia
- Search for the underlying cause of hypercalcemia, and remove or control it if possible.
- Discontinue all exogenous supplements containing calcium, phosphorus, and vitamin D, and remove horses from pastures containing *C. diurnum.*
- Emergency treatment is indicated in the care of patients with cardiac disease, severe renal decompensation, and systemic disease with hypercalcemia in the 15- to 20-mg/dL range.
- Administer 0.9% NaCl IV to expand the extracellular fluid volume and increase the glomerular filtration rate. Potassium (20 mEq/L) and magnesium (10 g/L, *not* to exceed 25 to 30 g over 30 minutes) supplementation of the intravenous fluids should be administered more slowly or be added to oral fluids.
- Begin diuretic therapy with a calciuric diuretic such as furosemide, 1 to 2 mg/kg q12h, and keep intravenous fluid maintenance levels at 5 mL/kg/h, or at least equal to urine output.
- Administration of corticosteroids may reduce calcium concentrations and decrease the likelihood of soft tissue and cardiac mineralization by decreasing calcium loss from bone, decreasing intestinal calcium absorption, and possibly increasing renal excretion of calcium. **Note:** Steroid-responsive forms of hypercalcemia include lymphoma, lymphosarcoma, leukemia, multiple myeloma, thymoma, vitamin D toxicity, granulomatous disease, and hyperadrenocorticism.
- Treatment with salmon calcitonin may be indicated if severe, prolonged hypercalcemia is present.

Congestive Heart Failure
- Congestive heart failure has a multitude of causes in horses, both congenital and acquired (Figure 17-31).
- Most equine patients with congestive heart failure have acquired cardiac disease:
  - Valvular heart disease
  - Myocardial disease
  - Both
- Severe cardiac arrhythmias, such as ventricular tachycardia, also can cause congestive heart failure.
- Severe congenital cardiac disease is an uncommon cause of congestive heart failure in horses. Congestive heart failure in these individuals may develop slowly over a

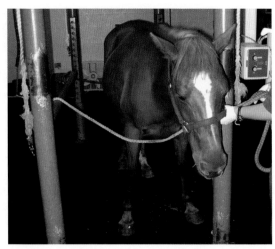

Figure 17-31 Severe pectoral edema and depression in a 9-year-old horse with congestive heart failure.

Box 17-5	Clinical Signs and Physical Examination Findings in Horses with Acute Mitral or Aortic Regurgitation

- Murmur: Systolic or diastolic
- Tachycardia: Heart rate usually ≥60 beats/min
- Irregular rhythm present or absent: Usually atrial fibrillation but may have atrial or ventricular premature contractions or both
- Loud third heart sound
- Tachypnea: Respiratory rate usually ≥24 breaths/min with increased respiratory effort, flared nostrils, and prolonged recovery after exercise
- Coughing: At rest or during or after exercise
- Expectoration of foamy fluid may or may not occur
- Exercise intolerance or poor performance
- Syncope: Rare
- Harsh inspiratory and expiratory vesicular sounds
- Crackles or moist sounds: Rare

prolonged period or suddenly and require emergency intervention.
- ***Practice Tip:*** *Horses with severe primary myocardial disease, acute onset of severe valvular heart disease (mitral, including ruptured chordae tendineae, or aortic [Box 17-5]), or multifocal ventricular tachycardia are most likely to have clinical signs of acute, left-sided heart failure and need emergency treatment.*

Left-Sided Heart Failure
- Clinical signs include anxiety, tachypnea, dyspnea, tachycardia, coughing, foamy nasal discharge, expectoration of a foamy fluid, lethargy, and exercise intolerance
- Diagnosis often is missed because of the subtlety of clinical signs in many horses.
- ***Practice Tip:*** *Rupture of mitral valve chordae tendineae is the most likely cause of acute fulminant pulmonary edema in individuals with primary valvular heart disease.*
- Patients with bacterial endocarditis also may have acute left- or right-sided heart failure because of rapid destruction of the valve apparatus by the vegetative lesion.

Practice Tip: *The most common site of endocarditis in the horse is the mitral valve, followed by the aortic valve.* Patients also may have fever, weight loss, and "shifting" leg lameness. Systemic septic emboli frequently occur.

- Acute severe myocarditis with severe left ventricular dysfunction is the most common cause of frank pulmonary edema in horses with primary myocardial disease. Many of these horses have a history of fever, often a suspected equine herpesvirus, influenza, or other viral infection, in the weeks or months preceding the signs of cardiac disease.
- Most horses with multifocal ventricular tachycardia and acute severe pulmonary edema also have severe myocardial disease.
- Weakness or syncope may occur, particularly with polymorphic or rapid monomorphic ventricular tachycardia.
- Patients with ventricular tachycardia also have frequent jugular pulses.
- Arterial pulses usually are weak, and extremities may be cool.
- Cyanosis at rest is rarely detected but occasionally is induced by exercise.

Auscultation

- Coarse breath sounds are heard over the entire lung field in most equine patients. Occasionally, horses also have crackles or moist sounds detected in the perihilar or ventral lung field. However, moist sounds are detected infrequently in horses with left-sided congestive heart failure because the edema is primarily interstitial.
- The abnormal lung sounds are most frequently detected when the horse is taking deep breaths in a rebreathing bag.
- Horses easily become distressed when breathing in a rebreathing bag or with breath holding, often cough, may expectorate foamy fluid, and have a prolonged recovery time to resting respiratory rate.
- Cardiac murmurs usually are heard if severe valvular or congenital disease is the cause of the congestive heart failure. Loud (grade 3/6 to 6/6), coarse, band-shaped, holosystolic, or pansystolic murmurs of mitral regurgitation are detected in most patients with acute left sided heart failure.
- Murmurs associated with ruptured mitral chordae tendineae usually are loud and honking initially. These murmurs might decrease in intensity with time if a ruptured chord dislodges.
- Most horses also have slightly quieter murmurs of tricuspid regurgitation.
- Occasionally, patients with bacterial endocarditis or myocardial disease do *not* have a murmur.
- A small number of patients in left heart failure have holodiastolic decrescendo murmurs of aortic regurgitation in addition to murmurs of mitral insufficiency.
- Murmurs associated with a congenital defect, such as a ventricular septal defect, are detected infrequently.
- The cardiac rhythm usually is rapid and regular, unless polymorphic ventricular tachycardia is the underlying cause of the congestive heart failure.

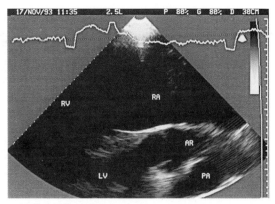

Figure 17-32 Long axis two-dimensional echocardiogram of a horse with right ventricular cardiomyopathy, syncope, and congestive heart failure. Evident are the greatly enlarged right atrium *(RA)* and right ventricle *(RV)* and the small pulmonary artery *(PA)* associated with severe pulmonary hypoperfusion. This echocardiogram was obtained from the right parasternal window in the left ventricular outflow tract position with a 2.5-MHz sector scanner transducer. The electrocardiogram is superimposed for timing. *AR,* Aortic root; *LV,* left ventricle.

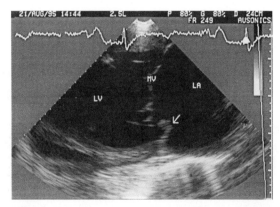

Figure 17-33 Long axis two-dimensional echocardiogram of a horse with ruptured chordae tendineae of the mitral valve *(arrow)* and acute left-sided congestive heart failure. This echocardiogram was obtained from the left parasternal window in the mitral valve position with a 2.5-MHz sector scanner transducer. An electrocardiogram is superimposed for timing. *LA,* Left atrium; *LV,* left ventricle; *MV,* mitral valve.

- Atrial fibrillation is more common among horses with chronic valvular regurgitation.
- Ventricular premature complexes or paroxysms of ventricular tachycardia may be present in horses with bacterial endocarditis of the mitral or aortic leaflets.
- Loud S_3 may be heard in association with ventricular volume overload.

Additional Diagnostics

- Obtain an ECG to establish the underlying cardiac rhythm.
- Obtain an echocardiogram to evaluate myocardial function (Fig. 17-32), determine the severity of underlying congenital or valvular heart disease (Figs. 17-33 and 17-34), and look for evidence of pulmonary hypertension (Fig. 17-35).
- A dilated pulmonary artery is compatible with significant pulmonary hypertension and the (low) possibility of impending pulmonary artery rupture (see Fig. 17-35).

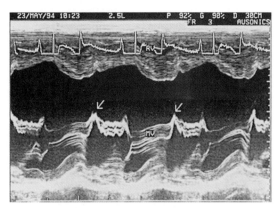

Figure 17-34 M-mode echocardiogram of a horse with acute, severe aortic regurgitation. Considerable separation between the mitral valve E point *(arrows)* and the interventricular septum is associated with significant left ventricular volume overload and dilatation of the left ventricular outflow tract and with the effect of aortic regurgitation on the septal leaflet of the mitral valve. The septal leaflet of the mitral valve has high-frequency vibrations caused by turbulence associated with the regurgitant jet. This echocardiogram was obtained from the right parasternal window with a 2.5-MHz sector scanner transducer. An electrocardiogram is superimposed for timing. *MV,* Mitral valve.

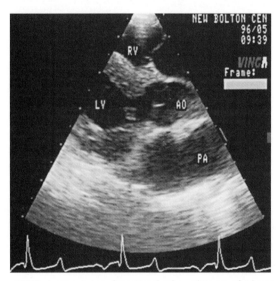

Figure 17-35 Long axis two-dimensional echocardiogram of a horse with ruptured chordae tendineae of the mitral valve and acute left-sided congestive heart failure. The small diameter of the aortic root *(AO)* and the larger diameter of the pulmonary artery *(PA)* are consistent with severe pulmonary hypertension. This echocardiogram was obtained from the right parasternal window in the left ventricular outflow tract position with a 2.5-MHz annular array transducer. An electrocardiogram is superimposed for timing. *LV,* Left ventricle; *RV,* right ventricle.

- Cardiac troponins, such as cardiac troponin I, might be elevated. Elevated troponin level is a sensitive and specific indicator of myocardial cell death; however, normal laboratory values do not exclude myocardial insult.
- Cardiac troponin I (cTn-I) is a more sensitive and specific indicator of myocardial cell death and damage than other cardiac isozymes such as creatine kinase (CK) MB. Normal values for horses are similar to those in humans and small animals, generally <0.1 ng/mL, depending on the assay. Different cTn-I assays have different reference ranges and cannot be compared.

- A chemistry profile, complete blood cell count, and measurement of total protein content and fibrinogen should be obtained to ascertain whether there is underlying disease and to evaluate the severity of any renal compromise (usually prerenal azotemia).

●❯ WHAT TO DO

Left-Sided Heart Failure

- Emergency management of pulmonary edema is instituted as soon as possible and includes furosemide, 1 to 2 mg/kg IV or 0.12 mg/kg/h as a constant rate infusion after a loading dose of 1 to 2 mg/kg IV. Dosing—increases or decreases—are dictated by respiratory rate and effort. There is *no* such thing as too much furosemide; the horse should be treated with whatever dose is needed to clear the pulmonary edema. Infusions result in increased diuresis with less renal damage than bolus dosing. Oral dosing of furosemide is shown to result in poor and variable absorption, so routes of administration other than oral are recommended. In an emergency, the intravenous route is used.
- ***Practice Tip:*** *Chronic administration of high doses of furosemide can lead to hypokalemic metabolic alkalosis.*
- Intranasal oxygen therapy is initiated with one or two nasal cannulas at 5 to 10 L/min.
- ***Practice Tip:*** *Drugs to reduce anxiety are administered if needed. Sedation should* not *be accomplished with alpha₂-adrenergic agonists such as xylazine and detomidine; these are vasoconstrictors that increase the regurgitant fraction and increase the workload of the heart. Instead, acepromazine is used for sedation and serves to decrease afterload.*
- Afterload reducers—vasodilators such as hydralazine, 0.5 to 1.0 mg/kg PO or 0.5 mg/kg IV q12h, or benazepril, 0.5 mg/kg PO q24h, if needed—are administered to patients with severe mitral or aortic regurgitation to improve cardiac output and reduce myocardial work. A single dose of enalapril, 0.5 mg/kg PO, the serum levels of enalapril and its active metabolite enalaprilat, were reported to be undetectable. Enalapril administration results in only a very mild decrease in angiotensin-converting enzyme (ACE) activity. Milrinone, 0.2 μg/kg IV, 10 μg/kg/min could be used for short-term management of CHF.
- If ventricular tachycardia is the cause of acute congestive heart failure, antiarrhythmic therapy is instituted as soon as possible. If the heart rate is >120 beats/min, ventricular tachycardia should be suspected. Selection of the appropriate antiarrhythmic drug depends on the severity of the arrhythmia and the associated clinical signs (see What to Do for Ventricular Tachycardia, p. 140).
- If sinus tachycardia, supraventricular tachycardia, or atrial fibrillation is present, positive inotropic support is instituted and consists of digoxin, 0.0022 mg/kg IV, or dobutamine, 1 to 5 mg/kg/min IV.
- Serum or plasma samples are obtained for measurement of digoxin concentration after several days of oral therapy to guide dosage adjustments.
  - Peak digoxin concentration is determined from a sample obtained 1 to 2 hours after oral digoxin administration.
  - Trough digoxin concentrations are measured and should fall within the therapeutic range of 0.5 to 1.5 ng/mL.
- Digoxin has a narrow therapeutic to toxic range; therefore, the patient is monitored for any signs of digoxin toxicity. Digoxin toxicity is reported in horses with digoxin concentrations >2 ng/mL.
- Anorexia, lethargy, colic, and the development of other cardiac arrhythmias are reported among individuals with digoxin toxicity.

- Hypokalemia potentiates the toxic effects of digoxin, yet digoxin toxicity can cause extracellular hyperkalemia by interfering with the sodium-potassium pump; therefore, careful monitoring of potassium status is important.
- Ectopic foci, usually atrial, develop with relatively small doses of digoxin in hypokalemic patients.
- The administration of digoxin is discontinued in the treatment of all horses when digoxin toxicity is suspected. A blood sample is obtained for measurement of serum or plasma digoxin, potassium, and creatinine concentrations.
- Digoxin toxicity is treated as follows:
  - Oral potassium supplementation, 40 g/450 kg PO, if the patient is hypokalemic, may be adequate if the clinical signs associated with digoxin toxicity are mild.
  - Intravenous potassium, 40 mEq/L, may be administered slowly in intravenous fluids to the hypokalemic patient if life-threatening arrhythmias are present.
  - Lidocaine, 20 to 50 µg/kg/min, is indicated for the management of ventricular arrhythmias associated with digoxin toxicity.
  - Phenytoin, 5 to 10 mg/kg IV for the first 12 hours, and then 1 to 5 mg/kg IM q12h or 1.82 mg/kg PO q12h is indicated in the management of supraventricular arrhythmias associated with digoxin toxicity. Side effects of phenytoin include a mild tranquilizing effect. Overdosing can lead to lip and facial twitching, gait deficits, and seizures. Do *not* use phenytoin in conjunction with other medications, particularly trimethoprim-sulfamethoxazole.
  - Administer cardiac glycoside–specific antibodies or their Fab fragment, Digibind. These agents bind excess circulating digoxin and prevent further development of digoxin toxicity. This treatment is reserved for patients with life-threatening digoxin toxicity because it is very expensive. In people with digoxin toxicity and hypokalemia, this treatment almost always results in a reversal of digoxin-induced cardiac arrhythmias.
  - Modify the dose of digoxin—increase dosing intervals to once daily or decrease dose—if prerenal azotemia is present.
- If the horse has bacterial endocarditis, broad-spectrum bactericidal intravenous antimicrobial therapy, both gram-positive and gram-negative coverage, are instituted after several blood cultures are obtained. A constant rate infusion administration of antimicrobials is performed initially, if possible. Aspirin therapy, 20 mg/kg PO or per rectum q24 to 48h, is also instituted to discourage the septic thrombus from increasing in size.
- Patients with bacterial endocarditis involving the pulmonic or tricuspid valve may have severe pneumonia or pulmonary thromboembolism because of septic emboli. Tricuspid valve endocarditis has frequently been associated with septic thrombophlebitis of the jugular vein.
- Clinical improvement within several days usually occurs with this treatment regimen. However, because of the severity of the underlying cardiac disease in most horses with clinical signs of congestive heart failure, the improvement usually is of short duration, 2 to 6 months.

Right-Sided Heart Failure
- *Practice Tip: Patients with long-standing congenital, valvular, or myocardial disease that gradually leads to congestive heart failure frequently have little in the way of clinical signs referable to the respiratory system. These horses usually have clinical signs of right-sided congestive heart failure and rarely need emergency treatment.*

- Horses may have tachypnea at rest, an occasional cough, prolonged recovery times to resting respiratory rate after exercise, and biventricular failure or a large pleural effusion associated with right-sided heart failure.
- The veterinarian usually is consulted because the horse has preputial, pectoral, or ventral edema.
- Generalized venous distention and jugular pulsations usually are present.
- Syncope may be present in patients with severe right-sided congestive heart failure and decreased pulmonary blood flow.

Auscultation
- Coarse vesicular sounds at rest or with a rebreathing bag and crackles or moist sounds are rarely detected.
- Dullness may be detected in the cranioventral lung field on auscultation or percussion associated with pleural effusion.
- In rare instances, the heart may sound muffled because of a small pericardial effusion.
- Murmurs of mitral and tricuspid valvular regurgitation are detected frequently.
- Some affected horses also have murmurs of aortic regurgitation or a ventricular septal defect or another, usually complex, congenital defect. The murmurs associated with complex cardiac defects do *not* have to be impressive.
- The heart rate usually is elevated and irregular if atrial fibrillation is present.
- Patients with monomorphic ventricular tachycardia and congestive heart failure usually have a more rapid (>120 beats/min) and regular rhythm but have similar clinical signs.
- These horses should be treated with antiarrhythmic drugs to cardiovert ventricular tachycardia (see Ventricular Tachycardia, p. 139).
- A loud S_3 may be associated with ventricular volume overload.

WHAT TO DO

Right-Sided Congestive Heart Failure
- Treatment with furosemide, positive inotropic drugs (usually digoxin), and vasodilators (hydralazine, benazepril) as indicated before, should be started.
- Clinical improvement usually is noticed within 24 hours (see Table 17-6).

Pericarditis and Pericardial Effusion
- Pericarditis is uncommon in horses, but it usually manifests as an emergency with clinical signs of cardiovascular collapse.
- Concurrent or historical respiratory tract disease is present in approximately 50% of patients with pericarditis.
- *Practice Tip: Transportation, fever, exposure to large number of horses, and high prevalence of mare reproductive loss syndrome are risk factors for idiopathic pericarditis. Actinobacillus spp. is one of the most common organisms cultured from adult horses with septic pericarditis.*

- Arrhythmias are detected infrequently, usually are atrial if present, and indicate the presence of concurrent myocarditis.
- Horses with pericarditis, particularly those with septic pericarditis, may have mild anemia, neutrophilic leukocytosis, hyperproteinemia, and hyperfibrinogenemia.
- Cardiac tamponade can occur when fluid accumulates rapidly within the pericardial sac, impeding cardiac filling (particularly right sided) and causes a rapid decrease in cardiac output.
- The three determinants of the development of cardiac tamponade are
  - Distensibility of the pericardial sac
  - Rate at which fluid accumulation occurs within the pericardial sac
  - Amount of fluid present within the pericardial sac
- **Practice Tip:** *Cardiac tamponade should be suspected in any horse with increasing venous pressure, tachycardia, muffled heart sounds, systemic hypotension, and pulsus paradoxus.*
- **Definition:** Pulsus paradoxus is an inspiratory reduction in arterial blood pressure >10 mm Hg.
- Central venous pressures of up to 43 cm H_2O (normal central venous pressure, 5 to 15 cm H_2O) have been reported in patients with cardiac tamponade, large pericardial effusions, or constrictive pericarditis.
- Right atrial, right ventricular, and pulmonary arterial end-diastolic pressures may be increased in horses with cardiac tamponade.

Clinical Signs

- Many equine patients with pericarditis exhibit signs of discomfort that are initially interpreted as abdominal pain; they are therefore usually referred for colic.
- Physical examination findings include depression, tachycardia, generalized venous distention, pectoral, ventral, and preputial edema, and muffled heart sounds. Fever, lethargy, anorexia, jugular pulsations, weak arterial pulses, pericardial friction rubs, tachypnea, dullness in the cranioventral thorax, and weight loss also may be part of the clinical presentation.

Echocardiography

- **Practice Tip:** *Echocardiography is the diagnostic modality of choice for the assessment of the amount of pericardial fluid, its character, and the degree of cardiac compromise.*
- Fibrinous effusive pericarditis is most common in horses. The volume of fluid associated with pericarditis ranges from none detectable to >14 L (Fig. 17-36). Fluid within the pericardial sac usually is anechoic to slightly hypoechoic in horses with septic or idiopathic pericarditis. Sheets of fibrin with frondlike projections usually are imaged on the epicardial and pericardial surfaces. Compartmentalization of this fluid can occur, and walled-off areas develop in the pericardial sac. Concurrent pleural effusion often is present. Nonfibrinous effusive pericarditis is most common in patients with congestive heart failure, *not* in patients with primary pericardial disease. Hemopericardium has

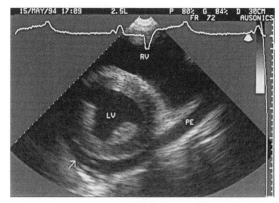

Figure 17-36   Short axis two-dimensional echocardiogram of a horse with pericarditis. The *arrow* points to some fibrin within the pericardial sac. This echocardiogram was obtained from the right parasternal window in the left ventricular position with a 2.5-MHz sector scanner transducer. An electrocardiogram is superimposed for timing. *LV,* Left ventricle; *PE,* pericardial effusion; *RV,* right ventricle.

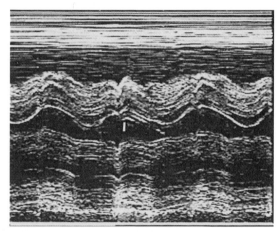

Figure 17-37   M-mode echocardiogram of a horse with idiopathic pericarditis and a fibrinous pericardial effusion demonstrating the swinging pattern of right ventricular free wall motion. The slight increase in right ventricular diameter is associated with inspiration *(I).* This echocardiogram was obtained from the right parasternal window in the left ventricular position with a 2.5-MHz sector scanner transducer.

been detected in several horses that have sustained thoracic trauma and in one foal with penetration of the right ventricular free wall by a broken and dislodged intravenous catheter. Blood within the pericardial sac looks like echogenic swirling fluid, and an organized thrombus may be seen in the space.
- Excessive motion or collapse of the right atrial and right ventricular free wall is detected by echocardiography in patients with pericardial effusion (Fig. 17-37).
- Diastolic collapse of the right atrial and right ventricular free wall occurs as the amount of pericardial fluid increases. This collapse is first pictured in the right atrium and right ventricular outflow tract because these areas have lower pressures and therefore are the easiest to compress.
- Early echocardiographic signs of cardiac tamponade include an inspiratory increase in the dimension of the right ventricle, an inspiratory decrease in the internal diameter of the left ventricle, and collapse of the right atrium (right atrial inversion).

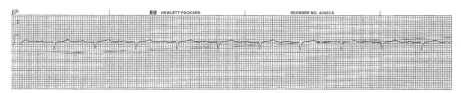

Figure 17-38 Base-apex electrocardiogram of a horse with pericarditis shows damping of the P waves, QRS complexes, and T waves from the pericardial effusion. Tachycardia is present (60 beats/min) and is a common finding in horses with pericarditis. The P-P interval and R-R interval are regular. This electrocardiogram was recorded at a paper speed of 25 mm/s with a sensitivity of 10 mm/mV.

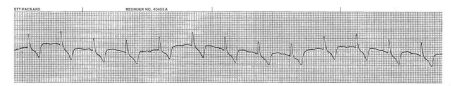

Figure 17-39 Base-apex electrocardiogram shows electrical alternans in a horse with pericardial effusion. The slight variation in the amplitude of the QRS complexes from 0.6 mV to 0.8 mV is evident. The amplitude of the P, QRS, and T complexes is damped. This electrocardiogram was recorded at a paper speed of 25 mm/s with a sensitivity of 10 mm/mV.

Electrocardiography

- ECG reveals small-amplitude P, QRS, and T complexes caused by damping of the electrical impulse by the surrounding pericardial fluid (Fig. 17-38).
- Electrical alternans, a cyclic variation in the size of the QRS complexes, is reported in horses with pericardial effusion but is seen infrequently (Fig. 17-39). Electrical alternans is believed to be caused by the swinging motion of the heart in the pericardial fluid.

- A globoid cardiac silhouette is detected during thoracic radiography. This sign usually is accompanied by opacification of the ventral thorax caused by concurrent pleural effusion. However, this radiographic appearance cannot be differentiated definitively from other forms of diffuse cardiac enlargement, and good-quality lateral thoracic radiographs cannot be obtained with portable radiographic equipment except in evaluation of foals.

●⟩ WHAT TO DO

Pericarditis

- Pericardiocentesis is the diagnostic and therapeutic tool of choice for horses with pericarditis, as long as there is enough pericardial fluid to perform this procedure safely.
- Echocardiography is used to reliably select a site for pericardiocentesis and placement of an indwelling tube, if considerable volume of pericardial fluid is imaged.
- In most patients with pericarditis, the ideal site is the left fifth intercostal space, above the lateral thoracic vein and below a line level with the point of the shoulder, over the left ventricular free wall and below the left atrium and AV groove.
  - **Practice Tip:** *Lacerations of the left atrium, coronary vessels, or right ventricle are avoided if this site is chosen for pericardiocentesis.*
- ECG monitoring (base-apex as rhythm strip is adequate) is performed during pericardiocentesis to monitor the patient for the development of arrhythmias induced by the procedure (Fig. 17-40).
- Place an intravenous catheter before pericardiocentesis is started for rapid venous access in case arrhythmias do develop.
- If a large number of ventricular premature complexes, ventricular tachycardia, or polymorphic ventricular complexes are detected, stop advancement of the pericardiocentesis catheter.
- If the ventricular arrhythmias do *not* disappear, institute intravenous administration of antiarrhythmic drugs or withdraw the pericardiocentesis catheter, depending on the severity of the arrhythmias detected. The catheter can be repositioned once the arrhythmia has resolved.

- Insert a large-bore (28F to 32F) Argyle catheter, using a trocar, as an indwelling tube if there is a large volume of pericardial fluid or if cardiac tamponade is present.
- This tube can be used for sample collection and pericardial drainage and lavage.
- Smaller-bore (12F to 24F) Argyle catheters containing a trocar are used if the volume of fluid within the pericardial sac is small.
- Submit the sample obtained for culture and sensitivity testing, cytologic evaluation, and viral isolation, if possible (Table 17-7).
- *Actinobacillus equuli* and streptococcal organisms are the most frequently isolated organisms from horses with septic pericarditis.
- Perform thoracocentesis if pleural effusion is present. Obtain a transtracheal aspirate if pulmonary disease is suspected. Request culture and sensitivity testing of both of these fluids; they may yield the causative agent responsible for the concurrent pericarditis.
- **Practice Tip:** *Lavage of the pericardial sac after drainage of the pericardial fluid greatly improves the prognosis for patients with pericarditis. Lavage the pericardial sac with 2 L of warm, sterile 0.9% saline solution.*
  - Infuse the lavage fluid and leave it in the pericardial sac for ½ to 1 hour. Drain the fluid and instill 1 to 2 L of sterile 0.9% saline solution with 10 to 20 × 10⁶ IU sodium penicillin/L or 1 g gentamicin/L.
  - Leave this infusate in the pericardial sac for the next 12 hours.
  - Repeat drainage, lavage, drainage, and instillation of sterile fluid until <0.5 L of pericardial fluid is retrieved at the time of the

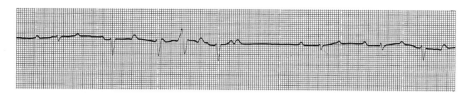

Figure 17-40   Lead II electrocardiogram obtained during pericardiocentesis of a horse with pericardial effusion. A paroxysm of ventricular premature depolarizations is evident. Two different morphologies of ventricular premature complexes are present in the paroxysm. The amplitude of the P, QRS, and T complexes is very damped. This electrocardiogram was recorded at a paper speed of 25 mm/s with a sensitivity of 10 mm/mV.

Table 17-7   Causes of Pericardial Effusions in Horses

Type of Effusion	Cause	Cytologic Finding	Culture Result	Treatment
Blood	Neoplasia	Neoplasia cells—usually red blood cells and lymphocytes	No growth	Drainage and corticosteroid therapy—symptomatic only
	Left atrial rupture (rare)	Blood	No growth	Intravenous fluids
	Aortic root rupture	Blood	No growth	Intravenous fluids
Trauma		Blood	No growth unless penetrating wound of the pericardium	Drainage if cardiac tamponade; intravenous fluid support
	Iatrogenic injury (intravenous or cardiac catheterization or cardiac puncture)	Blood	No growth unless iatrogenic contamination	Drainage if cardiac tamponade; intravenous fluid support
Transudate	Congestive heart failure		No growth	
	Hypoproteinemia		No growth	
Exudate	Idiopathic pericarditis	Lymphocytes, plasma cells, and red blood cells in large numbers	No growth, seroconversion to viral diseases possible	Drainage and lavage with sterile saline solution and instillation of broad-spectrum antibiotics, systemic broad-spectrum antibiotics until cytologic and culture results are negative for bacterial infection, then systemic corticosteroids
	Septic pericarditis	Neutrophils	± Positive culture (*Streptococcus* or *Actinobacillus* organisms)	Drainage and lavage with sterile saline solution and instillation of broad-spectrum antibiotics until the results of culture and sensitivity tests are available, minimum 4 weeks of antimicrobials

initial drainage or the pericardial catheter falls out and fluid does *not* reaccumulate.
- Administer broad-spectrum systemic antibiotics.
- Although not previously used in horses with this condition, instillation of tissue plasminogen activator (tPA), 6 to 30 mg, could be of value in decreasing fibrin production.
- Continue use of systemic and intrapericardial antimicrobial agents until results of the cytologic examination and culture and sensitivity testing have ruled out a bacterial cause of pericarditis.
- Although systemic concentrations of antibiotics are reached in the pericardial fluid with the administration of systemic antimicrobials alone, the use of intrapericardial antimicrobials increases threefold the concentrations of antimicrobials in the pericardial fluid. This local increase in antimicrobial concentration is helpful because of the fibrinous nature of pericarditis in horses and the rapid inactivation of many antimicrobial agents by fibrin.
- Long-term (4 to 6 weeks) systemic antimicrobial therapy is indicated in the care of horses with septic pericarditis.

- Intravenously administered fluids may be needed if the creatinine concentration is elevated to prevent or control renal failure.
- Patients with pericarditis should be given a guarded to fair prognosis initially, until response to treatment with pericardial drainage and lavage is detected, at which time the prognosis usually is changed to good for life and performance.
- Corticosteroids, dexamethasone, 0.045 to 0.09 mg/kg IV q24h for 3 days followed by a tapering dose, are indicated in the treatment of horses with idiopathic pericarditis (often lymphocytic plasmacytic) once a bacterial cause has been definitively excluded.
- Therapy for septic or idiopathic pericarditis should continue for several weeks after the patient is afebrile, the condition is clinically normal, and the pericardial effusion has resolved. During this time, the equine patient should be stall rested and hand walked, with turnout in a small paddock for an additional month.
- Echocardiographic reevaluation is indicated at that time to determine whether the horse is ready to return to work.

Myocarditis

- The origin of myocarditis may be viral (e.g., EHVI, influenza), immune mediated (e.g., purpura hemorrhagica), or toxic (e.g., monensin, blister beetle, snake bite). Myocarditis has also been linked to overdoses of clenbuterol; atypical myopathy; selenium deficiency or toxicity; glycogen branching enzyme deficiency of Quarter Horse foals; and doxorubicin, which is sometimes used for treating lymphosarcoma. *Borrelia* has *not* been documented to cause myocarditis in horses.
- Viral and immune-mediated myocarditis is associated with persistent fever, often of unknown origin, and tachycardia.

Clinical Signs

- Fever
- Lethargy
- Arrhythmias, especially ventricular tachycardia, are common.
- Signs of heart failure, right or left, may occur.

Diagnosis

- Echocardiography may demonstrate decreased cardiac function.
- An arrhythmia, ventricular tachycardia, may be seen on ECG.
- *Practice Tip: Cardiac troponin I is increased if there is myocardial necrosis or strain.*
- Fever that is *not* responsive to antibiotics is common.

Treatment

- Corticosteroids are indicated for clinically apparent myocarditis caused by viral or immune-mediated causes. Dexamethasone, 0.1 mg/kg, is recommended, followed by a tapering dose over 2 weeks with frequent follow-up echocardiography examinations.
- Prognosis is generally good if there are *no* signs of heart failure.

●〉 WHAT TO DO

Myocarditis

- Measure cTn-I to confirm there is myocardial cell disease.
- Perform echocardiography to confirm abnormally low cardiac contractility.
- Test for viral causes.
- Treat with dexamethasone: 0.05 to 0.1 mg/kg IV or IM.
- Monitor cTn-I and cardiac function.

Ionophore Toxicity

- *Practice Tip: Horses are uniquely sensitive to the cardiotoxic effects of several of the ionophores—monensin, salinomycin, and lasalocid. The median lethal dose of these ionophores in horses is much lower than that in other domestic species.*
- The ionophores, especially monensin, are primarily cardiotoxic, although other signs of systemic toxicity may be detected in exposed individuals. Horses of any age, breed,

or sex can be exposed to ionophore-contaminated feed. The contamination can come from feed accidentally contaminated at the feed mill or from accidental feeding of, or exposure to, ionophore-containing steer or poultry feed.
- Feed samples should be obtained for toxicologic analysis if ionophore exposure is suspected.
- Gastrointestinal samples from any horse that has experienced sudden death should be analyzed similarly.

Clinical Signs

- Sudden death often is the first indication of exposure to high doses of ionophores.
- Fever, depression, lethargy, restlessness, exercise intolerance, and profuse sweating are some of the signs first noticed by the owners or trainers of affected horses.
- Colic, anorexia, poor appetite, and feed refusal are common initial clinical signs because ionophore-contaminated feed is less palatable and, when eaten, changes the intestinal flora.
- Muscle weakness, trembling, and ataxia often occur.
- Affected horses may be polyuric and become oliguric or anuric. Diarrhea, colic, or ileus is reported frequently and usually precedes cardiac signs.
- Muddy or injected mucous membranes and thready arterial pulses may be detected initially.
- Cardiac arrhythmias may develop at any time after ionophore exposure but are most likely in the first few days to weeks after exposure.
- Generalized venous distention, jugular pulses, ventral edema, and murmurs of mitral or tricuspid regurgitation may develop weeks to months after ionophore exposure.
- Recumbency may occur without heart failure with any of the three ionophores.

Diagnosis and Prognosis

- *Practice Tip: Echocardiography is the diagnostic modality of choice in situations of suspected or known ionophore exposure to determine the severity of the myocardial injury in exposed horses.*
- Patients with normal left ventricular function and normal fractional shortening (30% to 40%) have an excellent prognosis for life and performance.
- Patients with slightly depressed fractional shortening have a good prognosis for life and a fair to good prognosis for performance. They should be able to perform successfully in lower levels of athletic work.
- The detection of a fractional shortening <20% in exposed horses is a poor prognostic indicator. Affected horses with a fractional shortening of >10% but <20% may initially survive monensin exposure but have persistent left ventricular dysfunction and exercise intolerance and may develop congestive heart failure over the subsequent weeks or months.
- Horses with a fractional shortening of <10% do *not* survive monensin exposure and are usually dead within days or

weeks after the echocardiographic examination (Fig. 17-41).

- ECG abnormalities can be detected in horses recently exposed to ionophores but are *not* good prognostic indicators of the severity of the myocardial injury.
- Axis shifts, ST segment depression, T wave changes, atrial and ventricular premature complexes, atrial fibrillation, ventricular tachycardia, and a variety of bradyarrhythmias are reported in horses exposed to ionophores (Fig. 17-42).
- Most horses exposed to ionophores in the field situation, however, do *not* have cardiac arrhythmias.
- Elevations in the level of cTn-I have been detected in horses exposed to ionophores.
- ***Practice Tip:*** *Cardiac troponin I is a sensitive and specific indicator of myocardial cell damage.* It has a short half-life so values may return toward normal range within 2 to 3 days following a severe, single-dose, ionophore exposure.
- Elevations in cTn-I may *not* occur for 18 to 48 hours after ingestion of the ionophore.
- Other clinicopathologic abnormalities that have been reported include elevations in hematocrit; total plasma protein concentration; osmolality; total bilirubin level; and serum levels of blood urea nitrogen, creatinine, aspartate aminotransferase, and alkaline phosphatase; and decreases in serum level of calcium and plasma level of potassium.

- The absence of abnormal clinicopathologic abnormalities, however, cannot rule out the diagnosis of monensin or other ionophore exposure.
- Toxic dose for an adult horse is 1.5 to 2.5 mg/kg but may be lower if monensin is ingested with a high-fat concentrate or if the stomach is relatively empty.

◉❯ WHAT TO DO

Ionophore Exposure/Toxicity

- Remove all suspected contaminated feed.
- Administer activated charcoal and magnesium sulfate to decrease further absorption of recently ingested feed. Absorption may be enhanced with vegetable oils.
- Administer large doses of vitamin E as soon as possible after exposure in an attempt to stabilize cell membranes and control peroxidation-mediated cell injury.
- Provide appropriate supportive care (Box 17-6).
- Keep exposed horses at stall rest for a minimum of 2 months.
- ***Practice Tip:*** *Digoxin is contraindicated in the management of acute monensin exposure because monensin and digoxin have an additive effect, causing calcium to flood into the myocardial cell.*
- The use of digoxin in a patient recently exposed to monensin can result in further overload of the intracellular calcium sequestration mechanisms and increase the amount and severity of myocardial cell injury and cell death.

Box 17-6	Approach to the Horse with Potential Ionophore Exposure

- Perform complete physical and cardiovascular examinations.
- Treat affected horses with antiarrhythmics as needed to control life-threatening arrhythmias.
- Pass a nasogastric tube and administer activated charcoal or mineral oil in attempt to prevent further absorption of the ionophore.
- Administer vitamin E or vitamin E with selenium as soon as possible.
- Keep exposed horses at stall rest and minimize stress.
- Do *not* administer digoxin, which is contraindicated if exposure is recent.
- Perform echocardiography:
  - Evaluate myocardial function carefully, looking for myocardial hypokinesis, dyskinesis, or akinesis.
  - Evaluate the myocardium for heterogeneity of muscle echogenicity (tissue characterization).
- Obtain blood for measurement of cardiac troponin I.
- Obtain an electrocardiogram, including 24-hour continuous ECG, if possible.

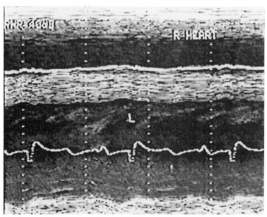

Figure 17-41   M-mode echocardiogram of a horse with monensin toxicosis. Systolic dysfunction is evident. This echocardiogram was obtained from the right parasternal window in the left ventricular position with a 2.5-MHz sector scanner transducer. An electrocardiogram is superimposed for timing. *L,* Left ventricle.

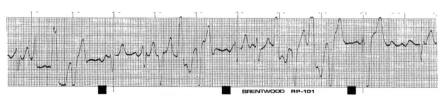

Figure 17-42   Lead II electrocardiogram of a horse with monensin toxicosis and polymorphic ventricular tachycardia. Considerably different QRS complexes are evident, and some are occurring in rapid succession. The ventricular rate is 110 beats/min. This electrocardiogram was recorded at a paper speed of 25 mm/s with a sensitivity of 5 mm/mV.

Aortic Root Rupture

- Aortic root rupture (ARR) in horses most frequently results in sudden death associated with massive hemorrhage into the thoracic cavity.
- If the aortic rupture is intracardiac rather than extrapericardial, the affected horse survives for a variable time.
- The life expectancy after ARR depends on the extent of the aortic rupture, the severity of the intracardiac shunt, the chamber or structure into which the rupture occurred, the severity of the resultant cardiac (ventricular) arrhythmias, the patient's myocardial function, and the presence or absence of other cardiac disease. Several horses with aortic rupture have lived for a year or more after the initial event. The longest survival time for a horse following documented aortic rupture is 5 years.
- ***Practice Tip:*** *Affected horses usually are male and primarily stallions, 10 years or older.*
- Recently, aortic rupture and aortopulmonary fistulation have been characterized in Friesians.
- The rupture in Friesians is of the aortic arch near the ligamentum arteriosum. Circumferential perivascular hemorrhage at the site and aortopulmonary fistulation is commonly found.

Clinical Signs at Time of Rupture

- Distress, interpreted initially as colic, tachycardia (rapid regular heart rates of 120 beats/min), jugular distention, and jugular pulsations are initial signs.
- The rapid regular heart rhythm and jugular pulsations suggest a rhythm of ventricular tachycardia.
- Acute death is common in both breeding stallions and Friesians, age range 1 to 20, median 4 years and both sexes.

Physical Examination Findings

- Bounding arterial pulses, loud continuous murmur with its point of maximal intensity in the right fourth intercostal space, and a loud S_3 occur.

- Systolic murmurs of tricuspid regurgitation have been reported in horses with aortic root rupture.
- *Friesians* with aortic rupture often have increased rectal temperature (reason unknown), peripheral edema, pale mucous membranes, tachycardia of ≥80 beats/min, increased jugular pulse and a bounding arterial pulse. In one report the circumferential accumulation of blood at the base of the heart caused massive peripheral edema, ascites, and pleural effusion due to obstruction of venous return.
- Auscultation of the abdomen usually reveals normal gastrointestinal sounds. A rectal examination yields normal findings.

Diagnosis

- ECG often exhibits uniform ventricular tachycardia (Fig. 17-43) with a heart rate of 120 to 250 beats/min; higher heart rates are possible but have *not* been recorded in horses with aortic root rupture.
- Echocardiographic examination might depict the rupture in the aortic root at the right aortic sinus or right sinus of Valsalva (Fig. 17-44).
- Aneurysmal dilatation and rupture of the right sinus of Valsalva (Fig. 17-45) are detected in approximately one half of affected horses, whereas in other horses, *no* preexisting aortic root disease is detected.
- The aortic root can dissect apically, down the interventricular septum (Fig. 17-46) with subsequent endocardial rupture into the right or left ventricle (most frequent) or rupture into the right atrium or tricuspid valve.
- Generalized cardiomegaly is common, and pulmonary artery dilatation is imaged in approximately one half of patients with aortocardiac fistulas from aortic root rupture.
- Aortic ruptures into the pericardial sac occur but are uncommon and are *not* localized to the right aortic sinus.
- In *Friesians,* the rupture often occurs near the ligamentum arteriosum and causes an aortopulmonary fistula. The

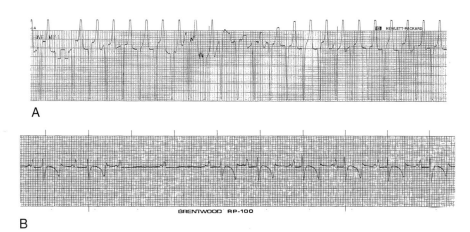

Figure 17-43   Lead aVf electrocardiograms of a horse with aortic root rupture and an aortic-cardiac fistula. Monomorphic ventricular tachycardia **(A)** is present at a ventricular rate of 160 beats/min, which is cardioverted successfully to sinus rhythm with second-degree AV block **(B)** after treatment with quinidine gluconate, lidocaine, MgSO$_4$, and procainamide. The horse was cardioverted to sinus rhythm with a rate of 60 beats/min with the procainamide infusion. This electrocardiogram was recorded at a paper speed of 25 mm/s with a sensitivity of 5 mm/mV.

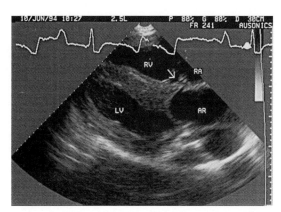

Figure 17-44 Two-dimensional echocardiogram of a horse with aortic root rupture and the presence of an aortic-cardiac fistula (same horse as in Fig. 17-43). The defect is evident in the right side of the aorta *(arrow)* just under the septal leaflet of the tricuspid valve. This echocardiogram was obtained from the right parasternal window just cranial to the left ventricular outflow tract view with a 2.5-MHz sector scanner transducer. *AR,* aortic root; *LV,* left ventricle; *RA,* right atrium; *RV,* right ventricle.

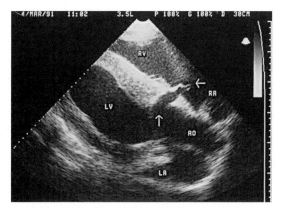

Figure 17-45 Two-dimensional echocardiogram of a horse with a ruptured sinus of Valsalva aneurysm. The communication *(vertical arrow)* between the aortic root *(AO)* and the right atrium *(RA)* is evident. Torn aneurysmal tissue *(horizontal arrow)* is floating in the right atrium. This echocardiogram was obtained with a 3.5-MHz sector scanner transducer from the right parasternal window slightly cranial to the left ventricular outflow tract view. *LA,* Left atrium; *LV,* left ventricle; *RV,* right ventricle.

continuous turbulent flow is imaged in the main pulmonary artery; the descending aorta cannot be seen on transthoracic echo.

- Pulsed wave, continuous wave, and color flow Doppler echocardiography and contrast echocardiography can be used to detect the intracardiac shunt flow and to attempt to semiquantify the severity of this shunt.

◉ WHAT TO DO

Aortic Rupture

- Correct the uniform ventricular tachycardia, as previously recommended, if the heart rate is greater than 100 beats/min, the horse has clinical signs of cardiovascular collapse, the rhythm is polymorphic (not reported), or an R on T is detected in the ECG (not reported).

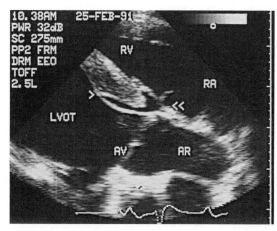

Figure 17-46 Two-dimensional echocardiogram of a horse with a ruptured sinus of Valsalva aneurysm and subendocardial dissection of blood down the interventricular septum (same horse as in Fig. 17-45). Dissection of blood down the left (primarily; *arrowhead*) and right side of the interventricular septum is evident. The aortic-cardiac fistula is between the right aortic sinus (see Fig. 17-45) and the right atrium *(double arrowhead).* This echocardiogram was obtained with a 2.5-MHz sector scanner transducer from the right parasternal window in the left ventricular outflow tract view. An electrocardiogram is superimposed for timing. *AR,* Aortic root *AV,* aortic valves; *LVOT,* left ventricular outflow tract; *RA,* right atrium; *RV,* right ventricle.

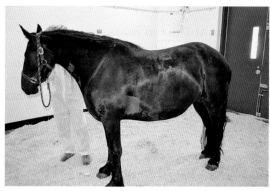

Figure 17-47 A 5-year-old Friesian horse with aortopulmonary fistulation and associated blood clots around the base of the heart, which caused signs of right-sided heart failure due to obstruction of venous return.

- Afterload reduction is indicated to help decrease the severity of the intracardiac shunt.
- Diuretics and positive inotropic drugs may be indicated if the horse has congestive heart failure.

Prognosis

- Affected individuals have a poor prognosis for life and should *not* be used for performance, even if the clinical condition or echocardiographic findings improve. These horses are always at increased risk of sudden death. In *Friesians,* death occurs acutely or within several days after clinical signs are noted (Figure 17-47).

References

References can be found on the companion website at www.equine-emergencies.com.

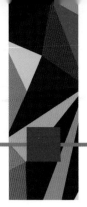

CHAPTER 18

Gastrointestinal System

DIAGNOSTIC AND THERAPEUTIC PROCEDURES

Barbara Dallap Schaer and James A. Orsini

Nasogastric Tube Placement

Placement of a nasogastric tube is used for the administration of large volumes of enteral medication(s), fluids, and electrolytes. This is also an important diagnostic and therapeutic procedure in the evaluation and treatment of a horse with signs of colic. Nasogastric intubation, followed by creation of a siphon, is performed to evacuate any accumulated fluid or gas in the stomach due to functional or mechanical proximal obstruction of the gastrointestinal tract. Fluid is removed to alleviate gastric pain caused by visceral distention, and most importantly to prevent gastric rupture. Nasogastric intubation is indicated in suspected cases of esophageal obstruction to confirm the diagnosis and relieve the esophageal obstruction. Nasogastric tubes are commercially available that are specifically designed for treatment of esophageal obstruction (directions included with tube).[1] Every clinician develops his or her own technique for passing a nasogastric tube. The following description may be useful for the less experienced.

Equipment
- Nasogastric tube (sized appropriately)
- Bucket half-filled with warm water
- 400-mL nylon dose syringe, *or*
- Veterinary injection pump (fluid pump)[2]

Procedure
- Immerse the nasogastric tube in warm water until it is clean and flexible.
- Adequately restrain the horse. This may require a chain shank over the nose or under the lip, a twitch, chemical restraint, or a combination thereof.
- Stand on the horse's left side, place the right hand over the nose, and use the thumb to reflect the alar fold of the left nostril dorsally. Do not obstruct airflow in the right nostril. Apply pressure to the bridge of the nose so that the head is flexed more ventrally to promote swallowing of the tube.

- Using the left hand, guide the tube ventrally and medially along the ventral nasal meatus. The middle nasal meatus is immediately dorsal and must be avoided.
- Advance the tube slowly, and refrain from forcing the tube if excessive resistance is encountered. If the patient is tossing its head, hold the tube in the nostril using the thumb of the right hand. Mild sedation with an α_2-agonist (e.g., xylazine, detomidine) can be used as an adjunct to physical restraint.
- The tube encounters some resistance as it reaches the epiglottis. Many horses swallow the tube immediately, but it may be necessary to rotate the tube approximately 180 degrees to facilitate passage into the esophagus. Gently "bumping" the epiglottis with the end of the tube, or blowing into the tube may encourage some patients to swallow. Try to pass the tube on the patient's first swallow because subsequent attempts to stimulate swallowing become progressively more difficult. If no swallow reflex is elicited, attempt to pass the tube using the opposite nostril.
- Be absolutely certain the tube is in the esophagus and not in the trachea. There are several ways to ensure correct placement. ***Important:*** *All must be confirmed before the tube is advanced farther and before any medication is delivered:*
  - Resistance is encountered when the tube moves down the esophagus. The tube passes down the trachea relatively easily, and the tube passing over the tracheal rings is palpable.
  - Negative pressure (aspiration is not possible) is obtained with suction if the tube is in the esophagus because the lumen collapses. Suction on the end of a tube in the trachea does not result in negative pressure.
  - The end of the tube is seen advancing down the neck to the left of midline when in the esophagus. The tube is not seen if it is in the trachea. The tube should be palpated as it passes toward the thoracic inlet, or more easily, as it rests beside the proximal trachea (usually to the left). Exact tube placement is confirmed by gently pushing the trachea dorsally with one hand while using the fingertips to feel the tube in the esophagus. This is the most reliable assessment of correct tube placement. In a small percentage of horses, the tube in the esophagus is palpated on the right side.
- Blow into the tube to facilitate advancement through the cardia into the stomach. Once the tube is in the stomach, gas that smells like ingesta is emitted.

[1]Rüsch esophagus flush probe, Oesophagus-sprelsonde (Willy Ruesch AG, Kernen, Germany).
[2]Veterinary injection pump (Nasco, Inc., Fort Atkinson, Wisconsin).

- Attempt to obtain reflux before administering large volumes of fluid. ***Practice Tip:*** *To obtain reflux, create a siphon by establishing a column of water between the stomach and the free end of the nasogastric tube.* Administer one or two dose syringes full of warm water to fill the tube, aspirate a small amount of fluid, detach the syringe, and lower the tube end. Several attempts are often needed before gastric fluid is successfully siphoned off the stomach. If there is high index of suspicion of gastric distention, ultrasound evidence of the stomach imaged at the most caudal intercostal space, or clinical signs of proximal obstruction (high heart rate, small intestinal distention on abdominal palpation per rectum, etc.), be persistent in attempting to decompress the stomach.
- If no net reflux is obtained after an appropriate number of attempts, it should be safe to administer enteral medication or fluid. Lift the tube end above the patient's head to complete delivery of the medication. Before removing the tube, lower the tube end to ensure that there is not excessive pressure on the stomach. Evacuate the contents of the tube before removing the tube.
- Crimp the tube or leave the dose syringe attached during removal so that fluid does not drain into the pharynx or nasal passage.

    A normal horse usually has gastric reflux of less than 2 L of fluid. To determine the amount of reflux, measure the total volume obtained minus the volume started with in a single bucket. Alternatively, total volume obtained minus the amount used to create the siphon can be calculated if two buckets are used.

- ***Important:*** *Do not administer enteral fluids to patients with significant reflux.* It is *not* absorbed and increases the likelihood of gastric rupture. Excessive reflux is often the result of proximal intestinal obstruction, either mechanical or functional. Patients with a large quantity of reflux should have a nasogastric tube left in place and secured to the halter in an attempt to prevent gastric rupture. The tube should have a Heimlich valve placed over the end to allow fluid and gas to escape. Retrieval of reflux should be repeated every few hours in these cases.

Complications

- Accidentally administering a large volume of fluid into the lungs of a patient can be fatal. For this reason, one must literally "see, feel, smell, and hear" the tube in the correct position. If a large volume of fluid is accidentally administered into the trachea, immediate communication with the owner followed by prompt medical attention is warranted. Extreme caution should be used with enteral administration of mineral oil; mineral oil aspiration is often fatal.
- Bleeding from the nose is an occasional complication. The conchal mucosa is extremely vascular and easily injured. Most nosebleeds eventually stop without serious consequences.
- If a nosebleed occurs prior to reaching the stomach, rinse the tube and attempt to pass it gently through the other nostril.

- A smaller diameter tube is less likely to damage the mucosa. Make sure the tube has no nicks or sharp edges that could cause mucosal injury. If bleeding continues for more than 10 to 15 minutes or is believed to be excessive, an intranasal spray of 10 mg phenylephrine hydrochloride diluted in 10 mL of sterile saline solution infused through a nasal catheter may help to stop the nose bleed.

Abdominocentesis

Peritoneal fluid analysis can be a useful tool in evaluating the patient with acute gastrointestinal disease, intermittent abdominal pain, diarrhea, or chronic weight loss (see p. 159).

Equipment

- Twitch or possibly sedation, if necessary
- Clippers
- Material for sterile scrub
- Sterile gloves
- Sterile 18- to 22-gauge, $1\frac{1}{2}$-inch (3.8-cm) needles, metal teat cannula (3.75 inches [9.4 cm] long), $3\frac{1}{2}$-inch spinal needle, or metal bitch urinary catheter (10.5 inches [26.3 cm] long) (the latter two may be necessary for larger or obese horses)
- 2% local anesthetic (with 25-gauge needle and 3-mL syringe)
- #15 blade if using a cannula or urinary catheter
- Sterile gauze sponge
- Tubes containing ethylenediaminetetraacetic acid (EDTA) and plain Vacutainer tubes for analysis
- Sterile vial, Port-a-Cul culture and transport system, or blood culture bottle for culture and sensitivity

Procedure

- Choose an area in the most dependent portion of the abdomen (usually directly on the midline 5 cm caudal to the xyphoid). A right paramedian approach may be used to avoid the spleen. Alternatively, ultrasonography can be used to gauge the depth of the peritoneum and to attempt to position the abdominocentesis site in a location away from viscera.
- Clip the area chosen for abdominocentesis.
- Perform an aseptic scrub and perform a local block under appropriate restraint if using anything larger than a 25-gauge needle.
- Properly restrain the horse using twitch, lip chain, sedation, or a combination thereof.
- Don sterile gloves and maintain sterility throughout the procedure. If using a teat cannula or bitch catheter, incise through the skin and subcutaneous tissues at anesthetized site using #15 scalpel blade.
- While standing next to the patient, select insertion site for needle or teat cannula. Position your body to avoid injury from patient reaction to needle insertion. Insert the needle with a controlled, quick movement through the skin only, and then advance it gently through the muscular layers and peritoneum. If using a teat cannula or bitch urinary catheter, insertion through a gauze sponge minimizes

contamination. If drops of abdominal fluid are not seen at the needle hub, reposition and rotate the needle or attach a syringe and aspirate. If necessary, place a second needle a few inches/cm from the first to release the negative pressure in the abdomen.

- Consider ultrasound examination to locate fluid pockets; however, peritoneal fluid can still be obtained even if *not* seen on ultrasonography.
- Once the end of the needle or cannula is in the abdomen, use caution when slowly redirecting and manipulating it to avoid penetrating viscera.
  - Allow the abdominal fluid to drop directly into the EDTA Vacutainer tube. If clinically indicated, fluid may be also submitted for microbiologic culture and sensitivity and peritoneal lactate and glucose concentrations.
- ***Practice Tip:*** *Most horses react to the needle or cannula penetrating the peritoneum (the response can vary from twinging to kicking) and a difference in resistance is felt between penetrating the muscle and peritoneum.*

Complications

- Cellulitis or abscess formation can occur after a break in aseptic technique or during sampling of heavily contaminated peritoneal fluid. Accidental enterocentesis (aspiration of bowel contents) is *not* uncommon, but rarely causes a problem other than sample contamination. If an enterocentesis occurs, the area should be carefully monitored for 3 to 5 days; swelling with pain may indicate septic cellulitis requiring antibiotic therapy. A blunt-tipped cannula decreases the likelihood of bowel puncture, but caution is advised as puncture can still occur if the bowel wall is diseased or weighted ventrally along the abdominal wall (i.e., with sand impaction). Ultrasound-guided abdominocentesis is useful in foals to decrease the risk of intestinal laceration.

- Accidental splenic aspiration causes sample contamination, or in rare severe cases, significant hemorrhage.
- Omental herniation has been reported to occur in foals after abdominocentesis performed with a teat cannula in the rostral to middle abdomen. If this occurs, transect the omentum at or near the body wall, close aseptically prepared skin/subcutaneous tissues, apply an antiseptic cream or ointment, and cover with an abdominal bandage.

Peritoneal Fluid Analysis

Changes in peritoneal fluid are recognized fairly quickly after the onset of gastrointestinal disease (Table 18-1). In cases of acute strangulating obstruction, changes in peritoneal fluid are often seen within hours of the onset of clinical signs. More insidious lesions, such as nonstrangulating obstruction, enteritis, and peritonitis, may produce less dramatic changes in peritoneal fluid concurrent with the progression of clinical signs. Inguinal herniation, intussusception, and entrapment

Table 18-1	Correlation of Peritoneal Fluid Parameters and Intraperitoneal Disorders			
Condition	**Appearance***	**Total Protein* (g/dL)**	**Total Nucleated Cells/L***	**Cytologic Findings***
Normal†	Yellow, clear	<2.0	$<7.5 \times 10^9$	40%-80% neutrophils 20%-80% mononuclear
Nonstrangulating obstruction	Yellow, clear to slightly turbid	<3.0	$<3.0\text{-}15.0 \times 10^9$	Predominantly neutrophils (well preserved)
Strangulating obstruction	Red-brown, turbid	2.5-6.0	$5.0\text{-}50.0 \times 10^9$	Predominantly neutrophils (degenerate)
Proximal duodenitis-jejunitis	Yellow-red, turbid	3.0-4.5	$<10.0 \times 10^9$	Predominantly neutrophils (well preserved)
Bowel rupture	Red-brown, green, turbid with or without particulate matter	5.0-6.5	$>20.0 \times 10^9$ $(20\text{-}150 \times 10^9)$	>95% neutrophils (severely degenerate); intracellular and extracellular bacteria, with or without plant matter
Septic peritonitis	Yellow-white, turbid	>3.0	$>20.0 \times 10^9$ $(20\text{-}100 \times 10^9)$	Predominantly neutrophils (degenerate)
Postceliotomy	Yellow-red, turbid	Variable	Variable	Predominantly neutrophils (slightly to moderately degenerate); no intracellular bacteria
Enterocentesis	Brown-green, with or without particulate matter	Variable	$<1.0 \times 10^9$	Free bacteria, few cells, plant matter
Intraabdominal hemorrhage	Dark red	Initially similar to peripheral blood, WBC count increases with time		PCV less than PCV of peripheral blood, erythrocytophagia, few to no platelets

WBC, White blood cell; *PCV,* packed cell volume.
Note: Absence of gross or cytologic abnormalities in the peritoneal fluid does not rule out compromised intestine.
*Most common findings; exceptions can occur.
†Including peripartum mares.

of bowel in the omental bursa may initially result in local peritonitis with normal peritoneal fluid.

- Normal peritoneal fluid is clear and light yellow, with a specific gravity of approximately 1.005 mg/dL.
- Turbidity results from increased protein or cellular content, which may be caused by septic peritonitis or inflammation of a segment of intestine. The color of the fluid can reflect the type of cells present. Cloudy white-to-yellow or even orange fluid represents large numbers of white blood cells, as in septic peritonitis.
- In strangulating obstruction, segments of bowel become compromised following arterial occlusion and diminished venous and lymphatic drainage from the affected segment. Initially, red blood cells and protein leak out of vessels resulting in a modified transudate. An increased total protein level and red blood cell count (serosanguineous fluid) may be seen early in the disease process. Peritoneal fluid becomes increasingly turbid as bowel ischemia progresses and white blood cells migrate.
- Necrotic bowel leaks bacteria and endotoxin, accelerating chemotaxis of white blood cells into the peritoneal cavity. Red-brown or green-colored fluid may indicate rupture of the stomach or intestine; peritoneal fluid obtained in these cases contains plant material and large numbers of several types of bacteria.
- Nucleated cell counts may be increased in the case of gastrointestinal rupture, but in the face of large volumes of free water and plant material, cell lysis may dramatically decrease nucleated cell count numbers. A low cell count in the face of grossly appearing abnormal peritoneal fluid does not rule out gastrointestinal rupture, particularly if the index of clinical suspicion is high.
- Dark red fluid may be obtained when a vessel or the spleen is entered. In rare instances, hemoperitoneum results from rupture of a vessel; the sample contains no platelets and may have evidence of erythrophagocytosis. The packed cell volume (PCV) may be compared with that of a systemic sample to differentiate samples from the spleen (PCV is higher) and from a vessel (PCV is the same). Stippling of red color in the yellow peritoneal fluid generally indicates iatrogenic bleeding from the centesis.

Cytologic examination should include a white blood cell count and differential, total protein, evaluation of cellular appearance, and examination for the presence of bacteria or plant material. A direct smear is made with Wright or Gram stain or both.

- *Practice Tip:* White blood cell counts are normally lower in foals. A moderate amount of blood contamination in the sample (≤17%) should *not* affect any parameters except the number of red blood cells.
- *Practice Tip:* White blood cell count and total protein levels can be mildly increased in a patient that has undergone abdominal surgery even with manipulation of the intestines only. A sample with increased white blood cell numbers in which most neutrophils appear toxic and degenerate is evidence of septic peritonitis, even if the sample is obtained after celiotomy.

- *Practice Tip:* Peritoneal fluid lactate that is greater than plasma lactate may suggest strangulation or infarction of bowel.
- Peritoneal glucose concentrations that are less than blood glucose can occur with septic peritonitis.

Cecal or Colonic Trocarization

Cecal trocarization can be performed to decompress the cecum in patients with cecal tympany; colonic trocarization may be necessary as a salvage procedure or in an emergent situation in which the degree of colonic distention seems to be significantly contributing to rapid physiologic deterioration. In most cases, trocarization is performed in situations in which surgical intervention is not a viable option or in cases in which the degree of large bowel distention appears life-threatening in the face of prolonged transport time to a surgical facility.

Cecal gas distention is suspected in patients with colic when a "ping" is heard on simultaneous percussion and auscultation in the right paralumbar fossa and is confirmed with rectal palpation. Cecal tympany can be a primary or secondary disorder. Decompression might stimulate cecal motility and relieve the pain caused by distention. The procedure can be performed in patients with extreme abdominal distention before surgery if difficulties with ventilation or compromise of venous return are a concern once the patient is anesthetized. Cecal or colonic decompression in these patients may decrease intraabdominal pressure and improve venous return and ease of ventilation. If the patient is not a surgical candidate, trocarization might resolve colic in cases of tympany or simple colonic displacements. Cecal trocarization is not without risk, and the procedure should be performed only in situations in which there appears to be an obvious clinical benefit outweighing the risks.

Equipment
- Twitch
- Clippers
- Material for aseptic scrub
- 2% local anesthetic, 5-mL syringe, and 22-gauge, 1½-inch (3.8-cm) needle
- Sterile gloves
- 14- or 16-gauge, 5-inch (12.5-cm) pliable intravenous catheter
- 30-inch extension set
- Small cup of tap water

Procedure
- Consider using a twitch if the patient is not sedated. Sedation is *not* always necessary but may minimize risk to patient and personnel.
- Clip an area in the right paralumbar fossa where the "ping" is best heard, or alternatively in cases of severe colonic distention, on the left side where the ping is heard or gas distention is palpated per rectum.
- Infiltrate 3 to 5 mL of local anesthetic subcutaneously and in the underlying muscle at the trocarization site.

- Perform aseptic scrub.
- Wearing sterile gloves, insert the catheter and stylet through the skin, subcutaneous tissue, and abdominal muscle. The catheter should remain perpendicular to the skin. Remove the plastic cap on the catheter; if the catheter is in the cecum, gas escapes. When the catheter is in the cecum, remove the stylet entirely or withdraw the stylet approximately one-half inch to prevent collapse of the catheter by the abdominal wall.
- Attach the extension set and place the free end in the cup of water. Bubbles are produced as long as gas is escaping from the cecum; suction may be used if available.
- If gas is no longer retrievable, withdraw the catheter; *do not* attempt to redirect.
- Administer antibiotics (e.g., 300 mg [3 mL] gentocin or 750 mg [3 mL] amikacin) through the catheter as it is being removed.

Complications

- Low-grade, localized peritonitis, which can affect peritoneal fluid parameters, is expected to occur after this procedure.
- Clinical evidence of disseminated peritonitis and subsequent complications related to cecal or colonic wall trauma are rare but can occur. Abdominal wall abscessation at the puncture site may occur; however, this is unusual.
- Signs of infection should raise suspicion of a more serious problem and be managed promptly with the appropriate therapy. Injecting antibiotics through the catheter during removal may minimize this complication and is recommended.
- Repeat trocarization is *not* recommended because clinical peritonitis can develop.
- Local cellulitis or abscess can occur at the trocarization site. The inflammation is usually self-limiting but should be monitored and managed appropriately.

Transrectal Trocarization of the Large Colon

- Dr. Massimo Magri in Italy recently reported a transrectal technique for decompressing the colon when there is severe colonic distention. ***Note:*** *The technique appears to have merit in horses with severe abdominal distention, providing relief from severe pain. This permits a more complete examination to be performed, and in some cases, resolution of the distention allows intestinal motility to resume and/or the colon to fall in a more normal position (if displaced). It can be curative in some horses if there is* not *a strangulating lesion.* Buscopan can be given before the procedure if there are strong rectal contractions on the initial abdominal palpation per rectum. The procedure appears to be safe and quick but requires mechanical suction to remove the gas. Dr. Magri has developed a special cylinder that encloses the needle so that there is no danger of the needle puncturing the rectum until it is placed against the distended colon; the device is then activated as it enters the colon. The other end of the instrument is connected to suction.

Information is available in Equine Veterinary Education Journal [Eq Vet Ed April 2013; 25(4):184-188].

Complications

- Problems associated with transrectal trocarization of the large colon are similar to those listed for the transcutaneous procedure. (See previous section, p. 160.)

Esophagostomy

Esophagostomy is used for the placement of an indwelling feeding tube. Most commonly the procedure is performed with the horse standing under sedation and local anesthesia. Depending on the temperament of the patient, the type of obstruction, financial concerns, and the surgeon's preference, the procedure may also be performed under general anesthesia. Placement of a nasogastric tube before surgery is recommended to identify the esophagus and minimize the dissection of surrounding tissues. A ventrolateral approach is used most commonly when an esophagostomy is performed for placement of a feeding tube. This approach typically provides improved access to the middle and distal cervical esophagus as opposed to a ventral approach. A surgeon experienced in other esophageal approaches should be consulted if another procedure is contemplated for feeding tube placement.

Equipment

- Twitch
- Clippers
- Material for aseptic scrub
- 2% local anesthetic, 5-mL syringe, and 22 guage, 1½-inch (3.8-cm) needle
- Sterile gloves
- Small surgical pack
- Appropriate suture material as needed
- Penrose drains, ½-inch (1.27 cm)
- Stomach tube in the esophagus to identify the esophagus in the surgery field

Procedure

- An approximately 5-cm incision is made ventral to the jugular vein at or near the junction of the middle and distal cervical esophagus (Fig. 18-1, *A-C*).
- Separate the sternocephalicus and brachiocephalicus muscles.
- Identify and gently retract the carotid sheath, which contains the vagosympathetic trunk and recurrent laryngeal nerve and artery.
- ***Practice Tip:*** *The vagosympathetic trunk and recurrent laryngeal nerve must be identified and avoided during the surgical procedure.*
- Incise the deep cervical adventitia overlying the esophagus; elevation of the esophagus with two ¼″ Penrose drains or Allis tissue forceps may aid in the dissection.
- Once an appropriately sized lumen into the esophagus has been created, the original stomach tube can be retracted, and the selected feeding tube can be inserted into the newly created esophagostomy. Depending on surgeon

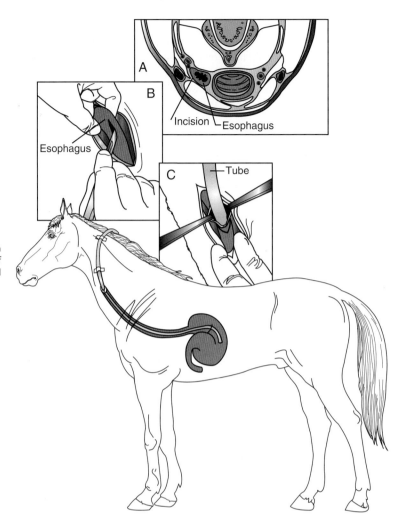

Figure 18-1 Technique of esophagostomy for placement of an indwelling feeding tube. **A,** Location of esophagus on left side of neck. **B,** Incision into esophageal lumen. **C,** Feeding tube passed normograde to stomach.

preference and suspected duration of the esophagostomy, mucosa may be sutured to the skin to minimize subcutaneous contamination. The tube should be firmly secured in place, often with tape and skin sutures.

Complications

- Even with delicate tissue handling, laryngeal hemiplegia from damage to the recurrent laryngeal nerve can be a sequela to the surgery.
- Further complications can include esophageal stricture and dissecting infections while the tube is in place or following tube removal.

AGING GUIDELINES

David L. Foster

- Aging of horses by the teeth becomes less exact as the individual advances in years.
- Bracketing age into 0 to 2 years, 2 to 5 years, 5 to 10 years, 10 to 20 years, and >20 years is generally a useful starting point.
- Specific aging of the horse is accomplished by the following:

- Noting the eruption of the deciduous incisors
- Shedding of the juvenile incisors
- Eruption and wear of the permanent incisors

Once the deciduous incisors are shed and the permanent incisors are erupted, aging is less clear with advancing age. The degree of wear, general shape, length, and other features contribute to suggest an "approximate" age. As the horse ages, small variations of the teeth, oral configuration, and diet contribute to the appearance, angulation, and wear of the teeth.

- General guidelines are described as follows:
  - Foals use the "rule-of-8":
    ○ First incisors erupt at 8 days.
    ○ Second incisors erupt at 8 weeks.
    ○ Third incisors erupt at 8 months.
  - Two-year-olds shed the central deciduous incisors.
  - Three-year-olds shed the second deciduous incisors.
  - Four-year-olds shed the third deciduous incisors.
  - Five-year-olds have all permanent incisors.
  - Seven-year-olds have all the incisors erupted, and the corner mandibular incisors (303/403) have their table surface in wear and a large central "cup."
  - Ten-year-olds: Galvayne's groove appears on 103/203 (maxillary I3); 301/401 and 302/402 have developed a

Box 18-1	Thoroughbred Tattoos
A = 1971, 1997	N = 1984, 2010
B = 1972, 1998	O = 1985, 2011
C = 1973, 1999	P = 1986, 2012
D = 1974, 2000	Q = 1987, 2013
E = 1975, 2001	R = 1988, 2014
F = 1976, 2002	S = 1989, 2015
G = 1977, 2003	T = 1990, 2016
H = 1978, 2004	U = 1991, 2017
I = 1979, 2005	V = 1992, 2018
J = 1980, 2006	W = 1993, 2019
K = 1981, 2007	X = 1994, 2020
L = 1982, 2008	Y = 1995, 2021
M = 1983, 2009	Z = 1996, 2022

"round" table surface. All cups are lost from the mandibular incisors.

- At greater than 10 years of age, it becomes increasingly more difficult to determine age accurately by dental examination.
- The length, angulation, degree of wear, and shape of incisors are "markers" of an individual's age but become increasingly unreliable with advancing age.

Using Tattoos and Brands to Age Horses

Several horse breed registries mark the year of birth in the tattoo or freeze brand applied to their horses.

Thoroughbreds

- All racing Thoroughbreds in the United States receive a lip tattoo.
- A letter followed by four or five numbers (representing the registration number) completes the tattoo.
- The letter denotes the year of birth: A—1971 through Z—1996; all letters of the alphabet are used.
- The alphabet is repeated every 26 years; all Thoroughbreds born in 1997 are tattooed beginning with the letter A; 1998, B; 1999, C, to the end of the alphabet (Box 18-1).
- An exception is made for foreign-bred horses that, once properly identified, receive a lip tattoo beginning with an asterisk followed by a number and no letter; this serves as the full registration number.

Standardbreds

- The Standardbred tattoo system can be used to determine the year of birth. However, it is an idiosyncratic system and is difficult to apply in the field without a tattoo list.
- In the United States, a system is used that records the full registration number, a letter to denote the year of birth, and four more characters, one of which may be another letter (Table 18-2).
- Standardbreds rotate the year of birth letter from the first position to the last in the tattoo character series once all letters are used. Not all letters of the alphabet are used in any given series.

Table 18-2	Standardbred Tattoos		
Born in 1981 or Earlier	**Born in 1982 or Later**		
First three digits are numbers. The fourth can be a letter or a number. The fifth is a letter indicating year of foaling. *The letters M, N, O, Q, and U are not used.*	The first character is a letter, indicating year of foaling. The second can be a letter or a number. The last three digits are numbers. *The letters I, O, Q, U, and Y are not used.*		
A = 1961	A = 1982	A = 2003
B = 1962	B = 1983	B = 2004
C = 1963	C = 1984	C = 2005
D = 1964	D = 1985	D = 2006
E = 1965	E = 1986	E = 2007
F = 1966	F = 1987	F = 2008
G = 1967	G = 1988	G = 2009
H = 1968	H = 1989	H = 2010
I = 1969	J = 1990	J = 2011
J = 1970	K = 1991	K = 2012
K = 1971	L = 1992	L = 2013
L = 1972	M = 1993	M = 2014
P = 1973	N = 1994	N = 2015
R = 1974	P = 1995	P = 2016
S = 1975	R = 1996	R = 2017
T = 1976	S = 1997	S = 2018
V = 1977	T = 1998	T = 2019
W = 1978	V = 1999	V = 2020
X = 1979	W = 2000	W = 2021
Y = 1980	X = 2001	X = 2022
Z = 1981	Z = 2002	Z = 2023

- Any Standardbred born after 1995 may have its identification markings as a lip tattoo or a freeze brand applied to the upper right side of the neck.
- For example, 4321A could be a lip tattoo assigned to a horse born in 1961.
- A Standardbred born in 1995 could have a lip tattoo or a freeze brand of P4321.

Arabian Horse Registry of America/U.S. Bureau of Land Management Registry

- Registry uses a freeze-brand encryption to identify full- and partial-bred Arabian horses and mustangs (Fig. 18-2).
- The first figure represents the breed.
- If the figure is rotated to the right (clockwise), it represents a half-breed.
- The next stacked figures represent the year of birth and are followed by the horse's registration number.

Racing Quarter Horses

- Racing Quarter Horses are identified by lip tattoos, but they do *not* indicate the year of birth as in Thoroughbreds and Standardbreds.

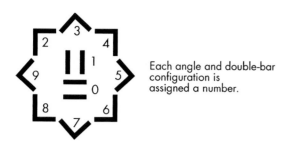

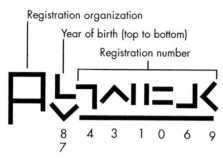

Registration organization

Year of birth (top to bottom)

Registration number

8 4 3 1 0 6 9
7

Figure 18-2 Freeze branding system for breed registration can be useful in individual age identification. A number is assigned to each angle or double bar configuration *(top)*. Sample registration is depicted below the freeze branding system. (Courtesy Michael Q. Lowder, DVM, MS.)

Equine Dental Nomenclature

Two nomenclature systems are used for horses:
- Anatomic descriptive system (Fig. 18-3)
- Triadan (numeric) nomenclature system (Fig. 18-4)

The use of a concise nomenclature system promotes communication between professionals; accurate record keeping; and organized oral examinations. In the anatomic system (see Fig. 18-3), a letter defines the type of tooth being described. All lowercase letters used denote deciduous teeth, capital letters permanent teeth: I, incisors; C, canines; P, premolars; and M, molars. A number then is assigned to the letter that denotes the location of the tooth in the oral cavity (e.g., first molar and second incisor). The oral cavity is divided into four quadrants. The horse's right maxillary arcade is the first arcade. The other three quadrants are assigned sequentially in a clockwise manner from the examiner's position facing the horse. The anatomic letter then has the positional number placed around the letter to represent the location of the tooth. For example, a right mandibular second incisor would be defined as $_2$I; a left maxillary second incisor would be defined as I^2.

The right mandibular arcade of an adult male would be noted in the anatomic system as follows: $_1$I, $_2$I, $_3$I, $_1$C, $_2$P, $_3$P, $_4$P, $_1$M, $_2$M, $_3$M (assuming that the first premolar is *not* present).

The Triadan digital nomenclature system assigns a three-digit number to each tooth (see Fig. 18-4). The first number defines the quadrant in which the tooth resides. The quadrants are numbered one through four starting with the horse's right maxillary arcade and progressing clockwise relative to the examiner facing the horse, as is the case for the anatomic nomenclature system. The following two numbers in this system define the position of the tooth relative to the centerline of the oral cavity. The first or central incisor is assigned "01," the next (middle) incisor "02," and so on. The right

mandibular arcade of an adult male would be described in the Triadan system as follows: 401, 402, 403, 404, 406, 407, 408, 409, 410, 411. This supposes that 405 (the lower first premolar or wolf tooth) is *not* present.

Dental Radiology Ambulatory Techniques

Edward T. Earley

Extraoral Radiographs

Refer to Table 18-3.

Dorsal Ventral View (DV)
- A 14- × 17-inch cassette is recommended (Fig. 18-5).
- Center the beam on the rostral aspect of the facial crest (Fig. 18-5).
- Bungee cords can be used to support the cassette (Figs. 18-6 and 18-7).

Lateral View (LAT)
- A 14- × 17-inch cassette is recommended (Fig. 18-8).
- Opened-mouth technique is recommended (Fig. 18-9).
- Center the beam at the rostral aspect of the facial crest (Figs. 18-9 and 18-10).

Lateral 30-Degree Dorsal–Lateral Oblique (L 30-Degree D-LO) or (D OBL)
- A 10- × 12-inch cassette is recommended.
- The film is oriented to the side of the lesion.
- The cassette is positioned slightly ventral to accommodate the oblique image (Fig. 18-11).
- The view is taken at 30° dorsal to the lateral view.
- The image is focusing on the maxillary arcade corresponding to the same side as the cassette (Fig. 18-12).
- An opened-mouth technique helps separate the arcades (Fig. 18-13).

Lateral 45-Degree Ventral Lateral Oblique (L 45-Degree V-LO) or (V OBL)
- A 10- × 12-inch cassette is recommended.
- The film is oriented to the side of the lesion (Fig. 18-14).

View	Distance (cm)	kV	mA	Time (second)	mA-s
Dorsal ventral	40-50	78	25	0.04	1
Lateral	40-50	74	25	0.04	1
D OBL rostral cheek teeth	40-50	70	25	0.03	0.75
D OBL caudal cheek teeth	40-50	74	25	0.04	1
V OBL rostral cheek teeth	40-50	74	25	0.04	1
V OBL caudal cheek teeth	40-50	80	25	0.05	1.25-2.0

Table 18-3   **Extraoral Technique Chart**

Cassettes: 10 × 12 inches and 14 × 17 inches with rare earth intensifying screens.
Film: Green, 400 speed.
D, Dorsal; *OBL*, oblique *V*, ventral.

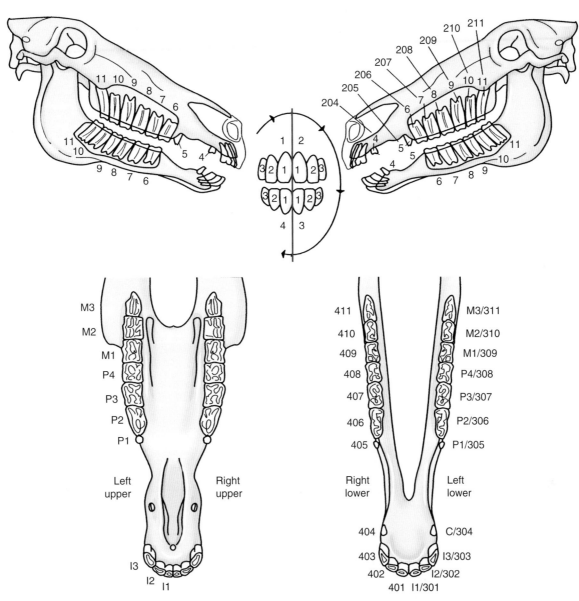

Figure 18-3 Numbering and anatomic descriptive systems used to identify equine teeth.

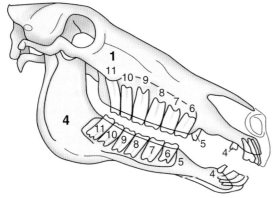

Figure 18-4 In the Triadan system, juvenile or deciduous teeth are identified by replacing the first digit with 5, 6, 7, or 8. For example, 203 for the permanent tooth would be identified by the number 603 for the deciduous tooth.

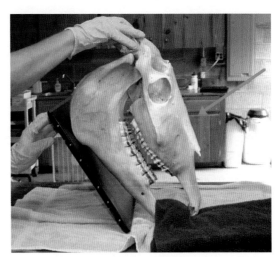

Figure 18-5 Dorsoventral positioning.

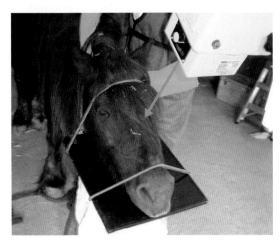

Figure 18-6   Dorsoventral position with bungee cords.

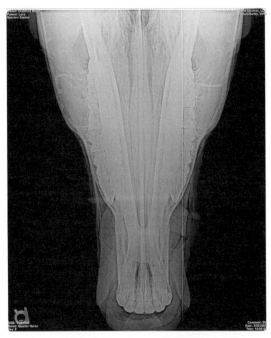

Figure 18-7   Dorsoventral radiograph.

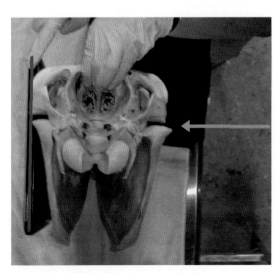

Figure 18-8   Lateral positioning.

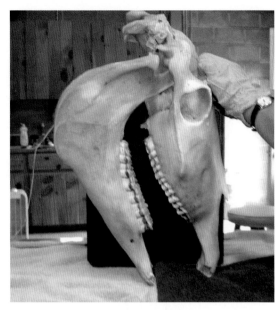

Figure 18-9   Lateral view.

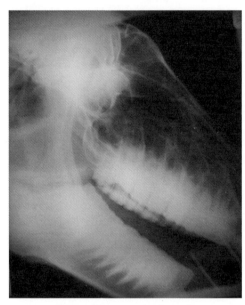

Figure 18-10   Lateral radiograph.

- The cassette should be positioned slightly dorsal to accommodate the oblique image (Figs. 18-15 and 18-16).
- The view is taken at 45° ventral to the lateral view.
- The image is focusing on the mandibular arcade corresponding to the same side as the cassette (Figs. 18-17 and 18-18).
- An opened-mouth technique helps separate the arcades.

Opened-Mouth Techniques

- The mouth can be held open with a small section of polyvinyl chloride pipe placed between the incisors (3 to 4 inches in length and $1\frac{1}{2}$ to 2 inches in diameter; Figs. 18-19 and 18-20).
- A Stubbs full-mouth speculum[3] can be used to hold the mouth open and to support the cassette. Use of a longer

---

[3]Stubbs Equine Innovations, Inc., Johnson City, Texas.

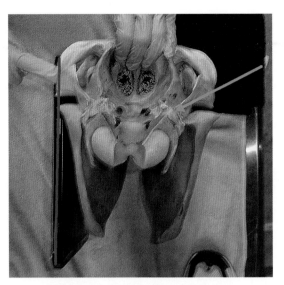

Figure 18-11   Dorsal oblique positioning.

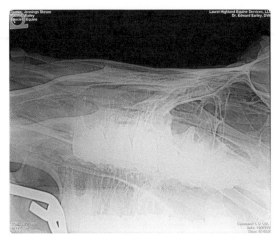

Figure 18-13   Lateral dorsal oblique radiograph.

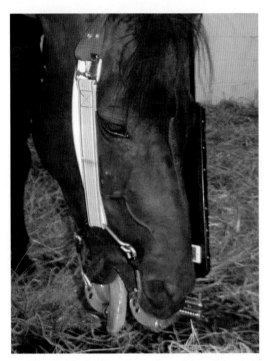

Figure 18-12   Positioning for an opened-mouth lateral dorsal oblique.

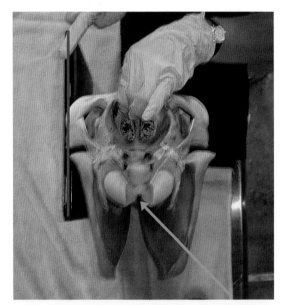

Figure 18-14   Ventral oblique positioning.

elastic strap (draft poll strap) is best so that the buckle is placed up near the poll/ear and out of the radiographic view (Figs. 18-12, 18-21, 18-22, and 18-23).

Radiograph Orientation

- When identifying multiple views of dental radiographs, it is recommended to orient the radiographs in a fashion so that each view is instantly recognizable.
- Using a technique that is common for small animal and human dental radiology leaves *no* room for confusion between the left and right arcades.
- The viewing technique always orients the radiograph in the same plane as viewing the horse from that position (see Fig. 18-23).

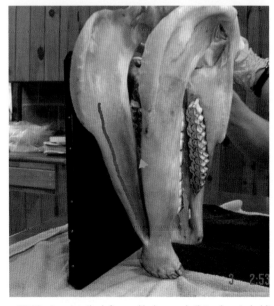

Figure 18-15   Imaging the left mandibular arcade (lateral ventral oblique).

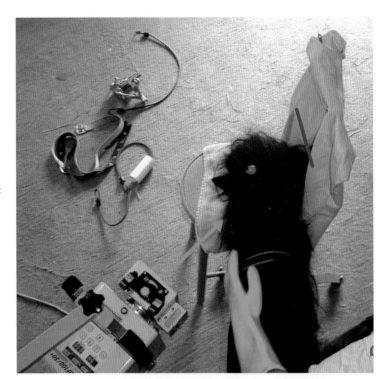

Figure 18-16 Positioning for the right mandibular arcade (right ventral oblique).

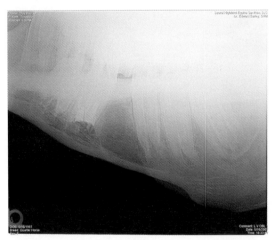

Figure 18-17 Technique for the rostral cheek teeth.

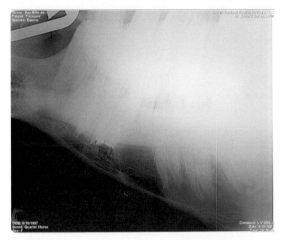

Figure 18-18 Technique for the caudal cheek teeth.

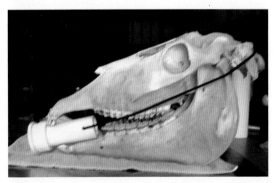

Figure 18-19 Adapted polyvinyl chloride pipe with an elastic strap.

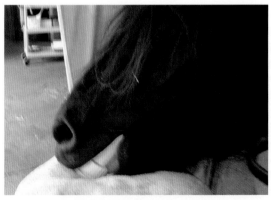

Figure 18-20 Adapted polyvinyl chloride pipe in use.

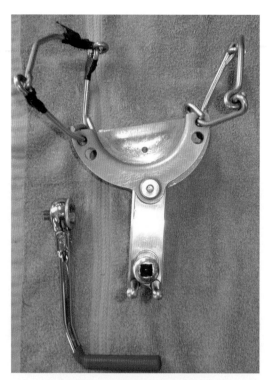

Figure 18-21   Stubbs full-mouth speculum.

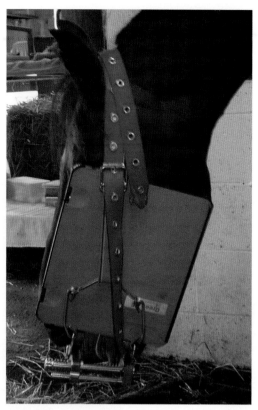

Figure 18-23   Placement of the cassette using the Stubbs full-mouth speculum.

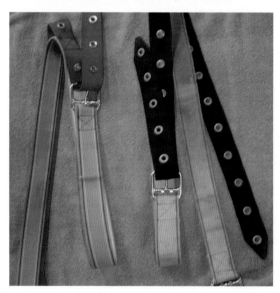

Figure 18-22   Elastic "draft poll strap" *(left)* and an elastic "regular poll strap" *(right).*

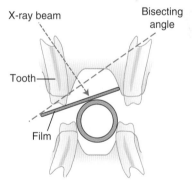

Figure 18-24   Bisecting angle. (Courtesy Dr. Dave Klugh.)

- When viewing a radiograph of the left arcades (200 and 300 arcades), the nose would always be facing the left (see Figs. 18-13, 18-17, and 18-18).
- When viewing a radiograph of the right arcades (100 and 400 arcades), the nose would always be facing the right (see Fig. 18-10).
- A DV image is facing the horse from the front. As a result, the right side of the horse is always oriented to the left on a DV radiograph.

Intraoral Radiographs

Refer to Table 18-4.

Bisecting Angle Technique: Maxillary Cheek Teeth

- Place a flexible cassette[4] in the mouth over the tongue against the palate.
- Estimate the angle between the maxillary cheek teeth and the film.
- Estimate an angle that "bisects" or "equally splits" the angle of the maxillary cheek teeth and the film.
- The line drawn at 90° to the bisecting angle is the projection needed for the radiograph (Fig. 18-24).
- If the angle is too steep (acute), the image of the tooth is shortened (Fig. 18-25).
- If the angle is too flat (obtuse), the image of the tooth is lengthened (Fig. 18-26).

[4]Diagnostic Imaging Systems, Inc., Rapid City, South Dakota.

Table 18-4   **Intraoral Technique Chart**

View	Distance (cm)	kV	mA	Time (second)	mA-s
Maxillary cheek teeth	30-40	60-70	30	0.02	0.60-0.70
Maxillary incisors	30-40	60	30	0.02	0.60
Mandibular incisors	30-40	60	30	0.02	0.60

Flexible cassettes with screens (100 or 200 speed); 200 speed is used most commonly.
Film: Green, 400 speed. Cut 8- × 10-inch film into 4- × 8-inch strips.

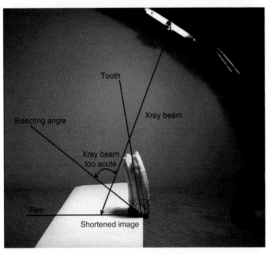

Figure 18-25   Shortening of the tooth image. (Courtesy Dr. Robert Baratt.)

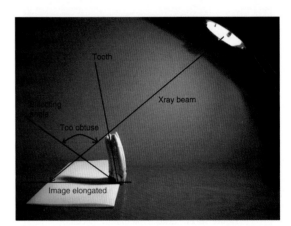

Figure 18-26   Lengthening of the tooth image. (Courtesy Dr. Robert Baratt.)

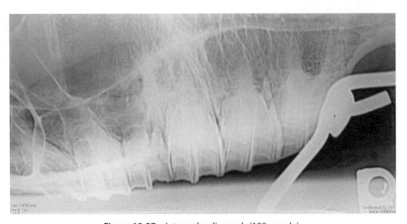

Figure 18-27   Intraoral radiograph (100 arcade).

- Fig. 18-27 demonstrates the resulting intraoral radiograph of the 100 arcade with proper placement of the flexible cassette.
- Fig. 18-28 demonstrates the proper orientation of the x-ray beam for a bisecting angle technique.
- The Stubbs full-mouth speculum works well for this radiograph because there is minimal obstruction of the view from the metal cheek piece (Fig. 18-29).

Bisecting Angle Technique: Maxillary Incisors
- Place the flexible cassette (film side up) above the tongue, between the maxillary and mandibular incisors (Fig. 18-30).

- Estimate the angle between the maxillary incisors and the flexible cassette (the angle of the incisors flattens with age).
- Approximate the bisecting angle and align the x-ray beam at 90 degrees to the bisecting angle.
- Align the x-ray beam at 90° to the bisecting angle.

Bisecting Angle Technique: Mandibular Incisors
- Place the flexible cassette (film side down) under the tongue, between the maxillary and mandibular incisors (Fig. 18-31).
- Estimate the angle between the mandibular incisors and the flexible cassette.

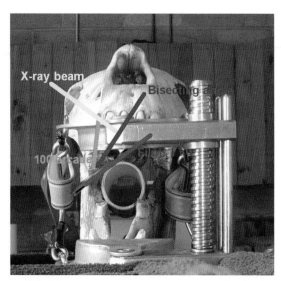

Figure 18-28 Bisecting angle technique using a Stubbs full-mouth speculum.

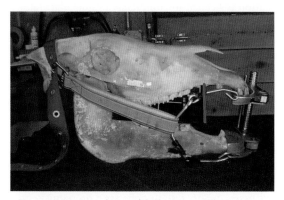

Figure 18-29 Lateral view of the bisecting angle technique.

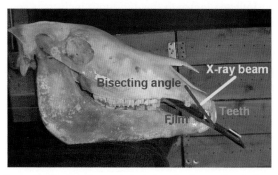

Figure 18-30 Bisecting angle technique for the maxillary incisors.

- Approximate the bisecting angle and align the x-ray beam at 90 degrees to the bisecting angle.
- Align the x-ray beam at 90° to the bisecting angle.

Radiograph Orientation

- When viewing the incisors, the same dental techniques are applied as with the cheek teeth. The right arcade is always oriented on the left side of the radiograph.
- The maxillary incisors are directed in a downward orientation (Fig. 18-32).
- The mandibular incisors are directed in an upward orientation (Fig. 18-33).

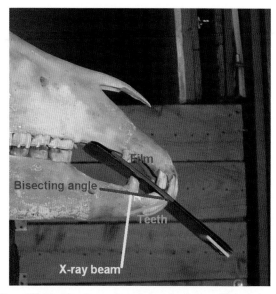

Figure 18-31 Bisecting angle technique for the mandibular incisors.

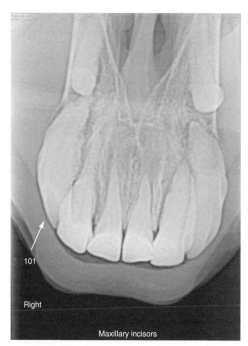

Figure 18-32 Orientation of maxillary incisors.

UPPER GASTROINTESTINAL EMERGENCIES

Teeth

Edward T. Earley, David L. Foster, and James A. Orsini

- The nomenclature used for the mouth is a mixture of classic, archaic, and modern systems. A consistent, coherent nomenclature improves communication between veterinarians and assists in maintaining records. Most veterinarians use the Triadan nomenclature system (see "Equine Dental Nomenclature" earlier in text, p. 164, and Fig. 18-3) because it is specific and understandable.

UPPER GI

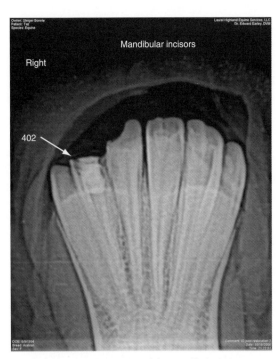

Figure 18-33 Orientation of the mandibular incisors.

- No oral examination is complete unless a full-mouth speculum is used to see and safely palpate the horse's mouth. A good light source, examination mirror, and a dental probe are also necessary.
- Only severe oral problems prevent a horse from eating.
- Drooling or quidding should alert the clinician to an oral emergency.
  Practice Tip: *Rabies and other neurologic diseases such as botulism and tetanus must be considered in differential diagnoses in a horse with clinical signs of drooling or quidding! Proper safety precautions should be taken to protect the examiner and assistants.*
- Vaccination history, physical examination, gloves, and eye protection are essential for performing a safe oral examination.
- Examine the ventral aspects of the tongue and the caudal buccal tissues, which are frequently overlooked.
- Fractured teeth may have exposed pulp tissue that requires vital pulpotomy. This procedure needs specialized equipment not commonly available in the field. Removing the tooth is an alternative but is complicated by the loss of exposed crown resulting from the fracture.

Emergency Care: Dental-Oral

Tongue Lacerations
- Most emergencies are traumatic.
- Lacerations are cleaned, anesthetized, debrided, and apposed with absorbable suture material such as polydioxanone.[5]

---

[5]PDS (Ethicon, Somerville, New Jersey).

- Supportive treatment decreases healing time: anti-inflammatory drugs (phenylbutazone or flunixin meglumine), antibiotics, and oral flushes with 1% chlorhexidine diacetate (Nolvasan) diluted to 1:200 (5.0 mL/L) in water q12h.
- Lacerations of the tongue are occasionally seen. These can be transverse lacerations caused by inappropriate use of a bit, linear lesions produced by instruments during routine dental care, wounds caused by mandibular tooth fragments, incomplete shedding of the mandibular premolars, sharp edges of the lingual aspect of the mandibular cheek teeth, or wounds that occur when horses bite their tongues while racing and jumping.
- ***Practice Tip:*** *An infected deep laceration of the tongue causes severe pain and manifests with the chief complaint of difficulty eating, drooling, quidding, and depression.*
- Clinical signs vary from bleeding, sialorrhea/ptyalism, protruding tongue, fever, malodor from the mouth, poor or no appetite, and dysphagia.
- Sedation is needed to completely evaluate lacerations and injuries involving the mouth.
- Fresh lacerations are primarily repaired and older wounds are best left to heal by secondary intention.

Injury to the Incisor Teeth
This section serves as a reference for colleagues presented with incisor fractures as an emergency. Our intent is not to give detailed instructions on how to perform these procedures. If a fracture is diagnosed that requires special treatment, it is recommended that one refer the case to an equine practitioner with advanced training in dentistry. In all incisor fracture cases, quality radiographs are a prerequisite to determine treatment options and prognosis.
- Self-inflicted injury to the deciduous incisors is common in young horses.
- Avulsions of the juvenile teeth occur when the teeth are "caught" on a relatively immovable object such as a stall guard, webbing, feed tub, or bucket. The individual panics and pulls back with partial avulsion of the incisor teeth.
- The injuries may *not* be noticed for hours or even days.

Presentation
- Juvenile teeth displaced rostrally
- Torn mucosal border of the lingual/palatal aspect of the affected teeth
- Contaminated exposed root area of the affected teeth

First Priority
Consider the viability of the permanent incisors originating below the deciduous teeth. Aggressive debridement and repositioning of the deciduous teeth can injure the developing permanent teeth. Removal of the juvenile teeth is best, rather than risking damage to the permanent tooth buds while attempting a repair of the injury. The delicate tooth buds frequently are injured by the sharp, apical edges of the unstable, partially avulsed deciduous teeth.
- Radiographs of the affected incisors are recommended (see p. 164).
- Remove the unstable juvenile teeth.

- Debride the wound edges.
- Allow the wound to heal by secondary intention, using analgesic, antibiotic, and oral flushes as necessary.

Often the permanent teeth develop and erupt without problems. Young horses missing several deciduous incisors rarely have difficulties, whereas the loss of permanent incisors over the many years these teeth are in service causes significant incisor malalignment requiring dental care to maintain incisor balance.

- *Practice Tip: Trauma to the incisors produced by an external source (e.g., kicks and collisions) typically drives the teeth into the oral cavity. If this occurs in the juvenile incisors, injury to the permanent incisors is more likely than if the trauma is produced by an outward rotation of the incisors.*
- *Practice Tip: Use a pair of bungee cords placed under the lips and attached to the halter to retract the lips and better expose the injury.*

●❯ WHAT TO DO

Injury to the Incisor Teeth
- Restrain and sedate the patient.
- Support the head with a head stand or overhead device.
- Desensitize the area with either local infiltration or a regional block.
- Examine the injury.
- Radiographs are usually indicated in such injuries.
- Extract nonviable teeth and debride the wound.
- Suture soft tissue if possible (usually not possible).
- Administer analgesics, antibiotics, and oral flushes postoperatively.

Stabilization via Cerclage Wire
- Severe destabilization limited to a portion of the incisors may be treated with the use of stabilizing wires. If the repair can be achieved without incorporating the cheek teeth into the repair, the treatment can be performed successfully in the standing horse. However, if the cheek teeth are required to be incorporated into the repair, general anesthesia is indicated.
- Sedate and restrain the patient.
- Radiograph the injury.
- Administer local anesthesia.
- Debride the occlusal fragments of any fractured crowns. Treat the exposed pulps of any fractured teeth that are intended to be saved. Otherwise, remove the tooth. *Do not* attempt to wire teeth with deeply fractured crowns; they *do not* survive.
- Reduce the fracture and return the teeth to their normal orientation.
- Stabilization of the injury via cerclage wire requires the passing of the wire through the interdental space of a stable tooth that is not involved in the fracture.
- Use a small ASIF (Association for the Study of Internal Fixation) drill bit and a hand chuck or drill. Take care *not* to enter the pulp chambers of any teeth while drilling the pathway for the wire.
- Direct the drill through the interdental space at or just below the gingival border.
- Insert a 14-gauge needle into the drill hole to serve as a wire guide.
- Healthy canine teeth may be incorporated into the repair, and slight notching of the crown provides the wire some purchase on the conical tooth.
- Once the cerclage wire is in place, tighten it by twisting the free ends of the wire. Then cut the wire and bend the free ends inward.

It is recommended to apply a protective covering to the wire ends to prevent oral trauma (e.g., dental acrylic or polymethyl methacrylate).
- When appropriate, bonding agents may be incorporated into the repair to stabilize the repair further.
- Six-month follow-up radiographs are necessary posttreatment to evaluate the health of the teeth.

External trauma to the deciduous incisors caused by kicks, collisions, and falls is treated as described for self-inflicted injury. Generally, these injuries almost always result in injury to the permanent tooth buds. Gentle debridement of the wound and anatomic replacement and stabilization of the teeth with stainless steel wires may correct incomplete or minor avulsion of the teeth.

If the avulsion involves permanent incisors, a more aggressive attempt to "rescue" these teeth is needed. Debridement of the contaminated wound followed by repositioning and stabilization of the area with cerclage wire can reclaim some of the teeth.

Note: It is important to determine whether the permanent incisors are fractured and, if so, to remove the fractured ends and evaluate the remaining apical portion of the tooth for viability.

Practice Tip: *Geriatric horses with newly fractured incisors often have a history of a sleep disorder and have fallen on their muzzle after "passing out."*

Regional and Local Anesthesia of the Incisors
- Use 5 to 10 mL of lidocaine with a $1\frac{1}{2}$-inch, 22-gauge needle.
- Local infusion of the lidocaine in the loose mucosa on the labial, palatal, or lingual aspect of the affected teeth successfully desensitizes the teeth.
- Regional anesthesia of the incisors is achieved by blocking the mental foramen (mandibular incisors) or the infraorbital foramen (maxillary incisors).

●❯ WHAT TO DO

Fractured Incisors—Other Management Principles
Vital Pulpotomy
- A *vital pulpotomy* refers to the surgical removal of a portion of the pulp in a vital tooth.
- The diseased portion of the pulp is removed down to the healthy pulp.
- A thin layer of $Ca(OH)_2$ is applied to help initiate the formation of a dentinal bridge.
- Next, a glass ionomer is applied as an attempt to create a permanent seal over the pulp canal.
- Following the glass ionomer, a flowable composite is used to help restore part of the crown.
- The vital tooth continues to erupt. Fig. 18-34 demonstrates the eruption of 201 (see p. 164 for Triadan terminology) over a 14-month period (compared with Fig. 18-35 at the time of the injury).
- The radiograph of 101 at 14 months postprocedure shows that the pulp horn is still viable (Fig. 18-36).
- A remnant of 202 was removed at the time of the vital pulpotomy.
- As the tooth continues to erupt, the exposed crown could have an additional restoration performed using a compactable composite.

Crown Restoration
- A chronic crown fracture can develop a caries lesion that slowly erodes the enamel and dentin.
- Fig. 18-37 involves 402 with a crown fracture at the mesial border and a caries lesion on the labial aspect of the tooth.

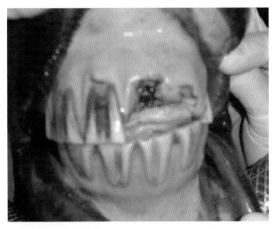

Figure 18-34   Fractured 201 with an acute pulp exposure.

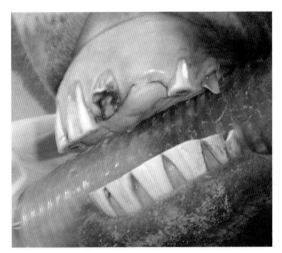

Figure 18-35   Fourteen months after vital pulpotomy.

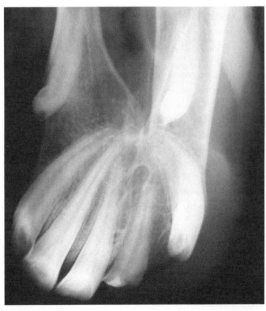

Figure 18-36   Intraoral radiograph of the maxillary incisors at 14 months after vital pulpotomy.

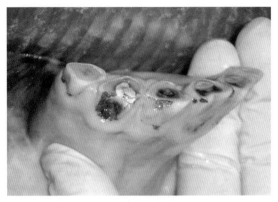

Figure 18-37   Initial presentation of 402.

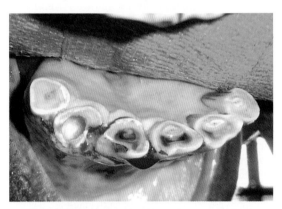

Figure 18-38   Fractured and necrotic crown removed.

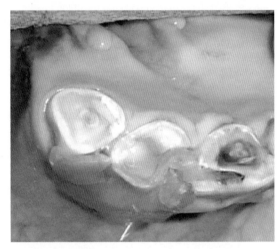

Figure 18-39   Baseplate wax used as an abutment.

- The pulp was exposed to $Ca(OH)_2$ 6 months before, and as a result, a strong dentinal response was seen clinically and radiographically.
- The necrotic and fractured portion of the crown was removed, and part of the gingival margin was removed on the labial aspect of 402 (Fig. 18-38).
- The tooth was etched and bonded. An initial layer of a glass ionomer was applied.
- Following the glass ionomer, baseplate wax was used to form an abutment for the restoration (Fig. 18-39).
- Next, a flowable composite was used to help fill in the irregularities of the damaged crown.
- Following the flowable composite, a compactable composite was applied in two layers in order to build the restoration to the same level as the original crown.

- Next the baseplate wax was removed, and the composite was reduced to the mesial and distal edges of the original crown (Fig. 18-40).
- A postoperative radiograph shows the restoration of 402 (Fig. 18-41).

Periodontal Splinting

- Periodontal splinting with polyethylene fibers is used for support until the periodontal ligaments reattach to the damaged tooth.
- This example involves 101, in which a partial enamel and dentin fracture occurred at the level of the reserve crown (Fig. 18-42).
- The pulp canal is *not* involved with the fracture.
- An initial gingival incision was made to remove the fragment.
- Following removal of the fragment, the damaged portion of 101 was restored with a flowable composite.
- The polyethylene fibers were bonded to 101 and the two neighboring incisors (102 and 201) (Fig 18-43).
- A flowable composite was worked into the fiber in an effort to strengthen the splint.
- A radiograph demonstrates the restoration and splint 6 months following the procedure (Fig. 18-44).

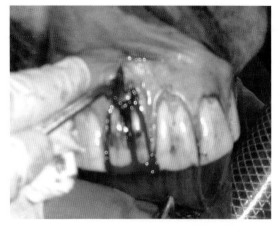

Figure 18-42 Small fracture of the reserve crown of 101 removed.

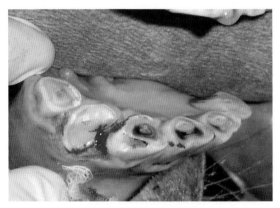

Figure 18-40 Final restoration.

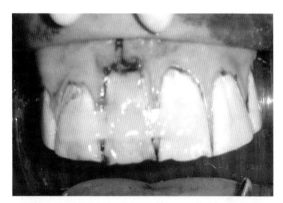

Figure 18-43 Periodontal splinting using polyethylene fibers and composite.

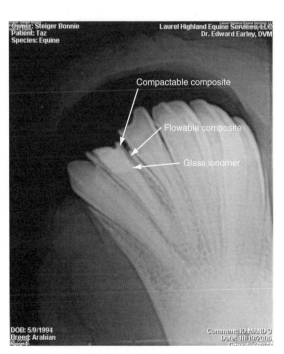

Figure 18-41 Postrestoration radiographs.

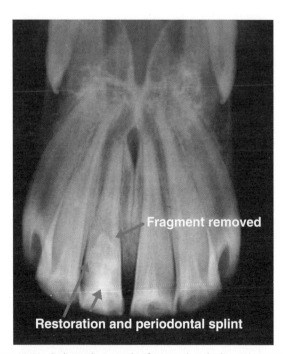

Figure 18-44 Radiographs 6 months after periodontal splint and restoration.

Acute Salivation (Ptyalism)

Thomas J. Divers

- Acute salivation (ptyalism/sialorrhea) can be caused by the inability to swallow normally produced saliva (i.e., choke, see p. 177; neurologic disorders, particularly botulism; equine protozoal myeloencephalitis [EPM]; and guttural pouch mycosis) or from injury to the mouth or pharynx.
- Ptyalism can be caused by excessive production of saliva, most commonly from red clover toxicity (slaframine), mouth injury/irritations, and gastric ulcers with esophagitis in foals.
- A thorough physical examination and history are important to differentiate local causes from a focal manifestation of a generalized disease (i.e., red clover toxicity) to arrive at an accurate diagnosis.
- ***Practice Tip:*** *The most common causes of ptyalism are choke and red clover poisoning in some geographic areas in adults. In foals, the most common cause is gastric and esophageal ulceration (see p. 182).*
- The cause of salivation can be determined by oral examination in some cases. Evaluate the entire oral cavity, looking for a laceration, ulcerations, vesicular disease, foreign body (especially in the tongue or caught between the upper dental arcade), tooth root or soft tissue abscess, a fractured tooth (see p. 173), injury to the palate, strangles, or evidence of chemical injury. Kicks to the incisors and head or catching the mouth on bucket handles, for example, are all common causes of mouth injury. Tongue injuries are often self-inflicted in horses with cerebral disorders. Stomach tube injury or irritation may cause ptyalism. Sedation (detomidine with butorphanol) and the careful use of an equine mouth speculum may be needed to allow a safe and complete examination of the mouth.
- ***Practice Tip:*** *Without proper sedation, the mouth speculum becomes a dangerous weapon to the examiner if the patient "tosses" his head.*
- Excessive biting on the speculum also can result in a tooth fracture. General anesthesia may be required to perform a complete oral examination in some horses, particularly those with foreign bodies and injury to the caudal pharynx.

Localized Causes of Salivation

- The most common equine foreign bodies are a wooden stick large enough to lodge between the upper arcade of teeth, a small stick penetrating the soft tissues of the pharyngeal cavity or soft palate, and a metallic foreign body in the tongue or pharynx. Reaction to oral medications is a common cause of mouth irritation.
- Evaluate the tongue for blisters, ulceration, foreign body, or cellulitis.
- Burrs or grass awns (e.g., Foxtail, sandbur, cheat grass, tickle grass [see www1.extension.umn.edu/agriculture/horse/pasture/mouth-blisters/docs/mouth-blisters.pdf

for pictures]) can become stuck in the mouth while eating hay contaminated with these plants and cause salivation. This may be a problem of a particular farm or batch of hay.
- Patients that have licked mercury blister compounds are prone to severe oral erosions; this product is rarely used today. Enrofloxacin (Baytril 100) causes severe stomatitis in some horses. A pharmaceutical procedure for mixing the drug in a gel is reported to reduce the likelihood of oral irritation; however, stomatitis may still occur in a few horses. Oral metronidazole may cause excess salivation but it does *not* cause oral erosions. Nonsteroidal anti-inflammatory drug (NSAID) therapy, on occasion, may cause oral ulcers; however, excessive salivation from these drugs is uncommon.
- Most vesicular lesions in the mouth are idiopathic, but one must consider vesicular stomatitis, which appears more commonly in New Mexico and Colorado every few years. Suspicious oral ulcers should be reported to the state veterinarian. Immune-mediated pemphigus vesicular formation in the oral cavity occurs but is unusual.
- *Actinobacillus lignieresii, Actinomyces* spp., and *Corynebacterium* spp. infection can cause wooden tongue and/or mandibular region abscesses in horses.
- Consider also sialadenitis (inflammation of a salivary gland), sialolith in horses and donkeys, fractured teeth, or fractured bones of the mouth, hyoid apparatus or temporohyoid. Primary pharyngitis or acute epiglottitis, retropharyngeal lymphadenopathy, guttural pouch empyema, pharyngeal edema, and esophageal obstruction are other causes of ptyalism.
- Swelling of the tongue caused by tumors (rhabdomyosarcoma, squamous cell carcinoma), foreign body, injury, or eosinophilic myositis may cause salivation and some dysphagia.
- Facial paralysis and masseter myopathy (selenium deficiency) are other causes of salivation. With facial paralysis or brainstem disease affecting the cranial nerves V or VII, horses may pack food in their cheek on the affected side. With masseter myopathy the tongue may protrude.

Neurologic or Toxic Causes of Salivation

- Neurologic causes of excessive salivation include:
  - Botulism
  - EPM
  - West Nile virus (WNV)
  - Rabies
  - Other encephalitides
  - Moldy corn poisoning
  - Yellow star thistle
  - Ivermectin toxicity
  - Propylene glycol toxicity
  - Hepatic encephalopathy (see specific neurologic diseases, Chapter 20, p. 277)
- Cantharidin (blister beetle) toxicity may cause both local irritation and systemic effects—colic, hematuria, etc. (see Chapter 34, p. 584).

- Iatrogenic bethanechol administration (a parasympathomimetic)
- Pasture-associated salivation (slobbers) most commonly caused by ingestion of white or red clover infected with *Rhizoctonia leguminicola:*
  - Most common in the southeastern United States and some areas of South America
  - Has also been reported with feeding of alfalfa
  - Black spores can be seen on the leaves of the infected plant (see Chapter 34, p. 587).
  - Clinical disease occurs mostly in grazing horses but can occur from feeding stored hay.
    - Toxin is slowly degraded in hay stored for several months.
  - Lacrimation, frequent urination, and diarrhea may also occur as a result of cholinergic activation.
  - Signs may start within 30 minutes of ingesting the toxin.
  - Signs generally resolve within 1 day of removing affected horses from pasture.

Diagnosis

Ancillary diagnostic tests include radiography, ultrasonography, and endoscopy of the mouth and pharyngeal area. Ultrasonography may define an area that can be sampled for cytologic examination and culture. Radiographs are helpful in identifying a foreign body or diseased tooth. Observe from a distance whether the ability to prehend, masticate, and swallow is retained. In some cases, a complete oral examination with the horse under general anesthesia may be necessary before an etiology is determined. When multiple horses have oral vesicular lesions, testing for vesicular stomatitis is performed (serology and aspiration of a vesicle for virus isolation). Outbreaks of vesicular lesions in horses may occur unrelated to vesicular stomatitis; the cause usually is not identified in those outbreaks. For toxin-related causes, an index of suspicion regarding possible exposure to toxins or chemical irritants that may have been ingested is important.

WHAT TO DO

Diseases of the Mouth Causing Excessive Salivation
Treatments may include the following:
- Removal of foreign bodies—radiographs may be needed to localize the foreign body
- Extraction of diseased tooth causing clinical signs
- Remove from pasture if clover associated "slobbers" is the cause
- Antibiotics for infection-related cause (i.e., wooden tongue)
- Intravenously administer fluids if dehydrated and unable to swallow normally
- NSAIDs for mouth wounds or fractures
- Other symptomatic treatment:
  - Nolvasan mouth wash (mix 1 part of 2% chlorhexidine gluconate [Durvet[6]] with 10 parts water), colloidal or chelated silver mouth rinse solution, or 2% potassium permanganate as a

[6]Information available at durvet.com.

mouth disinfectant/antiseptic wash. Nolvasan wash is good for foals with mouth "thrush" (*Candida*) also.
- Furacin (nitrofurazone) in a prednisolone spray for pharyngeal edema, inflammation, and epiglottitis. Penicillin is often the first-choice antibiotic for mouth wounds/infections because many commensal oral organisms are sensitive to penicillin. Some patients may need a tracheostomy (see Chapter 25, p. 456) if laryngeal-pharyngeal swelling is compromising the airway. ***Practice Tip:*** *Fluid therapy—it is important to remember that in horses, the anion of highest concentration in saliva is chloride and there is a relatively low concentration of bicarbonate. On rare occasion, horses have an acid-base disturbance caused by saliva loss; hypochloremic metabolic alkalosis may occur (if acid-base changes are present they are generally mild). For those cases, fluid therapy consisting of 0.9% sodium chloride and 20 mEq/L KCl is usually recommended.*

WHAT TO DO

Systemic Causes of Excess Salivation
Treatment for the specific disease (see neurologic disorders or toxicities p. 176).

Esophagus

- The most common clinical problem affecting the esophagus of a horse is obstruction of the esophageal lumen (choke). This disorder occurs as a single acute episode or as a chronic, intermittent problem. In either case, these conditions are emergencies. If the condition recurs, a diverticulum or stricture should be considered as a possible cause.
- ***Practice Tip:*** *Megaesophagus and chronic choke are common in Friesians and carry a poor prognosis for long-term survival; Friesian horses may also have gastric emptying problems.*

Esophageal Obstruction

- Esophageal obstruction, most often acute, results from obstruction of the esophageal lumen with food (e.g., dried beet pulp, hay, pellets, wood chips, or bedding). These problems occur among horses with ravenous eating habits, especially older horses being fed pelleted feed.
- Other risk factors are immediately feeding the nervous and excited horse upon arrival at a hospital or exhausted horses at rest stops. Occasionally, choke occurs when a heavily sedated horse is permitted to eat. Most cases of esophageal choke are in adult horses, but it may occur in younger horses.
- ***Practice Tip:*** *Geriatric horses are predisposed to choke because of decreased saliva production and sometimes poor mastication of feed.*
- The most common clinical signs of esophageal choke are excessive salivation, retching, coughing with saliva, and food dripping from the nostrils. In most instances, if the obstruction is in the cervical region (the most common sites for obstruction are proximal esophagus and just cranial to the thoracic inlet) and of recent origin, enlargement of the esophagus can be palpated.

UPPER GI

- Over time, swelling and muscle spasm in this region make it difficult to delineate the mass. The likelihood that the obstruction is in the cervical portion of the esophagus increases if the patient "retches" immediately after attempting to swallow. There is a 10- to 12-second delay between the swallow and the onset of retching if the obstruction is in the distal esophagus.

Diagnosis of Choke

- History and clinical signs are nearly diagnostic but in most cases the obstruction is confirmed by passing a nasogastric tube and encountering an obstruction in the esophagus.
- *Practice Tip: The initial aim of treatment is to reduce the patient's level of anxiety, allow the esophageal muscles to relax, and to adequately hydrate the horse.*

●〉 WHAT TO DO

Medical Management of Esophageal Obstruction

- Tranquilize the patient with acepromazine and/or additional sedation with xylazine to relax the entire esophagus and lower the horse's head.
- *Important:* If choke is suspected, advise owners to remove hay and water immediately. These conservative treatments frequently are enough to relax the esophagus and allow the obstruction to pass on its own within 4 to 6 hours.
- *Practice Tip: If the horse has choked previously or there is a belief that the choke is of longer than 6 hours' duration, it is considered a medical emergency.* Most veterinarians upon arrival prefer to pass a stomach tube following tranquilization, not only to confirm the diagnosis but also to provide a gentle water lavage at the level of the obstruction *while the horse's head is kept down* along with very gently "pushing" the obstruction. This is recommended on the first visit unless you believe the obstruction is *very proximal,* just caudal to the larynx. In this situation, if there is *no* evidence of laryngeal obstruction and it is a first-time choke, administer a tranquilizer, withhold feed and water, and allow 3 to 4 hours for this to resolve before attempting lavage.
- N-butylscopolammonium bromide (Buscopan), 0.3 mg/kg IV or IM (7 mL/450 kg), may also help resolve the obstruction by decreasing esophageal tone. Because of its anticholinergic effect, N-butylscopolammonium bromide given intravenously causes a transient (20 to 30 minutes) increase in heart rate. It is recommended for most cases, but because the most common site for choke, the proximal and mid-cervical area, involves skeletal muscle, the benefit is questionable.
- Oxytocin, 0.11 to 0.22 IU/kg IV q6h, is of questionable value, but it may help resolve the obstruction by decreasing esophageal smooth muscle tone. Smooth muscle constitutes only the distal third of the esophagus. Oxytocin administration may be associated with transient abdominal discomfort, sweating, and muscle tremors. **Note:** Oxytocin should *not* be administered to pregnant mares because of the potential abortifacient properties.
- If the above treatment is unsuccessful in relieving choke in 4 to 6 hours, consider lavage. With the patient sedated with xylazine or detomidine, causing the patient to lower their head, pass a stomach tube to the proximal limit of the obstruction; gently introduce a small volume of water through the tube and against the obstructing mass. This process should be repeated several times to break up the obstruction. As long as the head is kept low, large volumes of water can be pumped (stomach pump) into a medium-size stomach tube and against the obstruction.
- *Practice Tip: In the beginning and before a large volume of water is pumped, it is important to make sure the fluid is able to easily exit around the tube! Gently pressing the tube against the obstruction while flushing may cause the obstruction to move down the esophagus. Once a food obstruction begins to move, the choke is usually quickly resolved. If the obstruction is caused by a rope or another non-plant foreign body, pushing the object further down the esophagus may be contraindicated in case surgical removal is needed.*
- The Rüsch esophageal flush probe[7] for choked horses (Fig. 18-45) uses a pressurized water (room temperature-to-warm) source (hose/faucet). The operator needs to check that the primary tube through which choked material and water exit (egress) is *not* blocked, preventing overpressurization of the esophagus proximal to the obstruction! The valve between the water extension hosing and the proximal end of the ingress inner tube allows the water flow to be turned off at any time.
- Another aggressive lavage method is a warmed, cuffed endotracheal tube passed intranasally into the esophagus, providing the security of an inflatable cuff and preventing aspiration of water during lavage of the esophagus. Warming the tube before passage facilitates passage by making it more flexible. Fluid can be pumped through the endotracheal tube or through a small-diameter stomach tube that has been passed inside the larger endotracheal tube. The lavage solution is most commonly warm water.

Important: Careful manipulation is important to avoid esophageal injury and secondary stricture or esophageal perforation.

- An alternative procedure is to pass the endotracheal tube into the trachea and inflate the cuff to protect the trachea from aspirated material before flushing the esophagus.
- If the obstruction *cannot* be cleared or if the patient becomes unmanageable under sedation, general anesthesia, with the head positioned "down," is required for a more aggressive lavage. In the weanling or yearling that is difficult to restrain, this might be the easiest approach.
- *Practice Tip: If flushing is planned following short-acting anesthesia, always pass the nasogastric tube before general anesthesia; passing the tube into the esophagus of an anesthetized horse is difficult!*
- Intravenously administered fluids are an important supportive treatment in prolonged cases of choke to prevent dehydration and "drying" of the esophageal obstruction.
- Prophylactic antimicrobial agents are indicated for many choke cases because of the high risk of aspiration pneumonia. Antibiotics (e.g., penicillin G procaine, 22,000 IU/kg IM q12h and gentocin 6.6 mg/kg IV or IM q24h; ceftiofur, 2.2 to 4.4 mg/kg IM q12h; or trimethoprim-sulfamethoxazole, 20 to 30 mg/kg PO q12h) are usually administered for 5 to 7 days after relieving the obstruction. If the choke is of more than 6 hours' duration, the caretaker did *not* immediately remove hay and water, or if crackles are heard on thoracic auscultation, metronidazole (15 to 25 mg/kg PO or 25 to 30 mg/kg per rectum q8h) should be added to one of the above treatment protocols. If endoscopy is performed following relief of the choke and severe mucosal erosions are noted, metronidazole

---

[7]MEDVET (Kernen, Germany).

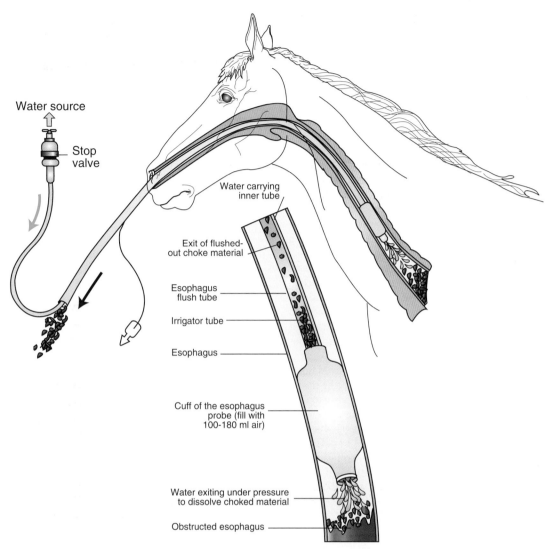

Water source

Stop valve

Water carrying inner tube

Exit of flushed-out choke material

Esophagus flush tube

Irrigator tube

Esophagus

Cuff of the esophagus probe (fill with 100-180 ml air)

Water exiting under pressure to dissolve choked material

Obstructed esophagus

Figure 18-45   Close-up, cross section of the Rüsch esophageal flush probe and its placement within the esophagus to treat "choke."

should be given per rectum; in these cases, sucralfate should also be administered PO.

- If there is concern that the choke has caused damage to the mucosa (based on the duration of choke, an effort is made to relieve the choke or irritating material causing the choke), the esophagus should be evaluated endoscopically in 24 to 48 hours and before refeeding.
- If there is concern about more severe aspiration than normal (most choke cases have some aspiration), a thoracic ultrasound should be performed 24 hours after alleviation of the choke (see p. 95).
- After relieving the choke, if a large amount of food is seen in the trachea during endoscopic examination and the horse is *not* coughing, the patient can be further tranquilized so that the head is positioned ventrally. Using a bronchoalveolar lavage (BAL) tube and with brief periods of suction (10 to 15 seconds at a time) gently lavage the trachea with small (30 mL) amounts of warm balanced crystalloid infused through the endoscope at the thoracic bifurcation of the trachea. If the initial lavage and suctioning do *not* yield particulate matter, *do not* continue the lavage.

- If they are known, correct the predisposing causes for the choke (e.g., improper feed and poor dentition).
- Once the obstruction is resolved, initially offer *only* water, because esophageal dilation after obstruction increases the likelihood of re-impaction for 48 hours. Recommend withholding feed for 48 hours or, if this is impractical, feed small amounts of a soft "soupy mash" diet to prevent recurrence of the obstruction. ***Note:*** Feeding mash is recommended for ponies and miniature horses at risk of hyperlipemia! Endoscopic examination, after the obstruction is relieved, provides evaluation of the esophageal mucosa and information concerning the likelihood of secondary complications (e.g., reobstruction, stricture, and perforation).

UPPER GI

▶️› WHAT NOT TO DO

Medical Management of Esophageal Choke

- *Do not* leave feed or water in the stall after choke is recognized!
- *Do not* use butorphanol, which may suppress the cough reflex.
- *Do not* use mineral oil as a lubricant for the esophagus; some will be aspirated and can cause severe granulomatous pneumonia.
- *Do not* be too aggressive in forcing the choke down the esophagus in the first 3 to 4 hours.
- *Do not* feed dried beet pulp or immediately feed a horse that has become excited or has received heavy sedation!
- *Do not* try to flush the esophagus without the head lowered!
- If the choke is a first time event and *cannot* be relieved after 1 hour of flushing, give the horse and yourself a break and try again later in the day or the following day as long as the horse can be tranquilized, food and water is removed, and IV fluids are being administered.
- *Do not* use atropine to relax the esophagus; use Buscopan instead.
- *Do not* forget follow-up care. Horses with esophageal obstruction of prolonged (>4 hours) duration, repeat offenders, and those *not* having hay and water immediately removed should be reexamined 24 hours after relieving the choke and ideally have both ultrasound examination of the lungs and endoscopy of the esophagus performed.
  - If the horse has an increase in respiratory rate 12 to 24 hours following relief of the obstruction, the patient should be closely examined and may need antibiotic treatment for pneumonia!
- *Do not* refeed too soon.
  - Begin refeeding with a gruel (thoroughly soaked and watery mash or pellets).
  - Ponies, miniature horses, and pregnant mares may need nutritional support (IV dextrose and/or amino acids) if feed is withheld or cannot be consumed for more than 24 hours; monitor triglyceride values in these cases.

▶️› WHAT TO DO

Surgical Management

If all attempts to dislodge the obstruction are unsuccessful, surgical intervention is indicated. Although several procedures are used to manage strictures, diverticula, tumors, and other rare causes of obstruction, cervical esophagotomy is the only emergency procedure.

- Cervical esophagotomy is performed with a nasogastric tube placed in the esophagus and the horse under local or general anesthesia. The anesthesia protocol depends on the temperament of the patient, the type of obstruction, cost, and the surgeon's preference. Make an incision on the midline or ventral to the left jugular vein over the obstruction. Once the obstructed portion of the esophagus is identified, attempt extraluminal massage and manual breakdown of the mass before entering the esophageal lumen. If this maneuver is unsuccessful, make a 2-cm longitudinal incision distal to the obstruction on the ventral or ventrolateral aspect of the esophagus (see p. 161). These sites are used to aid in ventral drainage if the incision is left open to heal by secondary intention or if dehiscence of the primary incision occurs. A ½-inch Penrose drain is used to occlude the esophagus distal to the esophagotomy, and a stallion catheter is introduced retrograde into the esophageal lumen. Gentle intermittent pressure lavage is attempted to retropulse the obstruction into the pharynx. If retrograde pulsion fails, the esophagotomy incision is extended, and sponge forceps are used to remove the obstruction.

- A stomach tube is passed, normograde and retrograde, to ensure a patent lumen. Suture the esophagus in a simple continuous pattern using 3-0 monofilament polydioxanone (PDS, Ethicon) or polypropylene suture placed in the mucosa and submucosa with the knots in the lumen of the esophagus. Close the muscular layer of the esophagus using an interrupted pattern of absorbable material. Position a suction drain adjacent to the esophagus and close the subcutaneous tissues. The suction drain remains in place for 48 hours, all food is withheld, parenteral nutrition is provided, and fluids are administered intravenously. Feed the patient a slurry of pelleted feed for 8 to 10 days, beginning on postoperative day 5.

- An alternative is to use a second esophagotomy distal to the site of the obstruction to feed the patient a gruel and water mixture through an indwelling stomach tube sutured in place. This tube can be used for 10 days to allow the sutured proximal esophagotomy time to heal by primary intention. If dehiscence occurs, a traction diverticulum can develop but usually is associated with few complications.

- If necrotic tissue is debrided at the obstruction site, a stomach tube is recommended. Suture the tube in place and feed the individual a gruel and water mixture through the tube for 10 days. The stoma is left to heal by secondary intention after tube removal.

Prognosis and Complications

The prognosis for survival with simple esophageal obstruction is excellent. The prognosis is favorable for horses with pulsion diverticula but poor if strictures occur that require resection and anastomosis of the esophagus. Aspiration pneumonia is a serious sequela, to be recognized early and managed aggressively. Use clinical examination and ultrasonography to determine the severity of aspiration pneumonia. The incidence of these complications seems related to the time to resolution of the primary obstruction and whether feed and water were properly withheld. Treat the patient aggressively with particular care to avoid possible iatrogenic complications. Choke in miniature horse foals is relatively common and can be difficult to relieve.

Esophageal Perforation

Causes for esophageal perforation (rupture) include the following:

- Chronic obstruction
- Swallowed perforating foreign body such as a needle or thorn
- Penetrating external wounds, even rarely a misguided needle puncture
- Repeated or traumatic nasogastric intubation
- *Note:* Horses that are extremely difficult to tube and then have a large tube left in for several days sometimes have pressure necrosis of the most proximal dorsal esophagus. Rarely following nasogastric tubing does esophageal perforation occur, but if it occurs and is *not* recognized for several days, a communication with the mediastinum may result in fatal pleuritis.
- Extension of infection or injury (e.g., kick) from surrounding tissues
- Clinical signs vary from a fistula draining saliva and feed material with open perforations to severe cervical

swelling, cellulitis, abscessation, and subcutaneous emphysema with closed esophageal perforation. Dyspnea may develop and necessitate emergency tracheotomy.

• Confirm the diagnosis with endoscopy, radiography, or contrast radiography. *Small perforations are difficult to detect with endoscopy.* Survey radiographs may reveal subcutaneous emphysema, and positive-contrast studies may demonstrate leakage of fluid and gas medium into the surrounding tissues.

WHAT TO DO

Esophageal Perforation

• Acute (6 to 12 hours) perforations can be debrided and closed primarily if sufficient viable esophageal tissue is present.
• Maintain affected horses with nothing by mouth for 48 to 72 hours after surgery to allow time for mucosal healing and to minimize postoperative fistula formation.
• Administer broad-spectrum antimicrobial therapy. Antimicrobial combinations commonly used include the following:
  • Na$^+$/K$^+$ penicillin, 22,000 to 44,000 IU/kg IV q6h, and aminoglycosides: gentamicin, 6.6 mg/kg IV q24h, or amikacin, 19.8 mg/kg IV q24h
  • Metronidazole 25 to 35 mg/kg per rectum q6h, for anaerobes
• Administer intravenous, balanced, polyionic fluids to correct electrolyte and acid-base abnormalities, or if aminoglycosides are being administered, to preserve sufficient renal perfusion.
• Administer NSAIDs.
• Administer tetanus prophylaxis.

• If primary closure is *not* possible, which is usually the case, establish adequate ventral drainage to minimize extension of the cellulitis along fascial planes, which could result in septic mediastinitis and pleuritis. The wound is left to heal by second intention.
• Nutritional supplementation through an esophagostomy and indwelling nasogastric tube distal to the site of perforation, or total parenteral nutrition, may be needed during the convalescent period.
• If severe nonperforating tears are noted on endoscopy, these can be managed with intravenous nutrition until salivation is no longer present, after which a gruel can be fed. The value of sucralfate in these cases is unproven but it is often used.

Prognosis

• The prognosis for acute esophageal perforation is fair if prompt, aggressive therapy is instituted and primary closure of the defect is possible.
• In chronic cases, the prognosis is guarded because of the high probability of secondary complications such as esophageal stricture, reobstruction, and septic mediastinitis or pleuritis.

Stomach and Duodenum
Gastric Ulcers
James A. Orsini and Thomas J. Divers

For information regarding clinical signs of gastric ulcers and guidelines for their diagnosis, see Tables 18-5 and 18-6.

Table 18-5	Clinical Signs of Gastroduodenal Ulceration in Horses
Adults	**Foals**
Poor appetite	High-risk group: 1 to 4 months of age
Depression or other behavioral changes	Bruxism/odontoprisis (teeth grinding)
Poor performance, which might be related to decreased feed consumption, anemia, decreased stride length, or chronic pain/stress	Ptyalism (hypersalivation) generally indicates an outflow problem and esophagitis
Mild to moderate signs of abdominal pain	Rolling onto back, especially after nursing
Poor hair coat	Other signs of abdominal pain
Loss of body weight, body condition score <5/9	Poor appetite
Positive response to ulcer treatment	Interruption of nursing (discomfort)
	Diarrhea or history of diarrhea

Table 18-6	Diagnosis of Gastric Ulcers
Adults	**Foals**
Clinical Signs: See Table 18-5.	Clinical Signs: See Table 18-5.
Endoscopy is the only reliable diagnostic tool to confirm a presumptive diagnosis of gastric ulcers. For video or fiber-optic endoscopy, use a 200- (minimum) to 300-cm length scope.	Ancillary Tests:
Grades of gastric ulceration (Fig. 18-46):	Gastroduodenal endoscopy (see Fig. 11-24)
Grade 0/normal—epithelium intact	Barium contrast radiography
Grade 1/mild ulceration—reddening, hyperkeratosis, and single or multifocal ulcer lesions	Occult fecal blood tests are *not* sensitive; a negative result does not rule out gastroduodenal ulceration.
Grade 2/moderate ulceration—large or multifocal lesions or extensive superficial lesions	
Grade 3/severe ulceration—extensive, coalescing lesions and deep lesions	

Gastric Ulceration in Adult Horses*

Table 18-7

Therapeutic Goals	Specific Treatment Options

Suppress Gastric Acid Secretion	Proton pump inhibitors:
	  Omeprazole (Gastrogard, Ulcergard): 2-4 mg/kg PO q24h
	  Omeprazole (Losec): 0.5 mg/kg IV q24h
	  Esomeprazole sodium: 0.5 mg/kg IV
	Pantoprazole 1.5 mg/kg IV q24h
	Histamine (H_2) receptor antagonists:
	  Cimetidine (Tagamet): 16-25 mg/kg PO or 6.6 mg/kg IV q6-8h
	  Ranitidine (Zantac): 6.6 mg/kg PO or 1.5 mg/kg IV q8h
	  Famotidine (Pepcid): 2.8-4 mg/kg PO or 0.23-0.5 mg/kg IV q8-12h

Protect the Ulcerated Mucosa	Mucosal protection/repair:
	  Sucralfate (Carafate): 20-40 mg/kg PO q6-8h
	  Misoprostol (Cytotec): 2.5-5 µg/kg PO q12-24h (**Note**: May cause diarrhea)
	Antacids (buffer already secreted acid):
	  $Mg(OH)_2$ and $Al(OH)_3$ must be given PO q2-4h
	  If severe colic is present, add 30-40 mL of 2% lidocaine to the above for a 500-kg horse.

Stimulate Gastric Emptying	Gastric prokinetics include bethanechol, metoclopramide, erythromycin, and cisapride. *Do not use if outflow obstruction is present or suspected.*
Prophylaxis	Omeprazole: 1-2 mg/kg PO q24h

Gastroduodenal Ulceration in Foals*

Table 18-8

Situation	Treatment Recommendations
Subacute or chronic ulceration (mild to moderate clinical signs)	1. Administer oral sucralfate *plus* an acid blocker (H_2 receptor antagonist or proton pump inhibitor): • Use adult dosages (see Table 18-7) • Wait 1-2 hours between sucralfate and other oral meds • If *no* improvement after 3-5 days, consider outflow obstruction or other disorder • For foals unable to receive oral medication, use pantoprazole or ranitidine IV 2. Manage pain with xylazine or butorphanol: • *Do not* use NSAIDs unless absolutely necessary; even COX-2 selective NSAIDs may inhibit ulcer healing • If inadequate response, make an "antacid cocktail" (500 mL Pepto-Bismol or Mylanta + 100 mL Maalox liquid + 4 sucralfate crushed tablets + 1 cup activated charcoal powder + 500 mL warm water) and give via soft NG tube to sedated foal • May also add 15 mL of 2% lidocaine to cocktail for rapid pain relief 3. Provide supportive care as needed: • Fluid therapy for diarrhea, for example • Give misoprostol (see Table 18-7) if ulcers were caused by NSAIDs Be aware of possible complications/sequelae, including gastric or duodenal perforation, duodenal stricture, cholangitis, and aspiration pneumonia.
Emergency care (acute, severe clinical signs)	1. Follow care as outlined for subacute/chronic cases, but give ulcer meds IV. 2. If severe gastroesophageal reflux, marked salivation, esophageal distention, and esophageal ulceration, give one of the following prokinetics until signs improve: • Bethanechol: 0.03-0.04 mg/kg IV or SQ q6-8h • Metoclopramide (Reglan): 0.25 mg/kg *slowly* over 1 hour IV q4-8h; can be given SQ • Lidocaine: 1.3 mg/kg bolus IV, followed by constant-rate infusion at 0.04 mg/kg/h IV; use of this dose in foals less than 3 weeks old could result in increased risk of toxicity because of delayed hepatic metabolism
Prophylaxis	1. Minimize risk factors where possible (e.g., minimize NSAID use, use COX-2 selective NSAIDs when necessary, promptly treat diarrhea). 2. Give antiulcer meds to stressed foals: • Use oral sucralfate, an acid inhibitor, or both. • Sucralfate may be used alone in recumbent, critically ill foals or in foals at increased risk of nosocomial enteric infections. • An acid inhibitor should be added once the foal is able to stand. 3. Check for duodenal stricture if the problem is not acute.

COX, Cyclooxygenase; *NG,* nasogastric; *NSAID,* nonsteroidal anti-inflammatory drug.

*Clinical response to H_2 receptor antagonist or proton pump inhibitor should occur in 3 to 5 days after starting treatment. If *not*, consider other differential diagnoses, such as outflow problems and inadequate treatment.

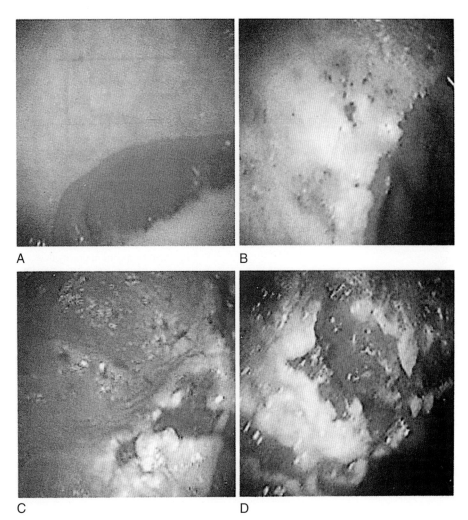

Figure 18-46 **A,** Grade 0 ulcer (normal). Intact mucosal epithelium (may have reddening and/or hyperkeratosis). **B,** Grade 1 ulcer (mild). Small single or multiple ulcers. **C,** Grade 2 ulcer (moderate). Large single or multiple ulcers. **D,** Grade 3 ulcer (severe). Extensive (often coalescing) ulcers with areas of deep ulceration.

Duodenal or Gastric Perforation

Duodenal or gastric perforation usually occurs in foals younger than 8 weeks.

- Risk factors include the use of NSAIDs and stresses to the foal, including diarrhea.
- Many cases occur with minimal warning signs of gastric ulceration.

Common Clinical Signs

- Foals often are found acutely depressed or "colicky" with a tense/guarded abdomen.
- Foals have increased heart and respiratory rates.
- Foals may have a high fever, yet they may continue to nurse.
- Often, diarrhea accompanies duodenal perforation; the diarrhea is often present before the perforation or as a consequence of endotoxemia.

Diagnosis

- Clinical signs
- Ultrasonography: large amounts of flocculent fluid are seen
- Abdominocentesis: may confirm septic peritonitis

◉› WHAT TO DO

Duodenal or Gastric Perforation

Humane destruction is generally the outcome, except for those patients with a small duodenal perforation that may be found at exploratory surgery and sealed by the omentum. Acute gastric perforations in young foals with milk found in the abdomen have been successfully repaired.

Prevention

- NSAIDs should be administered to young foals *only* when absolutely necessary, as in the management of endotoxemia or colic, especially in foals with diarrhea.
- If an NSAID has been administered to a foal, initiate treatment with omeprazole, 2 to 4 mg/kg PO q24h.
- *Practice Tip: Do not rely on sucralfate alone to prevent ulcers if NSAIDs are being used.*
- *Practice Tip: Firocoxib, 0.09 mg/kg IV q24h; meloxicam 0.6 mg/kg PO or IV q12 to 24h; and carprofen, 1.4 mg/kg q12 to 24h PO or IV, may be the safest NSAIDs to use when more long-term therapy for skeletal disorders is required in foals.*

Acute Grain Overload

Clinicians often are called in an emergency to examine and treat a horse that has accidentally ingested a large quantity of grain (a commercially prepared concentrate or a cereal grain hay such as barley).

●❯ WHAT TO DO

Acute Grain Overload

If the patient has *no* abnormal clinical signs at examination, the following treatment is recommended:

- Pass a stomach tube and check for gastric reflux; if there is *no* reflux, use gravity flow (funnel) to administer 1 lb (450 g) Epsom salts ($MgSO_4$) or 1 lb (450 g) activated charcoal, or half of each, mixed in 1 gallon (3.8 L) warm water (per 500-kg adult).
- Administer 1 mg/kg followed by 0.3 mg/kg flunixin meglumine IV or PO q8h for 48 hours.
- Administer diphenhydramine 1.0 mg/kg IM q12h or 0.5 mg/kg doxylamine succinate SQ q6h for 24h; other antihistamines may be substituted.
- Remove all feed for 24 hours.
- Cryoprophylaxis for laminitis should be performed if there is an increased risk for the disease (see Chapter 43, p. 712).
- Di-trioctahedral (DTO) smectite (Biosponge), 0.5 to 3 lb/1.1 to 6.6 kg per 450 kg, PO or NG tube q12-24h; gastrointesintal adsorbent.

Prognosis

Prognosis should be excellent if treatment is given before clinical signs develop.

Symptomatic Grain Overload

- The clinical signs most frequently seen with symptomatic grain overload are
  - Colic
  - Significant abdominal distention
  - Severe lameness (laminitis)
  - Trembling
  - Sweating
  - Polypnea
  - Less frequently, diarrhea
- Clinical findings include:
  - Bright red to purple membranes
  - Tachycardia
  - Absence of intestinal sounds (some pings may be heard on simultaneous auscultation and percussion of the abdomen)
  - Gastric reflux
  - Colonic distention with tight bands palpated on rectal examination
- CBC usually reveals severe polycythemia, neutropenia with a left shift, and vacuolization of neutrophils (toxic changes).

●❯ WHAT TO DO

Symptomatic Grain Overload

- Give intravenous fluid therapy. Administer hypertonic saline solution initially, but this must be followed within 1 to 2 hours by administration of a polyionic fluid at 2 to 4 L/h for the adult; 500 mL of 23% calcium borogluconate, can be administered but must be diluted with several liters of the polyionic fluids. Add KCl, 20 to 40 mEq, to each liter of fluid after urination is documented. ***Practice Tip:*** *A ratio of 10:1 of polyionic fluid:hypertonic fluid is the accepted rule-of-thumb when using hypertonic saline as part of fluid replacement therapy.*

- Administer plasma if possible (2 to 4 L for an adult). Hyperimmune plasma containing antibodies against endotoxin is preferred but is not essential.
- Administer flunixin meglumine 1 mg/kg IV q12h initially and 0.3 mg/kg q8h after signs of colic are no longer evident.
- Administer lidocaine (1.3 mg/kg as a slow bolus IV followed by 0.05 mg/kg/min) to improve intestinal motility, provide analgesia, and to impair neutrophil margination that may be a trigger factor for laminitis.
- Pass a nasogastric tube and leave it in place to relieve gastric distention. If there is *no* gastric reflux, administer ½ lb (225 g) of charcoal and ½ lb of magnesium sulfate in ½ gallon (1.9 L) warm water (per 500-kg adult) by means of gravity flow.
- Polymyxin B, 2000 to 6000 IU/kg IV q12h for 1 to 2 days, can be used to bind circulating endotoxin if renal function is normal.
- Pentoxifylline, 10 mg/kg PO or IV q12h, may be administered:
  - If there is no gastric reflux
  - Administer slowly intravenously as a compounded solution
  - It may inhibit inflammatory cytokine production
- Administer aggressive and early therapy for laminitis if signs of founder are present (see Chapter 43, p. 709).
  - Remove feed, bed heavily, apply dental packing or pads to the feet.
  - **Ice legs and feet for a minimum of 2 days or until clinical signs resolve, using ice boots or equivalent cyrotherapy.**
- If there is considerable cecal or colonic distention, perform trocarization (see p. 160) and infuse 1×10^6 units of penicillin into the cecal/colon lumen. Penicillin preparation instilled is not important for the antimicrobial effect targeting *Streptococcus bovis*.

Prognosis

- The prognosis, if there are moderate to severe clinical signs, is poor. If severe abdominal pain and significant abdominal distention are present, affected patients usually die within 24 to 48 hours even with the most aggressive therapy.
- If signs of laminitis occur before signs of the presence of intestinal disease abate, the prognosis is grave.

Acute Gastric Dilation
P.O. Eric Mueller, John F. Peroni, and James N. Moore

- Primary gastric dilation is believed to be associated with:
  - The ingestion of highly fermentable feed, such as grass clippings
  - The ingestion of excessive amounts of corn or other grain
- Secondary gastric dilation occurs when fluid from the small intestine accumulates in the stomach because of:
  - Ileus
  - Obstruction of the small-intestinal lumen
  - Strangulating obstruction involving the small intestine
  - Severe inflammation of the small intestine
- In one study of 50 horses with gastric rupture, horses drinking water from a bucket, stream, or pond were at

greater risk of gastric rupture than were those with access to an automatic waterer.

- Foals with duodenal/pyloric obstruction have significant gastric dilation; however, because of the gradual obstruction and dilation, abdominal pain (colic) is *not* pronounced.
- Horses exhibit signs of severe pain and increased heart and respiratory rates caused by pain and diaphragmatic pressure.
- If the dilation is primary, the mucous membranes are pale, and on rectal examination, the spleen can be palpated because it is displaced caudally by the enlarged stomach. *Practice Tip: Ultrasound examination of the left side of the abdomen is helpful in imaging the size of the stomach. It is abnormal if the stomach extends to the caudal limits of the last rib!* If the dilation results from a problem involving the small intestine, the patient may exhibit signs of toxicity, the peritoneal fluid may reflect intraabdominal ischemia (discoloration with erythrocytes, increased WBC count and protein concentration), and several loops of distended small intestine may be palpable on rectal examination.
- In some cases, spontaneous regurgitation may occur immediately before the stomach ruptures along its greater curvature.

●〉 WHAT TO DO

Acute Gastric Dilation

- For acute abdominal pain, the primary goal is to relieve intragastric pressure by passing a medium or large-bore stomach tube. Lidocaine may be needed to relax the cardiac sphincter; it may be necessary to create a "siphon" effect to ensure that all excess fluid is removed from the stomach (see p. 157).
- Once emergency care is given, perform a complete physical examination to determine the cause. In primary dilation, the patient should remain pain-free once the intragastric pressure is relieved.
- If the dilation results from a small-intestinal problem, relief is transient. Intravenous lidocaine (1.3 mg/kg as a slow IV bolus followed by 0.04 mg/kg/min CRI [constant rate infusion]) and polymyxin, 2000 to 6000 IU/kg IV q8h, are used for gastric dilation caused by nonobstructing small-intestinal disease such as proximal enteritis.
- If the stomach ruptures, the patient immediately appears comfortable, but then rapid deterioration occurs as the result of endotoxic and cardiovascular shock. Ingesta are evident in the peritoneal fluid, and the serosa of the intestines is roughened on rectal examination. Humane destruction is recommended.

Prognosis

- The prognosis for primary dilation is excellent, provided intragastric pressure is rapidly relieved.
- The prognosis for secondary gastric dilation depends on the underlying disease and the duration of the condition before treatment is started.

Gastric Impaction

Gastric impaction occurs infrequently. The most common causes are the following:

- Grain overload
- Dry, impacted ingesta
  - Poor dentition
- Squamous cell carcinoma of the stomach
- Ingestion of persimmons
- Severe hepatic disease

If the impaction is associated with causes other than squamous cell carcinoma, the patient may show signs of moderate to severe pain. Most often these patients do *not* show evidence of systemic toxicity unless the grain overload has progressed, resulting in signs of acute laminitis. Gastroscopic examination and ultrasound (finding an enlarged stomach) are helpful procedures in making the diagnosis; on extremely rare occasions, the stomach may be palpated rectally with gastric impaction. Horses with impacted ingesta in the stomach may be in uncontrollable pain, which necessitates immediate exploratory surgery. The diagnosis in these cases is made at surgery. Horses with more chronic impactions may have mild to moderate pain. The diagnosis can be made by ultrasound examination, demonstrating an enlarged stomach and gastroscopic examination, showing large amounts of feed present after *not* being fed for more than 16 hours.

Practice Tip: Friesians may be genetically predisposed to both esophageal and gastric motility disorders.

●〉 WHAT TO DO

Gastric Impaction

- For severe impactions, surgery is recommended. At surgery, administer 2 to 3 L of water through a 3-inch (7.5-cm) intraabdominal needle placed through the gastric wall. Redirect the end of the needle, infiltrating different areas of the mass, and gently massage the impaction.
- Postoperative care includes:
  - Lavage of the stomach
  - Drainage through a large-bore gastric tube

If persimmon impaction is suspected, or visualized on gastroscopic examination, repeated administration of Coca-Cola (1 L) by nasogastric tube has been reported to be effective.
- For horses with milder pain and less severe distention, based upon ultrasound examination, withhold food and administer 6 L of isotonic electrolyte via gravity flow every 6 to 12 hours.

Prognosis

- Guarded for horses with acute severe pain.
- Much better for horses with more mild pain—a recent report from Finland (Vainio et al., 2011) even suggests it is good.
- Poor for horses with liver failure and gastric impaction.

Acute Abdomen—Colic
Classification and Pathophysiology of Colic

A variety of enteric diseases can result in the manifestation of abdominal pain (colic) in horses. Abnormalities of the equine gastrointestinal tract are broadly classified as physical or functional obstructions. With a nonstrangulating physical obstruction, the mesenteric blood supply is intact, but the bowel lumen is occluded. This can be caused by intraluminal masses or reduction of the lumen by intramural thickening or extramural compression. Strangulating obstruction implies luminal occlusion and reduction or occlusion of the mesenteric blood supply. Incarceration of the intestine through internal or external hernias, intussusception, or a greater than 180-degree twist of a segment of intestine on its mesentery can result in a strangulating obstruction.

Functional obstruction, referred to as adynamic or paralytic ileus:

- Can be idiopathic
- Can result from inflammatory disease (e.g., duodenitis/proximal jejunitis and colitis)
- Can be caused by serosal irritation from surgical manipulation

Intestinal obstruction prevents the aboral movement of gastrointestinal contents and results in distention of the intestine. As the distention increases, venous drainage from the intestinal wall is impaired, and the mucosa becomes congested and edematous. If the obstruction persists for a prolonged time (>24 hours) significant compromise of intestinal vascular integrity can result in mucosal ischemia. With progressive distention, gastric, cecal, or colonic rupture can result. In strangulating obstruction, these events are combined with rapid tissue hypoxia and ischemia of the affected segment and lead to necrosis and transmural leakage of bacteria and endotoxin. Cardiovascular deterioration rapidly follows transperitoneal absorption of endotoxin, resulting in hypovolemia and endotoxic shock.

Diagnosis

Early History

- Previous episode of colic, duration of colic, recent changes in management (feed, water, deworming, medication, exercise routine), breeding, pregnancy

Recent History

- Degree of and change in pain (looking at flank, pawing, kicking at abdomen, rolling), last defecation, sweating, treatment, and response to treatment

Physical Examination

Assess the following parameters immediately and completely during initial examination of the patient with a history of acute abdominal pain:

- Attitude
- Abdominal shape (distention)
- Body temperature, pulse, and respiratory rate
- Skin turgor, mucous membrane moisture and color, and capillary refill time (CRT)
- Abdominal auscultation and percussion
- Nasogastric intubation—quantity and characteristics of fluid
- Abdominal palpation per rectum

The physical examination starts with observation of external appearance and attitude. Abdominal distention is generally a sign of large-intestinal disease in adult horses, but it can occur with severe small-intestinal distention, especially in

foals. Multiple abrasions, particularly around the periorbital area, indicate that the patient recently experienced severe abdominal pain. Recent enlargement of an umbilical or abdominal hernia, or of the scrotum may indicate intestinal incarceration with obstruction or strangulation. Rectal temperature of 39° C (102° F) or greater may be suggestive of colitis or peritonitis; if possible, the rectal temperature should be taken in all colic cases prior to abdominal palpation per rectum. Assess the degree of pain with the patient in a quiet environment.

Signs of Abdominal Pain in Order of Severity—Severe to Most Severe

- Lying down for long periods
- Inappetence
- Restlessness
- Quivering of the upper lip
- Turning the head toward the flank
- Repeated stretching as if to urinate
- Kicking the abdomen with the hind feet
- Crouching as if wanting to lie down
- Sweating
- Dropping to the ground and rolling
- ***Practice Tip:*** *Severe, unrelenting pain may require analgesics before examination* (Table 18-9).

Consider previous treatment by the owner, trainer, or RDVM when assessing the severity of abdominal pain. Depression with mild to moderate abdominal pain and fever may indicate an inflammatory condition (enteritis or colitis). In the absence of extreme muscle exertion, suspect inflammatory disease (enteritis, colitis, peritonitis) as the cause of abdominal pain accompanied by fever. Loud "fluid and bubbling" sounds can be heard on abdominal auscultation in some patients with impending colitis. Ultrasound examination can be helpful in delineating enteritis (distended, thickened small intestine with increased motility) from strangulating obstruction (distended small intestine with no motility).

Tachycardia and tachypnea can serve as indicators of abdominal pain, cardiovascular shock, and endotoxemia.

Skin turgor, mucous membrane moisture and color, and CRT can aid in assessment of dehydration resulting from intestinal dysfunction. Mucous membrane moisture and color change from moist and pale pink to dry and red with a decrease in circulating blood volume. With the onset of shock and endotoxemia, mucous membrane color can progress to reddish blue or purple (cyanosis).

Auscultate for intestinal borborygmi in all abdominal quadrants. Pain and inflammation related to the gastrointestinal tract result in decreased borborygmi. Increased borborygmi can be present early with enteritis or colitis, only to progress to ileus and cessation of the sounds as the bowel becomes progressively inflamed and distended. Increased borborygmi are present early in patients with intestinal obstruction, but intestinal sounds decrease as the obstruction becomes complete. Simultaneous auscultation and percussion may reveal high-pitched sounds (pinging) caused by cecal (right flank) or colonic (left flank) tympany. A sound

Table 18-9	Analgesics and Relative Efficacy for Control of Acute Abdominal Pain		
Analgesic	**Trade Name**	**Dosage**	**Efficacy**
Flunixin meglumine	Banamine	0.25-1.1 mg/kg IV	Excellent
Detomidine hydrochloride	Dormosedan	10-40 µg/kg IV or IM*	Excellent
Xylazine hydrochloride	Rompun	0.2-1.1 mg/kg IV or IM*	Good
Butorphanol tartrate	Torbugesic	0.02-0.08 mg/kg IV or IM†‡	Good
Ketoprofen	Ketofen	1.1-2.2 mg/kg IV	Good
N-butylscopolammonium bromide	Buscopan	0.3 mg/kg IV (7 mL/450 kg)§‖	Good
Morphine sulfate		0.3-0.66 mg/kg IV‡¶	Good
Pentazocine	Talwin	0.3-0.6 mg/kg IV‡	Poor
Chloral hydrate		30-60 mg/kg IV titrated	Poor
Dipyrone	Novin	10 mg/kg IV or IM	Poor
Phenylbutazone	Butazolidin	2.2-4.4 mg/kg IV	Poor

*Repeated administration may compromise cardiac output and colonic motility.
†Doses in upper range may cause ataxia.
‡Indicates a controlled substance.
§Causes transient increase in heart rate.
‖Available in Europe as a compositum with dipyrone.
¶*Use only with xylazine* (0.66 to 1.1 mg/kg IV) to avoid central nervous system excitement.

similar to an ocean wave can be heard in some patients with sand impaction; if a sand impaction is suspected, perform auscultation of the rostral-ventral abdomen for 5 minutes listening for the characteristic sound.

Perform nasogastric intubation immediately when a patient demonstrates abdominal pain. Gastric decompression is essential to determine whether gastric distention is present and to provide relief to patients with primary or secondary gastric distention. Nasogastric reflux can be caused by small-intestinal obstruction or secondary ileus from large-intestinal disease. Horses with proximal enteritis characteristically have large volumes of reflux (10 to 20 L). Blood-tinged, foul-smelling reflux fluid may indicate small-intestinal strangulating obstruction or severe proximal enteritis. If small-intestinal obstruction or enteritis is suspected, it is important to leave the tube in place to prevent spontaneous gastric rupture and subsequent death.

A careful rectal examination is mandatory when examining a horse that has abdominal pain. The rectal temperature should be taken before the rectal examination. Before beginning the abdominal palpation per rectum, note the amount and consistency of fecal material in the rectum. Absence of fecal material or the presence of dry, fibrin- and mucus-covered feces is abnormal and suggests delayed intestinal transit. Fetid, watery fecal material often is seen in horses with colitis. Examination should be performed in a consistent, systematic manner to minimize missing a lesion. Intraabdominal structures palpable in a normal horse (Fig. 18-47), starting in the left cranial abdominal quadrant and progressing clockwise, are subsequently identified.

Palpable Intraabdominal Structures
- Caudal border of the spleen
- Nephrosplenic (renosplenic) ligament
- Caudal pole of the left kidney
- Mesenteric root
- Ventral cecal band (no tension)

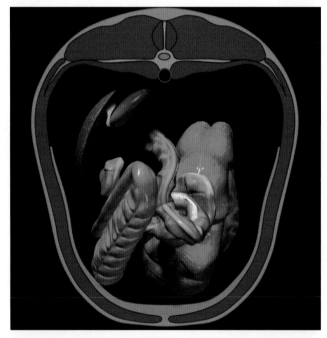

Figure 18-47 Caudal view of a standing horse shows the abdominal structures palpable in normal patients during rectal examination. Beginning in the left dorsal abdominal quadrant and progressing in a clockwise direction, palpable structures include the caudal border of the spleen, nephrosplenic ligament, caudal pole of the left kidney, small colon containing fecal balls, root of the mesentery, cecal base and ventral taenia, portions of the left ventral and dorsal colon, and the pelvic flexure.

- Cecal base (empty)
- Small colon containing distinct fecal balls
- Pelvic flexure

The small intestine is *not* palpable, except for the infrequent and chance palpation of the ileum in some horses or unless an underlying abnormality exists. Determination of the presence of bowel distention of any form is important in formulating a working diagnosis.

Abnormal Rectal Examination Findings

- Cecal distention
- Gas- or ingesta-distended small intestine (Fig. 18-48), large colon (Fig. 18-49), or small colon
- Significant intramural or mesenteric edema
- Bowel malposition (see Fig. 18-49)
- Herniation
- Impaction
- Intussusception
- Intraabdominal mass, abscess, or hematoma
- Enterolithiasis
- Volvulus of the mesenteric root

Always examine the internal inguinal rings, urethra, and bladder (male) and reproductive tract and bladder (female). Sequential rectal examinations are often helpful in determining the rate and severity of disease and the need for surgical intervention.

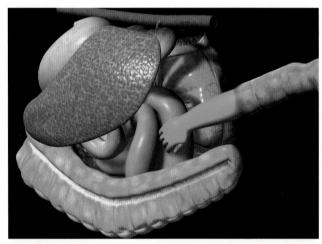

Figure 18-48   Caudal view of a standing horse shows severe small intestinal distention. Multiple loops of gas- and fluid-distended small intestine are palpable.

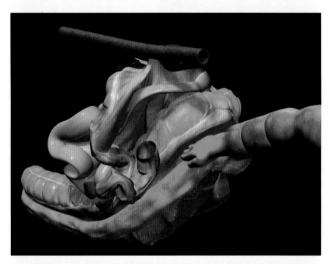

Figure 18-49   Caudal view of a standing horse reveals right dorsal displacement of the large colon. The left ventral and dorsal colons are displaced lateral to the cecum. The colon and associated taenia are palpated immediately cranial to the pelvic canal, coursing from the right caudal abdomen, transversely across the abdomen, and then continuing beyond the examiner's reach toward the left cranial abdomen.

Ultrasonography

Ultrasonography is an important component of the examination and is covered in detail in Chapter 14, p. 85).

Response to Analgesics

The degree of pain demonstrated by a horse with gastrointestinal disease is variable and depends on the characteristic "pain threshold" of the individual horse and the severity of disease present. ***Practice Tip:*** *In general, the greater the pain, the more severe the disease. In the later stages of disease, abdominal pain may be replaced by considerable depression and cardiovascular deterioration as a result of bowel necrosis and systemic endotoxemia.* Pain control is accomplished with gastric decompression through a nasogastric tube and administration of peripherally and centrally acting analgesics (see Table 18-9). Assessment of a patient's response to analgesics is helpful in determining the severity of disease and likelihood of successfully treating the patient with medical management alone. Horses demonstrating unrelenting pain *not* responsive to analgesics require immediate surgical exploration or humane destruction.

Clinicopathologic Evaluation

- PCV
- Total plasma protein (TPP)
- Complete blood count (CBC)
- Blood gases
- Electrolyte determination
- Lactate

Packed Cell Volume and Total Plasma Protein

Hypovolemia resulting from intestinal dysfunction results in dehydration. The PCV and TPP are the most accurate measurements to support a clinical assessment of dehydration in most patients with abdominal pain.

	PCV (%)[8]	TPP (g/dL)
Mild dehydration	45-50	7.5-8.0
Moderate dehydration	50-60	8.0-9.0
Severe dehydration	60	9.0

Practice Tip: *Significant increases in PCV without corresponding increases or decreases in TPP may indicate protein loss into the intestinal lumen, peritoneal cavity, or sympathetic and endotoxin-induced splenic contraction.*

Complete Blood Count

Most simple or strangulating obstructions do *not* cause a significant change in the white blood cell (WBC) count until the terminal stages of diseases. Acute inflammatory diseases (enteritis, colitis), however, often cause leukopenia (<4000 cells/μL) with a left shift and toxic changes noted in the neutrophils. Significant leukopenia (<1000 cells/μL) also occurs with fulminant septic peritonitis resulting from acute bowel rupture. Mature neutrophilia and high TPP and fibrinogen levels may indicate chronic peritonitis caused by abdominal abscessation.

---

[8]These values are not relevant to nursing foals, which generally have lower PCV and protein values.

Blood Gases

Acidemia may be seen with advanced hypovolemic shock. Evaluation of blood gases is important for appropriate management of severe acid-base abnormalities, especially in patients who need general anesthesia and surgical treatment. Patients with simple colon displacements may have an insignificant base excess, whereas patients with strangulating obstruction usually have an obvious base deficit.

Lactate

Blood and peritoneal lactate is an important laboratory test in the evaluation and monitoring of the acute abdomen.

- Blood and peritoneal fluid lactate determinations can be performed stall-side.
- Elevated blood lactate concentration suggests a global decrease in perfusion (hypotension/dehydration) and/or local ischemia or strangulation.
- **Practice Tip:** *The initial value of the blood lactate is* not *as important prognostically as the change in lactate after early treatments; absence of a decline in blood lactate 2 to 4 hours after aggressive treatments, including resuscitation with hypertonic saline and/or polyionic crystalloids, is suggestive of a serious and possibly strangulating condition.*
- **Practice Tip:** *More significant elevations in peritoneal fluid in comparison to blood lactate is highly suggestive of a strangulation obstruction.*

Electrolytes

Measurement of serum electrolytes rarely is helpful in making a diagnosis. A rare exception is acute abdominal pain caused by hypocalcemia and ileus (synchronous diaphragmatic flutter may be present).

- Electrolyte determinations are vital for appropriate management before, during, and after surgical treatment.
  - Hyponatremia and hypochloremia may suggest impending colitis.

Abdominocentesis

Abdominocentesis (see p. 158) is a useful diagnostic tool for assessment of intestinal compromise. Abdominocentesis is performed with an 18-gauge, sterile hypodermic needle or a blunt cannula (teat cannula or canine female urinary catheter). Collect fluid in a sterile tube containing EDTA for cytologic analysis of the fluid and into a second sterile tube without additives for culture and sensitivity, if indicated. Fluid analysis includes specific gravity and protein determinations and cell types, numbers, and morphology (see Table 18-1). Ultrasonography may be useful in locating peritoneal fluid. Use caution in performing abdominocentesis on foals; needle perforation of the bowel can cause adhesions, and using the teat cannula method can result in herniation of omentum unless performed in the most caudal part of the abdomen.

Normal peritoneal fluid is
- Odorless
- Nonturbid
- Clear to pale yellow
- The nucleated cell count should be less than 3000 to 5000 cells/μL, with a total protein concentration less than 2.5 g/dL.

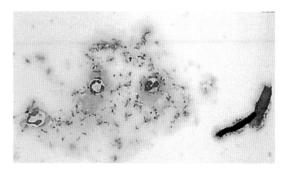

Figure 18-50   Peritoneal fluid (×400). Ruptured intestine.

- In early, simple obstruction of the small or large intestine, peritoneal fluid typically remains normal.
- In a strangulating obstruction or severe intestinal inflammation, the peritoneal fluid can become serosanguineous with increases in nucleated cell count and total protein concentration.
- Dark, turbid fluid with the smell of ingesta, increased nucleated cell counts, and increased protein concentration signifies bowel necrosis and leakage.
- The presence of plant material and intracellular bacteria indicates bowel rupture (Fig. 18-50). (If this material has been collected by needle aspiration, it should be repeated with a teat cannula before the diagnosis of ruptured viscus is made.)
- The presence of blood-tinged fluid indicates:
  - Splenic puncture
  - Intraabdominal hemorrhage
  - Iatrogenic hemorrhage
  - Intestinal necrosis

Practice Tip: *With splenic puncture, the PCV of the fluid is greater than the peripheral PCV, and the fluid contains large numbers of small lymphocytes. Fluid from intraabdominal hemorrhage reveals a PCV less than that of peripheral blood, erythrocytophagia, and few to no platelets.*

Important: The absence of gross or cytologic abnormalities in the peritoneal fluid does *not* exclude the presence of compromised intestine.

- Some strangulating lesions, such as intussusception, external hernia, and epiploic foramen incarceration may *not* demonstrate abnormalities in the peritoneal fluid because of sequestration of the fluid in the omentum, intussuscipiens, or hernial sac.
- If sand impaction is suspected or if considerable cecal or colonic distention is present, abdominocentesis should be performed only to confirm suspected bowel rupture.

Practice Tip: *If physical examination reveals other findings consistent with a surgical lesion and referral for surgery is considered, abdominocentesis should* not *be performed in the field because of the risk to the patient and the examiner.*

Medical Versus Surgical Management

Considerations in determining the need for exploratory surgery are as follows (Box 18-2):
- Pain
- Response to analgesic therapy

GI:COLIC

| Box 18-2 | Indications for Exploratory Celiotomy in Horses Demonstrating Acute Abdominal Pain |

Severe, unrelenting abdominal pain*
Pain refractory to analgesics*
Abnormal rectal examination†
Abnormal ultrasonographic examination†
Increased heart rate†
Large quantities of gastric reflux†
Absence of borborygmi†
Serosanguineous abdominal fluid with increased protein and
    nucleated cell count†

*These parameters alone are indications for emergency exploratory celiotomy.

†These parameters are NOT sole indications for emergency exploratory celiotomy but must be evaluated in view of other clinical findings.

- Cardiovascular status
- Blood and peritoneal fluid lactate evaluation (see p. 189)
- Rectal examination findings
- Ultrasonographic findings
- Quantity of gastric reflux
- Abdominocentesis results

A history of abdominal pain often requires reassessment of these parameters over time. A change in one or more clinical criteria may determine the need for surgical or medical management. *Practice Tip: Manifestation of pain and the response to analgesic therapy are the most valuable measurements in assessing the need for surgical intervention. Patients demonstrating unrelenting pain or recurrent pain after administration of analgesics are considered surgical candidates.*

Rectal examination is the *second* most valuable criterion for surgery. Demonstration of pain concurrent with abnormal rectal examination findings is a strong indicator. Failure of medical therapy, abnormalities identified during ultrasound examination of the abdomen, systemic cardiovascular deterioration, increases in blood lactate or peritoneal fluid lactate higher than blood lactate and/or changes in peritoneal fluid (color, protein, etc.) results supporting intestinal degeneration are additional justification for surgical intervention.

●» WHAT TO DO

Medical Versus Surgical Management— Acute Abdomen

Treatment of horses demonstrating acute abdominal pain is directed at the following:
- Pain relief
- Stabilization of cardiovascular and metabolic status
- Minimizing the deleterious effects of endotoxemia
- Establishing a patent and functional intestine. This can be accomplished with one or more of the following therapeutic modalities:
  - Analgesic therapy (see Table 18-9)
  - Fluid therapy and cardiovascular support
  - Laxatives and cathartics
  - Antiendotoxin therapy
  - Therapy for ischemia-reperfusion injury
  - Antimicrobial therapy
  - Nutritional support
  - Surgical intervention

Analgesic Therapy
Pain relief is accomplished by means of gastric decompression with a nasogastric tube and administration of peripherally and centrally acting analgesics (see Table 18-9). Perform gastric decompression (see p. 157) q2h using an indwelling nasogastric tube; it may be necessary to repeat up to q2h to prevent distention, which can potentially lead to pain, gastric rupture, and death. Patients being referred for possible exploratory surgery should have an indwelling nasogastric tube in place during transport to the referral facility if there has been a need for repeated gastric decompression.

Fluid Therapy and Cardiovascular Support
Intravenous administration of polyionic, balanced electrolyte solutions is necessary to maintain intravascular fluid volume. Administration of colloid solutions such as hydroxyethyl starch (6% Hetastarch,[9] 5 to 10 mL/kg IV) improves systemic blood pressure and cardiac output. Hypertonic saline solution is the ideal resuscitation crystalloid but *must* be followed by adequate fluid replacement with balanced crystalloid solutions (ideally within 1 hour after administration of the hypertonic solution). *Practice Tip: The ratio of crystalloid to colloid solution (ratio of saline to 7% hypertonic) should be 10:1 (10 L saline or other crystalloid to 1 L of hypertonic saline).* Monitor hydration status with clinical assessment and measurement of PCV and TPP. Monitor blood gas and serum electrolyte values, and adjust the intravenous solutions to correct the deficits.

If the plasma protein concentration is <4.5 g/dL and the patient is dehydrated, administer plasma (2 to 10 L IV slowly), 25% human albumin, or a synthetic colloid (Hetastarch or VetStarch/Abbott Labs, up to 10 mL/kg) to maintain plasma oncotic pressure and avoid inducing pulmonary edema during rehydration with intravenous fluids.

Laxatives
Laxatives are used to increase gastrointestinal water content, soften ingesta, facilitate intestinal transit, and manage impaction of the cecum and large and small colons. For maximal effect, oral and intravenous fluids should be administered concurrently. Do *not* administer laxatives orally to patients with nasogastric reflux.

Commonly Used Laxatives
- Mineral oil (6 to 8 L/500 kg body mass) can be administered to facilitate manure passage after the impaction begins to resolve; however, mineral oil is *not* useful for penetrating or hydrating the primary impaction.
- Magnesium sulfate (Epsom salts, 500 g diluted in warm water per 500 kg body mass, daily). *Do not* use for longer than 3 days or to treat patients with decreased renal function in order to avoid enteritis and possible magnesium intoxication. Its use is preferred for large-colon impactions.
- Psyllium hydrophilic mucilloid (Metamucil, 400 g/500 kg body mass q6-12h) until the impaction resolves. Especially useful for sand impaction.

---

[9]6% Hetastarch (Braun Medical, Irvine, California).

- ***Practice Tip:*** *Mixing psyllium with water makes a thick paste that clogs the pump and tube. Alternatively, mix psyllium with mineral oil for easier administration.*
- Dioctyl sodium sulfosuccinate (DSS, 10 to 20 mg/kg up to 2 doses, 48 hours apart). Can cause mild abdominal pain and diarrhea.

Antiendotoxin Therapy

Antiserum (500 to 1000 mL) directed against the gram-negative core antigens of endotoxin[10] can be administered intravenously diluted in balanced electrolyte solution. Endoserum should be slowly warmed to room temperature and administered slowly to avoid undesirable side effects, such as tachycardia and muscle fasciculations. Hyperimmune plasma,[11] directed against the J-5 mutant strain of *Escherichia coli,* or normal equine plasma (2 to 10 L), administered intravenously slowly, can be equally as or more beneficial, supplying protein, fibronectin, complement, antithrombin III, and other inhibitors of hypercoagulability. Polymyxin B,[12] 2000 to 6000 IU/kg IV q12h for 24 to 48 hours, binds and neutralizes circulating endotoxin and may be beneficial in the management of systemic endotoxemia.

Pentoxifylline (Trental) is used to treat endotoxemia, 7.5 to 10 mg/kg PO, IV, q8-12h.

Therapy for Ischemia-Reperfusion Injury

If ischemia is suspected, dimethyl sulfoxide (DMSO), a hydroxyl radical scavenger, can be administered intravenously (100 mg/kg q8-12h) diluted to a 10% solution in a balanced electrolyte solution. Efficacy has not been verified. Kinetic studies support use every 12 hours at the anti-inflammatory dose.

Lidocaine infusion (1.3 mg/kg bolus followed by 0.05 mg/kg/min) has been shown to reduce bowel mucosal injury from repercussion injury when the lidocaine was given before the experimental injury occurred.

Antimicrobials

- Antimicrobial agents are not administered routinely to patients that demonstrate acute abdominal pain unless an underlying infectious agent is suspected. Broad-spectrum antimicrobials may be indicated if the patient has sepsis and neutropenia (<2000 cells/µL) to minimize bacteremia and organ colonization by enteric organisms and if the patient is undergoing exploratory celiotomy.
- Penicillin (22,000 to 44,000 IU/kg IV q6h or IM q12h) and metronidazole (30 mg/kg per rectum q8h or 15 mg/kg IV q8-12h) often is administered to patients with duodenitis or proximal jejunitis. The suspected targeted agent is *Clostridium perfringens* type A.

Nutritional Support

See Chapter 51, p. 768.

Horses demonstrating abdominal pain should have hay and grain withheld for at least 12 to 18 hours. If they *do not* have gastric reflux, they should be allowed free-choice water

and should have access to trace mineral salt. A patient that responds to initial medical treatment should be returned gradually to a normal diet over 24 to 48 hours (moist bran and alfalfa pellet mash, grazing grass, hay, then grain). Patients being referred for possible exploratory surgery should *not* be fed during transport to the referral facility.

Surgical Intervention

Candidates for exploratory celiotomy (see Box 18-2) have the following signs:

- Unrelenting pain
- Recurrent pain after administration of analgesics
- Palpable abnormalities detected on rectal examination
- Ultrasonographic findings demonstrating an obstructive pattern or intussusception
- Systemic cardiovascular deterioration
- Changes in peritoneal fluid results indicating intestinal degeneration
- Failure of medical therapy

Ventral midline celiotomy is the surgical approach of choice. Specific treatments are discussed with each gastrointestinal disorder.

LOWER GASTROINTESTINAL EMERGENCIES

For gastric diseases causing colic, see p. 181.

Disorders of the Small Intestine

Intussusception

Small-intestinal intussusception usually occurs in younger horses and involves an invagination of a segment of intestine *(intussusceptum)* and mesentery into the lumen of an adjacent distal segment of intestine *(intussuscipiens).* Continued peristalsis draws more intestine and its mesentery into the intussuscipiens, causing venous congestion, edema, infarction, and necrosis of the involved segment. Small-intestinal obstruction and strangulation result. Intussusception results from alterations in intestinal motility.

Predisposing Factors

- Enteritis, especially foals
- Maladjustment of septic foals in intensive care units
- Abrupt dietary changes
- Heavy ascarid *(Parascaris equorum)* or tapeworm *(Anoplocephala perfoliata)* infestation
- Anthelmintic treatment
- Intestinal anastomosis
- In most cases, *no* specific factor is identified.
- ***Practice Tip:*** *Jejunojejunal and jejunoileal intussusception are more common in foals, whereas ileocecal intussusception is more common in adults.*

Diagnosis

- Clinical signs of jejunojejunal and ileocecal intussusception vary with the degree and duration of the condition.

[10]Endoserum (Immvac, Columbia, Missouri).
[11]Polymune-J (San Luis Obispo, California) or Foalimmune (Lake Immunogenics, Inc., Ontario, New York).
[12]Polymyxin B (Bedford Laboratories, Bedford, Ohio).

- Most commonly, intussusception leads to complete intestinal obstruction and strangulation of the intussusceptum, causing an acute onset of unrelenting abdominal pain, although it may rarely be a cause of a more chronic colic.
- Nasogastric reflux develops, and progressive dehydration and hypovolemia rapidly follow.
- Rectal examination reveals loops of distended small intestine, and occasionally the intussusception can be palpated. With ileocecal intussusception, a turgid segment of bowel may be palpable within the cecum.
- Increased peritoneal protein concentration and nucleated cell count reflect devitalization of the affected bowel. Changes in the peritoneal fluid, however, may not accurately reflect the degree of intestinal compromise because of isolation of the devitalized intussusceptum within the intussuscipiens (see p. 159).
- In foals, jejunal intussusception is usually identified with ultrasound.
- Chronic ileocecal intussusception with partial obstruction causes the following:
  - Intermittent or continuous abdominal pain
  - Weight loss
  - Poor general physical condition
  - Varying degrees of anorexia
  - Depression
- Chronic ileocecal intussusception can continue for weeks to months and eventually leads to an acute episode of severe abdominal pain compatible with a complete obstruction of the intestine.

▶▶ WHAT TO DO

Intussusception
Initial Therapy Is Supportive
- Gastric decompression
- Balanced polyionic intravenous fluids, such as lactated Ringer's solution
- Analgesics such as xylazine, butorphanol tartrate, or flunixin meglumine
- Monitoring of physiologic and clinical parameters:
  - Pain
  - Nasogastric reflux
  - Heart rate
  - Mucous membranes
  - Hematocrit, PCV/TPP
  - Borborygmi
- Surgical exploration is indicated if intussusception is suspected.

Exploratory Surgery
- Ventral midline exploratory celiotomy
- Manual reduction of the intussusception
- Resection and anastomosis of the affected intestine
    Some intussusceptions *cannot* be reduced because of the length of bowel involved, venous congestion, and edema. These cases require en bloc resection and anastomosis. Even if the intestinal segment appears viable, consider resection and anastomosis because of the possibility of mucosal necrosis, serosal inflammation, and postoperative adhesion formation.

Prognosis
Prognosis is good with early diagnosis and surgical repair but poor if the intussusception is advanced and irreducible because of the likelihood of ileus, peritonitis, and postoperative adhesion formation.

Volvulus
- Volvulus is the rotation of a segment of intestine around the long axis of its mesentery.
- Although most cases are *not* accompanied by a predisposing lesion, the following can lead to volvulus:
  - Adhesions
  - Infarction
  - Intestinal incarceration
  - Pedunculated lipoma
  - Mesodiverticular bands
- Abrupt dietary changes and verminous arteritis also have been implicated.
- The length and segment of the intestine involved are variable.
- The ileum is frequently included because of its fixed attachment at the ileocecal junction.

Diagnosis
- Acute onset of progressive, moderate to severe, continuous pain that may initially respond to analgesics.
- Analgesic efficacy rapidly decreases as the disease progresses.
- Rapid, progressive cardiovascular deterioration occurs as evidenced by poor peripheral perfusion (rapid, weak pulse; hyperemic or cyanotic mucous membranes; and a prolonged CRT).
- Hypovolemia and hemoconcentration develop rapidly.
- Nasogastric reflux often is present, but decompression may *not* provide pain relief as it does in simple obstruction.
- Rectal examination usually reveals moderate to severe small-intestinal distention (see Fig. 18-48) and occasionally a tight mesenteric root. Placing mild tension on the mesentery may elicit a pain response.
- Lack of palpable small-intestinal distention does not rule out the possibility of a strangulating lesion because the distended intestine may be beyond the reach of the examining arm.
- Abdominal ultrasonography reveals dilated, nonmotile small intestine.
- Abdominocentesis may yield normal or serosanguineous fluid with increased peritoneal protein concentration (>3.0 g/dL) and nucleated cell count (>5000 cells/µL). The devitalized portion of intestine may be isolated from the peritoneal cavity (e.g., a volvulus within the omental bursa), and results of peritoneal fluid analysis therefore may not accurately reflect the degree of intestinal change.
- Peritoneal fluid lactate is elevated, often higher than blood lactate. Serial sampling of peritoneal lactate demonstrates increased lactate concentrations over time.

●› WHAT TO DO

Volvulus
Initial Therapy Is Supportive
- Gastric decompression
- Balanced polyionic intravenous fluids (e.g., lactated Ringer's solution) with plasma
- Analgesics (e.g., xylazine, butorphanol tartrate, and/or flunixin meglumine)
- Monitoring of physiologic and clinical parameters:
  - Pain
  - Nasogastric reflux
  - Heart rate
  - Mucous membranes
  - Hematocrit, PCV/TPP
  - Borborygmi
- Surgical exploration if volvulus is suspected

Exploratory Surgery
- Perform a ventral midline exploratory celiotomy.
- Identify the strangulated portion of intestine.
- Determine the direction of rotation of the affected segment by means of palpation of the mesentery.
- After correction, evaluate intestinal viability and perform resection and anastomosis if needed.

Prognosis
- Prognosis depends on the duration of illness and amount of intestine involved in the volvulus.
- Prognosis is good with early detection and rapid treatment.
- For patients with long-standing strangulation, postoperative peritonitis, ileus, and adhesion formation are common sequelae.
- *Practice Tip: When resection of more than 50% of the small intestine is needed, there is a high incidence of postoperative complications (malabsorption, weight loss, and liver damage).*

Herniation
- Herniation of the small intestine is classified as:
  - Internal
  - External
- Internal hernias occur within the abdominal cavity and do *not* involve a hernial sac. Examples are:
  - Displacement of the small intestine through the epiploic foramen
  - Mesenteric defects
  - Rents in the gastrosplenic and broad ligaments
- External hernias extend outside the limits of the abdominal cavity and include:
  - Inguinal
  - Umbilical
  - Ventral abdominal
  - Diaphragmatic

Epiploic Foramen Herniation
- The epiploic foramen is a potential opening, approximately 4 to 6 cm in length, separating the omental bursa from the peritoneal cavity.

- The foramen is bounded dorsally by the caudate lobe of the liver and caudal vena cava and ventrally by the right lobe of the pancreas and the portal vein.
- The epiploic foramen is limited cranially by the hepatoduodenal ligament and caudally by the junction of the pancreas and mesoduodenum.
- *Practice Tip: Adults (older than 8 years) may be predisposed to epiploic foramen entrapment because of enlargement of this space caused by atrophy of the right caudate lobe of the liver.*
- Aerophagia (wind sucking) has also been associated with a predisposition to herniation through the epiploic foramen.
- Herniation through the foramen occurs more commonly from left-to-right (from the medial side) displacement but may also occur from right-to-left (from the lateral side) displacement.
- Gastrosplenic ligament herniation may appear clinically similar to epiploic herniation.

Diagnosis
- Acute onset of moderate to severe pain that may initially be responsive to analgesics.
- The effectiveness of analgesics decreases as the disease progresses.
- Rapid cardiovascular deterioration occurs, with hypovolemia and hemoconcentration.
- Nasogastric reflux is usually present, but decompression may not provide pain relief.
- Rectal examination reveals moderate to severe small-intestinal distention (see Fig. 18-48) in most cases.
- Some horses may have mild signs of pain with no nasogastric reflux or palpable intestinal distention. The lack of palpable small-intestinal distention does *not* rule out a strangulating lesion because the distended intestine may be beyond the reach of the examiner.
- Ultrasonography generally reveals distended nonmotile small intestine.
- Abdominocentesis is useful in determining the severity of the lesion and the need for surgical intervention.
- Peritoneal fluid analysis may reveal normal or serosanguineous fluid with increased protein concentration (>3.0 g/dL) and nucleated cell count (>5000 cells/μL). Lactate is increased in peritoneal fluid but may be within normal range in plasma on rare occasion. The devitalized portion of intestine within the omental bursa may be isolated from the rest of the peritoneal cavity. Therefore, fluid obtained at abdominocentesis may *not* accurately reflect the severity of intestinal compromise.

●› WHAT TO DO

Epiploic Foramen Herniation
Initial Therapy Is Supportive
- Gastric decompression
- Balanced polyionic intravenous fluids (e.g., lactated Ringer's solution)
- Analgesics (e.g., xylazine, butorphanol tartrate, and/or flunixin meglumine)

GI:COLIC

- Monitoring of physiologic and clinical parameters:
  - Pain
  - Nasogastric reflux
  - Heart rate
  - Mucous membranes
  - Hematocrit, PCV/TPP
  - Borborygmi
- Surgical intervention if epiploic entrapment is suspected

Exploratory Surgery
- Surgery frequently is needed to confirm the diagnosis.
- Perform a ventral midline exploratory celiotomy.
- Perform decompression of the bowel, careful manual dilation of the foramen, and reduction of the hernia.
- **Important Note:** Traumatic dilation of the foramen can result in life-threatening rupture of the caudal vena cava or portal vein.
- Evaluate intestinal viability, and perform resection and anastomosis if necessary.

Prognosis
Prognosis depends on the duration of illness, the length of intestine requiring resection, and difficulty encountered reducing the hernia.

Gastrosplenic Ligament Incarceration
- Incarceration of the small intestine through the gastrosplenic ligament is uncommon.
- Anatomically, the ligament attaches the greater curvature of the stomach to the hilum of the spleen and continues ventrally with the greater omentum.
- Defects in the ligament are generally acquired as the result of trauma.
- The distal jejunum is most commonly involved, with herniation occurring in a caudal to cranial direction.

Diagnosis
Clinical signs are similar to those of epiploic foramen herniation:
- Acute onset of severe abdominal pain, nasogastric reflux, small-intestinal distention on rectal examination, and rapid systemic deterioration occur.
- Distended small intestine may *not* be palpable early in the disease because of the cranial location in the abdomen.
- Abdominal ultrasonography generally reveals distended nonmotile small intestine in the left cranial abdomen, between the spleen and left body wall.
- Abdominocentesis may yield normal to serosanguineous fluid with an increased total protein and nucleated cell count. The severity of the signs depends on the location, duration, and extent of the lesion.
- Exploratory celiotomy is frequently needed for a definitive diagnosis.

⦿› WHAT TO DO

Gastrosplenic Ligament Incarceration
Initial Therapy Is Supportive
- Gastric decompression
- Balanced polyionic intravenous fluids (e.g., lactated Ringer's solution)

- Analgesics (e.g., xylazine, butorphanol tartrate, and/or flunixin meglumine)
- Monitoring of physiologic and clinical parameters:
  - Pain
  - Nasogastric reflux
  - Heart rate
  - Mucous membranes
  - Hematocrit, PCV/TPP
  - Borborygmi
- Surgical intervention if strangulating obstruction is suspected

Exploratory Surgery
- Perform a ventral midline exploratory celiotomy.
- Reduce the hernia.
- The ligament is relatively avascular, and digital enlargement of the rent facilitates reduction of the incarceration with minimal risk of life-threatening bleeding.
- Resection and anastomosis of devitalized bowel is performed.
- The defect in the ligament is *not* closed.

Prognosis
Prognosis depends on the duration of illness and length of intestine resected.

Mesenteric Defects
- Defects or rents in the *mesentery, broad ligaments, or greater omentum* produce a potential space for intestinal incarceration or strangulation.
- Mesenteric defects most often occur in the small-intestinal mesentery (Fig. 18-51), and less commonly, in the large and small colon mesentery.
- Defects commonly are acquired as a result of blunt abdominal trauma or surgical manipulation of bowel and mesentery. A segment of intestine may pass through the defect and become incarcerated or strangulated.
- A mesodiverticular band, a congenital remnant of a vitelline artery and its associated mesentery, extends from one side of the mesentery to the antimesenteric border of the jejunum or ileum and is a common site of incarceration. This tissue normally atrophies during the first trimester. Failure to atrophy results in formation of a triangulated mesenteric sac. A loop of intestine can become incarcerated in the sac; the result is mesenteric rupture, herniation, and strangulation.

Diagnosis
Clinical signs are similar to those of volvulus:
- Acute onset of abdominal pain.
- Nasogastric reflux with small-intestinal distention on rectal examination.
- Abdominal ultrasonography generally reveals distended nonmotile small intestine.
- Systemic cardiovascular deterioration.
- Abdominocentesis reveals normal to serosanguineous fluid with increased protein concentration, nucleated cell count, and lactate.
- The severity of the signs depends on the location, duration, and severity of the lesion.

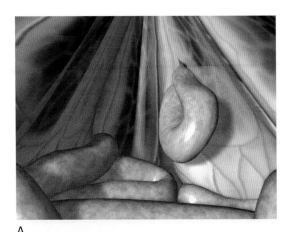

A

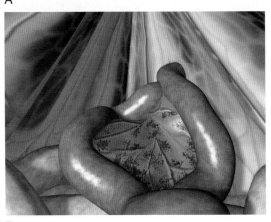

B

Figure 18-51   A, Intraabdominal view of a loop of jejunum passing through a mesenteric rent. **B,** Strangulation of the loop of small intestine occurs as the thicker-walled ileum becomes lodged in the mesenteric rent, thereby impairing blood flow in the affected intestine.

●》 WHAT TO DO

Mesenteric Defects

Initial Therapy Is Supportive
- Gastric decompression
- Balanced polyionic intravenous fluids (e.g., lactated Ringer's solution)
- Analgesics (e.g., xylazine, butorphanol tartrate, and/or flunixin meglumine)
- Monitoring of physiologic and clinical parameters:
  - Pain
  - Nasogastric reflux
  - Heart rate
  - Mucous membranes
  - Hematocrit, PCV/TPP
  - Borborygmi
- Surgical intervention if a strangulating obstruction is suspected

Exploratory Surgery
- Surgery is needed for definitive diagnosis.
- Ventral midline exploratory celiotomy is performed.
- The incarceration is reduced.
- The hernial ring may require manual dilation to reduce the hernia.
- The mesenteric defect is closed.
- Resection and anastomosis of devitalized bowel is performed.

- **Important Note:** Defects near the root of the mesentery are difficult to close because of limited exposure.
- **Practice Tip:** *Dorsally located mesenteric defects that cannot be closed may be repaired at a second surgery using a standing laparoscopic approach.*

Prognosis

Prognosis depends on the duration of illness and the length of intestine that requires resection. The prognosis is poor if difficulty is encountered reducing the hernia and closing the defect.

Inguinal Hernia

- Acquired inguinal hernias in stallions are associated with breeding or strenuous exercise and cause acute abdominal pain.
- A sudden increase in intraabdominal pressure or an enlarged internal inguinal ring may predispose to inguinal hernia.
- Inguinal hernias are commonly unilateral and occur frequently among Standardbred, Saddlebred, and Tennessee Walking horses.
- Inguinal herniation and evisceration can also occur as a sequela to castration!
- Congenital inguinal hernias in foals usually close spontaneously as the foal matures and only occasionally require surgical correction if the hernia *cannot* be reduced or if it is very large.
- Scrotal herniation may require surgical correction when the intestine ruptures the parietal tunic.

Diagnosis

- Acquired inguinal and scrotal herniation in a stallion can produce acute intestinal obstruction that necessitates emergency surgical intervention.
- Incarcerated bowel is strangulated; hypovolemic and endotoxic shock occur and cause systemic cardiovascular deterioration.
- The hernia is usually indirect and unilateral, with the incarcerated intestinal segment descending through the vaginal ring and contained within the tunica vaginalis.
- Affected horses have a rapid onset of moderate to severe abdominal pain.
- Palpation of the scrotum may reveal a firm, swollen, cold testicle on the affected side, but early in the disease process scrotal swelling may be absent.
- A swollen and slightly turgid tail of the epididymis may be palpated in early cases owing to passive congestion.
- The loop of herniated small bowel may be palpable per rectum passing through the internal inguinal ring. Palpate just below the brim of the pelvis and to each side.
- Ultrasonography generally reveals distended nonmotile bowel within the inguinal ring or scrotum.
- Signs of strangulating obstruction are the following:
  - Tachycardia
  - Dehydration
  - Endotoxemia

- Cardiovascular deterioration, which develops with time
- Abdominocentesis reveals fluid with an increased total protein level and nucleated cell count. Peritoneal fluid analysis may not accurately reflect the severity of intestinal compromise because of sequestration of fluid within the scrotum.
- Herniation and rupture of the vaginal tunic in newborn foals can cause mild to more severe pain and depression, local edema, and subsequent abscessation.

◉〉 WHAT TO DO

Inguinal Hernia
Initial Therapy Is Supportive
- Gastric decompression
- Balanced polyionic intravenous fluids (e.g., lactated Ringer's solution)
- Analgesics (e.g., xylazine, butorphanol tartrate, and/or flunixin meglumine)
- Monitoring of physiologic and clinical parameters:
  - Pain
  - Nasogastric reflux
  - Heart rate
  - Mucous membranes
  - Hematocrit, PCV/TPP
  - Borborygmi
- Surgical intervention if inguinal or scrotal herniation is suspected in adult horses

Exploratory Surgery
- Ventral midline exploratory celiotomy.
- Inguinal incision is used to achieve adequate surgical exposure and reduction.
- Reduction, resection, and anastomosis of the affected bowel are performed.
- Unilateral castration and inguinal herniorrhaphy are usually required.
- ***Practice Tip:*** *Inguinal herniation in newborn colts may be contained in the vaginal tunic or may rupture the tunic and lie subcutaneously. Those within the vaginal tunic may be manually reduced and generally correct spontaneously. Those that rupture the tunic or those that are large and cannot be reduced, require immediate surgical repair through inguinal and scrotal incisions.*

Prognosis
- Prognosis is good if reduction and repair are performed within hours of herniation before strangulation occurs.
- The prognosis worsens with increasing duration before correction.
- The prognosis for breeding soundness is good if only one testicle is involved.

Diaphragmatic Hernia
- Diaphragmatic hernia can be congenital or acquired and is an unusual cause of abdominal pain in horses.
- Most often it results from strenuous exercise, a hard fall, hitting something while running, or being hit by a car.
- Pregnant or periparturient mares also are at risk.

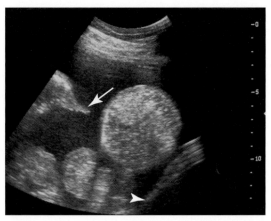

Figure 18-52 Ultrasound of the thorax of a 20-year-old gelding with mild pain, sternal edema, and thoracic effusion. The 5-mHz scan shows multiple loops of thickened small intestine and fluid in the thoracic cavity. To the middle left of the image, a caudal tip of consolidated lung is present *(arrow)*, and to the bottom right of the image, diaphragm *(arrowhead)*.

Diagnosis
- Clinical signs of diaphragmatic hernia include abdominal pain, tachypnea, and dyspnea.
- The severity of signs depends on the size of the hernia opening and degree of visceral herniation.
- The presence of viscera within the thoracic cavity may reduce the intensity of lung sounds and cause dullness on percussion.
- Radiography or ultrasonography (Fig. 18-52) is helpful in finding thickened or ingesta-filled loops of intestine in the thoracic cavity (finding bowel on both sides of the diaphragm).
- Blood gas measurement may indicate respiratory compromise and hypoxemia.
- Thoracocentesis and abdominocentesis may yield blood-tinged fluid with an increased total protein level and nucleated cell count, which are evidence of the presence of devitalized bowel. Be *cautious* performing a thoracocentesis if a diaphragmatic hernia is suspected; the bowel could be entered.
- Exploratory celiotomy often is necessary for a definitive diagnosis.

◉〉 WHAT TO DO

Diaphragmatic Hernia
Initial Therapy Is Supportive
- Gastric decompression
- Balanced polyionic intravenous fluids (e.g., lactated Ringer's solution)
- Analgesics (e.g., xylazine, butorphanol tartrate, and/or flunixin meglumine)
- Supplemental oxygen therapy if necessary
- Monitoring of physiologic and clinical parameters:
  - Pain
  - Nasogastric reflux
  - Heart rate
  - Mucous membranes
  - Hematocrit, PCV/TPP
  - Borborygmi

Exploratory Surgery

- Ventral midline exploratory celiotomy
- Reduction, resection, and anastomosis of the affected bowel
- Closure of the diaphragmatic defect by suturing or use of a synthetic mesh (Marlex,[13] Proxplast,[14] high-density polyethylene [HDPE][15])

Prognosis

The prognosis is guarded to poor because of difficult surgical exposure and a high incidence of postoperative complications, including septic pleuritis, implant failure, and hernia recurrence. The prognosis is better in young horses as a result of the improved surgical exposure.

Pedunculated Lipoma

- Pedunculated lipoma is a common cause of small-intestinal strangulation or obstruction in horses older than 10 years.
- Lipomas attach to the mesentery by a fibrovascular stalk of variable length.
- They are frequently incidental findings at exploratory surgery or necropsy.
- These masses have the potential to incarcerate a segment of small intestine (or rarely small colon) and produce strangulating obstruction (Fig. 18-53).

Diagnosis

Practice Tip: Pedunculated lipoma should always be considered in the differential diagnosis when a horse older than 10 years has signs of small-intestinal obstruction.

- Acute abdominal pain
- Hemoconcentration
- Decreased borborygmi
- Nasogastric reflux usually is present but may be absent early in the disease. Multiple loops of small intestine are palpable on rectal examination (see Fig. 18-48) or are evident on abdominal ultrasonographic examination. Increases in peritoneal total protein concentration and nucleated cell count reflect the degree of intestinal compromise.

●» WHAT TO DO

Pedunculated Lipoma

Initial Therapy Is Supportive

- Gastric decompression
- Balanced polyionic intravenous fluids (e.g., lactated Ringer's solution)
- Analgesics (e.g., xylazine, butorphanol tartrate, and/or flunixin meglumine)
- Monitoring of physiologic and clinical parameters:
  - Pain
  - Nasogastric reflux
  - Heart rate
  - Mucous membranes

- Hematocrit, PCV/TPP
- Borborygmi
- Surgical intervention if a strangulating obstruction is suspected

Exploratory Surgery

- Ventral midline exploratory celiotomy
- Ligation and transection of lipoma
- Resection and anastomosis of the affected intestine
- Removal of any lipomas found at surgery to minimize recurrence

Prognosis

Prognosis is often favorable with early diagnosis and prompt treatment. If devitalized intestine *cannot* be resected or if peritonitis is severe, the prognosis is guarded to poor.

Ileal Impaction

- The ileum is the most common site of small-intestinal intraluminal impaction (Fig. 18-54). The incidence varies with geographic location.
- This condition is more common in Europe and the southeastern United States; the cause is unknown.
- An association with fine, high-roughage forage and coastal Bermuda hay has been implicated.

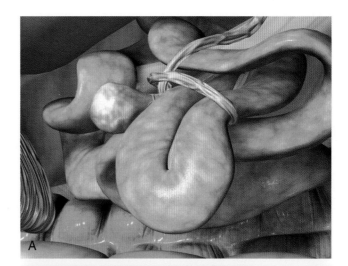

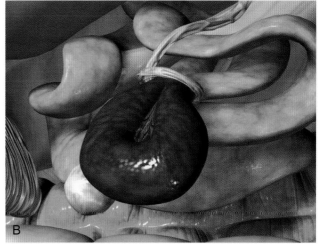

Figure 18-53 A, Movement of a loop of jejunum into a half-hitch formed by a pedunculated lipoma on its stalk. **B,** Strangulation of the loop of jejunum by the pedunculated lipoma.

---

[13]Polypropylene (Davol A Bard Company, Warwick, Rhode Island).
[14]Plastics (Goshen Laboratories, Goshen, New York).
[15]HDPE (MEDPOR, DermNet, New Zealand).

GI:COLIC

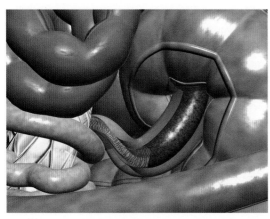

Figure 18-54   Obstruction of the lumen of the ileum by ingesta. The wall of the ileum has been rendered transparent to facilitate visualization of the impaction.

- Ingesta accumulate in the ileum causing obstruction. Spasmodic contraction and absorption of water from the ileal lumen exacerbate the impaction.
- Mesenteric vascular thrombotic disease, tapeworm infestation *(A. perfoliata)*, and ascarid impaction *(P. equorum)* are less common causes.
- ***Practice Tip:*** *Ileal hypertrophy should be considered in older horses with a history of chronic colic.*
- On the rare occasion, idiopathic hypertrophy of large portions of the small bowel may cause chronic colic. The hypertrophy in these cases can be easily seen on abdominal ultrasound examination. Prognosis is guarded in these cases and are best managed by dietary (low roughage) control.
- Focal or diffuse eosinophilic inflammatory disease of the small intestine and left dorsal colon may also present with thickened bowel and either acute or chronic colic.
- Of the inflammatory bowel disorders (lymphocytic-plasmacytic, eosinophilic, granulomatous, lymphosarcoma, etc.) eosinophilic cases seem to have the highest incidence of colic as a clinical sign. Medical management (corticosteroids) for eosinophilic enteritis has a fair to guarded outcome although for focal disease surgical removal is usually successful.

Diagnosis

Clinical signs are variable and depend on the duration of the impaction:

- Moderate to severe abdominal pain is caused by focal intestinal distention and spasmodic contraction around the impaction. Affected horses usually have a transient response to analgesics.
- Rectal palpation reveals multiple loops of moderately to severely distended small intestine (see Fig. 18-48). Early examination may reveal 5- to 8-cm diameter, firm, smooth-surfaced ileum originating at the cecal base and coursing from the right of the midline obliquely downward and to the left side.
- Abdominal ultrasonography generally reveals distended nonmotile small intestine.

- Nasogastric reflux may be absent in the early stages. During the 8 to 10 hours after the initial episode of colic, small intestinal and gastric distention develops and results in recurrence of signs of pain and progressive dehydration.
- Gastric decompression often provides temporary pain relief. Borborygmi diminish or disappear, and intestinal distention without motility is seen on ultrasound examination.
- CBC, electrolytes, blood gases, and findings at abdominocentesis frequently are within normal limits.
- Hemoconcentration and increased total peritoneal protein level and nucleated cell count may occur with long-standing impaction.

⦿❯ WHAT TO DO

Ileal Impaction

Initial Therapy Is Supportive
- Gastric decompression
- Balanced polyionic intravenous fluids (e.g., lactated Ringer's solution)
- Analgesics (e.g., xylazine, butorphanol tartrate, and/or flunixin meglumine)
- Monitoring of physiologic and clinical parameters:
  - Pain
  - Nasogastric reflux
  - Heart rate
  - Mucous membranes
  - Hematocrit, PCV/TPP
  - Borborygmi
- The impaction may respond to medical therapy (one to three doses of xylazine may resolve the impaction based on its use in several horses), and is believed to cause relaxation of the intestine; N-butylscopolammonium bromide (Buscopan) may have a similar effect.
- 6 to 8 L of water via nasogastric tube if *no* net reflux
- If medical therapy is unsuccessful, surgical intervention is necessary.

Exploratory Surgery
- Ventral midline exploratory celiotomy
- Reduce the obstruction by extraluminal massage
- Mix the impaction with jejunal fluid or infuse of the impaction with sterile saline solution or sodium carboxymethylcellulose with or without 2% lidocaine to facilitate reduction
- With significant mural edema and congestion, jejunal enterotomy may be necessary to facilitate emptying of the ileal contents without excessive manipulation of the bowel
- Resection and anastomosis (ileocecostomy or jejunocecostomy) is rarely necessary but may be required if additional problems exist, such as ileal hypertrophy or mesenteric vascular thrombotic disease.

Prognosis

Prognosis is good for both medical and surgical treatment if no concurrent abnormalities exist (e.g., ileal hypertrophy) and is guarded if ileocecostomy or jejunocecostomy is needed because of postoperative ileus and the high incidence of intraabdominal adhesions.

Ascarid Impaction

- Heavy ascarid *(P. equorum)* infestation can lead to intra-luminal obstruction in foals, weanlings, and yearlings.
- Affected horses have a history of a poor parasite control program leading to heavy infestation with ascarids.
- ***Practice Tip:*** *Impaction commonly follows (24 to 48 hr) after treatment with an anthelmintic (e.g., pyrantel, ivermectin), tranquilizers, or general anesthetics.*
- Fenbendazole, although a highly effective anthelmintic, is *not* commonly implicated in the development of ascarid impaction.
- Intestinal rupture, peritonitis, and intussusception are possible sequelae.
- Foals develop immunity to the parasite by 6 months to 1 year of age. Consequently, this condition is uncommon in adults.

Diagnosis

Clinical signs depend on the duration and degree of small-intestinal obstruction and include the following:

- Unthriftiness
- Poor hair coat
- Mild to severe abdominal pain
- Nasogastric reflux that usually is present and may contain ascarids
- Rectal examination and abdominal ultrasonography that reveal multiple loops of distended small intestine. Ascarids may be seen within the lumen on ultrasound examination (Fig 18-55, *A* and *B*).
- ***Practice Tip:*** *The final diagnosis is based on signalment, history, and the presence of signs of small-intestinal obstruction.*

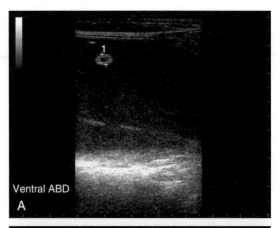

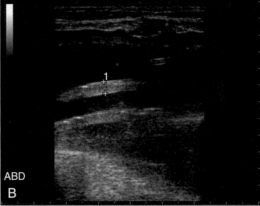

Figure 18-55   A, Ultrasound image of the ventral abdomen of a 3-month-old foal with colic and distended small intestine because of a *Parascaris equorum* impaction. The hyperechoic circle is a *Parascaris equorum* seen on cross section. **B,** The same foal as in Fig 18-54; Three *Parascaris equorum* parasites are seen longitudinally. The foal was dewormed the previous day.

●〉 WHAT TO DO

Ascarid Impaction

Partial Obstruction of the Intestine with Ascarids

- Intestinal lubricants (e.g., mineral oil)
- Balanced polyionic intravenous fluids (e.g., lactated Ringer's solution)
- Analgesics (e.g., xylazine, butorphanol tartrate, and/or flunixin meglumine)
- Low-efficacy or slow-onset anthelmintics (fenbendazole, ivermectin), which are preferred to prevent future recurrence

Ventral Midline Exploratory Surgery to Relieve the Obstruction

- Surgery is required with complete obstruction or if medical therapy is unsuccessful.
- Multiple enterotomies (Fig. 18-56) may be needed to remove the ascarids, although massaging the parasites into the cecum may improve the prognosis

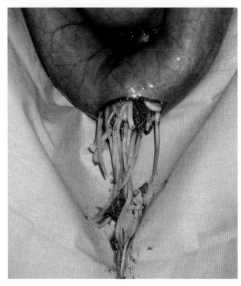

Figure 18-56   Intraoperative image demonstrating a small intestinal enterotomy in a weanling to facilitate removal of an ascarid impaction.

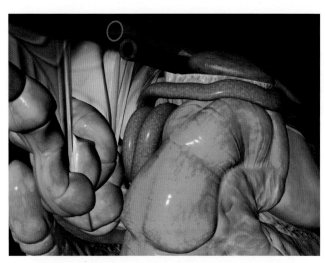

Figure 18-57   Caudal right view of inflammation and distention of the duodenum and jejunum caused by proximal enteritis.

GI:COLIC

Prognosis

Prognosis is good if medical treatment is successful and guarded if surgery and multiple enterotomies are performed because of the high occurrence of intraabdominal adhesions.

Duodenitis and Proximal Jejunitis

- Duodenitis and proximal jejunitis are characterized by transmural inflammation, edema, and hemorrhage in the duodenum and proximal jejunum (Fig. 18-57).
- The stomach and proximal small intestine are moderately distended with fluid, whereas the distal jejunum and ileum usually are flaccid.
- Histologic lesions include hyperemia and edema of the mucosa and submucosa, villous epithelial degeneration and sloughing, neutrophil infiltration, hemorrhage in the muscular layer, and fibrinopurulent exudation on the serosa.
- The cause of this extensive intestinal damage is unknown; *Clostridium perfringens* and *Clostridium difficile* are presumed causative agents and frequently can be cultured from the gastric reflux.
- *Salmonella* is rarely cultured from gastric contents.
- Proximal small-intestinal distention, gastric reflux, dehydration, and hypovolemic and endotoxic shock result from the intestinal damage. The inflammation and damage can alter intestinal motility, causing adynamic ileus.

Diagnosis

Clinical Signs

- Acute abdominal pain
- Large volumes of nasogastric reflux fluid (red to greenish brown; spontaneous reflux may even be seen in a few cases)
- Absent borborygmi
- Tachycardia
- Dehydration
- Slight increase in body temperature (38.6° C to 39.1° C [101.5° F to 102.4° F])

- Hyperemic mucous membranes
- Increased hematocrit
- Moderate to severe small-intestinal distention on rectal examination; early in the disease, small-intestinal distention may be absent
- Distended proximal small intestine with thickened wall and mild to moderate motility at ultrasound examination

Clinical Laboratory Findings

- Increased PCV and TPP (hemoconcentration)
- Increased creatinine concentration indicating prerenal or renal azotemia
- Increased peritoneal total protein concentration
- Mild to moderate increase in nucleated cell count (5000 to 25,000 cells/mL) in peritoneal fluid
- Hypokalemia
- Occasionally, metabolic acidosis
- CBC that may reveal a normal, increased (neutrophilia caused by inflammation) or decreased (neutropenia and left shift caused by endotoxemia and consumption) WBC count
- Gram stain of the gastric reflux fluid that shows a large number of large gram-positive rods (Fig. 18-58)
- *Practice Tip: The clinical findings can be confused with those of strangulating or nonstrangulating obstruction. After nasogastric decompression, abdominal pain usually subsides and is replaced by depression in patients with duodenitis and proximal jejunitis. The presence of persistent abdominal pain with serosanguineous abdominal fluid supports the diagnosis of strangulating obstruction, but serosanguineous abdominal fluid can also be present with proximal enteritis.*

⬤ WHAT TO DO

Duodenitis and Proximal Jejunitis

- Voluminous gastrointestinal reflux is produced for 1 to 7 days, requiring gastric decompression through an indwelling nasogastric tube every 2 hours to prevent distention, pain, and gastric rupture.
- Food and oral medication are withheld until small-intestinal borborygmi return.
- Intravenous administration of a balanced crystalloid solution is required to maintain intravascular fluid volume.
- Monitoring of blood gases and serum electrolytes (Na^+, K^+, Cl^-, HCO_3^-, Ca^{2+}) daily and adjustment of the intravenous solution are necessary to correct any deficiencies.
- Administer low-dose flunixin meglumine, 0.25 mg/kg IV q8h, to minimize the adverse effects of arachidonic acid metabolites (thromboxane A_2 and prostaglandins).
- Antiserum (Endoserum) directed against gram-negative core antigens (endotoxin) is administered intravenously diluted in a balanced electrolyte solution. Hyperimmune plasma directed against the J-5 mutant strain of *E. coli* (Polymune-J or Foalimmune) or normal equine plasma (2 to 10 L) administered intravenously slowly may be equally beneficial, supplying protein, fibronectin, complement, antithrombin III, and other inhibitors of hypercoagulability.
- Polymyxin B, 2000 to 6000 IU/kg IV slowly q12h as needed, if the horse shows evidence of significant toxemia and after urination is seen.
- Nonfractionated heparin, 100 U/kg SQ q12h, or preferably low-molecular-weight heparin, 50 to 100 U/kg SQ q24h, may decrease the incidence of laminitis.

- DMSO 10% solution can be administered intravenously (100 mg/kg q8h or q12h) but efficacy is in question.
- Na$^+$ or K$^+$ penicillin (22,000 to 44,000 IU/kg IV q6h) or procaine penicillin (22,000 to 44,000 IU/kg IM q12h) can be administered, in addition to metronidazole (30 mg/kg per rectum q8h or 15 mg/kg IV q6h) for *C. perfringens* or *C. difficile,* as the suggested causative pathogen.
- Motility modifiers can be useful in reducing gastric reflux and may decrease the cost of treatment and complications associated with frequent passage of the nasogastric tube.
- Recommendations for motility modifiers are as follows:
  - 2% lidocaine, slow intravenous bolus, 1.3 mg/kg (approximately 30 mL/450-kg adult) followed by 0.05 mg/kg per minute infusion; the motility modifying effect is believed secondary to the anti-inflammatory effect.
  - Cisapride, 0.1 to 0.2 mg/kg IV q8h, 0.3 mg/kg PO q8h; adverse effects can occur with the IV administration
- Monitor serum creatinine concentration and urine output after fluid therapy because secondary renal failure is common.
- Laminitis is a common complication. The feet should be monitored, and treatment should be incorporated in the medical therapy, including the following (see Chapter 43, p. 709):
  - Ice distal limbs and feet with ice boots for 48 hours or until toxic neutrophils and band cells are *no* longer present in the CBC.
  - Heavily bed the stall with shavings or sand.
  - Removing shoes, trim and balance feet, and apply Styrofoam, dental putty, or other hoof and frog support to enlist mechanical support of the entire foot.
  - Apply lower limb support bandages.
  - Administer phenylbutazone, after discontinuing flunixen meglumine, (2.2 to 4.4 mg/kg PO or IV q12h) if laminitis develops.
  - Administer acepromazine (0.02 mg/kg IM q8h) for its vasodilatory properties.
  - Administer DMSO intravenously as listed before.
  - Pentoxifylline (Trental), 7.5 to 10 mg/kg PO, IV, q8-12h; recommended for endotoxemia, laminitis, vasodilator and rheologic effects.
- With prolonged (>7 days) nasogastric reflux, bowel decompression or intestinal bypass through a standing right flank laparotomy or ventral midline celiotomy can be used to augment medical therapy.
- Some surgeons, particularly in the United Kingdom, believe that immediate exploratory laparotomy and decompression results in a more rapid recovery.

Prognosis

- With aggressive medical management, the disease resolves in most cases.
- Sequelae that adversely affect the prognosis include:
  - Laminitis
  - Renal failure
  - Intraabdominal adhesion formation
  - Pharyngeal or esophageal injury
  - Gastric rupture
- ***Practice Tip:*** *Patients with red gastric reflux fluid appear to be more prone to complications than are horses without such reflux.*

Nonstrangulating Infarction

- Nonstrangulating infarction is an inadequate blood supply (necrosis caused by loss of blood supply) of the intestine without a strangulating lesion.
- Postmortem examination commonly reveals the cause to be thrombus formation at the cranial mesenteric artery from damage by migration of the fourth and fifth stages of *Strongylus vulgaris* larvae.
- Infarction is hypothesized to be the result of hypoxia induced by vasospasm.

Diagnosis

A poor parasite control program may predispose horses to nonstrangulating ischemia and infarction. The disease also occurs in horses regularly treated with anthelmintics. Clinical signs of variable severity range from depression to moderately severe abdominal pain:

- Heart rate, respiratory rate, and body temperature may be normal or increased.
- Hyperemic mucous membranes suggest endotoxemia or inflammation caused by migrating parasites.
- Rectal examination and abdominal ultrasound examination findings may be normal or include distended small intestine.
- Pain, fremitus, or thickening is commonly evident on palpation of the mesenteric root.

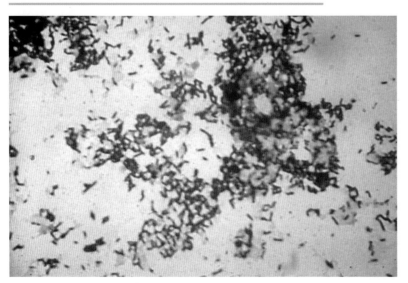

Figure 18-58   Gram stain of gastric fluid from a horse with proximal duodenitis-jejunitis that demonstrates many large gram-positive rods (compatible with *Clostridium perfringens*).

- Auscultation of the abdomen may reveal normal, increased, or decreased borborygmi.
- Gastric reflux may be present because of functional obstruction of the intestinal segment.
- PCV, TPP, and creatinine level may be increased because of dehydration.
- Peripheral blood examination may reveal a normal, decreased (neutropenia with a left shift resulting from endotoxemia), or increased (neutrophilia resulting from inflammation) WBC count.
- TPP may be increased because of chronic inflammation caused by parasites or decreased as a result of protein loss through damaged intestinal mucosa.
- Abdominal fluid may be normal or contain an increased amount of total protein (>3.0 mg/dL), and the WBC count can be as high as 200,000 cells/μL.

WHAT TO DO

Nonstrangulating Infarction

- Balanced crystalloid intravenous fluids to correct dehydration and enhance reperfusion of the affected intestinal segments
- Maintain gastric decompression
- Broad-spectrum antimicrobial drugs, K⁺ penicillin, 22,000 IU/kg IV q6h; gentamicin, 6.6 mg/kg IV q24h, if peritonitis is present
- Flunixin meglumine, 0.25 mg/kg IV q8h, to reduce thromboxane production and increase mesenteric perfusion
- DMSO 10% solution, 100 mg/kg IV q8-12h, to decrease superoxide radical injury during reperfusion
- Aspirin (20 mg/kg PO every other day) and fractionated heparin (40 to 100 IU/kg IV or SQ q6-12h) or preferably low-molecular-weight heparin (40 to 50 U/kg IM) to diminish and/or prevent thrombosis. Monitor the hematocrit closely for red blood cell agglutination and declining hematocrit resulting from nonfractionated heparin administration.
- Pentoxifylline (Trental), 7.5 to 10 mg/kg, PO, IV, q8-12h to treat endotoxemia, vasodilator and rheologic properties
- Exploratory surgery for patients unresponsive to medical therapy

Prognosis

- Prognosis is poor for patients that need surgery for intestinal resection.
- Ischemia that is *not* obvious at the time of exploratory surgery may progress to infarction.
- Ileus and adhesions are common postoperative complications.
- Large segments of affected intestine may be too extensive for resection.
- Identification and resection of diseased small- or large-intestinal segments sometimes is successful with fluorescein dye, Doppler ultrasonography, or surface oximetry to determine intestinal viability.

Acute Ileus of the Small Intestine

- Acute colic caused by ileus of the small intestine and stomach is occasionally seen, mostly in postparturient mares.

- Affected horses are generally very painful and both ultrasound and rectal examinations confirm small-intestinal distention without motility (ultrasound exam).
- Peritoneal fluid and blood lactate measurements are suggestive of a nonstrangulating lesion.
- Hypocalcemia may be the cause in some cases with demonstrated serum hypocalcemia; otherwise the cause of the disorder is unknown.

WHAT TO DO

Small-Intestinal Ileus in the Postparturient Mare

- Pass a nasogastric tube to prevent gastric rupture.
- Provide intravenous fluids with calcium as required.
- Administer analgesics, preferably NSAIDs (which have minimal effect on intestinal motility) to control abdominal pain that can be severe.
- Administer lidocaine CRI.
- If severe colic continues and small-intestinal distention does not improve after the previous actions, surgical decompression may be required.
- Prognosis is good if appropriate treatment is begun before gastric rupture.

Eosinophilic Enteritis Causing Intestinal Obstruction

- There are several infiltrative or inflammatory bowel diseases (either small intestine or large intestine) of the horse.
- Eosinophilic infiltration is the most common one to cause colic and sometimes may cause focal obstruction of the small intestine or left dorsal colon.
- Diagnosis can occur based on histopathology of resected tissue taken at surgery, or based on response to corticosteroid treatment.
- Horses with focal lesions have been shown to also have eosinophilic infiltrates in the normal appearing intestine.

Disorders of the Large Intestine
Cecal Impaction

- Cecal impaction generally occurs as the result of other diseases, especially those associated with:
  - Endotoxemia
  - Surgery
  - Chronic pain, secondary to septic metritis, infectious arthritis, fractures, and corneal disease
  - Cecal impaction can also be a sequelae of stall rest in a horse previously in a high level of work.
- Most cases have large amounts of dry ingesta in the cecum (true impaction), whereas other cases have a large volume of fluid contents (cecal dysfunction).

Diagnosis
Clinical Findings

- Anorexia
- Reduced fecal output or smaller than normal fecal balls
- Mild to severe abdominal pain

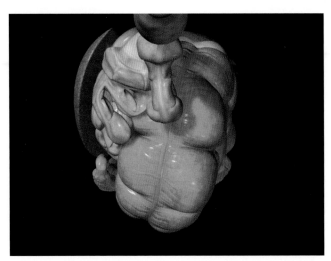

Figure 18-59 Caudal view of the abdomen demonstrating cecal distention caused by a cecal impaction.

- **Practice Tip:** *Occasionally, there are few prodromal signs, such as only slight depression.*
- Abdominal distention may be present but is often absent.
- With severe impaction, abdominal auscultation reveals a high right-sided "cecal ping."
- Heart rate varies with the severity of pain, and mucous membranes usually are pink and tacky.
- Nasogastric reflux is unusual unless the impaction is of prolonged duration or cecal dysfunction results in ileus of the small intestine.
- PCV, TPP, and creatinine levels are increased as a consequence of dehydration.
- In cases of cecal perforation, peritoneal total protein concentration and nucleated cell count are increased.
- The diagnosis is confirmed on rectal examination; the ventral cecal taenia is tight and displaced ventrally and medially. Dry ingesta are palpable in the body and base of the cecum, and moderate amounts of gas fill the base (Fig. 18-59). Cecal distention can make the dorsal and medial cecal taeniae readily palpable and leave the left colon and small colon empty.

●》 WHAT TO DO

Cecal Impaction

Medical Management of Mild to Moderate Cecal Impaction

- Give nothing by mouth ; water is fine if there is *no* gastric reflux.
- Administer three times the daily maintenance requirement of fluid (60 to 90 L/450 kg/day), balanced crystalloid solutions with 20 mEq/L KCl IV, and water orally to rehydrate the impaction: 6 to 8 L of water/500 kg q2h through an indwelling nasogastric tube. Administer intravenous lidocaine (1.3 mg/kg slow bolus followed by 0.05 mg/kg/min CRI) to enhance motility, especially for cecal dysfunction.
- Administer laxatives to facilitate rehydration of impacted material (see Laxatives, p. 190)
- Reintroduce feed slowly to avoid recurrence.
- Feed grass, water-soaked pellets, and bran mashes for the first 24 to 48 hours after feed is reintroduced.

Conditions Requiring Surgical Management
- Uncontrollable pain
- Severe impaction (extremely tight medial cecal band)
- Unsuccessful medical therapy
- Characteristics of peritoneal fluid suggesting cecal compromise
- The surgical options through ventral midline celiotomy include the following:
  - Extraluminal massage
  - Typhlotomy and evacuation (most commonly performed)
  - Partial or complete typhlectomy
  - Cecocolic anastomosis
  - Ileocolic anastomosis
  - Jejunocolic anastomosis

  Practice Tip: *Jejunocolic or ileocolic anastomosis is considered superior to cecocolic anastomosis because it has fewer long-term sequelae. Complete typhlectomy through a right paralumbar laparotomy is difficult, and fecal contamination of the abdomen is a complication.*

Prognosis

- Prognosis is good for patients with mild to moderate cecal impaction without underlying cecal dysfunction.
- Severe cecal impaction necessitating surgical treatment is complicated by peritonitis, adhesions, perforation, and death.
- The prognosis for severe impaction is guarded.

Important Note: Cecal distention with "fluidy" contents may also occur and cause a similar clinical condition. This appears to be a primary motility disturbance and is often more troublesome than "dry" cecal impaction.

Cecal Perforation

The site is generally the medial or caudal surface of the base owing to excessive tension on the cecal wall as a result of severe impaction. Perforation also is associated with late gestation and parturition. The pathogenesis remains unknown; tapeworm (*A. perfoliata*) infestation has been implicated.

Diagnosis

- The horse has signs of cardiovascular shock resulting from septic peritonitis.
- The rate of deterioration is related directly to the degree of peritoneal contamination.
- Rectal examination reveals enlargement of the cecum with emphysema and roughening of the serosa of the cecal base.
- The peritoneal fluid, obtained with a teat cannula, has an increased or a decreased nucleated cell count and increased total protein concentration; degenerative WBCs and intracellular and extracellular bacteria and plant material are present.

●》 WHAT TO DO

Cecal Perforation—Symptomatic Only

- Balanced, polyionic, intravenous fluids
- Broad-spectrum antimicrobial agents
- Flunixin meglumine

Prognosis

Prognosis is poor and may be grave if fecal contamination occurs due to resulting septic peritonitis and endotoxic shock.

Large Colon Impaction

- Large colon impaction most commonly occurs at two sites of narrowing:
  - Pelvic flexure
  - Transverse colon
- At these locations, retropulsive contractions (propagation in an oral direction) retain ingesta for microbial digestion. These contractile patterns can contribute to impaction.

Predisposing Factors

- Poor dentition
- Ingestion of coarse roughage
- Inadequate fluid intake
- Stress associated with transportation
- Intense exercise resulting in hypomotility
- Inadequate water intake
- Excessive fluid loss through sweating

Diagnosis
Clinical Findings

- Anorexia
- Abdominal distention
- Decreased fecal output
- Mild, initially intermittent, to severe abdominal pain
- Heart rate varying with the degree of pain; pink and tacky mucous membranes
- Nasogastric reflux is uncommon unless ileus of the small intestine or compression of loops of small intestine occurs.
- PCV, TPP, and creatinine concentration are increased when clinical dehydration is present.
- With complete luminal obstruction, abdominal distention is significant.
- Rectal examination reveals impacted ingesta with varying degrees of distention of the pelvic flexure and ventral colon; in severe cases, the colon is palpable in the pelvic canal.
- Impaction in the transverse colon is *not* palpable.
- In chronic, severe cases, distention of the colonic wall can cause pressure necrosis of the intestinal wall and peritonitis. The peritoneal fluid protein level and nucleated cell count reflect intestinal compromise. Abdominal pain usually is severe and unrelenting, and signs of toxemia (hyperemia, cyanotic mucous membranes, or both), tachycardia, and tachypnea are apparent.

◆》 WHAT TO DO

Large Colon Impaction

- Withhold food to prevent continued accumulation of ingesta.
- Allow access to water if there is *no* nasogastric reflux.
- Provide medical management:
  - Patients with mild impaction respond to administration of water and mineral oil, magnesium sulfate (preferred), or DSS and electrolytes through a nasogastric tube.

- Intravenous fluids (4 to 5 L/h per 450 kg) and laxative therapy are needed for moderate to severe colon impaction.
- Administer analgesics as needed. N-butylscopolammonium bromide (Buscopan) is used successfully along with laxatives by many clinicians, although there remains some controversy with this treatment.
- Surgical decision based on the following:
  - Unsuccessful medical management
  - Unrelenting abdominal pain
  - Rectal examination that reveals large colon displacement
  - Endotoxemia, cardiovascular deterioration
  - Changes in peritoneal fluid indicating intestinal compromise
- Ventral midline exploratory celiotomy:
  - Defines extent of impaction
  - May reveal other abnormalities: e.g., colon displacement, enterolith
  - Perform a pelvic flexure enterotomy
  - Lavage the lumen of colon to evacuate ingesta

Prognosis

- Prognosis is good for medical management of mild-to-moderate severe large colon impaction.
- Prognosis is fair to good for surgical correction of severe impaction, unless necrosis of the intestinal wall or colonic devitalization results in intestinal perforation.

Sand Impaction

- Ingestion of sand while grazing or eating hay, or especially grain spillage on closely grazed pastures in areas with sandy soil, may result in sand impaction.
- The ingested sand settles in the large colon, where it accumulates and eventually results in a nonstrangulating luminal obstruction.

Diagnosis
Clinical Signs

- Clinical signs are similar to those of large colon impaction; the signs of pain are frequently acute. The horse may have a history of chronic colic or diarrhea.
- Auscultation of the cranial ventral abdomen, for 4 to 5 minutes, may reveal a sound similar to an "ocean wave."
- Sand may be palpated on rectal examination and found in feces placed in water; the ingesta floats in water, and the sand settles to the bottom of the container.
- The impaction is commonly palpable on rectal examination in the pelvic flexure or cecum, whereas impaction in the right dorsal (most common) or transverse colon is *not* palpable.
- *Practice Tip: The lack of sand found on rectal examination or in manure does not rule out a diagnosis of sand impaction, as in severe impactions no sand is moving aborally.*
- *Practice Tip: Abdominocentesis, if performed, should be done with extreme caution to avoid enterocentesis caused by the location of the sand-filled colon on the ventral abdominal floor.*
- Abdominal radiographs may be helpful. The radiographic pattern has been described by Kendall et al. (See online Bibliography for complete citation.) The irritating effect of

the sand on the colonic mucosa can cause diarrhea or low-grade fever.
- Under the weight of the sand, degeneration and necrosis of the bowel wall can result in endotoxemia and peritonitis.

WHAT TO DO

Sand Impaction
Medical Management
- Horse frequently responds to early administration of fluids and laxatives (mineral oil). Psyllium hydrophilic mucilloid (Metamucil) is the most effective laxative: 400 g/500 kg q6h until the impaction resolves. *Practice Tip: Once in contact with cold water, the mucilloid forms a gel that can be difficult to pump through a nasogastric tube; therefore, the tube must be in place and the mixture administered immediately. The gel lubricates and binds with the sand, moving it distally and relieving the obstruction. Alternatively, mixing the psyllium with mineral oil instead of water maintains the psyllium in solution, thereby facilitating easier administration by nasogastric tube.*
- Continue psyllium treatment at 400 g/500 kg once a day for 7 days to remove residual sand. Alternating psyllium and mineral oil may prevent obstruction associated with retrograde movement of sand and psyllium.

Surgical Management
- Perform a ventral midline exploratory celiotomy for patients that do *not* respond to medical treatment or have other abnormalities, such as colonic displacement.
- Remove sand through a pelvic flexure enterotomy.
- Sand can cause extensive damage to the colonic wall, leading to postoperative complications such as postoperative ileus, intestinal wall degeneration, and peritonitis.

Preventive Management
- *Do not* overgraze pastures.
- Provide a hay supplement when needed, and *do not* place feed on the ground.
- Add prophylactic psyllium treatment to feed to remove sand from the colon: Administer psyllium, 400 g/500 kg once a day for 7 days, for preventive treatment every 4 to 12 months, depending on sand exposure risk.
- Consider using flavored or soluble psyllium, which may be more palatable than unflavored forms.

Prognosis
- Prognosis is good for mild to moderately severe sand impaction.
- The surgical prognosis for severe sand impaction is good unless necrosis or devitalization of the intestinal wall results in rupture of the colon.

Cecocolic Intussusception
- Cecocolic intussusception is an unusual cause of intestinal obstruction that results from invagination of the apex of the cecum through the cecocolic orifice into the right ventral colon.
- The entire cecum can invaginate into the colon and become strangulated.

- The cause is unknown; however, conditions causing aberrant intestinal motility, such as parasite infestation, diet changes, impaction, mural lesions, and the presence of motility-altering drugs, have been implicated.
- *Practice Tip: Cecocolic intussusception is more common among horses younger than 3 years.*

Diagnosis
- Patients with strangulating intussusception may show signs of acute, severe abdominal pain.
- In contrast, affected horses with chronic nonstrangulating intussusception may have mild to moderate abdominal pain; depression; weight loss; and scant, soft feces.
- The intussusception is frequently palpable per rectum as a large mass in the right caudal abdomen; if the ileum is involved, distended small intestine is palpable.
- In some cases, the intussusception may be observed on ultrasound examination
- The presence of a firm mass palpable in the cecal base or the right ventral colon is confirmatory.
- Abdominocentesis reveals increases in peritoneal total protein and nucleated cell count. These changes may *not* be evident until late in the disease because the cecum is sequestered within the ventral colon.
- Failure to respond to medical therapy leads to exploratory surgery and a definitive diagnosis.

WHAT TO DO

Cecocolic Intussusception
- Perform a ventral midline exploratory celiotomy.
- Reduce the intussusception—this can be difficult because of mural edema and adhesions between the serosal surfaces.
- If extraluminal reduction is successful, assess cecal viability and, if required, perform complete or partial typhlectomy.
- Reduction and resection of the devitalized portion of cecum can be performed through an enterotomy in the right ventral colon if extraluminal reduction is impossible.

Prognosis
- Prognosis is fair if the apex of the cecum is involved and extraluminal reduction is possible.
- Prognosis is poor if reduction requires enterotomy or the entire cecum is involved due to the risk of septic peritonitis.

Large Colon Displacement
- The left ventral and dorsal colons are freely movable, allowing for intestinal displacement and volvulus.
- The cause is unknown, with the following implicated:
  - Alterations in colonic motility
  - Excessive gas production
  - Rolling resulting from abdominal pain or dietary changes
  - Excessive concentrate intake
  - Grazing lush pastures
  - Parasite infestation
- Generally, *no* causative factor is identified.

GI:COLIC

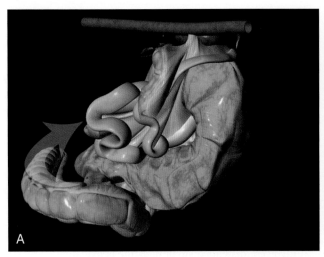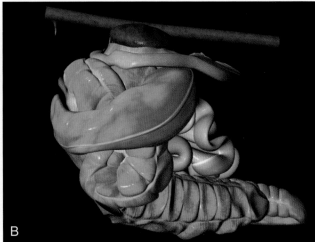

Figure 18-60   A, View of an early stage in the development of right displacement of the colon. The colon has begun to move caudally ventral to the cecum. **B,** Final stage of right displacement of the colon in which the colon is positioned caudal to the cecum and has rotated such that the ventral colon is dorsal and the dorsal colon is ventral.

- *Practice Tip: Large colon displacement is more common in geldings.*
- Right dorsal displacement of the colon is displacement of the left colon lateral to the cecum between the cecum and the right body wall (Fig. 18-60). The pelvic flexure commonly moves lateral to the cecum, in a cranial to caudal direction, and rests at the sternum. Displacement may be accompanied by a variable degree of volvulus.
- Left dorsal displacement of the colon is a displacement of the left colon to a position between the dorsal body wall and the nephrosplenic (renosplenic) ligament (Fig. 18-61). The large colon is hypothesized to pass through the nephrosplenic space from a cranial to caudal direction or migrates dorsally, lateral to the spleen.

Diagnosis
Clinical Signs
- Signs include abdominal pain and abdominal distention, the severity of which depends on the duration and amount of colonic tympany. The signs generally develop rapidly and are more severe than with impaction because of tension on the mesentery and greater colonic tympany.
- The displacement may occasionally place pressure on the duodenum and cause nasogastric reflux.
- Peritoneal fluid usually is normal in the early stages of displacement; with chronic displacement, the amount of peritoneal fluid, total protein, and nucleated cell count may be increased.
- Right dorsal displacement is characterized on rectal palpation by mild to severe gas distention of the cecum, colon, or both, with large colon taeniae palpable lateral to the cecum or horizontally crossing the pelvic inlet (see Fig. 18-49).
- *Practice Tip: Gamma-glutamyltransferase and direct bilirubin may be greatly increased with right dorsal displacement because of biliary obstruction. For other gastrointestinal (GI) displacements to cause these changes is unusual.*

- Ultrasound examination of the mid to lower right abdomen in horses with right dorsal displacement may reveal distended vessels within the displaced and rotated right colon (see Chapter 14, p. 86).
- Left dorsal displacement is characterized on rectal palpation by mild to severe gas distention of the cecum, colon, or both, with palpable large-colon taeniae coursing cranially and to the left, dorsal to the nephrosplenic ligament.
- Signs of pain are elicited when the nephrosplenic area is palpated per rectum and the spleen is displaced caudally, away from the left body wall because of tension on the ligament.
- Ultrasound examination of the upper left abdomen in horses with left dorsal displacement reveals colonic gas such that the left kidney and dorsal edge of the spleen *cannot* be visualized. If the colon is rotated slightly, mesenteric vessels may be seen (see Chapter 14, p. 87).
- Several loops of moderately distended small intestine may be palpable if the small intestine is involved secondarily.
- Decompression of the stomach and cecum provides temporary pain relief.

Prevention of Reccurence
Surgical prophylactic procedures are recommended in horses with recurrent left dorsal displacement (two or more occurrences):
- Colopexy or partial resection of the large colon at the time of the initial celiotomy
- Standing laparoscopic ablation of the nephrosplenic space with suture or mesh at a subsequent surgery

Prognosis
Prognosis is good to excellent for complete recovery. The incidence of adhesions and laminitis with large colon displacement is low.

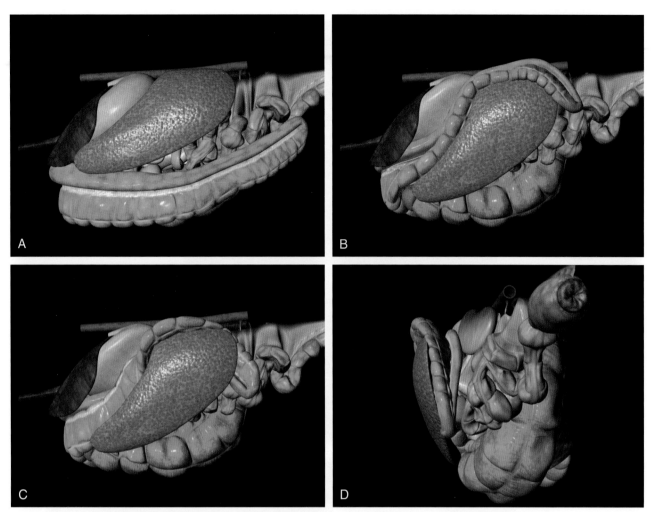

Figure 18-61   A, View from the left side of the horse with the ascending colon in its normal position. **B,** Displacement of the ascending colon over the dorsal edge of the spleen, with rotation of the colon on its long axis. **C,** A final stage in displacement of the colon over the nephrosplenic ligament. Weight of the displaced colon borne by the ligament impedes venous blood flow from the spleen, thereby causing the spleen to engorge. **D,** Caudal view of the final stage of the displacement, with the colon entrapped over the nephrosplenic ligament and engorgement of the spleen.

⬤⟩ WHAT TO DO

Large Colon Displacement

Right Dorsal Displacement
- If abdominal pain is *not* severe, withhold feed and administer, to an adult horse, 6 L q4h of electrolyte solution by nasogastric tube; correction may occur in 24 to 36 hours.
- Ventral midline exploratory celiotomy if surgical exploration is indicated (see Box 18-2).
- Examine the colon for volvulus and correction of the displacement.
- Enterotomy is not always necessary and is at the surgeon's discretion. If the colon is secondarily impacted, an enterotomy is recommended.

Left Dorsal Displacement: Nonsurgical Correction
- The two most common nonsurgical methods are oral fluids and withholding feed as described earlier or to administer phenylephrine (8 to 16 mg/450 kg in 1 L of 0.9% sodium chloride slowly IV over 15 minutes):

- To contract the spleen
- Follow the phenylephrine with light exercise for 5 to 10 minutes
- Repeat a rectal examination
- Repeat ultrasound examination to confirm the abnormality is corrected.
- **Practice Tip:** *Do not use the phenylephrine treatment protocol for severely volume-depleted patients, those with cardiovascular instability, or horses more than 16 years of age.* Significant pressor effect and reflex bradycardia may cause severe hypoperfusion in severely dehydrated horses. In aged horses, phenylephrine administration may result in significant internal hemorrhaging.
- If unsuccessful, the phenylephrine treatment may be repeated several times and is reported to have a success rate of 70% to 90% in patients with a stable cardiovascular system and without severe colonic distention or devitalization.
- Proper rolling procedure (Fig. 18-62):
  - Administer general anesthesia with the patient positioned in right lateral recumbency.

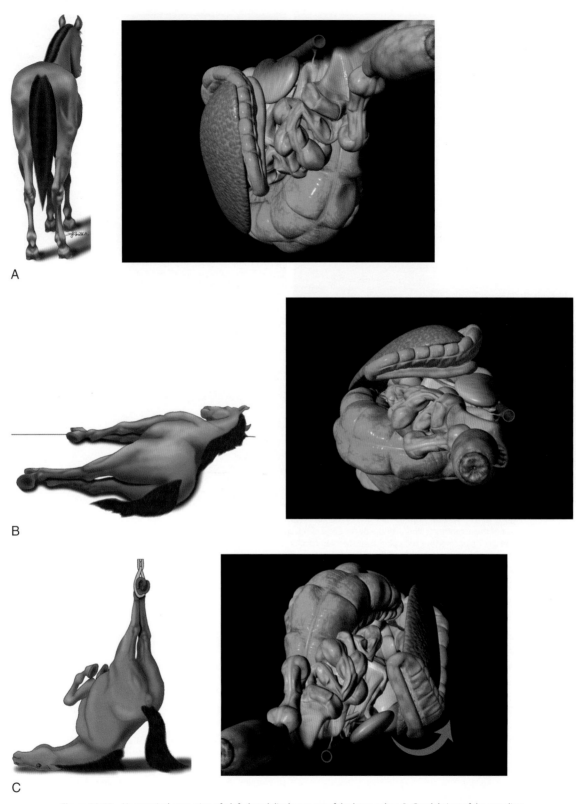

Figure 18-62   Nonsurgical correction of a left dorsal displacement of the large colon. **A,** Caudal view of the standing horse with the left ventral and dorsal colons entrapped over the nephrosplenic ligament. **B,** The patient is anesthetized and placed in right lateral recumbency. **C,** Hobbles are placed on the pelvic limbs, and the patient is positioned in dorsal recumbency; the pelvic limbs are lifted to raise the hind end off the ground; the large colon falls cranially, lateral, and to the right *(arrow)*.

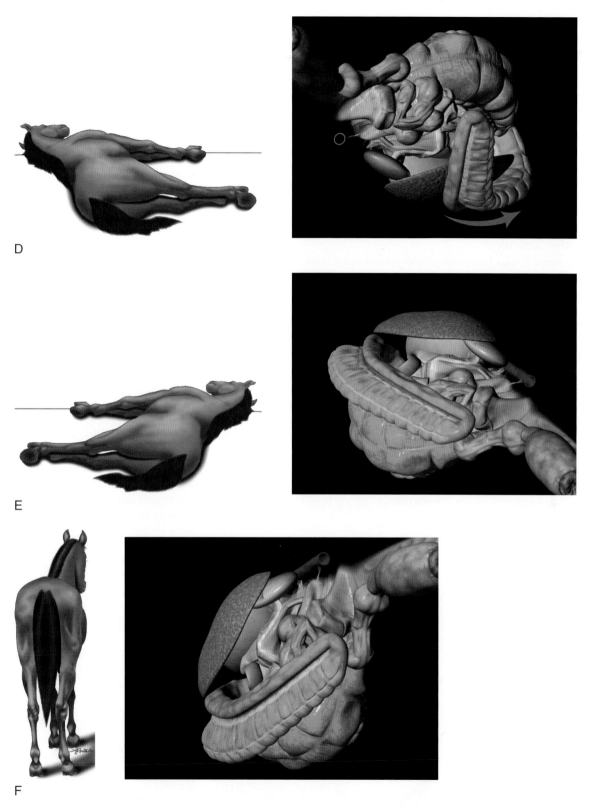

Figure 18-62, cont'd   D, The patient is then positioned in left lateral recumbency; this allows the colon to continue to fall ventral and lateral to the spleen *(arrow).* **E,** The 360-degree rotation is then completed by rolling the patient into sternal recumbency (not shown) and then back to right lateral recumbency, with the colon coming to rest in a position medial to the spleen. **F,** The patient is allowed to recover; if the procedure is successful, the colon assumes a position ventral and medial to the spleen. Rectal palpation is performed to assess the position of the colon.

GI:COLIC

- Place hobbles on the pelvic limbs, and position the patient in dorsal recumbency.
- Lift the pelvic limbs to raise the hind end of the patient off the ground; vigorously perform ballottement of the abdomen.
- The large colon falls cranially and to the right.
- The 360 rotation is completed by rolling the patient into sternal recumbency and then back to right lateral recumbency.
- When in right lateral recumbency, the colon should rest in a position medial and ventral to the spleen. Allow the horse to recover.
- Rectal palpation is performed to assess the position of the colon with the patient in lateral recumbency or after recovery.

Large Colon Volvulus

- Large colon volvulus is rotation of the ventral and dorsal colons on their long axes and frequently includes the cecum.
- Viewing the left ventral and dorsal colon from behind, or with the horse in dorsal recumbency, the colons usually twist in a counterclockwise direction (Fig. 18-63).
- The large colon and cecum can rotate on the vertical axis of the mesentery (volvulus).
- Rotation of 360 degrees causes the colon to lie in an apparently normal position with the mesenteric root occluded.
- ***Practice Tip:*** *Large colon volvulus is one of the most severe acute abdominal emergencies in horses.*
- The cause is unknown, but hypomotility caused by dietary changes, electrolyte imbalances, and stress can predispose the colon to excessive gas accumulation and volvulus.
- A higher incidence of colonic volvulus occurs among periparturient mares.

Potential Complications of Nonsurgical Correction (Rolling)
- Worsening or recurrence of displacement
- Iatrogenic colonic or cecal volvulus, splenic vessel rupture, and internal hemorrhage
- Cecal or colonic rupture

Left Dorsal Displacement
Surgical correction is performed in the following cases:
- Marked colonic distention with persistent and severe pain
- Evidence of intestinal devitalization is found during peritoneal fluid analysis.
- Increased risk is present for colonic or cecal rupture and the resulting fatal peritonitis.

- Large colon volvulus recurs in 20% to 30% of corrected cases.

Diagnosis
- Colonic volvulus (>180 degrees) causes an acute onset of severe abdominal distention and continuous abdominal pain only mildly responsive to or refractory to analgesic therapy. Xylazine or detomidine alone or in combination with butorphanol provides transient pain relief.
- Tachycardia, tachypnea, and blanched or congested mucous membranes are usually clinically evident.
- Respiratory acidosis can develop if colonic distention impairs normal respiratory function.
- Serosanguineous peritoneal fluid with an increased total protein concentration and nucleated cell count reflect the presence of intestinal ischemia and necrosis.
- Rectal palpation reveals severe colonic distention, frequently accompanied by mural and mesenteric edema

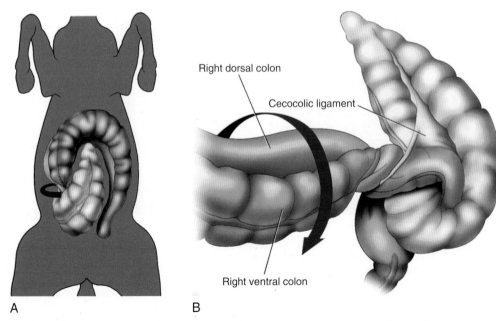

Right dorsal colon

Cecocolic ligament

Right ventral colon

A   B

Figure 18-63   Large colon volvulus. **A,** Ventral view of a horse in dorsal recumbency with a 360-degree *counter-clockwise (arrow)* volvulus of the large colon. **B,** Right lateral view of a horse in dorsal recumbency with 180-degree counterclockwise *(arrow)* volvulus of the large colon.

resulting from venous congestion. Taeniae traversing the abdomen may be palpable, but a comprehensive rectal examination is frequently impossible because of the considerable colonic distention and degree of pain.

- Rotations (twists) between 180 degrees and 270 degrees may manifest as moderate pain only and slow deterioration.

Large Colon Volvulus
- Successful treatment requires early diagnosis and emergency surgical correction.
- Ventral midline exploratory celiotomy is performed.
- Decompression and enterotomy often are necessary to facilitate correction.
- Affected colon typically appears bluish gray initially and becomes red to black after reperfusion.
- Nonviable colon requires resection or humane destruction of the horse.
- Up to 95% of the ascending colon may be resected without adversely affecting colonic function.
- Plasma, DMSO, and heparin may be useful in attenuating "reperfusion injury."

Prevention of Recurrence
- In brood mares or nonperformance horses, colopexy, or suturing the lateral taenia of the left ventral colon to the abdominal wall, is performed by some surgeons to reduce the risk of recurrence.
- Tearing of the adhesion, suture failure, and colonic rupture are reported complications of this procedure.
- *Practice Tip: Elective colonic resection is performed to minimize the likelihood of recurrence; this procedure is preferred for performance athletes.*

Prognosis
- Prognosis depends on early diagnosis and surgical intervention.
- Intestinal ischemia and necrosis rapidly progress to hypovolemia, endotoxemia, peritonitis, and irreversible shock.
- The prognosis is poor unless surgery is performed within a few hours of the onset of clinical signs.
- In some patients, postoperative absorptive dysfunction, diarrhea, and protein-losing enteropathy occur and may be short-lived or permanent.

Atresia Coli
- Atresia coli is congenital absence or closure of a portion of the intestine. It manifests in three forms:
  - Membrane atresia: A tissue diaphragm occludes the lumen of the colon or rectum.
  - Cord atresia: A fibrous cord connects the noncommunicating ends of the colon.
  - Blind-end atresia: The most common type; there is *no* connection or mesentery between noncommunicating ends of colon.

- Atresia coli results from ischemia of the affected segment during development; the condition is believed to be hereditary.
- Lethal white foal disease is an autosomal recessive pigmentary disorder in which newborn paint foals have albinism coupled with congenital defects of the intestinal tract, most commonly atresia coli. These defects are *not* compatible with life.

Diagnosis
- Abdominal pain in the newborn during the first 12 to 24 hours of life and lack of meconium stool are the first signs.
- Digital palpation of the rectum reveals mucus and no meconium.
- Abdominal radiography may reveal an enlarged segment of colon with no obvious obstruction; contrast radiography is needed to confirm the diagnosis.
- Abdominal distention and pain are indications for surgical exploration.
- Meconium impaction is the primary condition to rule out (see Disorders of the Small Colon and Rectum, in the following section).

Atresia Coli
- Surgical correction is the only treatment.
- Ventral midline exploratory celiotomy is performed.
- The distance and size disparity between the affected bowel segments make anastomosis difficult.
- The aboral segment often is too small for end-to-end anastomosis. Side-to-side anastomosis may be needed but often is *not* possible because of the excessive distance between the proximal and distal intestinal segments; therefore, euthanasia is recommended.

Prognosis
Prognosis is guarded because of the difficult technical aspects of performing the anastomosis in this part of the intestine.

Nonstrangulating Infarction
See Disorders of the Small Intestine, p. 191.

Ulcerative Colitis (NSAID Toxicity)
See p. 232 and Appendix 6, p. 823.

Disorders of the Small Colon and Rectum
Small Colon Impaction and Foreign Body Obstruction
- Inflammatory bowel disease frequently predisposes the colon, especially the small colon, to impaction and may be associated with positive fecal cultures for *Salmonella* organisms. In many cases, a predisposing factor is never identified.
- Dehydration of fecal matter can cause impaction of the small colon, and a foreign body or an enterolith (see Enterolithiasis, p. 212) can cause an obstruction.

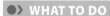

- Complete obstruction causes severe abdominal pain; tympany and secondary ileus of the proximal small and large colons result from the obstruction.

Diagnosis

- The diagnosis is confirmed on rectal examination with palpation of the impaction or gas-distended loops of small colon. The small colon is identified on rectal examination by its characteristic single, wideband on the antimesenteric surface and ropelike mesenteric band.
- Foreignbody impaction occurs more commonly among horses younger than 4 years of age because they are curious. For example, they eat portions of hay nets, rubber fencing, bits of rope, and string.
- Impaction is sometimes accompanied by inflammatory bowel disease, such as salmonellosis.
- If impactions are recurring, myenteric ganglionitis should be considered.
- ***Practice Tip:*** *Small colon impaction is common among miniature horses and is generally* not *associated with an inflammatory/infectious disease.*

●⟩ WHAT TO DO

Small Colon Impaction and Foreign Body Obstruction

Medical Management

- Analgesics
- Large volumes of balanced, polyionic intravenous fluid
- 6 to 8 L of water or magnesium sulfate in water q2h through an indwelling nasogastric tube if *no* gastric reflux is recovered
- Warm water enemas or gravity administered (by soft tube) electrolyte solution to soften the fecal material
- Misoprostil (2.5 to 5 μg/kg PO, q12-24h) has been used to increase perfusion to the bowel and fluid secretion into the colon in cases where surgery is *not* an option. Do *not* administer to pregnant mares; pregnant women should not handle the drug.
- ***Caution:*** Use extreme care to prevent rectal perforation during administration of enemas.

Surgical Management

- Needed with unrelenting pain, severe gas distention, or failure of medical treatment
- Perform a ventral midline exploratory celiotomy.
- Use enemas and extraluminal massage of the small colon to break down the impaction.
- Perform an enterotomy to remove a foreign body or enterolith.
- Perform pelvic flexure enterotomy and evacuation of large colon ingesta
- Patients with small colon impaction frequently have culture results positive for *Salmonella* organisms. The condition of these horses can become endotoxic with secondary laminitis, peritonitis, and adhesions. The role of *Salmonella* infection in the development of the impaction is unknown.

Prognosis

- Prognosis is fair to good for patients with foreign body obstruction or simple impaction of the small colon.
- Prognosis is guarded if the culture result for *Salmonella* organisms is positive.

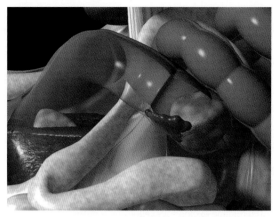

Figure 18-64 Obstruction of the descending colon by a polyhedral-shaped enterolith. Note the presence of an additional enterolith in the lumen of the right dorsal colon. The wall of the colon has been rendered transparent to facilitate visualization of the enteroliths.

- Rectal examination of horses with small colon impaction presents greater risk of iatrogenic perforation.

Enterolithiasis

- Enteroliths are concretions of magnesium and ammonium phosphate crystals deposited around a nidus, frequently a piece of wire, stone, or nail.
- There may be one or multiple concretions, and they do *not* cause a surgical problem until they become lodged in the transverse or small colon (Fig. 18-64).
- The specific geographic distribution of the condition—California, Florida, Indiana—has led to speculation that undetermined constituents of the soil and water in these areas may be inciting causes.
- ***Practice Tip:*** *Enterolithiasis is seen most commonly in middle-aged horses (5 to 10 years of age), and the condition is overrepresented in Arabians and miniature horses.*

Diagnosis

- Affected horses may have a history of chronic weight loss and recurring acute bouts of mild to moderate abdominal pain or acute, severe abdominal distention and pain with *no* history of colic.
- The obstruction most commonly is at the proximal small colon or transverse colon. Smaller enteroliths can be located distally in the small colon. When the obstruction is complete, pain is severe, and distention of the colon is considerable.
- With complete obstruction, heart and respiratory rates are increased, and mucous membranes are pink.
- Rectal examination reveals colonic and cecal distention.
- Peritoneal fluid is generally normal unless the wall of the colon is compromised.
- Abdominal radiography may confirm the diagnosis of enterolithiasis, but in the field, imaging can be performed only on miniature horses.
- Patients with chronic enterolithiasis often have concurrent gastric ulcers, which can confound the diagnosis.

●〉 WHAT TO DO

Enterolithiasis

- Perform ventral midline exploratory celiotomy.
- Decompress the distended colon and cecum.
- Remove small, freely movable enteroliths through a pelvic flexure enterotomy.
- Remove large enteroliths in the transverse colon and proximal small colon through a large colon enterotomy at the diaphragmatic flexure.
- ***Practice Tip:*** *If an enterolith has a polyhedral shape, multiple enteroliths are present.*

Prognosis

Prognosis is good; the survival rate is 65% to 90%.

Meconium Impaction

- A common cause of acute pain in newborn foals is retention of meconium in the small colon and rectum.
- Impaction occurs more frequently in males, weak newborns after a dystocia, and foals born at more than 340 days of gestation.

Clinical Signs

- Acute abdominal pain during the first 24 hours after foaling
- Tachycardia
- Repeated attempts to defecate
- Rolling
- Abnormal stance (back arched dorsally)
- Swishing the tail
- Abdominal tympany if obstruction of the small colon is complete (Fig. 18-65)
- The foal appears transiently normal for short periods and nurses. The diagnosis often is confirmed with digital palpation of meconium impaction in the distal small colon and rectum.
- The impaction may be seen on either radiographs or abdominal ultrasound in many cases.

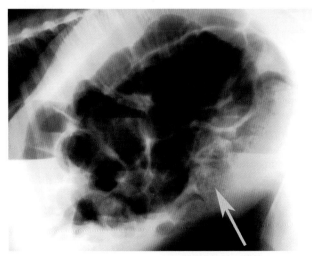

Figure 18-65 Radiograph demonstrates the abdomen of a 2-day-old foal with meconium impaction of the colon causing severe gas distention *(arrow)*. Surgery was needed to correct the problem.

Diagnosis

- Repeated attempts to defecate without producing stool
- Digital palpation of the meconium impaction
- Radiographic or ultrasound confirmation

●〉 WHAT TO DO

Meconium Impaction

- Enemas with warm, soapy water (500 to 1000 mL) delivered by means of gravity flow through a soft rubber tube. Fleet enemas may also be used (4 ounces) but are more irritating and, with repeated use, may cause hyperphosphatemia.
- Acetylcysteine enema—the foal must be adequately sedated with valium (5 to 10 mg IV/50-kg foal). A soft Foley catheter is inserted 2 to 3 inches inside the rectum and the balloon distended with 30 mL of air. One hundred to 200 mL of a 4% acetylcysteine solution is slowly infused without pressure into the rectum through the Foley catheter and left in place for 30 minutes before the balloon is deflated and the catheter is removed.
- N-butylscopolammonium bromide can be used in the enema (0.3 mg/kg) or intravenously (0.2 mg/kg) to relax the bowel.
- Administer intravenous, balanced polyionic fluids.
- Administer mineral oil by nasogastric tube.
- Administer sedatives as needed.
- Perform ventral midline exploratory celiotomy for refractory patients and for those with proximal impaction, accompanied by enemas and extraluminal massage of the affected colon.
- Small colon enterotomy rarely is necessary.
- ***Important Note:*** Repeated enemas or enemas with caustic solutions result in rectal edema and irritation and a syndrome that mimics meconium impaction. Foals receiving several enemas often become very toxic because of injury of the rectal mucosa.

Prognosis

Prognosis is excellent.

Mesocolic Rupture

- Mesocolic rupture affects mares during parturition and results in tearing of the mesentery of the small colon (Fig. 18-66).
- The condition is a complication of prolapse of the rectum and may be accompanied by prolapse of the bladder, uterus, vagina, small intestine, or a combination of these organs.

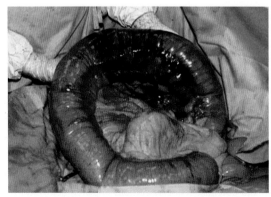

Figure 18-66 Intraoperative photograph demonstrating a rupture of the small colon mesentery in a mare after a severe rectal prolapse during foaling.

- Multiparous mares older than 11 years of age are at greatest risk.
- Clinical signs of abdominal pain develop during the first 24 hours postpartum and are complicated by intraabdominal bleeding and peritonitis.
- The mare's clinical condition deteriorates rapidly if the blood supply to the small colon is compromised or the intestine is entrapped in the mesocolic rent.
- Rectal examination reveals impaction or tympany of the small colon.

●> WHAT TO DO

Mesocolic Rupture
- Perform ventral midline exploratory celiotomy.
- Perform resection and anastomosis of the affected small colon.
- A colostomy will be necessary if the tear involves the mesorectum.

Prognosis

Prognosis is poor because of ischemia of the small colon, difficult surgical exposure, and complications associated with the colostomy, such as prolapse of the proximal small colon through the colostomy stoma and adhesions.

Rectal Tear

- **Practice Tip:** *A complication of performing a rectal examination is the risk of a rectal tear.*
- The incidence is highest among young, nervous, anxious equine patients; older horses with a weakened or edematous rectal wall, such as those with small-colon impactions; and patients that strain during rectal examination.
- The incidence is higher among Arabians than it is among other breeds, presumably because of the smaller size of Arabians.
- Stallions and geldings are at greater risk than are mares. The tears most often occur at the 10 to 12 o'clock position 25 to 30 cm from the anus.
- The tear is most often longitudinal and is hypothesized to occur where blood vessels penetrate the intestinal wall.

- Spontaneous tears or impaction of a segment of the rectum can occur.
- Rectal tears are classified as follows:
  - *Grade I:* Mucosa or submucosa
  - *Grade II:* Muscular layer only
  - *Grade III:* Mucosa, submucosa, and muscular layers without serosal penetration (3a), including mesorectum (3b)
  - *Grade IV:* Tears involving all layers and extending into the peritoneal cavity
- ***Important Note:*** Grades III and IV are life-threatening, with cellulitis, abscessation, and acute septic peritonitis as sequelae. The diagnosis is confirmed with careful examination of the tear after the patient is sedated and the rectum evacuated. Intraluminally administered lidocaine gel or epidural anesthesia facilitates rectal examination.

Clinical Signs

- Blood on rectal sleeve up on withdrawal of the examining arm
- Sudden relaxation of the rectum while the horse is straining
- Hemorrhagic feces or straining to defecate
- Idiopathic tears—immediate clinical signs may *not* be apparent. Signs of abdominal pain, endotoxemia, and depression may develop within 2 to 3 hours after rectal examination.

Diagnosis

- Confirmation of a suspected rectal tear is based on the clinical signs.
- Careful examination of the rectum under sedation or epidural anesthesia
- Endoscopic (proctoscopy) of the rectum if physical examination does not confirm diagnosis (use sedation or epidural anesthesia)
- Immediate referral to a surgical facility for follow-up diagnostic procedures

●> WHAT TO DO

Rectal Tear
- Immediately begin administration of broad-spectrum antimicrobial agents.
- Include metronidazole, 15 to 20 mg/kg PO q8hr, or suppository q6h for anaerobes.
- Provide intravenous, balanced polyionic fluids.
- Administer NSAIDs.
- Adequately restrain and sedate the horse, administer N-butylscopolamine bromide (Buscopan, 0.3 mg/kg IV) and 50 mL of 2% lidocaine in 120 mL of lube per rectum. With a well lubricated bare arm, determine the location (distance cranial to the anus) and severity of the tear.
- Gently evacuate feces from the rectum and tear.
- Inform the owner about the possible occurrence of a rectal tear and the potential sequelae without implying admission of guilt or wrongdoing

Grade I Tears
- These tears are managed conservatively unless the tear can be sutured easily with 2-0 or 0 polydioxanone (PDS, Ethicon) in a simple continuous pattern.
- These tears heal with minimal or *no* complications.

Grade II Tears
- Because of the lack of frank blood in the lumen of the rectum, grade II tears frequently are *not* diagnosed at the time of injury.
- These tears are identified weeks later when a perirectal fistula or abscess develops.

Grade III or IV Tears
- Administer Buscopan to reduce peristalsis.
- Administer epidural anesthesia (xylazine, 0.17 mg/kg in 6 mL saline) to minimize straining.
- Pack the rectal lumen from the anus to cranial to the tear (moistened rolled cotton or gauze packing suitable).

GI:COLIC

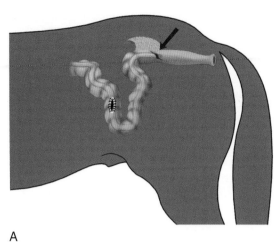 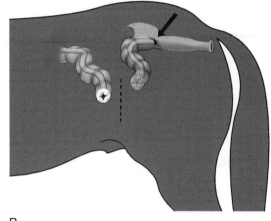

A   B

Figure 18-67 Colostomy technique. **A,** Loop colostomy. **B,** Diverting colostomy positioned in the left flank. *Arrows* indicate the location of the rectal tear. Loop colostomy is performed at the initial flank incision. The diverting colostomy is performed in a separate incision, cranial to the initial flank incision *(dotted line)*.

- Transport to a surgical referral facility for primary suture repair and/or a diverting colostomy.
- A rectal liner[16] or primary surgical repair of the tear is used in the management of grade III lacerations to bypass the site of injury and potentially avoid the need for a colostomy.
- A colostomy may be performed to divert feces from the site and prevent peritoneal contamination.
- ***Important Note:*** Grade IV tears often necessitate a colostomy. For most grade III tears, a colostomy is recommended (Fig. 18-67).
- Loop colostomy is performed with the patient under general anesthesia or under sedation and local anesthesia. The colostomy exits through the left flank (Fig. 18-67, *A*).

- An alternative is to oversew the proximal end of the distal small colon; the distal end of the proximal small colon exits from the flank as a diverting colostomy (Fig. 18-67, *B*).
- If the patient is placed under general anesthesia, large colon enterotomy is performed to reduce fecal bulk exiting from the colostomy.
- A rectal liner[16] or primary surgical repair of the tear is used in the management of grade III tears to bypass the tear and potentially avoid the need for a colostomy.
- Grades III and IV tears heal by secondary intention; the loop colostomy is reversed after the tear heals.

Prognosis
- Prognosis is excellent for grades I and II rectal tears.
- Prognosis is guarded for grade III tears.
- Prognosis is guarded to poor for grade IV tears.

Rectal Prolapse
- Rectal prolapse is caused by straining because of constipation, obstipation, dystocia, colitis, urethral obstruction, or foreign body impaction of the distal small colon or rectum.
- In some cases *no* known predisposing cause can be identified.
- The condition occurs more commonly in mares and is classified according to severity as follows:
  - Type I prolapse involves only the rectal mucosa and submucosa and appears as a large circular anal swelling.
  - Type II involves the entire rectal wall and is called "complete" prolapse; the ventral portion of prolapsed tissue is thicker than the dorsal portion.
  - Type III includes invaginated peritoneal rectum or small colon and is difficult to differentiate from type II prolapse.

- Type IV involves intussuscepted peritoneal rectum or small colon beyond the anus. A palpable invagination adjacent to the intussuscepted intestine differentiates type IV from type III prolapse.

Important Note: Internal rupture of the small colon mesentery should be suspected in type IV rectal prolapse involving greater than 30 cm of rectum (see Mesocolic Rupture, p. 213).

●› WHAT TO DO

Rectal Prolapse
Type I or Type II Prolapse
- Identify and correct underlying cause of prolapse if possible.
- Reduce the edema in the tissues with topical application of glycerin or dextrose and apply petroleum jelly (Vaseline).
- Reduce the prolapse under epidural anesthesia. An indwelling epidural catheter may be needed.
- Tranquilize the patient unless contraindicated.
- Administer Buscopan
- Place a purse-string suture in the anus.
- Administer stool softeners, such as mineral oil.
- Perform submucosal resection if medical treatment is unsuccessful.

---

[16]Rectal Ring (Regal Plastic Co., Detroit Lakes, Minnesota).

Type III or IV Prolapse
- Perform celiotomy to reduce the intussusception.
- Perform colostomy for type IV prolapse if the blood supply to the affected bowel is compromised.

Prognosis
- Prognosis is good for types I and II prolapse.
- Prognosis is guarded to poor for types III and IV.

Colic in the Late-Term Pregnant Mare
- Colic in a mare during the last trimester of pregnancy often is a diagnostic challenge.
- GI disorders must be ruled out with careful clinical examination, but the large, gravid uterus often prevents a complete rectal examination.
- The effect of the colic episode on the fetus is always of concern because abortion can result in substantial emotional and financial loss.
- The overall postcolic abortion rate among mares is between 16% and 18%.
- Endotoxemia and intraoperative *hypoxia* or *hypotension* during colic surgery in the last 60 days of gestation have been associated with a higher incidence of abortion.
- Causes of colic in late-term pregnant mares *not* associated with the GI tract include the following:
  - Abortion and premature parturition
  - Uterine torsion
  - Hydrallantois
  - Ruptured prepubic tendon
  - Uterine artery bleed

●〉 WHAT TO DO

Colic in the Late-Term Pregnant Mare
- Pregnant mares with colic and endotoxemia during the first 2 months of pregnancy may benefit from treatment with progestin supplementation, altrenogest (22 to 44 mg PO q24h for a 450-kg adult) or injectable progesterone (150 to 300 mg/450 kg IM q24h) for 100 to 200 days of pregnancy. Although the benefit of this treatment in late pregnancy is not evidence based, it is generally used.
- Administration of NSAIDs may alleviate the adverse effects of endotoxemia in pregnancy.
- Glucose should be administered to late pregnant mares recovering from colic or surgery.

Abortion and Premature Parturition
- Mares may have signs of mild to moderate abdominal pain and minimal udder development. Vaginal examination reveals loss of the cervical plug and relaxation of the cervix.
- This finding alone does *not* indicate impending abortion because similar findings occur in many normal mares days or weeks before delivery.
- Rectal examination often reveals the fetus to be positioned within the birth canal.

●〉 WHAT TO DO

Abortion and Premature Parturition
- Treatment is supportive and is directed at an uncomplicated delivery and postpartum care of the mare.
- Postmortem examination of the aborted fetus and placenta may determine the cause of the abortion, such as equine herpesvirus 1 (see Abortion Evaluation, Chapter 24, p. 433). The mare should be isolated until the results of the examination are available.

Uterine Torsion
- Uterine torsion can be a cause of colic in late-term pregnant mares.
- Uterine torsion usually occurs between 8 months of gestation and term, but rarely at term.
- Unlike the case in cows, in which the torsion most often is diagnosed at term, mares affected usually are *not* in labor when clinical signs are first evident.
- Also unlike the disorder in cows, torsion in mares is usually cranial to the cervix and vagina, thereby minimizing the benefit of a vaginal examination in making the diagnosis.
- The degree of torsion ranges from 180 to 540 degrees and occurs in either direction with equal frequency.
- Uterine rupture can occur as the result of torsion but is an uncommon complication.

Diagnosis
- Mild to moderate intermittent abdominal pain is the most consistent sign; however, some mares may demonstrate severe, unrelenting pain.
- A mild increase in heart and respiratory rates also may be present.
- Diagnosis is made with the signalment, history, and findings on rectal examination.
- Rectal palpation of the broad ligaments reveals the ligaments to be tight as they cross the caudal abdomen below and above the cervix.
- Palpation of the dorsal-most ligament, and occasionally the body of the uterus, indicates the direction of the torsion (Fig. 18-68, *A*).
- In clockwise torsion, as viewed from behind, the left broad ligament is pulled tight over the uterus and courses to the right in a horizontal to oblique direction (Fig. 18-68, *B*). The right broad ligament is pulled ventrally and diagonally to the left, and because of its more ventral and caudal position in the abdomen, may be the easier of the two ligaments to identify during rectal palpation.
- In counterclockwise torsion, the opposite is true (Fig. 18-68, *C*).

●〉 WHAT TO DO

Uterine Torsion
- Early recognition and intervention are imperative for a successful outcome for the mare and the foal.
- The optimal method of correction depends on the condition of the mare and fetus and the stage of gestation.

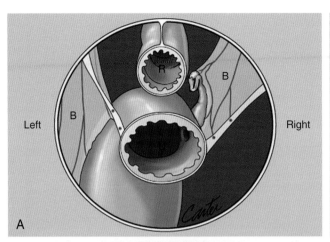

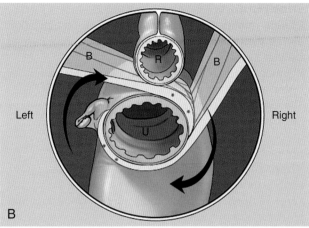

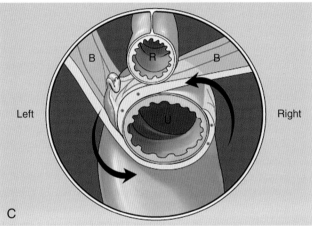

Figure 18-68 **A,** Normal orientation of uterus and broad ligament. **B,** Clockwise uterine torsion. **C,** Counterclockwise uterine torsion. (Art by Kip Carter [The University of Georgia], © University of Georgia Research Foundation, Inc. Used under license.)

Nonsurgical Correction: Rolling
See Chapter 24, Fig. 24-10.

Surgical Correction (Preferred)
Flank Celiotomy
- Flank celiotomy provides the least stress for the foal and mare, and it can be performed during any stage of gestation.
- The procedure is performed with the standing mare under sedation (xylazine or detomidine with or without butorphanol) and local anesthetic infiltration along the proposed incision site.
- Controversy exists as to the preferred side of entry relative to the direction of the torsion. Many surgeons prefer to enter the abdomen from the side to which the torsion is directed (e.g., right flank for clockwise torsion).
- If the abdomen is entered from the side to which the torsion is directed (e.g., right flank for clockwise torsion), the surgeon's hand is passed ventrally to the uterus, and the uterus is lifted and rotated upward to correct the torsion.
- If the abdomen is entered on the side opposite that to which the torsion is directed (e.g., left flank for clockwise torsion), the surgeon's hand passes dorsally to the uterus, and the uterus is pulled toward the surgeon to correct the torsion.
- Alternatively, in late-term pregnancies, a left and right flank incision may be made simultaneously with two surgeons to facilitate reduction.
- Correction can be facilitated by means of grasping the limbs of the fetus through the wall of the uterus and gently "rocking" the uterus to gain enough momentum for complete rotation and final correction.

Ventral Midline Celiotomy
- Ventral midline celiotomy provides the best exposure for assessment and manipulation of the gravid uterus.
- Indications for ventral midline celiotomy include uterine rupture, uterine tearing, and uterine devitalization.
- This approach also allows identification and correction of concurrent intestinal disorders.
- The procedure can be performed during any stage of gestation.
- Standard ventral midline celiotomy is performed.
- If hysterotomy is indicated, the ventral midline approach provides the best surgical exposure.
- Ventral midline celiotomy should be reserved for cases *not* amenable to nonsurgical correction or flank celiotomy because of the associated risks of general anesthesia to the mare and foal.

Prognosis
- Prognosis is good to excellent for complete recovery and future breeding soundness of the mare with uterine torsion.
- Fetal viability depends on the duration and degree of torsion.
- The abortion rate after uterine torsion is reported to be between 30% and 40%.
- Prognosis for both the mare and foal is more favorable if uterine torsion occurs before the last 30 days of gestation.

Uterine Rupture

- Uterine rupture can be a complication of manipulation during dystocia or can occur during apparently normal foaling.
- Rupture also can be a sequela to uterine torsion or hydrallantois.
- The tear usually occurs at the dorsal aspect of the uterus (see Chapter 24, p. 444).

Diagnosis

- Suspect uterine rupture in any mare demonstrating post-partum abdominal pain.
- Large ruptures may result in significant blood loss and produce signs of hemorrhagic shock.
- Diagnosis is confirmed on vaginal and uterine examination.

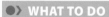

➧ WHAT TO DO

Uterine Rupture

- If a uterine tear is suspected, irrigating solutions should *not* be infused into the uterus.
- Administer the following:
  - Broad-spectrum antimicrobial agents
  - Balanced, polyionic intravenous fluids
  - Plasma or synthetic colloids
  - NSAIDs
  - Peritoneal drainage
- Allow small tears to heal by secondary intention.
- Close large tears primarily; general anesthesia and ventral midline celiotomy may be necessary.
- Cervical tears may be repaired under standing epidural anesthesia.

Prognosis

- Prognosis depends on the size of the tear, duration before recognition and treatment, degree of peritoneal contamination, and nature of the intrauterine contents.
- Prognosis is good for small tears recognized early and poor for large tears with an emphysematous fetus and gross peritoneal contamination.

Hydrallantois

See Chapter 24, p. 436.

Ruptured Prepubic Tendon

- The prepubic tendon is a strong, thick, fibrous structure that attaches to the cranial border of the pelvis and provides attachment for the rectus abdominis, oblique abdominis, gracilis, and pectineus muscles.
- The tendon forms the medial borders of the external inguinal rings.
- Hydrallantois, twins, or fetal giants may predispose to prepubic tendon rupture.

Diagnosis

- Prepubic tendon rupture must be differentiated from ventral hernia, which also occurs most frequently in late-term pregnant mares.

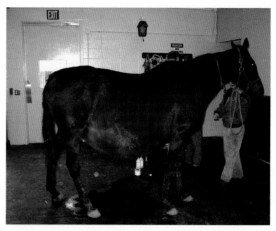

Figure 18-69 Photograph demonstrating a prepubic tendon rupture in a horse. (Courtesy Dr. Stefan Witte.)

- Ventral hernia may respond favorably to surgical repair; however, the prognosis for prepubic tendon rupture is poor.

Clinical Signs

- Severe, progressive, ventral abdominal swelling and edema with the pelvis tilted cranially and ventrally (Fig. 18-69). The mammary gland also assumes a more cranioventral position.
- *Practice Tip: Mild to moderate abdominal pain usually is apparent, and the mare is reluctant to walk. In contrast, mares with a ventral hernia are not reluctant to walk, and the pelvis and mammary gland are in a normal position.*
- Identification of the defect by means of external palpation may be difficult because of excessive edema formation.
- Rectal examination and ultrasonography are helpful in differentiating prepubic tendon rupture from ventral herniation.

➧ WHAT TO DO

Ruptured Prepubic Tendon

- In mares near term, early induction of parturition and assisted foaling may be required. For pregnancy >315 days, give 100 mg of dexamethasone daily for 3 days to "speed" maturation of the foal.
- Exploratory celiotomy and cesarean section should be performed immediately on mares that demonstrate intractable pain or systemic deterioration or in which a concurrent incarcerating intestinal lesion is suspected.
- Stabilized mares should be confined to stall rest, placed in abdominal support bandages, and administered NSAIDs.
- Low-bulk, pelleted feed should be fed to decrease the volume of ingesta.
- These mares may foal normally; however, they should be observed closely and assisted with foaling if necessary.

Prognosis

- Stabilized mares not in pain may raise a foal successfully but should *not* be used for breeding.
- The likelihood of long-term survival is poor.

Abdominal Pain After Foaling

- Abdominal pain is common in mares and is usually mild and associated with bruising of the pelvic canal and secondary ileus.
- More serious conditions include:
  - Uterine hemorrhage
  - Small colon impaction
  - Rupture of the small colon mesentery
  - Large colon volvulus
  - Ruptured uterus, cecum, and/or bladder
- These problems must be ruled out by clinical, laboratory, and ultrasound examination and must be surgically corrected if necessary.
- Peritoneal fluid analysis in normal post foaling mares can occur and is similar to normal horse laboratory values
- Medical therapy alone may be appropriate for small colon impaction and occasionally small dorsal tears of the uterus and/or bladder.

Peritonitis

- Peritonitis, inflammation of the peritoneal cavity, is classified according to the following:
  - Origin: primary or secondary
  - Onset: peracute, acute, or chronic
  - Extent of involvement: diffuse or localized
  - Presence of bacteria: septic or nonseptic
- Peritonitis usually is acute, diffuse, and results from GI compromise or infectious disease.
- Severity depends on the causative agent, virulence of the organism, host defenses, extent and site of involvement, recognition of problems, and treatment.
- Generally the aboral sites, cecum to small colon, contain more bacteria and anaerobes and therefore are associated with more severe disease.
- The organisms frequently cultured are enteric aerobes (*E. coli, Actinobacillus* organisms, *Streptococcus equi, S. zooepidemicus,* and *Rhodococcus* organisms) and anaerobes (*Bacteroides, Peptostreptococcus,* and *Clostridium*), and in rare cases, *Fusobacterium* organisms.

Causes

- Idiopathic
- Perforation of the GI or genitourinary tract
- ***Practice Tip:*** *Infectious disease* (Actinobacillus) *is a common cause of peritonitis in adult horses without known predisposing causes. Some horses may even have repeat occurrences separated by months or years.*
- Trauma
- Iatrogenic after abdominal surgery

Diagnosis

- Clinical signs depend on the causative agent and the extent and duration of disease.
- Local peritonitis has minimal systemic signs.
- Diffuse peritonitis has signs of endotoxemia and septicemia, abdominal pain, pyrexia, anorexia, weight loss, and diarrhea.

- Peracute peritonitis resulting from intestinal rupture causes severe signs of endotoxemia, depression, and rapid cardiovascular deterioration; severe abdominal pain, sweating, muscle fasciculations, tachycardia, red to purple mucous membranes with increased CRT; and dehydration.
- In acute diffuse peritonitis, death occurs 4 to 24 hours after the primary insult.
  - Fever and abdominal pain may *not* occur and depend on the stage of endotoxic shock.
  - Ileus and gastric reflux may develop as the result of peritoneal and serosal inflammation.
  - Rectal examination may yield normal findings or dry, emphysematous, "gritty" serosa and peritoneum and distention of the large and small intestine from ileus.
- Affected horses with localized, subacute to chronic peritonitis have signs of depression, anorexia, weight loss, intermittent fever, ventral edema, intermittent abdominal pain, and mild dehydration. Usually large amounts of echogenic fluid are found within the abdominal cavity on ultrasound and there is thickening of the intestinal walls.

Clinical Laboratory Findings

- Increased PCV
- Increased (hemoconcentration) or decreased (protein loss into the peritoneal cavity) TPP concentration
- Hyperfibrinogenemia
- Increased creatinine concentration: prerenal or renal azotemia
- Metabolic acidosis

Results of Complete Blood Count

- Significant leukopenia: neutropenia and left shift caused by endotoxemia and consumption in peracute and acute peritonitis
- Leukocytosis: neutrophilia caused by inflammation with hyperfibrinogenemia in chronic peritonitis

Peritoneal Fluid Analysis

- Collect peritoneal fluid in an EDTA tube for cytologic examination, measurement of total protein, and WBC count. Collect samples for bacterial culture in a sterile tube (see p. 158).
- Total protein concentration and nucleated cell count is increased: 20,000 to 400,000 cells/µL
- Cytologic examination shows free or phagocytized bacteria in leukocytes.
- Perform Gram stain for initial evaluation and selection of antimicrobial agents while awaiting culture and susceptibility results.

●▶ WHAT TO DO

Peritonitis

- Prompt and aggressive treatment is needed.
- Perform the following:
  - Manage the primary disease; however, with *Actinobacillus* peritonitis there is usually *no* other disorder and antibiotics with even low-level supportive care results in a rapid recovery.

GI:ENT

- Provide analgesics.
- Reverse the endotoxic and hypovolemic shock.
- Correct metabolic and electrolyte abnormalities.
- Correct dehydration.
- Correct hypoproteinemia.
- Administer broad-spectrum antimicrobial therapy.
- Administer intravenous balanced electrolyte solution to maintain intravascular fluid volume.
- Hypertonic saline solution (7% NaCl, 1 to 2 L IV) improves systemic blood pressure and cardiac output. Hypertonic saline solution administered initially must be followed by adequate fluid replacement with a balanced crystalloid solution (see Chapter 32, p. 567).
- A TPP concentration <4.5 g/dL necessitates administration of plasma, 2 to 10 L IV slowly, to maintain plasma oncotic pressure and minimize pulmonary edema during rehydration with intravenous fluids.
- Antiserum (Endoserum) against gram-negative core antigens (endotoxin) can be administered intravenously diluted in a balanced electrolyte solution. Hyperimmune plasma directed against the J-5 mutant strain of *E. coli* (Polymune-J, Foalimmune) or normal equine plasma (2 to 10 L) administered intravenously, slowly, may be equally beneficial for supplying protein, fibronectin, complement, antithrombin III, and other inhibitors of hypercoagulability.
- Administer polymyxin B, 2000 to 6000 IU/kg IV q12h as needed.
- Administer flunixin meglumine, 0.66 to 1.1 mg/kg IV q12h, or low dose, 0.25 mg/kg IV q8h, to reduce the adverse effects of arachidonic acid metabolites. NSAIDs should be used with caution in the care of hypovolemic, hypoproteinemic patients to avoid GI and renal toxicity.
- Monitor blood gas and serum electrolyte levels and correct deficiencies.
- Start antimicrobial therapy immediately after a peritoneal fluid sample has been obtained for culture and susceptibility.
- Antimicrobial combinations commonly used include the following:
  - Na$^+$/K$^+$ penicillin, 22,000 to 44,000 IU/kg IV q6h, and
  - Aminoglycosides: gentamicin, 6.6 mg/kg IV q24h; or amikacin, 15 to 25 mg/kg IV q24h; or enrofloxacin, 5.0 mg/kg q24h IV or 7.5 mg/kg q24h PO.
  - Metronidazole, 15 to 25 mg/kg PO, or suppository q8h for anaerobes
- Duration of antimicrobial therapy depends on the following:
  - Severity of the peritonitis
  - Causative agent
  - Response to treatment
  - Complications: thrombophlebitis, abdominal abscessation
- After stabilization, perform surgical intervention to correct the primary problem (if known) and reduce peritoneal contamination by abdominal drainage, peritoneal lavage, and peritoneal dialysis.
- Use clinical signs and sequential evaluation of clinicopathologic parameters and peritoneal fluid to assess response to treatment. Generalized septic peritonitis may necessitate 1 to 6 months of antimicrobial therapy.

Prognosis

- Prognosis depends on:
  - Severity and duration of the disease
  - Primary causative agent
  - Complications, which include:
    - Intraabdominal adhesion formation
    - Laminitis
    - Endotoxic shock

- Prognosis is fair to good in mild, acute, diffuse peritonitis if prompt, aggressive management of the underlying problem is successful or if it is unknown.
- Prognosis is good in *Actinobacillus* peritonitis.
- Prognosis is poor if there is significant abdominal contamination or intestinal perforation.

ACUTE DIARRHEA

Diarrhea in Nursing Foals

Nathan Slovis

Necrotizing Enterocolitis

- Necrotizing enterocolitis is a common cause of diarrhea and colic in foals, usually during the first week of life. The diarrhea can be hemorrhagic.

Causes

- Cases of necrotizing enterocolitis generally are considered to be caused by perinatal asphyxia syndrome, the anaerobic bacteria *C. difficile*, *C. perfringens* type C, or *Bacteroides fragilis*.
- *Practice Tip: Recumbency and feeding milk replacer are considered to increase the risk of acquiring the disease. Cases of clostridial diarrhea frequently become a farm problem.*
- Perinatal asphyxia syndrome (PAS) produces hypoxic ischemic encephalopathy (HIE) resulting in neurologic deficits ranging from hypotonia to grand mal seizures. Foals affected with perinatal asphyxia also experience gastrointestinal disturbances ranging from mild ileus and delayed gastric emptying to severe, bloody diarrhea and necrotizing enterocolitis (NEC).
- It has been postulated that when the preterm infant is stressed by periods of hypoxia or hypotension, blood flow is redistributed, via input from the adrenergic system, away from the splanchnic bed. During the period of reperfusion, oxygen free radicals are generated; these free radicals can cause the tissue damage that is typically seen with reperfusion injury.
- If the hypoxic event is severe enough, then NEC can occur resulting in:
  - Bloody diarrhea
  - Pneumatosis intestinalis
  - Ascites
  - Intestinal perforation
- *Practice Tip: A diagnosis of hypoxic ischemic ileus is presumptive when the patient has a history of:*
  - *Peripartum asphyxia (placentitis, premature placental separation)*
  - *Negative fecal diagnostics for infectious diseases*
  - *Abdominal ultrasonography reveals distended small intestine with decreased motility*
- *C. difficile* produces several toxins; only the effects of toxin A and B are well known.
  - When established in the colon, pathogenic strains of *C. difficile* produce toxins that cause diarrhea and

colitis. **Note:** Strains that do not produce these toxins are not pathogenic.

- **C. perfringens** produces four major toxins, with one relatively newer toxin identified (β_2).
  - Recently an unassigned type of *C. perfringens* that produces alpha toxin and the newly discovered β_2-toxin was described. The toxin was isolated from piglets with necrotic enterocolitis and was also found in horses with enterocolitis. Because the alpha toxin, produced by all types of *C. perfringens* including nonpathogenic type A strains, is not considered a primary cause of digestive lesions, it was suggested that the β_2-toxin, which is present in this new type of *C. perfringens,* is responsible for the lesions.
  - *C. perfringens* diarrhea in foals is considered to result from infection with type C (beta toxin) (sporadic cases) or enterotoxin from *C. perfringens* type A, which may be associated with a high morbidity.

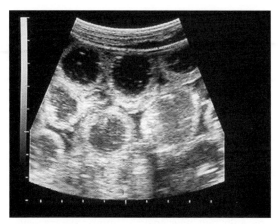

Figure 18-70 Foal diarrhea: Ultrasound finding in a 3-day-old foal with hemorrhagic diarrhea due to *Clostridium perfringens* type C. The same organism was cultured from the feces and blood. With antibiotic and supportive treatments the foal recovered in 3 days.

Clinical Signs

- Colic that frequently precedes the production of diarrhea by several hours
- Abdominal distention
- Fever
- Potentially hemorrhagic diarrhea (not noted in most type A cases but common in type C cases)

    Practice Tip: C. perfringens type C cases usually have normal IgG, bloody diarrhea, and are almost always in foals younger than 8 days of age and sporadic in occurrence as opposed to the sometimes outbreak of presumed C. perfringens *type A and* Clostridium difficile *diarrhea in neonatal foals, which often do* not *have bloody feces.*

- Anorexia

Diagnosis

- Clinical signs
- Rule out other causes of abdominal pain (see p. 185).
- Meconium impaction and enteritis are the most common causes of colic in foals.
- Perform abdominal ultrasonography:
  - Enterocolitis leads to hypomotile, thickened loops of small intestine (Fig. 18-70), whereas a physical obstruction (Fig. 18-71) typically does *not* demonstrate diffuse amotility, and the walls are not as thick.
  - One may see "pneumatosis intestinalis," intramural gas echoes in the small or large bowel wall.
- Perform abdominal radiography (85 kVp, 20 mA-s, rare earth screens) if necessary.
  - Similar to ultrasonography, radiography shows more diffuse gas distention of the small bowel as opposed to a smaller area of distention seen with problems such as intussusception.
- Abdominocentesis should be performed only in cases with difficulty differentiating surgical from medical problems.
  - Use a teat cannula or bitch catheter rather than performing a needle aspirate.

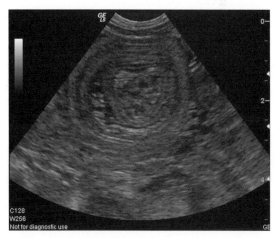

Figure 18-71 Classic sonographic view of an obstructive intestinal lesion, which was a midjejunal intussusception.

- Indiscriminant "centesis" is fraught with complications including enterocentesis and peritonitis.
- Use ultrasound to identify an area to sample.
- Clinical pathology results are as follows:
  - Blood cultures frequently are positive for *C. perfringens* in foals with severe clostridial enteritis. They may also be blood culture positive for *Enterococcus* spp.
  - CBC generally reveals a leukopenia with toxic neutrophils.
  - Serum chemistry showing hyponatremia, hypochloremia, and frequently a low total CO_2 is indicative of acidosis.
  - Hypoproteinemia is secondary to the effects of clostridial toxins leading to extravasation of plasma proteins.
  - Metabolic acidosis is also consistent with clostridial enterocolitis and hypovolemia or gastrointestinal tract loss of bicarbonate.

- Hyponatremia may also be attributable to the gastrointestinal tract losses, as well as to an excess of free water associated with water or milk consumption by these foals.
- Fecal diagnostics for clostridial enteritis are as follows:
  - Direct fecal smear with Gram stain
    - A presumptive diagnosis may be made (until culture and toxin analysis) by demonstration of abundant gram-positive bacteria in a fecal smear.
    - However, this test may not be sensitive because *C. perfringens* was isolated from 59% of samples in which no gram-positive rods were seen.
  - *C. difficile* toxin assays: toxin types A and B. More recently two new enzyme immunoassays have been introduced that:
  - Detect toxin A/toxin B (*C. difficile* TOX A/B test[17])
  - Detect antigen of *C. difficile* and toxin A (TRIAGE Micro[18])
    - These tests have a good sensitivity (69% to 87%) and specificity (99% to 100%).
    - *C. difficile* TOX A/B test, Techlab has been validated for use in feces of horses.
    - ***Practice Tip:*** Do not *use* Styrofoam cups *to submit a fecal sample because they can bind the clostridial toxins. Fecal samples can be stored for up to 72 hours between 2° and 8° C.*
    - Most cases appear to be positive for toxins on examination of a single fecal sample although repeat testing may further improve sensitivity.
  - The toxin must be demonstrated in feces to confirm diagnosis.
  - The presence of *C. difficile* in culture is not diagnostic because many strains do *not* produce toxin or disease
  - Some healthy foals may have *C. difficile*–toxin positive stool.
- *C. perfringens* toxin assay: enterotoxin assay
  - Enzyme-linked immunosorbent assay (ELISA) is commercially available for *C. perfringens* enterotoxin (Tech Lab).
    - Labile-toxin assay must be run within one-half hour of sample collection or sample should be frozen for testing.
  - Obtain a fecal anaerobic culture.
  - Commercial anaerobic kits are available[19]; it is best to use anaerobic blood plates.
- Pure growth of *C. perfringens* is *indicative* of disease, but toxin must be identified to confirm disease.
- Polymerase chain reaction (PCR):
  - Incorporated primers for *C. difficile* toxin A and B
  - Incorporated primers that allowed for classification of *C. perfringens* types A, B, C, D, and E, as well as genes for β_2-toxin and enterotoxin (CPE)

[17]TOX A/B test (Techlab, Blacksburg, Virginia).
[18]TRIAGE Micro (BIOSITE, San Diego California, 1-888-BIOSITE).
[19]BD GasPak EZ (Becton, Dickinson and Company, Sparks, Maryland).

- PCR testing of feces would be needed to confirm *C. perfringens* type C. One option for testing is at Iowa State University Diagnostic Laboratory (515-294-1950).

Prognosis
- Initially, the prognosis is considered guarded because the intestinal necrosis may progress rapidly. (This is especially true with the infrequent and sporadic cases of *C. perfringens* type C.)
- If the foal survives the initial 48 hours, the prognosis generally improves significantly.

WHAT TO DO

Clostridial Diarrhea
Pain Relief
- Attempt to control pain *without* the use of high doses of flunixin meglumine; a single full dose is many times necessary to control the pain.
  - Dipyrone, 3 to 5 mL IV; xylazine, 0.6 to 1.0 mg/kg IV; butorphanol, 0.02 to 0.04 mg/kg IV or IM; or ketoprofen, 1 mg/kg IV. Meloxicam 0.6 mg/kg IV is another more COX-2 selective option but is expensive in the United States.
  - If the foal remains painful and is gas-distended *and* obstructive disease is ruled out, administer neostigmine, 0.2 to 1 mg SQ (total dose) q1h for 3 treatments then q6h along with analgesics or sedation.

Antibiotics
- Sodium or potassium penicillin, 22,000 to 44,000 IU/kg IV q6h
- *Note:* The most common organism cultured from the blood of neonatal foals with enterocolitis is *Enterococcus* spp. (fecal streps). These are gram-positive facultative anaerobic cocci found in the intestinal tract that are resistant to most cephalosporins (therefore, ceftiofur is *not* a good choice for treating septic foals with enterocolitis); ampicillin (15 mg/kg q8h IV) is preferred over penicillin for enterococci but *not* as good as penicillin for *Clostridium* spp.
- Amikacin, 21 to 25 mg/kg IV q24h (Use *only* when urine production is normal.)
- Metronidazole, 15 mg/kg PO q8 to 12h or 10 mg/kg IV q6 to 8h; use if abundant gram-positive rods are found on fecal smear or *C. difficile* toxins are identified.

Intravenous Fluids
- Continual administration is unlikely if the mare is in the same stall as the foal. One to 2 L of fluids can be administered, as a bolus, over 20 to 30 minutes q4h to q12h a day.
- Lactated Ringer's solution, Normosol-R, or Plasma-Lyte preferred
- If severe, acute hyponatremia is present, correction of sodium to 125 mEq/L can be rapid, but further correction should be gradual to prevent neurologic signs.
  - Potassium chloride, 20 mEq/L if foal is urinating: Most foals on large volumes of IV fluids require supplemental potassium, particularly if they are anorectic.
  - Sodium bicarbonate: based on results of a clinical chemistry TCO_2 or blood gas and *only* after correcting dehydration.
  - Dextrose solution: If the foal appears weak and serum glucose measurement cannot be obtained, add 55 mL of 50% dextrose to 1 L of fluid for a 2.5% solution; 110 mL for a 5% solution.

- Plasma, 2 L or more IV
  - Hyperimmune for endotoxin is preferable.
  - A hyperimmunized *Clostridium difficile Toxin A and B* plasma is currently available.[20]
  - Oral and IV administration of *C. perfringens* type A, C, and D hyperimmunized plasma may be given to the neonate.[21]
  - The oral dosage ranges from 50 to 100 mL every 6 hours for 48 to 72 hours.
  - If the foal is severely ill, use nasogastric intubation with 250 to 500 mL of the hyperimmunized plasma. Subjectively, foals given the hyperimmunized plasma have formed feces quicker than the foals not treated with the plasma.
- *Note*: The efficacy of the plasma in treating diarrhea/toxic insult is currently anecdotal.

Intestinal Protectants

- Lactaid[22] (1 tablet every feeding or q2h), lactase,[23] or yogurt (1 to 2 oz q6h): foals are likely to be lactose intolerant with clostridial infection.
- Di-tri-octahedral smectite, Bio-Sponge[24] or Anti-Diarrhea Gel[25]
  - Studies have shown in vitro adsorption of clostridial toxins by these products.
- Bentonite clay can also be used for treatment because it adsorbs *C. perfringens* alpha, beta, and beta-2 exotoxins without interfering with absorption of equine colostral antibodies or metronidazole.
- Bismuth subsalicylate, 30 to 60 mL PO q2-6h
- Probiotics: clinical evidence is in question; *Lactobacillus pentosus* WE7 may actually be detrimental to recovery. Following omeprazole or ranitidine treatment, to raise gastric pH, fecal transfaunation from a healthy foal or the mare may be indicated.
- Gastric ulcer prophylaxis:
  - Sucralfate, 22 mg/kg PO q6h *and*
  - Omeprazole, 1-4 mg/kg PO q24h *or*
  - Ranitidine, 1.5 mg/kg IV(expensive) or 6.6 mg/kg PO q8h *or*
  - Famotidine, 0.23 to 0.5 mg/kg IV q8 to 12h or 2.8 to 4 mg/kg PO q8 to 12h

Supportive Care

- Keep the foal dry and warm.
- Apply a desiccant to the hind quarters; frequently wash and dry the tail.

Prevention

- Numerous prophylactic measures can be instituted on farms with a history of *C. perfringens*–associated enterocolitis in foals.
- Institute optimal hygienic efforts to ensure a clean foaling stall, and at parturition, clean the mare's udder before and after birth and the perineal and hind limb area to reduce exposure of the foal to fecal pathogens.
- Some farms have eliminated foal diarrhea outbreak by foaling the mares out on pasture.

[20]Lake Immunogenics *Clostridium difficile* Toxin A and B Antibody Select HI Plasma (Ontario, New York 14519).
[21]Lake Immunogenics *Clostridium perfringens* Type A, C, and D Antibody Select HI Plasma (Ontario, New York 14519).
[22]LACTAID (McNeil Consumer Healthcare, Fort Washington, Pennsylvania 19034).
[23]Lactase enzyme (6000 Food Chemical Codex units/50-kg foal) orally every 3 to 8 hours (McNeil Consumer Healthcare, Fort Washington, Pennsylvania 19034).
[24]Bio-Sponge (Platinum Performance, Buellton, California 93427).
[25]Anti-Diarrhea Gel (Hagyard Medical Institute, 4250 Iron Works Pike, Lexington, Kentucky 40511-8412).

- Oral administration of *Lactobacillus acidophilus* (found in yogurt and commercial probiotics) have been successfully used in chickens to minimize the overgrowth of *C. perfringens*.
- Prophylactic use of metronidazole (10 mg/kg PO q12h) has also been instituted after birth with reports of mixed results.
- In mares with a history of good milk production, feed a ration containing low to moderate amounts of digestible energy 1 week before parturition and 1 week after parturition to reduce excessive milk production, and therefore, excessive milk intake by the foal. Use this only on farms with high morbidity of disease.
- Specific preventative methods addressing *C. perfringens* include: immunization of mares with a toxoid vaccine (aluminum hydroxide adsorbed culture supernatant PLUS recombinant beta-2 toxoid. Vaccine strain is *C. perfringens* type A and carries genes for alpha, beta-2, and CPE) recently developed (2007) by Hagyard Equine Medical Institute (www.hagyardpharmacy.com).
  - Other oral enteric protectants include the oral and/or IV administration of hyperimmunized plasma, previously mentioned.
  - Specific immune treatments for *C. perfringens* types C and D provide some protection against alpha toxin; it is generally believed that this protection is inadequate against *C. perfringens* type A organisms.
- If clostridial disease is a historical problem on a farm, administration of the following has occasionally appeared to be of clinical benefit:
  - Prophylactic treatment of all newborns with penicillin G procaine, 22,000 units/kg IM q12h for 3 days, or combined with metronidazole, 15 mg/kg PO q12h for 3 to 5 days
- Strict isolation protocol of affected individuals
- Barrier protocol for handlers
- Disinfect stalls using:
  - Hypochlorite and phenolic compounds. **Important:** Hypochlorite is *not* effective in organic debris so must clean with detergent first.
  - *C. perfringens* types C and D antitoxin is available for other large animal species, but safety and efficacy in foals are not well documented.

Foal Salmonellosis

Clinical Signs

- Variable diarrhea that may be scant or profuse, watery, or hemorrhagic
- Fever, usually >103° F, anorexia, tachycardia, tachypnea, and abdominal pain
- These signs are often related to bacteremia/endotoxemia rather than electrolyte derangements and dehydration
- Other signs of bacteremia include the following:
  - Green-tinted iris (presumed septicemia-induced uveitis), injected sclera and mucous membranes
  - Lameness associated with septic arthritis or physitis
  - Abnormal lung sounds associated with pneumonia of hematogenous origin
  - Lethargy, stupor, or seizures associated with meningitis or from severe electrolyte derangements (e.g., hyponatremia)

Laboratory Findings

- Leukopenia as a result of neutropenia is common.
  - Neutrophils frequently demonstrate toxic changes.
- Fibrinogen concentration may be elevated.

- Low platelet count may indicate the presence of disseminated intravascular coagulation.
- *Practice Tip:* *Hyponatremia, hypochloremia, acidosis, and azotemia are the most common laboratory findings with salmonellosis and most other causes of infectious diarrhea.*
  - Acidosis may mask life-threatening hypokalemia by raising the plasma potassium at the expense of total body potassium.
  - Low serum potassium may result from a combination of decreased intake, increased loss in diarrheic feces, fluid therapy causing kaluresis and polyuric acute renal failure.

Diagnosis

- For *Salmonella* spp., fecal cultures use selective media and selenite enrichment media.
- Other organisms of possible significance for foal diarrhea include *E. coli, Aeromonas hydrophila, Yersinia psuedotuberculosis, Enterococcus* spp., *Campylobacter* spp., *Streptococcus* spp., *Clostridium* spp., coronavirus, rotavirus, and *Pseudomonas* spp.
- Blood cultures frequently are positive (BBL, Becton, Dickinson and Company) in foals with salmonellosis.
- PCR
- *Practice Tip: The Enhanced rapid test system (Reveal[26] 2.0* Salmonella *test system) for the detection of* Salmonella *spp. should be performed on suspicious cultures (black or green colonies noted on Hektoen agar).*

WHAT TO DO

Foal Salmonellosis
- Treatment emphasis is on fluid therapy, antibiotics, and nursing care.

Fluid Therapy
- Polyionic fluids, Lactated Ringer's, Normosol-R and Plasma-Lyte are the best choices because sodium chloride is an acidifying solution.
- Use hypertonic saline only if polyionic fluids do *not* alleviate hypotension associated with severe disease *or* it can be administered in 1- to 2-mL/kg boluses at 30- to 60-minute intervals for severe hyponatremia.
- Goal for initial correction of severe hyponatremia should be sodium concentration of 125 to 130 mEq/L, *no higher.* **Practice Tip:** *Chronic (days) hyponatremia should be corrected more slowly.*
- Add potassium chloride to fluids; 20 mEq/L, if foal is urinating and serum potassium <3.5 mEq/L.
- **Note:** Potassium administration should *not* exceed 0.5 mEq/kg/h.
  - Two tablespoons of Lite Salt (50% KCl) can be added to a pint of yogurt to safely assist in providing potassium to foals.
- If acidosis persists in the face of adequate fluid therapy and normal L-lactate (the metabolic acidosis is believed to be due to either D-lactate production or bicarbonate loss in the feces), add sodium bicarbonate to fluids.

[26]Reveal (Neogen, Lansing, Michigan 48912).

- Use an isotonic solution or 12.5 g baking soda added to a gallon of sterile water; be careful of too rapid correction of hyponatremia.
- General rule in bicarbonate administration is to give as a bolus half of the calculated deficit and then to correct remaining deficit over 12 to 24 hours.
- If sodium bicarbonate is used, more potassium supplementation is necessary!

Antibiotic Therapy
- Ticarcillin/clavulanic acid, 44 mg/kg IV q6h; or ceftiofur, 5 mg/kg IV q8h; or ceftazidime, 20 to 40 mg/kg IV q6 to 8h, often combined with:
  - Amikacin, 21 to 25 mg/kg IV q24h; *do not* administer amikacin until the foal has been observed to urinate a normal volume.
  - Enrofloxacin, 6 mg/kg IV q24h or 7.5 mg/kg PO q24h for resistant strains of salmonellosis; risk of drug-induced joint disease limits this treatment to foals with life-threatening and highly drug resistant salmonellosis! Marbofloxacin 2 mg/kg q24h PO can be used as a replacement for Enrofloxacin.
    - Monitor foals for joint effusion (nonseptic synovitis), lameness, flexoral laxity, or anemia because these can be commonly encountered when using this medication.
    - Empirical treatment with Adequan, 1 vial IM every 3 days, has helped decrease the incidence of synovitis.

Additional Therapy
- Endotoxemia treatment:
  - A minimum of 1 L of hyperimmune (to endotoxin) plasma
  - Consider low-molecular-weight heparin, 50 units/kg SQ q24h, if evidence of disseminated intravascular coagulation exists (i.e., decreased platelets, prolonged clotting profile, decreased antithrombin III activity).
  - Flunixin meglumine, 0.25 mg/kg IV q8h, *only* with serious endotoxemia and after initiation of intravenous fluid administration
- Ulcer prophylaxis *and*
  - Sucralfate, 22 mg/kg PO q6h
  - Omeprazole, 4.0 mg/kg q24h *or*
  - Ranitidine, 1.5 mg/kg IV or 6.6 mg/kg PO q8h *or*
  - Famotidine, 0.7 mg/kg IV q24h or 2.8 mg/kg PO q24h
- Intestinal protectants
  - Di-tri-octahedral smectite (Bio-Sponge) or (Hagyard Anti-Diarrhea Gel), yogurt, bismuth subsalicylate, or activated charcoal may be beneficial.
- Nursing care
  - Keep foal clean; apply petroleum jelly to perineal region.
  - Wrap tail with plastic bag and Elasticon (around base of tail with separate piece extending dorsally up to midsacral region).
  - *Do not* wrap tightly; monitor for frequent slipping.
  - *Do not* use Vetwrap.
- For abdominal pain, use the following:
  - Dipyrone, firocoxib and reportedly carprofen are considered less ulcerogenic than flunixin meglumine and can be used when several treatments with NSAIDs are needed.
  - Dipyrone, 4 to 10 mL IV; xylazine, 0.3 to 1.0 mg/kg IV; butorphanol, 0.02 to 0.04 mg/kg IV or IM; ketoprofen, 1 mg/kg IV. The continuous administration of lidocaine, IV, can also be used, although in young foals, hepatic metabolism can be delayed.
  - If ileus is clinically present *and* obstructive disease is ruled out, administer neostigmine, 0.2 to 1 mg SQ q1h for 3 treatments then q6h along with analgesics or sedation.
- For uveitis, use topical ophthalmic corticosteroid with or without antibiotic (if no corneal ulcer) and atropine.

- Keep the mare and foal together; the mare is likely fecal positive for *Salmonella* spp., and separation creates extra stress on the foal and the mare.
- Follow strict isolation protocol!

Prevention

- Prevention of *Salmonella* consists of proper hygiene. Before the foal is able to nurse, the udder and perineal regions of the mare are to be thoroughly washed with dilute chlorhexidine or Ivory soap and water.
- During an outbreak, at risk foals should also be intubated with 6 to 8 oz of colostrum before contact with the mare.
- An experimental inactivated bacterin (*Salmonella typhimurium* and *newport*) vaccine has been developed by Hagyard Equine Medical Institute and Dr. John Timmoney at the Gluck Research Center in Lexington, Kentucky. This vaccine is currently being used on endemic farms since 2007.

Prognosis

- The prognosis is considered fair *if* the foal responds positively to initial therapy over the first 48 hours.
- If the foal continues to deteriorate during the first 48 hours in spite of aggressive therapy or septic foci develop in joints, lungs, or meninges, the prognosis is guarded.
- *Practice Tip: It is unusual for both the mare and foal to have diarrhea associated with* Salmonella *spp., but it is likely that the mare cultures fecal positive for the organism.*
- Keep the pair isolated from other horses on the farm.
- Generally, a minimum of three, and preferably five, negative cultures should be obtained from the mare and foal before reintroducing the pair to the general herd.

Rotavirus Diarrhea

- *Practice Tip: This is the most common infectious diarrhea in nursing foals (group A rotavirus).*
- Rotavirus causes diarrhea in foals up to 6 months of age but is more common in younger foals.
- The virus is associated with an increased incidence of gastric ulceration.
- The virus is highly contagious; often several foals on a farm are affected simultaneously.

Clinical Signs

- Watery yellow to yellow-green diarrhea
- Nonfetid diarrhea with a distinctive odor
- Lethargy, anorexia frequently observed before the onset of diarrhea
- Neonates may become tympanic and colicky

Diagnosis

- ELISA (Virogen rotatest, Rotazyme[27])
  - Foals that have had diarrhea for several days may have negative results.

- PCR
  - There is documented analysis of several equine samples positive for rotavirus by PCR that tested negative in an immunoassay with human rotavirus specificity. ***Practice Tip:*** *This underscores the importance of equine–specific test reagents for veterinary medicine and the risk of false-negative results when using nonspecies-matched reagents.*
  - Sequences showed 98% identities to equine rotavirus isolates deposited in GenBank.
  - These results suggest that the immunoassay with human specificity *does not* detect all equine isolates.
- Laboratory findings usually are relatively mild compared with *Salmonella* spp.
- For CBC, toxic neutrophils and the presence of band neutrophils are not common.
- Serum chemistry reveals hypochloremia, hyponatremia, hypokalemia, and acidosis.

⟫ WHAT TO DO

Rotavirus Diarrhea
- Gastric ulcer prophylaxis is indicated.
- May be self-limiting
- Monitor hydration status and laboratory parameters for indications to initiate fluid therapy.
- See previous section on fluid therapy for foal diarrhea.
- Intestinal protectants are necessary (see previous section for dosages):
  - Bismuth subsalicylate
  - Di-tri-octahedral smectite (Bio-Sponge)
  - Hagyard Anti-Diarrhea Gel
  - Yogurt
- Lactaid should be administered because rotavirus-infected foals are likely to have maldigestion.
- Lactase[28] 6000 Food Chemical Codex (FCC) lactase U/50 kg PO q3 to 8h for 10 to 14 days has also been used to improve digestion of milk lactose.

Prevention

- Take measures to prevent spread of the disease.
  - Isolate all affected foals.
  - Control the entry of birds and pets into the barn.
  - Personnel should enter stall last during daily cleaning and feeding.
    - Wear boots, coveralls, and gloves when entering the stall.
    - *Do not* share buckets and utensils between stalls.
    - If possible, assign one person to care only for affected foals.
    - Provide foot-baths outside stall using phenolic compounds or hypochlorite.

---

[27]Rotazyme (Abbott Laboratories, Diagnostics Div., North Chicago, Illinois).

[28]Lactase enzyme (6000 Food Chemical Codex units/50-kg foal) orally every 3 to 8 hours (McNeil Consumer Healthcare, Fort Washington, Pennsylvania 19034).

- Vaccination of brood mares confers moderate protection and is considered at least to decrease the severity of the disease.
- **Practice Tip:** *On rare occasion with rotavirus and other causes of foal diarrhea, the foal becomes bloated and colicky following nursing; use lactaid, lidocaine CRI if possible, and restrict the amount of time the foal nurses for a couple of days (if required).*

Prognosis

Prognosis is considered good to excellent.

Enterotoxigenic *Escherichia Coli*

- Usually affects a single foal on the farm
- Infection with pili-positive and enterotoxin-positive *E. coli*

Clinical Signs

- Watery diarrhea, usually not fetid
- Moderate to severe depression
- Fever not typically present
- Signs of gastric ulceration usually present

Diagnosis

- Laboratory findings typically demonstrate acidosis.
- Rule out other causes of diarrhea.
- Aerobic fecal culture shows heavy growth of mucoid colonies.
- Submit culture to a laboratory that tests for *adhesion* and *enterotoxin*.

●▶ WHAT TO DO

E. Coli Diarrhea

- Treatment is similar to other causes of foal diarrhea with consideration that *E. coli* or *Enterococcus* spp. may become bacteremic.
- Amikacin use should be limited to foals producing normal volumes of urine.
- *E. coli* antibody specifically against K99 pili is commercially available as an oral paste[29] for foals, but field value is not well documented.

Cryptosporidiosis

- **Practice Tip:** Cryptosporidium *is a protozoal pathogen with significant zoonotic potential.*
- Oocysts are infective when shed.
- Zoonotic potential exists.
- Diarrhea is a result of infection with *Cryptosporidium parvum* and typically occurs in immunocompromised (often hospitalized) foals, although *C. parvum* has been associated with diarrhea in otherwise healthy foals.
- Infection often is noted in Arabian foals with combined immunodeficiency.
- Infection may occur in foals that have secondary immunosuppression associated with chronic, catabolic disease or another enteric pathogen.

[29]Equine Coli Endotox (Novartis Animal Health US, Inc., 800-843-3386).

- Diagnosis is based on detection of oocysts in fecal samples.
- Kinyoun acid-fast stain, immunofluorescence, PCR and flow cytometry are useful.
- **Note:** *Cryptosporidium* can also be found in the feces of normal foals.
- *Eimeria* and *Giardia* spp. may be noted in samples; the pathogenicity of these organisms in the horse has not been conclusively documented.

●▶ WHAT TO DO

Cryptosporidiosis

- Supportive care—fluids and nutrition!
- Total parenteral nutrition (TPN) may be required.
- Administer paromomycin, 100 mg/kg PO q24h for 5 days or nitazoxanide (NTZ) 2 g PO q12h for 3 days. (The equine product is no longer available; however, for valuable foals, NTZ, approved for human use, can be acquired.)
- Efficacy and safety have *not* been proven in foals but nitazoxanide is effective in calves.
- Transmission is from foal to foal.

Prevention

- Use barrier precautions with patients.
- Extreme heat and cold are considered the best methods to kill oocysts.
- Concentrated hypochlorite solutions may be used.

Fetal Diarrhea

- It is *not* unusual to deliver a newborn and see the foal covered in amniotic fluid stained with fetal diarrhea.
- **Practice Tip:** *This problem generally signifies an unthrifty newborn that is at high risk for the development of aspiration pneumonia.*

Clinical Signs

- Foals may be clinically normal, but typically they are depressed, demonstrate poor suckle reflex, and may exhibit signs of ischemic-hypoxic encephalopathy.
- Foals are reluctant or unable to stand and nurse.
- Signs of sepsis may be severe.
- Toxic mucous membranes and poor perfusion are evident.

●▶ WHAT TO DO

Fetal Diarrhea

- Suction the trachea for 10-second intervals at a time, while administering intranasal oxygen, to remove meconium-stained amniotic fluid.
- Administer broad-spectrum antibiotics (see *Salmonella* spp., p. 223).
- Administer IV fluids and plasma.
- Give colostrum orally.
- If respiratory signs begin to worsen, administer the following:
  - Dexamethasone, 0.1 to 0.25 mg/kg IV once, or prednisolone sodium succinate, 100 mg IV once.
  - The dose may be repeated for 2 to 3 days if there is a positive response to the initial dose.

⬤〉 WHAT NOT TO DO

Meconium Aspiration from Fetal Diarrhea

- *Do not* suction trachea for prolonged periods without supplemental oxygen.

Enterococcus Durans (Previously Group D Streptococcus)

- *Enterococcus durans* is a gram-positive coccus in the alimentary tract that has been implicated as a cause of enteritis in foals, piglets, calves, and puppies. *E. durans* has been reported as a cause of diarrhea in 5 of 7 foals that developed diarrhea during the first 10 days of life.
- In one Australian study, *E. durans* was isolated from a foal that had severe diarrhea, then used to experimentally infect 7 foals by stomach tube exposure. All 7 foals developed profuse watery diarrhea within 24 hours of inoculation with varying degrees of depression, anorexia, abdominal tenderness, and dehydration.
- The pathogenesis of diarrhea and enteric disease remains unknown. Diarrhea induced by *E. durans* is *not* associated with enterotoxin production or substantial mucosal injury.
- Decreased activity of brush border digestive enzymes, such as lactase and alkaline phosphatase, suggests there is a direct mechanical interference with digestion and absorption at the brush border.

⬤〉 WHAT TO DO

Enterococcus Durans Diarrhea

- Subjectively, systemic treatment with some β-lactams appears to decrease the diarrhea duration (ampicillin or penicillin). The organism is highly resistant to cephalosporins.
- The ideal treatment is to improve husbandry on the farm.

Coronavirus

- Equine coronavirus (ECoV, a beta coronavirus) was isolated and characterized only recently but was described as an infectious agent in sick foals in 1976.
- Several studies and case reports have identified coronaviruses in foals with enteric disease but the pathogenicity and etiologic role in enteric disease have *not* been examined. A recent prevalence study in central Kentucky clearly shows that healthy foals without signs of GI disease are equally infected with equine coronavirus as sick animals. This finding suggests low pathogenicity of ECoV in foals. However, when analyzed as a coinfecting agent, ECoV is significantly associated with diseased foals; all ECoV infections in the GI diseased group were associated with coinfections (15 of 15) while foals in the healthy group were mostly monoinfected (8 of 10). ***Practice Tip:*** *This finding supports the theory that (certain) viruses primarily act as immune-suppressing agents allowing opportunistic infections to take place.*
- Opportunistic infections can be of different origin, including bacterial or protozoal, as shown in the study.

Coinfection data in piglets clearly indicate that coronavirus and bacterial coinfections have a significant effect on the magnitude of the inflammatory immune response and the amount of tissue damage compared with single infected foals. Furthermore, in young turkeys, coronavirus and enteropathogenic *E. coli* (EPEC) were shown to synergistically interact and cause severe growth depression and high mortality when compared with monoinfected turkeys.

- These observations suggest a role for coronavirus in foals and the diagnostic value of detecting ECoV in apparently healthy foals to assess their potential susceptibility for coinfections.
- In coronavirus-infected healthy foals, the focus should be directed toward epidemiologic aspects to reduce the likelihood of coinfections. Additional information is needed to determine equine coronavirus virulence factors and the relative importance as a coinfecting agent contributing to GI disease in foals.

Diagnosis

- PCR, virus isolation, or electron microscopy of fecal sample.

⬤〉 WHAT TO DO

Coronavirus Diarrhea

- See treatment under Rotavirus Diarrhea, p. 225.
- Currently there is an ultrapurified Bentonite clay that is available for use in horses that has the same composition as a product being investigated in humans suffering from rotavirus or coronavirus gastrointestinal infections.[30]

Lactase Deficiency (Dietary)

- Lactose intolerance has been diagnosed in foals as either:
  - Lactose malabsorption
    - Physiologic problem that arises from the consumption of too much lactose and the capacity for lactase to hydrolyze it to glucose and galactose.
    - An example is overfeeding or incorrectly prepared milk replacer.
  - Secondary lactase deficiency
    - For example, a lactase deficiency that is the result of injury of the brush border (location of lactase enzyme) during enterocolitis.
  - Primary lactase deficiency
    - These foals have low or completely absent lactase concentrations.

Diagnosis

- Based on response to treatment and/or the lactose tolerance test.
  - Lactose monohydrate (1 g/kg body weight in a 20% water solution) is administered by nasogastric tube

---

[30]Bentonite clay (Hagyard Pharmacy, 4250 Iron Works Pike Lexington, Kentucky).

after fasting for 4 hours; plasma glucose concentrations are monitored.

- ***Practice Tip:*** *Fluoride oxalate may need to be used as an anticoagulant if the sample cannot be immediately cooled and there is more than 1 hour between collection and submission of the sample before dosing; monitor every 30 minutes for 2 hours.*
- Normal digestion of lactose results in a doubling of the normal glucose concentration in 60 to 90 minutes.

●〉 WHAT TO DO

Lactase Deficiency
- Supplement with lactase enzyme (6000 Food Chemical Codex units/50-kg foal) orally every 3 to 8 hours or a tablet of Lactaid.

Acute Pancreatitis in the Neonatal Foal

- Acute onset of diarrhea almost immediately followed by signs of septic shock and gross hyperlipemia with marked elevations in amylase and lipase are characteristic of pancreatitis in foals.
- The cause of the pancreatitis is unknown but most foals are approximately 3 days of age and were healthy and vigorous nursers on days 1 and 2.
- The first sign is often diarrhea. Abdominal ultrasound may reveal increased peritoneal fluid and an abnormal appearing mass in the area of the pancreas.
- Peritoneal fluid is inflammatory, with both hemorrhage and lipids causing a milky pink color, and may have higher amylase and lipase than values in plasma.

●〉 WHAT TO DO

Acute Pancreatitis in the Neonatal Foal
- IV fluids
- Systemic antibiotics
- Plasma
- Low-molecular-weight heparin
- Selenium and vitamin E
- Flunixin meglumine
- Parenteral nutrition (excluding lipids)

    Note: One foal survived the acute disease and was treated with oral pancreatic enzymes and milk feeding and succumbed to fibrinous peritonitis due to the inflammatory pancreatitis.

Diarrhea in Weanlings and Yearlings

Thomas J. Divers

Proliferative Enteropathy: *Lawsonia Intracellularis*
- Affects many mammals, including foals most commonly 4 to 7 months of age.
  - The organism can be found in the feces of normal foals and adult horses (especially on farms that have had clinical cases).
- Worldwide distribution
- Obligate intracellular bacterium

- Different strains of the organism; the "pig" strain appears to be relatively nonpathogenic in foals while strain(s) isolated from some wild animals may be pathogenic to foals.
- ***Practice Tip:*** *Hypoproteinemia is the hallmark laboratory finding.*

Clinical Signs
- Rapid weight loss, often in the face of a normal appetite
- Poor hair coat and a pot-bellied appearance
- Ventral edema and lethargy
- Diarrhea in approximately 50% of cases and abdominal pain in 10% to 15%
- Fever is rare
- Uncommonly, an acute necrotizing form of *Lawsonia* occurs with acute, severe systemic inflammation, necrosis of the bowel, and secondary bacterial invasion may be a clinical presentation.

Laboratory Findings
- CBC results are variable; most common abnormalities are low total protein, leukocytosis, and anemia
- Serum chemistry: classically hypoproteinemia caused by *hypoalbuminemia*
- May have electrolyte abnormalities from diarrhea or edema: hyponatremia, hypochloremia
- Increased creatinine kinase

Diagnosis
- Fecal PCR for the organism is the *best* test.
  - Multiple fecal samples or fecal sample and rectal swab together may improve sensitivity
- Serum neutralization titer: potentially evaluate acute and convalescence titers
- Abdominal ultrasonography: "wagon-wheel" small-intestinal wall edema is the characteristic appearance (Fig. 18-72)
- Postmortem: Warthin-Starry silver stain of affected tissues

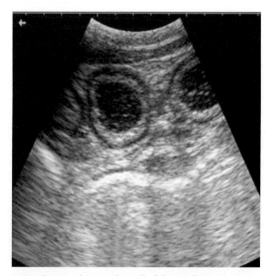

Figure 18-72   Severe edema in the wall of the small intestine in a weanling with diarrhea and hypoproteinemia that was fecal positive by polymerase chain reaction for *Lawsonia intracellularis.*

WHAT TO DO

Lawsonia

- Antibiotic therapy usually is indicated for at least 21 days:
  - Oxytetracycline, 6.6 mg/kg IV q12h or 10 mg/kg IV q24h—the primary and preferred treatment by clinicians, although an invitro sensitivity on swine isolates suggests that macrolides have better activity.
  - **Note:** Serum creatinine should be monitored with tetracycline treatment. **Practice Tip:** *Many Lawsonia foals are dehydrated and because of the low albumin, there is more non-bound/free tetracycline in the plasma, both of which may increase risk of renal failure!*
  - Doxycycline, 10 mg/kg PO q12h or minocycline, 4 mg/kg PO q12h, are the secondary preferred treatment. **Note:** The absorption of doxycycline varies in individual horses but is likely higher in foals than adult horses
  - It is common practice to start treatment with oxytetracycline IV and then switch to doxycycline or minocycline PO.
  - Chloramphenicol, 44 mg/kg PO q6 to 8h
  - Azithromycin, 10mg/kg PO q24h for 5 days then EOD (every other day) with or without rifampin, 5 mg/kg PO q12h.
- Supportive care:
  - Administer IV fluid therapy in cases with severe diarrhea to correct electrolyte imbalances and dehydration (p. 222).
  - For severe hypoproteinemia, consider oncotic support.
    - Hetastarch, Vetstarch or Pentastarch, 7 to 10 mg/kg IV
    - May consider IV plasma, a minimum of 2 L
  - For ulcer prophylaxis, see p. 223.
  - Foals with *Lawsonia* infection and acute severe systemic inflammation should be treated for septic shock as detailed under treatment of systemic inflammation (see Chapter 32, p. 567).

Prognosis

- Prognosis is considered favorable with appropriate therapy in most cases; the physical appearance of the foals may take *months* to improve.
- There are a small number of foals that do not respond to treatment.
- A vaccine approved for swine has been used rectally on farms with endemic disease caused by *Lawsonia*.

Rhodococcus Equi Enterocolitis

- *Rhodococcus equi* may cause diarrhea in foals from approximately 3 weeks of age up to 9 months of age.
  - Infection is of the lymphoid tissue (Peyer's patches) in the intestinal mucosa.
  - May present as insidious onset of diarrhea, often with fever that is persistent.
  - Fever, marked leukocytosis, and high fibrinogen are *not* found as commonly as with *R. equi* pneumonia.
  - Usually one foal is affected at a time, although outbreaks may occur.
- Other organ systems *may* be infected simultaneously.
  - Pulmonary tissue demonstrates pyogranulomatous pneumonia.
  - Lymphoid tissue in the intestinal tract demonstrates ulcerative enterocolitis.

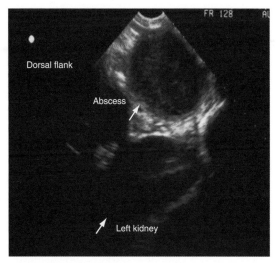

Figure 18-73 Abdominal abscess in the region of the mesenteric root caused by infection with *Rhodococcus equi*.

- Abdominal abscessation is associated with the mesenteric lymph nodes (Fig. 18-73).
- Septic physitis and osteomyelitis can occur.
- Uveitis or synovitis may be noted.

Diagnosis

- If diarrhea is the only syndrome caused by *R. equi*, the diagnosis is more difficult.
- Perform radiography/ultrasonography of the thorax and abdomen to evaluate for changes associated with *R. equi*. Negative results *do not* rule out *R. equi* enteritis.
- Tentative diagnosis is based on ruling out other causes of diarrhea plus the following:
  - Findings show 10^5 organisms per gram of feces or 100 colonies of *R. equi* per plate from a fecal swab.
  - Additionally, the pathogenicity of the organism can be documented based on detecting the presence of virulence-associated antigen plasmids (VapA-P).
  - Many strains of *R. equi* are *not* virulent.
  - Healthy foals frequently have positive fecal cultures for *R. equi*: The combination of high numbers of *R. equi* colonies combined with the presence of VapA-P and other indications of *R. equi* infection (e.g., synovitis) helps guide therapy.

WHAT TO DO

Rhodococcus *Equi* Enterocolitis

- Clarithromycin, 7.5 mg/kg PO q12h, or azithromycin, 10 mg/kg PO q24h for 5 to 10 days, followed by 10 mg/kg q48h; either one is combined with rifampin, 5 mg/kg PO q12.
- Ideally, the rifampin should be given 2 hours after the macrolide treatment to decrease competition for intestinal absorption.
- Fluid therapy and intestinal protectants as for Salmonellosis (see p. 224)

GI:ENT

Prognosis

- Prognosis varies.
- Prognosis is fair to good with appropriate treatment.
- The prognosis worsens if there is concurrent bone infection or abdominal abscessation!
  - *Practice Tip: Foals that have signs of weight loss before the development of diarrhea frequently have abdominal abscessation.*

Antibiotic-Induced Diarrhea

- Antibiotic-induced diarrhea most commonly is associated with the administration of macrolides, or less commonly, trimethoprim-sulfamethoxazole or rifampicin.
  - Foals tend to tolerate macrolides fairly well while nursing, but in transition to a more functional cecum and colon and adult diet, erythromycin, azithromycin, and clarithromycin may cause colic, severe diarrhea, and toxemia in older foals and weanlings.
  - Most antibiotic-associated diarrhea cases occur in the first 2 to 6 days of therapy.
  - A common scenario is that an older foal (>3 months) develops pneumonia and treatment for *R. equi* pneumonia is begun; two days later the foal is colicky, sometimes bloated, toxic (endotoxemic), and has diarrhea.
  - *Practice Tip: Always be sure of the diagnosis of* R. equi *in foals over 3 months of age before beginning macrolide treatments;* R. equi *pneumonia is rare in foals over 4 months of age!*
  - *C. difficile* infection is the cause of the diarrhea in some of the cases. In milder cases, it appears to be more of a dysbiosis.

Clinical Signs

- Abdominal distention and colic generally precede the onset of diarrhea.
- Signs of endotoxemia may be severe.
  - Injected mucous membranes and sclera are evident.
  - Tachycardia and tachypnea are present.
  - Extremities may be cold.

Laboratory Findings

- Nonspecific findings associated with dehydration are as follows:
  - Elevated PCV and serum creatinine
  - Hypochloremia and hyponatremia
- Possibly leukopenia or leukocytosis
  - Neutrophils frequently toxic

Diagnosis

- Submit feces for culture.
  - *Salmonella* spp. and *R. equi*
  - Anaerobic culture
- Submit feces for toxin assays.
  - *C. difficile* and *C. perfringens*

●〉 WHAT TO DO

Antibiotic-Induced Diarrhea

- Provide pain relief:
  - Avoid full-dose flunixin meglumine if possible; use dipyrone, 22 mg/kg IV; butorphanol, 0.05 mg/kg IV or IM; or xylazine, 0.5 to 1.0 mg/kg IV.
    - *Do not* use NSAIDs in excess as right dorsal colitis (RDC) can occur in weanlings although it is *not* nearly as common as in adult horses.
- Provide IV fluids: Plasma-Lyte, Normosol-R, Lactated Ringer's solution; *volume replacement is the most important consideration.*
  - Supplement volume replacement with 20 mEq/L of KCl unless the following are true:
    - The patient is oliguric, the serum creatinine concentration >5 mg/dL, or the serum potassium >5.0 mEq/L.
- Supplement with bicarbonate if the horse is acidotic (pH <7.1) and does *not* respond to initial therapy.
- Treat endotoxemia (see p. 224).
  - Administer plasma, 1 to 2 L IV, to improve hemodynamics.
    - Endotoxin hyperimmune plasma is preferred.
  - Administer flunixin meglumine, 0.25 mg/kg IV q8h if colic present.
- Administer antibiotics:
  - Metronidazole, 15 to 25 mg/kg PO q8h to q12h
  - If no improvement occurs in 3 to 4 days, discontinue oral antibiotics.
- Bacteriotherapy:
  - Bacteriotherapy is transfaunation. The donor intestinal fluid is best if it is taken from the cecum of a horse that is being humanely destroyed for noninfectious causes, is *Salmonella* culture negative, and has a normal appetite (e.g., laminitis case).
  - Fecal collection from the rectum of a healthy, properly dewormed horse would be second best choice.
  - One to 2 L of fluid can be collected from the cecal contents or feces collected from the rectum and placed in a warm balanced electrolyte solution so that 1 to 2 L of fluid can be collected; these can be given via nasogastric tube; once is often sufficient if cecal contents are used.
  - The transfaunation fluid can be kept in a refrigerator (ideally in a glass bottle with air evacuated but with a pressure release valve!) or frozen if there is a several day delay in treatment or if it needs to be repeated.
- Provide supportive care:
  - Ulcer prophylaxis including sucralfate (see p. 223).
  - Intestinal protectants:
    - Treat with di-tri-octahedral smectite (Bio-Sponge)
    - Bismuth subsalicylate

Salmonellosis

●〉 WHAT TO DO

Salmonellosis

- Treat weanlings as you would treat a foal (see p. 223) with Salmonellosis.
- Treat yearlings as you would an adult horse (see p. 235) with salmonellosis.
- Lesions in the colon of a weanling with salmonellosis can be severe, with marked thickening noted on ultrasound exam (Fig. 18-74).

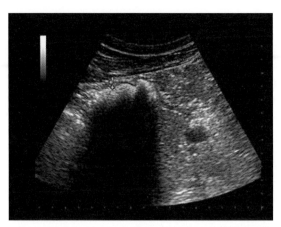

Figure 18-74 Marked thickening of the colon in a 6-month-old Thoroughbred filly that did *not* survive *Salmonella* diarrhea in spite of intensive therapy, including parenteral nutrition.

Other Causes of Diarrhea in Weanlings

- *Neorickettsia risticii:*
  - There are no studies to confirm the frequency of Potomac horse fever in weanlings.
  - The diagnosis and treatment are the same as in adult horses (see the following).
- *Listeria* species:
  - This bacterium is a sporadic cause of diarrhea in nursing up to weanling foals.
  - In younger foals, bacteremia and shock may occur, whereas in older foals the disease does not appear to be as severe.
  - Treat with penicillin 22,000 units/kg IV q6h.
  - Supportive intestinal treatments are recommended.
- *Brachyspira pilosicoli:*
  - This is an uncommon cause of diarrhea (mostly chronic) in weanlings.
  - The anaerobic bacteria damage the brush border of the colon causing diarrhea. Infection may occur from contaminated water.
  - Diagnosis includes ruling out other more common causes, histologic finding on postmortem samples, and fecal PCR testing.
  - Treatment is metronidazole, 15 to 20 mg/kg PO q8h.
- Parasites:
  - Acute heavy infection with *Parascaris equorum* or *Strongylus* spp. may cause diarrhea but diarhea is uncommon with even heavy infection from these parasites!
    - Unthriftiness and colic are the more common clinical signs.
    - In yearlings, weight loss and protein-losing enteropathy may occur.

Acute Infectious and Toxic Diarrheal Diseases in the Adult Horse

J. Barry David and Thomas J. Divers

- Acute diarrhea in the adult horse often presents as a medical emergency.

- The horse sometimes exhibits signs of abdominal pain, which may initially be difficult to differentiate from a surgical colic.
- A complete history and physical examination including abdominal ultrasound examination and analysis of the laboratory measurements of a CBC and serum chemistry are important in the workup of a horse with acute colitis.

Presentation

- Abdominal pain, lethargy, and fever are common signs that may precede the production of diarrhea in adult horses with colitis.
- Occasionally, the patient may present with a colonic impaction and fever.
- ***Practice Tip:*** *Acute infectious diarrhea in adult horses is considered a medical emergency.*
- Elevations of heart and respiratory rates are common, as is the appearance of dark or injected mucous membranes accompanied by the typical signs of dehydration.
- The findings of abdominal auscultation generally are those of hypomotility, decreased frequency and intensity of borborygmi or an increase in gas/fluid interface sounds.
- ***Practice Tip:*** *Any form of colitis may result in laminitis.*

Causes of Acute Colitis in Adult Horses

Potomac Horse Fever (PHF)

- *Neorickettsia risticii* infection
- A common cause of fever in endemic areas with approximately 20% of cases developing diarrhea and/or laminitis
- Seasonal occurrence in endemic areas—more common in June to November in the Northeast, North Central, and Mid-Atlantic regions of North America. It also causes disease in some South American countries.
- Infection may occur in pastured or stabled horses.
  - In pastured horses, infection may result from *N. risticii*–infected trematodes (cercariae) of fresh water snails released into water or in the pasture near a wet area (as snail slime trails).
  - This may be especially common during hot weather and may occur during droughts as wet areas in the pasture concentrate both the available grass and either snails or especially aquatic insects, which may have ingested the *N. risticii*–infected metacercariae, that die in the pasture.
  - These aquatic insects are responsible for transporting *N. risticii* to feed buckets when they are attracted to light in the stables at night.
- After infection, presumably by ingestion, infected horses may become febrile within 1 to 3 days. This fever often goes unnoticed and most horses never show clinical signs.
- Approximately 20% of horses a second fever, leukopenia, toxemia, and sometimes diarrhea develop 5 to 7 days later as the organism moves from the blood to the colon (trophism) and causes colitis.
- No stress factors are required for this cause of colitis.
- Vaccine efficacy is in question because there appear to be a number of strains of this intracellular bacteria.

- Clinical signs are often indistinguishable from *Salmonella* spp.
- ***Practice Tip:*** *Except for more pronounced colic with both right dorsal colitis and blister beetle toxicity, most causes of acute colitis in horses have a similar clinical and clinical pathology presentation.*
- ***Important:*** Laminitis appears to be more commonly associated with PHF than other causes of colitis.
  - Laminitis may occur with only fever and protein-losing enteropathy without diarrhea in some PHF cases!

Diagnosis and treatment for all causes of colitis are listed on pp. 233-237.

Salmonellosis

- May be associated with stress
- 1% to 5% carriers in most studies
  - Closer to 1% except for colic cases
- Other risk factors for disease include:
  - Off feed, abdominal surgery
  - Housed on large brood mare farms
  - Antibiotics (both oral and systemic)
- Dose and gastric pH are also important in determining disease risk
- Virulence of serovar seems to be of some importance in determining disease; *S. typhimurium, S. agona,* and *S. newport* seem to be especially prominent causes of clinical diarrhea in the horse although many other serovars have caused salmonellosis in horses. There is *no* recognized correlation between multi-drug resistant (MDR) strains (i.e., DT-104) and virulence.
- Rarely bloody diarrhea
- May be a farm problem
  - It is *not* unusual to have a farm problem involving mostly foals or mostly adults.
  - One age group is clinically ill while the accompanying foal or mare is culture positive and often not ill.

Diagnosis and treatment for all causes of colitis are listed on pp. 233-237 .

NSAID Toxicity

- Phenylbutazone and flunixin meglumine have been implicated in causing the disease.
  - The drugs *may* have been administered in appropriate dosages to uniquely sensitive or dehydrated horses and ponies or may have been overdosed.
- Phenylbutazone is generally considered to have the highest tendency to create GI problems but flunixin may pose an equal risk.
- NSAIDs may cause the problem when administered orally or intravenously.
- Patients typically develop *hypoproteinemia* as a result of *hypoalbuminemia* early in the course of the disease. ***Note:*** It would be difficult to diagnosis RDC in a horse unless the plasma protein is low.
- The most severe form of the disease affects the right dorsal colon and the diarrheal/colic disease associated with

NSAIDs is often referred to as right dorsal colitis (RDC). The mechanism for this is unknown.

Diagnosis and treatments are listed on pp. 233-237.

Cyathostomiasis

- Occurs most commonly in yearlings or young adults
- Generally poor body condition patients with a questionable history of parasite control
- Most commonly occurs in October through April
- Often insidious in onset of diarrhea without fever or may occur after deworming

Diagnosis and treatment are listed on pp. 233, 234.

Antibiotic-Associated Colitis

- Illness generally occurs 2 to 6 days after start of antibiotic administration.
  - Almost any antibiotic can cause the problem; there may be some differences based on geographic location: ceftiofur (both Naxcel and Exceed), trimethoprim-sulfamethoxazole, oral penicillin V, Quartermaster in the guttural pouch, macrolides (especially when given to horses >4 months of age), rifampicin, and less commonly oxytetracycline/doxycycline, and enrofloxacin.
- Decreased roughage consumption and switching from intravenous to orally administered antibiotics may predispose the patient to antibiotic-associated colitis.
- Illness is believed to result from the death of beneficial GI flora, allowing an overgrowth of toxigenic *C. difficile* and/or *C. perfringens,* or in many cases, a dysbiosis (change in normal intestinal flora). Horses with dysbiosis without clostridiosis are generally *not* as sick but may be totally inappetent.

Diagnosis and treatments are listed on pp. 233-237.

Colitis X

- Acute colitis and associated endotoxemia and anaphylaxis may have multiple causes including anaphylaxis, acute clostridiosis, or rapid overgrowth of other pathogenic bacteria such as some strains of *E. coli, Proteus* spp., *Enterococcus* spp., and/or *Pseudomonas* spp.
- Colon wall edema is a characteristic finding and sometimes hemorrhagic regions are noted during postmortem examination.
- Aerobic and anaerobic cultures should be performed.

Coronavirus

- There have been several outbreaks of beta coronavirus-associated fever; leukopenia; anorexia; and sometimes, diarrhea or colic in adult horses.
- The incidence of diarrhea in horses is approximately 20%. On one farm, nine horses were infected—all with fever, anorexia, and leukopenia but no clinical diarrhea.
- The degree of anorexia is marked in many cases.
- Diagnosis is based on PCR-positive coronavirus feces and ruling out other causes.
- Nasal swabs do *not* detect coronavirus-infected horses. The PCR testing can be performed by IDEXX (diarrhea

panel) or other molecular laboratories such as U.C. Davis or Cornell University Diagnostic Laboratory that have experience in testing horses for the virus.

- Treatment is generally supportive and prognosis is good.
- Coronavirus is highly contagious in horses; quarantine for 2 weeks is recommended plus fecal PCR testing.

General Diagnostic Tests for Adult Colitis

- Perform a complete physical examination: a horse presenting with acute abdominal pain and fever is likely to have an early case of colitis or, less likely, peritonitis.
- Obtain a detailed history, including vaccinations, deworming, antibiotic administration, NSAID use, the presence of other clinical cases of diarrhea on the farm, previous cases of salmonellosis and PHF on the farm, types of feeds and changes in the feeding program, and the duration of the signs.
- Most cases of *C. difficile* colitis occur 2 to 5 days after starting antibiotic treatment. Antibiotic dybiosis can occur almost immediately after beginning antibiotics.
- Isolate the patient from herd mates until the results of fecal diagnostics are known and/or the clinical signs have resolved.
- Perform general diagnostic tests for acute colitis:
  - Whole blood and serum for a CBC, serum chemistry, and other diagnostic analyses.
  - Ancillary stall-side tests may include serum lactate, electrolytes, creatinine, and blood gas with ionized calcium.
  - If you are located in an endemic area of PHF, submit serum samples for serologic testing and whole blood for PCR. Whole blood PCR is most useful in the early stages of the disease.
  - If coronavirus is suspected, fecal PCR testing is recommended.
  - Submit fecal cultures for *Salmonella* spp.
  - Submit fecal samples for detection of clostridial diseases (toxin assays): Tox A and B for *C. difficile* and enterotoxin and beta-2 toxin gene for *C. perfringens* type A.[31]
- Abdominal ultrasonography should be performed.
  - Edema or thickness of the bowel wall may be visualized in some cases, especially in horses with NSAID toxicity (RDC) (Fig. 18-75 and 18-76, *B*). The right dorsal colon can usually be identified between the 11th to 13th intercostal spaces against the liver, duodenum, dorsal to the right ventral colon, which has increased numbers of sacculations.
  - With RDC, the hypoechoic layer is bordered by a hyperechoic layer on both the serosal and mucosal sides and the thickened hypoechoic layer is less echogenic than liver. The thickness of the hypoechoic layer is usually 50% to 75% of total mural thickness of the right dorsal colon.
  - Frequently, ingesta of a nearly homogeneous fluid nature are observed swirling in the large colon (Fig. 18-76) of horses with colitis. Normal colonic sacculations with an air interface are lost.

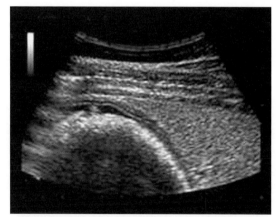

Figure 18-75 Ultrasound examination of the right abdomen at midlevel of an adult horse with right dorsal colitis demonstrates marked edema of the colon wall. The liver is to the right.

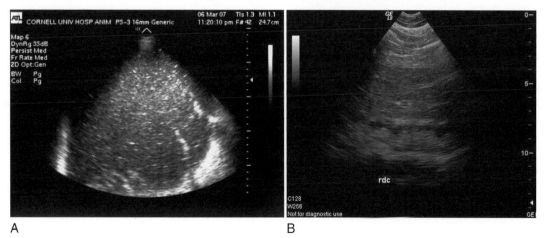

A   B

Figure 18-76 **A,** Homogeneous appearing, fluid-filled large intestine seen on an ultrasound examination of a horse that developed diarrhea 4 hours later. **B,** Edema of the right dorsal colon associated with an overdose of phenylbutazone in a 2-year-old Thoroughbred filly.

[31]Department of Veterinary Science and Microbiology, University of Arizona, Tucson, Arizona.

- Palpation per rectum is not generally needed, unless the horse is distended and/or is painful. In fact, palpation may initiate rectal prolapse in some colitis cases.
  - Edema or thickness of the colon wall may be appreciated.
  - Early in the course of disease mild to moderate impaction may be part of the clinical presentation.
- Abdominocentesis is not routine for colitis cases because it may enhance the formation of ventral edema sometimes leading to scrotal cellulitis in stallions. Perform *only* if peritonitis is suspected.
  - Elevated protein is typical in peritoneal fluid samples from horses with colitis.
- Routine blood work includes the following:
  - CBC
    - Leukopenia with toxic appearing neutrophils is commonly seen.
  - Serum chemistry panel
    - Hyponatremia, hypochloremia, and azotemia are common findings in acute cases.
    - Hypoproteinemia and hypoalbuminemia are manifestations of significant disease.
    - Hyperammonemia (overproduction of ammonia in the gut) may sporadically occur with any of the infectious causes of diarrhea.
  - Use serial serum lactate concentration as a prognostic indicator.
    - Look for at least a 30% reduction in 4 to 8 hours or a 50% reduction in 24 hours after initiation of treatment for an improved prognosis.

Laboratory Testing for Specific Diseases

Potomac Horse Fever

- An (IFA) titer >1:640 is somewhat diagnostic in an unvaccinated individual; >1:2560 is often diagnostic in a vaccinated individual.[32] Sensitivity and specificity of these numbers are unproven.
- Remember that values may be low in an acute case, as seroconversion may occur later in the course of the disease.
- Potomac horse fever PCR requires a whole blood sample (EDTA tube) shipped on ice overnight to one of several laboratories in the country. The PCR may be negative in many cases as the organism has moved from the blood to the colon.
  - The PCR is available at Cornell Diagnostic Laboratory, University of California—Davis, University of Connecticut, and other laboratories

Salmonella

- *Salmonella* spp. fecal cultures generally are performed in multiple cultures (3 to 5 days in a row).
  - Do *not* refrigerate samples; transport them in selenite or Ames transport media.
  - If samples are cultured in-house, use selective media.
  - Positive culture provides species for basic epidemiologic studies and the capability to perform antibiotic sensitivity studies.
  - *Citrobacter* spp. in the feces may require extra steps of testing to differentiate from salmonella.
- Serotype data, antimicrobial resistance patterns, and Pulse-Field-Gel-Electrophoresis (PFGE) can be used to determine epidemiology of an outbreak.
- *Salmonellae* spp. PCR testing is available through an Enhanced Rapid Test System (Reveal 2.0 *Salmonella* test system[33]) for the detection of *Salmonella* spp. A culture would need to be performed to determine antibiogram.
  - PCR is performed on suspicious cultures (black or green colonies noted on Hektoen agar).
  - This testing is especially useful during outbreaks for both early detection of infected horses and environmental culturing and quickly separates *Salmonella* and *Citrobacter* spp.

Clostridiosis

- Clostridial disease frequently is implicated as the causative agent of antibiotic-induced colitis.
- Gram stain on direct fecal smear may show an overwhelming number of gram-positive rods, which may be *indicative* of clostridial colitis although sensitivity of the Gram stain is likely low.
- The definitive diagnosis of *C. difficile* requires identification of the presence of clostridial toxins in the feces.
- A commercial ELISA assay for toxins A and B has been studied and is considered reliable and adequate for use in the horse.[34]
- For the diagnosis of *C. perfringens,* pure growth in anaerobic fecal culture is considered *suggestive* that the organism is the cause of disease.
  - Commercial enterotoxin assay is available (see p. 222) and is required for a more definitive diagnosis.
    - Because the toxin is considered labile, the assay must be performed within a half-hour of collection of fresh manure or the manure sample must be frozen within a half-hour and kept frozen until testing. PCR testing is also available at some laboratories.

NSAID-Induced Colitis

- Ultrasonography of the abdominal cavity *may* demonstrate bowel wall edema of the right dorsal colon (see Fig. 18-75). The thickness of the RDC may vary from dramatic to subtle. There is a commercial fecal test for albumin loss (SUCCEED Equine Fecal Blood Test[35]), but sensitivity/specificity data from independent scientific publications are needed.

Cyathostomiasis

- Fecal test for parasites is generally recommended but seldom reveals a cause for the diarrhea. Identifying

---

[32]There may be an increase in control (background) IFA values in recent years, and it is possible that the titers have lost accuracy in confirming a diagnosis.

[33]Neogen (Lansing, Michigan 48912).
[34]Tox A/B test (Techlab, Blacksburg, Virginia).
[35]SUCCEED Equine Fecal Blood Test (Freedom Health, LLC, Aurora, Ohio).

cyathostome larvae on a rectal mucosal biopsy or appearance of the adults in the manure is supportive of cyathostomiasis.

Coronavirus
- Feces should be submitted for PCR testing at a laboratory that is experienced in the testing (e.g., U.C.-Davis, Cornell diagnostic laboratory, or other locations).

●❯ WHAT TO DO

General Therapy for Colitis, Regardless of the Cause
- Crystalloid fluids: the hallmark of therapy
  - Plasma-Lyte, Normosol-R, and lactated Ringer's solution are preferred in most cases.
    - KCl, 20 to 40 mEq added to each liter: the *safe* rate of KCl administration is 0.5 mEq/kg/h.
    - Most horses with diarrhea are expected to have a total body decrease in potassium regardless of the plasma K^+ concentration. If the plasma K^+ is above 6 meq/L, this could be an indication of acute renal failure.
- Hypertonic saline, 4 mL/kg IV bolus for hypovolemic shock
  - Follow the administration of hypertonic saline immediately with crystalloid therapy in a 10:1 ratio; 10 L crystalloid for each liter of hypertonic saline.
  - Sodium bicarbonate: Use *only* if the patient is severely acidotic (pH <7.1) and hypertonic saline followed by large volume lactated Ringer's or Plasmalyte have *not* corrected the metabolic acidosis but the L-lactate is decreasing. This scenario could indicate an intestinal overproduction of D-lactate.
- Treat endotoxemia:
  - Plasma: Administer a minimum of 2 L.
    - Plasma contains several opsonins such as fibronectin and antithrombin III, in addition to antibodies.
    - Hyperimmune plasma from horses exposed to endotoxin is preferred.
  - Plasma also provides oncotic support if the patient is hypoproteinemic.
  - Flunixin meglumine, 0.25 mg/kg IV q8h—*except in cases of RDC.*
    - Continue administration until signs of endotoxemia are alleviated.
  - Pentoxifylline, 10 mg/kg PO or IV q12h
    - Shown in vivo to decrease cytokine production during endotoxin challenge (if given before endotoxin challenge) and protects against multiple organ injury
    - May cause red blood cells to be more deformable
  - Polymyxin B sulfate, 6000 units/kg IV q12h if renal function is normal
    - Considered to directly bind endotoxin and may provide an initial notable clinical response.
  - Clopidogrel (Plavix), 4 mg/kg PO q24h on day 1 and 2 mg/kg PO q24h on subsequent treatments may inhibit platelet activation and may decrease the likelihood of laminitis and colon and jugular venous thrombosis; the absorption of the drug in horses with colitis is unknown.
- Treatment of hypoproteinemia:
  - Plasma: A significant amount of plasma is required to increase plasma oncotic pressure.
  - Hydroxyethyl starch (Hetastarch, VetStarch or Pentastarch), 5 to 10 mL/kg IV
    - Increases colloid oncotic pressure
    - Synthetic colloid may "plug" leaky endothelial cell gaps
    - May assist in reducing bowel wall edema

- Intravenous multiple B-vitamins can be given daily but must be administered slowly.
- Intestinal protectants should be administered in most cases.
  - Di-tri-octahedral smectite (Bio-Sponge[36]) is most commonly used for clostridial diarrhea. Bismuth subsalicylate and/or activated charcoal may be beneficial.
- Unless patient is clinically painful, provide free-choice water and offer an additional electrolyte bucket:
  - Add a commercial electrolyte mixture per label directions, *or*
  - Add to each 1 to 2 L of water the following:
    - 30 mL of 50% dextrose
    - 12 g baking soda
    - 10 g KCl
- *Prophylaxis for laminitis*: cryotherapy is the *only* proven method of prevention. This can be performed using 5-L fluid bags attached to the feet and/or commercially available boots that fit over the coronary band; both filled with *crushed* ice slurry (see Chapter 43, p. 712). The top of the bag can be taped to the fetlock area using Elasticon or duct tape. For horses with larger feet or those that "walk out" of the 5-L fluid bags, commercial boots can be purchased and filled with *crushed* ice slurry.
- Provide a highly digestible fiber (low-residue) feed, if possible, particularly with NSAID toxicity.
  - A complete pelleted ration with the addition of 1 to 2 oz of dietary linseed or corn oil is an option.
  - Most importantly, keep the horse eating unless bloated, gastric reflux, or "colicy."
  - Offer the horse pasture/grass, if available.
- Minimize risk of thrombophlebitis:
  - Use polyurethane catheters.
  - Sample blood from vessels other than the jugular veins.
  - Monitor catheter site frequently; alternate catheter sites.
- Prevent exposure to other horses; isolate the patient if possible.
- Wrap tail; use caution to not wrap the tail too tight. *Do not* use Vetwrap.

●❯ WHAT TO DO

Specific Treatments for Adult Colitis
Salmonellosis
- Administration of antibiotics is of questionable clinical benefit in adult horses. Although no evidence indicates that they help this condition, most clinicians prefer parenteral administration; there can be translocation of other organisms from the diseased intestine.
- If possible, choose antibiotic based on fecal culture and sensitivity report.
- Risks associated with antibiotic use include the following:
  - Fungal pneumonia and colitis, further dysbiosis
  - Nephrotoxicity associated with aminoglycosides and decreased renal blood flow because of hypovolemia and endotoxemia
  - Outcome in adult horse salmonellosis does not appear to be affected by antibiotic use. Enrofloxacin, 7.5 mg/kg IV q24h is frequently used.

Potomac Horse Fever
- Oxytetracycline, 6.6 mg/kg IV q12h or 10 mg/kg IV q24h
  - **Caution:** May be nephrotoxic in dehydrated horses!
- Better prognosis when administered early in the course of the disease.

[36]Bio-Sponge (Platinum Performance, 90 Thomas Road, PO Box 990, Buellton, California 93427).

Antibiotic-Associated Colitis
- Metronidazole, 15 to 25 mg/kg PO q6 to 8h; it is very rare for metronidazole to cause diarrhea
  - Improvement should occur within 3 days; consider discontinuing antibiotic therapy if clinical improvement is not seen.
- Di-tri-octahedral smectite (Bio-Sponge), generally 3 lb administered by nasogastric tube 2 to 3 times, 8 hours apart.
- Administer commercial plasma with antibodies targeting *Clostridium difficile* toxins.
- Bacteriotherapy using the cecal contents of healthy recently euthanized horses has caused a marked improvement in horses with antibiotic-induced diarrhea; the feces returning to normal "overnight"; one treatment is often sufficient. Fecal transfaunation can be performed if cecal contents are not available, but it does not seem as successful as a cecal transfaunation. This treatment is recommended for either clostridial diarrhea or dybiosis.

NSAID Toxicity
- Plasma: 4 to 8 L IV
- Hetastarch, VetStarch, or Pentastarch: 7 to 10 mL/kg IV
- Sucralfate: 22 mg/kg PO q6 to12 to 24h
- Misoprostol: 2 to 4 µg/kg PO q12h to q24h
  - Mild diarrhea, increased rectal temperature, and mild colic have been reported after administration.
  - The drug is associated with abortion. ***Do not* use misoprostol in the pregnant mare, and it must *not* be handled by pregnant women!**

Cyathostomiasis
- Moxidectin[37]: 400 to 500 µg/kg PO once, along with dexamethasone 0.04 mg/kg IV or IM q24h for 3 days
- Fenbendazole: 10 mg/kg PO q24h for 5 successive days is frequently used but efficacy is questionable.
- Corticosteroids used in combination with moxidectin may improve recovery.

Coronavirus
- No specific treatment

>> WHAT TO DO

Abdominal Pain Associated with Acute Colitis
- Rule out obstructive GI tract disease:
  - Nasogastric intubation: evaluate for gastric reflux.
  - Abdominal ultrasonography
  - Abdominocentesis and palpation per rectum if colitis is not the obvious diagnosis
- Treat ileus:
  - Calcium borogluconate 23%: 500 mL added to 10 L of crystalloid fluids
  - Lidocaine: 1.3 mg/kg as a slow IV bolus followed by a constant rate infusion of 0.05 mg/kg/min

Analgesics
- NSAIDs: Flunixin meglumine and possibly ketoprofen *initially* at the recommended full dose, except in cases of NSAID-induced colitis.
  - Firocoxib (0.09 mg/kg IV) is the safest selection for NSAID use in horses with colitis; however, even COX-2 specific inhibitors may slow healing of the damaged bowel. If firocoxib is used to control pain in horses with colitis, a low dose (0.3 mg/kg) of flunixin may be added to the treatment to inhibit thromboxane.

[37]Moxidectin (American Cyanamid, Wayne, New Jersey).

- It is generally recommended to decrease the dosage of NSAIDs early in the treatment of the infectious diarrheal disease to protect the GI mucosa. There is no evidence that NSAID use prevents laminitis in these cases.
  - Concurrent treatment with lidocaine CRI and flunixin meglumine is reported to lessen the negative effects of NSAIDs on bowel healing.
- Sedatives: xylazine, detomidine, and butorphanol may be used on a short-term basis.
- If the patient is distended because of colonic gas and remains nonresponsive to standard analgesic regimens, consider the following:
  - Cecal or colonic decompression (see p. 160) if "ping" is present in right dorsal abdomen (cecal) or marked gas distention of the colon is found on rectal examination
  - Neostigmine, 0.005 to 0.01 mg/kg SQ q1h, for 3 to 5 treatments to stimulate colonic motility
  - Chloral hydrate for narcosis and as a last resort to control the "colicky" horse, administered to effect, generally 30 to 60 mg/kg IV.
  - Butylscopolammonium bromide (Buscopan, 0.3 mg/kg IV) decreases pain associated with intestinal distention but inhibition of motility and delayed passage of the soft feces may worsen ileus and toxemia.

Prognosis for Acute Colitis in Adult Horses
- The prognosis for acute colitis in adult horses is variable.
- Factors that worsen the prognosis include the development of laminitis, renal failure, and systemic inflammatory response syndrome.
- The prognosis for a performance horse is considered poor if laminitis occurs and is not markedly improved after 3 days of treatment.
- The presence of scant, watery diarrhea for more than 24 hours and purple mucous membranes indicate a less favorable prognosis.
- Patients with a PCV >65% or refractory erythrocytosis may recover but often fail to gain weight, founder, or cascade into renal failure.
- The majority of cases are azotemic, which is generally a prerenal cause.
- The patient's serum creatinine concentration and serum potassium concentration should move rapidly toward the normal range within the first 36 hours of fluid therapy or primary renal failure should be considered.
- If blood lactate and cTn-I concentrations do not decrease after resuscitation therapy, the prognosis is guarded.
- If urine production is *not* seen after the administration of several liters of intravenous fluids or after the administration of 2 L of hypertonic saline and the serum potassium concentration is >5.5 mg/L, the patient is likely in acute renal failure (see Chapter 26, p. 489).
- The prognosis for acute renal failure is fair if the patient becomes polyuric with continued intravenous fluid administration.

Toxic Causes of Acute Colitis/Diarrhea in Horses
- There are many causes of acute diarrhea and most cause additional clinical signs other than diarrhea:

- Ionophore toxicity (see Chapter 34, p. 602)
- Hoary alyssum (see Chapter 34, p. 600)
- Clover poisoning (see Chapter 34, p. 604)
- Sand or gravel ingestion (see p. 204)
- Anaphylaxis (see Appendix 4, p. 814)
- Endotoxemia (see p. 235)
- Acute grain overload (see p. 184)
- Dietary changes and excitement may also cause acute diarrhea; however, these horses are generally *not* ill.
- Perhaps the most severe toxin affecting the horse's intestinal tract causing both colic and diarrhea is blister beetle poisoning.

Cantharidin Intoxication (Blister Beetle Poisoning)
Presentation
- Elevated heart rate and respiratory rate are associated with the most common clinical sign of abdominal pain.
- The severity of the signs is directly related to the degree and duration of intoxication.
- Oral ulcers/erosions are frequently noted; the horse may appear to play in the water.
- Horses experiencing cantharidin intoxication are typically anorexic, lethargic, and may exhibit signs of urinary tract dysfunction such as pollakiuria, hematuria, and stranguria.
- Signs associated with profound hypocalcemia include a stiff, stilted gait and thumps (synchronous diaphragmatic flutter).
- Severe cases may have neurologic signs or acutely die.

Cause
- Cantharidin is a toxin found in the hemolymph and gonads of the male *Epicauta* spp. beetles (Fig. 18-77).
- The beetles are most common in the Southwest, and they swarm in alfalfa fields when mating in mid- to late summer.
- Modern hay harvesting methods of cutting and crimping hay in a single pass kills swarms of beetles.
- Cantharidin creates mucosal lesions throughout the GI tract, and it is rapidly excreted by the kidneys, which in turn leads to renal parenchymal damage and hemorrhagic cystitis.
- Myocardial damage occurs by an unknown mechanism.
- ***Practice Tip:*** *As few as 5 to 10 beetles may be fatal to a horse.*

⏩ WHAT TO DO

Blister Beetle Intoxication
- Supportive treatment:
  - Provide pain relief
    - Flunixin meglumine, 1.1 mg/kg IV q12h
    - Butorphanol, 0.04 to 0.1 mg/kg IV or IM or consider a constant rate infusion of butorphanol or lidocaine
  - Evacuate GI tract:
    - Mineral oil by nasogastric intubation provides laxative effects and binds the lipid-soluble toxin; but recent work suggests it also increases absorption and toxicity. Therefore,

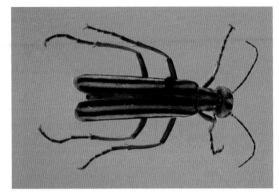

Figure 18-77   Three-striped blister beetle. (Courtesy Dr. David Schmitz, Texas A&M College of Veterinary Medicine.)

administration of activated charcoal or smectite in addition to magnesium sulfate would seem more appropriate.
- Establish diuresis and base choice of fluids on serum chemistry results and urine production.
  - Cases are frequently hypocalcemic and hypomagnesemic.
    - Administer 500 mL of 23% calcium borogluconate diluted in 5 to 10 L of intravenous fluids.
    - Administer 5 to 10 g of magnesium sulfate diluted in fluids.
- Administer anti-inflammatory agents:
  - Dexamethasone, 0.1 to 0.2 mg/kg IV once
- Provide ulcer prophylaxis:
  - Sucralfate 20 mg/kg PO q6 to 12h and
  - Ranitidine, 6.6 mg/kg PO q8h
    or
  - Omeprazole 4 mg/kg PO q24h
- Administer broad-spectrum antibiotics:
  - Avoid aminoglycosides and sulfonamides

Diagnosis
- Submit several hundred milliliters of stomach contents and urine to Texas Veterinary Medical Diagnostic Lab, College Station, Texas, or other labs that assay the toxin.
- Examine hay for the presence of *Epicauta* spp.
- Submit GI contents and kidneys from postmortem samples.

Prognosis
- The prognosis for cantharidin intoxication is considered guarded in most cases.
- Clinicopathologic findings that worsen the prognosis include:
  - Azotemia
  - *Markedly* elevated cardiac troponin I (cTn-I) concentrations or concentrations that do not decrease with therapy
- The risk of intoxication can be reduced by feeding only alfalfa hay harvested before June (first cutting). **Important:** Storing or pelleting hay *does not* denature cantharidin.
- Client education for those producing their own hay is essential to minimizing exposure to blister beetles.

References
References can be found on the companion website at www.equine-emergencies.com.

GI:ENT

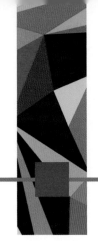

CHAPTER 19

Integumentary System: Wound Healing, Management, and Reconstruction

Christine L. Theoret and Ted S. Stashak

The Skin
Anatomy
- The skin is the largest and one of the most important organ systems.
- The primary function is to protect against wear and bacterial invasion and to maintain homeostasis of the underlying structures via thermal regulation and the prevention of water loss.
- The average thickness of the skin is 3.8 mm.
- The skin is derived from two embryonic germ layers:
  - Epidermis, from ectoderm, has the ability to regenerate.
  - Dermis (corium), from mesoderm, cannot completely regenerate.
- *Practice Tip: Cleavage lines: Langer's lines of tension are parallel to the long axis of the limbs, head, and torso but are perpendicular to the long axis of the neck and flank. Wounds parallel to these cleavage lines heal best.*
- Skin is nourished by two types of blood vessels:
  - Musculocutaneous vessels, which perforate the body of underlying muscle
  - Direct cutaneous arteries, which reach the skin by passing between muscle bodies
- In horses with loose-fitting skin, the direct cutaneous vessels predominate. They run subdermally, in association with the *panniculus* muscle, parallel to the skin surface. Smaller vessels branch off these cutaneous arteries and arborize within the dermis to supply it and the adnexal structures of the skin by forming three closely interconnected plexuses:
  - The deep subcutaneous plexus
  - The middle cutaneous plexus
  - The superficial subpapillary plexus

Epidermis
- Epidermis is made up of five stratified squamous cell layers (Fig. 19-1).
  - Stratum *basale* (base layer) has two nucleated cell types:
    - Keratinocytes constantly reproduce and push upward toward the surface to replace cells that have sloughed off the surface.
    - Melanocytes are responsible for producing the melanin that gives hair and skin their color.

- Stratum *spinosum* (prickle-cell layer): Cells in this layer are nucleated and become activated to reproduce when the outer epidermal layers are stripped off.
- Stratum *granulosum* (granular cell layer): The cells in this layer are in the process of dying, with nuclei that are shrinking and undergoing chromatolysis.
- Stratum *lucidum* (clear cell layer): This layer is composed of nonnucleated keratinized cells and is only present in hairless areas of the body.
- Stratum *corneum* (horny cell layer): This layer is composed of fully keratinized dead cells that are constantly being shed from the surface as scales. This layer forms a barrier that protects the underlying tissue from irritation, bacterial invasion, and noxious substances, as well as from fluid and electrolyte losses.
- Nourishment is by diffusion of fluids from the capillary beds in the dermis.

Dermis
- Dermis is made up of two main layers:
  - The papillary layer lies below the epidermis.
  - The reticular layer extends from the papillary layer to the subcutaneous tissue.
- It contains a rich supply of blood vessels, lymphatic vessels, hair follicles, sebaceous and apocrine sweat glands, and sensory nerve endings (Fig. 19-2).
- Fiber types include collagenous, reticular, and elastic.
- Cell types include fibroblasts, histiocytes, and mast cells.

Wound Repair
- There are three phases (Fig. 19-3):
  - Acute inflammation
  - Repair or proliferative phase
  - Maturation or remodeling phase

Acute Inflammatory Phase
- Acute response is proportional to the severity of the injury.
- The objective of inflammation is to cleanse the wound and amplify the subsequent repair phase.
- Inflammation is characterized by vascular and cellular responses that protect the body against excessive blood loss and invasion by foreign substances.

- Factors affecting duration of the inflammatory response are the following:
  - Degree of trauma
  - Nature of injury
  - Presence of foreign substances
  - Infection
- Vascular response consists of immediate yet temporary vasoconstriction followed by longer-lasting vasodilation

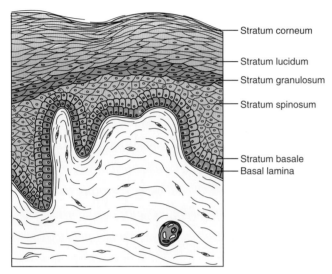

Figure 19-1 The layers of the epidermis. (Modified from Stashak TS. In Jennings PB, editor: *The practice of large animal surgery,* Philadelphia, 1984, Saunders.)

that promotes the passage of cells, fluids, and protein into the wound space.

- Cellular response involves principally the platelet and inflammatory leukocytes.
  - Platelets aggregate to form a clot that seals the wound to prevent further bleeding and functions as a scaffold for the migration of inflammatory and mesenchymal cells. Finally, the clot dehydrates superficially to form a scab, which acts like a bandage to protect the wound from external contamination.
  - Platelets also promote inflammation via the release of potent chemoattractants and mitogens that serve as signals to initiate and amplify the repair phase. Cytokines secreted from platelets also mobilize phagocytic cells, antibodies, and complement; the latter provide an immune response.
  - Leukocytes (mainly neutrophils and monocytes) are recruited to the site of injury by vasoactive mediators and chemoattractants released during the vascular response.
    - Neutrophils act as first line of defense by destroying debris and bacteria through phagocytosis and subsequent enzymatic and oxygen-radical mechanisms.
    - Neutrophils aid mononuclear cells in further breakdown of dead tissues via the release of degradative proteinases.
    - Monocytes differentiate into macrophages upon entering the wound; they phagocytize debris and bacteria via mechanisms similar to those used by the neutrophil.

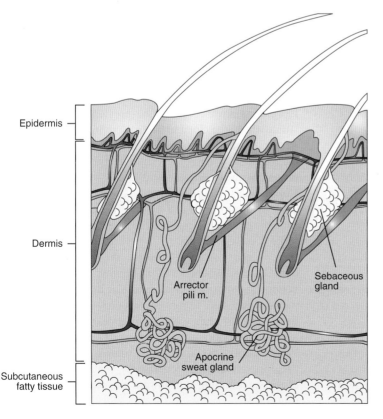

Figure 19-2 The epidermal and dermal layers of the skin. Dermal adnexa also are illustrated.

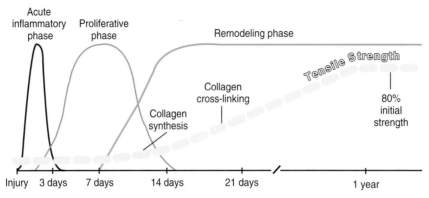

Figure 19-3   Generic temporal profile of synchronized phases and gain in tensile strength of tissue repair process in mammals; superimposed profile specific to healing of skin wounds in the horse limb. (Modified from Theoret CL: *Clinical Techniques in Equine Practice,* 3:110-122, 2004.)

- ○ Important functions of the monocyte include the production of cytokines and growth factors essential to the recruitment and proliferation of mesenchymal cells. In this manner, the activated macrophage participates not only in debridement but also in the subsequent phase of repair, via the induction of angiogenesis, fibroplasia, and epithelialization.
- Although inflammation is essential to the normal outcome of wound repair, perpetuation of this response (as can be the case in limb wounds of horses) may contribute to the pathogenesis of diseases characterized by excessive fibrosis or scarring.

●〉 WHAT TO DO

Acute Inflammatory Phase
- Clinicians have the greatest influence on this phase: proper surgical debridement and wound irrigation, good hemostasis, and adequate drainage can greatly hasten wound healing.

Repair Phase
- The provisional clot from the acute phase is replaced by granulation tissue during this phase.
- Granulation tissue is formed by three elements that move into the wound space simultaneously: macrophages, fibroblasts, and new blood vessels.
- Granulation tissue formation in an open wound is beneficial.
  - It provides a surface for migrating epithelial cells.
  - It resists infection as a result of the excellent blood supply.
  - It carries the fibroblasts responsible for collagen formation.
  - It facilitates wound contraction (via the myofibroblast).
- Healing of wounds on the distal extremities of horses is often excessive, tending toward abnormal repair that can result in the formation of exuberant granulation tissue.

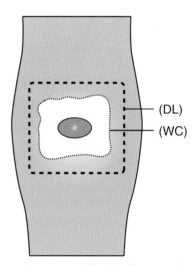

Figure 19-4   Wound contraction. The dashed line *(DL)* indicates the original size of the wound. *WC* indicates the extent of the wound contraction, and the white zone represents the extent of epithelialization.

Fibroplasia
- Mesenchymal cells transform into immature fibroblasts. Fibroblasts advance along the previously formed fibrin lattice within the clot and begin secreting the extracellular matrix (ground substance). The extracellular matrix is composed of glycoproteins (fibronectin and laminin) and proteoglycan (hyaluronic acid).
- Collagen is synthesized by the fibroblasts predominantly from hydroxyproline and hydroxylysine.
- Immature (type III) collagen fibrils are replaced by mature (type I) collagen fibers.
- As collagen content increases, the ground substance decreases and wound strength improves with maturity.
- Following deposition of extracellular matrix, protein synthesis slows and fibroblasts acquire contractile ability (myofibroblast phenotype) or disappear by apoptosis.

Wound Contraction
- Wound contraction is a process whereby wound edges are progressively brought together by centripetal movement of the surrounding skin toward the center of the wound (Fig. 19-4).

- Contraction is attributed to cells combining the characteristics of fibroblasts and smooth muscle cells, referred to as myofibroblasts, and "piling up" of the collagen into smaller units. Wound contraction is a critical determinant of the speed of second intention healing and the final cosmetic outcome.
- This process typically involves three clinical phases:
  - Immediate retraction (wound size increases)
  - Rapid contraction
  - Slow contraction
- In regions of the body with loose skin, wound contraction usually is sufficient to bring about complete closure of the wound with minimal scar formation.
- Where skin is firmly attached (e.g., distal region of the limb), a wider scar forms.
- Wound contraction is impeded by the following:
  - Persistent inflammation
  - Exuberant granulation tissue
  - Full-thickness skin grafts applied to the wound bed before 5 days
  - CO_2 laser excision (the laser reduces the wound myofibroblast number and function)

Epithelialization

- Basal epidermal cells at the wound margin begin to separate and migrate toward areas of cell deficit within hours of injury.
- Epidermal cells migrate beneath the scab and detach it by secreting proteolytic enzymes.
  - Epidermal cells continue to migrate on the surface of a wound until like cells are contacted, at which point the dissected scab falls off.
- Basal epidermal cells proliferate at the wound margin, 1 to 2 days after injury, in order to replenish the migratory front.
- The monolayer of cells attaches to the new basement membrane and differentiates into a stratified epidermis; this is a lengthy process, resulting in the maintenance of a thin and fragile neoepidermis for prolonged periods.
- Important factors that arrest epithelialization include the following:
  - Chronic infection
  - Fibrin remnants of the clot
  - Exuberant granulation tissue
  - Repeated dressing changes
  - Extreme hypothermia
  - Desiccation of the wound
  - Reduced oxygen tension
- Epithelialization can be accelerated by the application of certain cytokines/growth factors and by the use of semi-occlusive or occlusive dressings that keep the surface moist.

Maturation Phase

- Proteoglycans replace hyaluronan in the extracellular matrix to improve resilience.

- Collagen type I gradually provides the wound with tensile strength as deposition peaks between 7 and 14 days.
- The maturation phase is characterized by a reduction in fibroblast numbers with an equilibration of collagen production and collagen lysis, via a fine balance of matrix metalloproteinases and their inhibitors (tissue inhibitors of metalloproteinases [TIMPs]). Despite the reduction in fibroblasts, blood vessels, and collagen fibrils, the tensile strength of the wound increases as a result of the following:
  - Alignment of collagen fibers along lines of tension
  - Collagen cross-linking
  - Formation of collagen bundles
  - Bonding of collagen bundles and new collagen to the ends of old collagen fibers

---

●〉 WHAT TO DO

Maturation Phase
- Skin grafts may be useful in cases in which epithelialization and wound contraction are insufficient to close the wound.

Principles of Wound Management and Selected Factors That Affect Wound Healing

Anemia and Blood Loss

- Normovolemic anemia unrelated to malnutrition or chronic disease does not appear to affect wound healing until the packed cell volume (PCV) drops below 20%.
- Hypovolemic anemia caused by blood loss with vasoconstriction can impair wound healing. Reduced oxygen tension renders the wound more susceptible to infection by altering phagocytic mechanisms. Normal oxygen tension is also necessary for collagen synthesis.
- Wound healing should progress normally if the following are corrected:
  - Anemia with PCV <20%
  - Chronic infection
  - Malnutrition
  - Hypovolemia

●〉 WHAT TO DO

Anemia and Blood Loss
- Correcting hypovolemia, and possibly the use of hyperbaric oxygen therapy, should reduce the incidence of infection and allow healing to progress.
- There is an increased susceptibility to infection in the anemic equine patient. Use of regional perineural or line blocks should be performed distant to the injury for wound repair.

ITEG

●> WHAT NOT TO DO

Anemia and Blood Loss

- Do not use local anesthetics with epinephrine when debriding and repairing a wound.

Blood Supply and Oxygen Tension

- Healing wounds depend on adequate microcirculation to supply nutrients and oxygen.
- Oxygen is needed for cell migration, multiplication, and synthesis of collagen and protein in healing wounds.
- Alteration in the microcirculation can result from the following:
  - Tight bandages or casts
  - Seroma formation
  - Tight sutures
  - Local trauma
  - Use of local anesthetics with vasoconstrictive agents

●> WHAT TO DO

Blood Supply and Oxygen Tension

- Avoid placing bandages too tightly, particularly in those regions overlying the wound.
- Use cast padding (e.g., Custom Support foam[1])
- Drain any seromas
- Place sutures just tight enough to appose the tissues

Temperature and pH

- Wounds heal faster at higher temperatures and lower pH.
- Healing is accelerated at an ambient temperature of 30°C (86°F) rather than 18° to 20°C (64.4° to 68°F).
- Lower temperatures (12° to 20°C; 53.6° to 68°F) reduce tensile strength in wounds by 20%. Alternating warm and cold temperatures delays wound healing.
  - The inhibitory effect of decreasing temperature is a result of reflexive vasoconstriction and reduction of local blood flow.
- Warm hydrotherapy accelerates healing of sutured wounds and is beneficial during the inflammatory/debridement phase of open wounds.
  - Moist heat greater than 60°C (140°F) causes thermal injury to cells.
  - Moist heat greater than 49°C (120.2°F) is optimum for accelerating hemostasis in a newly incised wound.
  - Warm hydrotherapy accelerates healing by increasing blood flow.
- Acidification of a wound promotes healing by increasing the release of oxygen from hemoglobin.
- Bandaging is beneficial in increasing the wound surface temperature and decreasing the loss of CO_2 (alkalinity results from the loss of CO_2).

●> WHAT TO DO

Temperature and pH

- Bandaging, although beneficial in the early phase of healing, may promote the development of exuberant granulation tissue in distal limb wounds if used beyond the repair phase. Proper wound preparation, the selection of an appropriate wound dressing and protection, and immobilization of the wound site reduce the risk of exuberant granulation tissue developing.
- Discontinue the use of hydrotherapy when a healthy granulation bed develops.

Malnutrition and Protein Deficiency

- Wound healing can be impaired with mild to moderate short- or long-term protein/energy malnutrition.
- The patient's metabolic trend (positive or negative) at the time of injury or surgery is important.
- Hypoproteinemia adversely affects wound healing by impairing the following:
  - Fibroplasia
  - Angiogenesis
  - Matrix remodeling
- Plasma protein concentration <6 g/dL greatly retards healing.
- Impairment in wound healing is easily reversed with adequate nutrition.
- Horses with Cushing's Disease (pituitary pars intermedia dysfunction) are at increased risk for delayed or impaired wound healing because of immune suppression associated with the disease.

●> WHAT TO DO

Malnutrition and Protein Deficiency

- Offer adequate balanced nutrition before elective surgery and/or after injury and emergency surgery.
- Feeding DL-methionine to protein-deficient patients reverses the retardation in wound healing. DL-methionine converts to cysteine, which serves as an important cofactor in collagen synthesis and disulfide cross-linking as collagen matures.
- Vitamin deficiencies are not usually a problem except when the patient is chronically debilitated and undernourished; consider vitamin (A, C, and E) supplementation.

Nonsteroidal Anti-inflammatory Drugs

- Because inflammation is a part of the normal wound healing process, anti-inflammatory drugs such as phenylbutazone, aspirin, indomethacin, and flunixin meglumine can negatively affect wound healing if administered during the acute inflammatory phase.
- These drugs may be useful because they:
  - Diminish pain related to inflammation
  - Improve overall well-being
  - Encourage ambulation, resulting in improved circulation
  - Reduce the adverse effect of endotoxins on wound repair
- Conversely, it has been shown that horses suffer from a weak inflammatory response to trauma, which could hinder wound repair.

---

[1]3M Animal Care Products, St. Paul, Minnesota.

●❯ WHAT TO DO

Nonsteroidal Anti-inflammatory Drugs

- Administer the lowest dosage for the desired effect, and use only when necessary for pain control.

Corticosteroids

- Administered in moderate to large amounts within 5 days of injury, corticosteroids greatly retard wound healing by stabilizing the lysosomal membrane and preventing release of enzymes responsible for initiating the inflammatory response.
- Corticosteroids also suppress the following:
  - Fibroplasia
  - Angiogenesis
  - Collagen formation
- Corticosteroids also retard the following:
  - Wound contraction
  - Epithelialization
  - Gain in tensile strength

Trauma

- Excessive trauma within the wound or from other sites (e.g., multiple lacerations or fractures) does the following:
  - Prolongs the acute inflammatory phase
  - Makes the wound more susceptible to infection
  - Decreases the gain in tensile strength during the remodeling phase (proportional to the degree of trauma)
  - Results in excessive scar production
- Tissue trauma can be reduced by:
  - Debriding the wound thoroughly
  - Reducing surgery time
  - Using isotonic or isosmolar irrigation solutions
  - Maintaining hemostasis
  - Apposing tissues using proper tension and nonreactive suture material
  - Administering systemic antibiotics and nonsteroidal anti-inflammatory drugs (NSAIDs)

Dehydration and Edema

- Dehydration of the wound surface delays epithelialization by desiccating the marginal epithelial cells, slowing their migratory ability.
- Poor perfusion of peripheral tissues in a dehydrated patient is believed to delay wound healing.
- The cause, extent, and location of the edema determine its effect on healing:
  - Mild to moderate dependent edema, not associated with chronic disease or infection, has little harmful effect on wound repair.
  - Severe edema alters the vascular dynamics within a wound and impairs wound repair.
- Treatments with NSAIDs, pressure bandages, sweats under a bandage, and hydrotherapy are most beneficial in the management of edema associated with the limbs. Hand-walking exercise may be beneficial in the reduction of edema in regions of the upper body that cannot be bandaged.

Wound Infection

- Wound infection is defined as the presence of replicating microorganisms within a wound leading to host/tissue injury. Whether infection develops depends on the following:
  - Dose of microorganisms remaining in the wound. *Note:* Clinicians/surgeons can greatly influence this with proper wound care (see p. 245).
  - Virulence of the organisms
  - Wound microenvironment/contamination. *Note:* Clinicians and surgeons can profoundly improve the wound environment.
  - Functional capacity of the patient
  - Mechanism of injury
- Wound infection results when the number of microorganisms exceeds 10^6 per gram of tissue or per milliliter of fluid in an open wound or 10^5 per gram of tissue or per milliliter in a closed wound.
- Virulence factors include the following:
  - Secretion of adhesins (causes adherence of host cells)
  - Formation of bacterial cell capsules, which protect against phagocytosis
  - Formation of a *biofilm*, which protects and ensures bacterial replication
  - Release of enzymes and toxins
- Infection is a major factor in the following:
  - Delayed wound healing
  - Reduced gain in tissue tensile strength
  - Dehiscence following wound closure
  - Formation of exuberant granulation tissue
- Infection delays healing by:
  - Mechanically separating the wound edges with exudate
  - Releasing endotoxins, which inhibit cytokine/growth factor and collagen production
  - Reducing the vascular supply (as a result of mechanical pressure and a tendency to form microthrombi in small vessels adjacent to the wound)
  - Prolonging debridement
  - Producing proteolytic enzymes that digest collagen and damage host cells
  - Causing vascular and cellular responses typical of inflammation
  - Favoring the excessive deposition of granulation tissue, which slows wound contraction and epithelialization, delaying closure
- Infection rates in veterinary medicine:
  - Wound infections develop in approximately 5% to 5.9% of small animal surgical patients overall, and in approximately 2.5% of patients undergoing clean elective procedures. These rates are comparable to those reported in human beings.
  - Infection occurs in approximately 10% to 28% of equine orthopedic surgical patients overall and 8% of the orthopedic patients undergoing clean surgical procedures. Higher infection rates are thought to reflect the exclusive use of orthopedic patients in these studies.

- Contaminated wounds with lesser concentrations of microorganisms can become infected when the following occur:
  - Presence of foreign bodies
  - Excessive necrotic tissue in the wound
  - Hematoma formation
  - Impaired local tissue defense (burn or immunosuppressed patients)
  - Altered vascular supply
- Dirty wounds have a twenty-fivefold greater infection rate than do clean wounds.
  - Wounds contaminated with dirt have a higher risk of infection given the presence of specific infection-potentiating factors (IPFs) residing predominantly in the clay (inorganic) or organic fractions. These IPFs:
    - Decrease the effect of leukocytes
    - Decrease activity of humoral factors
    - Neutralize antibodies
    - Allow as few as 100 microorganisms to cause infection
  - Wounds contaminated with feces are highly susceptible to infection; feces can contain as many as 10^{11} microorganisms per gram.
- Hemorrhage: hemoglobin liberated after bleeding in a wound suppresses local wound defenses. The ferric ion from hemoglobin:
  - Inhibits the natural bacteriostatic properties of serum
  - Inhibits the intraphagocytic killing capabilities of the granulocyte
  - Can increase the virulence and replication of infecting bacteria
  - *Note:* Hematoma formation is considered a leading factor in decreasing local wound resistance to infection.
- Mechanism of injury
  - The cause of injury influences the patient's susceptibility to infection.
  - Lacerations caused by *sharp* objects such as metal, glass, and knives generally are more resistant to infection.
  - Shear wounds from barbed wire, sticks, nails, and bites are more susceptible to infection because of the degree of soft tissue injury.
  - Soft tissue trauma from entanglement/entrapment or impact with a solid object and/or a kick is more susceptible to infection because of the degree of soft tissue injury and resultant reduction in blood supply.
  - The greater the magnitude of energy on impact, the more severe the soft tissue damage and the greater the alteration in blood supply. Wounds created by impact injury are reported to be *100 times* more susceptible to infection compared with wounds caused by shearing forces.
  - Susceptibility to infection increases in *multiple trauma patients* even though the injury(ies) occurs at a site other than the surgical site; reduced tissue perfusion is believed to be the cause.

Infection in a Surgical Wound

WHAT TO DO

Infections in Surgical Wound

- Anesthesia:
  - Reduce the depth of anesthesia. Excessive depths of anesthesia cause reduced tissue perfusion leading to reduced oxygen tension, acidosis, and impaired resistance to infection.
  - Reduce the length of anesthesia. Prolonged anesthesia impairs alveolar macrophage function, slows leukocyte chemotaxis, and depresses neutrophil migration and function. Wound infection rates increase by 0.5% per minute after the initial 60 minutes of anesthesia, which translates to a 30% increased risk of postoperative infection for each additional hour of anesthesia.
  - Ensure proper hydration to enhance tissue and organ perfusion.
  - Avoid propofol. Propofol is shown to increase postoperative infection rates 3.8 times in clean wounds.
- Clipping:
  - Two comprehensive small animal studies found that clipping (#40 blade) the patient before induction of anesthesia increased the risk of infection. Patients having their hair clipped <4 hours or >4 hours before induction of anesthesia were 3 times more likely to develop surgical infections. Clippers nip the skin at the creases, producing gross cuts in which bacteria colonize. ***Recommendation:*** Clip hair after induction of anesthesia if possible.
  - When clipping the hair, protect the wound with sterile moist gauze sponges; clip a wide area of hair around the wound. *Dampen the hair with water or coat lightly with K-Y water-soluble jelly to prevent hair from falling into the wound.* Sponges used to pack the wound are discarded and replaced by new ones.
- Shaving:
  - Shaving before induction of anesthesia is associated with a higher infection rate (6%) compared with an infection rate of 1.9% when the patient is shaved after the induction of anesthesia. ***Recommendation:*** Shave hair after the induction of anesthesia and use a razor with a guarded head.
- Surgical technique:
  - Limit the use of electrocautery. Excessive use of electrocautery is shown to double infection rates. However, if bleeding vessels are grasped with fine nonserrated tissue forceps and electrocautery is used, infection rate is not increased over that of other methods of hemostasis.
  - Decrease surgery time. Wound infection rates double after 90 minutes of surgery and nearly triple when it exceeds 120 minutes.
  - Use aseptic technique.
  - Provide meticulous hemostasis.
  - Eliminate dead space and use a suction or gravity drain if necessary.
  - Use nonreactive sutures and proper suturing techniques.
- Antimicrobials:
  - Generally, antimicrobials are not recommended for patients in good health with a functional immune system if the surgery lasts <60 minutes and is done in a clean environment.
  - Generally, antimicrobials are needed in cases with tissue ischemia, if an enterotomy is performed, and if surgery >60 minutes.
- Patients in which antimicrobials are administered within 2 hours of surgery, and for 24 hours after surgery, have a 2.2% infection rate compared with those not receiving antimicrobials, who have a 4.4% infection rate. Patients receiving antimicrobials within 2 hours of surgery and for periods longer than 24 hours postoperatively, have a 6.3% infection rate, whereas patients in whom antimicrobials are started after surgery have an 8.2% infection rate.

Infection in a Traumatic Wound

◉› WHAT TO DO

Infection in Traumatic Wounds

- Clinical principles are the same as for elective surgery.
- Patient sedation and wound analgesia are as follows:
  - Some patients require sedation before wound preparation.
  - Avoid using phenothiazine tranquilizers in hypovolemic patients.
  - Regional perineural anesthesia is useful for wounds of the distal extremities, whereas regional infiltration of a local anesthetic is used elsewhere.
  - Direct infiltration of the wound with a local anesthetic (not containing epinephrine), while not ideal, is acceptable only after the wound is cleaned.
- Wound cleaning:
  - Cleaning is one of the most important components of effective wound management.
  - In acute wounds <3 hours in duration, water or saline may be all that is needed for adequate wound cleansing.
  - ***Practice Tip:*** *For field use, saline solution can be made by adding 10 mL (2 tsp) salt to 1 L boiling water or 40 mL (8 tsp) to a gallon (3.8 L) of boiling water.*
  - Commercial wound cleaners are recommended when enhanced wound cleaning is needed. Most products, however, contain surface active agents (surfactants) to improve removal of wound contaminants. Surfactants have been shown to be toxic to cells, delay wound healing and inhibit the "bodily defense against infection," and therefore should not be used. The two products shown to be the least cytotoxic are Constant-Clens[2] and Equine Vet.[3] The latter contains a wound stimulant, acemannan hydrogel, which is the active ingredient of Aloe Vera. Both products can be delivered to the wound surface at 12 psi when the spray container is held 6 inches (15 cm) from the wound. Antiseptics should not be added to wound cleanser because they increase the cytotoxic effects.
  - Vetericyn VF,[4] a relatively new wound product, has many of the attributes of an ideal wound cleanser. It is a superoxidized solution with a neutral pH, with a broad antimicrobial spectrum against bacteria, fungi, viruses, and spores and reportedly has a 30-second kill effect. Vetericyn VF also has a shelf life >24 months.
  - Lacerum Wound Cleanser[5] is a tissue-friendly solution that contains an antibacterial and antifungal agent (cetylpyridinium chloride) that kills microorganisms and encourages new cell growth. It is shown to be effective against certain organisms including *E. coli, Salmonella, Streptococcus pyogenes* and *equi, Candida albicans, Proteus vulgaris, Shigella, Pseudomonas, Klebsiella,* and most species of *Staphylococcus,* including *S. aureus.*
  - Use smooth sponges to scrub the wound. Wounds scrubbed with coarse sponges are significantly more susceptible to infection.
  - Scrubbing the wound with antiseptic soaps is not recommended because they are cytotoxic. Additionally, povidone-iodine surgical scrub is ineffective in reducing bacterial levels in wounds.

- Wound irrigation:
  - In acute wounds <3 hours in duration, irrigation effectively reduces the number of bacteria that reside on the wound surface. As time passes, bacteria invade the wound tissues and therefore are not removed with irrigation alone; debridement is required.
  - Because bacteria adhere to the wound surface by an electrostatic charge, irrigation solutions are most effective when delivered by a fluid jet of at least 7 psi at an *oblique angle* to the wound surface. Pressures of 10 to 15 psi have been shown to be 80% effective in removing soil-potentiating factors and adherent bacteria from a wound.
  - ***Practice Tip:*** *Wounds should not be irrigated with fluids delivered at pressures >15 psi; greater pressures cause fluid to penetrate deeper into the wound tissues along with any pathogens.*
  - A pressure of 7 to 15 psi can be achieved by forcefully expressing irrigant solutions from a 35-mL or 60-mL syringe through an 18-gauge needle, using a spray bottle, a "WaterPik" or a Stryker InterPulse irrigation system.[6]
- Sterile isotonic saline or lactated Ringer's solutions are commonly used. Tap water delivered from a hose can be used initially for large wounds. *Discontinue when granulation tissue develops.* Solutions are often combined with antiseptics/antimicrobials.
- Antiseptics used for wound lavage/irrigation:
  - Povidone-iodine (PI) solution (10%)
    - PI is a commonly used wound irrigant because of its broad antimicrobial spectrum against gram-positive and gram-negative bacteria, fungi, and *Candida* organisms. Bacterial resistance has not been identified.
    - Diluting the solution uncouples the bond, making more free iodine available for antimicrobial activity. ***Practice Tip:*** *0.1% and 0.2% (10 to 20 mL/1000 mL) concentrations are recommended.* Bactericidal effect is 15 seconds.
    - PI (1%) solution used for irrigation of abdominal incisions after closure of the peritoneum is *significantly superior to saline* in reducing postsurgical wound infection.
    - Disadvantages include the following:
      - PI is inactivated by organic material and blood; therefore, it is not effective when used to soak a gauze dressing.
      - Less than 0.1% concentrations are inactivated by large number of neutrophils.
      - Concentrations >1% are required to kill *Staphylococcus aureus.*
      - The disadvantages do not diminish the benefits seen with dilute PI irrigation of wounds.
  - Chlorhexidine diacetate (CHD) solution (2%)
    - CHD has a broad antimicrobial spectrum. **Note:** CHD is not effective against *fungi* and *Candida* organisms, and *Proteus* and *Pseudomonas* organisms have developed or have an inherent resistance to CHD.
    - CHD is still commonly used for wound irrigation.
    - When CHD is applied to intact skin, its antimicrobial effect is immediate and has a lasting residual effect caused by its binding to protein in the *stratum corneum.*
    - Currently, 0.05% CHD (25 mL of 2% CHD/975 mL) solution is recommended for wound irrigation. Greater concentrations can be harmful to wound healing.

---

[2]Covidien Animal Health/Kendall, Dublin, Ohio.
[3]Carrington Laboratories, Inc., Irving, Texas.
[4]Oculus Innovative Sciences, Inc., Petaluma, California.
[5]Rood & Riddle Veterinary Pharmacy, Lexington, Kentucky.

[6]Med-Vet Innovations, Inc., Penrose, Colorado.

- Dilution in a sterile electrolyte solution results in precipitation within 4 hours. *This does not affect the antibacterial effects of CHD.*
- A CHD solution of 0.05% has greater bactericidal activity against *Staphylococcus aureus* than 0.1% PI.
- CHD has continued activity in the presence of blood and pus; therefore, it is effective when used to soak a gauze dressing.
- Disadvantages include the following:
  - CHD is toxic to the eyes.
  - Full-strength CHD delays wound healing to a greater extent than does alcohol.
  - Greater than 0.5% solutions inhibit epithelialization and granulation tissue formation.
  - Less than 0.05% concentration results in significant *S. aureus* survival.
  - CHD has a narrow margin of dilution safety.
  - Ointment (2% Chlorhexidine gluconate) appears to inhibit wound healing.
- **Note:** for PI and CHD:
  - In an in vitro study, low-pressure irrigation (14 psi) with dilute solutions of PI or CHD resulted in almost complete removal of all bacteria adhering to bone. The antiseptics were found to exert a nineteen-fold decrease in bacterial numbers compared with low-pressure irrigation with saline controls.
  - **Practice Tip:** *Faster wound contraction can be expected in wounds irrigated with dilute CHD or PI compared with saline controls.*
- Hydrogen peroxide (3%):
  - Narrow antimicrobial spectrum
  - Damaging to tissues and cytotoxic to fibroblasts and causes thrombosis in the microvasculature
  - *Not recommended for wound care/irrigation*
- Sodium hypochlorite solution (0.5%; Dakin's solution):
  - Release of chlorine and oxygen kills bacteria
  - Dakin's solution is more effective than PI and CHD in killing *S. aureus*
  - Cytotoxic to fibroblasts and retards epithelialization
  - Decreases blood flow in microvessels
  - Chemically debrides the wound
  - Recommended use is one-quarter strength (0.125%) for wound treatment
  - **Note:** In a pinch, dilute 5% sodium hypochlorite diluted 40× with tap water achieves a 0.125% solution.
- Conclusions on antiseptics:
  - Antiseptics kill surface bacteria only and cannot kill bacteria imbedded in tissue.
  - Antiseptics are most effective in reducing bacterial numbers in acute contaminated wounds and not in chronic wounds or wounds with established infection.
  - Wounds with established infection should be treated by debridement and systemic and topical antimicrobials.
- Antimicrobials used for wound lavage/irrigation:
  - The addition of antimicrobials to the lavage solution greatly reduces the number of bacteria in a wound.
  - One percent neomycin solution is effective in preventing infection in wounds experimentally contaminated with feces.
  - **Practice Tip:** *Penicillin "sprayed" on a wound before closure reduces the chance of infection by 75%.*
  - **Note:** Biologically oriented surgeons never select a wound irrigation solution that they are not willing to put in their own conjunctival sac.

- Amount of fluid for irrigation:
  - Depends on the size of the wound
  - Depends on the degree of contamination
  - At a minimum the gross contaminants must be removed
  - Discontinue use before the tissue becomes waterlogged
- Antiseptics for skin preparation:
  - The two most commonly used surgical scrubs for skin preparation are povidone-iodine (Betadine) and chlorhexidine (Hibiclens).
  - Rinsing with saline or 70% isopropyl alcohol does not make a difference in antimicrobial effect for PI. **Note:** *Rinsing with 70% alcohol, however, reduces the residual effect and antiseptic quality of Hibiclens.*
  - A disadvantage of Betadine is the occurrence of skin reactions, particularly in small animals. Occasionally, horses treated with PI may develop an acute skin reaction.
    - Skin reactions are more common in the horse after clipping, scrubbing, and rinsing with 70% alcohol, spraying with PI solution, and bandaging.
    - Skin reactions include subcutaneous edema and skin wheal formation.
  - A disadvantage to using Hibiclens is that even short exposure to the eye, even in small concentrations, results in corneal opacification and ocular toxicity.
  - **Note:** Even with the high kill rate of these antiseptics, 20% of the bacterial population in the skin resides in protected hair follicles, sebaceous glands, and in crevices of the lipid coat of the superficial epithelium.
- Surgeon hand and arm preparation:
  - Hand cultures immediately following standard surgical hand preparation and 4 hours in surgical gloves showed that alcohol (70% ethyl) and chlorhexidine (4%) were effective surgical scrubs with good residual effect. *Betadine was found to have little residual effect.*
  - Conclusions:
    - Chlorhexidine preparations are superior.
    - Betadine has poor prolonged effect.
    - Triclosan is not effective in most trials.
    - Seventy percent ethanol (v/v) has low antibacterial effectiveness. Seventy percent ethyl alcohol is superior.
    - Waterless skin preparation:
      - A blinded study comparing Avagard[7] to 4% chlorhexidine gluconate (CHG) or Betadine for hand and arm preparation over a 5-day period and under surgical gloves for 6 hours found that Avagard is superior in antiseptic quality and is less irritating than the Betadine or CHG.
- Wound exploration:
  - After the wound is cleaned and free of devitalized tissue and debris, digitally explore it using sterile gloves. *Make sure to first rinse the talcum powder from the outer surface of the gloves.*
  - A sterile probe is useful in identifying the depth of the wound, whether a foreign body is present, or whether bone is contacted, and it can be used in conjunction with radiography (Fig. 19-5).
  - Normal synovial fluid is identified by stringing it between the thumb and forefinger (normal viscosity), and if questions remain (fluid is thin/watery), a fluid sample should be submitted for cytologic examination and culture/sensitivity.
  - If synovial cavity penetration is suspected, place a needle in the synovial cavity at a site remote to the wound (Fig. 19-6). If synovial fluid can be retrieved, submit it for cytologic examination

[7]3M Center, St. Paul, Minnesota.

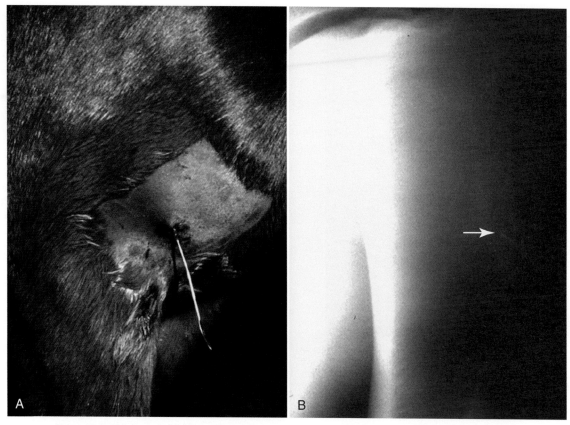

Figure 19-5   This horse had a history of sustaining a puncture wound 2 months earlier. The wound would break open and drain periodically. **A,** A metal probe is used to identify the direction and depth of the wound and determine if bone is contacted. **B,** Radiograph of the humerus identifying focal osteitis of the deltoid tuberosity *(tip of metal probe, arrow).*

and culture/sensitivity. After aspirating, inject sterile saline solution into the synovial structure; if the joint capsule has been breached, fluid is seen exiting the wound. If a synovial structure is involved, irrigate it with 3 to 5 L of sterile saline or crystalloid solution. Some clinicians follow the crystalloid joint lavage with 1 L of a 10% dimethyl sulfoxide (DMSO) solution. Intrasynovial instillation of antimicrobials also is recommended.
- Radiographic examination includes:
  - Standard
  - Contrast/fistulography
- Ultrasound examination can document injury to tendons, ligaments, and joint capsules. Ultrasound can identify foreign bodies that are not apparent on radiographs, gas accumulation, and muscle separation (Fig. 19-7).
- Arthroscopy can be helpful in identifying radiographically occult lesions, particularly those involving cartilage, and in identifying foreign bodies within the joint (e.g., hair, dirt, or other foreign bodies; (Fig. 19-8). Arthroscopy also improves visualization during debridement and large volume lavage.
- Wound debridement:
  - Debridement reduces the number of bacteria and removes contaminants (dead tissue, foreign bodies) that alter the local defense mechanisms, thereby improving vascularity.
  - The standard approach is sharp debridement, converting a contaminated wound to a clean wound. The types of debridement include:
    - Excisional (layered; Fig. 19-9)
    - En block

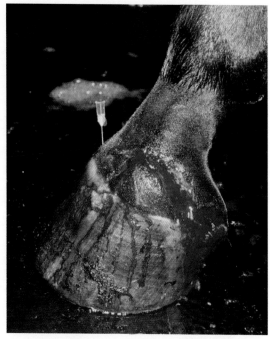

Figure 19-6   An example of a needle placed in the distal interphalangeal (coffin) joint at a site remote to the wound. (From Stashak TS: *Proceedings of the American Association of Equine Practitioners* 52:270-280, 2006.)

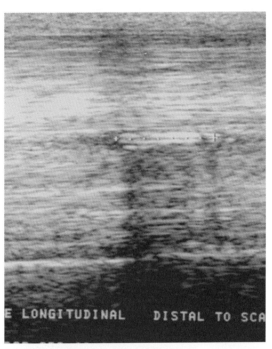

Figure 19-7 A longitudinal ultrasound examination identifying a piece of wood *(cursors)* located at the distal extent of the carpal canal at the attachment of the carpal check ligament to the deep digital flexor tendon. (From Stashak TS: *Proceedings of the American Association of Equine Practitioners* 52:270-280, 2006.)

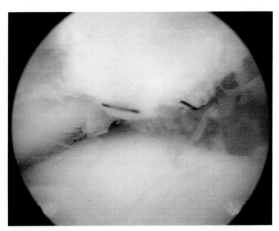

Figure 19-8 Arthroscopic view of the distal interphalangeal (coffin) joint. Note the hair (dark particles) in the joint. This horse had sustained a puncture wound to the cornet band region 1 week earlier. (From Stashak TS: *Proceedings of the American Association of Equine Practitioners* 52:270-280, 2006.)

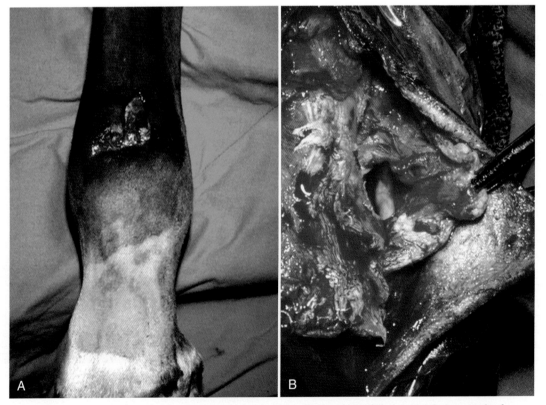

Figure 19-9 **A,** A 6-hour-duration entrapment injury involving the dorsolateral fetlock region. **B,** An example of extensive layered debridement of this wound. Note that the damaged joint capsule was also debrided, exposing the joint.

- Simple or piecemeal (used for very large wounds of the body; Fig. 19-10)
- Staged (done over a number of days): This approach avoids the inadvertent removal of viable tissue. Governing criteria are color and attachment. White, tan, black, or green tissue that is poorly attached is debrided. Pink to dark purple tissue that is well attached is left in place.
- ***Note:*** If exposed ischemic, contaminated cortical bone is debrided (partial decortication) sufficient to reach bleeding/serum oozing bone, granulation tissue proliferates from the bone surface. Partial decortication can be best accomplished with a pneumatic driven burr, a bone rasp, and/or bone curette (Fig. 19-11). Hydrogel wound dressings containing acemannan, CarraSorb Carra Vet[8] reportedly help accelerate the migration of granulation tissue over exposed bone.
- Hydrosurgical debridement:
  - Utilizes a high velocity stream of sterile saline, which creates a localized vacuum (Venturi effect)
  - Causes less tissue damage
  - Removes only devitalized tissue
  - Combines sharp debridement and irrigation
  - Is believed to be more effective in removing bacteria
- CO_2 laser:
  - Reduces the bacteria numbers but does not sanitize the wound
  - Causes contracture of collagen fibers, and decreases the fibroblast number, which diminishes wound contraction
  - Photoablates exuberant granulation tissue, reduces postoperative pain, and causes minimal bleeding

[8]Carrington Laboratories, Inc., Irving, Texas.

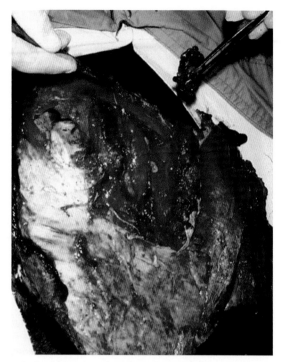

Figure 19-10   A large wound involving the lateral thoracic region is a good example of where piecemeal debridement can be used. (From Stashak TS: *Proceedings of the American Association of Equine Practitioners* 52:270-280, 2006.)

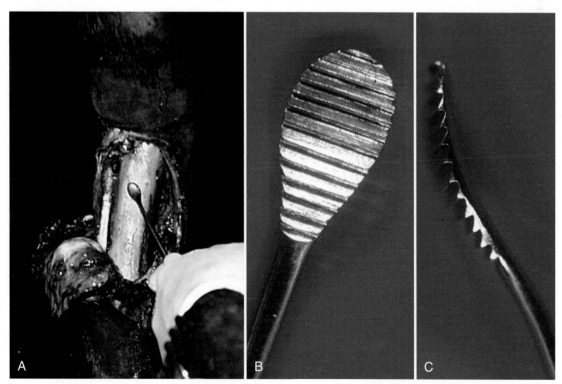

Figure 19-11   A, A large degloving injury of the dorsal metatarsal region with exposed ischemic bone (chalky appearance). The bone is being partially decorticated (debrided) with a hip arthroplasty rasp. **B,** Bottom view of the spatula-shaped head of the rasp. **C,** Lateral view showing the curved head of the rasp. (**B** and **C** from Stashak TS: *Proceedings of the American Association of Equine Practitioners* 52:270-280, 2006.)

- Enzymatic:
  - Wound surface coagulum and bacterial biofilm encompass contaminants and bacteria, thus preventing access of topical antimicrobials/antiseptics and systemic antibiotics.
  - Proteolytic enzymes degrade the coagulum and biofilm.
  - Indications: When surgical debridement is contraindicated because it could result in damage to or removal of tissue needed for wound reconstruction and when a wound approximates nerves and vessels.
  - Products include the following:
    - Pancreatic trypsin (Granulex[9])
    - Streptodornase and streptokinase (Varidase[10])
    - Collagenases, proteinases, fibrinolysin, and deoxyribonuclease (Elase ointment[11])
    - **Practice Tip:** *Collagenase ointment (Santyl[12]) has the highest proteolytic activity and the greatest likelihood of achieving a clean wound.*
- Debridement dressings include the following:
  - Adherent open mesh gauze (e.g., 4- × 4-inch gauze sponges)
  - Wet-to-dry dressings using 4- × 4-inch mesh gauze or sheet cotton
  - Kerlix AMD[13] is an excellent choice because it contains a broad-spectrum antiseptic and kills bacteria on the surface of the wound and prevents "strike through" (penetration through the dressing).
  - Occlusive dressings are autolytic. Good choice for an acute clean wound.
- Systemic antimicrobials:
  - Decision is easy; selection depends on type and location of wound.
  - Pulse dosing improves antimicrobial penetration
  - **Practice Tip:** *Parenteral administration is recommended initially. Intravenous (IV) administration is preferred because its effects are predictable. Intramuscular absorption often is prolonged and variable and depends on the site selection and amount of exercise.*
  - Oral administration is used after adequate blood levels are achieved
- Antimicrobial choices[14]:
  - For *superficial wounds,* antimicrobials generally are not needed in clean wounds <3 hours in duration that are sutured or left to heal by second intention. Generally, antimicrobials are needed for heavily contaminated wounds >3 hours in duration. Useful antibiotics include: penicillin (22,000 to 44,000 IU/kg IV or IM q6 to 12h) alone or in combination with trimethoprim-sulfadiazine (15 to 25 mg/kg PO q12h). Alternatively, topical application of an antibiotic can be used alone.
  - *Deeper wounds* including synovial cavities require penicillin (22,000 units/kg IM or IV q 6h) or ampicillin (6.6 to 11 mg/kg IM or IV q8-12h), or cefazolin (11 mg/kg IV or IM q6 to 8h) in combination with an aminoglycoside.
    - Gentamicin (6.6 mg/kg IV, IM or SQ q24h) or amikacin (15 to 25 mg/kg IV or IM q24h) may be used.

- Ceftiofur (adults, 1-5 mg/kg IV, IM, q6-12h; foal, 2-10 mg/kg IV, IM, q6-12h) or enrofloxacin (5 mg/kg IV q24h or 7.5 mg/kg PO q24h; *not recommended for foals*), which are reserved for bacteria resistant to previous drug regimens, may be used.
- For deep fascial cellulitis/septic myositis caused by *Clostridium* spp. or pyonecrotic processes:
  - High doses of penicillin, ampicillin, or cefazolin and metronidazole (15 mg/kg PO q6 to 8h) or rifampin (10 mg/kg PO q12h) or ceftiofur
  - Penicillin and metronidazole are recommended as the first choice combination; tetracycline and metronidazole as a second choice combination, based on the response to treatment in other species
  - Incision and drainage (I&D) may be used when and where appropriate; ultrasound may assist in the decision for I&D
- Duration of antimicrobial therapy:
  - Minimum course: 3 to 5 days
  - Established soft tissue infection: 7 to 10 days
  - Established synovial infection: 10 days if regional limb perfusion (RLP) was used and 21 days if RLP was not used.
  - Established bone infection: 3 to 6 months. The duration of treatment may be shortened if an antimicrobial perfusion technique (intravenous or intraosseous) is used. See regional limb perfusion, Chapter 5, p. 16.
  - **Note:** Wounds contaminated with 10^9 microorganisms per gram of tissue develop infection despite antimicrobial treatment.
- Topical antibiotics:
  - Topical antibiotics, especially some ointments or creams (e.g., nitrofurazone [Furacin] and gentamicin cream), can retard wound healing.
  - Solutions are most effective when applied to wounds before closure or when used as an irrigation solution.
  - Creams and ointments that remain in contact with the wound longer prevent desiccation of the wound surface and are best used under bandages or on exposed wounds.
  - Topical antibiotics are most effective when applied within 3 hours of injury. However, if a wound >3 hours or a chronically infected wound is debrided, a new wound is created, justifying topical antibiotic use. In the latter case, systemic antimicrobials also are recommended.
  - Three out of four human wounds did not become infected when penicillin was sprayed on wounds before closure compared to no antibiotic.
  - *Triple antibiotic ointment* (bacitracin, polymyxin B, and neomycin) has a wide antimicrobial spectrum but is ineffective against *P. aeruginosa*. The zinc component of bacitracin stimulates epithelialization (a 25% increase) but can retard wound contraction. Triple antibiotic ointment is poorly absorbed; therefore, toxicity is rare.
  - *Silver sulfadiazine (SS)* has a wide antimicrobial spectrum, including *Pseudomonas* organisms and *fungi*. SS has been shown to increase epithelialization by 28% in some studies, and in others it slows epithelialization. In a study performed in horses, SS did not accelerate wound healing.
  - *Nitrofurazone ointment* has a good antimicrobial spectrum against gram-positive and gram-negative organisms but has little effect against *Pseudomonas* organisms. *However, nitrofurazone ointment has been shown to decrease epithelialization by 24% and decreases wound contraction in horses.* The antimicrobial nitrofurazone, not the vehicle, is responsible for the delay in wound healing and its carcinogenic properties.

---

[9]www.vetrxdirect.com.
[10]www.Drugs.com
[11]Pfizer Pharmaceuticals Group, New York, New York.
[12]HEALTHPOINT, Ltd. www.healthpoint.com.
[13]Covidien Animal Health/Kendall, Dublin, Ohio.
[14]All dosages are from the JLV-VTH Formulary, Colorado State University, 2009 edition.

- *Gentamicin sulfate* has a narrow antimicrobial spectrum, but it may be applied to wounds infected with gram-negative bacteria, particularly *P. aeruginosa*. Treatment with 0.1% oil-in-water cream base slows wound contraction and epithelialization.
- *Cefazolin* is effective against gram-positive and some gram-negative organisms. When applied at 20 mg/kg, cefazolin surpasses minimal inhibitory concentration (MIC) in the wound fluid for longer periods than does systemically administered cefazolin at the same dose. The powder form provides a more sustained tissue concentration than does the solution. Because of this property, cefazolin may be effective in the management of established infections.
- *Note:* Multiple antimicrobial-resistant bacterial strains continue to be a major health concern; therefore, new emphasis is being placed on the development and use of alternative wound care products, particularly those with no known induction of bacterial resistance.
- Management of synovial penetration:
  - Acute penetration <6 to 8 hours' duration:
    - Broad-spectrum systemic antimicrobials
    - Synovial irrigation
    - Intrasynovial antimicrobials
    - Wound debridement
    - Wound closure
  - Systemic broad-spectrum antibiotic therapy is considered one of the cornerstones of treatment of synovial infections.
    - A study of experimental infectious arthritis found that increasing the dose of antibiotic from one to two times a day, regardless of the method of drainage, significantly reduced the isolation rate of *S. aureus*.
    - Combination antibiotic treatment is preferred.
  - Synovial irrigation:
    - Use sterile salt solution (1 to 3 L) plus 10% DMSO (1 L)
    - Advantages of arthroscopy/tenoscopy include:
      - Allow direct visualization to:
        - Assess damage (Fig. 19-12)
        - Remove foreign bodies/material (see Fig. 19-8), free fibrin, and fibrin strands, which may form adhesions within a sheath (Fig. 19-13), and remove pannus (fibrocellular clot over the cartilage). Both fibrin and pannus impede treatment by protecting foreign material, and can act as a medium for bacterial growth.
  - *Note*: A clinical study of contaminated and infected synovial cavities found 40% of the synovial cavities examined by endoscopy contained foreign material, which had been predicted in only 15%, based on preoperative diagnostics.
  - Intrasynovial antimicrobials:
  - Intrasynovial injection of antimicrobials: Administer less than one systemic dose every 24 hours.
  - The bactericidal effects of aminoglycosides are concentration dependent. High peak concentration is also associated with longer postantibiotic effect (PAE).
    - Amikacin (250 mg): Amikacin has good activity against most pathogens found in orthopedic infections in horses, and resistance to amikacin is less likely compared with gentamicin.
    - Gentamicin (200 to 500 mg): Gentamicin is effective against 85% of the bacterial isolates obtained from musculoskeletal infections in the horse. Gentamicin also has been shown to be active in infected equine synovial fluid. Intraarticular administration of 150 mg of gentamicin resulted in peak concentrations of 4745 mg/mL compared with 5.1 mg/mL

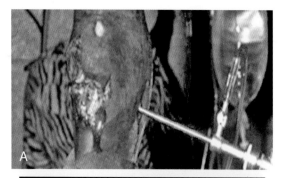
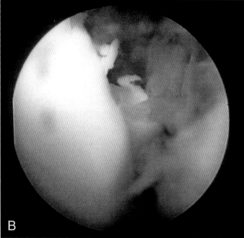

Figure 19-12 A, A 3-hour-old wound that involved the tendon sheath and the metatarsophalangeal joint. **B,** Arthroscopic view of the metatarsophalangeal joint; note the osteochondral fragments originating from the abaxial surface of the proximal sesamoid bone and the fibrin surrounding the fragments.

when given systemically at 2.2 mg/kg. The concentration remained significantly higher than the MIC for *Escherichia* for more than 24 hours.
  - Penicillin: 5×10^6 IU
  - Ceftiofur (150 mg): One study found that intrasynovial treatment with 150 mg of ceftiofur resulted in synovial fluid concentrations that were significantly higher than those found after IV administration of 2.2 mg/kg. Synovial fluid concentration following intrasynovial administration remained above MIC for 24 hours; following IV administration, concentration remained above MIC for only 8 hours.
- *Practice Tip:* Regional limb perfusion allows delivery of an antimicrobial into normal, inflamed, infected ischemic tissue and exudates at very high concentrations, greater than that achieved by the parenteral administration. Perfusion is done IV or intraosseously (see pp. 253). Antimicrobial doses reported include the following:
  - Amikacin, 500 to 700 mg and up to one third the parenteral adult dosage. *Note:* A study showed that antimicrobial concentrations did not attain MIC in synovial fluid, subcutaneous tissue, or bone marrow of horses following IV delivery of 250 mg amikacin, 30 minutes after release of the tourniquet. The conclusion is that a dose >250 mg is recommended to attain effective tissue and synovial fluid concentrations of amikacin.
  - Gentamicin, 500 mg to 1 g and up to one third the parenteral adult dosage. *Note:* Doses >1 g may result in soft tissue sloughing, and doses >3 g have resulted in loss of blood

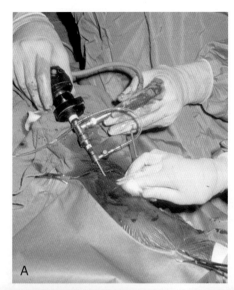

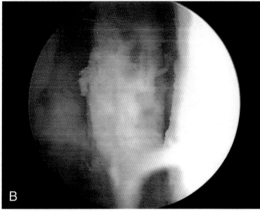

Figure 19-13   A, Arthroscope placed in the carpal canal sheath. **B,** Arthroscopic view identifying a piece of wood and fibrin within the carpal canal.

supply to the phalanges (Fig. 19-14); 500 mg to 1 g of amikacin or gentamicin is generally used clinically.

- Enrofloxacin was shown to cause vasculitis in 3 of 7 horses following IV regional limb perfusion. Nonetheless, concentrations above MIC were maintained for 24 to 36 hours in bone and synovial fluid when enrofloxacin was delivered at 1.5 mg/kg.
- The technique is primarily used for treatment of septic osteitis/osteomyelitis and for septic synovial structures of the distal extremities (including the carpus and tarsus) (see Fig. 19-16). An Esmarch bandage may be used to remove blood at the site to be treated, after which a tourniquet, either cuffed or surgical rubber tubing, is placed proximal to the site for the phalanges and proximal and distal to the site if the carpus or tarsus is involved. Alternatively the Esmarch bandage can be left in place and tied at a site proximal to the phalanges or distal and proximal to the carpus and tarsus, after which it is separated to expose the carpus or tarsus. A recent study found the Esmarch was more effective in preventing loss of amikacin from the distal limb than was a pneumatic tourniquet. Subsequently, 30 to 60 mL of a sterile balanced electrolyte solution containing the antibiotic is delivered under pressure over a 1- to 10-minute period by the intraosseous or the intravenous route. The tourniquet is removed after 30 minutes.
- IV delivery involves placing an IV catheter of an appropriate size[15] in the lateral palmar/plantar digital vein at the level of the proximal sesamoid bone for the digit (Fig. 19-16), the cephalic vein for the carpus, and the saphenous vein for the tarsus.
- Advantages to IV delivery:
  - Slightly higher antibiotic concentrations are observed in the synovial compartment than achieved with the intraosseous approach.
  - It is quick and simple to perform.
  - It requires no special equipment.

---

[15]Butterfly catheter.

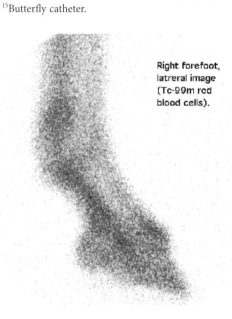

Left forefoot, lateral image (Tc-99m red blood cells).

Right forefoot, latreral image (Tc-99m red blood cells).

A   B

Figure 19-14   Horse presented for non–weight-bearing lameness left forelimb following the administration of 3 g gentamicin intraosseously on two occasions. **A,** Nuclear medicine vascular phase study of left forelimb showing loss of blood supply to the mid- and distal phalangeal region. **B,** Control right forelimb.

○ Disadvantages to IV delivery:
  - Di Vein identification can be difficult in cases in which there is significant swelling associated with the region and multiple IV injections.
  - Maintaining an IV catheter is difficult because of the tendency to develop venous thrombosis. **Note:** Using a smaller gauge butterfly catheter and diluted antimicrobial reduces the osmolality of solution and phlebitis as a sequela of the IV infusion.
  - A "cutdown" procedure may be required to gain access to the vein.
• *Intraosseous delivery:* A 4-mm-diameter hole is drilled into the medullary cavity of the distal third of the metacarpal/metatarsal III. A centrally cannulated (bored out) 4.5 mm or 5.5-mm ASIF (Association for the Study of Internal Fixation) cortical screw, with a Luer-lock head is placed into the marrow cavity. If the screw is not self-tapping, a tap is used to create threads in the cortex before screw placement (Fig. 19-15). Alternatively, the male adaptor end of an IV delivery set can be used; it is wedged into the 4-mm diameter bone hole with needle holders using a to-and-fro rotating motion (our preference).
  ○ Advantages to intraosseous delivery:
    - It is easier to perform than IV perfusion if there is soft tissue swelling at the site.
    - It avoids repeated venipuncture; permits frequent local perfusion even in the standing horse, with minimal adverse effects.
  ○ Disadvantages of intraosseous delivery:
    - There is some leakage of the perfusate around the cortical hole, particularly when the IV extension set method is used. This can be avoided if the male adaptor is seated firmly in the hole.

  - The procedure is more involved than IV perfusion.
  - An indwelling cannulated screw is exposed at the skin and is therefore a potential source of infection of surrounding bone and medullary cavity. **Note:** An indwelling cannulated screw needs special attention in management.
• *Antimicrobial-impregnated beads:*
  ○ Are made from polymethylmethacrylate (PMMA) or hydroxyapatite cement

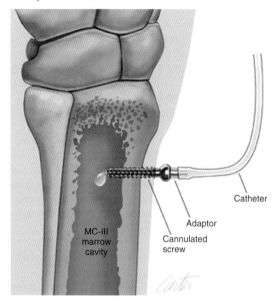

Figure 19-15   Intraosseous perfusion of the metacarpus. (Courtesy Dr. James A. Orsini; reprinted from Orsini JA: *Clinical Techniques in Equine Practice,* 3[2]:225, 2004.)

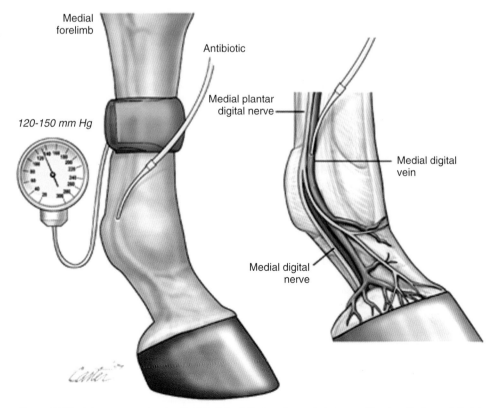

Figure 19-16   Intravenous regional perfusion of the fetlock region wond phalanges. (Courtesy Dr. James A Orsini; reprinted from Orsini JA: *Clinical Techniques in Equine Practice,* 3[2]:225, 2004.)

- Polymer is mixed with antimicrobial
- **Practice Tip:** *Rule of thumb for the quantity of antimicrobial used is 5% to 10% the weight of PMMA: 0.5 g to 2 g for every 10 to 20 g of PMMA cement.*
- Local concentrations of the antimicrobial are increased 200 times that achieved by systemic administration.
- MIC persists for up to 80 days after implantation.
- Serum levels do not reach toxic levels.
- Gentamicin and amikacin are used most often.
- **Practice Tip:** *Ceftiofur-impregnated beads are unlikely to provide long-term bactericidal concentrations.*
- This method is not used routinely in horses with chronic synovial infection unless other methods have failed.
- The authors have not placed PMMA beads within high motion synovial cavities because of the risk of iatrogenic damage to the articular cartilage and synovia.
- Gentamicin-impregnated collagen sponge[16] with 130 mg gentamicin:
  - The sponge is used commonly in humans for soft tissue surgery and injury with good results.
  - Reportedly higher concentrations of the antibiotic are achieved for 3 days (first day, 15 times; third day, 2 times) in wound exudate than with polymethylmethacrylate beads.
  - Collagen sponge is absorbed within 12 to 49 days depending on the vascular supply to the region
  - Seven of eight horses with moderate to severe traumatic septic synovial cavities (arthritis and tenosynovitis) responded favorably to this treatment. The collagen sponges were implanted in the synovial cavity through the arthroscope cannula.
  - A bovine type 1 collagen sponge with 130 mg gentamicin increases the antibiotic concentration >20× MIC within 3 hours in the tarsocrural joint.
- Open synovial drainage for nonresponsive cases
  - In an experimental study, arthrotomy for joint infection was more successful in eliminating infection than were arthroscopy and synovectomy. However, it was associated with higher risk of ascending contamination and wound healing problems. This has not been our experience when utilizing antiseptic dressing (e.g., Kerlix AMD[17]) in the postoperative period.
  - A clinical study found that open drainage for joint and tendon sheath infection was very successful in eliminating the infection, with few complications.
- Ingress/egress joint lavage:
  - The preferred approach is synovial irrigation using a fluid pump with intermittent synovial cavity distention. Distention of the synovial cavity allows the irrigation solution and subsequent intrasynovial antibiotic delivery to reach all areas. An ingress multifenestrated tube is placed in the synovial cavity and secured with sutures. A fluid pump (preferred), or hand-held bag that can be pressurized, is used to deliver fluid into the synovial structure. A gloved hand with sterile gauze is used to plug the distal egress wound site to distend the synovial cavity (Fig. 19-17). Following appropriate treatment, the egress tube is rinsed with full strength heparin to prevent fibrin from plugging the fenestrations.

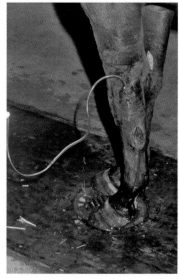

Figure 19-17   Open synovial irrigation of the carpal canal sheath with an ingress irrigation cannula in place. A fluid pump is used to irrigate the sheath while a gloved hand and sterile gauze are used to plug the distal egress wound site to maximize distention of the tendon sheath.

- Continuous intrasynovial infusion:
  - There have been several reports using this method to treat chronic refractory synovial infections.
  - In a research trial, a catheter plus balloon infuser was placed in the tarsocrural joint.
    - Gentamicin dosage of 0.02 to 0.17 mg/kg/h for 5 days resulted in concentrations 100 times the MIC for common equine pathogens.
    - Complications seen with the catheter system included: failure of the infuser balloons (rupture or leakage) and blockage due to either an air lock in or collapse of the flow control tubing.
  - Two clinical reports used a Joint Infusion System[18] and the On-Q Painbuster[19] postop pain relief system. The system was used in a variety of synovial cavities in both foals and adults, and results appear to be comparable to those obtained with other techniques.
- Annular ligament/retinacula release:
  - Annular ligaments associated with the digital sheaths and retinacula within the carpal and tarsal sheaths create an inelastic canal through which the associated tendons glide.
  - With chronic infection, the canal may become constricted because of secondary tendonitis, swelling of the synovial lining, and pannus formation. Subsequent movement of the tendon through the narrowed canal can be painful, leading to lameness that contributes to patient morbidity.
  - The canal can also become so narrow that it creates a compartmentalization of the synovial cavity proximal and distal to the ligament or sheath, thus making drainage difficult. In such cases, the annular ligament or retinaculum should be transected to alleviate pain and allow for improved drainage.
  - These procedures are usually reserved for horses with a chronic, established infection that has not responded favorably to conventional therapy.

---

[16]Collatamp G (Schering Corporation, United Kingdom).
[17]Kendall Health Care, Mansfield, Massachusetts.
[18]Mila International, Florence, Kentucky.
[19]I-Flow Corp., Lake Forrest, California.

Approaches to Wound Closure and Healing

Primary closure is performed within several hours after injury and is used for the following:

- Fresh, minimally contaminated wounds, with a good blood supply

Delayed primary closure is performed before the formation of granulation tissue and is used for the following:

- Severely contaminated, contused, or swollen wounds and for many wounds that involve a synovial structure

Secondary closure is performed after the formation of granulation tissue and is used for the following:

- Chronic wounds with a compromised blood supply (the wound is closed after a healthy bed of granulation tissue develops)

Second intention healing wounds are closed by epithelialization and wound contraction. It is relied on for the following:

- Large wounds involving the body, neck, and upper limb regions (Fig. 19-18).
- Extensive degloving and avulsion wounds of the limbs (see Fig. 19-11, *A*)
- *Skin grafting* is used when tissue deficits exceed the capability of wound contraction and epithelialization. *Reconstructive surgery* is used for a better cosmetic and functional end result in a healed wound.

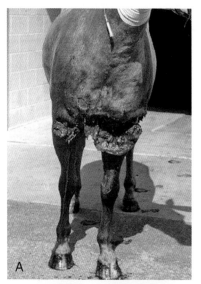
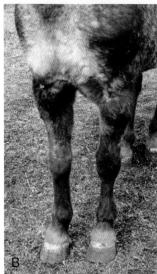

Figure 19-18 A, Large wound involving cranial extensor muscles of the antebrachium and cranial pectoral muscle region that healed by second intention. **B,** The wound after 3 months.

●〉 WHAT TO DO

Wound Closure

- Primary closure is appropriate for acute cases <6 hours' duration that are clean and wherein the synovial cavity is free of foreign material.
  - These wounds should be closed only after performing arthroscopy or tenoscopy and regional limb perfusion.
- For wounds >6 hours' duration:
  - Use delayed closure
  - Healing by second intention is most common
- Chronic cases >6 to 8 hours' duration:
  - All of the above actions are recommended except for wound closure
  - Perform regional limb perfusions
  - Use open synovial drainage for nonresponsive cases
  - Ingress/egress drainage can be performed
  - Can use annular ligament/retinacula release procedures

●〉 WHAT TO DO

Local Anesthetics and Wounds

- Regional anesthesia is best. Intralesional injection of 2% solutions is acceptable but not ideal.
- To avoid potential negative effects on healing, dilute with sterile water to achieve 0.5% concentration. Apparently no reduction in the anesthetic effect is observed after diluting.

●〉 WHAT NOT TO DO

Local Anesthetics and Wounds

- Avoid using epinephrine with the local anesthetics.

Local Anesthetics

Effects

- Intralesional injection of 2% concentrations of lidocaine and carbocaine were evaluated in many the studies:
  - Inhibits platelet aggregation, ground substance formation, and collagen synthesis. Epinephrine exacerbates this inhibition via vasoconstriction.
  - Results in reduced wound breaking strength in rats
- Intralesional injection of 0.5% lidocaine has no effect on wound healing compared with saline controls.

Suturing Techniques and Suture Material

- Suturing technique and the material chosen influence wound healing.

- Synthetic monofilament sutures are superior; they are less reactive and stronger, and if absorbable, they are absorbed at a constant rate.
- Simple interrupted sutured skin wounds, compared with simple continuous sutured skin wounds, have been shown to have the following characteristics:
  - Less edema
  - Increased microcirculation
  - 30% to 50% greater tensile strength after 10 days
- In horses, simple interrupted sutured *linea alba* compared with continuously sutured *linea alba* have the following characteristics:
  - Greater bursting strength at 5 to 10 days
  - No difference in bursting strength at 0 and 21 days
- Simple interrupted suture patterns cause less inflammation than vertical mattress and far-near near-far patterns
- ***Practice Tip:*** *Use interrupted sutures where impaired healing is anticipated and excessive tension is present.*
- Loosely approximated wounds are stronger at 7, 10, and 21 days postoperatively than wounds tightly closed with sutures.

●❯ WHAT TO DO

Suturing Techniques and Suture Materials
- Appose wound edges anatomically. Overreduction of tissues should be avoided.
- Use the least number of sutures required to close the wound. Increased number of sutures equals increased infection rates.
- Deep suture only fascial planes, tendons, and ligaments.

Tension Sutures
- These patterns are used to reduce tension on the primary suture line.
- Widely placed vertical mattress sutures without or with supports, using buttons, gauze, or rubber tubing, are effective in reducing tension on the primary suture line (Fig. 19-19, *A* and *B*).
- Sutures with supports are used in areas that cannot be effectively bandaged (e.g., upper body and neck regions; Fig. 19-19, *C*).
- Sutures without supports are used in areas that are bandaged or to which a cast is applied.
- Tension sutures are removed in 4 to 10 days, depending on the appearance of the wound, and staggered removal is preferred (removing half the sutures initially and the remaining half later).
- Of the appositional tension suturing patterns, the far-near near-far suture pattern is superior. The far component reduces tension while the near component holds the tissues edges in apposition (Fig. 19-20).

Hematoma and Seroma
- Hematoma formation is considered a leading factor in decreasing local wound resistance to infection.
- Collection of blood or serum in tissues delays healing by mechanically separating the wound edges.
- If expanding fluid pressure is significant, it can alter the blood supply to the wound margins.
- Blood/serum provides an excellent media for bacterial growth.

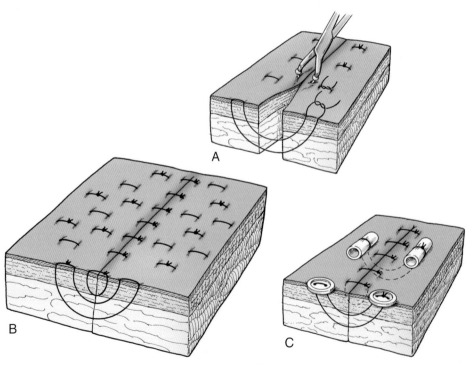

Figure 19-19   A, Taking up skin tension with towel clamps for placement of vertical mattress tension sutures without supports. **B,** The use of several rows of vertical mattress tension sutures to close an undermined wound. **C,** The use of vertical mattress tension suturing with supports. (Modified from Stashak TS: *Equine wound management*, Philadelphia, 1991, Lea & Febiger.)

- Hemoglobin inhibits local tissue defenses, and iron is necessary for bacterial replication because the ferric ion plays a role in increasing bacterial virulence.

Drains

- Used when a large dead space remains after suture closure
- Must be maintained in a sterile environment
  - Use a sterile bandage for the extremities
  - Use a sterile stent bandage for the upper body
- Drains should be buried and sutured dorsally/proximally and either of the following:
  - Traverse a wound that is parallel to the long axis of the limb adjacent to but not directly underlying the sutured skin edges and exit adjacent to the distal extremity of the wound (Fig. 19-21)
- Cross underneath sutured transverse wound edges and exit ventrally or distally
- Placed underneath a skin flap
- Drains should exit from a separate incision adjacent to the wound edge and be sutured in place. (This placement of the drain reduces the chances of retrograde infection directly involving the suture line [Figs. 19-21 and 19-22].)
- Drains usually are left in place for 24 to 48 hours but may remain longer if drainage is continuous and does not decrease in volume.
- *Note:* Drains are a two-way street, and meticulous postoperative care of the drain exit site is essential to decrease the risk of retrograde infection.
- The use of drains is somewhat controversial because they represent a foreign body within the wound; however, if

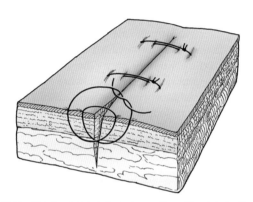

Figure 19-20 The far-near near-far suture pattern. (Reprinted with permission from Stashak TS and Theoret CL, editors: *Equine wound management,* ed 2, Ames, IA, 2008, Wiley-Blackwell, p. 211.)

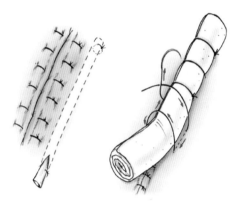

Figure 19-21 *Left,* The proper use of a drain and its relationship to a sutured wound oriented parallel to the long axis of the limb. *Note:* The proximal end of the drain is buried and sutured, and the distal end of the drain is sutured to the exit site. *Right,* A sterile stent bandage is being sutured over the wound and drain to cover/protect them.

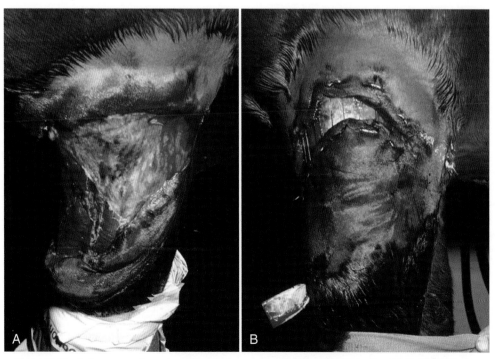

Figure 19-22 **A,** A transverse laceration of the upper cranial antebrachium (forearm) with a skin flap. **B,** Illustration of proper placement of a drain under the skin flap.

ITEG

drainage of a hematoma from "dead space" is needed, *the consequences of not using a drain are considerably more serious than the potential complications that may arise from using a drain.*

Bandaging
Advantages
- Protection from further contamination
- Exerted pressure reduces edema
- Absorption of exudate
- Increased temperature and reduced loss of CO_2 from the wound surface reduce pH
- Immobilization of a structure and reduction of additional trauma (e.g., a wound on the dorsal surface of the hock)
- *Practice Tip: Bandaged distal extremity wounds heal 30% faster than do nonbandaged wounds.*

Disadvantages
- Wounds on the distal extremities may develop exuberant granulation tissue under a bandage.

Wound Dressings
- A wide variety of wound dressings are available, ranging from passive adherent/nonadherent to interactive and bioactive products that contribute to healing.
- Most of the newer dressings are designed to create "moist wound healing," which allows wound fluids and growth factors to remain in contact with the wound, therefore promoting "autolytic debridement" and subsequently accelerating wound healing.
- Despite substantial advancements in wound dressings, *no single material produces the optimum microenvironment for all wounds or for all the stages of wound healing.* Consequently, the selection of a wound dressing should be dictated by an understanding of the stages of wound healing and the condition, location, and depth of the wound.
- Wound dressings have been broadly classified as adherent, hydrophilic, nonadherent, and absorbent/nonabsorbent. Adherent dressings are frequently made from closely woven or widely open gauze, and under most circumstances, are considered passive; however, a few are considered interactive. Gauze dressings are generally highly absorbent and are still used for heavily contaminated exudative wounds.
- Hydrophilic dressings are made from materials that absorb a large amount of fluid from the wound's surface.
- Nonadherent dressings have variable absorbency and are subdivided into occlusive, semiocclusive, and biologic types.

Absorbent/Adherent and Nonadherent Dressing
Many, but not all, of the absorbent dressings adhere to the wound surface, affecting wound debridement. This section focuses on the types of dressing used most commonly in equine practice.

Gauze Dressings
- These dressings are used during the inflammatory phase of wound healing to assist with wound debridement. Wide mesh gauze usually promotes better adherence and wound debridement. The dressing may be applied dry or wet.
  - Dry dressings are used when wound fluids have a low viscosity.
  - Wet dressings are applied when the wound fluids have a high viscosity or a scab has developed. Sterile saline is often used as the wetting agent with or without the addition of soluble antiseptics, antimicrobials, or enzymes.
  - Wet dressings can be used for packing deep wounds.
  - Wet dressings are discontinued when a healthy bed of granulation tissue develops.
  - The dressing is usually changed after 24 hours, for 1 to 3 dressing changes total.
- *Curasalt,*[20] a hypertonic 20% saline dressing, appears to provide effective osmotic nonselective wound debridement. Curasalt is recommended for infected, necrotic, heavily exuding wounds only. The dressing is usually applied once and removed the following day.
- *Gamgee*[21] is used as a primary wound dressing while providing protection, support, and insulation.
  - Gamgee is highly absorbent and nonadherent; its proposed best use is for highly exudative limb wounds during the inflammatory phase of healing.
- *Antimicrobial gauze dressing (Kerlix AMD) and Poultice pad*
  - The characteristics and proposed best uses for these dressings are covered under Antimicrobial Dressings later in this section (see p. 262).

Hydrophilic Dressings
Particulate Dextranomers (PDs)
- PDs are available as beads (e.g., Debrisan[22]), flakes (e.g., Avalon[23]), and powders (e.g., Intrasite[24] and Intracell[25]).
  - They absorb the aqueous component, including prostaglandins, from wound exudate
  - They remove microorganisms from the wound bed, primarily by capillary action
  - They activate chemotactic factors that attract polymorphonuclear and mononuclear cells
- The best use for PDs appears to be for debridement of sloughing, exuding wounds. They should be discontinued when a healthy bed of granulation tissue develops and are contraindicated in dry wounds.
- *Note:* Because PDs are not biodegradable, they should be rinsed from the wound with saline or other sterile salt

[20]Covidien Animal Health/Kendall, Dublin, Ohio.
[21]3M Center, St. Paul, Minnesota.
[22]Johnson & Johnson, New Brunswick, New Jersey.
[23]Summit Hill Laboratories, Avalon, New Jersey.
[24]Smith & Nephew, Hull, United Kingdom.
[25]Macleod Pharmaceuticals, Inc., Fort Collins, Colorado.

solutions before the wound dries. Doing this avoids particulate residue buildup and the subsequent development of a granuloma.

Maltodextrin (MD)

- MD (Intracell)[25] is commercially available as a powder or gel containing 1% ascorbic acid.
  - The hydrophilic soluble powder has an affinity for fluids, "pulling" them up through the wound tissues and therefore bathing the wound from inside. These fluids encourage moist wound healing.
  - Intracell yields glucose from hydrolysis of the polysaccharide, providing energy for cell metabolism to promote healing.
  - Powder and gel are claimed to cause chemotaxis of macrophages, polymorphonuclear cells, and lymphocytes into the wound, thus enhancing the debridement process.
- The powder should be applied over the wound to a depth of approximately ¼ inch. A primary nonadherent semiocclusive dressing should be applied over the powder, followed by an absorbent wrap and tertiary bandage.
  - Bandages are changed daily, the wound is irrigated, and more powder is applied.
  - The proposed best use is for debridement to cleanse and promote healing in contaminated and infected wounds.
  - The powder is best used on exudative wounds, and the gel is best used for drier wounds.

Calcium Alginate (CA)

- CA is classified as a fibrous dextranomer.
- It is available from a variety of sources (Curasorb,[26] C-Stat,[27] Nu-Derm,[28] and Kaltostat[29]).
  - Made from salts of alginic acid obtained from Phaeophyceae algae found in seaweed
  - Can absorb up to 19 to 30 times its weight in wound fluid
  - Promotes a moist environment conducive to wound healing
  - Claimed to increase epithelialization and granulation tissue formation; this was not found in one study done in horses
  - Improves clotting
  - Activates macrophages within a chronic wound bed, which promotes granulation tissue formation
  - Some alginates have the ability to "kick-start" the healing cascade by causing lysis of mast cells, resulting in release of histamine and 5-hydroxytryptamine
- Because of these attributes, calcium alginate dressings are considered bioactive.

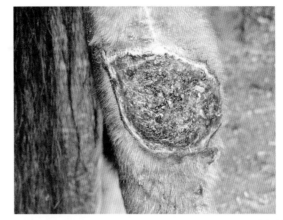

Figure 19-23   Example of a chronic wound on the dorsal surface of the hock/tarsal region that benefits from debridement and the application of a calcium alginate dressing. (Reprinted with permission from Stashak TS, Theoret CL, editors: *Equine wound management,* ed 2, Ames, IA, 2008, Wiley-Blackwell, p. 119.)

- Best use:
  - Moderate to heavily exuding wounds during the transition from the acute inflammatory to repair phases of healing
  - Wounds with substantial tissue loss, such as degloving injuries
  - Kick-starting the healing in a chronic wound bed
    - The dressing should be premoistened before application to a chronic dry wound that needs stimulation to proceed with the formation of granulation tissue. A better alternative is to first debride the wound, then apply the dressing without moistening it (Fig. 19-23 shows a dry wound of the dorsal hock). A semiocclusive nonadherent pad should be placed over the calcium alginate dressing, followed by secondary and tertiary bandage layers.

Freeze Dried Gel (FDG)

- A hydrophilic FDG containing acemannan is commercially available (CarraSorb[30]).
- It is shown to significantly accelerate healing in experimental wounds in rats.
- It has potent macrophage-activating properties and the ability to bind growth factors, prolonging their stimulating effect on granulation tissue formation.
- It has been shown to aggressively promote granulation tissue formation in open wounds and in wounds with exposed bone in dogs.
- It promotes moist wound healing and autolytic debridement.
- The dressing should be cut to conform to the wound and hydrated with sterile saline/water before application to a dry wound.

[26]Covidien Animal Health/Kendall, Dublin, Ohio.
[27]RS Jackson Inc., Alexandria, Virginia.
[28]Johnson & Johnson Products Inc., New Brunswick, New Jersey.
[29]Convatec ER Squibb and Sons, LLC, Princeton, New Jersey.

[30]Carrington Laboratories, Inc., Irving, Texas.

- Because of its ability to stimulate fibroplasia, it is recommended to only use it every 2 to 3 days.
- Best use:
  - During the early inflammatory phase, particularly for moderately exuding wounds and wounds with exposed bone
  - To reduce wound edema because of its hydrophilic action
  - Discontinue when granulation tissue fills the wound.

Chitin (C)
- C, a polymeric N-actyl-D-glucosamine, is a component of the skeletal material of crustaceans and insects.
- Various formulations are available: sponge, cotton, flake, and nonwoven fabric.
- A controlled study performed on canine full-thickness skin wounds found that the treated wounds tended towards greater epithelialization than did control wounds at 21 days.
- It is difficult to identify a best use for this product currently; it is not being used routinely for wound management in North America.

Occlusive Synthetic Dressings (OSDs)
- OSDs promote "moist wound healing" via nonporous materials with a low moisture/vapor transmission. A moist wound environment is rich in white blood cells, enzymes, cytokines, and growth factors beneficial to wound healing. Under these dressings, autolytic debridement usually occurs 72 to 96 hours after injury (assuming the dressing is applied at the time of injury), thus cleaning the wound in preparation for the repair phase. Fibroplasia and epithelialization are stimulated by cytokines and growth factors present in the moist wound. Proposed benefits to moist wound healing include:
  - Prevention of scab formation, which otherwise traps white blood cells preventing their participation in important wound healing functions
  - Reduction of the environmental pH, which improves oxygenation of the wound by shifting the oxygen-hemoglobin dissociation curve in favor of oxygen release from hemoglobin
  - Prevention of bacterial strike-through from the outside environment to the wound surface
  - Augmentation of epithelialization primarily by allowing epithelial cells to freely migrate over the moist wound surface
  - Enhancement of bacterial colonization but not infection. Reports in the equine literature do not, however, substantiate this latter claim; several studies indicate that the risk of developing infection is greater in wounds covered with occlusive dressings.
  - Additional benefits of moist wound healing include acceleration (shortening) of the inflammatory and proliferative phases with more rapid progression towards the remodeling phase.

- OCDs are considered interactive and are commercially available as:
  - Hydrogels
  - Hydrocolloids
  - Silicone dressings

Hydrogels (Polyethylene Oxide Occlusive Dressings)
- Hydrogels are a three-dimensional network of hydrophilic polymers with a water content between 90% and 95%.
- Hydrogels are available as sheets or gels.
  - Sheet hydrogels are believed to possess most of the properties of an ideal wound dressing (e.g., Tegagel dressing; Nu-gel[31]). When applied to a dry wound, they hydrate it, creating an environment for moist wound healing.
  - Amorphous hydrogels also possess a "moisture donor" effect for necrotic wounds that require debriding. By increasing the moisture content of the necrotic tissue and increasing collagenase production, hydrogels facilitate autolytic debridement.
- Hydrogels containing acemannan (CarraVet,[32] Carra-Sorb[32]) stimulate healing over exposed bone.
- Some hydrogels contain hyaluronic acid and chondroitin sulfate with a chemically cross-linked glycosaminoglycan hydrofilm (Tegaderm[33]). Addition of these substances reportedly increases epithelialization and granulation tissue formation compared with Tegaderm alone.
- Other products contain gauze impregnated with a hydrogel (e.g., FasCure[34]; Curafil[35]), and another contains 25% propylene glycol (Solugel[36]).
  - A study evaluating the effects of Solugel on second intention healing in horses found no beneficial effects compared with the control saline-soaked gauze dressing.
- In a study of equine limb wounds, the hydrogel sheet dressing generated excess exudate, increased the need to trim exuberant granulation tissue, and prolonged wound healing by more than twofold compared with controls. The persistent formation of exuberant granulation tissue was believed to be the result of continued application of the hydrogel sheet dressing during the repair phase.

● WHAT TO DO

Hydrogels
- The dressing should be applied within 6 hours of injury and continued for at least 48 hours before changing.
- The dressing should be discontinued at the earliest signs of granulation tissue formation.
- Before a sheet hydrogel dressing is applied, the skin around the wound should be cleaned and dried and the wound surface gently rinsed with a dilute antiseptic solution.

---

[31]Johnson & Johnson Products, Inc., New Brunswick, New Jersey.
[32]Carrington Laboratories, Inc., Irving, Texas.
[33]3M Center, St. Paul, Minnesota.
[34]Ken Vet, Greeley, Colorado.
[35]Covidien Animal Health/Kendall, Dublin, Ohio.
[36]Johnson & Johnson, Medical, North Ryde, Australia.

- The dressing is cut to the appropriate size and the thin sheet on one side is peeled off and the sheet is applied to the wound surface. The dressing is then covered with secondary and tertiary bandage layers. The dressing should be left in place for 2 days.
  - If the skin surrounding the wound begins to appear macerated because of excess moisture, the dressing should be replaced with a nonadherent semiocclusive dressing.
- These dressings are best used on clean acute wounds during the inflammatory phase of wound healing.

Vulketan Gels (VG)

- The active ingredient in Vulketan gel (VG) is a potent serotonin receptor antagonist, ketanserin.
- VG block the serotonin-induced macrophage suppression and vasoconstriction present in the early wound environment, thus allowing a strong and effective inflammatory response to occur within wounds. This action may translate into:
  - Superior infection control
  - Superior repair
- When VG was evaluated in a multicentric randomized controlled clinical study performed on equine distal limb wounds, it was found to be more effective than other standard treatments in preventing infection and the formation of exuberant granulation tissue.
- Because of its stimulating effect on the circulation, VG should not be applied to a fresh bleeding wound.

Hydrocolloid

- Hydrocolloid consists of an inner, often adhesive layer, a thick, absorbing hydrocolloid "mass," and an outer, thin, water-resistant and bacteria-impervious polyurethane film.
- Hydrocolloid is available as the following: Duoderm,[37] Dermaheal,[38] or carboxymethylcellulose particles embedded in an elastotic mesh (Comfeel[39]).
- Duoderm is oxygen impermeable, which is purported to promote the rate of epithelialization and collagen synthesis and to decrease the pH of wound exudate, thus reducing bacterial counts.
- Acceleration of epithelialization has not been documented in all studies.
- A study on horses found that Dermaheal or Duoderm dressings promoted the formation of granulation tissue directly from the surface of denuded bone and on the surface of frayed tendons and ligaments. This study also found that wound infection can develop under these dressings; when it does, application should be discontinued until the wound is healthy.
- The best use for these dressings in horses appears to be during the early inflammatory phase until granulation tissue fills the wound. The dressing should be applied to a clean wound, free of infection, and discontinued before the development of exuberant granulation.

Silicone Dressing

- A silicone dressing was investigated (Cica Care[40]) in experimental distal limb wounds in horses. It was observed that the silicone dressing greatly surpassed a conventional nonadherent absorbent dressing in preventing the formation of exuberant granulation tissue. Contraction and epithelialization progressed faster in the first 2 weeks of repair, possibly as a result of healthier granulation tissue. Furthermore, tissue quality exceeded that of wounds treated conventionally.

Semiocclusive Synthetic Dressings
Fabric Synthetic Dressings (FSDs)
- FSDs are commercially available as follows:
  - Petrolatum-impregnated gauze (NU Gauze sponges,[41] Vaseline Petrolatum Gauze,[42] Xerofoam,[42] Jelonet[43])
  - Petrolatum emulsion dressing (Adaptic[44]), oil emulsion knitted fabric (Curity[45]) and rayon/polyethylene fabric (Release[46]), petrolatum-impregnated gauze with 3% bismuth tribromophenate (Adaptic + Xerofoam[46])
  - Absorbent adhesive film (Mitraflex[47]).
  - Perforated polyester film filled with compressed cotton (Telfa[48])
- A study evaluating the effects of two semiocclusive dressings (Telfa and Mitraflex), a biologic dressing (equine amnion), and an occlusive dressing (Biodres—this dressing is no longer on the market) on the healing of experimental full-thickness distal limb wounds in horses found that wounds dressed with Biodres showed an increased need to trim exuberant granulation tissue, excess exudate, and prolonged wound healing by more than two times compared with the control Telfa. Wounds dressed with amnion required minimal trimming of the granulation tissue, and those dressed with Telfa healed the fastest.

Polyurethane Semiocclusive Dressings
- Polyurethane semiocclusive dressings are available as a film (e.g., Op-Site,[49] Tegaderm,[50] Bioclusive[51]) or foam (e.g., Hydrosorb,[52] Hydrosorb Wound Care Products,[53] Sof-Foam[54]).

[37]ER Squibb Inc., Princeton, New Jersey.
[38]Solvay Animal Health, Mendota Heights, Minnesota.
[39]Coloplast, Marietta, Georgia.
[40]Smith Nephew, Hull, United Kingdom.
[41]Johnson & Johnson Products, New Brunswick, New Jersey.
[42]Covidien Animal Health/Kendall, Dublin, Ohio.
[43]Smith & Nephew, Hull, United Kingdom.
[44]Johnson & Johnson Products, New Brunswick, New Jersey.
[45]Covidien Animal Health/Kendall, Dublin, Ohio.
[46]Johnson & Johnson Products, New Brunswick, New Jersey.
[47]Polymedica Industries Inc., Wheat Ridge, Colorado.
[48]Covidien Animal Health/Kendall, Dublin, Ohio.
[49]Smith & Nephew, Hull, United Kingdom.
[50]3M Center, St. Paul, Minnesota.
[51]Johnson & Johnson Products, New Brunswick, New Jersey.
[52]Ken Vet, Greeley, Colorado.
[53]Wound Care Products (Avitar, Inc., Canton, Ohio.
[54]Johnson & Johnson Products, New Brunswick, New Jersey.

- The *film* is transparent, waterproof, semipermeable to vapor, oxygen permeable, and adhesive to dry skin while nonadhesive to the wound, and has an analgesic effect.
  - Although these dressings are considered nonadherent, one product, Op-Site, has a tendency to strip newly formed epidermis from the surface of a healing wound.
  - Although the proposed best use for the sheet dressings in horses is during the repair phase, their unique characteristics allow them to be used during the entire healing period *of a clean wound.*
- The *foam* sponges come as sheet dressings, *in situ* formed foams, and adhesive foams (e.g., Tielle hydropolymer adhesive[54]).
  - They are highly conforming, vapor permeable, absorptive, and easy to apply and provide an effective barrier against bacterial penetration. Moisture is absorbed into the dressing, which reduces tissue maceration while providing a moist healing environment.
  - The proposed best use for the sponge is during the early inflammatory phase of healing, when there is considerable exudate in the wound. Under these circumstances, the bandage should be changed daily or as indicated according to the amount of fluid produced by the wound. Because of their semiocclusive nature, sponges are also indicated during the repair phase. An alternate use of the sponge is to deliver liquid medication or wetting agents to the wound by saturating the sponge before placing it on the wound. The same sponge, however, cannot be used for absorption and medication delivery.

Antimicrobial Dressings

- Infection and bacterial colonization remain important factors contributing to delayed wound healing. Because the widespread use of systemic and topical antimicrobials has resulted in increasing numbers of resistant bacterial strains (methicillin-resistant *S. aureus* [MRSA], vancomycin-resistant *Enterococcus faecalis* [VRE], and *Pseudomonas aeruginosa*), it has been suggested that the judicious use of antimicrobial dressings, notably those containing certain antiseptics, can be important in infection control and in promoting healing.

Iodine-Containing Dressing

- *Iodosorb*[55] is manufactured from cross-linked polymerized dextran that contains iodine. As the dressing hydrates in the moist wound environment, elemental iodine is released to exert an antibacterial effect and to interact with macrophages to produce tumor necrosis factor-alpha (TNFα) and interleukin-6, which can indirectly influence wound healing. Best use would be for contaminated wounds, early in the inflammatory phase of repair.
- *Iodoflex,*[56] a slow-release iodine dressing, has been reported to be effective in the treatment of extensive mycotic rhinitis

in dogs. The slow release is designed to maintain an adequate level of active iodine locally for at least a 48-hour period. It appears that the slow release of povidone-iodine (PI) in this product does not slow wound healing.
- A PI powder dressing[57] is also available. The product has 1.0% available iodine, a broad antimicrobial spectrum, and is also fungicidal.
- *Biozide Gel*[58] is a hydrogel containing a 1% available PI complex in a polyglycol base. A theoretical advantage to this product is that even though it is an occlusive dressing, it can be safely applied to a heavily contaminated or infected wound because of the antiseptic PI incorporated in the product.
- *Oxyzyme,*[59] a relatively new bioxygenating hydrogel dressing, which delivers both iodine (~0.04% w/w) and oxygen to the wound surface, was found in vitro to exert broad-spectrum antimicrobial activity, encompassing antibiotic-resistant organisms, anaerobes, and yeasts. The technology allowing delivery of both oxygen and iodine from this dressing involves a bilayered construction with an oxidase enzyme in the top layer and an iodide in the deeper layer. The oxidase enzyme reacts with oxygen in the air to generate hydrogen peroxide, which converts iodide to molecular iodine, which instantly converts hydrogen peroxide into dissolved oxygen; both are then delivered to the surface of the wound. Case studies in humans found the dressing to be effective in the treatment of venous leg ulcers.
  - At this time, this dressing is perceived to be of limited value in wound treatment in horses because it is recommended that it be applied without a secondary dressing to secure it.
- Objective studies attesting to the efficacy of any of these iodine-containing products on wound healing in horses are lacking. One objective study documented no delay in wound healing in horses treated with 10% PI ointment compared with another antimicrobial dressing.

Antimicrobial Gauze Dressing

- *Kerlix AMD*[60] is impregnated with 0.2% polyhexamethylene biguanide, which has a wide range of antimicrobial activities, including *P. aeruginosa,* while being more biocompatible to tissues than its close relative, chlorhexidine.
  - The dressing comes packaged as a sponge or roll, and the material can be applied wet or dry, as described for plain mesh gauze.
  - The proposed best use for this dressing is during the inflammatory phase of healing:
    - In wounds with a high concentration of bacteria
    - In wounds where there is an open synovial cavity (Fig. 19-24, *A*).

---

[55]Smith & Nephew, Hull, United Kingdom.
[56]Smith & Nephew, Hull, United Kingdom.

[57]PRN Pharmacal, Pensacola, Florida.
[58]Performance Products, Inc. www.mwivet.com.
[59]Colworth Science Park, Shambrook, Bedford, United Kingdom.
[60]Kendall Health Care, Mansfield, Massachusetts.

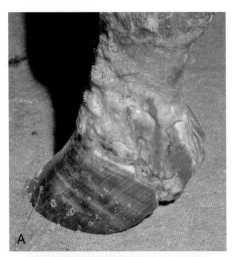

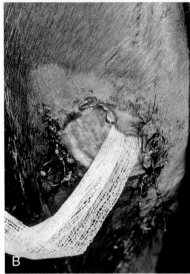

Figure 19-24   A, Example of a wound entering the distal interphalangeal joint that would benefit from being dressed with a Kerlix AMD dressing. **B,** Example of a large, undermined, heavily contaminated wound on the cranial surface of the pectoral region, packed with moistened Kerlix AMD gauze. (Reprinted with permission from Stashak TS, Theoret CL, editors: *Equine wound management*, ed 2, Ames, IA, 2008, Wiley-Blackwell, p. 127.)

- ○ The large roll is an ideal dressing for packing deep contaminated wounds associated with the body or upper limbs (Fig. 19-24, *B*). The packing is changed daily with progressively less gauze used to pack the wound.
- ○ Debriding wounds

Poultice Pad
- Animalintex Poultice and Hoof pad[61]
  - The pad is made of nonwoven cotton with a plastic backing.
  - The dressing contains boric acid (mild antiseptic) and tragacanth, which is a poultice agent, and the pad is shaped to fit the sole of the foot and as a non hoof-shaped bandage. The dressing can be applied hot, cold, or dry.

- The proposed best use is as follows:
  - Apply hot for infected hoof wounds (e.g., abscesses and dirty wounds); it can be used as a poultice for other regions of the body.
  - Apply cold for sprains and strains.

Silver Impregnated Dressings (SIDs)
- A range of SIDs (e.g., Silverlon,[62] Acticoat,[63] Actisorb,[64] Aquacel Silver,[65] PolyMem,[66] Urgotul SSD,[67] and Contreet[68]) are commercially available (see Table 2-1), but comparative data on their antimicrobial efficacies and effects on wound healing are limited. The silver that is released in variable concentrations from the dressing over time kills bacteria.
- Although SIDs are generally considered useful for control of bacterial infections (also fungal and viral), key issues remain, including the relative efficacy of different SIDs for wound uses and the existence of microbes that are resistant to silver. The perceived best use for these dressings is during the inflammatory phase through the beginning of the repair phase of wound healing.

Activated Charcoal Dressing
- Activated charcoal dressings are available (Activate[69] and Actisorb[70]). One of the dressings, Activate, is packaged as a multilayered, nonwoven, nonadherent material.
- Proposed advantages are the following:
  - Provide a moist wound healing environment for autolytic debridement
  - Effectively absorb bacteria
  - Prevent the formation of exuberant granulation tissue in horses
  - Reduce wound odor
- Best use is for the heavily infected wound during the inflammatory phase to the repair phase.
- Anecdotally, good healing has been seen in a limited number of cases through the repair phase of wound healing.

Antibiotic-Impregnated Collagen Sponges
These are discussed before under Management of Synovial Penetration (see p. 254).

Biologic Dressings
Biologic dressings are developed from natural products produced by the body. They can be made from body tissues (e.g.,

---

[61]3M Animal Care Products, St. Paul, Minnesota.

[62]Argentum, Lakemont, Georgia.
[63]Westaim Biomedical Corp., Fort Saskatchewan, AB, Canada.
[64]Silver 220 (Johnson & Johnson Products Inc., New Brunswick, New Jersey).
[65]Convatec, a division of ER Squibb and Sons, LLC, Princeton, New Jersey.
[66]Ashton Medical Products, Inc., Dayton, Ohio.
[67]Urgo, Chenove, France.
[68]Coloplast Corp., Minneapolis, Minnesota.
[69]3M Animal Care Products, St. Paul, Minnesota.
[70]Johnson & Johnson Products, New Brunswick, New Jersey.

amnion, peritoneum, or skin), engineered to form a biocompatible construct (e.g., extracellular matrix scaffold, collagen, etc.), or be derived from components of blood. Although tissue dressings enhance repair by providing an optimum environment for moist wound healing, most engineered dressings are designed to regenerate tissue components resulting in scar-free healing. Dressings made from cell-rich components of blood were developed to provide growth factors to stimulate healing. These dressings are considered bioactive.

Natural Tissue Dressings

Equine Amnion

Equine amnion, despite its occlusive properties, does not encourage exuberant granulation tissue formation nor does it promote more rapid healing in horses, except when it is used to dress pinch- and punch-grafted wounds. The proposed best use is to apply amnion to wounds of the distal extremities to suppress the formation of exuberant granulation tissue and to accelerate epithelialization in pinch- or punch-grafted wounds. Bandaging over the dressing is optional.

Equine Peritoneum and Split-Thickness Allogeneic Skin

A study done in horses found that wounds dressed with equine peritoneum or split-thickness allogeneic skin did not heal faster than similar wounds dressed with a control synthetic dressing.

Tissue Engineered Dressings

Collagen Dressing

Collagen dressings are made into gels (Collasate[71]), porous and nonporous membranes, particles (Collamend[72]), and sponges, and reportedly they enhance wound healing in human beings and in experimental animals. Studies evaluating bovine porous and nonporous collagen membranes or gel dressings in horses found no benefit of these dressings over semiocclusive control dressings. The fact that scabs formed in wounds dressed with porous bovine collagens indicates that the wound surface became dehydrated, and therefore the dressing was not acting as an occlusive or semiocclusive dressing.

Chemically Modified (Thiolated) Hyaluronic Acid (HA) Matrix

Chemically modified HA scaffolds (e.g., sheet dressing[73] and gel spray gel[74]) have been shown to accelerate and promote scar free healing in both experimental models and in clinical cases. A preliminary report suggests that cross-linked sheet dressing may accelerate the repair of limb wounds in horses. This controlled study, comparing the effects of EquitrX film (applied at bandage change) or a gel dressing (CantrX, applied either once or at every bandage change), to a control bandage

dressing, found that wounds treated with the films healed with superior tissue quality and cosmesis.
- Proposed best use:
  - Large degloving and avulsion wounds
  - Wounds where the best cosmetic outcome is desirable

Extracellular Matrix Scaffolds (ECMS)

ECMS are available as porcine urinary bladder lamina propria (ACell Vet Scaffold[75]) and porcine small intestinal submucosa (Vet BioSISt[76]). ECMS are described as having the capability of recruiting marrow-derived stem cells to migrate into the acellular scaffold, resulting in "*constructive remodeling*" of the severely damaged or missing tissue. The healed remodeled tissue has differentiated cell and tissue types including functional arteries and veins, innervated smooth muscle, cartilage, and specialized epithelial structures. Minimal scar tissue formation is found in the healed wounds.

Note: This is a new concept in wound healing.

Cell Rich or Cell Free Component Dressings

Solcoseryl

Solcoseryl is a protein-free, standardized dialysate/ultrafiltrate derived from calf blood (Solcoseryl[77]). In an equine study, Solcoseryl provoked a greater inflammatory response with faster formation and contraction of granulation tissue. Subsequently, Solcoseryl inhibited repair by causing a prolonged inflammatory phase of healing and delayed epithelialization. The perceived best use is for deep wounds during the early inflammatory phase; treatment should be discontinued at the first signs of epithelialization.

Platelet-Rich Plasma

Platelet-rich plasma (PRP) is, by definition, a volume of autologous plasma that has a platelet concentration well above baseline. While the normal platelet counts in whole blood average 200,000/mL, the platelet counts in PRP should average 1,000,000/mL. (*Note:* Lesser concentrations of platelets cannot be relied on to enhance wound healing, whereas greater concentrations have not currently shown to further enhance wound healing.) There are at least *four major groups of native growth factors* found in PRP with the potential to enhance wound healing. *Practice Tip:* PRP should only be made from anticoagulated blood since coagulation results in almost immediate release of growth factors. Within 10 minutes of coagulation, it is estimated that activated platelets release 70% of their stored mediators and close to 100% within the first hour. For this reason, clotting of the PRP (via addition of thrombin or $CaCl_2$) should be done just before its delivery to the surface of the wound.

●〉 WHAT TO DO

Dressing Selection to Promote Wound Healing

Dressing selection for promotion of healing during different phases of repair.

---

[71]PRN Pharmacal, Pensacola, Florida.
[72]Veterinary Products Laboratory, Phoenix, Arizona.
[73]SentrX Animal Care, Inc., Salt Lake City, Utah.
[74]Bayer, Animal Health, Shawnee Mission Parkway, Shawnee, Kansas.

[75]ACell, Inc., Jessup, Maryland.
[76]Cook Veterinary Products, Bloomington, Indiana.
[77]Solco Basle Ltd., Birsfelden, Switzerland

Inflammatory/Cellular Debridement Phase

- Use occlusive for clean or contaminated noninfected wounds until healthy granulation tissue forms.
  - Exceptions: Vulketan and Silicone gel can be used throughout the entire healing period
  - Promote autolytic wound debridement
- Use adherent, hydrophilic and antimicrobial dressings for heavily contaminated/infected exudative wounds. Discontinue when a healthy bed of granulation tissue has formed.
  - Gauze roll or strips can be used for packing tunneled and undermined wounds; the dressing is able to fill in the dead space and provide drainage.
- Use alginate dressings to "kick start" healing in chronic nonhealing wounds. Hydrate the dressing for dry wounds.
- Use acemannan-containing dressings to promote granulation tissue formation in wounds over exposed bone.
- Use protein-free dialysate of calf blood to promote granulation tissue and contraction in deep wounds. Discontinue at the first signs of epithelialization.
- Use oxidized regenerated cellulose/collagen dressing to promote healing in a chronic wound environment by inactivating matrix metalloproteinases and binding growth factors releasing them back into the wound in an active form as the gel is slowly broken down.

Repair Phase

- Use semiocclusive once granulation tissue develops
- Vulketan and Silicone gel can be also used

All Phases

- Vulketan and Silicone gel
- Liquid adhesives
- Biologic dressings
  - Chemically modified HA scaffolds
  - ECM: constructive remodeling of clean large avulsive wounds and tendon deficits
  - Autologous platelet-rich plasma gels

Topical Agents

Scarlet Oil (SO)

- Although SO has been used in the treatment of horse wounds for many years, there have been no controlled studies evaluating its effectiveness. The ingredients in SO are mineral oil, isopropyl alcohol (30%), methyl salicylate, benzyl alcohol (3%), pine oil, eucalyptus oil, parachlorometaxylenol, and biebrich scarlet red. Pine oil is used commonly as an antiseptic in household cleaning agents. SO can cause a painful contact dermatitis in some horses causing an objection to continued treatment. Some clinicians use this agent to stimulate granulation tissue formation in large upper body wounds. There are no data to prove that it is of any benefit and therefore the authors do not recommend its use.

Live Yeast Cell Derivative

- Live yeast cell derivative is a water-soluble yeast extract reported to stimulate angiogenesis, epithelialization, and collagen formation. It has been associated with improved wound healing in dogs. *Note:* In horses, however, the derivative prolonged wound healing and resulted in excessive granulation tissue formation.

Aloe Vera (AV)

- Reportedly AV has antithromboxane and antiprostaglandin properties that favor vascular patency and prevent skin ischemia.
- AV has been shown to stimulate wound healing; possess antibacterial, antifungal, and antiviral properties; act as an immune stimulant; have anti-inflammatory effects; and stimulate collagen production. It is also reported to be effective against *P. aeruginosa*.
- AV extract gel with acemannan has been shown experimentally to accelerate epithelialization and wound healing in open pad wounds in dogs at 7 days.
- Efficacy in horses has not yet been studied, and at least one study showed that AV delayed healing.

Honey

- Honey attracts tissue macrophages and is known to possess antibacterial activity.
- At the wound site, enzymes contained within the honey exert an antibacterial effect via acidification and the slow release of hydrogen peroxide, a mild disinfectant, and glucolactone/gluconic acid, a mild antibiotic.
- Honey provides antioxidants, which protect wound tissues from the damage imparted by free oxygen radicals released from inflammatory cells.
- Honey has been shown to up-regulate the expression of some inflammatory cytokines known to enhance fibroplasia and epithelialization.
- It accelerates wound repair in mammals, in particular laboratory rodents; however no published data to this effect exist for the management of wounds in horses.
- Honey used for treatment of wounds should ideally be unpasteurized and not heated above 37° C to prevent inactivation of glucose oxidase.
- Standardized honey products are commercially available for wound care (Manuka honey[78]-impregnated tulle dressing, Meloderm UMF,[79] 16+ irradiated active Manuka honey, Vetramil[80]).

Sugar

- Sugar is:
  - Bacteriostatic
  - Reduces edema
  - Attracts macrophages
  - Debrides the wound
  - Provides energy
  - Creates moist wound healing
- Sugar should be placed on the wound 1 cm thick and then covered with an absorbent dressing.
- Sugar is best used in necrotic, infected wounds.

[78]Advancis Medical, Nottingham, United Kingdom.
[79]UMF, Surrey, United Kingdom.
[80]BFactory BV, Wageningen, Netherlands.

Other Topical Agents

- *Vitamin E* is commonly used during the maturation phase of wound healing in horses, but clinical trials that examine its effects are lacking.
  - A study in humans found that 90% of treated wounds treated with Vitamin E had a poorer cosmetic outcome and 33% developed a contact dermatitis.
- *Lanolin:* has been used for centuries as a skin softener and moisturizer
  - In a controlled clinical trial evaluating partial-thickness wounds in piglets, it was found that lanolin cream alone significantly enhanced the rate of epithelialization and increased dermal thickness when compared with lanolin/human epidermal growth factor cream or gauze controls.
  - The proposed best use for lanolin is for abrasions and during the maturation phase of wound healing.
- *Tea tree oil (TTO):*
  - Products are nonirritating
  - Increases fibroplasia without causing the formation of exuberant granulation tissue
  - Encourages rapid healing
  - Is effective in controlling bacterial/fungal infections
  - The antifungal and antibacterial characteristics of TTO are well documented.
  - There is no scientific literature documenting the effects of TTO on wound healing in horses
  - The proposed best use of TTO is during the inflammatory through repair phases of wound healing
- *Gentian violet* has been shown to be carcinogenic.
- *Cut-Heal (CH):* contains fish oil, raw linseed oil, turpentine, balsam, fir and sulfuric acid
  - Sulfuric acid (aka, battery acid) and turpentine are recognized skin irritants
  - This product is commonly applied to wounds of horse by owners.
  - Its use is *not recommended.*
- *Alu-Spray (AS):*
  - Is indicated to create a physical barrier for protecting the wound from the surrounding environment
  - It does not come off with hot or cold water but can be washed off with soapy water.
  - The physical barrier can protect wounds from flies and gnats, which are common in the environment of horses
  - The perceived best use is for surgical sites that are not bandaged and for minor lacerations for open wound healing.
- *Red Kote:* is a germicidal, nondrying, softening wound dressing and healing aid
  - Indications:
    - Surface wounds
    - Cuts
    - Lacerations
    - Abrasions
  - No studies have been performed in horses
- *Amino Plex (AP):* is a solution made up of amino acids, trace minerals, peptides, electrolytes, and nucleosides
  - Reported properties are that AP reverses cell damage, increases glucose and oxygen uptake, enhances collagen synthesis, and accelerates epithelialization in human beings
  - No controlled studies have been done in the horse
- *Addison Lab-Zn7 Derm:* is a patented solution with a neutral pH
  - The solution enhances wound healing, promotes hair regrowth, and is antimicrobial
  - No controlled studies have been done in the horse
- *Tripeptide-copper complex (TCC):*
  - Is available as a topical or injectable medicant
  - Promotes neovascularization, epithelialization, and collagen deposition and enhances wound contraction
  - The topical form has been shown to enhance open wound healing in dogs while the injectable form stimulates type I collagen deposition in healing footpad wounds in dogs.
  - TCC has also been shown to enhance healing of chronic, ischemic wounds.
  - TCC is not commonly used in equine practice.
  - The proposed best use for TCC is during the repair phase of wound healing.
- *Granulex:* is an aerosol that contains trypsin (TR), Peru balsam, and castor oil
  - TR functions to liquefy fibrin and debride necrotic tissue.
  - Application of 1 mg of TR to a wound before topical application of antibiotic is ineffective in potentiating antibiotic activity.
  - Peru balsam contains cinnamic and benzoic acids, believed to act as irritants, resulting in enhanced blood flow by local stimulation of the capillary bed.
  - May also act as a mild antiseptic
  - Castor oil is a local protective agent that may promote epithelialization.
  - A prospective clinical trial in humans suffering from decubitus ulcers treated with Granulex revealed a faster healing rate than those with no direct medication of the ulcer.
  - Aspiration of Granulex spray is an important consideration if it is sprayed on or around the face because it is oil-based and may cause respiratory irritation.
- *Kinetic Proud Flesh Formula:* contains polyethylene glycol, nitrofurazone, dexamethasone, and scarlet oil
  - Recommended use is to apply to granulating wounds to suppress exuberant granulation tissue and treat superficial dermatitis.
  - No studies in horses are available.

Recombinant Growth Factors

- *Recombinant human transforming growth factor beta-1* was shown to exert no beneficial effects on experimental wound healing in ponies and horses at the doses used.
- *Recombinant platelet-derived growth factor*
  - Effective in the treatment of chronic nonhealing diabetic ulcers in human beings

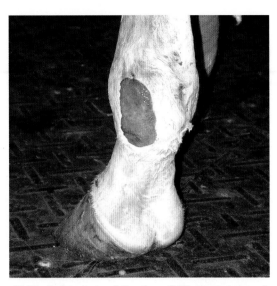

Figure 19-25 Exuberant granulation tissue (EGT), elevated above the skin edges and projecting over the advancing border of epithelium. (Photo courtesy Pr. Olivier Lepage, École Nationale Vétérinaire de Lyon.)

- No studies have been done in the horse.
- Platelet-derived growth factor is commercially available as Regranex.[81]
- *Practice Tip: It appears that a physiologically natural mix of cytokines and growth factors, such as that provided by platelet-rich plasma, is required to exert a beneficial effect on healing wounds, as a result of synergism between mediators.*

Exuberant Granulation Tissue (EGT)

- Wounds with large tissue deficits, located on the limb below the carpus or the tarsus, are predisposed to the development of exuberant granulation tissue (Fig. 19-25).
- Factors believed to encourage the formation of exuberant granulation tissue include:
  - Excessive contamination/chronic inflammation (often caused by the presence of a foreign body)
  - Increased movement (e.g., wounds located on the extensor and flexor surfaces of joints and in the heel bulb region)
  - Lack of soft tissue coverage (absence of an epithelial cover promotes the excessive formation of granulation tissue; EGT then physically and chemically impedes epithelialization, creating a vicious cycle)
  - Poor vascular perfusion/hypoxia leads to chronic inflammation, stimulates fibroblast proliferation, favors

[81]Ethicon Products, Somerville, New Jersey.

an imbalance in extracellular matrix remodeling towards increased synthesis and decreased turnover, and suppresses the differentiation of proliferating fibroblasts into a contractile phenotype (myofibroblast).
- Body size: Individuals >140 cm in height and weighing more than 365 kg seem predisposed; ponies have a more efficient inflammatory response to wounding, improved fibroblast orientation within the wound granulation tissue, and faster wound contraction.
- Aberrant cytokine profile, in favor of fibrogenic transforming growth factor beta$_1$ in wounds located on the distal limb: This growth factor stimulates fibroblast proliferation and synthesis of extracellular matrix components while limiting the disappearance of dermal fibroblasts by apoptosis (programmed cell death).
- The use of bandages and casts, which stimulate angiogenesis and fibroplasia, possibly via an effect on wound oxygen levels and cytokine profile

Prevention

- Careful examination of the wound is critical to exclude stimuli such as bone sequestrum or frayed tendon ends.
- Pressure bandages can be applied to young, edematous granulation tissue when the wound is located on the limb.

Treatment

- For newly formed granulation tissue:
  - Debride the wound and then apply a steroid-antibiotic ointment and a pressure bandage.
  - *Note:* One or two applications of the steroid-antibiotic ointment are usually all that is needed.
- Granulation tissue protruding above the surrounding skin surface forms a fibrogranuloma and is surgically excised; a pressure bandage or cast is applied.
- The silicone gel dressing effectively prevents the development of exuberant granulation tissue in experimental limb wounds.
- Caustics and astringents effectively remove and prevent the formation of granulation tissue through chemical destruction. However, chemicals are not cell selective and destroy the migrating epithelial cells, causing prolonged healing times, increased inflammation, and excessive scarring.

References

References can be found on the companion website at www.equine-emergencies.com.

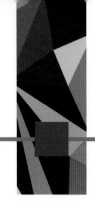

Liver Failure, Anemia, and Blood Transfusion

Thomas J. Divers

Icterus (Jaundice)

- Icterus usually indicates hemolytic disease, liver failure, or anorexia (Fig. 20-1).
- These entities usually can be separated with a well-taken history, clinical examination, and a few laboratory tests.
- **Practice Tip:** *If a problem is found in another organ system that might cause anorexia, icterus is probably physiologic icterus.*
- Physiologic icterus in adults is believed to result from:
  - Anorexia
  - Increased levels of plasma free fatty acids (FFA)
  - Competition between FFA and bilirubin for hepatic uptake
  - Decreased conjugation within the hepatocyte
- Icterus is common in young, septic foals and may be a result of several physiologic mechanisms.
- The best way to detect clinical icterus is by examining the membranes of the sclera, mouth, and vagina.

History

- If icterus is caused by anorexia, the history includes inappetence for more than 2 days.
- If neurologic signs, bilirubinuria, or photosensitivity are present, suspect liver failure.
- If the icterus is severe, suspect liver failure or hemolytic disease.
- During late summer and fall in the eastern United States, the incidence of both liver failure and hemolysis increases because red maple poisoning and Theiler's disease are more prevalent during this time.
- With liver failure or hemolysis, urine is dark red, bright red, black, or orange. With a severe myopathy it is usually dark red or black.

Diagnostic Tests

- If a urine sample is collected, a dipstick examination is helpful.
  - Physiologic icterus: no bilirubinuria
  - Liver failure: usually bilirubinuria (shaking may produce a green foam)
  - Hemolysis: strong reaction to occult blood and occasional reaction to bilirubin if the hemolytic disease is of several days' duration
- The best tests for determining the cause of icterus are the following:

- Packed cell volume (PCV) and total protein: Low PCV and normal to high total protein are most compatible with hemolysis. Pink plasma confirms intravascular hemolysis.
- Gamma-glutamyl transaminopeptidase (GGT): Elevations in the serum confirm liver disease.
- **Practice Tip:** *Bilirubin: Increases in direct and indirect bilirubin and bile acids with an elevation in GGT and a normal to high PCV indicate liver failure. (Conjugated bilirubin >0.5 mg/dL and plasma bile acids >25 μmol/L are together highly sensitive and specific for liver failure.) An increase in only indirect bilirubin with a lower than expected PCV indicates hemolysis.*
- Physiologic icterus: If suspected, manage the primary cause; physiologic icterus should resolve in 24 to 36 hours after a horse regains appetite. In rare instances, a healthy horse has persistent icterus and hyperbilirubinemia (indirect) associated with a conjugation defect.
- Hemolysis: If suspected, see p. 277.

Liver Disease and Failure

- Patients with liver failure may be examined on an emergency basis because of:
  - Bizarre, maniacal behavior—often head pressing
  - Blindness (cortical blindness—pupillary response to light usually present)
  - Ataxia
  - Severe depression
  - Acute dermatitis (photosensitivity)
  - Discolored urine (bilirubinuria)
  - Jaundice
- *Theiler's disease* is an example of a fulminant liver disorder necessitating emergency care. Affected horses may be maniacal or obtunded and may have signs of colic.
- **Practice Tip:** *Hyperlipemia in ponies and miniature equines is a common condition necessitating immediate medical care to prevent rapid progression of disease and death. Affected horses are generally depressed rather than maniacal, and edema of the ventral abdomen is a frequent finding.*
- Chronic active hepatitis and diseases that cause progressive fibrosis, such as pyrrolizidine alkaloid toxicosis, and cholangiohepatitis, can cause a sudden demise in which severe depression, yawning, maniacal behavior, colic, or sepsis from gastric rupture necessitates emergency care.
- Liver disease with elevations in serum hepatic enzyme activity is common with a large number of intestinal

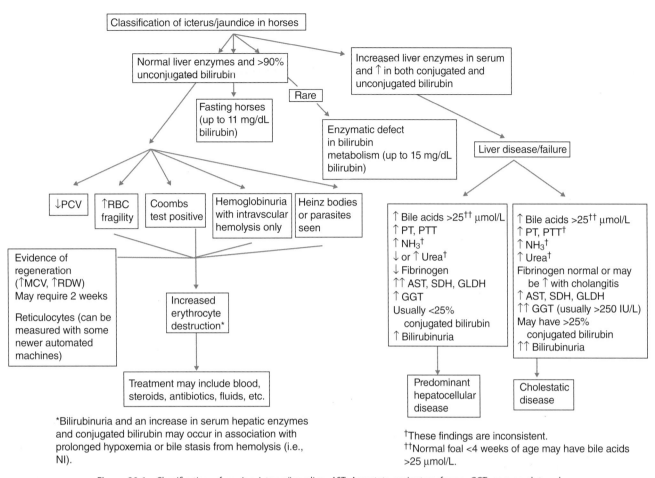

Figure 20-1 Classification of equine icterus/jaundice. *AST,* Aspartate aminotransferase; *GGT,* gamma-glutamyl transaminopeptidase; *GLDH,* glutamate dehydrogenase; *MCV,* mean corpuscular volume; *NH₃,* ammonia; *PT,* prothrombin time; *PTT,* partial thromboplastin time; *PCV,* packed cell volume; *RBC,* red blood cell; *RDW,* red cell distribution width; *SDH,* sorbitol dehydrogenase.

disorders (colic, diarrhea, and/or endotoxemia), but progression to liver failure is rare. The most common exception would be in horses with right colon displacements where obstructive hepatic failure may occur.

Disorders Causing Liver Failure
Theiler's Disease (Serum Hepatitis)
- Theiler's disease is a disease of adults. It is most likely caused by a hepatitis virus; an incriminating *Flavivirus* has recently been discovered. Additional research is needed to further confirm the association of this virus with Theiler's disease. A separate *Hepacivirus* has also been found in serum of presumably healthy horses that had samples submitted for routine Coggins testing. The clinical significance, if any, of this virus is unknown at this time.
- Theiler's disease (acute hepatitis) may be associated with the administration of an equine blood product 4 to 10 weeks earlier (serum hepatitis), but an identical clinical and pathologic disease also is observed without any history of blood product administration.
- Theiler's disease, especially the disease that occurs without a history of blood product administration, is most commonly seen during summer or fall.

- More than one horse on a farm may be affected over a period of several weeks.
- Affected horses may have a history of administration of tetanus antitoxin or equine plasma 4 to 10 weeks earlier.
- ***Practice Tip:*** *In many areas of the United States, if you are called in late summer or fall to examine an adult horse with signs of acute encephalopathy without fever, consider Theiler's disease.*

Clinical Signs
Encephalopathic Signs
- Neurologic signs may on rare occasion occur before jaundice
- Depression or bizarre behavior
- Blindness
- Ataxia

Icterus/Hyperbilirubinemia
- Icteric mucous membranes
- Discolored urine, which indicates bilirubinuria (with hemoglobinuria in some cases)

Colic Signs
- The reason for the colic signs is unknown but may be related to rapid change in liver size and gastric impaction that is commonly observed in equine liver failure.

Laboratory Findings

- Significant elevations in serum hepatocellular enzymes:
  - Aspartate aminotransferase (AST): usually >1000 IU/L; more than 4000 IU/L is a poor prognosis
  - Sorbitol dehydrogenase and glutamate dehydrogenase (GLDH): significant elevation
- Moderate increase in biliary-derived enzymes: GGT usually between 100 and 300 IU/L
- Bilirubinemia: Direct (conjugated) bilirubin concentration is increased, but the most dramatic increase is in unconjugated bilirubin. Conjugated bilirubin is usually less than 20% of total bilirubin.
- Prolongation of prothrombin time (PT) and partial thromboplastin time (PTT) (submit in blue-top/citrate tube with a control sample)
- Elevated levels of bile acids
- Increased blood ammonia (mildly elevated) or still within normal range, in some cases
- *Practice Tip: Only occasionally do adult horses with any liver disease develop hypoglycemia, but plasma glucose should always be monitored. If hypoglycemia is present, there could be dramatic improvement with glucose treatment.*
- *Practice Tip: Acid-base profile is variable. Most often the horse has severe metabolic acidosis! (Correction of metabolic acidosis should be attempted by administering an intravenous (IV) crystalloid, ideally Plasma-Lyte or another acetate buffer crystalloid—not sodium bicarbonate.)*

Diagnosis

- Ultrasound examination:
  - Because of an acute decrease in hepatic size with Theiler's disease, the liver often cannot be seen on the right side of the abdomen, but it can be seen at the seventh to eighth intercostal space low on the left side next to the diaphragm and spleen. The liver may look more anechoic than normal (see indications for biopsy of the liver, p. 276).

●》 WHAT TO DO

Liver Failure: Theiler's Disease

- Tranquilize the horse only if necessary to permit treatment. Use low doses of detomidine, 0.005 to 0.01 mg/kg, or xylazine, 0.2 mg/kg IV, as needed if the horse is maniacal. **Do not use xylazine or detomidine doses that cause the head to be lowered below the point of the shoulder. Prolonged lowering of the head may lead to cerebral edema and hypoxia.**
- Minimize stress and, if the horse is willing to eat, feed small amounts of grain (preferably grain with higher amounts of branched-chain amino acids; several commercial products are available) with a sorghum and corn base frequently, every 2 to 4 hours. Remove alfalfa hay and feed a lower protein and higher starch grass hay or "soaked" beet pulp. Grazing on late summer or fall nonlegume grasses is acceptable if it is done in the evening to prevent photosensitization. The size of the stomach should be determined by ultrasound examination prior to feeding if possible.

- IV fluid therapy: Give Plasma-Lyte with dextrose added to make a 1.0% or 2.5% dextrose fluid unless the horse's glucose is >150 mg/dL. Add 40 mEq/L KCl. If an acetate-buffered crystalloid is not available, use any crystalloid **but not sodium bicarbonate!** After volume deficits have been replaced, maintenance fluid rates should be 80 mL/kg per day or greater. In many cases, the PCV remains elevated despite apparent rehydration. Fluids containing acetate are preferred over lactate-containing fluids in the management of hepatic failure. Plasma (4 L) is often administered in addition to crystalloids for its colloidal, anti-inflammatory, and coagulation normalizing effects, and potential anti-apoptotic and antioxidant effects.
- **Practice Tip:** *Administer 4 to 8 mg/kg neomycin sulfate orally q8h mixed in molasses when hepatic encephalopathy is present or a concern. This treatment may be continued at a lower daily rate (2 to 4 mg/kg q12h for an additional 2 days. Diarrhea may result with too much oral neomycin.* Metronidazole, 15 mg/kg PO q12h, and/or lactulose, 0.1 to 0.2 mL/kg PO q8 to 12h, may be used in place of or in conjunction with neomycin if blood ammonia is markedly increased. Lactic acid–producing probiotics may also decrease intestinal ammonia production. Treatment preference is a combination of neomycin—day 1—plus lactulose and probiotics continued for 3 or more days. Any laxative effect of lactulose may be beneficial in addition to its ability to decrease ammonia absorption.
- For severe neurologic signs (ataxia or encephalopathy), mannitol, 0.5 to 1.0 g/kg, can be given; however, cerebral edema does not seem as pronounced in horses as in human beings with hepatic encephalopathy.
- Flunixin meglumine, 0.25 to 1.0 mg/kg q12h (high dose for only a single day), is routinely given because many horses with hepatic failure experience endotoxemia.
- For patients with severe or uncontrolled (no response to the preceding treatment) hepatic encephalopathy, flumazenil therapy (5 to 10 mg slowly IV to a 450-kg adult) or sarmazenil (0.04 mg/kg IV) can be attempted, but efficacy in human beings with hepatic encephalopathy is low, and the drugs are expensive.
- Administer B vitamins intravenously slowly and vitamin E orally.
- If there is no improvement in clinical signs following 12 hours of the above therapy, sterile (for nebulization) acetylcysteine IV (100 mg/kg mixed in 5% to 10% dextrose given over 4 hours) could be attempted in cases of acute fulminant and progressive liver disease with the goal of providing "powerful" antioxidant treatment.
- Pentoxifylline is used in most cases of liver disease: 10 mg/kg PO or IV (compounded) q12h for acute, severe hepatic disease or chronic, progressive disease.
- A nontoxic bactericidal antibiotic (e.g., ceftiofur) should be administered in all cases of acute liver failure to inhibit bacterial translocation from gut to blood.

●》 WHAT NOT TO DO

Liver Failure: Theiler's Disease

- *Do not* administer diazepam! If additional sedation is required, use pentobarbital or phenobarbital to effect, generally 5.0 to 11.0 mg/kg IV. Some prefer repeated administration of barbiturates, although detomidine continuous rate infusion of 0.6 µg/kg per minute decreased by 50% every 10 minutes can be used if needed to control maniacal behavior. The dose of either detomidine or barbiturates should be adjusted so that in the standing horse the head is not lowered below the point of the shoulder and respiration is not depressed.

- *Do not* administer bicarbonate. Rapid correction of acidosis can increase the level of ammonia and exacerbate central nervous system signs.
- *Do not* administer 5% dextrose as the sole source of fluid replacement because it does not sufficiently expand the intravascular space.
- *Do not* administer a large volume of fluids without appropriate potassium supplementation. Maintaining adequate serum potassium (K^+) concentration can be helpful in reducing hyperammonemia.
- **Practice Tip:** *When hepatic encephalopathy is a major concern, do not pass a nasogastric tube unless needed to administer oral medication. Bleeding and swallowing of blood can worsen hepatic encephalopathy. Medication (neomycin, etc.) can usually be given by dose syringe.*
- **Note:** An exception to this rule would be if ultrasound examination reveals a very large stomach (gastric impaction is occasionally seen with liver failure), in which case, a low-volume laxative (magnesium sulfate or mineral oil) needs to be administered via gravity flow.
- *Do not* leave affected horses outside in the sun.
- *Do not* stress the horse with long trailer rides, forceful nasogastric intubation, twitching, etc.

Cholangiohepatitis and Cholelithiasis

Signalment and Clinical Findings

- Cholangiohepatitis: Clinical findings most commonly include jaundice, fever, occasional colic, and anorexia. The condition is most common in adults. On rare occasions, there is a previous history of a possibly predisposing intestinal disease.
- Cholelithiasis: Recurrent episodes of signs of cholangiohepatitis occur, with more consistent colic; weight loss; and rarely, neurologic signs. Middle-aged or older horses with cholangiohepatitis are more likely to have stones than are younger horses. Fever is present in many cases because most, but not all, are associated with infection of the biliary system.
  - Persistent signs of colic or relapses following reasonably successful treatment for cholangiohepatitis suggest an obstructing stone is present.

Diagnosis

- Based on history, signalment, laboratory findings, and clinical signs

Laboratory Findings

- Significant elevation in GGT occurs: 300 to 3000 IU/L.
- Milder response in hepatocellular enzymes occurs, with AST usually <1000 IU/L.
- Liver function tests: Bilirubin is increased; often 30% or more is conjugated (direct) bilirubin. Serum bile acids are significantly increased (normal <12 mmol/L in a horse that is eating or <20 μmol/L in an anorectic horse). PT and PTT often are normal.
- Increases often occur in white blood cell and neutrophil counts, fibrinogen, and total protein.
- Biopsy reveals periportal fibrosis, dilation of bile ducts, and inflammation. Concentric fibrosis around the ducts is

present in some (but not all) cases with obstructing stones. Culture usually results in gram-negative enteric aerobic and gram-positive or gram-negative anaerobic organisms, if anything is isolated. Positive culture results are obtained in only 50% of cases.
- Aerobic and anaerobic cultures should be performed.
- Rarely, bile pigment and bacteria may be present in the peritoneal field.

Ultrasound Examination

- A subjectively enlarged liver is usually seen.
- Bile duct distention is present in some cases; however, many do not have ultrasound evidence of duct distention (Fig. 20-2).
- Possible acoustic shadows (stones) or "sludge are seen." *Important:* A large part of the liver cannot be visualized on ultrasound examination and sludge or stones are often *not* seen.
- Evidence of fibrosis can be severe in chronic cases and if severe is a poor prognostic finding.
- Gastroduodenoscopic examination may reveal a dilated bile duct opening and an obstructing stone (Fig. 20-3).

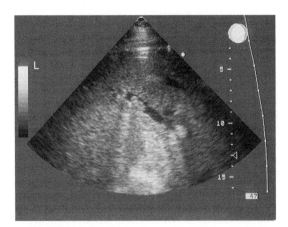

Figure 20-2 Sonogram of a horse with obstructed bile duct and sludge in the distended duct.

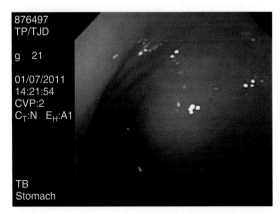

Figure 20-3 Endoscopic examination of the duodenum of a horse with a large stone obstructing the common bile duct. The "bulge" that is seen in this photo is the stone in the terminal common bile duct. Surgery was successful in forcing the stone out of the ducts; the horse completely recovered.

ICTERUS

ICTERUS

Cholangiohepatitis and Cholelithiasis

- Ceftiofur, 3.0 mg/kg IV or IM q12h, or trimethoprim-sulfamethoxazole, 20 to 30 mg/kg PO q12h, is a reasonable initial selection, pending results of culture and sensitivity from the liver biopsy. Unfortunately, biopsy cultures are only positive in <50% of cases.
- *Practice Tip: Selected antibiotics would best provide "coverage" for gram-positive enteric aerobes and anaerobes and gram-negative aerobic organisms.*
- Enrofloxacin, 5 to 7.5 mg/kg PO or IV q24h, has also been used successfully (generally in combination with metronidazole and/or penicillin) and would have better efficacy against enteric gram-negative organisms than either treatment above.
- Potassium penicillin and gentamicin (both IV) are a good option for hospitalized horses.
- Add metronidazole, 15 to 25 mg/kg PO q8 to 12h, to any of these regimens, especially if anaerobes are cultured.
- IV fluid therapy is necessary when affected horses have signs of colic and/or gentamicin is being used. Fluid therapy may help promote appetite, improve tissue perfusion, and promote bile flow.
- Administer vitamin K-1 IM or SQ for chronic and severe cholangitis. This is rarely needed. This agent may be ineffective if administered orally. *Do not administer intravenously!*
- *Practice Tip: Dimethyl sulfoxide (DMSO), 1 g/kg as a 10% solution administered IV q24h for 5 to 7 days, may help dissolve calcium bilirubinate stones.*
- Ursodeoxycholic acid should be used if other treatments are unsuccessful. This treatment has been used in several horses with severe chronic cholangiohepatitis and all have recovered.
- Administer pentoxifylline, 10 mg/kg IV or PO q12h.
- Administer S-adenosylmethionine (SAMe), 10 mg/kg PO q24h (efficacy unknown).
- For additional general therapy for liver failure (see p. 277).
- Nonsteroidal anti-inflammatory drugs (NSAIDs) can be administered for colic and inflammation.
- Two to 7 days of treatment are usually required to see both clinical and laboratory improvement. With persistent pain and limited improvement after 7 days of treatment, strong consideration should be given to an obstructing cholelith(s) that would require surgical intervention.

Cholangiohepatitis

- Hepatic encephalopathy is not as great a concern with cholangitis as it is in Theiler's disease.
- Some therapies for hepatic encephalopathy, such as oral neomycin, usually are not indicated in the management of cholangiohepatitis.
- Grazing should be encouraged to promote bile flow but *not* during peak sun exposure, or photosensitization may develop.

Hyperlipemia

- *Practice Tip: Hyperlipemia occurs mostly in ponies, donkeys, miniature equines, adults with pituitary adenoma, and less commonly in late-term pregnant and azotemic mares. In miniature horses, hyperlipemia can affect foals or adults.*

- In ponies, hyperlipemia is most common in pregnant or early-lactation mares. Hyperlipemia usually is a disease of well-conditioned or fat, middle-aged ponies and donkeys.
- The condition is characterized by fatty liver and serum that is cloudy or "milky" because of accumulation of lipids.
- Any condition that increases energy needs—for example, lactation or late pregnancy—or diseases that decrease appetite or result in catecholamine release and lipolysis can initiate hyperlipemia.

Clinical Signs

- Anorexia
- Depression
- Diarrhea
- Ventral edema
- Icterus

Diagnosis

- Increased triglycerides, >500 mg/dL (hyperlipidemia)
- Variable increases in hepatic enzymes, generally greatest in hepatocellular enzymes in the serum, but results of some liver function tests may not be abnormal
- Whitish discoloration of the serum or plasma (hyperlipemia)
- Azotemia frequently present

Hyperlipemia

- Enteral nutrition (unless esophageal choke is the predisposing event) via nasogastric tube feeding of a commercially available *low-fat* enteral feed (e.g., Critical Care Meals[1]) *or* a complete low-fat feed prepared as a gruel. There are several other enteral feeds formulated for horses that could be administered via feeding tube.
  - Mix some whey powder into the gruel (0.1 to 0.2 g whey/kg) twice daily. If blood ammonia is high, whey powder should be avoided or used at a lower amount.
  - Another option is using 0.5 g/kg glucose as a 15% solution, 10 to 20 g KCl, and a complete feed (low fat and <12% protein) gruel.
  - Calf electrolyte/energy replacements are acceptable, but sodium content may be too high for ponies with edema.
- For enteral treatment, an indwelling nasogastric tube with small-volume feeding every 2 to 4 hours is ideal
  - On day 1, give an adult patient 50 kcal/kg of a commercial enteral diet or home-prepared gruel.
  - If the feeds are well tolerated on day 1, increase to 75 kcal/kg on day 2.
  - Give 100 kcal/kg on day 3, if needed.
- If the patient does not tolerate enteral feeding (diarrhea or reflux), use intravenously administered parenteral nutrition if possible. This may be one of the few indications for the emergency use of total parenteral nutrition in the care of an adult equine.
  - Begin by placing a flexible polyurethane catheter in the jugular vein.

---

[1]MD's Choice, www.vetsupplements.com, Louisville, Tennessee.

ICTERUS

- The total parenteral nutrition solution[2] is a formulation of 50% dextrose and 4% branched-chain amino acids.
  - The final solution (with concurrent crystalloid IV fluids) should be <20% dextrose and should be administered at a lower-than-normal rate of 0.5 mL/kg per hour. In some cases, glucose is not well tolerated.
  - Do not use lipids in the parenteral nutrition.
- For miniature foals with hyperlipemia, administer mare's milk or mare milk replacer in small volumes every 2 hours (15% to 25% BW/day) through an indwelling 18F nasogastric tube (Ross Laboratories).
- If the affected pony or miniature horse is still eating, feed just about anything they show interest in eating (hand-picked grass if necessary), and use any "tricks" to increase appetite.
- Although principles for treating hepatic failure (see p. 277) need to be adhered to with hepatic lipidosis, it may not be necessary to limit high protein feeds because horses with hepatic lipidosis and hyperlipemia sometimes tolerate a high protein feed without causing hepatic encephalopathy.
- Alfalfa gruel has been used successfully.
- It is important that affected horses eat something, even if it is a higher-protein feed.
- In addition to enteral nutrition, the lipemic horse should be given intravenous polyionic fluids: 0.45 NaCl and 5% dextrose or Plasma-Lyte with 5% dextrose and additive KCl (20 to 40 mEq/L). *Practice Tip: Monitor plasma glucose level frequently both at the beginning of treatment and during either enteral or parenteral treatment; glucose should ideally be maintained at 90 to180 mg/dL in adult patients.*
- Supportive care with multiple B vitamins intravenously q24h and 2 to 4 g niacin per os q24h for adult ponies and donkeys may be beneficial and frequently is given.
- If there is persistent and severe hyperglycemia, insulin should be administered (start at 0.05 to 0.1 unit/kg per hour of regular insulin or administer compounded protamine zinc insulin, 0.4 IU/kg SQ q24h, or Ultralente insulin, 0.4 IU/kg IV q24h). If the animal is hyperglycemic and regular insulin is being used and plasma glucose does not decrease within 2 hours, the next dose should be doubled. *Important: When insulin is being used, blood glucose must be carefully monitored!*
- Administer flunixin meglumine, 0.25 mg/kg IV q8h, if needed for endotoxemia and to improve overall attitude. Ponies and miniature horses may be more susceptible to NSAID intestinal damage; *do not "overtreat" with NSAIDs!*
- *Practice Tip: Aggressively treat the primary disease; for example, use appropriate analgesics for laminitis and administer pergolide, 0.0017 to 0.01 mg/kg PO, to adults believed to have pituitary adenoma as an underlying cause. Higher doses of pergolide may suppress appetite. For lactating mares, switch the foal to a milk replacer until the mare is better.*

Prognosis

- Ponies or miniature horses that have no appetite and cannot receive adequate nutritional support or have a primary disease that is difficult to manage have a very guarded prognosis.

- Those that have severe ventral edema have a slightly more guarded prognosis because this may indicate a rapidly enlarging liver due to hepatic fat deposition.
- Horses with extremely high levels of plasma triglycerides (>1500 mg/dL) have a guarded prognosis; several cases have responded with triglycerides going from >2000 mg/dL to 100 mg/dL in 2 days using the above treatment regimen.

Pyrrolizidine Alkaloid Toxicosis

Geographic Incidence

- Predominately a disease of the western United States.
- The most common plants containing pyrrolizidine alkaloid are:
  - *Senecio jacobaea* (tansy ragwort)
  - *Senecio vulgaris* (common groundsel)
  - *Cynoglossum officinale* (hound's tongue)
  - *Amsinckia intermedia* (fiddleneck)
  - *Crotalaria* (rattlebox), a common plant of the southeastern United States, contains pyrrolizidine alkaloid but is rarely ingested by horses

Clinical Signs

- Although pyrrolizidine alkaloid toxicosis is a chronic disease, most affected horses have an acute onset of clinical signs.
- Central nervous system signs indicate acute hepatic encephalopathy: for example, depression, wandering, and yawning. Rarely, acute laryngeal paralysis is seen.
- Icterus is mild to moderate.
- Photosensitization is possible.
- Liver failure may result months after exposure to the toxic plant.

Diagnosis

Laboratory Findings

- The AST level usually is elevated. The GGT level is consistently elevated and may remain elevated for as long as 6 months after removal of horses (without symptoms) from exposure to the toxin.
- Bile acids are elevated.

Ultrasound Examination

- Increased echogenicity (fibrosis) of the liver is found.

⏩ WHAT TO DO

Pyrrolizidine Alkaloid Liver Failure

- Supportive therapy for fulminant liver failure and hepatic encephalopathy (see p. 277).
- Some of these horses with hepatic fibrosis and hepatic encephalopathy respond to general treatment for hepatic encephalopathy and fibrosis (pentoxifylline and SAMe) and remain clinically asymptomatic for several months.
- *Practice Tip: Make sure horses with hepatic failure are housed out of direct sunlight.*
- **Note:** What about other horses that have been exposed to pyrrolizidine alkaloids?

---

[2]Parenteral Nutrition Solution, BranchAmin (Clintec, Deerfield, Illinois).

ICTERUS

- Monitor GGT and bile acids to determine whether the disease is progressing. If the horses appear clinically normal 6 months after exposure and levels of GGT and bile acids are normal, the likelihood of development of hepatic failure from the exposure is minimal, and the horses can return to work. These horses can be treated with vitamin E, pentoxifylline, and SAMe. See supportive treatment for liver failure, p. 277.
- Find the contaminated hay, and do not feed it to horses.

⊚› WHAT NOT TO DO

Pyrrolizidine Alkaloid Liver Failure
- Do not stress the horse unnecessarily.
- Do not leave horse in the sunlight.
- Do not feed a high protein feed.
- Do not treat with colchicine; this drug inhibits mitosis, which might be contraindicated with megalocytosis, which is commonly observed in pyrrolizidine alkaloid toxicity.

Tyzzer's Disease (*Clostridium Piliforme*)
Signalment
- Disease affects 6- to 42-day-old foals.
- Usually only one foal on the farm is affected; however, farm problems occur in certain areas, such as Oklahoma.

Clinical Signs
- Immediate death
- Depression
- Anorexia
- Hyperthermia or hypothermia
- Jaundice
- Convulsions
- Shock
- Diarrhea

Diagnosis
- Based on age and clinical signs
Laboratory Findings
- Elevated AST and sorbitol dehydrogenase levels
- Abnormal results of liver function tests and bilirubinemia (direct and indirect fractions are increased)
- Hypoglycemia
- Severe metabolic acidosis
- Serologic testing for recovered and suspected cases
- Histopathologic examination of the liver or polymerase chain reaction (PCR) testing of fecal sample

⊚› WHAT TO DO

Tyzzer's Disease
- Provide supportive therapy for fulminant hepatic failure and hepatic encephalopathy (see p. 277).
- Administer antibiotics: penicillin, 44,000 U/kg IV q6h; gentamicin, 6.6 mg/kg IV q24h (if the foal is urinating and is being treated aggressively with intravenous fluids); and metronidazole, 15 to 25 mg/kg PO q6 to 12h.
- Provide aggressive management of septic shock.

- Normalize blood pressure with a nonlactate polyionic crystalloid solution and colloid (plasma) administered intravenously. If systemic arterial blood pressure cannot be normalized with fluid therapy and central venous pressure is elevated (>11 cm H_2O), use dobutamine, 5 to 10 µg/kg per minute. Finally, alpha-adrenergic drug therapy with dopamine, administered at 5 to 10 µg/kg per minute, or norepinephrine, 0.1 to 1.0 µg/kg per minute, may be used in an attempt to normalize arterial blood pressure.
- Administer hyperimmune plasma.
- Administer pentoxifylline, 10 mg/kg PO or IV q8 to 12h.
- Administer oxygen, 5 L/min, intranasally.

Prognosis
- Prognosis is grave.

Aflatoxicosis
- Aflatoxicosis is rarely reported among horses.

Leukoencephalomalacia (Moldy Corn)
- Leukoencephalomalacia is an uncommon cause of liver failure in horses; however, it frequently causes liver disease.
- Pasture-associated mycotoxins have been suspected in other cases of liver failure, but other than alsike clover–associated mycotoxin toxicity, no particular plant has a proven association.

Alsike Clover Toxicity
- Alsike clover poisoning is a cause of photosensitization and jaundice in horses in the northern United States and Canada.
- Outbreaks occur sporadically, likely associated with environmental conditions and increased growth of mycotoxin on the grass or a toxin (saponin) in the plant, and are usually associated with grazing and not hay.
- Significant elevations in GGT occur.

Panicum Spp. (Fall Panicum, Klein Grass) Toxicity
- *Panicum* spp. may cause liver failure in horses fed panicum hay; the condition may be a farm problem. Most cases have been in mid-Atlantic states (fall panicum), but they also occur in Texas (Klein grass).
- In mid-Atlantic area outbreaks, the condition has always been associated with feeding of current season hay in late fall and early winter.
- Hay looks perfectly normal and may have been fed from the same fields in previous years without problems.

Diagnosis
- Diagnosis is based on history and exposure, clinical findings of liver disease or failure, and ruling out other causes of hepatic failure.
- With fall panicum, Klein grass, or alsike poisoning, more than one horse on the farm may have increases in GGT although they may not have liver failure.
- Laboratory findings are similar to those of pyrrolizidine alkaloid poisoning (moderate increases in GGT and a mild to moderate increase in AST).

ICTERUS

●) WHAT TO DO

Alsike Clover or Panicum Grass Hepatotoxicity

• Supportive therapy and removal from the hay or pasture

Prognosis

• Prognosis is usually good for panicum and fair for alsike toxicity.

Iron Intoxication

• Iron intoxication may cause liver disease and rarely failure. It may result from parenteral administration of iron sulfate. It also may occur in a few horses because of abnormal liver uptake or storage (hemochromatosis) rather than excessive administration.
• Finding elevated iron concentration in the liver does *not* prove that it is the cause of liver disease. Many horses with liver failure resulting from multiple causes have increased serum iron concentrations.
• Treatment with deferoxamine in addition to therapy listed below for chronic active hepatitis can be attempted

Liver Failure in Foals Following Neonatal Isoerythrolysis

• Isoerythrolysis is an infrequent cause of liver failure in foals, but when it occurs, it often is associated with progressive fibrosis.
• Liver failure is most frequently observed following multiple blood transfusions but may rarely occur without a transfusion.
• Liver disease and function should be monitored with biochemical testing in foals with neonatal isoerythrolysis.
• If enzymes are increased and function tests are becoming increasingly abnormal, antioxidant and anti-inflammatory treatments (e.g., pentoxifylline and SAMe) and deferoxamine (1 g SQ twice daily for 14 days) should be initiated.

Chronic Active Hepatitis

• Hepatitis is a chronic inflammatory and possibly immune disorder. Horses are rarely presented as emergency cases.
• The diagnosis can be confirmed only after biopsy specimen examination. Prednisolone (1 mg/kg IM) or dexamethasone (0.06 mg/kg IV), colchicine (0.03 mg/kg q12 to 24h), SAMe (10 to 20 mg/kg q24h PO), milk thistle and pentoxifylline (10 mg/kg PO q12h) are used in the treatment, along with dietary management and avoiding sunlight. Ursodiol 15 mg/kg PO q24h, can be used if other treatments are not successful.

Drug-Induced Hepatic Disease

• Foals, especially those with gastrointestinal disease, that have been treated with a variety of ulcer medications and antibiotics occasionally develop increasing levels of liver enzymes, even as their primary disease is resolving.
• This elevation in liver enzymes resolves as medications are withdrawn.
• Doxycycline and rifampin, as combined therapy, may cause liver failure.

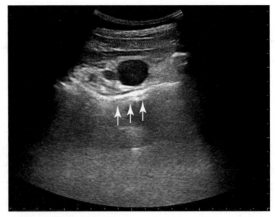

Figure 20-4   Ultrasound examination of the right abdomen of a horse with a colon displacement to the right. The large vessel seen on ultrasound appears to be present in approximately 50% of right colon displacement cases and results from rotation of the mesenteric side of the colon onto the abdominal wall so that the vessel can be seen. (Figure courtesy Dr. Sally Ness.)

Obstruction of the Bile Duct

• Unusual
• Colon displacement: If an adult has mild, persistent colic, no fever, normal serum globulin and plasma fibrinogen levels, abnormal results of a rectal examination, and a high bilirubin level (usually >12 mg/dL and GGT level usually >100 IU/L), suspect approximately 180 degrees of displacement or volvulus of the large colon. A displaced colon in the horse occasionally obstructs the bile duct. The displaced colon and enlarged colonic mesenteric vessels can sometimes be visualized on ultrasound examination of the caudal or midlateral right abdomen (Fig. 20-4).

●) WHAT TO DO

Colonic Obstruction of the Bile Duct

• Fasting in addition to administering oral electrolytes via nasogastric tube may allow the colon to return to normal position. If that does not correct the displacement in 2 to 3 days or the horse remains painful and peritoneal fluid lactate and protein increase, then surgery should be performed because there may be a rotation of the colon in addition to its displacement (see p. 205). Bilirubin and GGT levels should decrease within 24 to 36 hours, and no specific treatment of the liver disease is required.
• Obstruction of the bile duct also occurs among foals in association with healing duodenal ulcer and stricture.
  • Serum GGT concentration is increased and the foal may be icteric.
  • There is no retrograde movement of barium into the biliary ducts 2 hours after the oral barium study (1 L per foal) as occurs with duodenal stricture posterior to the opening of the bile duct.
  • The prognosis is very grave, although transposition of the bile duct and gastrojejunostomy or duodenojejunostomy are surgical options.

Portocaval Shunts

• Consider portocaval shunts if a foal, most commonly 6 weeks or older, has an acute onset of blindness, seizures, coma, or other signs of bizarre behavior.

ICTERUS

- Relapsing episodes are almost enough to confirm the diagnosis.
  - Rule out idiopathic Arabian foal and hypocalcemic seizures.
- Foals rarely have clinical signs unless they are eating sufficient amounts of grain, hay, or spring grass.
- Routine laboratory findings often are unremarkable; liver enzyme levels are typically normal; AST and creatine kinase levels may be increased because of seizure activity.
- Hypoglycemia may be present.
- Measurements of ammonia and bile acids in a blood sample are used to help confirm the diagnosis.
- Hepatic scintigraphy or ultrasound observation of air injected into the spleen bypassing the liver further confirms the diagnosis, but a portogram is needed if surgery is contemplated.

Important: Proper handling of the sample to measure blood ammonia level is critical. The blood should be collected carefully (hemolysis interferes with the measurement) in a heparin tube, kept on ice, and taken to a laboratory within 1 hour. If this is not possible, harvest the plasma within 30 minutes and freeze it at −4° F (−20° C) for measurement within 48 hours. Submission of a control sample collected from a horse of similar age and diet and sample handled in the same manner is ideal. Ammonia can be measured on some benchtop chemistry machines (IDEXX, see Chapter 15, p. 112).

●❭ WHAT TO DO

Portocaval Shunt

- Medical stabilization for hepatic encephalopathy, including polyionic crystalloid fluid therapy with 5 to 10 g dextrose added per liter.
- Neomycin mixed with Karo syrup and administered 3 times q12h apart may be effective in decreasing intestinal production of ammonia.
- Sedation with low-dose xylazine, 0.2 mg/kg, followed by pentobarbital or phenobarbital administration, 3.0 to 11.0 mg/kg or to effect, may be needed to sedate a foal having seizures.
- Surgical correction can be performed after diagnostic venography is performed to identify the shunt location.

●❭ WHAT NOT TO DO

Portocaval Shunt

Do not use diazepam for sedation because the treatment may worsen the neurologic signs!

Hyperammonemia without Liver Failure in Morgan Foals

- Hyperammonemia can occur in weanling Morgan foals (usually 3 to 10 months of age).
- This syndrome appears to be familial and may be associated with a metabolic defect in urea synthesis.

Diagnosis

- In the Morgan breed, clinical findings (often occurring after weaning) are diminished growth rate and depression,

moderately elevated liver enzymes, and normal or only mildly elevated bilirubin level.
- Blood ammonia levels are very high (>200 μmol/L).
- Terminal hemolytic anemia may occur in a few cases.

Prognosis

- Some horses have temporary improvement in clinical signs but die days or weeks later.

Primary Hyperammonemia in Adult Horses

- This condition may be seen in horses presented for abdominal pain.
- The horses exhibit cortical signs including blindness and have severe metabolic acidosis, hyperglycemia, and blood ammonia >200 μmol/L.
- Supportive treatment with fluids and neomycin orally is often successful, with recovery in 2 to 4 days.
- Sodium benzoate (250 mg/kg) mixed in 10% dextrose and given over 1 hour may have some benefit when the blood ammonia is >300 μmol/L.
- Sodium benzoate should *not* be used with liver disease!
- Approximately one half of these horses have complete recovery in 2 to 3 days with the above treatments; the others may have rapid progression to terminal coma.
- It is not unusual for the horse to have diarrhea or a decline in plasma protein for 1 to 3 days following the neurologic signs.

Hyperammonemia in Dysmature, Premature Foals

- Some dysmature, premature foals with persistent meconium impaction and/or constipation may develop high blood ammonia and worsening neurologic signs.

●❭ WHAT TO DO

Hyperammonemia in Dysmature, Premature Foals

- Enema and laxatives

Ultrasound Examination of the Equine Liver: to Perform or Not to Perform Biopsy

- Ultrasound examination of the liver is performed with a 5.0-MHz probe of the right abdomen beginning at the tenth intercostal space just above the point of the shoulder and continuing caudally and dorsally. Also, scan the left cranial quadrant of the abdomen at the seventh to ninth intercostal space in a line drawn from the point of the elbow and moving caudally.
- Liver biopsy or aspiration can be performed for diagnostic purposes, such as confirmation of pyrrolizidine alkaloid toxicosis or suppurative cholangitis and culture, or for prognostic purposes, such as assessment of fibrosis. These procedures rarely are needed as emergency procedures and are not necessary for proper management in most cases. The biopsy can be performed with a Tru-Cut biopsy needle introduced into a section of liver viewed at

ultrasound examination as relatively avascular (see p. 22) with local anesthesia.

General Management of Fulminant Liver Failure and Hepatic Encephalopathy

●》 WHAT TO DO

Liver Failure and Hepatic Encephalopathy

- Tranquilize the patient only if needed. Use low doses of detomidine, 0.005 to 0.01 mg/kg, or xylazine, 0.2 mg/kg IV, as needed. *Do not* use xylazine or detomidine doses that cause the head to be lowered below the point of the shoulder.
  - Persistent lowering of the head promotes cerebral edema.
- Minimize stress, and feed small amounts of grain (preferably grain with higher amounts of branched-chain amino acids, such as sorghum and corn) frequently.
- Remove alfalfa hay and feed grass hay or "soaked" beet pulp.
- Grazing on late summer or fall nonlegume grasses is acceptable if it is done in the evening to prevent photosensitization.
- Begin IV fluid therapy:
  - Give Plasma-Lyte if the horse is acidotic with enough added dextrose to make a 1.0% or 2.5% dextrose fluid unless the horse's glucose is already >130 mg/dL.
  - Add 40 mEq/L KCl. If an acetate-buffered crystalloid is not available, use the crystalloid that is available.
  - After volume deficits have been replaced, maintenance rates should be 80 mL/kg per day or greater. In many cases, the PCV remains elevated despite apparent rehydration.
  - Fluids containing acetate are preferred over lactate-containing fluids in the management of hepatic failure.
  - Plasma (4 L) is often administered in addition to crystalloids for its colloidal, anti-inflammatory, coagulation, and anti-apoptotic effects.
- Administer 4 to 8 mg/kg neomycin sulfate orally q8h mixed in molasses when hepatic encephalopathy is present or a concern. This treatment may be continued at a lower daily rate for 3 days. Diarrhea may result with excessive administration of neomycin. Metronidazole also may be used, 15 to 25 mg/kg PO q12 to 24h, and/or lactulose (0.1 to 0.2 mL/kg PO q8 to 12h) and lactic acid–producing probiotics. Preference is low-dose neomycin plus lactulose and probiotics. The laxative effect of lactulose is beneficial.
- ***Practice Tip:*** *Metronidazole is effective in decreasing enteric ammonia production, a good antimicrobial against anaerobic infections of the liver, and has anti-inflammatory and anti-endotoxin properties.*
- For severe neurologic signs (ataxia or encephalopathy), use mannitol, 0.5 to 1.0 g/kg IV; however, cerebral edema does not seem as pronounced in horses as human beings with hepatic encephalopathy.
- Flunixin meglumine, 0.25 to 1.0 mg/kg IV q12h (high dose for only a single day), is routinely given because many horses with hepatic failure experience endotoxemia.
- For patients with severe or uncontrolled (with the preceding treatment) hepatic encephalopathy, flumazenil therapy (5 to 10 mg slowly IV to a 450-kg adult) or sarmazenil (0.04 mg/kg IV) can be attempted, but efficacy in human beings with hepatic encephalopathy is low, and these drugs are expensive.
- Administer B vitamins intravenously slowly and vitamin E orally or intramuscularly.
- Consider parenteral nutrition for foals and adults with fulminant hepatic failure caused by acute disease. Use only formulations prepared for patients with hepatic failure (Heptamine[3]), in addition to 10% dextrose, and use a rate less than for routine total parenteral nutrition therapy. Experience with this form of therapy in the management of acute hepatic failure is limited to a few cases. Branched-chain aromatic amino acid supplements can be administered orally.
- S-adenosylmethionine (Denosyl-SDR or SAMe) 10 to 20 mg/kg q24h may provide antioxidant properties to the diseased liver.
- Sterile (for nebulization) acetylcysteine IV (100 mg/kg mixed in 5% to 10% dextrose and given over 4 hours) in cases of acute fulminant and progressive liver disease with the goal of providing powerful antioxidant treatment has also been used.
- Prednisolone (1 mg/kg IM) or dexamethasone (0.06 mg/kg IV) is used for relapsing chronic active hepatitis, drug-induced hepatopathy, or less commonly for acute progressive hepatic failure when more established therapy is not successful.
- Pentoxifylline is used in most cases of liver disease: 10 mg/kg PO or IV (compounded) qh for acute, severe disease and q12h for chronic, progressive disease.
- A nontoxic bactericidal antibiotic (e.g., ceftiofur) should be administered in all cases of acute liver failure to inhibit bacterial translocation (gut to blood).

●》 WHAT NOT TO DO

Liver Failure and Hepatic Encephalopathy

- *Do not* administer diazepam because it may worsen signs of hepatic encephalopathy. If sedation is needed, use pentobarbital or phenobarbital (generally 5 to 11 mg/kg to effect; start at a lower dose) or detomidine continuous rate infusion, starting at 0.6 μg/kg/min and decreasing the dose so that the horse's head is not below the point of the shoulder.
- When hepatic encephalopathy is a major concern, *do not* pass a nasogastric tube unless it is needed to administer oral medication. Bleeding and swallowing of blood can exacerbate hepatic encephalopathy.
  Important: An exception to this rule would be if ultrasound examination reveals a very large stomach (gastric impaction that is occasionally seen with liver failure), in which case a low-volume laxative (magnesium sulfate and mineral oil) is administered via gravity flow.
- *Do not* administer 5% dextrose as the sole source of fluid replacement because it does *not* sufficiently expand the intravascular space.
- *Do not* administer bicarbonate. Rapid correction of acidosis can increase the level of ionized ammonia and exacerbate central nervous system signs.
- Maintain adequate serum potassium (K^+) concentration because this is important in reducing hyperammonemia.
- *Do not* leave affected horses outside in the sun.

Hemolytic Anemia
General Diagnostic Considerations

- Collect blood in tubes containing ethylenediaminetetraacetic acid (EDTA) for a direct Coombs test if an immunologic reaction is suspected, as with isoerythrolysis or recent penicillin administration.

---

[3]Heptamine (B. Braun Medical, Inc).

- Request a new methylene blue stain if exposure to a plant toxin, such as red maple, is a possibility.
- Collect serum for a Coggins test and *Streptococcus M* protein antibody if edema and fever are present.
- In some areas of the United States and many parts of the world, *Theileria* should be considered and tested for by cytologic exam of a blood smear and PCR.
- Measure serum calcium if lymphoma is suspected.
- Examine the horse thoroughly for other diseases (e.g., clostridial myositis) that may cause hemolytic anemia.
- For classification of anemia in horses, see Fig. 20-5.

Toxic or Heinz Body Anemia

- Acute hemolytic anemia can be caused by plant toxins or occasionally can be a direct effect of intravenous administration of drugs (DMSO, tetracycline, propylene glycol).
- Acute hemolytic anemia also can occur in association with exposure to *C. perfringens* toxins or very rarely leptospirosis.
- Plants reported to cause intravascular hemolysis are wild onion and red maple.
- ***Practice Tip:*** *Red maple toxicity is most common during late summer and fall and results from ingestion of wilted leaves. Red maple toxicity often occurs 3 to 4 days after a storm. This disorder occurs in the middle or eastern United States, where red maple trees are present.*
- Garlic may also cause a hemolytic anemia if eaten in high amounts.

Red Maple Toxicity
Clinical Signs
- Depression
- Jaundice
- Discolored urine
- Colic: This is common, and is presumably due to intestinal ischemia.

Diagnosis
- History: The condition most commonly occurs following a storm and tree limbs blowing down and is much less common because of normal falling leaves. *Only* wilted leaves are toxic; green leaves are not. Toxicity from other maple trees has *not* been confirmed. Toxic dose is approximately 1.5 g/kg.
- Presentation: Late in the summer, methemoglobin production and acute death are not uncommon.

Diagnostic Tests
- PCV
  - The PCV often decreases to a life-threatening value (<14%) with red maple toxicity; this is rarely the case with onion toxicity.
- Total protein
- Bilirubin
  - The increase in serum bilirubin level is mostly indirect.
- Urinalysis
- Methemoglobin may cause the blood to appear a chocolate color. In some cases, the methemoglobin level may be very high (>50%), and death occurs rapidly without hemolytic anemia. The membranes are dark but not icteric, and the PCV may be normal with severe methemoglobinemia. Methemoglobin can be measured in many small animal, veterinary referral, or human hospitals.
- Heinz bodies may be found with meticulous searching if the horse has red maple poisoning. These structures are more commonly found with onion poisoning.
- Mean corpuscular volume (MCV) and mean corpuscular hemoglobin concentration (MCHC) may be increased, and the plasma protein (total solids) level is usually normal or increased.
- Mean corpuscular volume (MCV) and mean corpuscular hemoglobin concentration (MCHC) may be increased, and the plasma protein (total solids) level is usually normal or increased.
- Colic is common and renal failure and coagulopathy are less common.

●❯ WHAT TO DO

Red Maple Toxicity
- Blood transfusion if necessary (see p. 285)
- Vitamin C, 0.04 g/kg PO with fluids and electrolytes via nasogastric tube or 30 mg/kg mixed in IV fluids
- Provide a laxative, either mineral oil or magnesium sulfate, via nasogastric tube as more leaves may be in the colon
- Vitamin E and selenium IM
- Acetylcysteine (sterile nebulization solution), 20 to 50 mg/kg mixed in IV fluids may also be used in severe cases with multiple organ failure.
- Oxyglobin is currently unavailable but would be a great "band-aid" for the hypoxia that occurs with severe hemolysis and methemoglobinemia. Similar products could be reintroduced to the market.
- Analgesics if the horse is "colicky"
- Intranasal oxygen at a high rate may help some horses. Although normally only 2% of the available oxygen is free oxygen, this would be a higher percentage with severe hemolytic disease, and increasing free oxygen would help alleviate the tissue hypoxemia.

Immune-Mediated Hemolytic Anemia

- The condition may result from an autoimmune reaction or more commonly another disease (lymphoma, equine infectious anemia [EIA], *C. perfringens* or *Streptococcus* infection) or drug-induced hemolytic anemia (most commonly caused by intravenous administration of penicillin or ceftiofur).

Clinical Signs and Findings
- Lethargy
- Depression
- Edema, usually in the limbs and ventral body, that may be the result of sludging of red blood cell complexes in the microcirculation
- Jaundiced mucous membranes: The above signs are also found with *Anaplasma phagocytophilum,* but PCV is only mildly decreased in this disease.
- In a few cases, red urine and fever

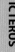

ICTERUS

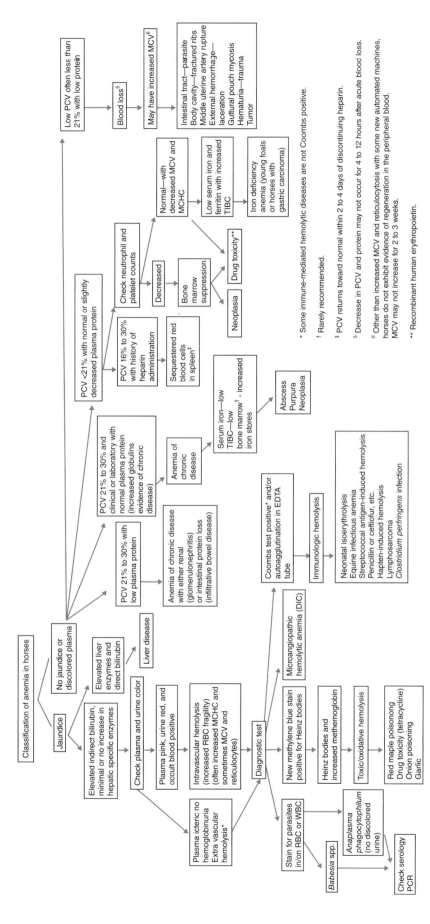

Figure 20-5 Classification of equine anemia. *DIC,* Disseminated intravascular coagulation; *MCHC,* mean corpuscular hemoglobin concentration; *MCV,* mean corpuscular volume; *RBC,* red blood cells; *TIBC,* total iron-binding capacity; *WBC,* white blood cells.
*Consider EIA, drug-induced causes, anaplasmosis, rarely neonatal isoerythrolysis.

ICTERUS

Diagnosis

- History of penicillin, ceftiofur, or other drug administration within past 1 to 2 weeks
- Recent infection with *Streptococcus* organisms or active *C. perfringens* type A myositis or cellulitis
- Suspicion of lymphoma

Laboratory Findings

- PCV is decreased.
- MCV and MCHC concentration may be increased. MCV may not increase for several days following hemolysis and regeneration.
- *Practice Tip: Look for severe autoagglutination in the EDTA sample; the plasma may be yellow or pink, depending on the duration of hemolysis and whether it is intravascular or extravascular.*
- Autoagglutination can be differentiated from normal rouleaux formation by means of dilution of the sample 1:3 with 0.9% saline solution.
- Increased reticulocyte numbers can be measured and would be expected to occur with regenerative anemia if some of the newer automated flow cytometry equipment is used.
- *Practice Tip: Internal bleeding can usually be ruled out with the history in addition there is no hemolysis noted in the plasma and a drop in both PCV and plasma protein with hemorrhage.*

Additional Tests

- EIA: Perform a Coggins test (serologic examination) and PCR.
- Coombs test (EDTA sample): If autoagglutination is obvious, there is no need to perform a Coombs test. A negative result does not rule out immune-mediated anemia.
- Antibody-coated RBCs may be detected with flow cytometry. (Dr. Wilkerson's laboratory at Kansas State University [785-532-4818] has performed most of these assays.)
- Heinz bodies may be seen with oxidant-induced hemolytic anemia but *not* with autoimmune hemolytic anemia. Echinocytes and spherocytes sometimes are seen with *C. perfringens* hemolysis.

◉〉 WHAT TO DO

Immune-Mediated Hemolytic Anemia

- Blood transfusion, if needed (see guidelines to determine need of transfusion on p. 285), from a compatible donor ideally determined by crossmatching; however, many times a healthy gelding of the same breed or a Quarter horse gelding who has never received a blood transfusion is a good donor.
- Administer dexamethasone, 0.04 to 0.08 mg/kg IV q24h.
- Intranasal oxygen to increase free oxygen is of some (but minimal) benefit.

Neonatal Isoerythrolysis

- Suspect neonatal isoerythrolysis (NI) in young foals, especially mule foals, younger than 7 days of age that have icterus, tachycardia, and weakness. In horse foals, 90% of cases are due to antibodies against Aa or Qa.

- The foal is usually a product of a multiparous mare. NI occurs in approximately 1% of horse foalings and nearly 7% of mule births.
- *Practice Tip: If a mare has received a previous blood transfusion, the foal should be considered at high risk of NI, and the mare's colostrum should be tested against the foals RBCs before nursing.* This can be done by diluting the mare's colostrum with saline (1:16) and mixing it with the foal's spun down RBCs and observation of agglutination (clumping). This may miss some cases that predominantly involve hemolysins. For high-risk mares (previous transfusion history), the mare should be checked for autoantibodies before foaling or simply find a colostrum replacement!
- Urine is usually discolored in peracute cases, usually light red (hemoglobin), although it can be brown (bilirubin) in chronic cases.
- Many causes of jaundice occur in young foals, such as sepsis. NI usually can be differentiated from other causes by means of measurement of the PCV, which usually is <20% in clinically ill foals with NI. NI is unrelated to the A or Q antigens in mules and is associated with antibodies against the donkey factor antigen. Commercial plasma is tested for antibodies against Aa, Qa, and donkey factor.

Diagnosis

- Use Coombs test with whole blood (EDTA) to help confirm an immune reaction. **Note:** Close examination of the sample may reveal autoagglutination (presence of clumps), in which case a Coombs test is not needed for confirmation.
- Liver function is frequently affected and *not* always correlated with severity of NI.
- Some cases, mostly those with one or more transfusions, may have progressive liver failure, possibly associate with iron overload, even after recovering from the hemolytic aspect of NI.

◉〉 WHAT TO DO

Neonatal Isoerythrolysis

- If the foal is less than 48 hours old, *do not* allow it to nurse unless the mare's colostrum/milk has a Brix refractometry score of <15%. If the foal needs to be refrained from nursing, this should be done with as little stress as possible to the foal; use a muzzle and if practical, *do not* physically separate the two. Continue to milk the mare.
- For peracute severe cases with PCV <20% within 24 hours, do the following:
  - For horse foals, perform a transfusion. A crossmatch (major and minor) is ideal.
  - If a crossmatch is not feasible, using an Aa/Qa-negative donor usually is safe and effective.
  - The mare's blood may be used if it is washed 3 times and suspended in saline solution before each transfusion, although it is time consuming.
  - Lastly, using a gelding of the same breed that has never received a transfusion is often successful.

- **Note:** If an oxyglobin product becomes available in the market, its ideal use would be in peracute cases of hemolytic anemia while whole-blood transfusion is being organized.
- Mule foals: Use a horse gelding or a female donor that has not been previously bred with a donkey.
- All equine practices should ideally have Aa/Qa-negative donors identified for emergency purposes. Blood typing can be performed by sending samples of acid-citrate-dextrose (ACD) anticoagulated blood to:
  - Veterinary Genetics Laboratory, School of Veterinary Medicine, University of California, Davis, CA 95616 (916-752-2211)
  - Equine Blood Typing Research Laboratory, University of Kentucky, Department of Veterinary Science, Lexington, KY 40546 (606-257-3022)
  - Donors should ideally be free of Aa and/or Qa antigens and hemolytic and agglutinating Aa, Qa antibodies, but these are hard to find.
- Administer intravenous fluids at maintenance level (approximately 60 mL/kg per day).
- **Important:** Administration of needed intravenous fluids decreases PCV but does not reduce the total numbers of RBCs and would be expected to improve oxygen delivery as long as viscosity is sufficient to maintain capillary pressure.
- Administer dexamethasone, 0.04 mg/lb (0.08 mg/kg IV), only in peracute cases (foals 2 days of age or younger with PCV <12%) if donor cells cannot be administered immediately or if compatibility is uncertain.
- Administer intranasal oxygen (5 to 10 L/min) bubbled through a nasopharyngeal tube if the foal is severely anemic. This will increase free oxygen in the plasma.
- Administer antibiotics to all foals with NI to minimize sepsis. Despite evidence of passive transfer of colostral antibodies, foals with NI can become septic. One reason for this is that the transfusion may cause immunosuppression. Also, some confirmed foals with NI have partial failure of passive antibody. Valuable foals should be administered a combination of intravenous penicillin and amikacin (if renal function is normal) or ceftiofur; less monetarily valued foals can be given a combination of trimethoprim-sulfamethoxazole, 20 mg/kg PO q12h, and penicillin 22,000 IU/kg IM q12h.
- Administer antiulcer medication: sucralfate, 1 g PO q6h, with or without a histamine-2 receptor blocker or proton pump blocker. Due to hypoxia and stress, the foals may be predisposed to gastric ulcers.
- Provide nutritional support (Land-O-Lakes) foal milk replacement, mare's milk, or goat's milk, at 15% to 20% of body weight per day during the time the foal is not allowed to nurse.
- Provide supportive care, such as keeping the foal warm but *not* hot.
- Expect a second decline in PCV 4 to 11 days after the transfusion.

WHAT NOT TO DO

Neonatal Isoerythrolysis
- *Do not* let a newborn foal nurse the mare's colostrum if the mare has ever had a whole blood transfusion.
- The foal should be 36 to 48 hours old before it is allowed to nurse a mare that has received a transfusion.
- An alternate source of colostrum should be provided and the foals IgG checked at 12 to 18 hours.

When to Administer Transfusions to Horses or Foals with Hemolytic Anemia
- **Practice Tip:** *There is no magical PCV that serves as a transfusion trigger. All of the following parameters should be used to make that determination.*
- Clinical signs: weakness, depression, pallor
- Clinical findings: tachycardia, tachypnea
- Hematocrit and hemoglobin level: Generally, hemoglobin values <5 g/dL should be considered as unable to support tissue oxygen requirements and maintain adequate blood viscosity. This cut-off level is probably higher for pregnant mares or horses with respiratory disease.
- Duration of the decline in hematocrit and hemoglobin level: The more acute the drop, the higher the probability a transfusion is needed.
- Blood lactate concentration >3 mmol/L would indicate inadequate oxygen delivery and possible need for transfusion.
- An additional test that is often overlooked and might be helpful is PvO_2 (partial pressure of venous oxygen), SvO_2 (venous oxygen saturation) measurement. Unless there is primary pulmonary disease or pulmonary shunting occurs, arterial samples may provide little or no information about need for a transfusion. A venous O_2 pressure <30 mm Hg in an anaerobic sample (heparinized syringe) collected from a vein that is only briefly held off and measured immediately (e.g., i-STAT), is a good laboratory determinant to suggest tissue oxygen deficit and time for transfusion. The same is true for SvO_2 <50%.
- **Practice Tips:**
  - *Perform transfusion if PCV decreases to <18% within 24 hours and hemolysis is ongoing.*
  - *In cases with a slower decline in PCV, transfusion can sometimes be postponed until the PCV is 12% or less.*

Supplements to Blood Transfusion
- Oxyglobin, 5 to 20 mL/kg, if available (currently not sold) could be used in peracute cases or in severe cases while whole-blood transfusion is being organized.
- Administer isotonic fluids if there is clinical evidence of hypovolemia. Although fluids decrease the PCV, they *do not* decrease oxygen-carrying capacity unless viscosity becomes very low. Fluid therapy may increase oxygen supply through an increase in perfusion as long as blood viscosity is adequate.
- Intranasal oxygen should be provided because this would increase free oxygen in the blood and have some mild positive effect on oxygen supply.
- Administer oral or intravenous vitamin C for oxidative disorders, 25 g q12h for 2 days.

Other Causes of Hemolysis in Adults
Babesia Infection: Piroplasmosis
- Also see diseases of South America, Chapter 40, p. 683, for more details.
- *Babesia caballi* and *Theileria equi* (*T. equi*)
- *T. equi* is more pathogenic.

ICTERUS

ICTERUS

- Found in South and Central America, including the Caribbean region, and in Europe, Russia, Asia, Africa, and the Middle East. *T. equi* infections have recently been documented in the southwest United States and to a lesser degree in some other regions of the United States.
- Affects horses, donkeys, mules, and zebras
- Incubation period approximately 7 to 22 days
- Multiple tick species (*Amblyomma* was the most common in the recent U.S. infections) are able to transmit the infection.

Clinical Signs

- All horses are susceptible; older horses are more severely affected. Once infected, most survivors are carriers unless cleared with imidocarb dipropionate.
- Fever 38.9° to 41.7° C (102° to 107° F)
- Hemolytic anemia
- Jaundice
- Hemoglobinuria
- Death

Generalized Signs

- Depression
- Anorexia
- Incoordination
- Lacrimation
- Mucous nasal discharge
- Eyelid swelling
- Petechiations on mucous membranes
- Increased recumbency

Differential Diagnosis

- Equine infectious anemia
- Liver failure
- Immune-mediated hemolytic anemia
- Less likely differentials include:
  - *Anaplasma phagocytophilum* (equine granulocytic ehrlichiosis) is mostly added to the differential list because fever, icterus, petechiations, edema, and incoordination are common to both diseases. It does not have recognizable hemolytic anemia although mild anemia is present.
  - *Purpura hemorrhagica* is characterized by fever, petechiations, and edema, but it does *not* have recognizable hemolytic anemia although mild anemia is present.

Diagnosis

- PCR is the best test for recent infection.
- Serologic tests: Competitive enzyme-linked immunosorbent assay (ELISA), complement fixation, indirect fluorescence antibody assays
- Cytologic identification of the organism can be made on a Giemsa-stained blood smear; however, the result may be negative in infected horses when the sample is drawn from a small-diameter vessel; the indirect fluorescence antibody test can distinguish between *B. caballi* and *T. equi*.

◑ WHAT TO DO

Piroplasmosis

- *T. equi* is more refractory to treatment than is *B. caballi* (see Chapter 40, p. 683).
- Imidocarb dipropionate[4]: For *B. caballi:* 2.2 mg/kg 2 treatments q24h; for *T. equi:* 4.0 mg/kg 4 treatments q72h.

◑ WHAT NOT TO DO

Piroplasmosis

- *Do not* treat donkeys at the higher Imidocarb dosage; death results. Imidocarb may cause signs of colic.

Prevention and Control

- Tick control is key.
- No effective vaccine is available.

Equine Infectious Anemia (EIA)

- Necrotizing vasculitis occurs in the horse, donkey, and mule.
- Outbreaks have been reported in North and South America, Africa, Asia, Australia, and Europe.
- Affected horses are carriers of the EIA retrovirus for life and may have periodic episodes of clinical signs.
- The virus is transmitted by the horsefly.
- Infected mares may abort at any stage of gestation.
- Clinical EIA may be recognized in different stages; it can be acute or chronic.
- Acute EIA is characterized by fever, depression, and petechiae. An acutely affected horse may die in a few days.
- *Important: EIA is a reportable disease.* It is most common in the south central United States (Fig. 20-6).

Clinical Presentation

- Signs of the acute form include fever, anemia, icterus, ventral edema, weight loss, depression, and petechiae.
- The incubation period is generally 1 to 3 weeks.
- Signs of the chronic form include depression, weight loss, anemia, weakness, and recurrent bouts of pyrexia.
- Many infected horses have *no* obvious clinical signs.

Diagnosis

- Agar-gel immunodiffusion (Coggins test): Serum antibodies to EIA retrovirus are found. Result may be falsely negative in first 2 weeks or more after infection. The result may be falsely positive in foals born to infected mares. Use a red-top tube (clot tube) sample for Coggins test. PCR is the most accurate test. An ELISA test is also available.
- Anemia can be marked and progressive; Coombs test result may be positive.
- Mild lymphocytosis and monocytosis occur.
- Thrombocytopenia is common during febrile episodes.

---

[4]Imidocarb dipropionate (Schering Plough Animal Health, Kenilworth, New Jersey).

Numbers displayed on each state represent
the number of positive cases/number of positive premises

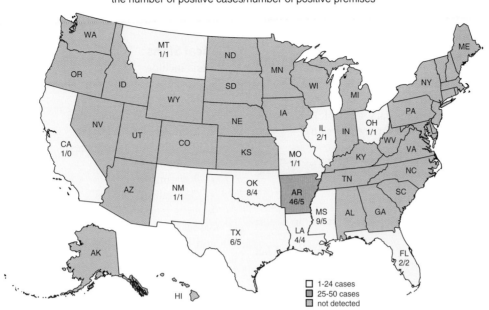

Figure 20-6   EIA distribution map 2010 from www.aphis.usda.gov/vs/nahss/equine/eia/eia_distribution_maps.htm.
Note: This is an excellent website for infectious disease surveillance in the United States.

● WHAT TO DO

Equine Infectious Anemia
- Isolate the horse as soon as possible in a screened stall (200 yards [180 m] from other horses).
- No treatment other than supportive care is successful if the horse is in the carrier state. No treatment or vaccination exists specifically for EIA.
- *EIA is a reportable disease.* Contact the state veterinary medical office. For requirements on Coggins test in each state, call the U.S. Department of Agriculture's toll-free number: 800-545-8732.

Equine Anaplasmosis (Previously Granulocytic Ehrlichiosis)

Granulocytic ehrlichiosis (*Anaplasma phagocytophilum*) is listed here as a differential diagnosis for babesiosis and equine infectious anemia because of many similar clinical signs even though it does *not* have obvious intravascular hemolysis!
- Granulocytic ehrlichiosis is a rickettsial disease caused by *Anaplasma phagocytophilum.*
- Recovery (without treatment) usually occurs within 2 to 3 weeks. Response to tetracycline treatment is rapid with resolution of fever in 12 to 36 hours and clearance of visible inclusion bodies in 1 to 2 days.
- The vector is a tick, *Ixodes* sp.
- The disease is not contagious, but multiple cases may occur on the same premises.
- The disease is mild in horses <4 years of age and clinically undetected in yearlings.
- Abortion is not an expected complication of granulocytic ehrlichiosis.

- The disease is common in northern California and in many parts of the eastern coast, Wisconsin and other surrounding states but has been reported in many states.

Clinical Presentation
- Signs include fever [38.9° to 41.7° C (102° to 107° F)], depression, anorexia, limb edema, mucosal petechiae, icterus, ataxia, reluctance to move (typically worse if horse is older than 3 or 4 years).
- Fever occurs 5 to 7 days after infection, often followed by development of the additional signs over the next 3 to 5 days if untreated.
- Clinical disease is most common in the fall and winter in California, and in the summer on the East Coast.

Diagnosis
- In many cases, clinical signs, geographic location, and thrombocytopenia support a tentative diagnosis without further testing.
- ***Practice Tip:*** *Cytoplasmic inclusions in neutrophils and eosinophils: Horses will usually have inclusions (morulae) by the third day of fever. PCR is the best test during the early fever stage.*
- Samples can be sent to:
  - The University of California—Davis Diagnostic Laboratory
  - Cornell Diagnostic Laboratory, Connecticut Veterinary Medical Diagnostic Laboratory
- Serologic test: The 4DX-SNAP test from IDEXX can test for *Anaplasma phagocytophilia* antibodies. Many horses during the acute febrile stage are negative, and with early

ICTERUS

treatment, antibody detection may be very weak or even undetectable.

- It may take untreated horses a week or more to seroconvert following infection.
- Leukopenia is mild to moderate
- Thrombocytopenia is often in 50,000/µl to 70,000/µl range, but may be even lower.
- Mild anemia is often present.
- Cerebrospinal fluid (limited data available) is usually normal, even with central nervous system signs.

●》 WHAT TO DO

Anaplasmosis
- Supportive therapy
- Oxytetracycline, 6.6 mg/kg IV q12 to 24h; shortens the disease course considerably
- Orally administered doxycycline or minocycline could be used, but would not be expected to be as effective as intravenously administered Oxytetracycline

Other Less Common Causes of Hemolysis and Icterus
See Discolored Urine in Chapter 26, p. 490.
- Hepatic failure (p. 268)
- Clostridial infection (Chapter 35, p. 618)
- Snake bite (Chapter 45, p. 724)
- Disseminated intravascular coagulation: Microangiopathic hemolytic anemia may occasionally occur with disseminated intravascular coagulation. Therapy is for the primary disease.
- Renal failure (p. 491)
- Burns
- Leptospirosis may rarely cause hemolysis or hematuria (p. 491).

Practice Tip: Nonfractionated heparin can cause an acute anemia in the horse. The PCV may decrease to as low as 14%. The anemia is a result of spurious lowering of the PCV and increased sequestration of the red blood cells by reticuloendothelial cells. Hemolysis does not occur, and PCV returns to the previous level within 2 to 4 days after discontinuation of heparin treatment. Low-molecular-weight heparin does not cause this problem.

Bleeding into a Body Cavity
- In adults, internal bleeding occurs most often into the abdomen. Hemorrhage can result from:
  - Trauma (ruptured spleen or liver)
  - Foaling (ruptured middle uterine artery or bleeding into the uterus)
  - Surgery (e.g., ovariectomy or enterotomy)
  - Idiopathic causes
  - Neoplasia (e.g., hemangiosarcoma)
- Idiopathic causes are common, especially bleeding into the abdomen among older horses.
- In the newborn foal, rib fractures and umbilical cord hemorrhage are most common.

- Acute hemorrhage into the thorax sometimes occurs in exercising horses without any preceding clinical signs of obvious disease.

Clinical Signs
- Signs include:
  - Abdominal pain (most common sign with abdominal hemorrhage)
  - Increased respiratory rate
  - Increased heart rate
  - Pale mucous membranes
  - Trembling
  - Sweating
  - Generalized distress
- Mucous membranes become pale pink after 20% to 25% blood loss (approximately 8 to 10 L for a 450-kg horse) and white if blood loss is 35% or more. Blood pressure decreases if there is 20% to 25% blood loss.

Diagnosis
Ultrasonography
- Perform ultrasound examination of the abdomen/thorax for detection of cellular fluid in the cavity. Carefully inspect the liver and spleen if trauma is suspected. Tears in the liver and spleen may be seen with ultrasound and usually require corrective surgery.

Abdominocentesis/Thoracocentesis
- Uniform stream of red fluid that does *not* clot, with a PCV often ranging from 8% to 20%, confirms the diagnosis of hemorrhage.
- Platelets usually are not seen in the fluid.
- Erythrophagocytosis may be present.

●》 WHAT TO DO

Bleeding into a Body Cavity
- Keep the patient quiet.
- Administer intravenous fluids (polyionic fluids), 20 to 80 mL/kg over several hours, depending on the degree of hypovolemia. Low to normal blood pressure should be maintained (permissive hypotension). *Do not* use hetastarch, but plasma is often given to replenish clotting factors.
- Administer epsilon-aminocaproic acid (Amicar), 30 mg/kg IV q6h, mixed in the intravenous fluids. Conjugated estrogen (Premarin 25 to 50 mg IV) diluted in 5% dextrose or crystalloids, may increase clotting factors and platelet aggregation and decrease antithrombin III in uncontrolled hemorrhage. ***Practice Tip:*** *Premarin is best used for uterine or urinary tract hemorrhage.*
- Administer analgesics as needed to control pain and anxiety: Flunixin and phenylbutazone have little effect on platelet function.
- Administer oxygen intranasally in severe cases.
- ***Practice Tip:*** *Perform a transfusion if PCV declines to <15% in subacute cases or chronic cases. In peracute cases, transfusion may be needed before any decrease in PCV. (See p. 285 for guidelines.)*

●) WHAT NOT TO DO

Bleeding into a Body Cavity

- Do not perform surgery unless the patient continues to deteriorate or an obvious reason is found on ultrasound examination for the hemorrhage (e.g., laceration of the liver, severe rib fracture displacement, etc.) because the abdominal bleeding is likely to stop in older horses with *no* history of trauma. If there is a history of trauma, surgery is more likely indicated.
- The blood should *not* be drained from the body cavity unless it is causing respiratory distress or abdominal discomfort. If blood is drained, it should be collected using aseptic technique in blood collection bags with two-thirds of the anticoagulant removed (see the following) in case an autotransfusion is needed.

General Considerations for Blood Transfusion: When to Perform Transfusion for a Bleeding Patient

There is no magical cutoff for PCV and plasma protein that definitely indicates a need for transfusion.

●) WHAT TO DO

Blood Transfusion

- *Practice Tip: Horses can generally lose 20% to 25% of their blood volume or 2% of their body weight without a significant change in blood pressure because of increased cardiac output, as well as pressor, renal, and endocrine responses.*
- If the hemorrhage has stopped, crystalloids are probably all that is needed to restore intravascular volume. As a general rule, crystalloids should be given at approximately 4 times the estimated blood loss. Blood transfusions should not be given unless there is an indication for whole blood (i.e., PCV is dangerously low, high plasma lactate that does not respond to fluid therapy, see p. 287.)
  - As fluid therapy is administered, blood pressure and the laboratory parameters listed for monitoring of transfusion (see p. 288) should be evaluated for markers of tissue hypoxia.
  - Unneeded transfusion may result in immunosuppression.
- Fresh-frozen plasma can and probably should be used in the management of ongoing hemorrhage with the goal of replacing depleted clotting factors. It does not contain intact platelets.
- *Practice Tip: Hetastarch should not be used in the presence of uncontrolled bleeding or disseminated intravascular coagulation.*
- Autotransfusion is used if it is reasonably clear that the bleeding is not associated with sepsis (e.g., traumatized bowel, liver abscess) or tumor.
- If bleeding into the abdomen or chest is so severe that it mechanically restricts ventilation, the blood should be removed. Otherwise, nonseptic blood should be left in the body cavity; the increased pressure helps promote clotting. The blood can be removed if immediate autotransfusion is required.

●) WHAT TO DO

Body Cavity Hemorrhage with Trauma

- Keep the patient quiet.
- Administer intravenous fluids (polyionic fluids), 20 to 80 mL/kg, over several hours or more, depending on the degree of hypovolemia and blood pressure.

- Administer epsilon-aminocaproic acid (Amicar), 30 mg/kg IV q6h, added to the intravenous fluids.
- Administer analgesics as needed to control pain and anxiety.
- Consider exploratory surgery. If a tear in the spleen is identified, splenectomy is possible. Gelfoam (gelatin foam sponge) may be used to manage liver lacerations. The prognosis is guarded with liver lacerations.
- Administer oxygen intranasally in severe cases.

●) WHAT TO DO

Middle Uterine Artery Rupture

- If the affected horse is very agitated, use acepromazine, 0.02 mg/kg, along with balanced crystalloids and blood transfusion.
- If the heart rate is >100 beats/min and the membranes are white, do not use acepromazine.
- Use hypertonic saline solution *only* if rapid deterioration appears imminent and temporary improvement in the blood pressure is needed to pursue blood transfusion or surgery.
- Treatments that maintain systolic pressure between 70 and 90 mm Hg are ideal (permissive hypotension).
  - Administer epsilon-aminocaproic acid (Amicar), 30 mg/kg IV q6h, added to the intravenous fluids and given over 60 minutes. There is also a dose for continuous rate infusion (CRI) (10-15 mg/kg/h).
- Other medical treatments such as Premarin and blood products should be considered if the above treatments are unsuccessful.
- If the mare is colicky or severely hypotensive, the foal should ideally be separated physically from the mare by a barrier that will allow the mare to touch and see the foal but will protect the foal if the mare falls.

Rib Fractures and Hemorrhage

General Considerations

- Hemorrhage into the thorax is common among foals with rib fractures.
- Any physical examination of a neonatal foal includes a careful examination of the thoracic wall. Rib fractures can cause severe pneumothorax, hemothorax, and rapid death.
- Look for evidence of pneumothorax. Provide oxygen intranasally, and perform thoracocentesis; apply a Heimlich chest drain if dyspnea is severe. Keep the foal or horse quiet, and start antimicrobial therapy with a broad-spectrum antibiotic.
- *Practice Tip: Rib fractures in foals are generally just caudal to the elbow, involve the ribs just behind the elbow, and are most commonly located on the left.*

Signs of Hemothorax

- Hemorrhagic anemia
- Dyspnea or rapid shallow breathing
- Sternal edema
- Painful chest, reluctance to move
- Decreased or absent ventral lung sounds, frequently recognized bilaterally
- Possible jugular distention or jugular pulses
- Jaundice can be present or absent

- Flail chest breathing (paradoxical respiratory movement) is common in foals when multiple ribs are fractured and displaced.

Diagnosis
- Perform physical and ultrasound examinations.
- Ultrasound examination of the thorax reveals swirling homogeneous cellular pleural fluid.
- Diaphragmatic hernia infrequently occurs simultaneously with hemothorax.
- Pleurocentesis reveals blood with no bacteria.

▶ WHAT TO DO

Rib Fractures and Hemorrhage
- *Important:* Keep the foal with fractured ribs quiet. Ideally, the foal is best lying on the fractured rib side to reduce fracture ends moving and potentially lacerating a coronary artery.
- *Important:* Surgery should be strongly considered if there is any displacement of the fracture and/or if flail chest or hemothorax are present.
- Administer intranasal oxygen; hemorrhage and hypoventilation may result in hypoxemia.
- Administer broad-spectrum antibiotics, especially if there is an open wound or evidence of pneumothorax.
- Closely monitor and consider blood transfusion (see p. 287).
- Pleurocentesis offers temporary improvement. The foal should be monitored carefully because the pleural cavity frequently fills with blood rapidly.
- Administer antiulcer medication (see p. 182).

Ruptured Aorta
- It is most common among older stallions during breeding.
- It often results in immediate death because of sudden exsanguination.
- Aortic rupture with pulmonary artery fistula can occur in adult Friesian horses.

Diaphragmatic Hernia
- Thoracic bleeding can occur with diaphragmatic hernia.
- Suspect diaphragmatic hernia if a colicky horse has "negative" (or empty-feeling) rectal palpation and evidence of respiratory compromise, especially if the lung sounds are quiet or absent.
- Diagnosis is made by means of ultrasound examination of the thorax. Be careful performing thoracocentesis because compromised bowel can be penetrated even with a teat cannula.

▶ WHAT TO DO

Thoracic Bleeding
- Treatment is stabilization and corrective surgery.

Other Sites of Internal Hemorrhage
- Thoracic lymphosarcoma commonly results in some hemorrhage into the pleural cavity, but rarely causes life-threatening anemia.

- Hemangiosarcoma may cause bleeding in muscle, body cavities, or both.
- Bleeding within the intestinal tract may occur in horses, and if the bleeding is in the small intestine (similar to hemorrhagic bowel in cattle) or small colon, intraluminal obstruction from the blood clots can be a problem.
- If there is bleeding is in the colon following an enterotomy, a transfusion may be needed because of volume depletion.
- Hemothorax develops in rare instances after exercise and pulmonary hemorrhage.
- Hemothorax may also occur following lung and liver biopsies, and following the administration of phenylephrine to older (>15 years) horses for colon displacements.
- Conservative management with intranasal oxygen, fluid therapy, and analgesics is often successful.
- Drainage of the blood is generally *not* needed unless severe respiratory distress is present.
- When a severe pelvic bleed occurs after foaling or when a fractured pelvis lacerates a large vessel, pain and pelvic deformity are the most common presenting clinical problems. There can be substantial blood loss requiring a transfusion or the horse can die if the pelvic hemorrhage is severe and sudden in onset.

External Hemorrhage
- Bleeding from a major vessel can be life threatening.
- This is most commonly a result of trauma, although cellulitis may occasionally erode through a large vessel causing life-threatening bleeding.

▶ WHAT TO DO

External Hemorrhage
- Whenever possible, apply a pressure bandage or suture the vessel to minimize additional blood loss.
- If the heart rate is elevated and the patient appears to be in hypovolemic shock, a blood transfusion and IV crystalloids are required. See p. 285.

Hemorrhage from the Guttural Pouch
- Bleeding from the guttural pouch is most often a result of a fungal infection and erosion of the external or internal carotid or maxillary arteries within the pouch.
- The presence of this condition should be confirmed by means of an endoscopic examination.
- Surgery is needed ASAP!
- Plans for a transfusion should be made as soon as the diagnosis is confirmed because acute, severe bleeding can occur at any time. Ligation of the common carotid artery on the affected side is usually of little benefit.
- Other causes of epistaxis should be ruled out; many require no specific treatment.
  - Some can be managed medically (e.g., thrombocytopenia with immunosuppression therapy: dexamethasone, 0.1 mg/kg, azathioprine, 3 mg/kg, and fresh whole blood transfusion collected in plastic).

- Some causes (i.e., ethmoid hematoma) are surgically corrected or treated with intralesional formalin injections if the cribriform plate is intact.

General Considerations in Blood Transfusion
When and How to Transfuse
- *Practice Tip: Perform blood transfusion in the following clinical situations:*
  - PCV decreases to <20% in the first 12 hours, and bleeding or hemolysis is ongoing.
  - PCV decreases to <12% over 1 to 2 days; hemoglobin of <5 g/dL generally has a detrimental effect on tissue oxygenation.
  - Elevated lactate and low PvO$_2$ and/or SvO$_2$ exists in addition to the above.
  - In peracute cases, death from hemorrhage can occur without a decrease in PCV. In these cases, the need for transfusion is based on:
    - The presence of severe tachycardia
    - White to gray mucous membranes
    - Signs of hypotension—-weak pulses, "cold sweat," general weakness, and evidence of severe bleeding

Choice of Donor
- More than 400,000 blood types are identified in the horse, and there is *no* universal donor.
- If time permits, choose a crossmatched donor. The primary goal is in the major testing—donor RBC collected in EDTA mixed with serum from the patient.
- If the donor has *not* been previously tested for isoantibodies, also perform a minor match— patient's RBCs collected in EDTA crossmatched with donor's serum.
- Most of the testing detects agglutination, although a few laboratories (e.g., University of California—Davis Laboratories) test for lysis using rabbit serum/complement. **Practice Tip:** *An onsite crossmatch can be performed if a centrifuge is available. Collect in EDTA and clot (red top) tubes a sample from both patient and potential donor.*
  - After centrifugation of tubes, use a pipette or syringe to extract 0.25 mL of packed RBCs from the spun EDTA tube of the potential donor (major crossmatch).
  - Mix with 4 mL saline and resuspend.
  - Centrifuge again and decant the supernate. (This can be repeated if time permits and the supernate is not colorless.)
  - Add 3 mL of normal saline to the packed and washed RBCs and resuspend.
  - In a plastic test tube or clot tube (red top); add 2 drops of the patient's serum (clot tube) followed by a drop of the washed and resuspended RBCs from the potential donor. Gently mix the two and maintain at near body temperature for 15 minutes; centrifuge for 3 minutes.
  - Carefully remove the tube and with good light, shake the tube several times as needed so that the RBC pellet moves.

- An alternative is to turn the tube from 12 o'clock to 3 o'clock and back as needed.
- If the pellet moves but does not break or breaks into several clumps, this would indicate severe agglutination (even small clumps should be considered agglutination) and an incompatible donor.
- If the RBCs resuspend into the saline without evidence of clumping this would suggest *no* agglutinating antibodies from the patient against the donor RBCs. Before disrupting the clot, the saline supernate should be clear because development of a pink discoloration indicates hemolysis; hemolytic antibodies cannot be ruled out without adding complement, but generally if there are no agglutinating antibodies "accept" the donor as compatible.
- If time does *not* permit, choose a gelding of the same breed, and/or mix a couple of drops of the donor RBCs (either spun or gravity separated) with two times the amount of patient serum (spun) or plasma (gravity separated) on a microscope slide and vice versa, to look for evidence of agglutination (clumping). This is a less refined but quicker assay than what is described above.
- Consider autotransfusion for body cavity bleeding without sepsis or neoplasia. Blood can be collected from the abdomen or chest via aseptic technique by using a teat cannula to collect the blood into a container with small amounts of ACD, approximately 1 mL 2.5% to 4% ACD per 18 parts blood.
- Store autologous blood for rare elective procedures (e.g., nasal surgery) in which severe hemorrhage is anticipated. Collect in citrate-phosphate-dextrose-adenosine (CPDA) rather than ACD. The blood can be stored at 4° C (39.2° F) for several days.

Collection and Administration
- Collect blood using aseptic technique in 2.5% to 4% ACD: 9 parts blood to 1 part citrate (9:1).
- *Practice Tip: Use a blood collection set; 15% to 20% of the blood volume (body mass in kilograms, 8% to 10% = liters of blood in the donor) of a healthy donor can be collected.*
- Autotransfusion (see previous discussion): Use approximately one third the normal amount of anticoagulant (ACD or citrate-phosphate-dextrose [CPD] or sodium citrate); if citrate is not available, use 1 unit heparin per milliliter of blood. Filters should be changed every 2 L during autotransfusion.
- Blood bags, evacuated bottles, administration sets, and anticoagulant can be purchased from Baxter Laboratories, see Web Appendix 1, Manufacturers. Bottles are faster but are not ideal if platelet replacement is important.
  - Various anticoagulants can be used and are listed below in order of ability to preserve red cells (least to greatest). This is generally *not* important unless storage of the red blood cells is planned.
    - Sodium citrate
    - ACD

ICTERUS

- CPD: Red cells can be stored at refrigeration temperature for 2 to 3 weeks. Platelets are viable for approximately 3 days (in a plastic container only).
- Citrate-phosphate-dextrose-adenine (CPDA): Cells may be stored at refrigeration temperature for 2 to 3 weeks. Platelets are viable for approximately 3 days (in a plastic container only).
- *Administration rate:* Administer whole blood with a blood administration set at a rate of 1 mL/kg for the first 30 minutes, followed by 10 to 20 mL/kg per hour with close monitoring of vital signs. Filters should ideally be replaced after 3 to 4 L. For rapid administration it may be necessary to inject some balanced crystalloid into the bottle to decrease viscosity. For bags, external pressure can be applied.
- Blood for transfusion should be warmed to body temperature.
- Packed RBCs (70%) can be used to manage euvolemic hemolytic anemia. For example, washed RBCs can be given to a foal with NI or an adult with congestive heart failure in need of a transfusion with normal or increased intravascular volume.

Side Effects

- If tachypnea, dyspnea, edema, restlessness, piloerection, and fasciculation occur, stop or slow the transfusion and administer diphenhydramine (Benadryl), 0.25 mg/kg IM.
- For severe anaphylaxis, administer epinephrine, 0.005 to 0.02 mL/kg of 1:1000 slowly IV.

How Much Blood to Administer

- *Practice Tip: For hemorrhage in an adult horse it is usually necessary to administer a minimum of 6 to 8 L in an adult or at least 30% to 40% of the estimated blood loss.*
  - *Note:* Decreases in CVP (jugular fill) and increases in blood lactate occur with 15% to 20% of blood loss, but heart rate increases and blood pressure changes may not occur until there is at least 20% of blood loss. A 500-kg horse has approximately 45 L of blood.
- Administer concurrent polyionic fluids and plasma.
- For hemolysis use the following equation to calculate blood volume needed:

$$\frac{\text{Desired PCV} - \text{PCV recipient}}{\text{PCV of donor}} \times (0.08 \times \text{Body weight in kilograms of recipient})$$
$$= \text{Liters of blood needed}$$

- There is no universal recommendation for an ideal PCV. A measurement of venous oxygen content (PvO_2), saturation (SvO_2), and lactate provides an estimate of oxygen deficiency. *Important:* An abnormally low PvO_2 or SvO_2 and elevated plasma lactate are indications of hypoxia.
- Expected life span of transfused compatible RBCs is as follows:
  - The mean life span of transfused compatible (crossmatched) allogeneic RBCs was recently reported to be 39 days.
- Blood collected in CPD maintains viable red blood cells for at least 2 weeks if refrigerated; transfusion of stored whole blood increases the risk of a reaction.

Other Therapy for Hemorrhage/Hemolysis

- For adults with immune-mediated hemolytic anemia: administer dexamethasone, 40 mg q24h. As the PCV stabilizes, the dexamethasone dosage can be decreased.
- For hypovolemic horses: administer isotonic fluids (up to 4 times the blood loss in shock). Although the PCV decreases, it actually improves oxygen-carrying capacity as long as the PCV does not become so low that there is not sufficient viscosity to keep capillaries open.
- For severe shock/hypotension: hypertonic fluids are recommended but should be used cautiously in horses with uncontrolled bleeding!
- For severely hypoxic horses: intranasally administered oxygen is indicated but 98% of the oxygen-carrying capacity in the horse is by hemoglobin.
- An alternative to whole-blood transfusion if a compatible donor could not be found, was bovine hemoglobin administered at 1 to 20 mL/kg. The half-life is approximately 2 days. *This product is currently unavailable.*
- For continued bleeding: perform surgery/bandaging!
- For uncontrolled bleeding: administer aminocaproic acid and maintain permissive hypotension (systolic pressure >70 mm Hg and urinating).

References

References can be found on the companion website at www.equine-emergencies.com.

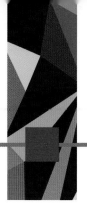

CHAPTER 21

Musculoskeletal System

Elizabeth J. Davidson and James A. Orsini

Diagnostic Analgesia for Lameness Evaluation

Diagnostic analgesia (nerve and joint blocks) is the most valuable tool for the localization of lameness. A thorough knowledge of applied neuroanatomy is required for accurate placement and interpretation of nerve and joint blocks. Perineural analgesia (nerve blocks) infiltrates the sensory nerve fibers and desensitizes corresponding anatomic regions. Intrasynovial analgesia is more specific and is used to localize lameness caused by disease of joints, tendon sheaths, and bursae.

Caution: If a fracture is suspected, radiography and/or nuclear scintigraphy is recommended before diagnostic analgesia procedures to rule out an incomplete fracture and prevent catastrophic bone failure after desensitization. In the severely lame (grades 4 to 5 out of 5) horse, local anesthesia may be used to localize the lameness by determining whether weight bearing or soundness at a slow walk is achievable. Stall confinement with or without mild tranquilization is necessary until the effects of the nerve or joint block wear off.

Equipment

- Twitch (optional)
- Material for sterile scrub (povidone-iodine or chlorhexidine and alcohol)
- Local anesthetics
  - 2% mepivacaine hydrochloride[1]: rapid onset of action and duration of 120 to 150 minutes
  - 2% lidocaine hydrochloride[2]: rapid onset of action and duration of 90 to 120 minutes; more irritating to tissues than mepivacaine
  - 0.5% bupivacaine hydrochloride[3]: intermediate onset of action (30 to 45 minutes) and duration of 3 to 6 hours; should be used when longer-lasting anesthesia is desired
- Sterile disposable 18- to 25-gauge, ⅝- to 3-inch (1.6- to 7.7-cm) needles
- An assortment of 3- to 60-mL syringes (not Luer-Lok); see the illustrations for exact needle and syringe size required for each block
- Sterile gloves for intrasynovial analgesia
- Clippers for intrasynovial analgesia (optional)

---

[1]Carbocaine-V (2% mepivacaine hydrochloride) (Upjohn Company, Kalamazoo, Michigan).
[2]Anthocaine (2% lidocaine hydrochloride) (Anpro Pharmaceutical, Arcadia, California).
[3]Marcaine (0.5% bupivacaine hydrochloride) (Abbott Laboratories, North Chicago, Illinois).

● WHAT TO DO

Perineural Analgesia

As a general rule, distal peripheral nerves are easily located and successfully anesthetized with small volumes (2 to 5 mL) of anesthetic. Nerve blocks above the carpus and tarsus require larger volumes of anesthetic (10 to 15 mL) because the nerves are surrounded by muscle and are difficult to palpate. Begin with the most distal peripheral nerve block and move proximally until the lameness is significantly improved or eliminated.

- See Figs. 21-1 to 21-4 for sites and landmarks for perineural analgesia, size of needle recommended, and amount of local anesthesia required.
- Scrub the injection site(s) to remove gross contamination and wash hands.
- Place twitch if needed. Sedation or tranquilization is not recommended because both may affect interpretation of the block.
- Identify the location of the nerve and quickly insert the needle through the skin at the desired location. If blood freely flows from the needle, redirect until no bleeding is noted.

- Attach the anesthetic-filled syringe to the needle, and inject anesthetic around the nerve. If injection resistance is encountered, the needle may be in a ligament, tendon, or intradermal tissue and should be repositioned.
- After perineural analgesia procedure(s), wipe the injection site(s) with alcohol.
- Allow 5 to 10 minutes before testing skin sensation for anesthesic effect.
- When appropriate, assess pain response associated with application of hoof testers, joint flexion(s), and deep palpation before and after nerve block procedure(s). Repeat the lameness examination and assess improvement (0% to 100%).
- Apply distal limb bandage (optional).

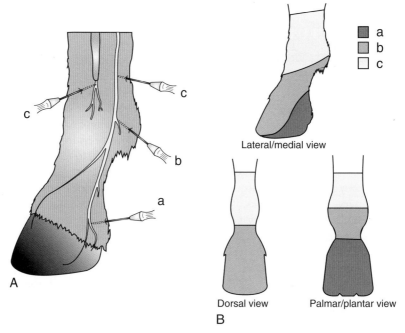

Figure 21-1
A, Sequential sites for perineural analgesia of the distal limb:
a. Palmar digital analgesia
   - 25-gauge, ⅝-inch needle; 1 to 2 mL of local anesthetic per site
   - The medial and lateral palmar digital nerves are located just palmar to their respective artery and vein and lie along the abaxial surface of the deep digital flexor tendon. With the limb held off the ground, insert the needle directly over the nerve, just proximal to the collateral cartilage. Direct the needle in a distal direction.
b. Abaxial sesamoid nerve block
   - 22- to 25-gauge, ⅝- to 1-inch needle; 1 to 3 mL of local anesthetic per site
   - This block can be performed with the horse standing or with the limb held off the ground. The palmar nerves are located along the abaxial surface of the proximal sesamoid bones and juxtaposed to the palmar artery and vein. The needle can be directed in a distal direction.
c. Low palmar analgesia
   - 20- to 22-gauge, 1- to 1½-inch needle; 2 to 4 mL of local anesthetic per site
   - Palmar metacarpal nerves—Insert the needle just distal to the bell of the medial and lateral splint bones to a depth of 1 to 2 cm.
   - Palmar nerves—Insert the needle subcutaneously in the groove between the deep digital flexor tendon and the suspensory ligament at a level just proximal to the bell of the splint bones. The injection site is just proximal to the distal digital tendon sheath. A prolonged scrub of this injection site should be performed in case there is inadvertent penetration of the sheath.
   - For low plantar analgesia—In addition, block the dorsal metatarsal nerve by inserting the needle in a dorsal direction starting at the bell of the lateral splint bone. Place a subcutaneous ring of anesthetic dorsal to the digital extensor tendons. Use a 22-gauge, 1½-inch needle and 2 to 6 mL of local anesthetic.
B, Colored areas represent the affected area of the distal limb.

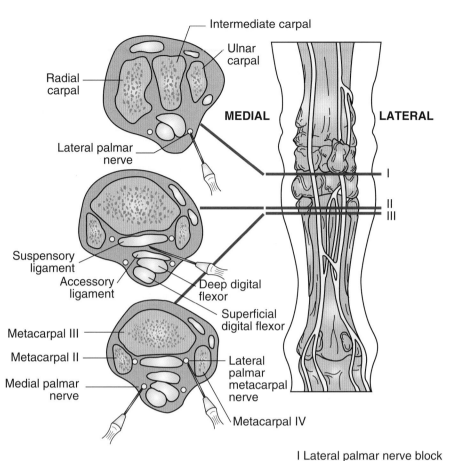
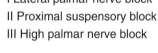

I Lateral palmar nerve block
II Proximal suspensory block
III High palmar nerve block

Figure 21-2 Sites for perineural analgesia of the proximal metacarpal region:
I. Lateral palmar nerve block
  • 22- to 25-gauge, $\frac{5}{8}$- to 1-inch needle; 5 to 6 mL of local anesthetic
  • Insert the needle perpendicular to the skin just distal to the accessory carpal bone. Deposit anesthetic in the dense connective tissue.
II. Proximal suspensory block
  • 22-gauge, $1\frac{1}{2}$-inch needle; 8 to 10 mL of local anesthetic
  • Insert the needle axial to the fourth metacarpal bone. Deposit anesthetic in a fan-shaped pattern, infiltrating the suspensory origin.
III. High palmar nerve block
  • 20- to 22-gauge, 1- to $1\frac{1}{2}$-inch needle; 3 to 5 mL of local anesthetic per site
  • Palmar metacarpal nerves—Insert the needle perpendicular to the skin, axial to the splint bones, abaxial to the suspensory ligament, and along the palmar cortex of the third metacarpus.
  • Palmar nerves—Insert the needle subcutaneously in the groove between the deep digital flexor tendon and the suspensory ligament.

Caution: Inadvertent analgesia of the carpal sheath or the palmar outpouchings of the middle carpal joint can occur. As a precaution, use an aseptic skin preparation and sterile technique when performing these blocks. If lameness is successfully eliminated with analgesia of this region, subsequent anesthesia of the middle carpal joint is indicated to rule out carpal joint disease.

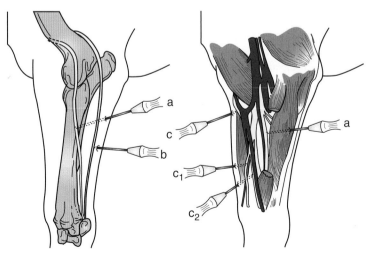

Figure 21-3 Sites for perineural analgesia of the antebrachium: These are the medial views of the antebrachium.
a. Median
  • 20- to 22-gauge, $1\frac{1}{2}$-inch needle; 10 mL of local anesthetic
  • Insert the needle medially, 5 cm distal to the elbow joint. The nerve is located along the caudal aspect of the radius.
b. Ulnar nerve block
  • 20- to 22-gauge, $1\frac{1}{2}$-inch needle; 10 mL of local anesthetic
  • Insert the needle in a groove between the flexor carpi ulnaris and the ulnaris lateralis, 10 cm proximal to the accessory carpal bone.
c. Musculocutaneous
  • 20- to 22-gauge, $1\frac{1}{2}$-inch needle; 3 to 5 mL of local anesthetic per site
  • Insert the needle subcutaneously on either side of the cephalic vein, about halfway between the carpus and elbow. (c_1 and c_2 are cranial and caudal branches of the musculocutaneous nerve.) Both branches of the nerve are anesthetized.

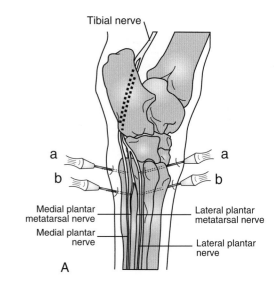

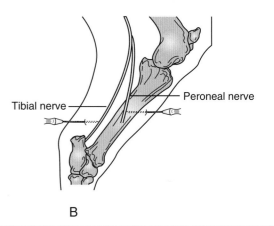

Figure 21-4   Sequential sites for perineural analgesia of the proximal hind limb:
A, Plantar lateral view of the proximal metatarsus; high plantar analgesia
- 20- to 22-gauge, 1- to 1½-inch needle; 3 to 5 mL of local anesthetic per site
    a. Plantar nerves—Insert the needle subcutaneously between the deep digital flexor tendon and the suspensory ligament both medially and laterally.
    b. Plantar metatarsal nerves—Insert the needle axial to the splint bones, abaxial to the suspensory ligament, and along the plantar cortex of the third metatarsus both medially and laterally.
    c. Dorsal metatarsal nerve—Make a circumferential subcutaneous ring along the dorsal proximal metatarsus.
B, Lateral view of the crus; tibial and peroneal analgesia
- 20- to 22-gauge, 1- to 1½-inch needle; 10 to 15 mL of local anesthetic per site
- Tibial nerve—Insert the needle 10 cm proximal to the point of the hock between the deep digital flexor and calcaneal tendons.
- Peroneal nerve—Insert the needle 10 cm proximal to the point of the hock in a groove between the long and lateral digital extensor muscles. Insert the needle until it contacts the tibia. Continuously deposit local anesthetic while withdrawing the needle.

●› WHAT TO DO

Intrasynovial Analgesia

Intrasynovial analgesia is relatively specific and it is *not* necessary to start with the distal limb. As a general rule, low-motion joints (e.g., tarsometatarsal, distal intertarsal, and pastern joints) are anesthetized with low volumes (3 to 5 mL) of local anesthetic. In high-motion joints, larger volumes (10 to 50 mL) of local anesthetic are required for complete analgesia. The procedure is similar to perineural analgesia, except aseptic technique and patient restraint are important for successful completion of the procedure.

- See Figs. 21-5 to 21-11 for sites and landmarks for intrasynovial analgesia, size of the needle recommended, and amount of local anesthetic needed for each synovial structure.
- Palpate the landmarks.
- Clip and shave the site for needle placement (optional).
- Perform an aseptic scrub at the site of injection.
- Wear sterile gloves to handle the syringe and needle and to palpate the landmarks.
- Use an unopened bottle of local anesthetic. One needle should be used to fill the syringe and another for synovial injection. Needles and syringes should remain sterile.
- Place a twitch for restraint.
- Once the synovial structure is identified, insert the needle into the selected synovial structure with a quick definitive puncture through

the skin. If the needle has been placed successfully, synovial fluid appears at the hub of the needle in most cases. Digital pressure on the joint capsule encourages synovial fluid to flow from the needle. Care should be used during needle placement to prevent damage to the articular cartilage and surrounding soft tissue.

- Collect and analyze synovial fluid. (See arthrocentesis procedure, p. 295.)
- Once the needle is inserted in the synovial structure, attach the syringe and inject the anesthetic. There should be minimal resistance. If resistance is encountered, detach the syringe and redirect the needle without exiting the skin. Holding on to the hub of the needle with one hand and injecting with the other facilitates rapid detachment of the syringe if the patient moves. An alternative technique is to attach an extension set to the needle and syringe to facilitate the injection.
- Allow 5 to 30 minutes before assessing the analgesic effect.
- Repeat the lameness examination and assess improvement (0% to 100%).
- For distal limb analgesia, gently rinse or spray the injection site with alcohol and apply a bandage (optional) after the injection.

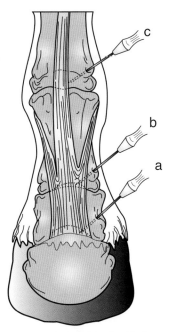

Figure 21-5 Intrasynovial analgesia of the distal limb:
a. Coffin joint
- 20-gauge, 1- to 1½-inch needle; 6 to 10 mL of local anesthetic
- Palpate a depression that is ⅝ inch dorsal to the coronary band and on midline. The needle may be inserted just medial or lateral to the common (forelimb) or long (hind limb) digital extensor tendon or directly on midline through the tendon. With the limb in a weight-bearing position, insert the needle in a distal and palmar/plantar direction to a depth of 1 inch.
b. Pastern joint
- 20- to 22-gauge, 1- to 1½-inch needle; 4 to 6 mL of local anesthetic
- The injection site is dorsal, just lateral to the common/long digital extensor tendon and at the level of or just distal to the palmar process of the proximal phalanx. With the limb in a weight-bearing position, insert the needle in a distal and medial direction.
c. Fetlock joint
- 20-gauge, 1-inch needle; 10 mL of local anesthetic
- The palmar/plantar pouch is located between the distal cannon bone and dorsal to the branches of the suspensory ligament. With the limb in a weight-bearing position, insert the needle perpendicular to the limb axis or in a slightly downward direction to a depth of ½ to 1 inch. Illustration shows intrasynovial analgesia by means of the dorsal approach, medial or lateral to the common/long digital extensor tendon, with the needle inserted almost parallel to the dorsal surface of the third metacarpal/metatarsal bone..

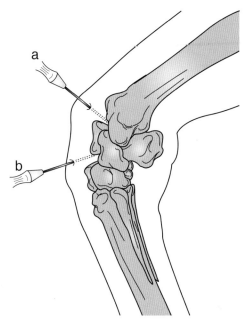

Figure 21-6 Intraarticular analgesia of the carpus:
- 20-gauge, 1-inch needle; 10 mL of local anesthetic per joint
- With the limb in a flexed position, injection sites are easily palpated. For the radiocarpal antebrachium joint *(a)*, locate the depression between the radius and the proximal row of carpal bones. For the middle carpal joint *(b)*, locate the depression between the proximal and distal row of carpal bones. For both joints, insert the needle medial to the extensor carpi radialis tendon or between the extensor carpi radialis tendon and the common digital extensor tendon, parallel to the proximal surfaces of the cuboidal bones, to a depth of 1 inch.

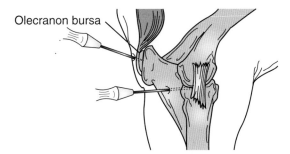

Figure 21-7 Intraarticular analgesia of the elbow joint:
- 18- to 20-gauge, 1½- to 3-inch needle; 20 mL of local anesthetic
- Palpate the elbow joint between the lateral humeral epicondyle and the lateral tuberosity of the radius. Insert the needle cranial or caudal to the lateral collateral ligament in a horizontal direction to a depth of 1½ to 2½ inches.
- Olecranon bursa: Insert needle between the tendon of the long head of the triceps and the palpable proximal olecranon. The bursa is enlarged if abnormal—"capped elbow" and needle placement is centered on the swelling in a lateral to medial direction.

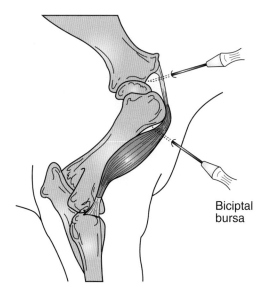

Figure 21-8 Intraarticular analgesia of the shoulder joint:
- 18- to 20-gauge, 3-inch needle; 20 to 30 mL of local anesthetic
- Access the joint at a site between the cranial and caudal prominences of the greater tubercle of the humerus. Direct the needle in a horizontal and slightly caudomedial direction to a depth of 2 to 3 inches.
- Bicipital bursa: Insert the needle ~4 cm proximal to the distal aspect of the deltoid tuberosity of the humerus or 3 to 4 cm distal and 6 to 7 cm caudal to the cranial process of the greater tubercle directing the needle in a proximal, medial, and somewhat cranial direction.

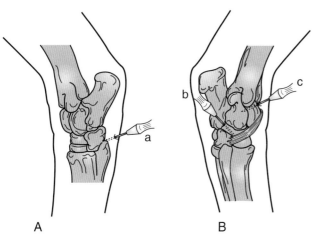

A   B

Figure 21-9   Intraarticular analgesia of the tarsus:
A, Lateral view of the tarsus.
a. Tarsometatarsal joint
   • 20- to 22-gauge, 1-inch needle; 4 to 6 mL of local anesthetic
   • Palpate a small depression proximal to the head of the lateral splint bone. Insert the needle in a horizontal and slightly distal and dorsomedial direction to a depth of 1 inch.
B, Medial view of the tarsus.
b. Distal intertarsal joint
   • 22- to 25-gauge, 1-inch needle; 2 to 3 mL of local anesthetic
   • On the medial aspect of the hock just proximal or distal to the cunean tendon, insert the needle in a lateral and horizontal direction between the third and central tarsal bones.
c. Tarsocrural joint
   • 20-gauge, 1- to 1½-inch needle; 20 to 30 mL of local anesthetic
   • Insert the needle in the dorsomedial pouch of the joint, distal to the medial malleolus and lateral or medial to the saphenous vein. The tarsocural joint communicates with the proximal intertarsal joint.

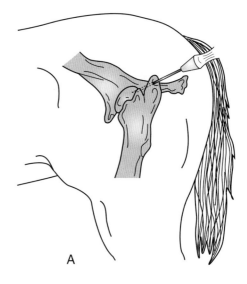

A

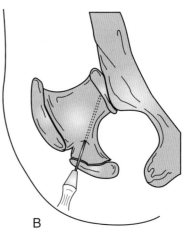

B

Figure 21-11   Intraarticular analgesia of the coxofemoral (hip) joint:
A, Lateral view of the hip.
B, Dorsal view of the hip.
   • 18- to 20-gauge, 6-inch needle with stylet; 25 to 30 mL of local anesthetic
   • Insert the needle between the cranial and caudal process of the greater trochanter of the femur. Direct the needle in a slightly cranial, medial, and distal direction. This site is difficult to palpate because of the thick muscles covering the joint. Ultrasonography can be useful to identify injection site.

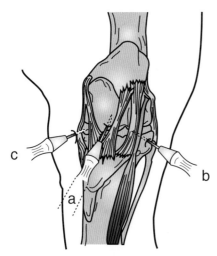

Figure 21-10   Intraarticular analgesia of the stifle:
a. Femoropatellar joint
   • 18- to 20-gauge, 1- to 1½-inch needle; 40 to 50 mL of local anesthetic
   • Proximal to the tibial crest, insert a needle lateral or medial to the middle patellar ligament. Direct the needle slightly proximally in the direction of the patella.
b. Lateral femorotibial joint
   • 18- to 20-gauge, 1- to 1½-inch needle; 20 to 30 mL of local anesthetic
   • Proximal to the lateral tibial plateau, insert the needle caudal to the long digital extensor tendon and cranial to the lateral collateral ligament. Direct the needle horizontally and slightly caudomedially.
c. Medial femorotibial joint
   • 18- to 20-gauge, 1- to 1½-inch needle; 20 to 30 mL of local anesthetic
   • Proximal to the medial tibial plateau, insert the needle between the medial patellar and medial collateral ligaments.

Evaluating Results of Local Analgesia

- It is important to test the efficacy of the diagnostic analgesic procedure:
  - Superficial pain is assessed by the horse's response to noxious stimulation of the skin when applying pressure with the tip of a pen or pinching with hemostats.
  - Deep pain can be assessed by application of hoof testers, limb flexion, or deep digital palpation.
- It is important to recognize that a larger region than expected may be desensitized because of proximal diffusion of local anesthetic.
- *Practice Tip:* Recognize the limitations of diagnostic analgesia:
  - Chronic diseases: Subchondral bone disease and diseases of a complex nature (e.g., proximal palmar metacarpal injury) may *not* "block out" 100%, and 70% to 80% improvement after block should be considered diagnostic.
  - Horses with lameness referable to multiple sites or multiple limbs may require multiple nerve or synovial blocks. In these horses, any improvement after blocking should be investigated further.

Caution: Anesthesia of a limb, especially with upper limb perineural analgesia, can result in loss of motor function and stumbling. Hence, lameness evaluation at high speeds while riding or driving after upper limb nerve blocks should be performed with extreme caution. After nerve or synovial blocks, lameness examination in hand (without a rider) should be assessed to determine if loss of motor function is present before high speed or evaluation under saddle is performed. If loss of motor function is noted, examination at speed or while riding or driving should *not* be attempted. The patient should be confined to a stall until the anesthetic effect is gone and the distal limb bandaged to prevent abrasions.

Complications

- After perineural analgesia, severe local tissue damage is unusual.
- Mild inflammation and swelling after injection, especially after proximal limb analgesia, may be noted.
- If a perineural vessel is inadvertently punctured, hematoma formation at the site of needle entry is common.
- Risks are minimized by proper skin preparation, correct and quick needle placement, minimal amount of local anesthetic, and adequate patient restraint.
- After the procedure, cleaning the area with alcohol and applying a distal limb bandage for 24 hours also lessens the risk of postinjection hematoma.
- Acute synovitis ("flare") and synovial infection are rare but potentially serious sequelae to intrasynovial analgesia.
- *Do not* place a needle through a contaminated wound or damaged skin; delay the procedure if periarticular cellulitis is present.
- Monitor the equine patient for pain and/or swelling for 2 weeks after the diagnostic procedure. If synovitis or lameness related to the block is seen, evaluation for possible iatrogenic infection is strongly recommended.

- Needle breakage is more likely in the proximal limb and/or when longer needles are used. Use the smallest-gauge needle possible and/or flexible (spinal needles) needles that bend rather than break. Adequate patient restraint minimizes this complication.
- Systemic side effects are extremely rare and include central nervous system signs such as muscle fasciculations, ataxia, and collapse. *Practice Tip: The maximum dose of local anesthetic recommended in a 500-kg horse is 300 mL of 2% lidocaine.*

Arthrocentesis and Synovial Fluid Analysis

Elizabeth J. Davidson and James A. Orsini

Arthrocentesis, followed by intraarticular medications, is commonly performed when diagnosing and treating joint disease. Synovial fluid analysis aids in the identification of joint disease and is critical in horses with septic arthritis.

Arthrocentesis

The landmarks for common sites of arthrocentesis are described earlier in this chapter. High-motion joints have large joint pouches and are easily entered. Low-motion joints are more difficult to enter. If the usual site of arthrocentesis is contaminated, an alternative site should be used.

Synovial Fluid Analysis

Synovial fluid is an ultrafiltrate of serum and alternations in its composition are a direct reflection of the synovial structure. Gross characteristics—color, clarity, volume, and viscosity—are immediately examined after collection. Normal synovial fluid is clear, slightly yellow, and completely free of particulate. Red streaks indicate bleeding that may be the result of trauma during needle placement or aspiration. A uniform red or amber tinge may be caused by chronic intraarticular injury. Turbid fluid or a dark yellow color is caused by inflammation. The presence of particles or purulent material indicates serofibrinous inflammation, which is often associated with infection (septic arthritis or tenosynovitis). Normal synovial fluid is highly viscous due to hyaluronan. Subjective assessment of viscosity is made by placing a drop of fluid between the thumb and finger. Normal fluid forms a 2- to 5-cm "string" between the thumb and finger. Diseased joints have a reduced amount and quality of hyaluronan and fail the "string" test.

Normal synovial fluid lacks fibrinogen and does *not* clot. Inflamed or diseased joints have elevated total protein levels. Cytologic analysis quantifies and characterizes the white blood cells. Gram-stained smear slides and bacterial culturing are essential if a septic process is suspected. Negative culture results *do not* rule out infection; bacteria are isolated in only 50% of samples. *Practice Tip: Polymerase chain reaction (PCR) techniques are used to identify bacterial DNA in many microbiology laboratories today.*

Attempts are made to correlate biochemical, immunologic markers, and breakdown products of the articular cartilage

MS

| Table 21-1 | Correlation Between Synovial Fluid Parameters and Intraarticular Disorders* |

Condition	Appearance	Viscosity	Volume	Total Protein (g/dL)	Nucleated Cells/µL	Cytologic Findings
Normal	Pale yellow, clear	High	Low	<2.5	<500	<10% neutrophils
Nonseptic synovitis	Yellow, translucent	Low	Generally increased	<3.5	<10,000	<10% neutrophils
Septic arthritis	Yellow-green, turbid	Increased	High	>4.0	>30,000	>90% neutrophils (degenerate) with or without intracellular bacteria
Degenerative joint disease (osteoarthritis)	Yellow, clear	Low (variable)	Low	<3.5	<10,000	<15% neutrophils

*Listed ranges are approximate. Considerable variability exists within the literature.

with joint disease. Changes have been documented with disease, but the accuracy of a single sample in a single patient is questionable.

Table 21-1 shows the correlation between synovial fluid parameters and specific equine joint disorders.

Equipment

- Sedative (intravenous xylazine and detromidine hydrochloride +/− butorphanol tartrate)
- Twitch
- Clippers (optional)
- Material for sterile scrub (povidone-iodine or chlorhexidine and alcohol)
- Sterile gloves
- 18- to 22-gauge needles
- 5- to 20-mL syringes (non–Luer-Lok)
- Blood collection tubes containing ethylenediaminetetraacetic acid (EDTA) and plain Vacutainer tubes[4]
- Culture material (Port-a-Cul,[5] blood culture bottles[6])

●》 WHAT TO DO

Arthrocentesis
- See Figs. 21-5 to 21-11 for sites and landmarks.
- Palpate the landmarks.
- Clip or shave the site for needle placement is preferred.
- Sedate the patient. Recommended dosage for adults is 0.3 to 0.5 mg/kg xylazine with 0.01 to 0.02 mg/kg butorphanol IV; for neonatal foals, 0.1 to 0.2 mg/kg diazepam IV *slowly*.
- Perform a sterile scrub at the site of needle placement.
- Wear sterile gloves to handle syringes and needles and to palpate the landmarks.
- Place a twitch for restraint (if needed).
- Once the synovial structure is identified, place the needle with a quick stick through the skin. *Do not* damage the articular cartilage

[4]Vacutainer tubes (Becton-Dickinson Vacutainer Systems, Rutherford, New Jersey).
[5]Port-a-Cul culture swab and transport system (Becton-Dickinson Microbiology Systems, Cockeysville, Maryland).
[6]Septi-check, BB blood culture bottle (Roche Diagnostic Systems, Indianapolis, Indiana).

and surrounding soft tissue with the needle. Synovial fluid appears at the hub of the needle in most cases. Digital pressure on the joint capsule encourages synovial fluid to flow from the needle.
- If synovial fluid freely drips from the needle, the fluid may be collected directly into the collection tubes. A second nonsterile assistant removes the top of the tube and collects the fluid as it drips.
- Or, attach a syringe to the needle and aspirate fluid and transfer to collection tubes or to culture media.
- Analyze synovial fluid:
  - For *culture,* use a plain tube or Port-a-Cul or blood culture bottle.
  - For *cytologic* evaluation, use an EDTA (purple top) tube.
- ***Caution:*** Do not place the needle through an open or contaminated wound or in an area of possible infection. Determination of joint involvement after trauma or infection often requires alternative needle placement if the usual site for joint access is contaminated in any way.

Complications
- The most common complication is failure to obtain synovial fluid.
  - Placement of the needle within or adjacent to surrounding soft tissue structures, such as tendon or ligaments, or placement of the needle within cartilage or synovial lining is frequently the cause of this.
  - Redirecting or rotating the needle without exiting the skin can be attempted. If the needle is plugged with tissue during placement, arthrocentesis with a new needle or an alternative entry site should be used.
- Bacterial cultures on synovial fluid are often unrewarding. Negative culture results should *not* negate appropriate treatment.
- Also, see Intrasynovial Analgesia, Complications, p. 295.

Temporomandibular Arthrocentesis

James A. Orsini and Elizabeth J. Davidson

Synovial fluid is obtained from the temporomandibular joint (TMJ) by means of arthrocentesis. As with other joints, analysis of synovial fluid may be useful for determining the pathologic features of disease. Arthrocentesis is also used to administer intraarticular medications or to perform intrasynovial analgesia.

Note: The following descriptive procedure has *not* been studied in foals or in young horses that have immature bone growth. Anatomic variations in the young horse do *not* correlate directly with the following topographic anatomy to identify the TMJ.

Equipment
- Sedative (intravenous xylazine and detomidine hydrochloride +/- butorphanol tartrate)
- Clippers (optional)
- Sterile scrub materials (povidone-iodine or chlorhexidine and alcohol)
- 20-gauge, 1½-inch (3.8-cm) needles and syringes (3, 6, or 12 mL)
- EDTA and plain Vacutainer tubes
- Culture material

MS

●》 WHAT TO DO

Temporomandibular Arthrocentesis
- Clip an area bordered by the lateral canthus of the eye and the base of the ear and from the facial crest to the zygomatic process of the temporal bone (optional).
- Sedate the patient. Recommended dosage for adults are as follows: 0.3 to 0.5 mg/kg IV xylazine or detomidine at 3 to 6 microgram/kg IV; butorphanol can be added at a dosage of 0.01 to 0.02 mg/kg IV.
- Scrub the area.
- Maintain aseptic technique.
- Palpate the TMJ by placing the first digit of the hand at the lateral canthus of the eye and the fifth digit at the base of the ear. With the middle three digits flexed, the third digit marks the lateral aspect of the mandibular condyle.
- Palpate the zygomatic process of the temporal bone, which is 1 to 2 cm dorsal to the condylar process of the mandible (Fig. 21-12).
- A soft depression should be palpable midway between the condylar and zygomatic processes and 0.5 to 1.0 cm caudal to the imaginary line between the two bony structures.
- Insert a 20-gauge, 1½-inch (3.8-cm) needle into the TMJ beginning perpendicular to the skull and directing the needle slightly rostral (approximately 15 degrees). The needle may have to be directed slightly ventral, depending on the patient.
- Advance the needle ½ to 1½ inches (1.6 to 3.8 cm) into the joint until synovial fluid appears. If bone is encountered, withdraw the needle and redirect it ventrally or dorsally to enter the joint.
- Collect samples into EDTA and red-top (no additive) Vacutainer tubes for cytologic examination and culture. If the sample is *not* to be processed within 12 hours, place it in a blood culture bottle or a Port-a Cul transport system.

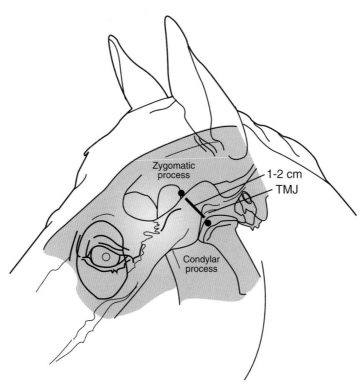

Figure 21-12 Location of zygomatic process of the temporal bone. *TMJ*, Temporomandibular joint.

Complications
See Intrasynovial Anesthesia, Complications, p. 295.

Endoscopy of the Navicular Bursa
James A. Orsini

- Penetrating wounds to the sole of the hoof often result in infectious navicular bursitis because the foreign object tends to be directed toward the concave surface of the coffin bone. *This type of injury is an emergency and aggressive treatment is needed as soon as possible after the injury for the best prognosis.* Endoscopy of the navicular bursa offers an alternative surgical treatment to the traditional "street nail" procedure and results in a better outcome in most cases. The prognosis for puncture wounds resulting in sepsis of the navicular bursa is guarded; however, the use of an arthroscope to debride the navicular bursa is the most appropriate treatment. The technique for evaluation of the navicular bursa is useful for examination of the following:

- Navicular bursa
- Insertions of the navicular suspensory ligaments
- T and impar ligaments
- Navicular bursal synovium (bursa podotrochlearis)
- Dorsal surface of the deep digital flexor tendon

The technique facilitates the following procedures:
- Navicular bursa lavage
- Pannus debridement
- Synovial resection
- Debridement of lesions of the navicular bone and deep digital flexor tendon

Equipment
- General anesthesia equipment
- Arthroscopy equipment: 4-mm 25- to 30-degree forward oblique arthroscope[7]
- 18-gauge, 3½-inch needle
- EDTA and plain (no additive) Vacutainer tubes
- Culture material (Port-a-Cul, blood culture bottles)

---

[7]Karl Storz Veterinary Endoscopy-America, Inc., Goleta, California.

●》 WHAT TO DO

Endoscopy of the Navicular Bursa
See Fig. 21-13.
- Administer general anesthesia with the patient in lateral recumbency with affected limb uppermost.
- Support the limb proximal to the metacarpophalangeal/metatarsophalangeal joint with the distal limb free.
- Clip or shave the area from the metacarpophalangeal/metatarsophalangeal joint 360 degrees to coronary band.
- Clean and debride the sole and point of entry of the puncture wound.

- Maintaining aseptic technique perform an aseptic scrub of the puncture and surgical sites on the palmar/plantar aspect of the distal part of the limb.
- Collect fluid samples for cytologic examination and microbiologic cultures, and place the samples in an EDTA (purple-top) Vacutainer tube and Port-a-Cul tube.
- Make a 5-mm skin incision proximal to the lateral cartilage ungularis (collateral cartilage) on the abaxial margin of the deep digital flexor tendon and axial to the palmar/plantar digital neurovascular bundle.

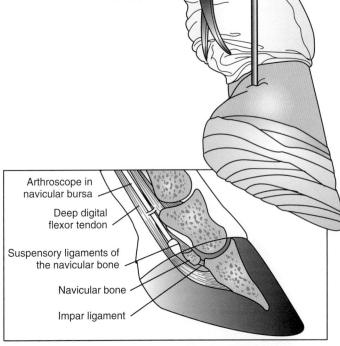

Arthroscope in navicular bursa

Deep digital flexor tendon

Suspensory ligaments of the navicular bone

Navicular bone

Impar ligament

Figure 21-13 Endoscopy of the navicular bursa.

- Direct the arthroscope cannula with a conical obturator through the skin incision and advance it distally and axially dorsal to the deep digital flexor tendon so that it enters the bursa at approximately the midpoint of the phalanx.

- After entering the bursa (loss of resistance), withdraw the obturator and replace it with a 4-mm, 25- to 30-degree forward oblique arthroscope.
- Suture skin portals after the arthroscopic procedure is complete.

Complications

Collateral damage to surrounding soft tissues can occur during insertion of the cannula caused by lack of "hands-on" training and practice with the arthroscope.

Cervical Vertebral Articular Process Injections

Elizabeth J. Davidson

- Neck pain is a cause of poor performance.
- A detailed clinical examination including physical, lameness, and neurologic evaluations, and good-quality radiography is recommended for appropriate diagnosis.
- In the past, treatments were limited to systemic anti-inflammatories and alternative medicine techniques, such as acupuncture therapy.
- Cervical facet arthrocentesis using ultrasonographic guidance is a technique that aids in the diagnosis and treatment of neck pain due to cervical facet joint pain.

Equipment
- Twitch (optional)
- Material for sterile scrub (povidone-iodine or chlorhexidine and alcohol)
- Sterile gloves
- Sterile disposable 18- to 20-gauge, 3½-inch spinal needle
- 10-mL syringes (non–Luer-Lok)
- Ultrasound machine equipped with 3.5- to 5-MHz micro-convex transducer
- Sedation: 0.3 to 0.5 mg/kg xylazine or 0.005 to 0.01 mg/kg detomidine
- Sterile acoustic gel
- Sterile cover sleeve for ultrasound transducer
- For diagnostic analgesia, 2% mepivacaine hydrochloride

◉》 WHAT TO DO

Cervical Vertebral Articular Process Injections
- Locate the general area of the cervical facet joints by palpating the neck. The cervical facet joints are located along the lateral and dorsal aspect of the cervical spine.
- Sedate the patient.
- Lower the head to the level of the point of the shoulder.
- Position the neck as straight as possible.
- Identify the joint using ultrasonographic guidance:
  - The articular processes are the most dorsolateral bony structures of the cervical vertebrae.
  - The joint space is located at the junction of the cranial and caudal processes, identified as an anechoic gap.
  - The articular processes form a characteristic "chair" sign (Fig. 21-14); the cranial articular process forms the seat and the

cranial aspect of the caudal articular process forms the chair back.
  - Color-flow Doppler imaging of the joint region is recommended to ensure the absence of the vertebral artery and its branches.
- Perform a sterile scrub at the site of injection.
- Wear sterile gloves to handle the spinal needle and syringe.
- Using aseptic technique, apply the sterile cover sleeve to the transducer. Apply a small amount of sterile acoustic gel between the transducer and the cover for improved imaging.
- Sterile acoustic gel or alcohol can be used on the skin at the injection site.
- Place a twitch for restraint (optional).
- Relocate the joint using ultrasonographic guidance.
- Infiltrate the site of needle entry with 1.5 mL of 2% mepivacaine hydrochloride local anesthetic (optional).
- Introduce the needle just cranial and parallel to the transducer, and direct it axially and caudally toward the joint space (Fig. 21-15).
- A properly placed needle casts a hyperechoic shadow (Fig. 21-16) from the skin edge to the joint.
- Remove the style and aspirate joint fluid.
- Joint fluid can be collected and analyzed.

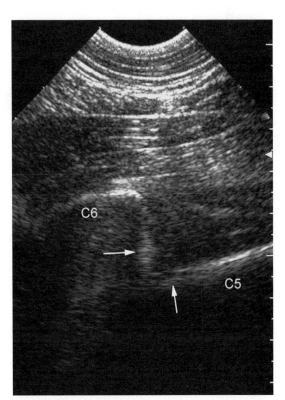

Figure 21-14 Ultrasound image of the right caudal cervical vertebrae of a 5-year-old Warmblood gelding with neck stiffness after falling. The characteristic "chair" sign is created by C5 as the seat and C6 as the back (*white arrows*). *C5,* Fifth cervical vertebra; *C6,* sixth cervical vertebra.

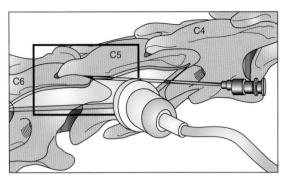

Figure 21-15   Right lateral view of the caudal cervical vertebrae. The ultrasound transducer is positioned over dorsal aspect of C5-6 articulation with proper placement of the spinal needle cranial to the joint.

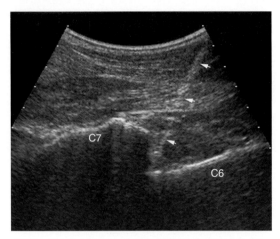

Figure 21-16   Ultrasound image of the right C6-7 articulation of a 10-year-old Warmblood with cervical facet osteoarthritis. A spinal needle *(arrows)* is inserted in the joint space. *C6,* Sixth cervical vertebra; *C7,* Seventh cervical vertebra.

WHAT NOT TO DO

Cervical Vertebral Articular Process Injections

- *Do not* puncture the vertebral artery. In the cranial neck the vertebral artery courses just ventral to the cervical facet joints.
- Avoid needle insertion in the ventral aspect of the joint because inadvertent penetration of the spinal canal can occur. If the spinal canal is entered, cerebral spinal fluid freely flows from the needle. *Do not* inject medications into the spinal canal.
- ***Practice Tip:*** *The procedure is challenging. Good-quality imaging, a skilled ultrasonographer, and a cooperative patient are imperative for success. The procedure may be performed by one person; however, it is easier with two: one ultrasonographer and one person performing the arthrocentesis.*

Complications

- As with any joint, infection after injection is a potential complication. Any increase in rectal temperature and neck swelling, stiffness, or soreness that was *not* present before the procedure should be investigated aggressively and treated appropriately.
- The spinal needle may bend or break during the procedure. Adequate sedation and restraint minimizes the risk.

Sacroiliac Injections

Elizabeth J. Davidson

- Sacroiliac joint pain is a cause of poor performance and hind limb lameness. Clinical and physical examination findings are variable.
- Diagnosis is difficult and it is often a diagnosis by exclusion.
- Intraarticular injection of the sacroiliac joint is nearly impossible because of its deep anatomic location and small size, yielding <1 mL of synovial fluid.
- Periarticular injection of the sacroiliac joint has been validated, and the medial approach is the preferred method.
- Infiltration of the sacroiliac region can aid in the diagnosis and management of sacroiliac joint injuries.

Equipment

- Twitch (optional)
- Material for sterile scrub (povidone-iodine or chlorhexidine and alcohol)
- Sterile gloves
- Sterile 3-mL syringe (non–Luer-Lok)
- Sterile 10-mL syringe (non–Luer-Lok) for diagnostic analgesia
- Sterile disposable 18-gauge, 6-inch spinal needle
- Sedation: 0.3 to 0.5 mg/kg xylazine or 0.005 to 0.01 mg/kg detomidine
- Stocks
- 2% mepivacaine hydrochloride

WHAT TO DO

Sacroiliac Injections

- Place horse in stocks for restraint.
- Sedate the patient.
- The horse should stand squarely on the hind limbs, bearing equal and full weight.
- Perform a sterile scrub at the tuber sacrale region.
- Wear sterile gloves to handle the spinal needle and syringe.
- Apply a twitch to the horse.
- Infiltrate the site of needle entry with 1 to 2 mL of 2% mepivacaine local anesthetic.
- Scrub the area again using aseptic technique.
- To inject the *right* sacroiliac joint region (Figs. 21-17 and 21-18), do the following:
  - Needle entry is slightly axial and 2 cm cranial to the *left* tuber sacrale.
  - Advance the needle across midline at a 45- to 60-degree angle to vertical and toward the *right* sacroiliac joint.
  - Advance the needle in a slightly caudal direction toward the cranial aspect of the *right* greater trochanter along the axial aspect of the *right* ilial wing.
  - Advance the needle until bone is encountered at the caudomedial aspect of the *right* sacroiliac joint region.
  - For diagnostic purposes, deposit 8 mL of 2% mepivacaine at the right sacroiliac joint region.
  - For therapeutic purposes, deposit medications at the right sacroiliac joint region.
- To inject the *left* sacroiliac joint, the needle entry is slightly axial and cranial to the *right* tuber sacrale. The needle should be directed in

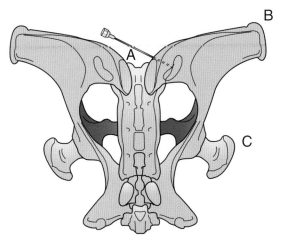

Figure 21-17 Dorsal view of the pelvis with a needle placement for injection of the right sacroiliac joint. *A*, left tuber sacrale. *B*, right tuber coxae. *C*, greater trochanter of the right femur.

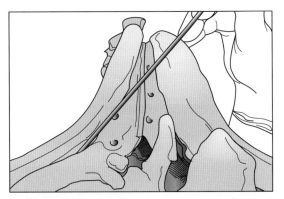

Figure 21-18 Cranial view of the sacroiliac region with the needle positioned adjacent to the right sacroiliac joint.

a similar fashion as previously mentioned until the bone along the axial aspect of the *left* ilial wing is encountered.

●〉 WHAT NOT TO DO

Sacroiliac Injections
- If bone is encountered shortly after needle placement, withdraw and reposition the needle. Most of the length of the needle is inserted before reaching the proper location.
- If the needle is inserted in an excessively ventral position, the sacrum and the dorsal branches of the sacral arteries and nerves may be encountered. Correct the needle placement by redirecting the needle with a greater angle to vertical.
- If the needle is inserted in an excessively horizontal position, the wing of the ilium is encountered. Correct the needle placement by redirecting the needle with a less angle to vertical, and slide it along the axial aspect of the ilial wing.
- Avoid the sciatic nerve and the cranial artery and nerve at the caudal aspect of the joint.
- ***Practice Tip:*** *In some horses, the dorsal spinous process of the sixth lumbar vertebra angles caudally and the dorsal spinous process of the first sacral vertebra angles cranially, creating a smaller interspinous space. If these normal anatomic variations are encountered, a second needle entry site just cranial or caudal to the initial entry site should be used.* ***Caution:*** Loss of cranial gluteal, sciatic, first sacral, femoral, and/or obturator nerve function may occur because of inadvertent

diffusion of the anesthetic agent. Affected horses have proprioceptive and motor deficits of the pelvic limb. Reduced weight-bearing ability to the point of falling over and prolonged recumbency may occur. Additionally, needle placement near midline can lead to migration of medications along the spinal nerve roots into the vertebral canal.

Complications
- Needle breakage can occur because of the length of the needle and the ligamentous tissues around the joint. Adequate sedation and restraint minimizes the risk.
- Hind limb ataxia or weakness after diagnostic analgesia is possible especially with caudally placed injections.
- Transient patchy sweating over the semitendinosus muscle and ipsilateral perineal paralysis have also been reported.

PEDIATRIC ORTHOPEDIC EMERGENCIES

Joanne Hardy

Acute Lameness in a Foal
Presentation
- Acute lameness in a foal is an important problem. Most owners assume that "the mare stepped on the foal," whereas in reality this is uncommon.
- ***Practice Tip:*** *The most common cause of acute lameness in a foal is septic arthritis/osteomyelitis.*
- Other causes of acute lameness include the following:
  - Long bone fractures
  - Physeal fractures
  - Foot abscesses
  - Muscle or tendon injuries

●〉 WHAT TO DO

Acute Lameness in a Foal
- Obtain a history on the foal's health up until presentation. Foals acquire septic arthritis by the hematogenous route; any history of prior or concurrent illness suggests septicemia.
- Perform a complete examination to determine whether any other problems such as pneumonia, diarrhea, or infected umbilical structures are present.
- Palpate the involved limb for evidence of joint effusion, crepitus, swelling, or instability. This includes placement of hoof testers on the foot.
- If any joint effusion is palpated, assume septic arthritis. (See the following section on septic arthritis/osteomyelitis, p. 302). ***Important:*** Remember that identification of joint effusion in the upper limbs, such as elbow, shoulder, and hip, can be difficult; arthrocentesis of these joints should be performed if an alternate source of lameness cannot be identified.
- In the case of vertebral osteomyelitis, *neurologic dysfunction* rather than lameness may be present. For example cauda equina syndrome, sciatic, or peroneal nerve dysfunction can be the only presenting sign.
- If swelling/instability is detected, obtain radiographs (see section on fractures, p. 304).

MS

MS

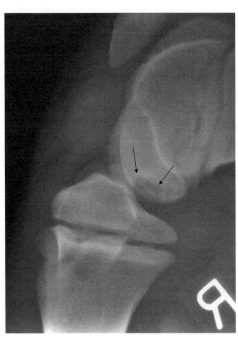

Figure 21-19   Radiograph of the stifle of a foal with type E osteomyelitis. Notice the lucency in the femoral condyle *(arrows)*.

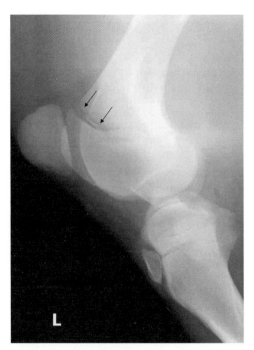

Figure 21-20   Radiograph of the stifle of a foal with type P osteomyelitis. Notice the widening of the physis *(arrows)*.

⊙⊃ WHAT NOT TO DO

Acute Lameness in a Foal
- Give it time and hope it gets better.
- Provide inadequate immobilization in the case of a fracture.

Septic Arthritis and Osteomyelitis

- Most foals with septic arthritis/osteomyelitis are, or have been, septicemic. Multiple joint involvements are identified in at least 50% of foals with septic arthritis. Foals may show systemic involvement or only have evidence of local infection.
- The classification of septic arthritis/osteomyelitis is as follows:
  - *Type S:* for synovial involvement (No osteomyelitis is identified.)
  - *Type E:* for epiphyseal involvement (Osteomyelitis of the epiphysis is identified (Fig. 21-19)
  - *Type P:* infection of the physis (Fig. 21-20)
  - *Type T:* infection of cuboidal bones in the tarsus or carpus; usually in immature foals (Fig. 21-21)
  - *Type I:* invasion of the joint from a periarticular infection/abscess

Diagnosis
- The diagnosis of septic arthritis/osteomyelitis is based on:
  - Arthrocentesis
  - Radiographs
  - Cultures
- In vertebral osteomyelitis, computed tomography or magnetic resonance imaging may improve diagnosis.
- In a foal with acute lameness, septic arthritis/osteomyelitis must be ruled out. With elbow, shoulder, stifle, or

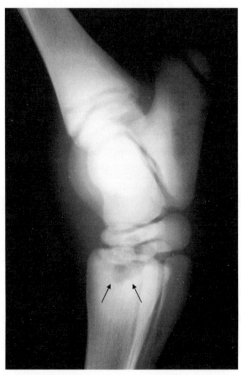

Figure 21-21   Radiograph of the tarsus of a foal with type T osteomyelitis. Notice the lucencies in the distal tarsal bones *(arrows)*.

coxofemoral joint involvement, arthrocentesis may be required because effusion of these joints may be difficult to palpate.
- With arthrocentesis, cytologic examination is necessary. (See p. 296 on cytologic examinations and procedure.)
  - Normal values: total protein <2.0 g/dL; white blood cell count <1000 cells/mL; neutrophil count <40%

- Septic arthritis: total protein >3 g/dL; white blood cell count >20,000 cells/mL; neutrophil count >80%; neutrophils may or may not be degenerate
- In septic physitis, if the infected physis is outside the joint, a sympathetic joint effusion may occur, with mild to moderate increase in total protein, white blood cell count, and percent of neutrophils.
- With arthrocentesis, culture is necessary. (See Chapter 9, p. 30, procedures for bacterial, fungal, and viral sampling.)
  - Synovial fluid should be placed in blood culture bottles to increase the likelihood of growth.
  - ***Practice Tip:*** *Twenty-five percent of synovial fluid that yields no growth is positive on Gram stain.*
  - Approximately 50% of cultures yield *no* growth. This does not mean that the joint is not septic.
- Additional information on culturing:
  - Blood cultures should be obtained.
  - Cultures from other infected sites should be obtained: blood culture, umbilical culture, transtracheal wash.
  - Bone biopsies in osteomyelitis can be obtained under radiographic or fluoroscopic guidance.
- Additional diagnostics:
  - Check the foal's immunoglobulin G level, and treat as needed.

●》 WHAT TO DO

Septic Arthritis and Osteomyelitis
- The principles of treatment of septic arthritis/osteomyelitis are as follows:
  - Broad-spectrum systemic antibiotics
  - Local drainage and lavage of affected joint(s)
  - Local antibiotics
- Broad-spectrum systemic antibiotics:
  - Antibiotics are best administered parenterally.
  - Include gram-positive and gram-negative organisms in the spectrum.
  - One third of septic foals have a gram-positive organism.
  - Two thirds of septic foals have more than one organism.
  - Table 21-2 lists common antimicrobials used for the treatment of sepsis in foals.
- Local lavage methods:
  - Through-and-through needle
  - Arthrotomy and teat cannula: if no response after 48 hours or if fibrin in the joint
  - Arthroscopy: for complex joints like the stifle, to obtain better debridement
- Local antimicrobial regimens:
  - Intraarticular injection
  - Regional intravenous injection (Fig. 21-22 and Box 21-1)
  - Intraosseous injection (see Chapter 5, p. 16, for procedures). This is particularly helpful for septic physitis.
  - Implantation of antibiotic-impregnated polymethyl methacrylate beads (Box 21-2)
  - Intraarticular catheter
- Adjunct treatments:
  - Nonsteroidal anti-inflammatory drugs
  - Other methods of pain control: fentanyl patches, butorphanol

Table 21-2	Antibiotic Therapy for Infection in Newborns and Foals	
Agent	**Dose**	**Route and Frequency**
Penicillin G procaine	22,000-44,000 IU/kg	IM q12h
Penicillin G sodium/potassium	22,000-44,000 IU/kg	IV q6h
Ceftiofur	2-10 mg/kg	IM, IV q6-12h
Gentamicin	6.6 mg/kg	IM, IV q24h
Amikacin	21-25 mg/kg	IM, IV q24h
Ticarcillin/clavulanic acid	50-100 mg/kg	IV q6h
Cefotaxime	30-50 mg/kg	IV q6h
Ceftazidime	30-50 mg/kg	IV q6h
Ceftriaxone	25 mg/kg	IV q12h
Cefpodoxime proxetil	10 mg/kg	PO q6-12h
Azithromycin	10 mg/kg	PO q24h
Clarithromycin	7.5 mg/kg	PO q12h
Rifampin	5-10 mg/kg	PO q12h

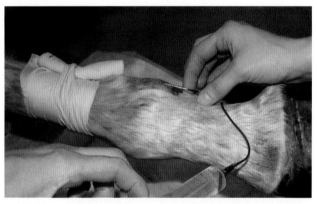

Figure 21-22 Regional perfusion of the distal limb in a horse. A tourniquet (Esmark bandage) has been placed on the metacarpus. The hair over the lateral digital vein has been clipped, and a 23-gauge butterfly catheter has been inserted in the vein. The antimicrobial, diluted in saline, is being injected.

Box 21-1	Regional Limb Perfusion/Pediatric Boxes and Figures

- Antimicrobials:
  - Amikacin: 500 mg diluted in 60 mL lactated Ringer's solution
  - Gentamicin: 1 g in 60 mL sterile water
  - Cefotaxime (Claforan): 2-g vial diluted in sterile water to 20 mL
- Place a tourniquet above and/or below the area to be perfused. A wide rubber tourniquet or a pneumatic tourniquet are preferred.
- Place a 23- to 27-gauge butterfly catheter into a vein or artery below or between the tourniquet(s).
- Once the catheter is in place, slowly inject the antimicrobial, being careful to remain in the vessel.
- Remove the catheter, and leave the tourniquets in place for 20 to 30 minutes.
  - Some horses are greatly bothered by the placement of the tourniquet. Regional analgesia before tourniquet placement alleviates this discomfort.

MS

Box 21-2	How to Make Antibiotic-Impregnated Polymethyl Methacrylate Implants

- Supplies: polymethyl methacrylate; a sterile plastic bowl and mixer; and if desired, sterile monofilament nonabsorbable suture material or stainless steel wire.
- Antibiotics in powder form are used in a ratio of 1:5 to 1:20 antibiotic to polymethyl methacrylate; liquids can also be used. Most antibiotics other than tetracyclines are acceptable.
- Prepare an aseptic work area, and use aseptic technique during preparation. Alternatively, the antibiotic-impregnated cement can be autoclaved when finished. Ideally, the implants should be made under a vacuum hood to evacuate the fumes. If unavailable, mixing should take place in a well-ventilated area.
- Open the package and place the powdered bone cement in the bowl. Place the selected antibiotic in the powder and add the liquid.
- Fashion into desired shape. Beads of 5- to 7-mm diameter are usually made, but oblong shapes may work better for placement in bone cavities. The beads may be attached to a suture strand for retrieval after placement.
- Allow to cure. Unused implants may be autoclaved.

- Support of the contralateral limb; in foals, lateral hoof extensions can help minimize the occurrence of varus deformity.
- Gastroprotective therapy: omeprazole (See p. 182 on gastric ulcers)
- Sterile bandage over the affected joint if arthrotomies are performed

Prognosis

- Always guarded
- Decreased prognosis if any of the following:
  - Systemic illness
  - Multiple joint involvement
  - Presence of osteomyelitis, particularly if it involves a weight-bearing surface
  - *Salmonella* positive
- Overall, 75% of patients are discharged from the hospital.
- Between 50% and 60% can go on to have an athletic career

Fractures

- ***Practice Tip:*** *Foals with fractures or luxations have an acute onset of severe lameness.*
- There may be associated crepitus, swelling, pain, and instability.
- Fractures of the pelvis or involving the proximal humerus can result in exsanguination accompanied by signs of hypovolemic shock.

⊙> WHAT TO DO

Fractures

- Obtain radiographs immediately. If the foal requires sedation, *do not* use heavy doses because ataxia may result.

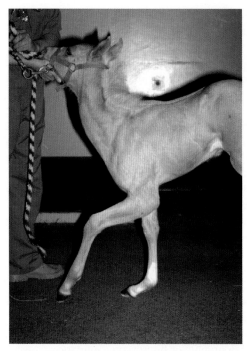

Figure 21-23 Foal with an olecranon fracture of 2 weeks' duration. The affected leg has contracture of the tendons. In addition, the contralateral limb is starting to break down, as manifested by the fetlock hyperextension.

- If the leg is clinically unstable, it may be better to apply external coaptation before obtaining a radiograph.
- If radiographic equipment is *not* immediately available or if the injury requires more sophisticated equipment, immobilization of the limb with external coaptation *must* be performed before moving the foal.
- If there is an open wound at the fracture site, parenteral antimicrobials should be administered.
- The principles of emergency treatment of orthopedic injuries parallel those for adults.
  - Sedate and tranquilize the patient.
  - Examine the injury.
  - Apply protective splints or bandages.
  - Consider the advisability of and options for further treatments.
- Fractures in foals respond to treatment better than those in adults and heal more rapidly.
- Internal fixation is more successful because of lower body weight. In general, a poorer prognosis is seen in foals >300 lb (135 kg).
- With open fractures or open wounds, foals may be prone to septicemia because of greater blood supply and immaturity of the immune system.
- Biaxial sesamoid fractures can occur in young foals, particularly if they have been stall confined and are turned out with their overly excited dam. These fractures with suspensory apparatus disruption are best managed conservatively with bandages and splints rather than surgical treatment.
- After fracture repair, foals can develop angular limb deformities (varus) of the contralateral leg if they are *not* fully weight bearing on the affected leg; this is in contrast to adults that develop support limb laminitis. Applying a lateral hoof extension can help support the limb and minimize the deformity.
- Foals that are *not* fully weight bearing in a front leg may also develop flexor contracture (Fig. 21-23). Application of a caudal splint may help prevent this complication.

WHAT NOT TO DO

Fractures

- Delay obtaining a diagnosis. **Important:** Eburnation of the bone ends may make fracture repair more difficult; increased soft tissue injury may compromise the blood supply to the fracture; and continued motion may result in comminution of the fracture.
- In the case of an olecranon fracture, delay may result in irreversible limb contracture if an appropriate splint is *not* applied.

Splints and Casts

- A splint for a foal can be constructed from a half-shell 2- to 3-inch-diameter PVC pipe applied over sufficient cotton wrapping. Alternatively, one can be made from fiberglass casting tape folded lengthwise.
- Remove and reset the splint q12h daily to avoid pressure sores.
- If a cast is used for angular limb deformities, it should allow continued weight bearing by leaving the foot free (tube or sleeve cast).
- Full-leg casts can result in osteopenia and severe flexor laxity.
- When rigid immobilization is *not* needed, use semirigid support.

Physeal Fractures

- The likelihood of physeal fracture depends on the individual closure time of each physis (see the accompanying website, www.equine-emergencies.com, Web Appendix 2).
- The radiographic appearance of the growth plate does *not* directly reflect the ability of the chondrocytes to proliferate.
- Injury to the growth plate can result in limb shortening and/or angular limb deformities.
- The physis is *weaker* than mature bone, joint capsule, ligaments, or tendons. Physeal fractures center on the germinal cells of the growth plate, resulting in failure of these cells to proliferate.
- Physeal fractures are the most common fracture type in foals.
- Physeal fractures can result in disturbed growth patterns or disruption of adjoining articular surfaces resulting in shortened limbs, angular limb deformities, or arthritis.
- The Salter-Harris classification is used to describe physeal fractures (Fig. 21-24).
- The prognosis worsens as the classification number increases, and other factors may help formulate a prognosis:
  - Severity of the trauma
  - Blood supply
  - Location of the physis
  - Foal's age
  - Time between injury and initiation of treatment
- ***Practice Tip:*** *Fracture types I and II are common in the distal metatarsal and metacarpal growth plate. These can be managed with external coaptation with or without internal fixation depending on the degree of displacement. The prognosis is good for future soundness.*
- Femoral capital physeal fractures are more successfully managed with internal fixation.
- Proximal femoral physeal fractures have a better prognosis than distal femoral physeal fractures because of the difficulty in reduction and plate contouring of the distal femoral physis.
- Younger foals have a better prognosis for soundness than older foals.
- Physeal fractures heal more rapidly than diaphyseal fractures.

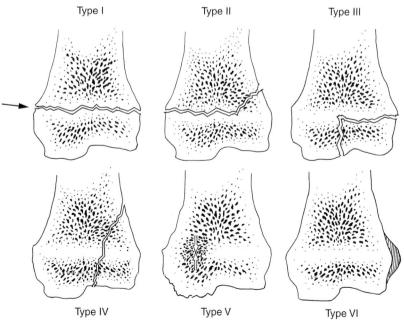

Figure 21-24 Salter-Harris fracture classification. *Arrow* at the point of the growth plate. (Adapted from Salter RB, Harris WR: Injuries involving the epiphyseal plate. In Stashak TS, editor: *Adam's lameness in horses,* Philadelphia, 1987, Lea & Febiger.)

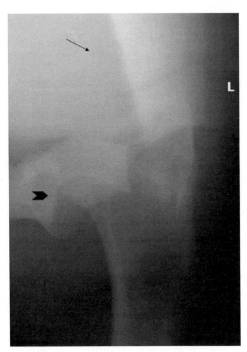

Figure 21-25   Radiograph of coxofemoral luxation in a foal. Note the position of the femoral head *(arrow)* cranial to the acetabulum *(arrowhead)*.

- Complications include the following:
  - Infection
  - Tendon contracture
  - Cast sores
  - Angular limb deformities
  - Tendon laxity
  - Angular limb deformity of the contralateral limb
  - Premature growth plate closure

Luxations

Patella

- Lateral luxation of the patella can be a congenital problem in foals.
- Luxation can be unilateral or bilateral. If luxation is bilateral, the foal is unable to stand.
- Luxation is more common in miniature horses and ponies.
- The diagnosis is made by palpation and radiography.
- Radiographs are important to determine whether there is hypoplasia of the lateral trochlear ridge or severe osteochondrosis with fragmentation of the lateral trochlear ridge.
- Successful treatment has been reported with recession sulcoplasty or lateral patellar release combined with medial imbrication.

Coxofemoral Joint

- Coxofemoral joint luxation in foals can result from a traumatic injury (Fig. 21-25).
- Coxofemoral joint luxation has been reported in foals after application of a full-limb cast.
- Coxofemoral joint luxation is also reported in one pony following upward fixation of the patella.

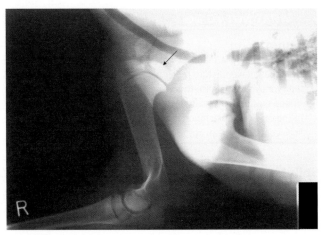

Figure 21-26   Radiograph of the right shoulder joint of a foal with scapulohumeral joint luxation *(arrow)*. Closed reduction and bandaging resolved the problem.

- Surgical repair can be attempted and is more likely to be successful in small breeds.
- Alternatively, femoral head excision can be performed in small breeds of horses (miniature horses and ponies).

Scapulohumeral Joint

- Scapulohumeral joint luxation can occur in foals that have considerable ligament laxity because of prematurity (Fig. 21-26).
- Reduction and external coaptation can be successful.
- Scapulohumeral joint arthrodesis has been reported in miniature horses and ponies.

Pastern Joint

- Bilateral subluxation of the proximal interphalangeal joints of the forelimbs has been reported in a foal following overexertion that resulted in rupture of the palmar supporting structures of the joint. Severe laxity of the flexor tendons is believed to be a predisposing factor.
- Foals with tendon laxity should be exercised gradually and with caution.

Tarsometatarsal Joint

- Traumatic tarsometatarsal joint luxation has been reported in foals.
- Closed reduction and cast immobilization is the most commonly used treatment.
- Alternatively, lag screws and pinning have been described.
- In one miniature foal, successful repair was obtained using closed reduction, internal fixation with Steinmann pins, and external coaptation.

Flexural Deformities

- Flexural deformities are conditions resulting in abnormal flexion or extension of the limbs.
  - Flexural deformities are divided into tendon laxity and contracture and can present from the time of birth in the case of laxity to 1 year old in the case of contracted tendon.

- These problems are frequently encountered in growing foals.

Tendon Laxity

- Tendon laxity is more common in premature foals. The most commonly affected joints are the fetlock and the carpus.
- Limb laxity can also develop when bandaging and splinting are used in a foal for the management of other orthopedic problems.

Fetlock Laxity

- Fetlock laxity is the most common flexural deformity in foals.
- Laxity is characterized by increased fetlock joint extension.
- Laxity may affect the forelimbs, the hind limbs, or all four limbs.
- In most cases, this problem is self-limiting and resolves as the foal gains strength.
- Exercise should be limited during this time, for excessive exercise may lead to sesamoid fracture.
- In severe cases, where the fetlock nearly or does touch the ground, applying heel extensions helps normalize weight bearing and tendon loading (Fig. 21-27).
- Extensions can be made of wood, plastic, or metal and can extend caudally to the end of the weight-bearing fetlock. Extensions should *not* be wider than the foot and can be taped or glued on the foot. However, the fixation should *not* be so rigid as to result in hoof wall avulsion should the foal step on the heel extension.

Carpal and Tarsal Laxity

- Carpal or tarsal laxity is observed in premature foals or in those that have been bandaged and/or splinted (Fig. 21-28).
- Radiography should be performed to evaluate the degree of carpal bone ossification (Fig. 21-29). Strict stall confinement and even forced recumbency should be mandated in foals with delayed carpal or tarsal bone ossification (see p. 309).
- Mild laxity usually self-corrects.
- If laxity is severe, bandaging and splinting without incorporating the fetlock into the bandage may help align the legs and avoid cuboidal bone injury. These splints can be placed for part of the day and removed to avoid pressure sores.
- Splinting the tarsus is more difficult, and tube casts may be easier to apply appropriately.

Tendon Contracture

- In the neonatal foal, tendon contracture is a congenital problem that can vary from mild to failure to fully extend the limb (Fig. 21-30). Severe contracture can be a cause of dystocia.
- When the carpus cannot be manually extended beyond 90 degrees, the prognosis is poor.
- *Practice Tip: In the neonatal foal, carpal contracture is the most common and is usually mild.*
- Treatment includes bandaging and splinting the affected limb.
- Administration of oxytetracycline (30 to 60 mg/kg IV diluted in 500 mL 0.9% saline for 1 to 3 treatments every other day) can also be used. **Important:** Renal function should be monitored because this drug has the potential to induce acute renal failure, particularly in the dehydrated foal.
- As soon as the contracture is resolved, splinting should be discontinued to avoid the development of excessive laxity.

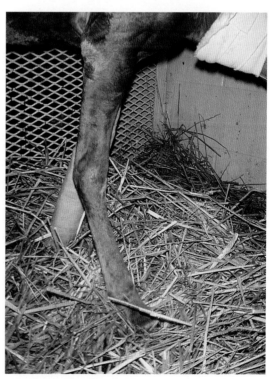

Figure 21-28   Premature foal with severe carpal laxity.

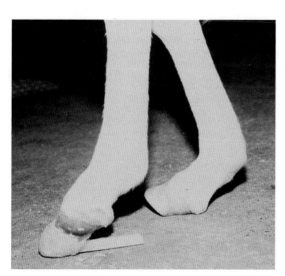

Figure 21-27   Foal with flexor tendon laxity showing improvement by applying a heel extension to one hoof.

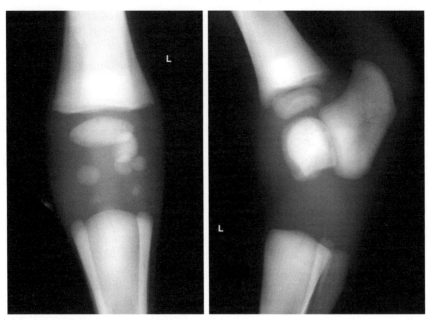

Figure 21-29   Radiographs of a foal with severe lack of ossification of the carpal *(left)* and tarsal *(right)* cuboidal bones.

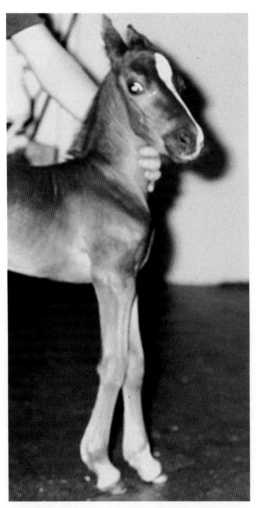

Figure 21-30   Mild carpal contracture in a foal.

Rupture of the Common Digital Extensor Tendon

- ***Practice Tip:*** *Foals with carpal contracture are at risk for the development of rupture of the common digital extensor tendon (CDET).* The rupture occurs on the lateral aspect of the carpus, within the synovial sheath, resulting in a fluctuant nonpainful swelling on the lateral aspect of the carpus (Fig. 21-31). This swelling should be differentiated from carpal joint effusion.
- Fetlock and pastern contracture can occur secondarily to rupture of the CDET.
- Affected foals knuckle over at the fetlock and can injure the skin on the dorsum of the fetlock.
- Application of a splint from the ground to the carpus helps prevent knuckling. Most foals learn to place their foot after a few days such that splinting can be discontinued.

Angular Limb Deformities

- Angular limb deformities are lateral or medial deviations of the limbs and described by naming the joint from which they arise and the direction of deviation of the limb distal to the joint:
  - Varus deformity describes medial deviation of the limb distal to the reference joint (Fig. 21-32).
  - Valgus deformity describes lateral deviation of the limb distal to the reference joint (Fig. 21-33).
- ***Note:*** It is important to recognize that rotational deformities, particularly of the metacarpus and metatarsus, can also occur.
- These problems are frequently encountered in growing foals.
- The three major types of angular limb deformities are the following:
  - Periarticular laxity
  - Incomplete ossification of the cuboidal bones

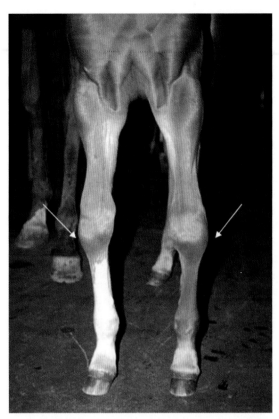

Figure 21-31 Bilateral rupture of the common digital extensor tendon in a foal *(arrows)*.

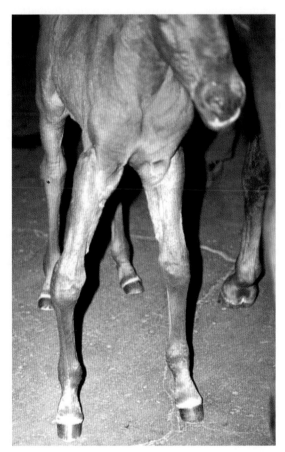

Figure 21-32 Carpal varus deformity of the right forelimb in a foal.

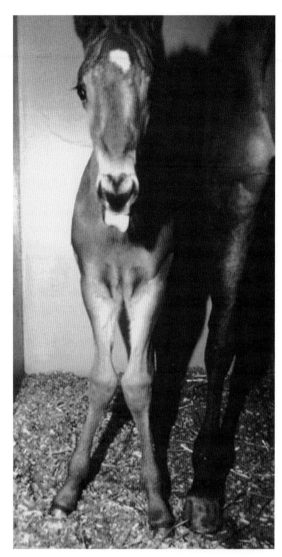

Figure 21-33 Bilateral carpal valgus deformity in a foal.

- Disproportionate growth of the epiphysis and metaphysis

Periarticular Laxity
- Valgus deformity is the most common laxity.
- Angular deformities resulting from periarticular laxity are most common in premature or dysmature foals.
- Radiographs are important to differentiate from incomplete cuboidal bone ossification.
- If there is complete ossification, moderate exercise can result in correction of the problem.

Incomplete Ossification of the Cuboidal Bones
- Incomplete ossification is most common in the premature or dysmature foal.
- Radiographs are essential for a diagnosis (see Fig. 21-29).
- Incomplete ossification most commonly involves the bones of the distal tarsus.
- Once identified, strict stall confinement and "forced" recumbency is critical to avoid permanent deformity.

MS

- In severe cases, external coaptation may be required but should be limited as much as possible because the laxity worsens.

Disproportionate Growth of the Epiphysis or Metaphysis

- Disproportionate growth can be differentiated based on radiographic evaluation.
- Disproportionate growth usually results in carpal or tarsal valgus, with delayed growth of the lateral growth plate.
- The treatment is a conservative approach for deformities that are less than 10 degrees.
- In moderate cases, growth acceleration can be achieved by periosteal release (stripping) on the side growing disproportionately slower; in severe cases growth retardation can be achieved by implant(s) (screw(s)/wire) on the side where growth retardation is needed.
- *Practice Tip: It is important to know the relative growth plate closure to allow early intervention. For example, active growth of the distal metacarpal physis occurs during the first 3 months of life. If growth "manipulation" of the physis is to be done, treatment should occur by 1 month of age. Active growth of the distal radial and tibial growth plates occurs up to 9 months of age. Therefore, growth "manipulation" should occur by 4 to 6 months of age depending on the severity of the deformity.*

Crooked Legs in a Foal
Presentation
- Owners may seek advice on a foal that has a "crooked leg."
- When faced with such an event, the veterinarian needs to determine whether the problem is the result of tendinous or ligamentous laxity or contracture or whether there is an angular limb deformity.
- In addition, a physical examination is important to determine whether the problem has resulted in systemic compromise of the foal because of the inability to nurse.

❱❱ WHAT TO DO

Flexural and Angular Limb Deformities
- Perform a complete physical examination to identify any systemic illness that may lead to weakness.
- A complete examination of the affected limbs should include radiographs if needed.
- It is particularly important to take radiographs for identification of incomplete ossification.
- Make a treatment plan that includes timely reevaluations.
- Use external coaptation carefully because foals are more prone to pressure sores and bandage-induced tendon laxity.
- Educate the client as to bandage care and daily removal.
- Use exercise carefully, and monitor the foal to avoid further injuries.

❱❱ WHAT NOT TO DO

Flexural and Angular Limb Deformities
- Forgo radiographic evaluations.
- Leave bandages on for prolonged periods without daily assessments.

Musculoskeletal Trauma
- Foals are susceptible to trauma, particularly during handling.
- *Caution* and adequate restraint should be used when working with foals, especially if they have *not* been handled routinely.

Rupture of the Gastrocnemius Tendon
- Rupture of the gastrocnemius is uncommon, and is reported in foals <3 weeks old in association with general weakness and struggling to rise. Rupture also occurs in adults as a result of injury.
- Rupture results from hyperflexion of the hock, with the hock flexed under the body during a fall.
- Rupture can also occur during recovery from anesthesia or following pressure necrosis after improper cast or bandage application.
- *Practice Tip: In foals, the rupture is usually at the musculotendinous junction, whereas in adults, avulsion of the origin is more common.*

Anatomic Review
- The gastrocnemius is the largest muscle of the caudal hind limb. Its theoretical action is to flex the stifle and extend the hock.
- Because of the anatomy of the peroneus tertius (fibularis tertius), the hock and stifle always flex or extend in unison, leaving the gastrocnemius with a primarily supportive role.
- The gastrocnemius is the most superficial muscle of its group and originates as two heads from the supracondylar tuberosities of the femur.
- The semitendinosus and semimembranosus muscles cover the gastrocnemius proximally.
- The two-headed unit forms a single strong tendon at the level of the midtibia, composing the major portion of the calcaneal tendon, and inserts on the point of the hock with the superficial digital flexor tendon winding around its medial surface.

Clinical Signs
- Hock flexion is possible without stifle flexion. Depending on the degree of injury, the hock is lower to the ground (Fig. 21-34). There may be lateral rotation of the calcaneus and medial deviation of the toe of the affected limb.
- Inability to weight bear occurs because the hock cannot be fixed.
- Swelling occurs on the caudal aspect of the thigh, behind the stifle.

Diagnosis
- Diagnosis is based on clinical appearance.
- Obtain an ultrasound of the caudal thigh.
- Use radiography to rule out avulsion fracture of the origin of the gastrocnemius. During healing, there may be calcification of the hematoma at the site of rupture.

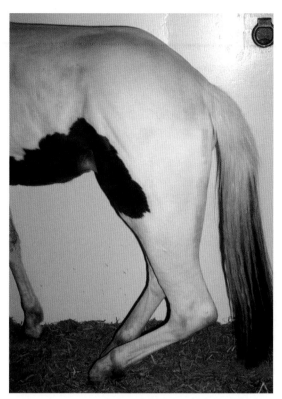

Figure 21-34 Young horse with incomplete rupture of the gastrocnemius muscle. Note that the hock is flexed while the stifle is in extension, and there is inability to bear weight because the hock and stifle cannot be fixed.

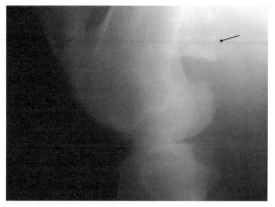

Figure 21-35 Healed gastrocnemius rupture at the origin. Note that there is a large calcification *(arrow)* at the site of previous rupture that resulted in a mechanical lameness.

Clinical Signs

- On endoscopy, pharyngeal collapse, pharyngeal spasm, pharyngeal edema, and displaced soft palate may be seen.
- Foals may present initially with upper airway signs and subsequently develop a HYPP episode. In most affected foals, intermittent laryngeal obstruction can be recognized from birth when the foal is restrained or excited.
- These episodes are characterized by muscle fasciculations, muscle twitching, myotonia, nictitans prolapse, and progress to recumbency.

Diagnosis

- The phenotype of the foal (heavy musculature) can lead to suspicion of genetic predisposition.
- Genetic testing is the most accurate way to confirm a diagnosis of HYPP and can be performed on hair or whole blood samples using an accredited laboratory. The American Quarter Horse Association can be contacted through their website at www.aqha.com (member services) to obtain a diagnostic kit.
- Alternatively, if the horse is *not* registered with AQHA, genetic testing can be performed at Veterinary Genetics Laboratory at the University of California, Davis, CA; 916-752-2211. Submit 5 to 10 mL of blood in an EDTA (purple top) tube (see p. 70).
- In the presence of an acute episode, a presumptive diagnosis can be made based on the phenotype and genetic history of the foal, combined with clinical signs.
- Measurement of serum or plasma potassium can help confirm the diagnosis; it is usually increased 5.0 to 11.7 mmol/L. However, the absence of hyperkalemia does *not* rule out a HYPP episode.
- In between episodes, electromyography can be performed. Complex repetitive discharges are the most consistent abnormal findings.
- In horses that die with signs consistent with HYPP, hair samples can be submitted for genetic testing. Increased aqueous potassium concentration can support a diagnosis of hyperkalemia, but the sample has to be collected soon after death.

◉⟩ WHAT TO DO

Rupture of the Gastrocnemius Tendon

- Mild gastrocnemius injuries in neonates can be managed with exercise restriction and forced recumbency. The foal should be assisted to stand and nurse and should be turned to avoid decubital injuries.
- More severe injuries can be managed with bandages and splinting. A modified Schroeder-Thomas splint is helpful to support the limb and should be removed when weight bearing is possible to avoid tendon contracture and soft tissue injuries. Alternatively, a splint can be applied on the caudal aspect of the limb extending from the ground to the tuber ischii.

Prognosis

- The prognosis is guarded for athletic function. In adults, fibrosis and calcification of the origin of the gastrocnemius may limit stifle movement (Fig. 21-35).

Myopathies

Hyperkalemic Periodic Paralysis

- Foals that are homozygous for the hyperkalemic periodic paralysis (HYPP) gene may present with signs of upper airway obstruction including inspiratory stridor.
- In homozygous individuals, onset of signs has been reported from birth to 3 years old.
- In homozygous foals, signs of upper airway dysfunction and myopathy are reported.

MS

- When obtaining a sample for potassium measurement, it is important to analyze the sample as soon as possible; potassium leakage from red blood cells falsely increases the potassium concentration (pseudohyperkalemia). If the sample CANNOT be immediately analyzed, it should be spun down and plasma or serum harvested and refrigerated or frozen for later analysis.

⊙ WHAT TO DO

Hyperkalemic Periodic Paralysis
- HYPP varies depending on the severity of signs.
- Severe progressive upper respiratory obstruction may occur with exercise. Therefore, in horses exhibiting signs of upper respiratory dysfunction, exercise should be stopped.
- Horses with mild signs, such as muscle fasciculations, may respond to the administration of glucose (corn syrup).
- In horses with more severe clinical signs, such as severe weakness or recumbency, treatment is aimed at lowering serum potassium or counteracting the effects of hyperkalemia:
  - Intravenous administration of 5% dextrose (4 to 6 mL/kg).
  - Although potentially beneficial, insulin administration should be done with *caution* to avoid hypoglycemia.
  - Intravenous administration of bicarbonate (1 to 2 mEq/kg).
  - Slow IV administration of 0.2 to 0.4 mL/kg 23% calcium gluconate diluted in 1 L of 0.9% saline.
  - Give only potassium-free fluids.
  - Administration of β-adrenergic agents by inhalation has *not* been evaluated in horses.
- Foals in severe respiratory distress may require a temporary tracheostomy.

Prevention/Prognosis
- Administer acetazolamide, 2 to 4 mg/kg PO q12h.
- Do not feed alfalfa hay products.
- Provide a salt supplement.
- Ensure a regular feeding and exercise schedule.
- Individuals that are homozygous may display more frequent episodes and therefore should be observed regularly, and performance should be limited.

Glycogen Branching Enzyme Disorder
- Glycogen branching enzyme disorder is a genetic, fatal glycogen storage disorder first identified in Quarter Horses and Paints.
- To date, heterozygote carriers have been found in 8.3% of Quarter Horses and 7.1% of Paints.
- It is reported that 1.3% to 3.8% of aborted fetuses of Quarter Horse lineage are homozygous for the mutant GBE1 allele.
- *No* homozygous mutant horses have lived more than 18 weeks.
- Clinical signs vary and include hypoglycemic seizures, progressive muscle weakness, respiratory failure, and sudden death.
- Most foals identified die or are euthanized by 8 weeks of age.
- Cases may also present as stillborn or aborted fetuses.

Diagnosis
- DNA analysis can allow determination of disease or carrier state.
- Hair sample analysis is preferred for determination of the carrier state. Information regarding sample submission and forms can be obtained from the Veterinary Genetics Laboratory at the University of California, Davis at www.vgl.ucdavis.edu (see p. 71).
- Liver or muscle samples can be submitted from foals at necropsy to the University of Minnesota Neuromuscular Diagnostic Laboratory. Information on sample submission and forms can be found at www.cvm.umn.edu/umec/lab/gbed/home.html.
- Muscle biopsies can also be submitted the Neuromuscular Diagnostic Laboratory from foals exhibiting signs of myopathy to differentiate from other types of muscle disease.

White Muscle Disease/Nutritional Myodegeneration
- The condition is more common in foals 2 to 6 months of age but may occur in newborn and older foals.
- The condition affects the myocardium, diaphragm, and respiratory muscles.

Clinical Signs
- In acute cases, the disease can result in rapid death from fatal arrhythmia, circulatory collapse, severe muscle swelling, limb edema, discolored urine and renal failure, and pulmonary edema.
- In less severe cases, weakness, inability to eat, lethargy, stiffness, and recumbency occur.
- Dysphagia is common.

Diagnosis
- Clinical signs
- Increased aspartate aminotransferase and creatine kinase
- Myoglobinuria: red or brown urine
- Decreased blood selenium, glutathione peroxidase (GSHPx), and vitamin E
- Response to vitamin E and selenium administration

⊙ WHAT TO DO

White Muscle Disease/Nutritional Myodegeneration
- Restrict activity.
- Give vitamin E and selenium supplementation by deep intramuscular injection.
- Provide daily oral vitamin E supplementation.
- Feed dysphagic foals by nasogastric tube.
- Fluid therapy to minimize renal damage is indicated if myoglobinuria is present.

Prevention
- Ensure adequate vitamin E and selenium intake in the brood mare.

Heat Stress

- Heat stress and heat stroke may occur in foals during hot summer months.
- Although heat stress may be primary, it usually results from an underlying disease process that has resulted in a fever during hot summer months.
- *Practice Tip: Heat stress can also be associated with administration of erythromycin or other macrolides.*
- Foals with wounds that result in subcutaneous emphysema may also be predisposed because the subcutaneous emphysema prevents appropriate heat dissipation.

Clinical Signs

- Patient has an elevated rectal temperature of >40° C (104° F).
- Severe rhabdomyolysis may be present with recumbency.
- Individual may have myoglobinuria.
- Because a fever may have precipitated the event, searching for an underlying problem is important.
- Seizures may be present in severe cases.

● WHAT TO DO

Heat Stress

- Move the foal to a shaded area; if possible move the individual to an air-conditioned environment.
- Cool the horse with water at room temperature, spraying the neck especially over the jugular veins and the extremities. The water should *not* be too cold because this causes surface vasoconstriction of the skin and prevents heat dissipation.
- Apply an alcohol bath.
- Start intravenously administered fluids to promote diuresis and prevent renal damage from pigmenturia.
- Monitor and treat electrolyte abnormalities related to muscle damage.

Other Injuries

Frostbite (also see Chapter 33, p. 576)

- *Practice Tip: At temperatures <10° C (50° F), wind speed increases the risk of cold-induced injuries. At a wind chill index of −25° C (−13° F), there is a risk of frostbite, and at a wind chill index of −45° C (−49° F), skin freezes in minutes.*
- Humidity increases the rate of skin cooling such that frostbite may occur with prolonged immersion in cold water at nonfreezing temperatures.
- The severity of frostbite injury correlates more with duration of exposure than temperature of exposure.
- Frostbite injury usually results in a prolonged reduction in tolerance to cold in the injured anatomic structure.
- *Practice Tip: Foals are at increased risk for frostbite because they have a higher ratio of body surface area to mass, leading to increased heat loss. In addition, hypoglycemia may decrease shivering and lead to weakness and recumbency.*
- *Important: At initial examination, frostbite injuries appear similar, and classification of frostbite is applied after rewarming. Even then, there is poor correlation between classification and long-term injury; therefore, prognosis should be reserved until after 3 to 4 weeks of the injury.*

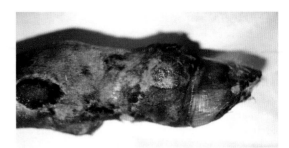

Figure 21-36 Distal limb of a foal with frostbite injury 3 days after the injury. The entire hoof sloughed 2 weeks after the injury.

- Although frostbite injuries can be classified into four categories; because of the low predictive value, the description of the frostbite injury is limited to "superficial" and "deep."
- In superficial injury, the rewarmed skin has clear blisters, whereas deep injuries have hemorrhagic blisters.
- Good prognostic indicators also include:
  - Retained skin sensation
  - Resilient pliable skin
  - Normal skin color
- Poor prognostic indicators include:
  - Firm, nonelastic skin
  - Dark blisters
- It is important to warn the owner that the extent of injury *cannot* be predicted, and it takes 3 to 4 weeks to be able to identify the extent of the damage (Fig. 21-36).

● WHAT TO DO

Frostbite

- Field care includes avoiding trauma and protecting the area with padding or bandages, particularly if there is loss of sensation, and avoidance of thawing if refreezing during transportation is a possibility. **Important:** Freeze/thaw cycles are more damaging to tissues than a single freeze cycle. **Practice Tip:** *Rubbing the skin should also be avoided because it causes mechanical trauma to the skin.*
- Once in a warm environment, rapid rewarming should be performed by immersion of the affected extremity in a water bath with a mild antiseptic at a temperature of 40° to 42° C (104° to 108° F) for 15 to 20 minutes.
- Supportive care, including fluid therapy, may be indicated if there is evidence of systemic illness.
- Tetanus prophylaxis should be instituted.
- Administration of aspirin and pentoxifylline may help reduce the risk of thrombosis in the affected parts.
- Local application of aloe vera may be beneficial as a thromboxane inhibitor.
- Broad-spectrum antimicrobials effective against aerobes and anaerobes should be administered as prophylaxis for gangrene.
- Wound debridement needs to be performed in the next 3 to 4 weeks, once the full extent of damage has occurred.
- It is important to warn the owner that the extent of the eventual tissue damage is *not* known until weeks after the injury has occurred.

Digital Arterial Thrombosis

- Thrombosis of peripheral arteries has been described in association with sepsis in foals.
- *Practice Tip: Foals at risk are those with sepsis accompanied by severe circulatory compromise (i.e., septic shock).*
- The diagnosis is made by identification of one or more cold digits. Eventually these digits slough, but this can take 7 to 10 days. This is *not* a painful condition, so foals continue to use the limb. Prevention of trauma to the area is important.
- The prognosis for survival in these foals is grave because loss of the hoof capsule usually results. Once this occurs, the likelihood of revascularization and regrowth of a new hoof is poor.
- Whether the preemptive use of anticoagulant therapy prevents this problem in septic foals is unknown.

Aortoiliac Thrombosis

- Aortoiliac thrombosis has been described in foals in association with diarrhea and sepsis.
- In foals with aortoiliac thrombosis, the limb is cold to the touch and lacks a palpable pulse. In addition, there is flaccid paralysis of the limb.
- Doppler ultrasound and nuclear angiography can be used to confirm the diagnosis.
- Reports of successful thrombolytic therapy are lacking at this time.

ADULT ORTHOPEDIC EMERGENCIES*

José García-López

Orthopedic and musculoskeletal emergencies in the adult equine include the following:

- Fractures
- Luxation of joints
- Luxation of the superficial digital flexor tendon
- Lacerations in general
- Lacerations of supporting structures
- Lacerations of vascular and nerve structures
- Lacerations/punctures involving synovial structures
- Lacerations/punctures to the hoof
- Sole abscess
- Laminitis, see Chapter 43, p. 697

In order to achieve a successful outcome when treating an equine orthopedic emergency, it is imperative for the ambulatory clinician to be able to identify the nature of the injury and recognize whether the problem can be self-managed or if referral to a hospital is necessary. For the latter cases, providing adequate first-aid care and initial management of these injuries often significantly affects the ability of future therapeutic/repair efforts. Because of the horse's inherent "fight or flight" response to trauma and pain, the horse frequently makes multiple or continuous attempts to use the injured limb, causing secondary soft tissue injury that potentially complicates repair efforts, and therefore the prognosis.

First Aid and Emergency Steps

●) WHAT TO DO

Emergency First Steps

- Make sure the patient is in the safest location possible. This may involve removing items and relocating other animals near the equine patient, rather than moving the injured patient.
- Perform a cursory examination to determine the physical status and general condition of the patient.
- Calm the patient using sedation, tranquilizers, and pain relief medications, being extremely careful not to make the patient too ataxic and using caution in horses with signs of sytemic shock. Use of a nose, shoulder, or eye twitch should also be considered to minimize the chance of "oversedation."
- Perform a brief initial examination of the injury to determine whether treatment options are feasible and whether additional diagnostic modalities are needed to better determine the prognosis for treatment.
- Clip, scrub, and debride any wounds as needed. In cases of open fractures or closed fractures that might become open, applying an antiseptic solution (e.g., chlorhexidine or Betadine-soaked gauzes) and/or antibiotic ointments (e.g., triple antibiotic[8]) to the area can be beneficial.
- If the horse is dehydrated or "shocky," administer intravenous fluids to correct deficits.
- Bandage and immobilize the injured limb using splints or a cast as applicable to the injury. Consider administering appropriate intravenous broad-spectrum antimicrobials before transporting to a referral center.
- Transport the equine patient to an equine hospital or referral facility; contact the referring veterinarian before shipping.
- When dealing with horses with forelimb fractures, consider transporting them facing backward to reduce the amount of stress in the forelimbs during vehicle braking.

Tranquilization, Sedation, and Pain Relief

●) WHAT TO DO

Medications

- Several sedatives and tranquilizers are available.
- Opioid medications may be combined with other drugs to provide added pain relief. An opioid agonist (morphine) and agonist-antagonist (butorphanol) are available.
- See Table 21-3.

---

*The author acknowledges and thanks Tamara M. Swor and Jeffrey P. Watkins, contributing authors in the third edition of *Equine Emergencies.*

[8]Triple Antibiotic Ointment (Perrigo, Allegan, Michigan; www.perrigo.com).

Table 21-3 Drugs and Dosages for Equine Musculoskeletal Emergencies

Drug	Dosage	Effects
Sedation		
Xylazine hydrochloride (Rompun)[1]	0.2-1.1 mg/kg IV	Sedation/analgesia for 20-30 min
Butorphanol tartrate (Torbugesic)[2]	0.02-0.04 mg/kg IV	Analgesia
Acepromazine maleate[3]	0.02-0.03 mg/kg IV	Sedation; vasodilation
Detomidine hydrochloride (Dormosedan)[4]	0.01-0.02 mg/kg IV	Sedation/analgesia for 50-60 min
Romifidine (Sedivet)[5]	40-100 µg/kg IV	Sedation with less ataxia

One can combine these drugs to achieve longer and more effective results.
Common combinations include the following:
Xylazine + butorphanol
Xylazine + acepromazine
Detomidine + butorphanol

Pain Management		
Phenylbutazone[6]	2.2-4.4 mg/kg IV	Analgesia
Flunixin meglumine (Banamine)[7]	1.1 mg/kg IV	Analgesia
Ketoprofen (Ketofen)[8]	2.2 mg/kg IV	Analgesia
Epidural morphine *plus*	0.2 mg/kg	Epidural catheter needed; analgesia
Xylazine hydrochloride (Rompun) OR	0.17 mg/kg	
Detomidine hydrochloride (Dormosedan)	0.03 mg/kg	
Fentanyl transdermal patches (Duragesic)[9]	2-3/100 µg/h per 500 kg	Replace every 2-3 days; need good skin contact (inner front leg, withers)

Continuous Rate Infusions		
Butorphanol	13 µg/kg per hour IV	Analgesia
Lidocaine	1.3 mg/kg IV loading dose 0.05 mg/kg IV maintenance	Analgesia
Ketamine	0.4-0.8 mg/kg per hour IV	Analgesia

Concentrations:
[1]Rompun, 100 mg/mL (Miles, Inc., Shawnee Mission, Kansas).
[2]Torbugesic, 10 mg/mL (Fort Dodge Animal Health, Fort Dodge, Iowa).
[3]Acepromazine maleate, 10 mg/mL (Vedco, St. Joseph, Missouri).
[4]Dormosedan, 10 mg/mL (Pfizer Animal Health, Exton, Pennsylvania).
[5]Sedivet, 10 mg/mL (Boehringer Ingelheim Vetmedica, Inc., St. Joseph, Missouri).
[6]RXV, 200 mg/mL (RX Veterinary Products, Westlake, Texas).
[7]Banamine, 50 mg/mL (Schering Plough Animal Health, Union, New Jersey).
[8]Ketofen, 100 mg/mL (Fort Dodge Animal Health).
[9]Duragesic, 100 µg/patch (Janssen Pharmaceutical Products L.P., Titusville, New Jersey).

Common Orthopedic Emergencies

●> WHAT TO DO

Common Orthopedic Emergencies
- Calm, sedate, and/or restrain the patient sufficiently to examine the injury and determine appropriate treatment options.
- Perform a cursory examination in order to stabilize the patient systemically and to determine the general category of injury.
- Decide whether the patient is able to bear weight on the injured limb, which may affect your decision for treatment.
  - If patient is non–weight bearing on the limb, consider the following possibilities:
    - Fracture
    - Luxation
    - Infection of a synovial structure
    - Penetrating foreign body, such as a nail, through the sole or frog
    - Sole abscess
  - If patient is weight bearing on the limb, consider the following possibilities:
    - Nondisplaced fracture
    - Laceration
    - Puncture wound

Long-Bone Fracture (General)
Presentation
The patient has an acute, severe, non–weight-bearing lameness of the affected limb. Moderate to severe soft tissue swelling is usually present. Equine fractures are often related to trauma from kicks or falls. Another common scenario is when the horse stumbles and a loud cracking sound is heard during athletic work (riding, longing). Fractures may be open or closed; fractures in areas of limited soft tissue coverage (e.g., metacarpal III) are commonly open. The patient often is extremely agitated and continues to place weight on the fractured limb. Laceration of major vessels and profuse bleeding are generally uncommon.

●> WHAT TO DO

Long Bone Fractures
- The patient should be immediately restrained and calmed.
  - Using a twitch can be helpful.
  - Sedatives and tranquilizers should be chosen carefully. Consider the systemic condition of the patient. The goal of sedation is to allow manipulation of the limb for stabilization and to prevent the horse from causing further injury to the limb.
  - Sedate cautiously and try not to cause unnecessary ataxia.
  - Butorphanol should be avoided with thoracic limb fractures because it causes the horse to lean forward and increases difficulty in standing.
  - If moderate doses of sedation are not adequate for intended purpose, do not give more, which could cause severe ataxia or recumbency. Instead, try a twitch or other physical restraint.
- External coaptation should be applied using appropriate splinting techniques. Specific splints are covered under specific fracture types.
- Obtain a complete history to determine cause and duration of fracture.

MS

- Determine tetanus toxoid immunization status and any other underlying health problems that may affect the patient's ability to resist infection or to impede fracture healing. A complete physical examination should be performed to determine the systemic physiologic stability of the equine patient.
- Administer intravenous fluids to correct for significant dehydration or in cases of hypovolemic shock before transporting. Intravenous fluid therapy also can be continued during shipping.
- Radiographs (two views as a minimum) should be obtained if appropriate. However, if not possible in a timely manner, the limb should be stabilized, the horse transported, and radiographs taken at the referral center. Radiographs may be essential to determine possible treatment options, appropriate splint lengths, and type of fracture.
- Fracture severity should be confirmed and treatment options determined. Categorize the fracture into type:
  - Distal limb fracture
  - Midlimb fracture
  - Upper limb fracture
  - Proximal limb fracture
- For open fractures and soft tissue wounds, perform the following:
  - If a wound is present, the fracture should be considered open.
  - Begin broad-spectrum systemic antimicrobials as soon as possible (Table 21-4).
  - Clean the wound carefully, use topical antimicrobials, and prevent further contamination of the wound with a bandage.
- Transportation:
  - Ideally, horses with thoracic limb fractures should be transported with the horse facing backward in the trailer.
  - Ideally, horses with pelvic limb fractures should be transported with the horse facing forward in the trailer.
  - The patient should be confined so that it cannot turn around and is tied loosely to allow the head to be used for balance.

- The patient should also be confined in the trailer so that the horse may lean on dividers for balance and support.
- The goals of emergency treatment are the following:
  - Minimize further soft tissue trauma
  - Decrease damage to ends of fractured bones and potentially eburnation of the fracture ends or comminution
  - Stabilizing the limb generally decreases patient anxiety
  - Prevent the fracture from becoming open
  - Prevent further stretching of blood vessels and nerves in the damaged limb
- Treatment options depend on fracture configuration and type and may include the following:
  - Internal fixation with compression plates and screws
  - Interlocking nails
  - Wires and pins
  - Transfixation pin casts, used alone or in combination with internal fixation
  - Cast treatment alone often does not provide sufficient stability for the fracture to heal primarily.

⬤〉 WHAT NOT TO DO

Long Bone Factures
- The patient should not be transported without proper external coaptation on the affected limb.
- Do not forget to treat systemic problems after stabilization of the affected limb. The patient may need intravenous fluid therapy for hypovolemic shock or to replace fluid losses due to excessive sweating.

Specific Points of Discussion for Long Bone Fractures

Dealing with a fractured limb in a horse is often challenging and difficult. Owners need careful counseling regarding treatment options and the expense involved with fracture repair. *Note:* It may not be in the best interest of the equine patient or owner to transport a horse with a fracture that is unrepairable or if the owner has serious financial constraints. It is recommended to consult the nearest surgical facility as soon as possible for an assessment of the prognosis for the specific type of fracture. Common complications after stabilization include implant failure during recovery or during the postoperative period, contralateral limb laminitis, cast sores, infection of implants, incisional infection, nonunion, or delayed union.

Prognosis depends on fracture location, whether it is open or closed, the mind-set of the horse and the ability to handle long-term external coaptation and exercise restrictions, the intended use of the horse, age of the patient, soft tissue associated trauma, the presence of intact blood and nerve supply, and the surgical expertise available. *Generally, prognosis for a successful outcome decreases as age and weight increase.* See Table 21-5.

Third Phalanx Fractures

Presentation

The patient has an acute and severe lameness in the affected limb and often is non–weight bearing. This injury often occurs when the horse kicks an immovable object or during athletic use. Lameness can increase during the initial 24 hours

Table 21-4	Common Antimicrobials for Musculoskeletal/Orthopedic Emergencies	
Drug	**Dosage**	**Route/Frequency**
Amikacin sulfate	21 mg/kg	IM, IV q24h
Ampicillin sodium	10-50 mg/kg	IM, IV q8h
Cefazolin sodium	11-25 mg/kg	IM, IV q6h
Ceftiofur sodium	2.2-4.4 mg/kg	IM, IV q12-24h
Doxycycline hyclate	10 mg/kg	PO q12h
Enrofloxacin	5 mg/kg 7.5 mg/kg	IV q24h PO q24h
Gentamicin sulfate	4-6.6 mg/kg	IM, IV q24h
Metronidazole	10-25 mg/kg	PO q8-12h
Penicillin sodium	10,000-44,000 units/kg	IM, IV q6h
Penicillin potassium	10,000-44,000 units/kg	IM, IV q6h
Penicillin G procaine	22,000-44,000 units/kg	IM q12h
Trimethoprim/sulfadiazine	15-30 mg/kg	PO q12h

One can combine these drugs to achieve synergism.
Common combinations include the following:
Ampicillin sodium + gentamicin sulfate or amikacin sulfate
Cefazolin sodium + gentamicin sulfate or amikacin sulfate
Penicillin potassium + gentamicin sulfate or amikacin sulfate
Penicillin G procaine + gentamicin sulfate or amikacin sulfate

Table 21-5	**Treatment and Prognosis for Return to Former Use for Various Equine Fractures**		
Fracture Location	**Fracture Type**	**Treatment**	**Prognosis**
Distal phalanx	Articular	Medical or surgical	Guarded
	Nonarticular	Medical	Good to very good
Middle phalanx	Comminuted	Medical or surgical	Guarded
Proximal phalanx	Comminuted	Surgical	Guarded to poor
	Noncomminuted	Medical or surgical	Good
Proximal sesamoids			
Apical	Small/large fragments	Surgical	Good
Midbody	Displaced	Surgical	Guarded
Abaxial	Small fragments	Surgical	Fair to good
Basilar	Small fragments	Medical/surgical	Guarded to poor
Comminuted/biaxial	Several fragments	Medical/surgical	Poor
Sagittal	Complete	Medical/surgical	Poor
Metacarpal/tarsal III			
Condyle (lateral)	Nondisplaced	Surgical	Good
	Displaced	Surgical	Guarded
Condyle (medial)	Articular	Surgical	Good
Dorsal cortical	Nonarticular	Surgical	Good
Transverse	Displaced	Surgical	Poor
	Nondisplaced	Surgical	Good
Small metacarpals and metatarsals	Distal	Surgical	Good to excellent
	Proximal	Surgical	Good
Carpal bones	Chip	Surgical	Guarded to excellent
	Slab	Surgical	Guarded to poor
Tarsal bones			
Talus	Trochlear ridges	Surgical	Good
	Sagittal	Surgical	Good
	Comminuted	Surgical	Poor
Calcaneus	Small/large fragments	Medical or surgical	Guarded
	Calcaneal tuberosity	Surgical	Guarded
	Comminuted	Medical or surgical	Fair
Central and third tarsal fractures	Slab	Surgical	Good
Ulna	Open	Surgical	Fair
	Closed	Surgical	Good
Radius	Open	Surgical	Poor
	Closed (<400 lb)	Surgical	Fair to good
	Closed (>400 lb)	Surgical	Poor
Humerus	Stress	Medical	Excellent
	Complete	Medical	Poor
Scapula			
Supraglenoid tubercle	Displaced	Surgical	Fair
Neck/body	Complete	Surgical	Grave
Tibia	Physeal	Surgical	Good
	Diaphyseal	Surgical	Guarded to poor
Patella			
Sagittal	Displaced	Surgical	Fair to good
Comminuted	Displaced	Surgical	Fair to good
Femur	Physeal	Medical or surgical	Guarded to poor
	Diaphyseal	Surgical	Guarded to poor

MS

MS

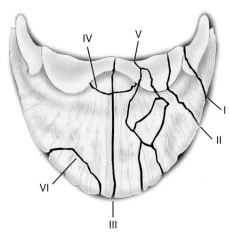

Figure 21-37 Classification of distal phalangeal fractures: I, Abaxial nonarticular fracture; II, abaxial articular fracture; III, axial and periaxial articular fracture; IV, extensor process fracture; V, multifragment articular fracture; VI, solar margin fracture.

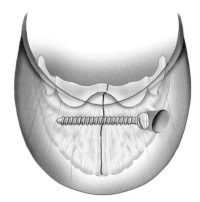

Figure 21-38 Illustration of a dorsoventral view of a type III fracture fixation using a cortical screw in lag fashion.

because swelling leads to increased pressure within the hoof capsule. Digital pulses are increased in the affected limb, and the entire hoof is often sensitive to hoof testers. Coffin joint effusion may be palpable if the fracture is articular. Forelimbs are affected in 80% of third phalangeal fractures.

Types of fractures are the following (Fig. 21-37):

I—Nonarticular; palmar or plantar process
II—Articular; palmar or plantar process
III—Articular; midsagittal
IV—Articular; extensor process
V—Articular; comminuted
VI—Nonarticular; solar margin

Other differential diagnoses to consider are:
- Sole abscess
- Puncture wound to the hoof
- Sole bruising
- Septic arthritis of the distal interphalangeal joint
- Septic navicular bursitis

◉〉 WHAT TO DO

Third Phalanx Fractures
- Take a complete history and perform a physical examination.
- Sedate and restrain the horse if needed (see Table 21-3).
- Examination with hoof testers may help localize the fracture. Clean and examine the sole of the hoof in order to rule out the presence of puncture wounds or sole bruises. These fractures are usually closed but can be associated with a puncture wound to the hoof.
- Radiographs should be taken if a fracture is suspected. Multiple views, including a 30-degree dorsopalmar, lateral, and both oblique views, allow for confirmation. If a fracture is not apparent but suspected, repeat radiographs in 7 to 14 days.
- Nuclear scintigraphy or advanced imaging modalities (computed tomography, magnetic resonance imaging) may aid in the diagnosis and characterization of the fracture.
- Local analgesia (unilateral or bilateral palmar digital nerve block, abaxial block) may be used to localize the lameness to the hoof (use caution: see "What Not to Do" below).

- Arthrocentesis of the distal interphalangeal joint with cytologic evaluation can be used to differentiate septic synovial infection from fracture if radiographs are not available or not diagnostic. ***Note:*** A fracture may cause the synovial fluid to be blood-tinged, requiring microscopic evaluation.
- Treatment depends on fracture type and age of the equine patient and may include the following:
  - Cast application
  - Bar shoes with 2 sets of side clips
  - Rim shoes
  - Surgical stabilization using a lag screw
  - Arthroscopy
  - Palmar/plantar digital neurectomy
- General treatment recommendations are as follows:
  - Type I, V, VI: conservative
  - Type II, III: conservative or surgical (lag screw fixation) (Fig. 21-38)
  - Type IV: surgical (arthroscopy with fragment removal; large fragments may require internal fixation [lag screw(s)])
- Regardless of treatment chosen, the patient should be confined to a stall for 3 to 6 months with restricted exercise (handwalking) for 4 to 12 months based on the type of fracture and severity of lameness.
- Conservative therapy consists of stall confinement and immobilization of the hoof using a foot cast or special shoe typically consisting of an egg bar shoe with 2 sets of side clips. Pain medications should be used as needed.
- In horses with articular fractures managed conservatively, treatment of the joint with hyaluronic acid may help reduce the degree of synovitis and subsequent development of osteoarthritis.
- If surgical referral is warranted, the horse should be transported as soon as possible for the best prognosis. The hoof wall acts as a splint, and additional external coaptation is not required before transporting.

◉〉 WHAT NOT TO DO

Third Phalanx Fractures
- Remember, do *not* use local analgesia/nerve blocks if a limb fracture is suspected and you are unable to localize the fracture to the hoof. Fractures involving the second and first phalanx may become displaced and result in additional injury if regional analgesia allows the horse to overuse the limb.

- Be careful interpreting/reading radiographs in the areas of normal bone irregularities, such as the crena (notch or cleft), vascular channels, palmar/plantar processes, or margins near the hoof wall. Fractures can be difficult to identify in these areas.
- If a fracture is not evident, do *not* forget to evaluate the synovial structures for possible infection.
- Do *not* fail to repeat radiographs at a later date if a fracture is suspected but *not* clearly identified initially.

Specific Points of Discussion for Third Phalanx Fractures

Fractures of the distal phalanx are uncommon and usually occur in equine athletes. Frequently the lameness improves in 3 to 4 weeks, and horses may be sound at the walk 4 to 8 weeks after injury. These fractures commonly heal with a fibrous union, and radiographs may always appear abnormal and show evidence of the fracture line. Some fractures may never heal completely. Persistent lameness may require a digital neurectomy for both pain relief and to allow the horse to return to use. Treatment depends largely on fracture type, and surgical treatment may greatly improve the comfort of the horse and shorten healing time. Osteoarthritis is a common sequela of articular third phalanx fractures and may be performance limiting. The horse may need bar shoes, side clips, and/or pads for the rest of their athletic career.

Distal Limb Fractures (Phalanges, Distal Metacarpus/Metatarsus)

Presentation

The patient usually has an acute, severe lameness in the affected limb. Soft tissue swelling may be present at the level of injury; and fractures may be open or closed. Typically, horses are non–weight bearing on the limb.

⦿⧽ WHAT TO DO

Distal Limb Fractures

- Patient restraint should be accomplished as previously discussed.
- Take a complete history, perform a physical examination, and treat any concurrent soft tissue wounds as previously described.
- External coaptation:
  - Pressure bandage/modified Robert Jones bandage
    - Bandage is used only for nondisplaced fractures that are stable (i.e., nondisplaced lateral condylar fracture).
    - Most fractures require more external coaptation than just a bandage.
    - The toe should be pointing toward the ground (equinus position) to align the dorsal cortices and assist in preventing further injury to the palmar/plantar vascular and nerve structures. The use of a roll of Elastikon tape placed under the heels is helpful in maintaining a proper hoof angle.
  - Splint:
    - Have an assistant hold and elevate the limb proximal to the carpus or tarsus.
    - Apply modified Robert Jones bandage (three to six layers) from the hoof to the carpus or tarsus (Box 21-3).
    - Apply a PVC (polyvinyl chloride) or wood splint to the dorsal surface of the thoracic limb (Fig. 21-39) or the plantar surface of a rear limb (Fig. 21-40).

> ### Box 21-3   Materials for a Robert Jones Bandage/Splint
> - 6 to 8 rolls of 1-lb roll cotton
> - 4 to 6 gauze bandages or elastic tape, 6-inch (15-cm)
> - 1 to 2 Ace bandages, 6-inch (15-cm)
> - 2 to 4 broom handles or wooden splints
> - Duct tape, 2-inch (5-cm)

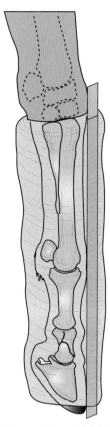

Figure 21-39 Splint-cast placement for a distal limb fracture of the thoracic limb. The splint is placed on the dorsal surface of the limb, over minimal padding, and secured with cast material.

- Apply a second splint at 90 degrees to the first splint if there is medial or lateral instability present.
- Secure the splint(s) with several areas of inelastic tape, placed 3 to 4 inches apart.
- Apply duct tape over the entire splint to minimize slippage.
- Cast:
  - A cast without a splint can be used; however, it is frequently difficult to maintain the limb in the ideal position without using a splint.
  - Apply a modified Robert Jones bandage (three to four layers) from the hoof to the carpus or tarsus.
  - Use four to six rolls of fiberglass casting tape, incorporating the hoof into the cast.
- Leg-Saver splint[9]
  - This splint is easy to apply.
  - It is a commercial aluminum brace with a dorsal bar that attaches to the limb with Velcro straps and aligns the dorsal cortices.

[9]Leg-Saver splint (Kimzey, Inc., Woodland, California; www.kimzeymetalproducts.com).

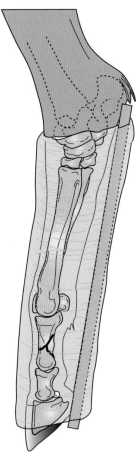

Figure 21-40   Splint-cast placement for a distal limb fracture of the pelvic limb. The splint is placed on the plantar aspect of the limb.

- Radiographs are recommended following splint application to assess fracture alignment.
- All horses with fractures should have anti-inflammatories, tetanus toxoid, and pain medications administered before shipping. Horses with open fractures or with compromised areas of skin should have broad-spectrum antimicrobials administered.

● WHAT NOT TO DO

Distal Limb Fractures
- Transporting a horse with a distal limb fracture without external coaptation decreases the chances of a successful repair.
- Closed fractures should *not* be allowed to become open.

Specific Points of Discussion for Distal Limb Fractures
Distal limb fractures often have the best prognosis for repair if appropriate first-aid treatment and stabilization of the limb are properly instituted. An initial cast, splint, or well-applied pressure bandage, placed immediately to protect the limb from further soft tissue damage, is imperative. Internal fixation may return some horses to athletic use. See Table 21-5 for specific fracture prognosis.

Midlimb Fractures: Midmetacarpus to Distal Radius; Midmetatarsus to Proximal Metatarsus

Presentation
The patient usually has an acute, severe lameness in the affected limb. Soft tissue swelling may be present at the level of injury. Fractures may be open or closed. Typically, horses are non–weight bearing on the limb.

● WHAT TO DO

Midlimb Fractures
- Patient restraint should be accomplished as discussed in the general long-bone fracture section (p. 315).
- Take a complete history, perform a physical examination, and treat any concurrent soft tissue wounds as previously described.
- External coaptation:
  - Place a modified Robert Jones bandage (see Box 21-3) on the limb.
    - A "true" Robert Jones bandage is 3 to 4 times the diameter of the limb when completed. This is often difficult without impeding the movement of the horse, so a modified version is preferred because it is smaller.
    - A pelvic limb modified Robert Jones bandage is less extensive than that on a thoracic limb.
  - Splint:
    - Thoracic limb:
      - Apply a PVC or wood splint to the caudal and lateral aspects of the limb.
      - The splint should extend from the elbow to the ground.
    - Pelvic limb:
      - Apply a PVC or wood splint to the plantar and lateral aspects of the limb.
      - The splint should extend from the top of the calcaneal tuber (calcaneus) to the ground.
    - The splints should be at right angles (90 degrees) to each other.
    - Secure splints to the bandage with inelastic tape.
- Radiographs may be obtained following splint application. If the patient is being transported to a surgical facility, it may be best to take radiographs at the referral facility.
- All fracture patients should have anti-inflammatories, tetanus toxoid, and pain medications administered before shipping. Horses with open fractures should also have broad-spectrum antimicrobials administered.

● WHAT NOT TO DO

Midlimb Fractures
- Transporting an orthopedic patient with a midlimb fracture without external coaptation significantly decreases the chance for a successful repair.
- Closed fractures should *not* be allowed to become open.

Specific Points of Discussion for Midlimb Fractures
Midlimb fractures are commonly open because of minimal soft tissue coverage in the area. The prognosis for successful internal fixation of these fractures is improved by rapid and correct first-aid treatment and stabilization of the limb. See Table 21-5 for specific fracture prognosis.

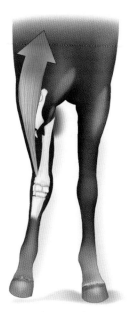

Figure 21-41 In the forelimb, all the muscles are arranged cranially, laterally, and caudally, resulting in a lateral deviation of the limb when the muscles contract, which can result in perforation of the skin at the medial aspect of the limb by sharp bone edges.

Upper Limb Fractures: Middle and Proximal Radius; Tibia and Tarsus

Presentation

The patient has an acute, severe, non–weight-bearing lameness. A horse with a fractured radius tends to abduct the limb because the majority of the musculature of the antebrachium is located on the lateral aspect (Fig. 21-41). ***Practice Tip:*** *The sharp fracture ends can easily penetrate the skin on the medial aspect of the limb. The same principle occurs in the pelvic limb with tibial fractures.* Stabilization of these types of fractures is difficult because the joints above the fracture cannot be adequately immobilized. Occasionally, small, incomplete radial fractures occur following a kick.

●▶ WHAT TO DO

Upper Limb Fractures

- Patient restraint should be accomplished as previously discussed (p. 315).
- Take a complete history, perform a physical examination, and treat any concurrent soft tissue wounds as previously described.
- External coaptation:
  - Place a modified Robert Jones bandage on the limb, extending from the foot proximally as high as possible.
  - Splint:
    ○ Thoracic limb (Fig. 21-42):
      - Place a PVC or wood splint from the foot to the height of the withers on the lateral side of the limb.
      - Place a second splint at a right angle (90 degrees) to the lateral splint on the cranial or caudal aspect of the limb.
    ○ Pelvic limb (Fig. 21-43):
      - Place a PVC or wood splint from the foot to the tuber coxae on the lateral side of the limb.
      - The position of the tarsus and stifle preclude placement of a second splint.
    ○ Secure splints to the bandage with inelastic tape.

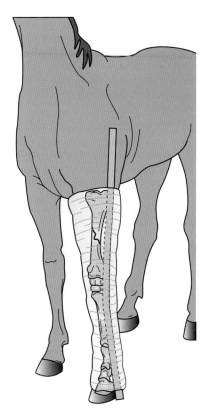

Figure 21-42 Robert Jones bandage with splint for an upper limb fracture of the thoracic limb. The extended splint helps reduce lower limb abduction.

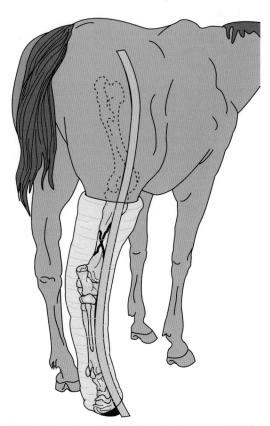

Figure 21-43 Robert Jones bandage plus splint for an upper limb fracture of the pelvic limb.

- Radiographs may be obtained following splint application. If the horse is being shipped to a surgical facility, it may be best to take radiographs at the referral facility.
- All equine fracture patients should have anti-inflammatories, tetanus toxoid, and pain medications administered before transportation. Horses with open fractures should also have broad-spectrum antimicrobials administered.
- Very small, incomplete nondisplaced radial fractures may be treated conservatively.
    - Extended stall rest and preventing the horse from lying down by keeping the equine patient cross-tied or with a pony on a rope, followed by sequential radiographs over several months can result in a successful outcome. There is always a chance that the fracture may progress and displace.

●› WHAT NOT TO DO

Upper Limb Fractures
- Transporting/Shipping a horse with an upper limb fracture without external coaptation can substantially decrease the chances of a successful repair.
- Closed fractures should *not* be allowed to become open.

Specific Points of Discussion for Upper Limb Fractures
In general, upper limb fractures in full-size horses (>500 lb or 227 kg) are difficult to repair. The prognosis for a successful outcome is guarded to poor because of complications and the significant mechanical forces placed by the horse on these bones. Similar repair of the same types of fractures in small horses or foals is possible. See Table 21-5 for specific fracture prognosis.

Fracture of the Olecranon

Presentation
The patient is non–weight-bearing lame on the affected limb in most cases but may be weight bearing and show only signs of severe lameness depending on the fracture configuration. Olecranon fractures are usually related to acute traumatic events, such as falling; a kick from another horse; and in young horses, during trailer loading or halter training, by flipping over backward. Fractures may be open or closed.

Commonly, horses display a classic "dropped elbow" presentation because they are unable to lock the carpus in extension because of loss of triceps muscle function. Extensive soft tissue swelling is often present in the region of the distal humerus and proximal radius.

Other differential diagnoses to consider include humeral fracture and radial nerve paralysis.
- Types of olecranon fractures (Fig. 21-44):
    - Type 1a
        - Fracture across the physeal plate
        - Nonarticular
        - Occurs in young horses
    - Type 1b
        - Fracture across the physeal plate and the proximal semilunar notch
        - Articular or nonarticular
        - Most often in younger horses
    - Type 2
        - Fracture that involves the semilunar notch
        - Articular
    - Type 3
        - Fracture across the proximal metaphysis
        - Nonarticular
    - Type 4
        - Comminuted fracture, involving the body of the olecranon
        - Articular
    - Type 5
        - Fracture of the ulna that breaks into the distal semilunar notch
        - Articular or nonarticular

●› WHAT TO DO

Fractures of the Olecranon
- Patient restraint should be accomplished as discussed previously (p. 315).
- Take a complete history, perform a physical examination, and treat any concurrent soft tissue wounds as previously described.
- External coaptation:
    - Apply a modified Robert Jones bandage from the foot to above the olecranon, going as high as possible (see Box 21-3).

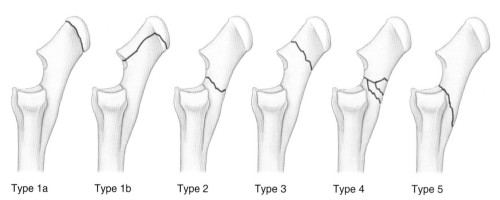

Type 1a   Type 1b   Type 2   Type 3   Type 4   Type 5

Figure 21-44   Classification of ulnar (olecranon) fractures.

- Apply a PVC or wood splint to the caudal aspect of the limb. This locks the carpus in extension, letting the horse bear weight on the limb and greatly decreasing the horse's anxiety and distress.
  - Secure the splint(s) with several areas of inelastic tape, placed approximately 3 to 4 inches apart.
  - Apply duct tape over the entire splint to minimize slippage.
  - Additional padding may be needed at the top of the splint.
  - A lateral splint should be applied also if there is any question of instability.
- Radiographs may be obtained following splint application.
- All horses with fractures should have anti-inflammatories, tetanus toxoid, and pain medications administered before shipping. Horses with open fractures should also have broad-spectrum antimicrobials administered.
- Most olecranon fractures require internal fixation to reestablish the triceps muscle function and for the best long-term prognosis.

WHAT NOT TO DO

Fractures of the Olecranon
- Transporting a horse with an olecranon fracture without external coaptation may decrease the chances of a successful repair.
- Closed fractures should *not* be allowed to become open.

Specific Points of Discussion for Fractures of the Olecranon
Prognosis for return to athletic function following an olecranon fracture depends on the fracture configuration and type. In general, horses do well following stabilization of this type of fracture. Young horses sustaining type 1b fractures and adult horses with type 5 fractures have a good prognosis for return to athletic use when treated with internal fixation. Complications include those discussed in the long-bone fracture section, as well as flexural deformities in the fractured limb and angular limb deformities in the contralateral limb of young horses, and osteoarthritis of the elbow joint. See Table 21-5 for specific fracture prognosis.

Proximal Limb Fracture (Above the Elbow Joint, Femur)
Presentation
The equine patient often has a severe, non–weight-bearing lameness. Occasionally, the triceps muscle is dysfunctional, resulting in a "dropped elbow" presentation much like that of an olecranon fracture. Severe soft tissue swelling is often present on the lateral aspect of the shoulder or the hip regions, making palpation of the area difficult. Crepitus and abnormal limb movement are often evident with limb manipulation. These fractures are seldom open because of the large muscle coverage.

WHAT TO DO

Proximal Limb Fractures
- Patient restraint should be managed as previously described (p. 315).
- Take a complete history, perform a physical examination, and treat any concurrent soft tissue wounds as previously described.

- External coaptation:
  - Humeral fractures should *not* be splinted, because the splint may act as a fulcrum at the level of the fracture and cause further damage.
  - Immobilization is not possible or helpful for proximal fractures.
- Radiographs are difficult to obtain in these areas. If the horse is being shipped to a surgical facility, it is more appropriate to take radiographs at the referral hospital.
- All fracture patients should have anti-inflammatories, tetanus toxoid, and pain medications administered before shipping. Horses with open fractures should also have broad-spectrum antimicrobials administered.
- Humeral and femur fractures are occasionally treated with conservative management (stall rest and anti-inflammatories) with guarded prognosis and a high incidence of complications.

WHAT NOT TO DO

Proximal Limb Fractures
- Cumbersome bandages make it more difficult for the horse to use the limb. Carpal extension bandaging is the only recommended form of external coaptation.
- The application of splints or casts should be avoided because these can cause additional injury.

Specific Points of Discussion for Proximal Limb Fractures
In general, proximal limb fractures in adult-size horses (>500 lb or 227 kg) are challenging or impossible to repair. The prognosis for a successful outcome is poor because of complications and the large biomechanical forces placed on these bones by the equine patient. Fracture repair of the same fracture in a smaller horse or foals is possible. See Table 21-5 for specific fracture prognosis.

Pelvic Fractures
Presentation
The patient presents acutely and severely unilaterally or bilaterally lame in the hind end, and frequently with a history of trauma. The pelvis may appear tipped, with one tuber sacrale higher than the other, or the tuber coxae appear uneven. The horse may be reluctant to walk forward or bear weight equally on the pelvic limbs. Occasionally, the equine patient can be in shock, with pale mucous membranes because of internal bleeding from a laceration of major blood vessels adjacent to the fractured ends.

WHAT TO DO

Pelvic Fractures
- Obtain a detailed history and perform a complete physical examination.
- Carefully palpate the tuber sacrale and tuber coxae.
  - Discrepancies in height if the horse is weight-bearing on both hind limbs generally support a diagnosis of pelvic fracture.
  - Displacement, heat, and pain on palpation of the tuber coxae support a "knocked down hip" or fracture of the tuber coxae.
    - These specific fractures are nonarticular and are treated conservatively with a good prognosis.

- Carefully perform a rectal examination.
  - A hematoma or unusual swelling may be palpated along the pelvic brim.
  - Crepitus on moving the pelvis may be appreciated.
  - Rocking the pelvis gently back and forth or walking the horse slowly forward during the rectal examination enhances abnormal bone movement.
- Radiographs (multiple views) are difficult to obtain in this region in the standing horse. General anesthesia is needed for a definitive diagnosis, although there are increased risks of fracture displacement during anesthesia recovery.
- Ultrasonographic examination both transcutaneously or per rectum aids in the diagnosis.
- ***Practice Tip:*** *Nuclear scintigraphy is currently the most common diagnostic modality, avoiding the risks of general anesthesia recovery.*
- Treatment:
  - Conservative:
    - Stall rest for 4 to 6 months
    - Anti-inflammatory medications
  - Surgical treatment is not possible in a full-sized adult horse; for foals it is possible but challenging.

WHAT NOT TO DO

Pelvic Fractures

- Do *not* forget to evaluate the systemic condition of the equine patient. Fluid therapy may be needed if hypovolemic shock is clinically suspected.
- If the patient shows signs of significant blood loss, *do not* transport until stabilized. Occasionally, large internal vessels may be lacerated by sharp fracture ends, resulting in rapid deterioration and death of the horse.

Specific Points of Discussion for Pelvic Fractures

Prognosis is generally good for survival of the patient if no blood vessels have been lacerated. Prognosis for return to athletic performance varies with the location of the fracture and degree of displacement. Fractures that involve the acetabulum have a poor prognosis for athletic use or soundness because osteoarthritis is generally a sequela. Fractures of the tuber coxae alone have a good prognosis for return to athletic function.

Nasofacial Fractures

Presentation

The patient usually has soft tissue swelling and evidence of trauma to the head and face, and epistaxis may be present. Direct trauma often causes fractures involving the paranasal sinuses and nasal passage. Fractures can also involve the nasal, frontal, maxillary, and lacrimal bones, leading to a facial deformity when viewed straight on or from the side. With severe, displaced fractures and significant soft tissue swelling, airway obstruction can occur, and the horse may have accompanying moderate to severe respiratory stridor.

WHAT TO DO

Nasofacial Fractures

- Obtain a complete history and perform a physical examination to assess the systemic stability of the patient. Look for other lacerations and soft tissue trauma. A neurological assessment should also be performed.
- Carefully palpate the head because the individual often is painful. Loss of bone continuity and subcutaneous emphysema (crepitus) are often part of the clinical findings.
- Nasofacial fractures should be considered open, even with intact skin, because of penetration of the paranasal sinuses and nasal mucosa by the fracture fragments.
- If respiratory compromise is severe, a temporary tracheostomy may be required to decrease the patient's anxiety.
- Radiographs of the head assist in determining extent and severity of fracture displacement.
- Endoscopic examination of the upper airway might be indicated, especially in cases of epistaxis in order to assess the guttural pouches and ethmoid region.
- Associated soft tissue lacerations should be routinely cleaned, debrided, and lavaged.
- Systemic antibiotics and anti-inflammatories (phenylbutazone or flunixin meglumine) are generally indicated.
- A tetanus toxoid booster should be administered if the patient has not received one in the past 6 months.
- Surgical reconstruction of the sinuses and nasal passages is preferred to help prevent chronic sinusitis, facial deformity, and bone sequestrum. Most surgeons use an open reduction technique for fracture repair because of expected better results.

WHAT NOT TO DO

Nasofacial Fractures

- Do not forget to examine the entire head for associated injuries and perform a neurological assessment.
- Severe facial deformity should receive surgical reconstruction to avoid sequelae and a compromised airway.
- If the patient has an increased respiratory effort or respiratory stridor, *do not* leave unattended or fail to refer such a patient; *do not* delay performing a tracheostomy, see Chapter 25, p. 456.

Specific Points of Discussion for Nasofacial Fractures

Facial fractures are common in the horse and most often involve the paranasal sinuses and nasal passages/cavity. The prognosis for full recovery is generally good; potential complications such as chronic sinusitis, bone sequestrum formation, and secondary nasal septal thickening, should be discussed with the owner. Permanent facial deformity may result if repair and stabilization of the fracture(s) are *not* performed. Repair of chronic fractures carries a guarded prognosis because of the difficulty in reestablishing the normal anatomy.

Incisive, Mandibular, and Maxillary Bone Fractures

Presentation

The equine patient often has soft tissue swelling at the fracture site. These fractures usually occur when the horse hangs onto an immovable object and pulls back or suffers trauma, such as a kick from another horse. Occasionally, these fractures are iatrogenic, associated with a tooth extraction, or pathologic, from chronic alveolar periostitis. ***Practice Tip:*** *Mandibular fractures are almost always open and communicate with the* *oral cavity and may be unilateral or bilateral. The interdental space is a common site for these fractures. Incisor bone fractures are commonly seen in young horses.* Food packs into the fracture line with an obvious odor originating from the mouth. Other clinical signs include tongue protrusion, inability to prehend food, excessive salivation (sialorrhea), dysphagia, malocclusion of the incisor teeth, crepitus, and pain on palpation.

●❯ WHAT TO DO

Incisive, Mandibular, and Maxillary Bone Fractures
- Obtain a complete history and perform a physical examination. Determine whether there is other associated head trauma.
- Administer a tetanus toxoid if the patient has not received one in the past 6 months.
- Carefully palpate the mandible and maxilla to determine whether more than one fracture is present. Determine whether the fracture is unilateral or bilateral. If there is a bilateral mandibular fracture, there is instability of the lower jaw.
- Obtain several radiographic views (minimum lateral and dorsoventral views) to assess the fracture and determine whether multiple fracture lines are present and whether tooth roots are involved. In cases of fractures involving the incisors, a dorsoventral projection with the cassette within the oral cavity is helpful to reduce superimposition.
- If feed material is packed in the fracture, lavage the fracture with water, saline, or other crystalloid solutions.
- Systemic antibiotics and anti-inflammatories (phenylbutazone or flunixin meglumine) are usually indicated.
- Unilateral, nondisplaced, or minimally displaced fractures can be managed conservatively because the other side of the jaw acts as an "external fixator." Conservative management consists of oral lavage several times per day, antibiotics, anti-inflammatories, and making forage readily available for the horse. The patient should *not* be allowed to rip and pull forage (i.e., hay nets and grazing should be avoided). At times, these fractures benefit from surgical stabilization consisting of intraoral wire fixation, with or without an intraoral acrylic splint, depending on fracture location and the degree of separation at the fracture site.
- Horizontal and vertical fractures are best treated conservatively because they are stabilized by soft tissues (masseter and pterygoid muscles).
- Comminuted, displaced, and bilateral fractures require surgical stabilization for the best functional and cosmetic outcome. Surgical techniques include intraoral wire fixation, orthopedic pins and wire, lag screw fixation, dynamic compression plating, intraoral acrylic splint, intramedullary pins, or external fixation device.

●❯ WHAT NOT TO DO

Incisive, Mandibular, and Maxillary Bone Fractures
- Do *not* use a speculum for oral examination because it may contribute to further displacement of the fracture.
- Do *not* let the patient graze or grab feed from a hay net or similar arrangement because this motion could cause fracture displacement.
- If tooth roots are involved, do *not* forget to reexamine the tooth/teeth several weeks later for viability.

Specific Points of Discussion for Incisive, Mandibular, and Maxillary Bone Fractures
Practice Tip: *The mandible is the most common skull bone fractured.* The prognosis is generally good to excellent for return to normal function. If the fracture involves tooth roots, the possibility of chronic dental infection requiring tooth removal several weeks to months later should be discussed with the owner. Chronic fractures and unstable fractures carry a poorer prognosis.

Temporomandibular Fractures

Presentation
The patient often has soft tissue swelling around the TMJ and is unable to open the mouth. Other clinical signs may include dysphagia, quidding, incisor malocclusion, and difficulty prehending food. Associated soft tissue lacerations and trauma are generally present with subcutaneous emphysema (crepitus). Chronic fractures often have masseter muscle atrophy and asymmetry.

●❯ WHAT TO DO

Temporomandibular Fractures
- Obtain a complete history and perform a thorough physical examination.
- Carefully palpate the temporomandibular area for signs of pain, heat, crepitus, and instability.
- Take multiple radiographic views to determine fracture configuration, comminution, and severity of displacement. Oblique views are the most useful.
- Ultrasonographic evaluation can also aid in the diagnosis.
- Most nondisplaced fractures are treated conservatively with anti-inflammatories (phenylbutazone or flunixin meglumine) and dietary modification.
- Surgical treatment is usually required if the fracture involves the joint; otherwise septic arthritis and osteoarthritis develop during fracture healing.
- Arthroscopic debridement and joint lavage may be needed if septic arthritis is diagnosed.
- Arthroscopic debridement may be needed if the articular disc (meniscus) is involved.
- A unilateral or bilateral mandibular condylectomy may be required for unstable fractures.

●❯ WHAT NOT TO DO

Temporomandibular Fractures
- Do *not* delay referring the patient to a surgical facility.

Specific Points of Discussion for Temporomandibular Fractures
Injury to the temporomandibular area is uncommon. The prognosis is guarded because of the high risk of secondary osteoarthritis developing as a sequela to fracture healing.

MS

Cranial Fractures

Presentation

Cranial injuries vary greatly in their presentation, from subtle neurologic changes to the comatose horse. Most cranial injuries are due to trauma. A young horse may fall over backward and strike the poll, or the horse may get kicked or run into a fixed object, injuring the frontal bones. Severe brain injury can occur in combination with fractures of the cranium or in the absence of a fracture because of the brain recoiling inside the cranial vault following impact—coup contusion or contrecoup contusion (see Chapter 22, p. 368). Clinical signs include bleeding from the nose and ears, ataxia, altered state of consciousness, neurologic deficits, stupor, disorientation, anisocoria, nystagmus, head tilt, bradycardia, and depressed respiratory system. A cranial fracture should be considered in any horse with acute neurologic deficits and concurrent bleeding from the ears, guttural pouches, or sinuses.

⏵ WHAT TO DO

Cranial Fractures

- Obtain a complete history and perform a physical examination to assess the systemic stability of the patient.
- Perform a complete neurologic examination.
- Standard radiographs, endoscopy, computed tomography, and magnetic resonance imaging are useful diagnostic imaging modalities to aid in the diagnosis.
- Initial therapy goals are to decrease cerebral edema and the intracranial pressure caused by edema and hemorrhage.
  - Nonsteroidal anti-inflammatory drugs
  - Steroids: 0.25 mg/kg aqueous dexamethasone IV
  - Dimethyl sulfoxide, 1 g/kg in a 10% to 20% solution in 0.9% saline IV
  - Hypertonic saline, 7.5%; 4 mL/kg IV
  - Broad-spectrum antimicrobials
- Establish an airway if necessary (temporary tracheostomy), and give the horse supplemental oxygen by insufflation if the patient is hypoxemic at a rate of 15 L/min.
- The rectus capitis ventralis muscle inserts on the basisphenoid and basioccipital bones (basilar bones), and avulsion fractures of the basilar bones often lead to fatal hemorrhage or bleeding into the guttural pouches that can be identified on endoscopy. Cranial nerves V, VII, VIII, IX, and X may also be affected, leading to neurologic signs that include dysphagia, decreased facial sensation, head tilt, leaning, or circling to the side of the lesion.
- Fractures of the dorsal or dorsolateral bones frequently show signs of depression, head pressing, impaired vision, decreased menace response, and may have epistaxis from the paranasal sinuses.
- Surgical treatment is attempted for closed, nondisplaced fractures with associated subdural hematomas or for open, displaced fractures requiring stabilization.
- If the fracture involves the petrous temporal bone, ceratohyoidectomy should be considered to reduce movement at the level of the fracture by the hyoid apparatus during food/water prehension and swallowing.
- Fracture classifications are as follows (Fig. 21-45):
  - Class I: bone disrupted without direct injury to brain parenchyma

- Class II: bone disrupted leading to laceration of the dura and resulting hemorrhage

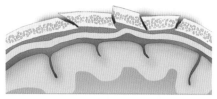

Class I

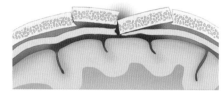

Class II

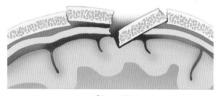

Class III

Figure 21-45 Cranial fracture classification.

- Class III: bone disrupted leading to penetration of the dura and laceration of brain parenchyma

⏵ WHAT NOT TO DO

Cranial Fractures

- Do *not* assume that inability to palpate a fracture means that there is not one present.
- Neurologic abnormalities may worsen after initial presentation. Do *not* delay discussing with the owner safety measures for the caretakers and the need for referral to a surgical facility.

Specific Points of Discussion for Cranial Fractures

The prognosis is guarded to poor, especially if surgical treatment is needed. Neurologic abnormalities may be permanent. The success of conservative treatment depends on the response to the initial treatment.

Orbital and Periorbital Fractures

Presentation

The patient has soft tissue swelling, pain, and heat around the head and eyes and often has associated lacerations. Crepitus may be present, and periorbital soft tissue structures may be distorted. A history of the patient running into a fixed object or a kick from another horse is common. These fractures are often depressed in the direction of the cranial vault, and the eye exhibits enophthalmos. Strabismus, chemosis, and subconjunctival hemorrhage may also be present. Retrobulbar bleeding and/or cellulitis can cause an exophthalmos.

● WHAT TO DO

Orbital and Periorbital Fractures

- Obtain a complete history and perform a physical examination to assess the patient systemically. Take care to identify any other lacerations or other areas of trauma.
- Carefully palpate the periorbital area. Determine whether the fracture is open or closed. Assess cranial nerve function.
- Radiographs (especially oblique projections) are helpful. Ultrasonographic evaluation may assist in identifying fractures and in evaluating the eye.
- Local anesthesia may be needed (auriculopalpebral nerve or infratrochlear nerve or retrobulbar blocks, see Chapter 23, p. 382).
- Stain the eye with fluorescein for corneal ulcers. The anterior and posterior chambers and retina should be examined for injury if possible. These problems may need special treatment.
- Gently clean soft tissue lacerations with sterile saline; open fractures require lavage. Remove small, unattached fragments of bone (ebonation).
- Systemic antibiotics and anti-inflammatory medications (phenylbutazone or flunixin meglumine) are indicated.
- Administer a tetanus toxoid if the patient has not received one in the past 6 months.
- If the fracture(s) are stable and there is no compression of the eye, soft tissue lacerations are routinely sutured.
- Treat stable, closed fractures without soft tissue laceration with anti-inflammatories, and monitor the eye for several days after injury for increased intraocular pressure or compression of the globe.
- Comminuted or depressed fractures frequently need to be managed at a surgical facility. Stabilization of fracture fragments, with sutures or metal implants, may be required to maintain a functional orbit. Surgical reduction may be performed using open or closed technique.
- Try to confine the patient to an area where there is a reduced chance of further damage to the periorbital area. Avoid narrow doorways, small feeding buckets, and hay feeders where the horse needs to place his head inside the feeder and risk bumping the periorbital area.

● WHAT NOT TO DO

Orbital and Periorbital Fractures

- Do *not* delay treatment if the eye is affected. Prolonged pressure on the eye may result in permanent damage.
- Do *not* fail to evaluate other structures of the head for injury.

Specific Points of Discussion for Orbital and Periorbital Fractures

In general, injuries to the head heal rapidly because of an excellent blood supply. Cosmetic appearance and functional use are generally good following this type of fracture. A more guarded to poor prognosis is given for injuries that result in severe trauma to the globe, neuropathies, fractures that injure the nasolacrimal system, unstable fractures that are not surgically repaired, and long-standing injuries

Luxation of a Joint

Presentation

Clinical signs depend on the joint involved and occur following disruption of one or more of the support structures of the joint. Signs range from complete joint instability and inability to bear weight on the limb to a horse that is weight bearing on the affected limb with minimal malalignment of the joint. Often the luxation is evident when the patient ambulates or on manipulation of the limb. Concurrent soft tissue wounds may be associated with the luxation, along with contamination of the affected joint. Luxations may spontaneously reduce and recur with movement or variable weight bearing. Subluxation or persistent luxation without reduction may also occur.

- Soft tissue structures commonly affected include:
  - Medial and/or lateral collateral ligaments
  - Fibrous joint capsule
  - Synovium
  - Intraarticular ligaments
- Other differential diagnoses to consider are the following:
  - Fracture
  - Septic arthritis

● WHAT TO DO

Luxation of a Joint

- Take a complete history and perform a complete physical examination to assess the patient systemically.
- Administer sedatives cautiously to calm the patient if needed.
- Carefully palpate the limb to determine whether the luxation is reducible.
- Use palpation to determine whether the luxation is occurring in a cranial, caudal, medial, or lateral direction.
- Plain and stressed radiographs are helpful to rule out concurrent fractures and help to determine soft tissue involvement. Ultrasonographic evaluation is also helpful to determine the condition of the affected soft tissue structures.
- Related soft tissue lacerations are handled in routine manner, with tissue debridement as needed. Administer a tetanus toxoid if the patient has not received prophylaxis in the past 6 months.
- If the joint is open, perform joint lavage, administer local and systemic antibiotics as soon as possible, and continue these until the joint is free of infection based on clinical response, culture, and laboratory tests. Regional limb perfusion is a useful adjunct treatment.
- Use external coaptation and stabilization of the dislocated joint when possible.
- Treatment with external coaptation may result in a functional athlete (full-limb cast or splint, incorporating the hoof). Osteoarthritis is a common sequela that may be performance limiting. With open joints, surgical access is needed to treat the joint, along with limb stabilization.
- Surgical stabilization is often necessary for the best outcome and may include casting, orthopedic implants, transfixation pin casting, and repeat surgeries if the joint is open.

● WHAT NOT TO DO

Luxation of a Joint

- Do *not* leave the patient untreated without some form of external coaptation.
- If the joint is closed, it is important to prevent further soft tissue damage that could lead to joint contamination.
- Do *not* assume that external coaptation results in a sound horse because osteoarthritis is a common sequela.

MS

MS

Types of Luxation
- Coxofemoral luxation
  - Coxofemoral luxation causes disruption of the joint capsule and the round and accessory ligaments of the femur.
  - General anesthesia is required for reduction, and it is difficult to maintain reduction.
  - There are some reports of successful surgical reduction and maintenance of stability in miniature horses using toggle pins and wires.
  - Osteoarthritis usually results in chronic lameness.
- Lower limb luxation (distal interphalangeal joint, proximal interphalangeal joint, metacarpal/metatarsal phalangeal joint)
  - These are common luxations; joint is usually open.
  - Luxation requires reduction.
  - Interdigitation of the metacarpal/metatarsal and first phalanx may present as stable in spite of severe soft tissue damage.
  - Stabilize the limb as for distal limb fractures.
  - Surgical arthrodesis of these joints can be performed.
  - Proximal interphalangeal (pastern) joint luxations can result in a comfortable horse and one that is potentially able to perform some level of athletic activity.
  - Coffin joint and fetlock joint luxations carry a guarded prognosis for soundness.
- Carpometacarpal/tarsometatarsal joint luxation
  - Luxation is very unstable.
  - Stabilize the limb as if treating a fracture.
  - Internal fixation, typically a total or partial arthrodesis, is often required to stabilize the lateral or medial aspects of the carpus or tarsus.
  - Osteoarthritis is a common sequela and is often performance limiting.
- Scapulohumeral joint luxation
  - This luxation is rare.
  - Soft tissue structures involved may include the biceps brachii, supraspinatus musculature, joint capsule, and infraspinatus muscle tendon of insertion.
  - Stabilization is difficult.
  - Spontaneous reduction may occur, and treatment is by confinement for several weeks.
- Stifle joint luxation
  - Luxation usually involves significant soft tissue damage, including one or more collateral ligaments, cruciate ligaments, and the meniscus.
  - Achieving limb stability is difficult.
  - Prognosis for athletic use is poor because of severe osteoarthritis and chronic instability.

Specific Points of Discussion for Luxation of a Joint
The prognosis depends on the joint involved, whether the joint is open or closed, and the degree of instability. Septic arthritis decreases the prognosis and increases the cost involved in treatment. Sequelae include the following:
- Osteoarthritis
- Mechanical lameness
- Persistent pain
- Chronic instability

If reduction of the luxation *cannot* be maintained, the joint becomes arthritic and nonfunctional. Closed luxation managed with long-term (12 to 16 weeks) external coaptation (cast) can have a successful outcome.

Luxation of the Hind Superficial Digital Flexor Tendon
Presentation
The patient usually has a sudden onset of acute, severe lameness in the affected limb, and soft tissue swelling is present at the level of the tarsus. The injury often occurs as the horse is in work. The tendon usually moves back and forth on the tuber calcanei and is in a normal position when the horse is standing still and bearing full weight on the limb. It may be necessary to walk the horse to observe the movement and instability of the superficial digital flexor tendon (SDFT). This tendon most commonly is displaced laterally and generally affects one limb. Subluxation, bilateral injury, medial SDFT displacement, and splitting of the SDFT (part of the tendon lays on the medial and lateral sides of the calcaneus) may occur.
- Other clinical signs include the following:
  - Pain on palpation of the affected area
  - Repeated attempts by the horse to kick out with the affected limb
  - A concurrent fetlock hyperextension related to chronic suspensory apparatus breakdown
- Other differential diagnoses to consider are the following:
  - Disruption of the gastrocnemius tendon
  - Desmitis of the plantar ligament

●▶ WHAT TO DO

Luxation of the Hind Superficial Digital Flexor Tendon
- Obtain a complete history and perform a physical examination to assess the patient systemically. Identify any concurrent lacerations or other areas of trauma.
- Carefully palpate the tarsal area.
- Ultrasonographic examination aids in the diagnosis of an abnormal position of the SDFT and the condition of the retinaculum.
- Sedation may be needed to calm the patient for examination (see Table 21-3).
- The severity of clinical lameness is reduced when the SDFT is dislocated.
- Conservative treatment requires an extended period of rest (6 months or more) to permit the soft tissues to fibrose/scar and stabilize the displaced tendon. The tendon is usually permanently displaced to the lateral or medial side of the calcaneus.
- For return to full athletic performance, surgical stabilization offers the best chance. Surgical treatment options include the following:
  - Stabilization of the tendon with suture
  - Orthopedic implants
  - Mesh
- A full-limb cast or bandage is often used with conservative or surgical treatment.

WHAT NOT TO DO

Luxation of the Hind Superficial Digital Flexor Tendon

- Avoid excessive anti-inflammatory medication because soft tissue swelling may help reduce tendon motion and improve stability.
- Do *not* allow the patient unrestricted exercise for a minimum of 6 months or more.

Specific Points of Discussion for Luxation of the Hind Superficial Digital Flexor Tendon

Prognosis for athletic performance is guarded because a mechanical lameness will likely exist. Medial luxation of the SDFT carries a poorer prognosis for return to soundness than lateral luxation. Successful surgical stabilization has been reported but generally is unrewarding.

Lacerations (General)

Presentation

Soft tissue trauma and damage are present. Location of lacerations may be anywhere on the horse, and evaluation of all involved structures is critical for assessment and treatment. Patients may be fractious and have other injuries such as fractures and luxations. Lacerations are one of the most common reasons for emergency care. For more information, see Chapter 19, p. 241.

WHAT TO DO

Lacerations

- Take a complete history and perform a physical examination.
- Administer tetanus toxoid if the horse has *not* had a booster within the last 6 months.
- Sedate and restrain the patient for close wound examination. See Table 21-3.
- It is important to identify the anatomic structures involved.
- Carefully palpate the affected limb, noting any joint effusion, synovial fluid staining the wound, or compromised vascular structures.
- Referral to a surgical facility is often warranted for lacerations needing special surgical treatment. These include lacerations involving the following:
  - Joints
  - Tendons and tendon sheaths
  - Bursae
  - Vessels and nerves
  - Coronary band and hoof wall
  - Extensive degloving injuries
  - Periosteum
- Lacerations that involve less critical structures are cleaned, debrided, and closed primarily if possible.
  - Use absorbable suture for the deep layers.
  - Use nonabsorbable or absorbable sutures for skin.
  - Skin staples may also be used.
  - Tension-relieving sutures are often necessary in areas with limited soft tissue coverage.
  - Stents or suture bolsters are used to reduce tension with tight closure.
  - Bandages or a form of external coaptation support and protect the suture line.
- Lacerations with significant contamination may be bandaged for several days and a delayed closure performed later.
  - Wet-to-dry bandages aid in wound debridement.
- Antibiotics and anti-inflammatories are warranted.
- See Chapter 19, p. 241, for more detailed information.

WHAT NOT TO DO

Lacerations

- Failure to identify all affected structures results in less than optimum first-aid and treatment.
- Do *not* assume that a superficial wound over a synovial structure does not involve the joint.

Specific Points of Discussion for Lacerations

Simple lacerations have a good prognosis for full return to athletic use and a good cosmetic result. Primary closure is always preferable to healing by second intention whenever possible. Lacerations that involve specific structures have a better prognosis if treatment is initiated early and aggressively.

Lacerations of Supporting Structures (Flexor and Extensor Tendons; Suspensory Ligament)

Presentation

Following an acute traumatic event with loss of function, there is often severe soft tissue injury. The wound depth often affects which support structures are injured or severed. Superficial lacerations frequently affect only the SDFT and the tendon sheath, and deeper lacerations affect the SDFT, tendon sheath, deep digital flexor tendon (DDFT), and suspensory ligament. Extensor tendons are typically affected at the level of the mid to proximal metatarsus or above the carpus; the extensor tendon also has a sheath that may be involved. It may not be possible to see the lacerated tendon on weight bearing because the laceration/injury occurred when the limb was elevated or flexed resulting in the injured structure now located below or above the skin laceration. Therefore ultrasound is often needed for these types of wounds to define the extent of the supporting structure injury. The alignment of the limb is useful in determining which structures are affected.

- Complete laceration of the following structures (at the level of the metacarpus/metatarsus) results in the following:
  - SDFT: slight dropping of the fetlock
  - SDFT and DDFT: dropped fetlock; toe dorsiflexion and elevation with weight bearing
  - SDFT, DDFT, and suspensory ligament: severe loss of fetlock support (fetlock may touch the ground, toe elevation)
- Extensor tendon: dorsal knuckling of limb; inability to place or difficulty in placing hoof

MS

● ▶ WHAT TO DO

Lacerations of Supporting Structures

- Take a complete history and perform a physical examination.
- Administer tetanus toxoid if the horse has not had a booster in the previous 6 months.
- Sedate and restrain the patient for complete wound examination.
- Clean and debride the laceration if possible.
- Stabilize the limb and obtain radiographs if indicated.
- For the DDFT, SDFT, and suspensory ligament, perform the following:
  - For conservative treatment, provide the following:
    - Daily wound care, regional limb perfusion, systemic antimicrobials
    - Splint or cast
  - If the tendon sheath is involved, it should be treated as discussed in the synovial structure laceration section (p. 332).
    - These types of lacerations are difficult to handle in the field, and horses should be transported to a surgical facility for the best prognosis.
    - Surgical treatment involves surgical wound debridement, tendon sheath lavage, reapproximation of tendon ends with suture, and external coaptation.
    - Start systemic antimicrobials and anti-inflammatories.
    - External coaptation is required before transporting to minimize further soft tissue trauma and neurovascular bundle damage. The patient needs to bear weight on the toe to protect the flexor tendons.
      - Cast:
        - Apply cast as described for distal limb fractures (p. 315).
      - Splint:
        - Kimzey Leg-Saver splint OR
        - Board splint (Box 21-4 and Fig. 21-46, *A*).
          - Place a light bandage on the limb from the coronary band to the carpus/tarsus.
          - Place hardwood board flat on the ground, drill through the hoof at the toe, and wire the toe to the board.
          - Flex the limb at the fetlock, and bring the board parallel with the palmar/plantar aspect of the metacarpus/tarsus.
          - Incorporate the board into the bandage with inelastic tape (Fig. 21-46, *B*).
- For the extensor tendon, perform the following:
  - Conservative therapy is often successful.
  - Apply a shoe with a toe extension in order to reduce the likelihood of knuckling. Alternatively you can use external coaptation consisting of a dorsal splint (see below and Fig. 21-47).
  - Perform daily wound care, regional limb perfusion, and administer systemic antimicrobials.

- Place a bandage.
- The extensor tendon sheath is often involved. This tendon sheath is difficult to lavage and usually does well with systemic antimicrobial therapy and wound care.
- Surgical treatment is generally required for extensive wound debridement. Reapposition of extensor tendon ends is seldom possible or necessary.
- External coaptation prevents knuckling of the hoof when weight bearing and allows the tendon to heal.
  - Bandage and PVC splint.
  - Extensor splint (Fig. 21-47).
    - Drill holes into the toe of the hoof.
    - Cut heavy PVC or a board the length (depends on the location of the injury) of the limb.

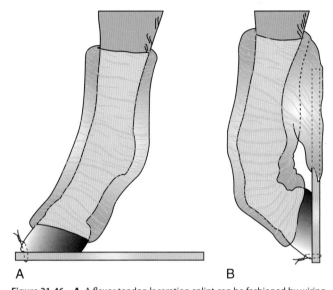

A   B

Figure 21-46   A, A flexor tendon laceration splint can be fashioned by wiring a hardwood board to the toe and flexing the limb to reduce tension on the severed tendon. **B,** The board then is incorporated into the bandage.

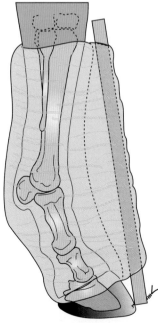

Figure 21-47 An extensor tendon laceration can be protected by means of wiring a polyvinyl chloride splint to the toe, extending the digit, and incorporating the splint into the bandage.

Box 21-4	Materials Needed for a Board Splint

- Leg bandages
- One roll of cotton padding
- Elastic tape
- One hardwood board, 40 cm long × 12 cm wide × 2 cm thick
- Hand drill
- Steel drill bit
- Heavy wire

- Toe to just below tarsus/carpus
- Toe to above carpus
- Drill holes in the end of the splint to match the hoof.
- Bandage the limb, and wire the splint to the toe.
- Attach the splint to the dorsal aspect of the bandage with inelastic tape.

●› WHAT NOT TO DO

Lacerations of Supporting Structures

- Do *not* transport the patient without external coaptation.
- Do *not* assume that the size of the wound equals the severity of tendon or ligament damage.
- Do *not* fail to provide adequate support for the limb, even with conservative therapy.

Specific Points of Discussion for Lacerations of Supporting Structures

The prognosis for lacerations of supporting structures depends greatly on the number of anatomic structures involved, the severity of injury, the amount of contamination, the duration of injury, and the owner expectations for the horse. Prognosis is improved if the vascular and nerve supplies are intact, the injury does not involve synovial structures, and contamination is minimal. Tendons require an extended healing period (6 to 8 months).

Practice Tip: In general, the more structures affected, the poorer the prognosis. The prognosis for survival is extremely poor if all supporting structures (DDFT, SDFT, suspensory ligament) and the tendon sheaths are involved. An open dialogue should be held regarding the expense in treatment for these patients and the high complication risk, including the following:

- Contralateral limb laminitis
- Adhesion formation
- Permanent lameness
- Persistent infection

Practice Tip: Lacerations to extensor tendons have a better prognosis for return to function than lacerations to flexor tendons and often do well with conservative therapy. Horses with extensor tendon damage often learn to place their foot in a normal position within a few days. Stringhalt is frequently a sequela of proximal metatarsal extensor damage.

Lacerations of Vascular and Nerve Structures

Presentation

The patient has a soft tissue wound and concurrent loss of large volumes of blood. Large pools of blood are often noted in the horse's surroundings. Arterial blood is often noticed "spurting" from the wound. It is often difficult to determine exactly which vessel is injured because of the continuous bleeding. It is possible, although uncommon, for exsanguination to occur if a large vessel in the distal limb is affected. A patient may exsanguinate quickly if large vessels (i.e., jugular vein, external carotid artery, femoral artery, or brachial artery) are transected. Nerve damage or transection results in the horse appearing less lame than expected or in loss of limb function.

●› WHAT TO DO

Lacerations of Vascular and Nerve Structures

- Take a complete history and perform a physical examination after controlling the bleeding.
- Administer a tetanus toxoid if tetanus prophylaxis is unknown or questionable.
- Control bleeding:
  - Apply pressure wraps, covering the area with heavy cotton padding followed by elastic tape.
  - After 20 to 30 minutes, remove the wrap and try to identify the source of bleeding.
  - Peripheral limb vessels are often ligated without any long-term complications.
  - Major feeding vessels to an area may need surgical repair under general anesthesia. Maintain pressure wraps during anesthesia induction to minimize blood loss.
  - The use of the antifibrinolytic drug aminocaproic acid (10 mg/kg IV diluted in 60 mL given over 5 minutes q6 to 24h), can be beneficial in cases of mild to moderate bleeding.
- Fracture-related vascular damage is usually unrepairable.
  - Fractures of the humerus or radius may result in lacerations of the brachial artery.
  - Fractures of the femur or pelvis can transect the femoral artery.
- Nerve laceration or damage:
  - Diagnosis is made by noting a change in limb carriage.
    - Radial nerve:
      - Clinical presentation is loss of triceps function leading to "dropped elbow"
      - Can be caused by humeral fracture, "paralysis" from blunt trauma, prolonged recumbency, or be idiopathic
      - Lower branch damage leads to stumbling and poor hoof placement
    - Antebrachial injury, radial physeal fracture with dorsal luxation present with the limb carried at an unusual angle, dropped elbow and nonweight-bearing lameness.
    - Femoral nerve:
      - Clinical presentation is loss of quadriceps function leading to inability to fix the stifle and bear full weight on the pelvic limb
    - Tibial/peroneal nerve:
      - Clinical presentation is stumbling and inability to extend the digit
- Distal limb nerve damage: common
  - Few complications other than neuromas, which may form during healing and cause lameness
  - Occasionally the hoof may slough
- Proximal limb nerve damage:
  - Often fracture-associated (femur or humerus)
  - These are not typically repaired
- Treatment:
  - Administer nonsteroidal anti-inflammatory medications.
  - Administer steroids.
  - Complete nerve transection is difficult to differentiate from neuropraxia (nerve trauma) that improves with time.
  - Neuropraxia improves with time (days to weeks).
  - External coaptation may be necessary to protect the limb.

MS

●› WHAT NOT TO DO

Lacerations of Vascular and Nerve Structures

- Do *not* leave the limb unsupported if nerve damage is suspected. As the patient attempts to use the impaired limb, further soft tissue and nerve trauma can occur.
- Do *not* forget to evaluate the systemic condition of the patient. Significant blood loss requires fluid therapy, blood transfusions, or supportive care.

Specific Points of Discussion for Lacerations of Vascular and Nerve Structures

The prognosis for vascular and nerve lacerations to the distal limb is good. Usually the horse has sufficient collateral circulation for adequate blood supply to the limb. Remember that blunt trauma to the limb may cause as much damage to the blood and nerve supply as transection of the structures would.

Large, major vessels and nerves transected or severely damaged have a guarded to poor prognosis for recovery. It is difficult to predict the time required for horses with neuropraxia to recover.

Lacerations/Punctures Involving Synovial Structures

Presentation

The patient has an acute wound/injury in which the soft tissue damage is located over or near a joint, bursa, or tendon sheath. Another common history is a horse that has sustained a laceration or puncture wound a few days before and is suddenly very lame (often non–weight bearing). Synovial fluid occasionally may be seen leaking from the wound, and sometimes bone or cartilage is noticed. Increased joint or tendon sheath effusion may be present. Lacerations involving joints or tendon sheaths are emergencies, and wounds near these structures are treated as such.

●› WHAT TO DO

Lacerations and Punctures of a Synovial Structure

- See Chapter 19, p. 251, for more information.
- Take a complete history, and perform a physical examination.
- Administer tetanus toxoid if the horse has not had a booster in the previous 6 months.
- Sedate and restrain the patient for a complete wound examination.
- Determine synovial structure involvement.
  - Radiographs:
    - Plain radiographs demonstrating gas in the joint indicate a communication with the skin.
  - Inject sterile contrast material into the synovial structure at a site distant from the wound, then take a radiograph focused on the lacerated area.
  - Arthrocentesis:
    - Surgically clip and prepare a site distant from the wound.
    - Insert a sterile needle and collect synovial fluid for cytologic examination and culture.
    - A white blood cell count of >30,000 cells/dL is presumptive evidence of infection.

- In chronic wounds, the synovial fluid may grossly be abnormal.
- Joint distention
  - From the arthrocentesis site, inject sterile saline and observe the wound for fluid leaking.
  - In cases of "dynamic" wounds, where the presence of several tissue planes between the skin surface and the joint move independently from each other (i.e., stifle region), active flexion and extension of the limb following joint distention is necessary to rule in or out joint involvement.
- Antimicrobial therapy within 24 hours greatly improves the prognosis.
- If the synovial structure is *not* involved, do the following:
  - Inject 250 to 500 mg sterile amikacin sulfate into the structure as prophylaxis to help prevent infection.
  - Suture wound primarily if possible.
- If the synovial structure is involved:
  - Start systemic broad-spectrum antimicrobials immediately.
  - Perform joint lavage standing in a tractable patient, or alternatively under general anesthesia. Appropriate local analgesia is needed for standing lavage.
  - Lavage of a tendon sheath is generally more difficult than a joint in a weight-bearing patient.
  - Following surgical preparation of a site distant from the open wound, place a large needle (14 gauge) intraarticularly.
  - A continuous ingress flow of sterile lactated Ringer's solution is recommended, with a minimum of 1 to 2 L of joint lavage.
    - Ten percent dimethyl sulfoxide may be added to the lactated Ringer's solution lavage.
  - Administer antimicrobials intraarticularly following lavage.
    - Antimicrobials with a low pH may irritate the synovial tissue.
    - Recommendations:
      - Amikacin sulfate (250 mg/mL): 250 to 500 mg per synovial structure
      - Gentamicin sulfate (50 mg/mL): 100 to 200 mg per synovial structure
  - Perform regional limb perfusion daily. Remember that regional limb perfusion is most effective using a concentration-dependent antimicrobial such as aminoglycosides or third-generation cephalosporins.
  - Apply topical antibiotic ointment to cover the wound, and place the limb in a sterile bandage. The affected synovial structure often needs daily lavage until the cytologic and culture results support no evidence of infection.
  - if there is not severe contamination of the joint and wound, suture the wound (complete or partial) to aid in reducing healing time and for protection of the synovial tissue. Leave a small opening for lavage fluid to exit, or use an egress needle.
  - A cast placed over the bandage is useful to immobilize the joint and increases the patient's comfort level. The cast is bivalved to allow daily access to the wound and secured with duct tape.

●› WHAT NOT TO DO

Lacerations and Punctures of Synovial Structures

- Do *not* assume that the synovial structure is unaffected at the time of the initial examination just because the patient is weight bearing.

- Potential involvement of synovial structures is determined at initial examination. Do *not* wait to see how the patient responds to conservative treatment.

Specific Points of Discussion for Lacerations and Punctures of Synovial Structures

The prognosis for open synovial structures is greatly improved if therapy is started within 24 hours of injury. Once an infection is established (>24 hours), clearing the infection is more difficult and prolonged, and chances of sequelae developing are greater. Potential sequelae include the following:

- Cartilage damage
- Osteoarthritis
- Persistent lameness
- Adhesions within the tendon sheath

Infection should be suspected in any patient who becomes more lame as the laceration heals. Open synovial structures carry a guarded prognosis, with early diagnosis and aggressive treatment resulting in the best chance of preventing the establishment of sepsis and ensuring recovery.

Lacerations Involving the Coronary Band and Hoof Wall

Presentation

Practice Tip: *Lacerations involving the heel bulb, hoof wall, and coronary band are common in horses.* The patient often has a history of the hoof trapped and then struggling to free it. This type of injury may also involve synovial structures, nerves, and blood vessels. Frequently the patient is weight bearing on the limb because of concurrent nerve injury, and there is often evidence of blood loss or vessel damage. Heel bulb lacerations are usually very contaminated because of their proximity to the ground.

●» WHAT TO DO

Lacerations of the Coronary Band and Hoof Wall

- Take a complete history and perform a physical examination.
- Administer tetanus toxoid if the horse has not had a booster in the past 6 months.
- Sedate and restrain the patient for a complete wound examination.
- Local anesthesia may be necessary to work on the foot. An abaxial nerve block or palmar/plantar digital nerve block (see Fig. 21-1) is usually adequate.
- Carefully examine and palpate the injury to identify potential structures that are involved and the depth of the laceration. Anatomic structures to consider include the following:
  - Coronary band
  - DDFT
  - Palmar/plantar support structures
  - Digital tendon sheath
  - Joints (proximal and distal interphalangeal)
  - Navicular bone and bursa
- Major lacerations involving one or more special structures may require shipping to a surgical facility. Place a foot bandage before shipping to minimize further contamination (Box 21-5). Start systemic antimicrobial administration if synovial structures are

Box 21-5 | Easy Foot Bandage

- Wrap a small baby diaper around the hoof.
- Secure diaper with a roll of self-retaining bandage, such as Vetrap. Be careful not to constrict the coronary band by placing Vetrap only on the hoof.
- Premake a duct tape patch by laying 4 to 6 strips of duct tape side by side; repeat this procedure, laying the additional strips at a right angle (90 degrees) to the first strips. Using scissors, cut into the corners several inches. Place the patch on the bottom of the hoof, over the Vetrap, and secure the corners by wrapping around the hoof.
- Prevent shavings and dirt from entering the top of the bandage with Elastikon.

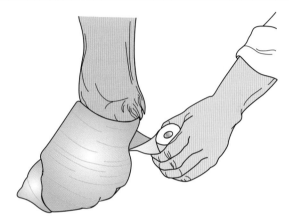

Figure 21-48 A short, slipper cast can be used to stabilize lacerations of the hoof wall or coronary band. The cast can be applied with the horse standing and should extend to just beneath the fetlock joint. Cast application follows the same procedural steps as for the application for a cast used for external coaptation.

involved. If you have time, perform a regional limb perfusion before shipping.
- Take radiographs to confirm that radiopaque foreign bodies are not imbedded in the wound (barbs, wire fragments).
- For simple lacerations, do the following:
  - Ensure no deeper structures are involved.
  - Clean and debride the wound.
  - Suture the wound primarily if possible because of the potential for contamination; leave an opening for drainage. Delayed primary closure may be elected.
  - Apply a foot bandage (Box 21-5) or foot/"slipper" cast (Fig. 21-48).
    - These wounds can be difficult to heal because of constant movement in this area.
    - A foot-cast or short-limb cast for 2 to 3 weeks allows granulation tissue to cover the tissue defect. The wound drains through the cast material.
    - ***Practice Tip:*** *Most clinicians prefer a foot cast whenever possible following adequate wound debridement in order to speed and support normal wound healing.*
- For coronary band laceration, do the following:
  - An interruption in coronary band integrity results in a permanent hoof wall defect.
  - Primary closure decreases the resulting defect.
    - Clean the laceration.
    - Use large horizontal or vertical mattress sutures using #1 or #2 nonabsorbable suture material.
  - Apply a foot bandage, foot-cast or short-limb cast.

◗ WHAT NOT TO DO

Lacerations of the Coronary Band and Hoof Wall

- An increase in lameness as the laceration heals is a warning sign! Do *not* delay reevaluation of the deeper anatomic structures.
- Do *not* delay removing the cast earlier than planned if the patient shows an increase in lameness.
- Do *not* forget that denervation may conceal the pain you would expect with involvement of deeper structures and extent of the injury.

Specific Points of Discussion for Lacerations of the Coronary Band and Hoof Wall

Simple hoof wall lacerations have a good prognosis for full recovery, although scarring often results at the coronary band with hoof wall defects as a sequela. Sometimes bar shoes are needed to provide several months of stability and comfort for the horse. A typical hoof wall laceration requires 4 to 8 months to heal with new hoof formation rather than by healing from side-to-side. Complicated lacerations that involve deeper important structures carry a guarded prognosis and require prompt attention and treatment as discussed in corresponding sections.

Lacerations: Degloving Injuries

Presentation

The equine patient has a large area of soft tissue loss to a limb. The superficial tissues tend to pull away from the underlying structures similar to removing a glove. A common history is falling through the bottom of a trailer or a trailer accident. The wound usually is contaminated with dirt and debris, and there may be concurrent fractures, injury to supporting tissues, and synovial structures involved.

◗ WHAT TO DO

Degloving Injuries

- Take a complete history and perform a physical examination.
- Administer tetanus toxoid if the horse has not had a booster in the past 6 months.
- Sedate and restrain the patient for comprehensive wound examination.
- Clean and examine the wound to determine anatomic structures involved. Assessment of tissue viability on initial examination is difficult. Often there is a large area of bone exposed, and the periosteum may be damaged concurrently.
- Wound debridement should be meticulous. General anesthesia may be required for extensive injuries.
- Radiographs are useful in bone evaluation. Radiographs may be repeated in 10 to 14 days in order to identify possible bone sequestrum.
- Perform primary wound closure where possible using tension-relieving sutures.
- Systemic antimicrobials and anti-inflammatory medications are usually indicated.
- Immobilization is needed for optimal healing and revascularization.
  - Apply a cast: Place a cast over a bandage and bivalve it for ease of removal, or apply a splint and bandage.

- After removal of the cast (7 to 10 days), devitalized tissue (dark brown or black, leathery) is often evident and can be removed at that time.

◗ WHAT NOT TO DO

Degloving Injuries

- Do *not* remove any viable tissue. If you are unable to determine tissue viability, leave the tissue in question intact and observe; it can always be removed later.
- Do *not* fail to take radiographs or reevaluate the wound if it has persistent drainage or is not healing properly. Bone sequestrum and foreign bodies are common delayed complications.

Specific Points of Discussion for Degloving Injuries

Potential complications with large tissue loss include the following:

- Bone sequestrum
- Osteomyelitis
- Osteitis
- Foreign bodies
- Loss of vessel and nerve supply
- Periosteal new bone
- Delayed wound healing
- Sloughing of the foot (rare)
- Formation of exuberant granulation tissue

Skin grafting may be needed, at a later date, to cover poorly epithelialized areas. These wounds are notorious for reopening after apparent healing and often require serial debridements. The prognosis varies and depends on the structures involved.

Puncture Wound to the Hoof

Presentation

The patient is very lame on the affected limb because of the penetration of a foreign body (usually a nail) into the sole. The puncture wound is often difficult to identify unless the penetrating object is still in place. Punctures into the caudal one third of the sole or frog are especially risky, with serious life-threatening consequences if they penetrate synovial structures. Structures in this area that may be compromised include the deep digital flexor tendon, digital flexor tendon sheath, impar ligament, third phalanx, navicular bone, navicular bursa, distal interphalangeal joint, distal second phalanx, proximal interphalangeal joint, and digital cushion.

Penetrating foreign bodies are often contaminated with fecal material or soil, resulting in life-threatening infections with gram-positive and gram-negative aerobic and anaerobic bacteria (*Clostridium* spp). The initial puncture wound closes rapidly and is difficult to find on examination. Drainage and local lavage is difficult to achieve. Puncture wounds to the hoof should be treated as emergencies because sequelae may be life threatening. Chronic infection of bone, soft tissue, and synovial structures may lead to persistent lameness and loss of athletic use of the horse.

●〉 WHAT TO DO

Puncture Wounds of the Hoof

- Obtain a detailed history, including the type of penetrating object (if known), duration of time since the foreign body penetrated the hoof, exact location of the penetrating foreign body (if removed), and degree of potential contamination.
- If the foreign body is still present in the hoof, it should be bent so that further penetration does *not* occur, and radiographs should be taken with the "object" still in place. This increases the ability to determine which structures are involved and the direction of the penetration. Most metallic foreign bodies are best seen on conventional radiographs. Radiolucent objects may require other imaging modalities (contrast study, ultrasound, magnetic resonance imaging [nonmetallic], computed tomography).
- If the penetrating object is not present, examine the sole for drainage and discoloration. A positive response to hoof testers may help in locating the point of entry of the object.
- The injection of contrast solution into the tract with subsequent radiographs can facilitate positive identification of the structures involved.
- Local anesthesia may be needed to examine the foot. An abaxial nerve block or palmar digital nerve block is recommended.
- Inspect the puncture wound and clean the sole. Removal of thin portions of frog or sole with a hoof knife may assist in wound debridement and provide ventral drainage. Lavage with sterile saline or other crystalloid solution.
- For deep wounds and those that are located near vital structures as described before, referral to a surgical facility where a more thorough debridement can be accomplished should be recommemded.
- If the wound occurred hours to 24 hours earlier, and the patient is severely lame, infection should be suspected until ruled out by culture, laboratory studies, and response to treatment. If deeper structures are affected, the response to routine treatment is generally poor.
- Place a foot bandage to minimize additional contamination. Cover the puncture site with topical triple antibiotic ointment before bandaging (see Box 21-5).
- Any foreign body still in the foot should be carefully removed before shipping the patient a long distance. Identify the point of entry with an indelible mark (circle); this helps the referring clinicians with future treatment.
- Administer tetanus toxoid if the patient has not received one within the last 6 months.
- If transporting to a referral facility, discuss with the referring clinician the initiation of antibiotic treatment or whether to delay starting treatment until culture samples have been taken from the deeper tissues.
- Administer anti-inflammatories (phenylbutazone or flunixin meglumine) for improved comfort.
- Foreign material may be difficult to find, and if exploration of the wound tract is planned, regional anesthesia may be needed for analgesia, ease of examination, and comfort of the patient.
- Discuss with the owner the importance of keeping the wound clean and looking for signs of infection (e.g., sudden or gradual change in lameness status). Stress that infection may develop days to weeks after the injury. If the patient becomes non–weight bearing or increasingly more lame in the affected limb, a veterinarian should be called immediately.
- In a very lame horse, perform arthrocentesis of any synovial structure—joint, bursa, sheath—in a severely lame horse and especially if there is a suspicion of penetration of a foreign body; fluid that appears septic (cloudy/turbid/discolored) may indicate penetration of the foreign body through the impar ligament and into the navicular bursa and coffin joint. Joint fluid should be submitted for analysis, culture, and susceptibility.
- Treatment is aggressive because of the life-threatening nature of the complications. Surgical debridement is often needed and should be performed in the acute stages to reduce the chances for chronic infection. Referral hospitals may use arthroscopy, bursoscopy (see p. 298), or a surgical approach through the penetrating tract/sole. These patients need long-term systemic antibiotics, regional limb perfusion(s), and local antibiotics, depending on the anatomic structures affected.
- Use care in inserting probes or flushing contrast material from the wound into the foot. You can increase the contamination or drive foreign material deeper into the foot or into structures not previously affected.

●〉 WHAT NOT TO DO

Puncture Wounds of the Hoof

- Do *not* be falsely assured that the wound is only superficial. Most entry wounds are small. Deeper foot structures affected may be difficult to determine. Foot soaks and local antibiotics are not prophylactic and are not a substitute for thorough debridement, drainage, and copious lavage and irrigation.
- Do *not* delay referral or treatment using arthroscopic lavage and debridement if there is any question of deeper structure involvement.
- A single debridement and lavage may be inadequate. Achieving ventral drainage is imperative.
- Do *not* rely on oral antibiotics alone. Daily or every-other-day regional limb perfusion and intraarticular treatments may be necessary.

Specific Points of Discussion for Puncture Wounds of the Hoof

Puncture wounds to the foot that are small, clean, and not located in the caudal third of the sole or frog often do well. Foreign bodies that are in the caudal foot and penetrate important deep structures are life-threatening emergencies with serious long-term sequelae. Management of these puncture wounds depends on the type of foreign body, location of the wound, depth of penetration, duration of time until treatment, and the general health of the patient. Puncture wounds that involve synovial structures are particularly serious and require immediate and aggressive treatment. Patients receiving early treatment have a better prognosis. Synovial structure infections and osteomyelitis have some of the most devastating and long-term complications. Any horse with a suspected penetration of the deep foot structures should be referred to a surgical facility as soon as possible.

Sole/Foot Abscess

Presentation

The patient has an acute, non–weight-bearing lameness similar to the severity of a horse with a fracture. The digital pulses are increased in the affected limb, and there often is generalized swelling of the distal limb. Hoof testers elicit an obvious positive response localized to the area of the abscess, and fluid or a moist "spot" may be noticed on the sole in the region. Occasionally, a tract leading to the abscess is easily identified.

- Other differential diagnoses to consider are the following:
  - Distal phalanx fracture
  - Septic distal interphalangeal joint
  - Septic navicular bursa
  - Sole bruise
  - Puncture wound to the hoof
  - Unilateral laminitis

WHAT TO DO

A Sole/Foot Abscess

- Obtain a detailed history and perform a complete physical examination.
- Administer tetanus toxoid if the patient has not received one within the last 6 months.
- Examine the bottom of the hoof for areas of drainage and discoloration. A positive response to hoof testers helps identify the affected region. Also, carefully palpate and examine the coronary band for drainage or soft areas where the abscess may be draining.
- Local anesthesia may be needed to debride the foot. An abaxial nerve block or palmar digital nerve block provides adequate anesthesia for the procedure.
- A hardened hoof may require removal of portions of frog or sole using a sharp hoof knife for evaluation.
- Soaking the foot overnight softens the keratinized tissue/hoof and aids in evaluation and localization of the abscess and establishment of ventral drainage. This is accomplished by using a wet-to-dry bandage or iodine-soaked bandage on the foot.
- It is best to remove the shoe to examine the hoof thoroughly, including the nail holes.
- Radiographs may help localize areas of excess fluid or gas and allow evaluation of the third phalanx if the abscess is chronic.
- If an abscess tract has been identified, remove all necrotic and undermined hoof/sole with a sharp hoof knife until normal bleeding tissue is reached. Minimize the size of the hole to avoid solar corium protrusion and prolapse. Flush the area daily with a dilute iodine or antiseptic (chlorhexidine or povidone-iodine [Betadine]) solution, and wrap it with a foot bandage (see Box 21-5). Another option, depending on the location of the abscess, is the use of a hospital plate instead of a foot bandage. An alternative to flushing is to soak the foot in a low-rimmed bucket or an empty intravenous fluid bag. Epsom salts (magnesium sulfate) may be added to the foot soak to treat the abscess. Discontinue the foot soaks once infection and inflammation are resolved. The affected foot can also be soaked in a sealed bag for 45 to 60 minutes with an oxyclorsine solution[10] (a chlorine-based compound).
- Should the abscess drain from the coronary band, establish ventral drainage if possible, and flush the tract from the coronary band distal, and then bandage as described.
- Replace the shoe once the sole is dry and cornified. Pads under the shoe may be used to protect the sole.
- If good ventral drainage is achieved and there are no other systemic signs, antimicrobials are often unnecessary. Systemic broad-spectrum antimicrobials are recommended if the patient has the following:

- Fever
- Cellulitis/swelling of the limb
- Other systemic signs (e.g., depression or anorexia)
- Crush and pack metronidazole tablets, 500 to 1000 mg, q24h, into the draining tract if anaerobic bacteria are suspected.
- Nonsteroidal anti-inflammatory drugs (phenylbutazone or flunixin meglumine) should be prescribed for pain management after opening and draining the abscess.

Note: The goals of treatment are as follows:
- Establish ventral drainage for the abscess.
- Keep the area clean and prevent recontamination using an impervious foot bandage, a shoe with a hospital plate covering the sole or similar arrangement.
- Remove and prevent recolonization of bacteria.
- Dry/desiccate the abscess cavity.
- Allow for new hoof growth.

WHAT NOT TO DO

A Sole/Foot Abscess

- Do *not* remove healthy tissue when exploring the infected site. If you are unable to identify the exact location, soak the foot overnight and reevaluate.
- Do *not* forget to rule out a fracture or septic synovial structure if an abscess is not identified.
- If the abscess is *not* found on initial examination, do *not* forget to reevaluate a second or third time in an attempt to create ventral drainage on the bottom of the hoof. Ventral drainage is always preferable to the abscess draining from the coronary band.
- Do *not* permit an abscess to go untreated because the third phalanx and distal interphalangeal joint may become secondarily infected should the abscess penetrate the deep hoof structures.

Specific Points of Discussion for Sole/Foot Abscess

Practice Tip: *Hoof abscesses are one of the most common causes for an acute and severe, non–weight-bearing lameness and have a wide variety of clinical signs.* Multiple causes permit bacteria to gain access to the hoof and include nails placed too close to or into the sensitive lamina (close nailing), small rocks that penetrate the sole, and sole bruises. Diagnosis and appropriate treatment in the acute stages helps prevent development of a chronic abscess, leading to chronic infection and osteitis. In general, the prognosis is good for an acute abscess, although it may take several weeks to heal completely. The prognosis is guarded if the bone or synovial structures are involved.

Take-Home Summary Points for Musculoskeletal Injuries

- Musculoskeletal injuries are common in the adult equine species.
- Many of these injuries become much more obvious as the patient bears weight on the affected limb.
- The injury may still be serious even if the patient is able to bear weight on the affected limb.
- Treatment must be initiated early for the best outcome.
- Figs. 21-49 and 21-50 provide guidelines for weight-bearing and non–weight-bearing injuries in adult horses.

[10]Clean Trax (Equine Technologies, Sudbury, Massachusetts).

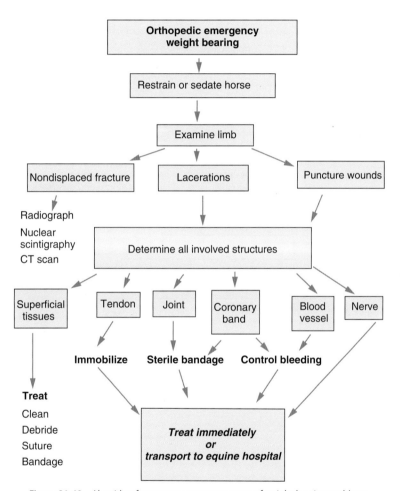

Figure 21-49   Algorithm for emergency management of weight-bearing problems.

MS

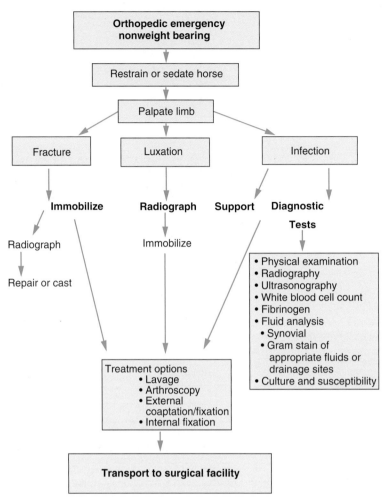

Figure 21-50   Algorithm for emergency management of non–weight-bearing problems.

References

References can be found on the companion website at www.equine-emergencies.com.

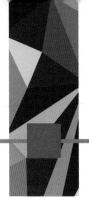

CHAPTER 22

Nervous System

DIAGNOSTIC AND THERAPEUTIC PROCEDURES

Amy L. Johnson

Cerebrospinal Fluid Collection

Cerebrospinal fluid (CSF) analysis is indicated whenever disease of the central nervous system is suspected. Analysis helps determine involvement of the central nervous system (CNS), and specific changes in the CSF might suggest certain types of infectious diseases. Fluid is most commonly acquired from two sites: the lumbosacral and the atlantooccipital (cerebellomedullary) cistern. Collection from the atlantooccipital cistern must be done under general anesthesia and might be contraindicated in patients with cerebral swelling. Ultrasound-guided cervical CSF centesis between C1 and C2 has also been described.

Equipment

- Twitch and/or sedation (detomidine and butorphanol)
- Clippers
- Material for aseptic preparation of site
- Sterile gloves
- 2% local anesthetic; 5-mL syringe; and 22-gauge, 3.75-cm (1½-inch) needle
- 15.2-cm (6-inch) or 20-cm (8-inch), 18-gauge spinal needle for lumbosacral aspirate or 9-cm (3½-inch), 18-gauge needle for atlantooccipital collection[1] (sterile)
- 3- and/or 10-mL slip-tip syringes (sterile); have several ready, and do not use Luer-Lok syringes
- Blood collection tubes containing ethylenediaminetetraacetic acid (EDTA) and plain Vacutainer tubes[2]
- CultureSwab[3] or Port-A-Cul[4] culture system
- Stool to stand on to reach lumbosacral puncture site
- Styrofoam shipping container with ice packs and appropriate address labels for sample submission by 1- or 2-day delivery to testing laboratory

---

[1]BD Spinal Needles (Becton, Dickinson and Company, Franklin Lakes, New Jersey); 20-cm needle is available from MILA International, Inc., Erlanger, Kentucky.

[2]BD Vacutainer tubes (Becton, Dickinson and Company, Franklin Lakes, New Jersey).

[3]BBL CultureSwab Collection & Transport System (Becton, Dickinson and Company, Sparks, Maryland).

[4]BBL Port-A-Cul Vial (Becton, Dickinson and Company, Sparks, Maryland).

Procedure

Collection from the Lumbosacral Space

- Restrain horse in stocks or perform the lumbosacral aspirate in a stall. Sedation is not always necessary but is strongly recommended if the patient tolerates it because it minimizes adverse physical reactions by the horse when the needle contacts the dura. Recommended dosage is 0.01 to 0.02 mg/kg detomidine with 0.01 to 0.02 mg/kg butorphanol intravenously (IV). Start at the lower end of the dosage range, particularly in severely ataxic horses. Consider applying a twitch as well.
- See Fig. 22-1 for landmarks for the lumbosacral tap.
- Clip and aseptically prepare a large square centered on midline at the cranial aspect of the tuber sacrale/caudal aspect of a line drawn across the back connecting the tuber coxae.
- Wear sterile gloves, and maintain sterility throughout procedure.
- Place a bleb of local anesthetic beneath the skin and 3 to 5 mL in the deeper muscle layers.
- With the patient standing squarely, insert a 15.2-cm/20-cm (6-inch/8-inch) spinal needle perpendicular to the midline. A 6-inch needle is long enough for most horses and easier to keep in a perpendicular plane than an 8-inch needle. The subarachnoid space is approximately 12 to 15 cm deep to the skin in the average adult. A loss of resistance is often felt as the needle passes into the subarachnoid space, and there is often sudden patient movement that varies from tail and hindquarter twitch or "tuck" (common) to more violent reactions (uncommon), including bucking, leaping, or falling. The likelihood of a violent reaction appears to be minimized with adequate sedation and restraint.
- Remove the stylet from the needle and check for fluid by aspirating any time a loss of resistance is felt at the appropriate depth, the patient appears to react, or bone is contacted.
- Fluid might appear at the needle hub soon after the subarachnoid space has been penetrated, although aspiration is the most definitive way to check for appropriate placement. If needed, occlude both jugular veins with digital pressure to increase intracranial pressure and improve CSF flow.
- If the initial sample appears blood contaminated, discard it and use another syringe for additional sampling. The use of 3 to 5 serial syringes, the use of small (3-mL) syringes, and aspirating slowly to minimize suction will minimize blood contamination in the final sample.

CNS

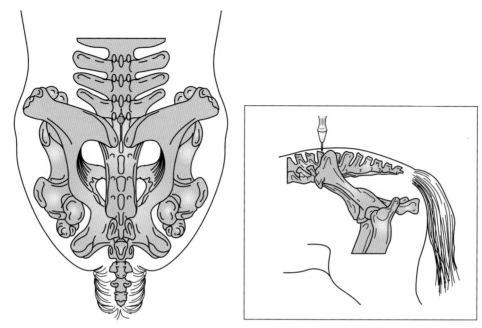

Figure 22-1 Needle placement for collection of cerebrospinal fluid from the lumbosacral (LS) space. The LS space is generally palpable as a depression caudal to the sixth lumbar spinous process. Palpate the caudal edge of each tuber coxa, and draw a line directly to midline to find the depression. This area *(inset)* is often 1 to 2 cm cranial to the prominence of each tuber sacrale. Angle the needle directly perpendicular to the vertebrae.

Figure 22-2 Needle placement for collection of cerebrospinal fluid from the atlanto-occipital space. Palpate the cranial borders of the atlas *(arrows)* and draw a line directly to midline. The site for puncture *(inset)* is on this line directly on the midline. Angle the needle perpendicular to the cervical vertebrae.

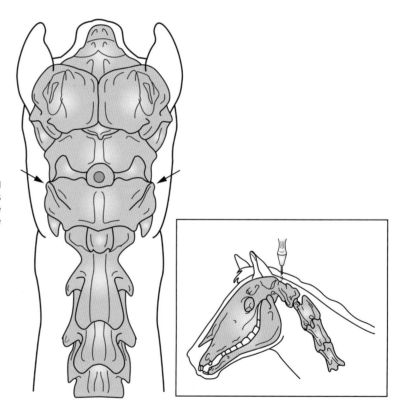

- After aspirating an adequate amount of fluid, place samples into EDTA and plain Vacutainer tubes, or onto a Culture-Swab or in a Port-a-Cul if culture is indicated.

Collection from the Atlantooccipital Space
- Place the patient under general anesthesia to prevent patient movement. This spinal tap is performed over the

proximal cervical spinal cord, and it is therefore possible to traumatize nervous tissue if the head or neck moves.
- Flex the patient's neck so that the head is at a right angle to the neck.
- See Fig. 22-2 for landmarks for atlantooccipital collection.
- Clip the area from the occipital protuberance to the cranial aspect of C2 and several inches on each side of midline

and perform a sterile scrub. Maintain sterility throughout the procedure.

- Wearing sterile gloves, insert the 9-cm (3½-inch) spinal needle to a depth of 5 to 6 cm or until loss of resistance is noted. ***Important:*** A loss of resistance is *not* always appreciable, so the safest way to perform this procedure is to check frequently for CSF when an appropriate depth is neared. Remove the stylet to determine correct placement in the subarachnoid space; fluid should flow spontaneously without aspiration. If fluid is not obtained, replace the stylet and advance the needle 3 to 4 mm before again checking for fluid.
- Once CSF appears at the needle hub, allow the CSF to flow into collection tubes. Aspiration is not required and might increase risk of blood contamination.
- Sample collection of CSF at C1-2 in the standing horse:
  - This is a relatively new procedure described by Dr. Pease at Michigan State University and reported in *J Vet Radiol Ultrasound* (53[1]:92-95, 2012).
  - The spinal cord is visualized using ultrasound at C1-2; the area is clipped and aseptically prepared.
  - The horse is sedated with 5 µg/kg detomidine and then administered 30 mg (for 500-kg horse) of morphine intravenously. Local anesthesia can be infiltrated subcutaneously, but generally is not required.
  - The ultrasound probe is placed dorsally to the spinal cord and directed ventrally so that the spinal cord and subarachnoid space are seen. With a continual image of the spinal cord using ultrasonography, a 3½-inch (8.9-cm) 18-gauge spinal needle is directed using the opposite hand or with the help of an assistant, such that it can be seen entering the subarachnoid space at a slightly dorsal angle (in case the horse moves). Once the needle is visualized in the space, the stylet is removed and CSF is gently aspirated.

Complications

- With the lumbosacral approach, the fourth and fifth sacral segments of the spinal cord are frequently penetrated by the needle with no noticeable neurologic impairment. The most likely (although still uncommon) complication is patient or clinician injury from a violent reaction of the horse to the procedure.
- With the atlantooccipital approach, trauma to the spinal cord or brainstem during needle placement could cause significant neurologic impairment. Perform this procedure under general anesthesia and advance the needle cautiously, frequently checking for fluid as an adequate depth of insertion is reached.
- With C1-C2 sampling, bleeding around the spinal cord can occur. Seizure activity has rarely been reported. Fever following the aspirate may also happen, but in most cases is self-limiting.
- Infection of the meninges, although rare, can be fatal; therefore, maintain sterile technique.
- Some horses appear depressed or appear to have a stiff neck after collection, particularly from the atlantooccipital

space. These clinical signs might be akin to the headache often reported by people after the similar procedure. Treatment with a nonsteroidal anti-inflammatory drug (flunixin meglumine or phenylbutazone) generally ameliorates the clinical signs.

Cerebrospinal Fluid Analysis

CSF is examined grossly for color, clarity, and particulate matter. Normal CSF is clear and colorless. An increase in turbidity or particles occurs with inflammation and infectious diseases. Red streaks in the fluid are caused by blood contamination during collection, whereas previous bleeding in the CNS produces a xanthochromic (yellow-colored) sample. Total protein measurement and cytologic evaluation (including total white blood cell and red blood cell counts, as well as differential cell counts) should be performed on every aspirate. Various changes in the cellular content are typical but not pathognomonic for specific disease processes. See Table 22-1 for correlation between abnormal values and CNS disease. Glucose level (normally between 50 and 70 mg/dL, or about 66% of blood glucose level) can be measured and might be lower than normal with inflammation or infection because of consumption by white blood cells and bacteria. Additionally, samples of cerebrospinal fluid and serum can be submitted for specific immunologic testing for diseases such as equine protozoal myeloencephalitis (EPM) and Lyme disease (neuroborreliosis).

NEUROLOGIC EMERGENCIES

Amy L. Johnson and Thomas J. Divers, with contributions from Alexander de Lahunta

Neurologic disorders frequently have an acute onset, can rapidly worsen, and often necessitate emergency diagnostics and therapeutics.

- The *first* goal of the examination is to determine that the nervous system is the origin of the clinical signs.
- The *second* goal is to determine the anatomic location of the abnormality within the nervous system; doing so shortens the list of differential diagnoses. Incoordination or ataxia usually suggests involvement of the long tracts in the spinal cord. Change in mentation indicates a cerebral or brainstem disorder. If the brainstem is involved, cranial nerve deficits and ataxia might be observed. Always consider metabolic disorders, such as hepatic encephalopathy, as a potential cause of change in mentation. ***Important:*** In the evaluation of horses with acute neurologic disorders, it is important to consider rabies. Weakness without ataxia causes a support problem and is characteristic of neuromuscular or lower motor neuron disease.
- The *third* goal is to be able to complete the examination and provide reasonable diagnostics and therapeutics without further bodily injury to the patient and personnel or damage to the facilities.

Condition	Appearance*	Total Protein* (mg/dL)	Total Nucleated Cells* (per µL)	Cytologic Findings
Normal	Clear, colorless	40-90 (some labs up to 100 or 120)	0-5	All mononuclear cells
Blood contamination	Red streaks of blood admixed	May be increased and not representative of actual level	May be increased and not representative of actual level	Increased percentage of neutrophils in proportion with peripheral blood
Bacterial infection	Yellow, orange, or red; often turbid	>100	>50 (often severely increased)	Primarily neutrophils or mixed pleocytosis (neutrophils + monocytes and macrophages)
Viral infection	Clear and colorless to yellow and slightly turbid	100-200	Normal to increased	Predominantly lymphocytes, although neutrophilic component possible
†Hemorrhage or trauma	Uniformly red‡ or yellow§	>100	Variable	Macrophages with erythrophagia and neutrophils
Fungal infection	Clear to yellow	100-200	>100	Mixed (neutrophils, monocytes, and macrophages)
Protozoal infection¶	Clear to yellow	40-200	0-40	Mixed macrophages, lymphocytes, and neutrophils

Table 22-1   Correlation of Cerebrospinal Fluid Parameters and Central Nervous System Disorders

*Characteristic finding but may vary.
†May be neutrophilic with severe and/or chronic disease.
‡Recent hemorrhage.
§Past hemorrhage.
¶Less than 15% of horses with equine protozoal myeloencephalitis have abnormal values.

Gait Evaluation

Unwilling or Unable?

Is the horse unwilling or unable? This is the first question to be answered in the examination of a horse with a gait abnormality. This is especially true when the horse is short-strided or does not support its weight on a limb. A loss of support from a femoral or radial nerve injury mimics a severe, painful disorder causing a reluctance to bear weight.

Patterns

With experience, clinicians recognize specific "patterns" in abnormal gaits that suggest the anatomic diagnosis. These patterns have five components: two qualities of paresis (weakness) and three qualities of ataxia (incoordination).

Paresis

In neurologic terms, paresis means deficiency in generation of gait or the ability to support weight. This definition covers the two qualities of paresis: lower motor neuron and upper motor neuron.

Lower motor neuron (LMN) paresis reflects degrees of difficulty in supporting weight and varies from a slightly shortened stride (easily mistaken for musculoskeletal lameness) to complete inability to support weight, which leads to collapse of the limb whenever weight is placed on it.

Upper motor neuron (UMN) paresis causes a delay in the onset of protraction, the swing phase of the gait. Usually the stride is longer than normal. Stiffness (spasticity) might be apparent in the stride. The UMN comprises numerous neuronal systems that initiate the gait through LMN recruitment and modulate muscle tone for normal posture and smooth locomotor function. In domestic animals, most of these neuronal cell bodies are located in the pons and medulla, and their processes descend the spinal cord in the lateral and ventral funiculi. Most lesions affecting these components of the UMN also affect the general proprioceptive sensory system and cause ataxia because the involved tracts are adjacent to each other.

Ataxia

Ataxia has three qualities that reflect the functional system involved: general proprioception, the vestibular system, and the cerebellum.

General Proprioceptive Ataxia

The general proprioceptive (GP) sensory system has its dendritic zones in specialized receptors in muscles, tendons, and joints. The GP system is responsible for "informing" the CNS of the degree of muscle contraction (tone) at any time. It tells the CNS where the animal's "parts" are in space at any instant. Loss of this system affects the gait by contributing to the delay in the onset of protraction. Loss also results in excessive adduction (swinging in) or abduction (swinging out) of the limb, and occasionally overflexion in the swing phase, scuffing/dragging of the hoof, and knuckling or standing on the dorsal aspect of the hoof.

The GP system and the UMN are affected by the same lesions because of their proximity.

Differentiation of UMN and GP signs is difficult and unnecessary.

Horses with UMN-GP deficits from a lesion anywhere between C1 and C6 have a tendency to overreach at the end of protraction; the result is a floating motion to the stride. This is referred to as a "UMN-GP deficit" because one does not know which system is responsible for preventing this action normally and because that differentiation is unnecessary to make the segmental anatomic diagnosis.

Neurologists do not try to differentiate conscious (cerebral) and unconscious (cerebellar) GP pathways. If an individual stands on the dorsal aspect of its digits, is this an LMN, UMN, conscious GP, or unconscious GP deficit? One cannot differentiate the latter three and must use other features of the examination to determine whether the deficit is LMN.

Vestibular (Special Proprioceptive) Ataxia

Vestibular ataxia reflects the loss of orientation of the head with the eyes, trunk, and limbs—a loss of balance. Lesions in this system cause the patient to lean, drift, or fall to one side, usually the side of the lesion. Vestibular ataxia generally is accompanied by a head tilt to that side and sometimes abnormal nystagmus.

These same signs result from a lesion in any part of the vestibular system: peripheral or central. The difference is in the other clinical signs exhibited by the patient. A horse with only vestibular ataxia and facial paralysis most likely has peripheral vestibular disease. These same signs with UMN-GP deficits and altered mentation indicate the presence of a central (brainstem) lesion.

Cerebellar Ataxia

Individuals with cerebellar disorders classically have dysmetria characterized by sudden bursts of motor activity with significant overflexion on protraction-hypermetria. This is accompanied by a stiff-spastic quality to the movement. The horse is unusual in that spasticity is much more pronounced than hypermetria. This is most obvious in the thoracic limbs, which are thrown forward on protraction with considerable extension of the limbs. This spastic overreaching movement differs in its degree and abruptness from the overreaching-floating that occurs with UMN-GP disorders. The cerebellum has several vestibular components, so there usually is some loss of balance. When the individual runs, it often swings its head and neck side to side with a stiff appearance. The presence of an obvious head tremor that might worsen with intention or loss of menace response also helps with the anatomic diagnosis.

Acute Ataxia
Evaluation and Management of Neurologic Conditions in Weanlings and Adult Horses

Ataxia (incoordination) results from loss of the ability to sense the position of the limbs in space. The most common type of ataxia in horses is general proprioceptive ataxia as a result of spinal cord disease.

Physical Examination
- Proceed with caution to avoid injury to the patient and personnel. An open grassy area with a slight incline is ideal.
- Observe the patient for inappropriate circumduction, adduction, or abduction of the limbs; base-wide stance; delay in protraction of the limbs; scuffing or abnormal wear of the hooves; and striking one limb with another. Tight circles, backing, and serpentines often exaggerate these deficits. The walk is the best gait to evaluate.
- Careful examination of the cranial nerves is helpful. If abnormalities are present, neuroanatomic localization shifts from spinal cord to brainstem, and differential diagnoses change.
- Is there a significant change in mentation (obtundation to stupor)? If so, neuroanatomic localization is most likely brainstem or forebrain.

Equine Protozoal Myeloencephalitis
- Equine protozoal myeloencephalitis (EPM) can manifest as acute onset of ataxia with, or more commonly, without cranial nerve deficits (vestibular disturbance, facial paresis, and dysphagia are the most recognizable cranial nerve deficits).

Signalment
- EPM can affect adults of any age; however, reportedly it is most common among horses between 15 months and 4 years of age. EPM is rarely diagnosed among individuals younger than 1 year.
- EPM appears to affect performance horses more frequently, seems more prevalent in the eastern United States, and is less common in the winter. *Rule out other common causes of CNS disease* by history, season of year, signalment, prevalence of CNS diseases in the area, appropriate diagnostic tests (survey cervical radiographs, myelography, guttural pouch endoscopy), and CSF evaluation when indicated. Response to therapy is a valuable diagnostic test for EPM.
- Confirm exposure to *Sarcocystis neurona,* the causative agent in most cases, as described under laboratory testing (see p. 344). (Also see Neosporosis (see p. 352); the occasional case of EPM is caused by *Neospora hughesi* rather than *S. neurona.*)

Clinical Signs (Acute Onset)
- Depression, if present, often serves to separate EPM from many other spinal cord diseases.
- Ataxia (often asymmetric) can progress to recumbency. In some cases the ataxia involves all four limbs and is symmetric, and then it is almost impossible at clinical examination to differentiate EPM from equine degenerative myeloencephalopathy (EDM) or cervical vertebral compressive myelopathy (CVCM).
- Trembling or muscle atrophy of a limb can be mild to severe (rare) and indicates LMN involvement. Trembling can be seen with acute disease, whereas noticeable atrophy requires 10 days or more.
- Head tilt and vestibular ataxia: Rule out temporohyoid osteoarthropathy (THO) with an endoscopic examination of guttural pouches.

- Facial paralysis: same as previous
- Difficulty swallowing: See Dysphagia, p. 375.
- Weak tongue tone, unilateral tongue muscle atrophy, tongue muscle fasciculations
- Dragging one or more limbs
- Blindness, which is rare but can occur
- Seizures: can occur as the only clinical sign
- Leaning or turning to one side without a head tilt (forebrain lesion)

Differential Diagnoses

- EPM can affect any part of the CNS—locally, regionally, or multifocally. Therefore, EPM can mimic virtually any other infectious or noninfectious neurologic disease, including cervical vertebral compressive myelopathy, equine degenerative myeloencephalopathy, equine herpesvirus 1, West Nile virus, neuroborreliosis, and rabies.

Diagnosis

- Definitive diagnosis can only be accomplished via post-mortem examination. Antemortem diagnosis is always presumptive and is most successful if three criteria are met:
  - Presence of compatable neurologic signs, history, and signalment
  - Exclusion of other likely differential diagnoses
  - Confirmation of exposure to the parasite via immuno-logic testing (see Laboratory Testing, later)
  - Confirmation of intrathecal antibodies

Laboratory Testing: Immunologic Findings

A serum or CSF sample or both can be sent to one of the following:

- Equine Diagnostic Solutions (EDS), LLC, (859-288-5255), 1501 Bull Lea Rd. Suite 104, Lexington, KY 40511. EDS offers antibody testing (SAG 2, 4/3 enzyme-linked immuno-sorbent assay [ELISA] and Western blot [WB]) on serum and CSF, as well as polymerase chain reaction (PCR) on CSF. The serum : CSF titer ratio using SAG 2, 4/3 ELISAs currently appears to be the most specific test for the diagnosis of EPM. The lower the serum : CSF ratio (<100:1 is the ratio considered positive for EPM), the more likely is the diagnosis of EPM. Note that PCR testing performed at any lab is a very insensitive diagnostic test for EPM and is *not* recommended.
- University of California, Davis, (530-752-7373), VMTH, Immunology/Virology Laboratory, 1 Garrod Dr. Room 1023, Davis, CA 95616. This lab offers antibody testing (indirect fluorescent antibody test [IFAT] and WB) on serum and CSF.
- Michigan State University Diagnostic Center for Population and Animal Health (DCPAH), (517-353-1683), 4125 Beaumont Road, Lansing, MI 48910. The DCPAH offers antibody testing (WB and IFAT) and PCR on serum and CSF.
- Neogen Corporation (800-477-8201) offers WB testing on serum and CSF.

- IDEXX Laboratories (800-621-8378) offers WB testing on serum and CSF.
- Pathogenes, Inc. (352-591-3221), 15471 NW 112th Ave, Reddick, FL 32686. This lab offers PCR and SAG-1, 5, and 6 ELISA antibody testing on serum and CSF.

A negative result of a serum or CSF antibody test generally has a very good negative predictive value as long as a test with high sensitivity (EDS) is used. However, several EPM-confirmed horses have had negative or very low positive serum test results using various tests, including the IFAT and SAG-ELISAs. The most common type of case to have a false-negative result is the acutely affected horse that might not have had time to seroconvert. Therefore, if clinical signs point toward EPM but initial test results are negative, a second test should be submitted 7 to 14 days after the first. A positive result on the second test is strong evidence of infection, whereas a negative result is strong evidence that EPM is not the cause of disease. In suspect cases with negative blood results, CSF analysis is recommended, as several EPM-confirmed horses have had detectable CSF titers despite negative serum results. Routine CSF cytology is often normal, although a mild to moderate pleocytosis, with a higher percentage of mononuclear cells than neutrophils occurs in some cases. If the WBCs are increased, then CSF protein is also likely to be increased.

Interpretation of positive results is more challenging. Positive serum antibody tests indicate exposure to the organism but do not have a strong predictive value for disease. Positive CSF tests are 30% more likely to predict disease but false-positive tests remain problematic; blood contamination of CSF or natural diffusion of antibodies across the blood-brain barrier lowers the positive predictive value of the CSF test for EPM.

Whenever possible, testing both serum and CSF is recommended so that an antibody ratio can be determined. Measurement of a ratio takes normal diffusion of antibodies into account and a positive result indicates proportionately higher antibody levels in CSF compared with serum, which is suggestive of the intrathecal antibody production that accompanies infection.

Treatment

- Treatment should be initiated immediately (before obtaining immunologic test results) for horses that develop acute or rapidly progressive signs that are compatible with EPM.

◗❯ WHAT TO DO

Equine Protozoal Myeloencephalitis

- Antiprotozoal therapy options:
  - Ponazuril, 5 or 10 mg/kg PO q24h for at least 28 days; the 5-mg/kg dosage that is approved by the Food and Drug Administration (FDA) for use in horses. This is best administered with 1 oz of corn oil.
  - Sulfadiazine (SDZ), 20 mg/kg PO q24h for at least 90 days, and
  - Pyrimethamine (PYR), 1 mg/kg orally q24h for at least 90 days (do not mix with feed or administer at time of feeding). The SDZ/PYR combination is available as an FDA-approved treatment

product. SDZ/PYR is best absorbed when not administered on a full stomach. This combination is normally administered for 3 to 6 months. Long-term use of SDZ/PYR is *not* considered safe in pregnant mares because of increased risk of fetal malformation and blood dyscrasia.
- Diclazuril, 1 mg/kg PO q24h for at least 28 days (FDA approved).
- Anti-inflammatory therapy:
  - Short-term corticosteroid treatment is most useful in acute, severe cases. Start with 0.05 to 0.2 mg/kg dexamethasone and perform a quick taper over 3 to 5 days. Long-term corticosteroid treatment might cause immunosuppression.
  - Flunixin meglumine 0.5 to 1.1 mg/kg q12 to 24h.

Clinical Note: If owners are willing and EPM is highly likely to be a cause of the neurologic signs, the use of ponazuril or diclazuril at higher than labeled dose with or without PYR is recommended for the treatment of EPM; the goal is to kill the organism as quickly as possible to decrease neuronal loss and relapse rates. A 2-mg/kg dosage of PYR for 1 to 2 weeks and/or a loading dose of ponazuril or diclazuril are often recommended. Loading doses of ponazuril or diclazuril generally consist of a 3× dose on day 1 (+/− day 2) or a 2× dose for 5 to 7 days. *These regimens would be extra-label use of FDA-approved drugs, and veterinarians must consider this in their prescribing practices.*

An additional combination treatment of decoquinate and levamisole (0.5 mg/kg decoquinate plus 1 mg/kg levamisole given orally q24h for 10 days) is offered by a compounding pharmacy. This combination is not FDA-approved at this writing. Decoquinate has been shown to have very high in vitro activity against *S. neurona*.

⬤▶ WHAT NOT TO DO

Equine Protozoal Myeloencephalitis
- Do *not* treat pregnant mares with SDZ and/or PYR for extended periods or at increased doses (>2 months).

Supportive Therapy for EPM
- Feed patients that cannot eat or drink with gruel at least twice a day by indwelling stomach tube or repeated nasogastric intubation (see Chapter 18, p. 157).
- Administer appropriate broad-spectrum antimicrobial therapy (penicillin + gentamicin + metronidazole or ceftiofur + metronidazole or TMS + metronidazole or chloramphenicol) if aspiration pneumonia is evident.
- Apply ophthalmic ointment 4 times a day to the eyes of patients with facial paralysis.
- Perform partial tarsorrhaphy if a corneal ulcer is already present (see Chapter 23, p. 394).
  - Corneal ulcers that develop as a result of facial nerve paralysis can be refractory to treatment.
- Consider administering levamisole, 1 to 2 mg/kg PO q24h, for 5 days followed by once weekly administration or EqStim[5] (4 to 5 mL on days 1, 3, 7, and weekly) as an immune modulator.

[5]EqStim 9 (Neogen Corp., 944 Nandino Blvd, Lexington, KY, 40511-12050).

- Administer vitamin E, 2000 to 10,000 units/day in feed, for nonspecific antioxidant properties.

Prognosis
- Prognosis is fair for return to function for horses receiving early and appropriate treatment.
- There should be a noticeable response within 2 to 5 weeks of treatment for acute-onset cases.

Cervical Vertebral Compressive Myelopathy ("Wobblers")
Horses with CVCM might be presented for emergency treatment because of a traumatic event that acutely worsens the underlying compressive disease.

Signalment
- Often a young, rapidly growing horse with a history of clumsiness, which suggests a preexisting condition.
- Trauma can exacerbate clinical signs to the point of severe ataxia or recumbency.
- Males are more commonly affected.
- "Wobblers" caused by severe osteoarthrosis is most common in older adults; however, younger horses can also be affected.
- Most common in Thoroughbred, Warmblood, and Tennessee Walking Horses.
  - Warmbloods are generally older at onset of signs than are other breeds.
- Horses with a history of racing or English performance are significantly more likely to be affected than those used for Western/pleasure activities in one study.

Clinical Signs
- Symmetric ataxia (in approximately 65% of cases) involves all four limbs. Asymmetry might be seen and does not preclude this condition. Deficits in the thoracic limbs might be subtle and are often a grade less severe than those in the pelvic limbs.
- Most patients are bright and alert with no depression.
- No cranial nerve deficits occur unless resulting from trauma.
- Neck pain is inconsistent but cervical hyperesthesia may be seen in nearly one half of cases; abnormal resistance to neck flexion is often seen in horses with osteoarthrosis. Horses (generally ages 5 and up) with caudal cervical osteoarthritis might be very resistant to elevation of the head and neck, lateral bending of the neck, or even lowering the neck.
- C6-T1 lesions often cause neck stiffness and more pronounced forelimb signs.
- Only rarely is focal muscle atrophy or anesthesia detected. Hyperesthesia of the affected site might also be noted.

Diagnosis
Survey radiographs might suggest CVCM characteristics: vertebral canal stenosis (minimum intravertebral sagittal diameter ratio <0.52 at C2-C6 and <0.56 at C7, determined

CNS

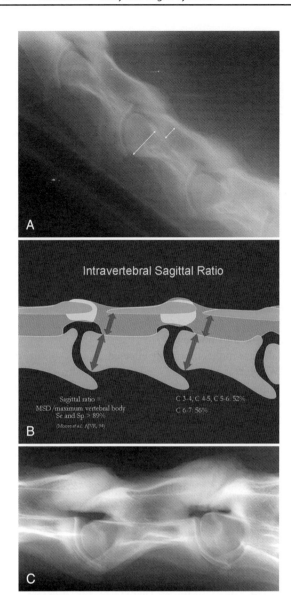

Figure 22-3 **A,** Cervical radiograph demonstrating areas of measurement for intravertebral sagittal ratios. **B,** Schematic drawing of the cervical vertebrae illustrating measurement of intravertebral sagittal ratio *(top red arrow,* measurement of spinal canal, divided by vertebral body, *bottom red arrow).* Normal ratio values are given. ***Note:*** The greater the number of vertebrae with abnormal ratios or the more abnormal any single ratio, the greater the accuracy of the test. **C,** Cervical radiographs of caudal C4, C5, and rostral C6. At C5-6 there is evidence of severe osteoarthropathy of the dorsal facets and malalignment of the vertebral bodies. **(B** photo courtesy Dr. J. van Biervliet.)

by comparing the narrowest dorsal-ventral measurement of the cranial vertebral canal with the widest dorsal-ventral measurement of the corresponding cranial vertebral body (Fig. 22-3, *A*). *As the ratio becomes <0.49 or if multiple vertebrae are abnormal, the accuracy of the test increases (Fig. 22-3, B).* Osteoarthritis of the articular processes, malalignment, and a ski jump appearance of the dorsocaudal vertebral body are also highly suggestive of the disease (Fig. 22-3, *C*).

- Obtain definitive diagnosis through myelographic demonstration of impingement on the spinal cord (>50% impingement of the dorsal column). *The 50% rule does not have a high specificity unless it is at C6-7 or it is on a mildly flexed or nonflexed view.* (**Note:** Make sure that 240-mg iodine

per milliliter iohexol is used for the myelogram. Large volumes of iohexol have been associated with seizures during recovery after a myelogram.)
- CSF usually is normal.

Differential Diagnoses
- EPM
- EDM
- Cervical trauma
- Space-occupying mass (spinal extradural hematoma, abscess, neoplasia)
  - ***Practice Tip:*** *Spinal extradural hematomas generally occur at C6-7 with an acute onset of tetra-ataxia and paresis without a known history of trauma. Horses with spinal hematomas frequently are clinically painful.*
- Cervical osteoarthrosis without cord compression—radiographic appearance of osteoarthritis at C5-6 and C6-7 is common in middle-aged to older horses. Enlargement of the joint capsules, changes in joint space, and synovial cysts can also occur. Some affected horses have neck pain, hypo- or hyperalgesia of the lower neck, and a gait abnormality that is difficult to characterize as lameness versus ataxia (see Chapter 21, p. 299).

➤➤ WHAT TO DO

Cervical Vertebral Compressive Myelopathy
- Dexamethasone, 0.1 to 0.2 mg/kg IV once per day for 1 to 2 days might provide transient improvement in cases made abruptly worse by trauma.
- Horses with cervical osteoarthrosis and clinical signs of cervical pain, forelimb lameness, and mild ataxia might show improvement (often for months) after ultrasound-guided intraarticular injection of the affected cervical synovial intervertebral articulations with corticosteroids—triamcinolone (8 mg) or methylprednisolone acetate (40 mg) (see Chapter 21, p. 299).
- Long-term dietary and exercise restrictions can help stop the progression of the disease in some young horses < 18 months of age. This technique is generally not successful for horses that have attained their approximate adult height.
- As for any traumatic CNS injury, antioxidant therapy (vitamin E, ubiquinone [coenzyme Q_{10}], thiamine) could be administered, although efficacy is unproven.
- Surgical arthrodesis benefits many patients but might not result in complete recovery: determination is made by age of the horse, intended use, neurologic status, number of vertebrae involved, myelographic findings, and duration of clinical signs.

Prognosis
- Prognosis is variable, depending on the degree of compression, number and location of compressed sites, age of the patient, severity of signs, and elected treatment.

Complications Following Myelography
Complications include seizures, blindness, prolonged recumbency, fever, and neck pain. These complications are not common other than fever, but when they occur, they are emergencies.

●›› WHAT TO DO

Seizures and/or Blindness (Cortical)

- Treat with anti-inflammatory drugs (dexamethasone, 0.1 mg/kg) and anticonvulsant sedatives (diazepam and/or phenobarbital intravenously) if seizure activity or agitation from blindness is present.

●›› WHAT TO DO

Horses That Cannot Rise

- Dexamethasone at 0.1 to 0.2 mg/kg can be given, and a lift sling can be used (see Fig. 37-5, p. 640). *Note:* Polysaccharide storage myopathy should be considered for Draft horses or Warmbloods that cannot rise and require treatment (see p. 360).

●›› WHAT TO DO

Fever and Neck Pain from Nonseptic Meningitis

- This is *not* an unusual complication; alert owner of risk before myelography procedure.
- Treat with nonsteroidal anti-inflammatory drugs (NSAIDs) or 0.05 mg/kg dexamethasone.

Neuroborreliosis

- Neuroborreliosis is caused by *Borrelia burgdorferi.*
- It may cause ataxia, muscle atrophy (symmetric or asymmetric), and less commonly, cranial nerve deficits.
- Diagnosis is based upon a rule-out of other diseases, evidence of intrathecal production of *B. burgdorferi* antibodies and most often a lymphocytic pleocytosis of the CSF. PCR for the organism in the CSF may sometimes be positive.
- Treatment is either intravenous tetracycline (6.6 mg/kg IV q12h) or minocycline 4 mg/kg PO q 12h.

●›› WHAT NOT TO DO

Neuroborreliosis

- Continuous treatment with oxytetracycline without monitoring serum creatinine

Equine Herpesvirus 1 Myeloencephalopathy

- Equine herpesvirus 1 (EHV-1), or rhinopneumonitis, causes respiratory disease and abortion, as well as neurologic disease. The neurologic form occurs sporadically, often as a sequela to one of the other two forms. *Important:* EHV-1 myeloencephalopathy is a reportable disease in most if not all states. When EHV-1 infection is suspected, immediately contact the state veterinarian or equivalent health official for further instructions regarding farm management and quarantine.

Signalment

- It is most common in adults >3 years of age (rarely occurs in foals).
- It is most common at the race track, breeding farm, boarding stable, or training facility.
- Often multiple cases occur on the same farm within a short time period; isolated cases have been reported.
- Although most cases seem to occur in January to July, no seasonality has been proven.

Clinical Signs

- Abrupt onset of (usually) symmetric ataxia and paresis that might progress rapidly to recumbency.
- Neurologic deficit of pelvic limbs is worse than thoracic limbs in most cases.
- Urinary bladder paralysis with urine dribbling is a common clinical sign.
- Hypotonic tail, decreased anal tone, and fecal retention occur in some cases.
- Horses rarely have vestibular signs and/or other cranial nerve deficits.
- Fever precedes and often then recurs at the same time as neurologic signs; biphasic fever. Individuals without neurologic signs on the same farm might have fevers. Initial fever generally occurs 1 to 3 days after infection, might subside, and then might return 5 to 7 days later around the time of neurologic signs. *Practice Tip: some horses are afebrile when neurologic signs are noted, and absence of fever is not a reason to rule out EHV-1 myeloencephalopathy!*

Differential Diagnoses

- For multiple horses with CNS signs and/or recumbency, consider the following:
  - Leukoencephalomalacia
  - Grass staggers
  - Ionophore toxicosis
  - Botulism
  - Viral encephalitis
  - Toxic hepatic failure
- For horses with fever and CNS signs, consider the following:
  - Viral encephalitis
  - Anaplasmosis

Diagnosis

- In the classic presentation, one or more horses from the same farm with a history of respiratory disease acutely develop fevers, pelvic limb ataxia, and bladder paralysis.
- In some outbreaks, there are no obvious respiratory signs.
- Hematology and serum biochemistry profile usually are unremarkable.
- CSF generally has an increased protein level with few nucleated cells (albuminocytologic dissociation). The CSF might be yellow (xanthochromia).
- PCR on whole blood and nasal swabs is the preferred antemortem test. Immunohistochemical (IHC) findings demonstrating herpes antigen in the CNS vascular endothelium or PCR on nervous tissues is the preferred postmortem test.
- PCR tests can distinguish between the "neuropathogenic" and "non-neuropathogenic" strains of EHV-1, which vary

by a single point mutation. Although outbreaks are more commonly associated with the "neuropathogenic" strain, "non-neuropathogenic" is a misnomer because this strain can also cause severe neurologic disease and neurologic outbreaks. *Cases and outbreaks of EHV-1 should be managed the same regardless of which strain is identified.*

- Fourfold increase in serum neutralization titer in samples drawn 10 days apart is highly suggestive of EHV-1 infection, but it is not always present in neurologically affected horses.

Treatment

The mainstay of treatment for EHV-1 myeloencephalopathy is supportive care. Anti-inflammatory and antithrombotic drugs are frequently used but are of uncertain benefit. Specific antiviral treatments are available, but their efficacy has not been definitively proven.

● WHAT TO DO

EHV-1 Myeloencephalopathy

- For cases with dysuria and bladder distention:
  - Perform urinary bladder catheterization and drainage 3 or 4 times per day in cases with dysuria and bladder distention.
  - Administer bethanechol (compounded), 0.04 mg/kg SQ q8h, to manage bladder distention. Injectable bethanechol is expensive and difficult to obtain and therefore is not an option in some cases. Bethanechol tablets for oral administration, 0.2 to 0.4 mg/kg PO q8 to 12h, are not as expensive but are not as effective as the parenteral product. Bethanechol powder can be easily dissolved and filtered through a 0.5-μm filter for intravenous or subcutaneous injection.
  - Administer antibiotics for cystitis, which is unavoidable with frequent or indwelling catheterization.
    - Trimethoprim-sulfamethoxazole, 30 mg/kg PO q12h, or ceftiofur, 2.2 mg/kg IV q12h.
    - Urine culture is recommended because resistant infections can develop despite antibiotic therapy. Enrofloxacin, 7.5 mg/kg PO or 5 to 7.5 mg/kg IV q24h, could eventually be needed.
- The potent anti-inflammatory effects of short-term (1 to 2 days) therapy with dexamethasone, 0.1 to 0.2 mg/kg IV, might prove lifesaving to a recumbent or rapidly progressing, nearly recumbent patient. Corticosteroids should be used only in patients with rapid progression of signs or acute recumbency. Don't administer steroids unless needed, *and* don't administer them too late!
- Valacyclovir, 20 to 40 mg/kg PO q8h. Whether antiviral therapy with valacyclovir improves the prognosis or shortens the recovery time is not clear. Valacyclovir might be of greater benefit in the early management of EHV-1 infection before neurologic signs develop. Ganciclovir, 2.5 mg/kg q8 to 12h IV, may be more efficacious.
- Aspirin 90 to 120 grains PO every other day and/or clopidogrel, 4 mg/kg PO as a loading dose followed by 2 mg/kg PO q24h might decrease vascular thrombosis.
- Supportive care: Provide protective leg wraps, intravenous or oral fluids to maintain hydration, topical care of decubital ulcers, and avoidance of urine scalding. Fecal evacuation, laxative treatment, and feeding low-residue diets (pellets) are recommended for patients with fecal incontinence (approximately 10% of cases).

- Use of a sling (Anderson or Davis quick lift sling; see Chapter 37, pp. 638 and 640) is recommended for recumbent horses. Horses that sustain pressure sores in the sling can be supported in a pool or, as a last resort and only if the horse is very calm, in a bovine float tank.

●〉 WHAT NOT TO DO

EHV-1 Myeloencephalopathy

- *Do not* overhydrate the horse, especially if there is bladder dysfunction.
- *Do not* forget to check on reportable disease status in your state/country.
- *Do not* forget to implement appropriate biosecurity measures!

Prognosis

- Prognosis is highly variable. Many individuals make a full recovery; others are left with residual deficits; some are euthanized because of paralysis and secondary complications. Nursing care can be very intensive, and full recovery can take months. Determining the prognosis at the beginning of the clinical course often is difficult, although *those that rapidly become recumbent rarely return to normal function.* Bladder dysfunction is the last clinical problem to resolve in many cases.

Management of an Outbreak

- Contact the state veterinarian ASAP to report suspicious cases.
- Quarantine the facility for at least 21 to 28 days after confirming the last case (infected/febrile horse).
- Stop movement of horses within the facility to avoid spread of the virus.
- Assign specific personnel to care for affected horses; these employees should not handle healthy horses.
- Monitor temperature q12h of all at-risk horses to detect a fever that generally precedes neurologic disease by 2 to 8 days. Maintain strict isolation of all febrile horses. It is also important that personnel taking the temperatures wear separate gowns and gloves for each horse and avoid contact with respiratory secretions. Valacyclovir (20 to 40 mg/kg 2 to 3 times daily for 5 days) might be most useful in horses with early fever.
- Use PCR testing of blood and nasal secretions to track infections.
- Steam cleaning and phenol- or iodophor-based disinfectants kill the virus.
- Vaccination in the face of an outbreak is of unknown benefit. Vaccination after clinical signs have resolved is recommended.
- There is no reported recurrence of the neurologic syndrome in a patient that has recovered from this disease.
- Individuals that have to be moved into a stable that has had EHV-1 should be vaccinated, but the vaccines might not protect against the neurologic form of EHV.
- Horses with suspected EHV-1 infection sent to referral hospitals should be isolated at the hospital.

West Nile Virus

Note: Although West Nile virus (WNV) is a viral encephalitic disease, it is listed under ataxia because the spinal cord signs are often more pronounced than the cerebral signs, which is dissimilar to eastern equine encephalitis (EEE).

Epidemiology

- WNV is a mosquito-borne flavivirus that affects horses in most areas of North America from late summer into fall in the northern half of the continent and nearly year-round in the southern-most parts. Dying birds usually precede equine outbreaks. Five percent to 10% of infected horses exhibit clinical signs, with 90% of cases being >1 year of age and most severe cases are >3 years of age.

Clinical Signs

- Ataxia (often more severe in the hind legs) and paresis are the most consistent signs. Although general proprioceptive (spinal) ataxia is most common, vestibular or cerebellar ataxia might also be seen.
- Fasciculations of facial and neck muscles are common and occur in approximately half of the cases.
- Hyperesthesia and hyperexcitability might be evident.
- Fever is only found at examination in 50% of the cases, although most probably have fever at some point in the disease process.
- Cortical signs are not as consistent with WNV as with EEE.
- Blindness (only occasionally) occurs.
- Stupor, anorexia, and lethargy are variable.
- Cranial nerve signs occur in a low percentage of cases.
- Approximately 25% to 30% of cases with neurologic signs become recumbent, and these have a poor prognosis for recovery.

Diagnosis

- Suspicion is based on geographic location, season of the year, history of birds dying with confirmed WNV, and clinical signs. See United States Department of Agriculture (USDA) monitoring and disease surveillance website www.aphis.usda.gov/vs/nahss/equine/index.htm for incidence of infectious diseases.
- Vaccination history is important because most cases occur in unvaccinated or improperly vaccinated horses.
- Serologic tests that measure immunoglobulin G (IgG) can be confounded by previous vaccination or exposure. Immunoglobulin M (IgM) capture ELISA is the most helpful test to identify horses with recent infection and has a reported sensitivity of 92% and specificity of 99%. However, a low percentage of clinically infected horses could be negative. There is no benefit to testing CSF over serum because sensitivity and specificity are identical.
- About 75% of cases have abnormal CSF: lymphocytic pleocytosis and increased protein occur in many, and xanthochromia occurs in about 20% of cases.

- Seek virus isolation, PCR analysis, or immunohistochemistry (sensitivity not 100%) of brain tissue to confirm disease in a euthanized horse.

● WHAT TO DO

West Nile Virus

- WNV antibody is commercially available[6] and is recommended in early cases based on evidence from human and rodent trials.
- Supportive care: provide fluids and nursing care, and maintain horse on good footing in a safe environment.
- Use NSAIDs for mild cases.
- For rapidly progressive or recumbent horses, treatment might include dexamethasone, 0.1 to 0.2 mg/kg q24h IV, and/or mannitol, 0.5 to 2 g/kg IV.
- Recumbent horses can be placed in a sling.

Prognosis

- Prognosis is variable, but apparent complete recovery occurs in approximately 60% of cases in the United States. Mortality rate has been reported at 28% to 33%.
- Affected horses either become rapidly recumbent or stabilize in 72 to 96 hours. Recumbent horses rarely recover enough to be usable.

Prevention

- Vaccines[7] are available and should be used!
- Provide mosquito control.

"Sidewinder" Syndrome

- "Sidewinder" syndrome occurs in older horses (usually late teens into twenties). Some cases appear to be caused by EPM, whereas other cases have no identifiable cause. Horses that develop this syndrome have an acute onset of an abnormal pelvic limb gait with relatively normal thoracic limb gait.

Clinical Signs

- Hindquarters are consistently shifted to one side of the horse's body so that the horse appears to be "crabwalking" or walking on 3 tracks (e.g., if shifted to the left, the left pelvic limb is placed laterally to the left thoracic limb, the right pelvic limb is placed in line with the left thoracic limb, and the right thoracic limb is on its own track).
- Hindquarters are shifted to one side regardless of whether the horse is standing or walking.
- Severely affected horses sometimes spin/circle in place, with their hindquarters "listing" to one side, and their thoracic limbs moving in a compensatory manner.
- The pelvic limbs show varying degrees of paresis and proprioceptive deficits; in some cases, there is no clinical evidence of ataxia.

---

[6]Lake Immunogenics, Inc., 348 Berg Road, Ontario, New York, 14519.
[7]Although vaccines are not approved for pregnant mares, adverse effects in pregnant mares have not been reported.

Diagnosis

- Because this is a descriptive syndrome, clinical signs allow diagnosis. Horses should be tested for EPM (see p. 344). Other diagnostic tests (such as nuclear scintigraphy and ultrasonography) to look for evidence of traumatic injury to the pelvis or tuber coxae have generally been unrewarding; a small number of cases have been found to have tuber coxae injury. Two horses have had lymphocytic neuritis (radiculitis) involving the thoracolumbar nerves. Neuroborreliosis should be considered as a possible cause in areas endemic for Lyme disease, although the association of a "sidewinder" and Lyme disease has not been confirmed.

●》 WHAT TO DO

"Sidewinder" Syndrome

- Treat for EPM if test results are positive.
- Anti-inflammatory medication (phenylbutazone, 2.2 mg/kg IV or PO q12h or flunixin meglumine, 0.5 to 1 mg/kg IV or PO q12 to 24h) rarely leads to clinical improvement. Severe cases might benefit from short tapering courses of dexamethasone (starting at 0.1 mg/kg, reducing the dose by 25% every 1 to 2 days).
- Minocycline, 4 mg/kg PO q12h and pregabalin, 2-4 mg/kg PO q8-12h, may be useful in treating Lyme disease or neuritis without an etiologic diagnosis.
- Spontaneous improvement might occur regardless of treatment but often is not sustained.

Prognosis

- Horses that are positive for EPM have a fair to guarded prognosis. Horses negative for EPM have a guarded to poor prognosis. Return to normal gait and previous level of work appears to be very unlikely. Some horses stabilize or improve at levels of function compatible with safe pasture turnout. It is not unusual for signs to improve and then worsen weeks to months later, frequently necessitating euthanasia. A definitive cause of the abnormal gait might not be found on postmortem examination.

Vestibular Disease

Clinical Signs

The vestibular system controls balance and maintains orientation of the head, eyes, and trunk.

- Head tilt
- Staggering, leaning, drifting sideways
- Abnormal nystagmus (most frequently with fast phase away from the affected side) observed only in the acute stages of vestibular disease in the horse
- Strabismus, especially ventral strabismus on the affected side when the head is elevated
- Loss of balance exacerbated by blindfolding
- Facial paralysis (cranial nerve VII deficit) might also be seen with peripheral or central vestibular disease.
- Other cranial nerve deficits, such as dysphagia, poor tongue tone, loss of facial sensation, and dropped jaw, can be seen with central vestibular disease.
- History of ear rubbing, head shaking, or difficulty chewing might accompany certain causes of peripheral vestibular disease.

- If severe, recumbency and inability to maintain sternal recumbency might occur
- If recumbent, patient might refuse to be positioned on side opposite the lesion

Vestibular disease can be due to peripheral or central problems. The distinction between a peripheral (outside the brainstem) and central (within the brainstem) lesion is as follows:
- Peripheral
  - Normal mentation
  - No general proprioceptive deficits
  - Normal strength
  - Possible involvement of the seventh cranial nerve
- Central
  - Depression, obtundation, or stupor
  - General proprioceptive deficits
  - Weakness/paresis
  - Possibly multiple cranial nerve involvement (other than cranial nerves VII and VIII)

Occasionally, a horse with a prosencephalic lesion on the ipsilateral side (frequently EPM) has an acute onset of body leaning or head and neck turn (with no head tilt) and drifting to that side.

Differential Diagnosis

- *Cranial trauma* (see Cranial Trauma, p. 368): basilar skull bone fractures are a common cause of central vestibular disease, whereas petrous temporal bone fractures cause peripheral vestibular disease
- *Temporohyoid osteoarthropathy (THO)* with (less common) or without (more common) otitis media and otitis interna: common cause of peripheral vestibular disease, but affected horses might be depressed and develop central signs because of inflammatory extension to dura mater
- *EPM:* common cause of central vestibular disease (see p. 343)

Other Less Common Causes

- Polyneuritis equi (cauda equina syndrome): peripheral vestibular disease
- Space-occupying mass: central vestibular disease
- CNS lymphosarcoma: central vestibular disease
- Encephalitis or encephalopathy: hepatic failure; viral or parasitic (*Halicephalobus*) encephalitis; central vestibular disease
- Lightning strike
- Guttural pouch mycosis with extension to the inner ear: peripheral vestibular disease
- Idiopathic vestibular disease: peripheral vestibular disease
- Cranial cervical lesion: can have vestibular signs with C1 spinal cord lesions

Diagnosis

- Palpate the base of the ear for any signs of pain. Investigate history of difficulty eating or abnormal head placement that might support the diagnosis of THO. Push up on the lingual process of the basihyoid bone in

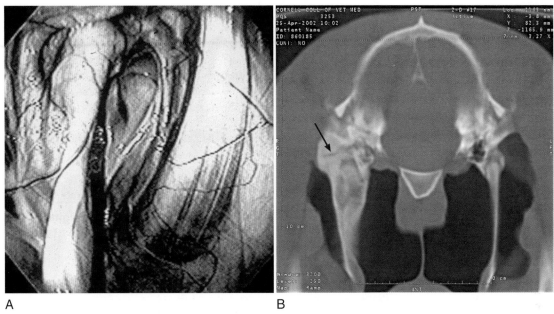

Figure 22-4 A, Temporohyoid osteoarthropathy. Endoscopic examination of the right guttural pouch of a 22-year-old Warmblood with acute facial paralysis and vestibular dysfunction. There is obvious proliferation of the most proximal part of the stylohyoid bone. Attempts at manual manipulation of the hyoid bone during endoscopy did not reveal movement of the stylohyoid bone at the temporohyoid junction, suggesting bony fusion. **B,** Computed tomography scan corresponding to endoscopy seen in part **A.** The right stylohyoid bone is thick and fused to the right temporal bone. Within the callus, there are incomplete fractures *(arrow)*.

the intermandibular space. This bony process should be easily movable in a vertical direction ($\frac{1}{2}$ to 1 inch "bounce").

- **Practice Tip:** *Horses with THO often have a rigid hyoid apparatus with minimal movement of the lingual process.*
- Perform endoscopic evaluation of upper airway and guttural pouch. In the guttural pouch, look for proliferative changes (bulging) of the proximal stylohyoid bone or the temporohyoid joint and lack of movement when external pressure is applied to the hyoid apparatus supporting THO (Fig. 22-4). Mycotic infections in the guttural pouch more commonly affect the vagus nerve but on rare occasion can affect the vestibular nerve if extensive enough to invade surrounding bony structures.
- Obtain skull radiographs: lateral, oblique, and ventrodorsal (most useful) views. Evaluate stylohyoid bones, tympanic bullae, petrous temporal bones, and guttural pouches. Lateral and oblique views might not be very sensitive.
- Use computed tomography (CT), which is excellent for evaluating lesions in this area.
- If the patient is compliant, perform an aural examination and culture of any exudate. Usually these are unrewarding. Few patients have drainage from the ear; those most often have *Staphylococcus aureus* infection. *Streptococcus* and *Actinobacillus* organisms also have been isolated from infected ears, and a rare case of mycotic inner ear infection has been seen.
- Obtain CSF analysis, including an *S. neurona* antibody titer to help rule out EPM. THO, trauma, and a rare case of EHV that causes vestibular signs could have discolored CSF.

◉⟩ WHAT TO DO

Temporohyoid Osteoarthropathy (THO)
- Trimethoprim-sulfamethoxazole, 30 mg/kg PO q12h, or enrofloxacin, 5 mg/kg PO q12h or 7.5 mg/kg q24h, or chloramphenicol, 50 mg/kg PO q6 to 8h, for 2 to 4 weeks. These are effective therapies for many staphylococcal infections in the horse and staphylococcus infection may be a secondary complication in THO.
- Phenylbutazone, 2.2 mg/kg PO once or twice daily, for 7 to 10 days.
- Corticosteroids: dexamethasone, 0.05 to 0.1 mg/kg IV q24h. Judicious use is advised but might be helpful for THO, trauma, or most vestibular diseases in which loss of balance is severe.
- Provide supportive care: *ophthalmic ointment and tarsorrhaphy (this is important; see Chapter 23, p. 394) for patients with facial nerve paralysis,* protective leg wraps, good footing, and easy access to food and water.
- Surgical resection of the ceratohyoid bone is recommended for cases of THO to improve chewing ability and to decrease risk of future fracture.

Prognosis
- Prognosis is fair to good for otitis media-interna.
- Prognosis is fair to good with THO, when clinical signs are caused by fracture of the fused bone; more than 50% have a good response to medical therapy. Unfortunately, it is difficult to predict outcome based on initial assessment. Improvement should be seen within 2 to 4 weeks; prognosis for complete recovery is more guarded but may still occur even after a year.
- Uncontrolled otitis interna or open fractures can progress to meningoencephalitis.
- Prognosis is fair to poor for central vestibular disorders.
- Rare cases of idiopathic vestibular disease resolve without treatment over several days.

Plant-Induced Ataxia

In certain areas of the United States (especially the South), during certain summers (probably associated with environmental conditions and proliferation of mycotoxins), ataxia can occur in one or more horses at pasture when grazing rye grass, Bermuda grass, or fescue grass.

Clinical Signs

- Affected horses usually are adults.
- Ataxia can be severe.
- Head tremors and hypermetria can occur.
- Ataxia occurs more commonly among individuals at pasture than those fed hay.
- Sorghum and Sudan grass and black locust bark also can cause ataxia.
- Distinctive clinical signs in addition to ataxia are as follows:

Sorghum or Sudan Grass	Black Locust Bark
Dribbling urine	Anorexia
Abortion	Depression
Arthrogryposis in utero	Mild colic
Stringhalt-like gait	Irregular heartbeat

●❯ WHAT TO DO

Plant-Induced Ataxia

- No specific therapy exists for mycotoxin, sorghum and Sudan grass, and black locust bark poisoning other than removal from the source of the poison.
- Consider treatment with dimethyl sulfoxide (DMSO), 1 g/kg IV as a 10% solution in saline solution or any isotonic fluid q24h for 3 to 5 days, or dexamethasone, 0.05 to 0.1 mg/kg q24h IV for 1 to 2 days with a tapering dose, or use both treatments.
- Horses affected with pasture-associated (mycotoxin) ataxia often return to normal within 5 days.

Other Causes of Acute-Onset Ataxia That Can Present with Ataxia as the Predominant Clinical Sign

- *Spinal cord trauma*: See p. 371.
- *Extradural hematoma*: Although this might be caused by trauma, it has been observed in several horses that had no history of trauma. The equine patients, all adults, were acutely ataxic and showed minimal improvement in neurologic status over several weeks. The dorsolateral aspect of C6-7 is the most common site for the hematoma. The hematomas are large enough that both sides of the cord are affected, causing tetra-ataxia. Myelograms reveal extradural compression; CSF is discolored in some cases and sometimes has an increase in protein and/or white blood cells. The affected individuals did not respond after several weeks of supportive therapy; the hematoma becomes organized and can have the appearance of a tumor at necropsy. It is possible that improvement might occur with more long-term anti-inflammatory/

antioxidant therapy or surgery; however, with prolonged spinal cord compression, complete recovery is unlikely.
- *Fibrocartilaginous emboli*: Emboli are rare but in adult horses can cause acute nonprogressive asymmetric hemiparesis or tetraparesis and ataxia without evidence of pain. The disease most commonly affects the cervical/thoracic intumescence in horses. Antemortem diagnosis is difficult, although a myelogram might show intramedullary swelling at the site. It is certainly possible that affected horses could improve after 7 to 10 days.

●❯ WHAT TO DO

Cervical Hematoma or Fibrocartilaginous Emboli

Antioxidants and anti-inflammatory drugs are used for suspect cases; however, efficacy is unproven.

- *Equine anaplasmosis* (formerly granulocytic ehrlichiosis; see Chapter 20, p. 283): Affected horses are occasionally ataxic (might rarely become recumbent), depressed, jaundiced, febrile thrombocytopenic, with petechiations. The organism is seen in neutrophils during febrile stages or is detected by PCR.

●❯ WHAT TO DO

Equine Anaplasmosis

- Tetracycline, 6.6 mg/kg q12 to 24h IV

- *Neospora-associated EPM:* The condition looks like *S. neurona* EPM except that the patients more commonly have nerve root signs (pain, hyperesthesia). *Neospora hughesi* does not cross-react serologically with the organism that causes EPM, so affected horses can have negative results on EPM serologic tests that identify antibodies against *S. neurona*. This disease appears to be more common in the western United States and is only occasionally documented in the eastern United States.
  - *Diagnosis:* Serologic tests for *N. hughesi* (IFAT at University of California, Davis—see p. 344)

●❯ WHAT TO DO

Neospora-Associated EPM

Treat as for EPM caused by *S. neurona*.

- *Postanesthetic hemorrhagic myelopathy* is a rare but fatal complication of horses positioned in dorsal recumbency for surgical procedures (mostly elective procedures such as bilateral hock arthroscopy). It appears to be most common among weanlings and young adults, particularly in horses of larger and heavier breeds (draft breeds and Friesians). There is generally complete paralysis of the rear limbs with areflexia of the pelvic limbs, tail, and anus. There is little or no response to stimuli of the pelvic limbs, tail, and anus.

●〉 WHAT TO DO

Postanesthetic Hemorrhagic Myelopathy

- Anti-edema, anti-inflammatory treatment (methylprednisolone sodium succinate, 30 mg/kg IV) can be tried; however, the prognosis is grave.
- Anesthesiologists have recommended preloading with fluids before surgery in at-risk horses to support systemic blood pressure and maximize perfusion to the spinal cord.

- *Spinal cord neoplasia* is a rare cause of acute ataxia. The most common extradural tumors include sarcomas and melanomas; lymphosarcoma is the most common intradural tumor.

Acute Ataxia in Foals

Causes

- Acute ataxia most commonly is a result of trauma (see Spinal Cord Trauma, p. 371).
- Congenital anomalies, such as spina bifida, should be considered when an ataxic newborn foal does not improve with standard anti-inflammatory and anti-edema therapy.
- Young foals, especially Arabian and Quarter Horse foals, with ataxia, extended neck posture, or a clicking noise caused by head movement should undergo radiography, CT, and/or fluoroscopy to rule out occipitoatlantoaxial malformation or subluxation or fractures of this area.

Vertebral Body Abscess

- Vertebral body abscess can cause acute pain and ataxia and paresis in foals.
- Affected foals are generally 2 to 8 months of age, and most appear healthy just before the onset of pain and neurologic signs.
- The clinical signs vary depending on the site of the infection.
- Sacrococcygeal abscesses causes decreased tail tone and ataxia and weakness in the hind legs (often asymmetric).
- Thoracolumbar lesions cause stiffness and UMN signs in the pelvic limbs.
- Cervical lesions cause neck pain, tetraparesis, and ataxia (worse in the front limbs if the lesion is in the caudal cervical region).
- The most common organisms are the following:
  - *Rhodococcus equi*
  - *Salmonella* organisms
  - *Streptococcus equi* subsp. equi and zooepidemicus
  - Rarely *Coccidioides* (coccidioidomycosis; mostly seen in Arizona and California)

Diagnosis

- Clinical examination and localization of site of pain
- Radiography
- Ultrasonography and guided aspirate for culture and/or direct staining
- CT
- Fecal or tracheal wash cultures or PCR for *Salmonella* or *R. equi* with history of exposure

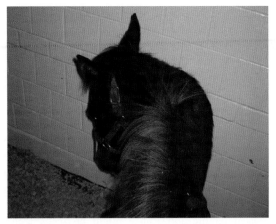

Figure 22-5 Cervical scoliosis in a young horse caused by dorsal horn necrosis from migration of *Parelaphostronglus tenuis*. The right side *(convex)* is the affected side, and analgesia was present over a four-vertebral area. The noticeable scoliosis was acute.

- Nasopharyngeal or guttural pouch culture or PCR for *S. equi* with history of exposure

●〉 WHAT TO DO

Vertebral Body Abscess

- Surgical curettage and/or drainage
- Antibiotics: Begin with penicillin potassium and amikacin (for suspected *Streptococcus* or *Salmonella*) or clarithromycin and rifampin (if *R. equi* is the more likely organism). Chloramphenicol can be used for long-term therapy. If surgery is performed, antibiotic-coated beads (erythromycin for *Rhodococcus* or *Streptococcus*) can be implanted.
- Nursing care (e.g., splints and physical therapy)

Cervical or Thoracic Scoliosis

Young horses (6 months to 3 years) in the eastern United States can have acute onset of cervical or thoracic scoliosis (Fig. 22-5). These horses are not painful, and the neck can be easily manually repositioned in the normal plane early in the course of the disease, particularly if the horse is sedated or anesthetized. Considerable hypalgesia of at least three cervical or thoracic segments exists over the scoliosis on the convex side. There might be mild ataxia ipsilateral to the convex side as well. CSF can be normal or have an eosinophilic/lymphocytic pleocytosis. This condition is caused by *Parelaphostrongylus tenuis* migrating through the dorsal gray column of the affected side.

●〉 WHAT TO DO

Cervical or Thoracic Scoliosis

- Ivermectin, fenbendazole, and corticosteroids are usually administered, but because of the severe necrosis of the affected segments of dorsal gray column, no horses have been reported to recover normal function.

Trembling in Horses

Causes of trembling include weakness, pain, shock, adverse drug reactions, hypothermia, and toxicity. *Diseases presented in this chapter are neurologic and neuromuscular problems that cause trembling.* Trembling may also occur from pain and shock.

Physical Examination

A careful physical examination indicates whether the trembling is a result of weakness, pain, shock, or other causes. In conditions with generalized weakness (e.g., botulism), the eyelids, tongue, tail, and anus all have reduced tone. ***Note:*** Botulism, equine motor neuron disease, and severe cachexia cause affected horses to stand with all four feet closer together than normal. If the weakness is a result of electrolyte abnormalities such as hypocalcemia or hyperkalemic periodic paralysis, a tetanic appearance might be seen. Trembling associated with abdominal pain or endotoxemia is common and can be detected with a complete clinical examination. Sweating can occur with weakness or pain. Trembling caused by a primary muscle disorder might be difficult to separate from other causes of trembling. Trembling in one limb also is common with EPM, vertebral osteomyelitis, myopathy, and any peripheral neuropathy.

Botulism

Botulism is caused by the neurotoxins of *Clostridium botulinum,* which inhibit release of acetylcholine at nerve terminals resulting in flaccid paralysis. *C. botulinum* is a gram-positive, spore-forming, obligate anaerobic bacterium. There are differences in the method of intoxication between foals and adults.

Signalment
Foals
- Often 2 to 8 weeks of age; most are 21 to 28 days of age
- Generally acquire toxicoinfectious botulism (ingestion of spores with subsequent germination and toxin production within the intestinal tract)
- Most common among foals in Kentucky, Maryland, Pennsylvania, and New Jersey
Adults
- Most often a result of ingestion of preformed toxin in forages
- Associated with a closed wound in rare instances
- Endemic in the mid-Atlantic states (*C. botulinum* type B is common in the soil) but seen in adult horses in many areas of North America. Horses on the West Coast are more likely to be exposed to *C. botulinum* type A (which is common in western soil).
- Outbreaks of *C. botulinum* type C have been reported in parts of the United States in association with contamination of feed with carrion.

Clinical Signs
- Generalized (and therefore symmetric) weakness in most, but not all, cases
- Decreased tail, anal, eyelid, and tongue tone (the tongue can easily be pulled from the mouth and held with two fingers)
- Trembling (often begins in triceps muscles) that is worse with exertion and subsides when horse becomes recumbent
- Excessive recumbency that can progress to total recumbency
- Dysphagia occurs in most but not all cases (may not occur in some type A cases); if the horse can swallow, it takes >2 minutes to consume 1 cup (approximately 140 g) of grain. Make sure a complete oral examination rules out other causes.
- Horses stand with all four limbs close together.
- The disease often progresses to severe paresis with inability to stand and subsequent respiratory failure.
- The onset usually is acute, with rapid progression within 18 to 48 hours, although some cases might progress more slowly or even stabilize without treatment.
- Mydriasis with slow pupillary light reflexes and ptosis might be evident.
- ***Note:*** Many horses with botulism are presented for colic because of clinical signs of inappetence, increased recumbency, trembling, and sweating.

Diagnostic Tests
- The diagnosis of botulism is made by consideration of the signalment, clinical signs, and geographic location.
- Consultation and diagnostic testing is available at the National Botulism Reference Laboratory at New Bolton Center (www.vet.upenn.edu/HospitalServices/Botulism Laboratory/tabid/2363/Default.aspx; 610-925-6383). Anaerobic culture of soil, feed, feces, gastrointestinal contents, or wound tissue for identification of *C. botulinum* and/or its toxin can be submitted to this lab to support the diagnosis in adult horses. Anaerobic conditions can be maintained by packing an airtight container full with the sample. Preformed toxin can be found in the intestinal content or feces of foals and feces, gastrointestinal contents, or feedstuff from some adult cases (keep contents frozen or ship chilled overnight). Spores found in intestinal contents of adult horses that die or in fecal samples (submit feces on 3 consecutive days; present in 30% of cases) can be strongly supportive of the diagnosis. In foals, the presence of the spore or toxin in the feces confirms the diagnosis if appropriate clinical signs are present.
- Muscle enzymes are normal or only slightly increased (unless the patient has been recumbent).
- Endoscopy often reveals a displaced soft palate, even in mild cases.
- Arterial or venous P_{CO_2} > 70 mm Hg suggests hypoventilation and a poor prognosis or need for mechanical ventilation.

◉〉 WHAT TO DO

Botulism
- Do not stress the horse; confine horse to a stall.
- Remove hay and water; muzzle the horse if patient attempts to eat the bedding.

- Administer botulism antitoxin *intravenously ASAP.*
  - Sources of antitoxin:
    - Lake Immunogenics, Inc.; www.lakeimmunogenics.com; 800-648-9990. Lake Immunogenics produces a trivalent antitoxin (effective against types A, B, and C).
    - Plasvacc; www.plasvaccusa.com; 805-434-0321. Plasvacc produces a monovalent antitoxin (effective against type B).
  - Signs can progress for 24 to 48 hours after administration of the antitoxin.
  - **Note:** Antitoxin administration binds circulating toxin but does not affect toxin already bound; therefore while it halts further deterioration, horses do not improve with administration.
- Give broad-spectrum antibiotics to prevent secondary complications such as aspiration pneumonia or infected pressure sores: ceftiofur, 2.2 mg/kg q12h IV, or trimethoprim-sulfamethoxazole, 30 mg/kg q12h PO (generally via nasogastric feeding tube).
- Metronidazole might be contraindicated. Debride the wound (in the unusual case of wound botulism).
- Supply feed and water or milk by means of nasogastric intubation (see Chapter 18, p. 151). In the care of acutely affected adults, passage of a nasogastric tube can be postponed until the antitoxin has been administered (at least 24 hours) to reduce stress.
- If laxatives are needed, mineral oil is preferred.
- If affected horses prefer to stand, provide stacked bales or similar arrangement on which the horse can rest its head.
- In foals, the standard maintenance feeding of approximately 22% of milk per kilogram of body weight per day usually is not required because the activity level of these foals is greatly decreased, and abdominal distention should be prevented. Milk should be fed at 10% to 15% per kg of body weight. Antiulcer medication is recommended.
- Provide supportive care: urinary catheterization if needed in the treatment of recumbent horses; good bedding and ventilation; ocular and wound care; turning of recumbent horses every 2 to 4 hours but only after placing in sternal recumbency for 5 minutes. Do not force horses or foals to stand.
- Clinical improvement will not be seen for 4 to 10 days until new motor end plates are regenerated.

► WHAT NOT TO DO

Botulism

- Penicillin procaine, aminoglycosides, and tetracycline should not be administered because of their effect on the neuromuscular junction. In cases with concurrent colic, avoid lidocaine and polymyxin B.

Prognosis
Foals

- Foals that can stand have a good prognosis with antitoxin therapy.
- Recumbent foals without respiratory distress have a good prognosis with adequate nursing care.
- Foals with respiratory distress and $P_{CO_2} > 70$ mm Hg have a poor prognosis without ventilatory support, which is expensive and requires 2 to 3 weeks of hospitalization. These foals should be maintained with intranasal tracheal intubation and an Ambu Bag until they can be admitted to an intensive care facility for ventilatory support. If intubation is not possible, they can be maintained with a foal resuscitator.[8] With appropriate ventilatory support, prognosis remains good.

Adults

- Adults that have a 3- to 5-day history of weakness and are still standing have a fair to good prognosis, sometimes even without antitoxin treatment.
- Adults that cannot stand or that have a peracute course of disease have a poor prognosis even with antitoxin administration unless prolonged and expensive hospital treatment is an option. Vaccination is not protective until three vaccines are received at appropriate intervals.

Equine Motor Neuron Disease

Equine motor neuron disease (EMND) affects adults, usually in a management situation in which there is little or no pasture (in Europe, EMND has been sporadically reported in horses with pasture but with low plasma vitamin E for unexplained reasons) and "less than green" hay, most commonly in the northeastern United States and Europe. *The disease is closely linked to prolonged (>17 months) deficiency of vitamin E.*

Clinical Signs

- Weight loss of more than 150 lb (70 kg)
- Trembling
- Weakness of the limbs and neck
- Generalized muscle atrophy
- Standing with all four limbs close together
- Increased periods of recumbency
- Good appetite
- No dysphagia, ataxia, or weak tail
- Raised tailhead in many cases
- Funduscopic changes—golden-brown lipofuscin deposits in reticulated pattern: Not all affected horses have visible changes, nor do all horses with these changes have EMND.

Definitive Diagnosis

- Clinical signs provide a tentative diagnosis.
- Laboratory test results are suggestive, not diagnostic. Serum creatine kinase (CK) level is mildly or moderately elevated (500 to 2000 IU/L) in approximately 90% of horses with EMND that are trembling.
- Measure plasma vitamin E; all horses with EMND have had levels <1 μg/mL if the sample is collected before supplementation.
- Perform muscle biopsy of the sacrocaudalis dorsalis medialis (tailhead) muscle. This is the most superficial muscle on either side of midline at the base of the tail. To perform the biopsy, sedate the horse with xylazine and infiltrate local anesthesia subcutaneously (not into the muscle). Make a 3-inch (7.5-cm) skin incision and dissect through any subcutaneous fat to the muscle. Make 2 parallel cuts in the muscle and undermine the isolated strip before cutting at each end to obtain a 1-inch-long by

---

[8]Foal resuscitator (MAI Animal Health, 605 Project Drive, Elmwood, Wisconsin, 54740-8716).

$\frac{1}{4}$-inch-wide (2.5- by 0.6-cm) specimen. Place the specimen in formalin after sticking it on a tongue depressor, and ship it to a pathologist experienced in the evaluation of equine muscle.

• Perform nerve biopsy of the ventral branch of the spinal accessory nerve (submitted in formalin). The results are approximately 94% accurate in predicting the presence of the disease, if the biopsy is interpreted by an experienced pathologist.

●〉 WHAT TO DO

Equine Motor Neuron Disease

• Vitamin E, 6,000 to 10,000 IU without added selenium PO q24h, should be supplemented indefinitely or until the diet has been adjusted to contain adequate amounts of vitamin E and blood levels are maintained in the normal range.
• Natural vitamin E supplements generally result in higher plasma levels and/or have greater activity than do synthetic vitamin E supplements, although the latter also raises plasma levels. Coenzyme Q_{10} administration has been advised, but efficacy is unproven.
• Provide green grass if possible.
• Prednisolone, 0.5 to 1 mg/kg PO q24h, appears to improve the signs in acutely, severely affected horses. Minocycline, 4 mg/kg PO q12h for 2 to 4 weeks, is theoretically of benefit against neuronal degeneration but has not been widely used for this purpose in horses.

Prognosis

• Prognosis is poor for return to previous function.
• The condition in more than half of affected horses begins to stabilize after 2 to 4 weeks.

Tetanic Hypocalcemia in Horses

Common Causes

• Lactation: more common in Draft horses and miniature horses
• Blister beetle toxicity (see p. 237)
• Colitis and colic in adults (see Chapter 18, p. 231)
• Exhaustion syndrome in endurance horses (see Chapter 33, p. 575)
• Excessive bicarbonate administration

Less Common Causes of Hypocalcemia in Adults

• Idiopathic
• Transport and stress
• Hypoparathyroidism: more common among foals (frequently 2 to 5 months of age); repeated episodes indicate a guarded prognosis unless prolonged supplementation is possible
• Farm problems can occur leading to signs in multiple foals, in which case low dietary magnesium as a cause of diminished parathyroid hormone (PTH) activity or vitamin D deficiency should be investigated

Clinical Signs

• Generalized stiffness
• Trismus
• Trembling

• Dysmetric flared nostrils
• Synchronous diaphragmatic flutter: common in adults with low ionized calcium
• Prolapsing third eyelids. Some of the signs of hypocalcemic tetany are similar to those of hyperkalemic periodic paralysis (HYPP).
• Respiratory distress
• Stringhalt or goose-stepping gait
• Recumbency
• Dilated pupils
• Sweating
• Tachycardia
• Hyperesthesia
• Choke
• Elevated temperature
• Seizures in foals
• Colic (often severe) caused by ileus. Colic can be the cause of the hypocalcemia, in which case hypocalcemia is generally mild, or a result of the hypocalcemia, in which case hypocalcemia is severe.

Laboratory Findings

• Calcium[9] usually <5.0 mg/dL (<1.25 mmol/L)
• Ionized calcium usually 2.4 mg/dL (<0.6 mmol/L)
• Magnesium usually <1.0 mg/dL
• Might be alkalotic and hypochloremic because of sweating, which further aggravates hypocalcemia

●〉 WHAT TO DO

Tetanic Hypocalcemia

• Administer 11.5 g (500 mL) 23% calcium borogluconate slowly IV over at least 15 minutes for a 450-kg adult. The calcium borogluconate can be mixed in 4 to 5 L of 0.9% NaCl and administered over 30 to 45 minutes. Adults in severe distress can be given 200 mL calcium borogluconate slowly IV without fluid dilution. Perivascular administration results in soft tissue inflammation and possible phlebitis.
• Monitor heart rate and rhythm.
  • The expected cardiovascular response is an increase in the intensity of heart sounds.
  • An infrequent extrasystole can be expected, *but* pronounced change in rate or rhythm is an indication to discontinue the treatment immediately.
• Complete recovery from hypocalcemia might require several hours to days. Treatment might have to be repeated. Foals often are more refractory to treatment.
• Also monitor and supplement serum magnesium as indicated.

Prognosis

The prognosis is good except for horses with hypoparathyroidism, which is more common among foals. Laboratory samples for PTH (to diagnose hypoparathyroidism) can be sent to the Endocrinology Section, Diagnostic Center for

---

[9]Conversion factor: milligrams per deciliter to millimoles per liter, divide by 4; millimoles per liter to milligrams per deciliter, multiply by 4.

Population and Animal Health, Michigan State University, Lansing, MI; 517-353-1683. Blood samples must be clotted, centrifuged, and sent overnight on ice. Normal values for individual laboratory tests should be reported. The prognosis is poor for foals with persistent hypocalcemia caused by hypoparathyroidism unless prolonged supplementation and treatment are provided.

Hyperkalemic Periodic Paralysis

HYPP is a defect in muscle membrane transport that is inherited through an autosomal dominant gene. Homozygous HYPP horses usually have more severe clinical signs than heterozygous HYPP horses.

Signalment
- Quarter Horses, Appaloosas, and Paints that are descendants of the Quarter Horse sire "Impressive."

Adults
- Typically, horses are 2 to 4 years of age at initial episode, and frequently the signs begin with onset of training.
- Some horses are younger or older when they first exhibit clinical signs.
- High-potassium diet, stress, or fasting can cause the onset of clinical signs.

Foals
- Patients can be neonates to weanling in age.
- Foals demonstrating clinical signs are usually homozygous for the condition.
- Dam might have no history of clinical disease.

Clinical Signs

Adults
- Patient has anxious attitude and remains alert.
- Episodic muscle tremors occur, often seen first in the muscles of the face and neck and then progressing to diffuse body tremors.
- Swaying and staggering are evident.
- Horse assumes dog-sitting posture (hindquarter paresis), which can progress to involuntary recumbency.
- Prolapse or "flash" of the third eyelid occurs.
- Usually individual is completely normal after recovery from an incident, and duration of clinical signs can vary from a few minutes to several hours.
- Signs can develop after a stressful event (e.g., colic), cold weather, anesthesia, or after feeding.
- Increased respiratory rate and upper airway noise are evident (snoring is present in homozygous HYPP horses and might be the only sign).
- Death can occur in a very low percentage of episodes, so this disease should be on the rule-out list for acute unexplained death.

Foals (see Chapter 21, pp. 311-312)
- Loud inspiratory noise
- Respiratory distress
- Collapse
- Most often exhibit respiratory signs when exercised, restrained, or nursing

Diagnosis
Signalment, clinical signs, endoscopy in foals, laboratory data, and response to treatment provide a tentative diagnosis. HYPP genetic testing leads to identification of homozygous and heterozygous individuals.

Laboratory Data
- Hyperkalemia, 5 to 12.3 mEq/L, is evident during an incident. Affected adults and foals rarely are reported to be normokalemic during clinical episodes.
- Muscle enzyme (CK and aspartate transaminase) levels are normal or only mildly elevated. Muscle biopsy does not provide a definitive diagnosis.
- HYPP testing is done by the Veterinary Genetics Laboratory at the University of California, Davis (530-752-9780), or several other laboratories in the United States, Canada, and Australia. Submit 20 to 30 hairs with roots or 5 to 10 mL of blood in an EDTA (purple top) tube (see p. 71).

●) WHAT TO DO

Hyperkalemic Periodic Paralysis
Foals
- Do not over-restrain the foal.
- Tracheotomy might be needed for foals with excessive pharyngeal collapse. If sedation is needed, diazepam (Valium) is better than an alpha-agonist because the latter increases upper airway resistance.

Adults and Foals
- Administer 23% calcium gluconate, 0.2 to 0.4 mL/kg, in 1 to 2 L of 10% dextrose *or* 250 mL 50% dextrose *or* sodium bicarbonate, 0.5 mEq/kg IV over 30 minutes. Calcium and glucose can be given together but not calcium and bicarbonate.
- Albuterol inhalant can be given if the foal is in respiratory distress.
- Milder cases respond to dextrose or Karo syrup with or without sodium bicarbonate (baking soda) administered orally or through a nasogastric tube. Sometimes light exercise (lunging) can alleviate clinical signs in these mild cases because epinephrine and beta-agonists increase intracellular potassium.
- Administer acetazolamide, 2.2 to 4.4 mg/kg PO q12h. This is a potassium-wasting diuretic used to lessen the incidence of clinical signs.
- Decrease potassium content of diet. Change from alfalfa to a *tested* grass hay but not brome grass. **Note:** Potassium in hay can vary widely. Another option is to reduce the alfalfa hay by mixing with a low-potassium grass hay or oat hay. Feed more oats and less sweet feed or pellets, but make sure the amount of calcium in the diet is adequate. Avoid supplements (e.g., molasses, "lite" salt, and kelp) that contain potassium. Provide consistent exercise.

Prognosis
- Acetazolamide therapy and dietary changes control clinical signs in most affected horses.
- Recurrent episodes are reported in some individuals that initially respond to treatment.
- Sudden death is occasionally reported.
- Discourage breeding of horses with positive genetic test results for the disease, even those horses with no clinical signs. This is controversial.

Tetanus

Tetanus is caused by an exotoxin produced by *Clostridium tetani* that blocks the release of inhibitory neurotransmitters and results in spasticity of skeletal muscles.

Signalment

- Any unvaccinated horse is susceptible.
- Clostridial organisms usually are introduced through a soft tissue or hoof wound.
- Disease generally develops 10 to 21 days following a wound.

Clinical Signs

- Initial signs are colic and vague stiffness.
- Trembling, spasm, and paralysis of skeletal muscles occur. Masseter muscles are commonly affected.
- Protrusion of the third eyelid occurs, especially when the horse is menaced.
- Eyelid retraction, flared nostrils, and erect ear carriage is evident.
- Sawhorse stance and stiff spastic gait, which can progress to recumbency
- Horse is unable to open jaw, has difficulty swallowing, and acquires aspiration pneumonia.
- Tailhead is raised.
- All of these signs are exacerbated by activity or excitement. Stimulation of a horse that has tetanus might precipitate panic, recumbency, and a long bone fracture or other secondary trauma.

Diagnosis

- Clinical signs occur in an unvaccinated horse; therefore, younger horses or foals are more commonly affected.
- There are no diagnostic blood tests.
- Anaerobic culture of *C. tetani* from the primary wound can be attempted.

Differential Diagnoses

- Most commonly severe neck pain
- Hypocalcemia
- Myopathy
- EMND
- Stiff horse syndrome
- Shivers
- Occasionally encephalitis

●▶ WHAT TO DO

Tetanus

- Provide a quiet environment with good footing and without barriers.
- Pad stall walls to reduce risk of injury.
- Minimize stimulation: Darken stall and stuff cotton in the ears.
- Provide deep bedding with straw, especially if the patient is recumbent.
- Provide muscle relaxation and tranquilization:
  - Administer acepromazine, 0.02 to 0.05 mg/kg q6h IM or IV. Increasing doses or shorter intervals might be required with time. Alternatively, use phenobarbital, 5 to 10 mg/kg slowly IV, followed by oral phenobarbital, 5 to 10 mg/kg q12h. Additional treatments that might be helpful include diazepam, 0.05 to 0.44 mg/kg IV, and methocarbamol, 40 to 60 mg/kg PO or 10 to 50 mg/kg IV q12-24h. These treatments might be required for days to weeks depending on the clinical course.
- Remove the source of infection:
  - Debride the wound; do not suture.
  - Infiltrate wound with penicillin procaine.
  - Administer penicillin potassium, 22,000 IU/kg q6h IV, for a minimum of 7 days. Note: addition of additional antimicrobials to provide broad-spectrum coverage should be considered for possible aspiration pneumonia.
- Neutralize unbound toxin:
  - Administer 100 to 200 U/kg tetanus antitoxin IV or IM, which should bind any residual circulating toxin but poorly crosses the blood-brain barrier to neutralize toxin in the CNS.
  - Consider intrathecal administration of antitoxin. Benefit has not been clearly demonstrated in horses but has been shown for people. Remove 50 mL of CSF by means of atlantooccipital aspiration (30 mL in a foal), and replace it with an equal volume of tetanus antitoxin. Anesthetize the horse for the CSF procedure. *This treatment can be considered for early cases that are still ambulatory and have mild to moderate clinical signs.*
  - ***Note:*** If the patient is severely affected—for example, sawhorse stance—intrathecal administration of antitoxin is *not* recommended because the individual might not be able to stand following the procedure (with lumbosacral administration the horse might collapse).
- Maintain hydration and nutritional status:
  - Place food and water off the ground in an easily accessible place.
  - Intravenous administration of fluids might be necessary to maintain hydration.
  - Oral fluids and gruel can be administered through a small-bore nasogastric tube in some cases. Intubation might be difficult because of muscle spasms and pharyngeal paralysis. Feed or intubate at peak tranquilization periods to reduce stress. Leave tube in place (see Chapter 18, p. 157).
- Establish active immunity: The amount of toxin necessary to produce disease often is insufficient to stimulate an immune response. Vaccinate with tetanus toxoid in a separate site from the antitoxin administration.

Prognosis

- Prognosis is fair to poor.
- Recovery is contingent on the severity of clinical signs and the attitude of the affected horse.
- Clinical signs can persist for weeks.
- Secondary complications include aspiration pneumonia, myopathy, and long-bone or pelvic fracture. Foals can develop a variety of orthopedic abnormalities.
- If the affected horse cannot stand, the prognosis is grave; if the horse is ambulatory after 5 days of clinical signs, the prognosis is fair to good.

Myopathy, Myositis

Trembling can occur with myositis or myopathy. These conditions include the following:

Non–Selenium-Deficient Tying-Up Syndromes

- Rule out polysaccharide storage disease especially if the patient is a Continental European Draft horse (Belgium or Percheron), Warmblood, or Quarter Horse (see Polysaccharide Storage Myopathy, p. 360). Ask about exposure to strangles and if the tying up has occurred previously in the horse or relatives. Rule in or out specific causes of myopathy.

Exertional Myopathy

- If the myopathy is believed to be caused by exertion or excitement preceding racing/training, treatment includes the following:

●》 WHAT TO DO

Exertional Myopathy

- Administer fluids to correct dehydration and electrolyte abnormalities. Remember, most horses with mild to moderate myopathy and exhausted horses are likely to be hypochloremic and alkalotic. Therefore, 0.9% NaCl with 20 to 40 mEq/L KCl often is the preferred fluid. Fluid diuresis might prevent myoglobinuric nephropathy. Hypertonic saline solution also can be used. In severe cases (myopathy, exhaustion, or both), acidosis might be present.
- Analgesic: phenylbutazone, 2.2 mg/kg IV q12h for 1 to 2 days
- Acepromazine, 0.02 to 0.04 mg/kg IV or IM q6h, *after* correction of fluid deficits
- Hot packs for affected muscles
- Methocarbamol, 10 to 50 mg/kg PO or IV q24h; only used when acepromazine does not cause sufficient relaxation
- Dantrolene or phenytoin can be used in Thoroughbreds and Standardbreds with sodium or calcium channel disorders instead of methocarbamol.

Atypical Myopathy

- This disease occurs in the United States; however, it is more common in Europe (see Chapter 40, p. 668).

Compartment Syndrome

- Compartment syndrome is associated with ischemia (localized myopathy from trauma).

●》 WHAT TO DO

Compartment Syndrome

- Treatment is similar to that used to treat exertional myopathy. If the disease is progressive and severe swelling occurs in areas of important nerves such as the radial nerve, perform fasciotomy to relieve the pressure.
- If one leg is involved, do not forget to support wrap the contralateral leg and supply additional frog and sole support to that foot if needed.
- If the horse tolerates a sling to decrease some weight bearing, this can be helpful in management.
- Some cases, especially of the triceps, might require several days for recovery.
- Antioxidant therapy, including vitamin E, coenzyme Q10, selenium, and DMSO might be useful for more severe cases.

Selenium-Deficient Tying-Up

- Consider this syndrome in certain areas of the United States (e.g., Northeast and North Central) and Canada,

especially (but not always) if the individual is poorly fed. Tying-up can affect limb muscles, tongue, heart, or just masseter muscles.
- For diagnosis and what to do, see the following section.

White Muscle Disease

- White muscle disease (selenium-deficient myopathy) most commonly occurs in foals from birth to 7 months of age but can occur in adults. The disease is most common in the northeast and northwest United States. If the cardiac muscle is affected, death might occur without clinical signs. With skeletal muscle involvement, dyspnea, dysphagia, recumbency, and stiff gait are typical. If the diaphragm is involved, acute and often progressive respiratory distress with respiratory acidosis might occur. Acute masseter myopathy with conjunctival bulging resulting from the swollen masseter and pterygoid muscles can occur in adult horses. Others are unable to keep the mouth closed and the tongue protrudes because of the masseter weakness. Hyponatremia, hypochloremia, hyperkalemia, and significant increases in muscle enzyme activity levels are typical biochemical abnormalities. The urine might be red or brown because of myoglobinuria.
- Diagnosis is based on clinical signs, increased serum muscle enzyme activities, myoglobinuria, and serum selenium (generally <7 µg/dL in affected adult horses and <5 µg/dL in affected foals).

Note: If selenium has already been administered and confirmation of the diagnosis is needed, blood can be collected in an anticoagulant tube and submitted to Michigan State University's Diagnostic Center for Population and Animal Health for measurement of glutathione peroxidase activity. After selenium administration, several days are required before the selenium molecule is incorporated into red blood cell glutathione peroxidase.

●》 WHAT TO DO

White Muscle Disease

- Repeated intramuscular injections of selenium, 0.06 mg/kg IM, might be needed for treatment.
- Supportive treatments to use include intravenously administered fluids, DMSO, vitamin E, NSAIDs, and gastric ulcer prophylaxis for foals.

●》 WHAT NOT TO DO

White Muscle Disease

- The authors prefer to never give selenium intravenously!

Purpura Hemorrhagica or Immune-Mediated Myositis
Clinical Findings

- Almost all cases of purpura have some increase in muscle enzyme activities.
  - In a few cases there is massive and rapidly progressive edema and inflammation of certain muscles, mostly in the hind legs. Affected horses can have an infarctive/ hemorrhagic myonecrosis of any skeletal muscle, plus

in rare cases, infarction of the bowel and/or lungs. Others have only severe myonecrosis and edema without infarction. The disorder is most common in Quarter Horses.
- A second and possibly related syndrome of rapid muscle wasting is also seen mostly in Quarter Horses infected with or exposed to *S. equi.*

Diagnosis
- Horse might have a history of exposure to *S. equi* or possibly other respiratory pathogens.
- High streptococcus M protein antibody level is found in many horses with the muscle wasting syndrome. Streptococcal organisms or M protein might be identified in the necrotic muscle of horses with the acute edema, myonecrosis, and/or infarction syndromes.
- Acute trembling, stiffness, muscle swelling, leg edema, and/or recumbency is present; with the acute edema and/or infarction syndrome, progression to recumbency can be rapid (hours).
- Increased levels of muscle enzyme activities (often significantly), neutrophilia, and increased fibrinogen and globulins are found in some cases.
- The horse might have other signs of purpura such as petechia, fever, and nondependent edema.
- Those with rapid muscle wasting show muscle loss mostly over the epaxial and gluteal muscles. Those with infarctive syndrome also have involvement of the hamstring muscles and pronounced leg edema.
- Edema and hemorrhage into muscle can be rapid and severe in the acute myonecrosis syndromes, and severe colic signs can be seen. Cardiac muscle may be involved, causing heart failure and acute death; cardiac troponin-I (cTnI) is markedly elevated in these cases. For acute painful swelling of muscles with fever, *Clostridium perfringens* myositis must be ruled out (see Chapter 35, p. 618).

● WHAT TO DO

Purpura Hemorrhagica Myositis
- See treatment of purpura hemorrhagica (Chapter 35, p. 615), and use the most aggressive treatment (e.g., high doses of corticosteroids, 0.1 to 0.2 mg/kg IV, for the acute myonecrosis syndrome) because this is often fatal. Horses with progressive atrophy syndrome usually respond to 0.06 to 0.1 mg/kg IV dexamethasone. Use *caution* in administering IV fluids if the heart muscle is affected.

Parasitic Myositis *(Sarcocystis fayeri)*
- Rare
- Present with trembling and stiffness
- Bloodwork changes include increased muscle enzyme activities; confirm diagnosis with muscle biopsy

● WHAT TO DO

Parasitic Myositis
- Phenylbutazone, 2.2 mg/kg PO q12-24h
- Trimethoprim-sulfamethoxazole, 30 mg/kg PO q12h

- Pyrimethamine, 2 mg/kg PO as a loading dose, and then 1 mg/kg PO q24h

Myopathy in American Miniature Horses
- Affected foal and adult miniature horses are described as having an unusual masseter myonecrosis with dysphagia, weakness, and trembling. Historically, affected horses and foals were fed a commonly used organophosphate fly control medication (tetrachlorvinphos). Whether the disease in the miniatures is due to the organophosphate or whether it might be compounded by marginally low selenium concentrations and/or genetic factors is unclear.

Polysaccharide Storage Myopathy
- Polysaccharide storage myopathy (PSSM) is a glycogen storage disease.
- The type 1 disease is common in Continental Europe breeds of Draft horses and Quarter Horses and only moderately common in Warmbloods (type 2 is more common in Warmbloods). It occurs less commonly in other breeds.
- Generally, the disease first occurs in young adults (3 to 7 years).
- Recurrent episodes of tying-up in Quarter Horses can sometimes be very severe, with greatly increased muscle enzyme activities.
- Trembling and stiffness can progress to recumbency and even death in susceptible Draft horses, many times with only mild increases in muscle enzyme activities.
- Serum selenium concentration can be normal or abnormal (often abnormal in Draft horses).
- There is no response to treatment with selenium.
- Recurrent episodes and persistent increase in muscle enzyme activities can occur in Quarter Horses.
- Muscle wasting, weakness in the hind limbs and even whole body trembling can be noted in a few cases, especially Draft horses. Some Draft horses have shivers and PSSM at the same time, resulting in a combination of weakness, spasticity, and painful clinical signs.

Diagnosis
- Diagnosis can be made via muscle biopsy or genetic testing.
  - There are two types of PSSM (type 1 and type 2).
  - Type 1 is caused by a known genetic mutation (in the glycogen synthase gene) and can be diagnosed by submission of blood (3 to 7 mL in EDTA tube) or 20 to 30 mane/tail hairs to the Neuromuscular Disease Laboratory at the Veterinary Diagnostic Laboratory, University of Minnesota, 1333 Gortner Avenue, St. Paul, Minnesota 55108 (612-625-8787).
- Both type 1 and type 2 PSSM horses may have high normal or slightly abnormal CK and AST at rest and cause similar muscle pathology and can be diagnosed via muscle biopsy of the semimembranosus or semitendinosus muscle.
  - Place the muscle biopsy on a tongue depressor, wrap it with a saline-moistened damp 4- × 4-inch sponge, place in a sealed plastic container (specimen cup),

and send overnight on ice packs to the University of Minnesota.

- Muscle enzyme activity is high in severely affected cases but might not be dramatically elevated in many Draft horses because this is not a myositis.

●〉 WHAT TO DO

Mild to Moderate Cases of Polysaccharide Storage Myopathy

- Give 2 cups (480 mL) vegetable oil q24h PO (in as low starch a feed as possible or through a nasogastric tube). Permanently adjust the diet so that it is relatively high-fat/low-starch (see www.cvm.umn.edu/umec/lab/PSSM/home.html#prevention).
- Provide analgesics.
- Gradually increase exercise after disease is no longer active and maintain a consistent exercise schedule.

●〉 WHAT NOT TO DO

Polysaccharide Storage Myopathy

- *Do not* exercise the horse during active disease.

●〉 WHAT TO DO

Severely Affected and Recumbent Cases of Polysaccharide Storage Myopathy

- Give 2 cups (480 mL) vegetable oil PO.
- Administer Intralipid, 0.2 g/kg IV, slowly over 1 to 2 hours.
- Provide analgesics.
- Provide supportive care (e.g., fluid therapy) and slinging support for down horses.
- Rice bran, 1 to 5 lb (0.45 to 2.25 kg) per day is an excellent source of fat. Most companies have a high-fat feed but it is essential to withhold carbohydrates in addition to feeding a high-fat diet.
- Maintain daily routine with respect to exercise once an episode is over.

Other Causes of Trembling

Many other causes of acute trembling exist besides those listed, including trauma, hypothermia, cachexia, and drug reactions.

White Snake Root Poisoning

- Signs of weakness leading to recumbency occur in horses eating white snake root. Increased frequency of urination is commonly seen (see Chapter 34, p. 594). Some of these cases might be *Atypical myopathy,* associated with exposure to maple or box elder seeds (see Chapter 40, p. 668).

Acute Lead Poisoning

- Trembling, depression, and ataxia (Chapter 34, p. 591) are signs. Laryngeal paralysis might be present with acute lead poisoning.
- Diagnosis is based on exposure, clinical signs, and blood lead concentration >0.3 ppm.

●〉 WHAT TO DO

Acute Lead Poisoning

- Administer calcium disodium EDTA, 110 mg/kg in 5% dextrose IV q24h for 2 days. Further interval treatment might be needed.

Ear Tick (*Otobius Megnini*) Infestation

- Muscle spasms, colic-like sweating, prolapse of the third eyelid, and colic-like signs have been associated with ear tick infestation. On percussion, some muscles have prolonged and severe contracture. Muscle enzyme activity levels are generally mildly to moderately increased. The spinose ear tick can be found in the ear of affected horses.

●〉 WHAT TO DO

Ear Tick Infestation

- Signs resolve within 24 to 96 hours after removal or treatment of the ticks with the pyrethrin piperonyl butoxide.

Aortoiliac Thrombosis (Saddle Thrombus)

- Although most cases are chronic and intermittent, a few individuals have acute onset of trembling of the hind limbs, violent shaking of the limbs, and/or weakness in the hind limbs. The diagnosis is established with transrectal ultrasonography. Palpation of limbs for decreased pulse yields inconsistent findings.

●〉 WHAT TO DO

Aortoiliac Thrombosis

- Pentoxifylline, 8.4 to 10 mg/kg PO q12h, can be attempted but is not proven; administer aspirin, 15 mg/kg PO, every other day or clopidogrel, 4 mg/kg PO as a loading dose followed by 2 mg/kg PO q24h. In the treatment of severely affected patients, surgical removal of the thrombus should be attempted by way of the femoral artery using a Fogarty venous thrombectomy catheter.[10]

Peripheral Neuropathy or Gray Matter Lesions

- Any peripheral neuropathy caused by trauma or inflammation (primary neuritis or more commonly resulting from vertebral osteomyelitis) can cause trembling in a leg. There are reports of rare cases of inflammatory neuritis with constant pawing, trembling, and atrophy of a limb that were responsive to corticosteroid therapy only. *Signs such as hyperesthesia and sweating in a focal area can result from an injury/injection and sympathetic nerve injury. Ipsilateral sweating caudal to a point on the body suggests involvement of the descending sympathetic tract in the spinal cord at the origination point. Focal gray matter lesions, such as EPM, also can cause shaking in one or more legs.*

Any Cause of Meningitis Can Cause Trembling

- Covered under specific disease

---

[10]Fogarty venous thrombectomy catheter (Edwards Lifesciences, Irvine, California).

Horner Syndrome

- Horner syndrome is most often caused by the following:
  - Perivascular injections along the jugular vein *with ipsilateral sweating rostral to C2.*
  - A C1-T2 spinal cord disease with ipsilateral sweating over the whole side of the body.
  - A cranial thoracic mass with ipsilateral sweating over the head, neck, and shoulder.
- Abnormal sweating is the most obvious sign of Horner syndrome in horses.
- Nasal edema, snoring, and/or ptosis of the eye on the affected side might also be noticeable.
- Horses do not get Horner syndrome with inner/middle ear disease and only rarely is it associated with guttural pouch mycosis or temporohyoid osteoarthropathy.

● ❯ WHAT TO DO

Horner Syndrome

For perivascular injections causing Horner syndrome, treatment is as follows:
- Administer anti-inflammatory therapy systemically (dexamethasone unless contraindicated) and topically (DMSO with dexamethasone and/or diclofenac [Surpass]).
- Horner syndrome caused by perivascular administration of xylazine or detomidine will resolve within several hours without treatment in many cases.

Change in Mentation

A change in the demeanor or behavior of a horse might be the first neurologic clinical sign recognized by an owner and suggests cerebral or (less commonly) brainstem dysfunction. Erratic behavior or depression combined with ataxia or apparent blindness can be a sign of an infectious or metabolic disease that affects the CNS.

Hepatic Encephalopathy

Hepatic encephalopathy is one of the most common causes of acute cerebral signs in adults (see Chapter 20).

Primary Hyperammonemia Associated with Intestinal Disease

Hyperammonemia in the absence of hepatic disease is an increasingly recognized cause of acute behavior change, blindness, circling, and seizure activity in the adult horse. Colic usually precedes the CNS signs by 12 to 24 hours, and diarrhea often occurs during recovery of CNS signs. The pathogenesis is not fully known but is thought to involve overproduction of ammonia in the gastrointestinal tract or increased absorption of ammonia that overwhelms hepatic metabolism.

Diagnosis

- History of gastrointestinal signs immediately before CNS signs
- Classic triad of laboratory findings:

- Hyperglycemia
- Metabolic acidosis
- Hyperammonemia >150 μmol/L
- Normal liver enzyme activities
- Normal hepatic function tests

● ❯ WHAT TO DO

Primary Hyperammonemia
- Sedation with phenobarbital, 5 to 10 mg/kg IV
- Neomycin, 20 mg/kg PO q6h plus lactulose 0.2 mL/kg PO q12h
- Normosol-R or Plasma-Lyte-A intravenously
- *No* sodium bicarbonate!
- Magnesium sulfate, 1 g/kg PO
- Sodium benzoate, 250 mg/kg IV over 1 hour, is used for primary hyperammonemia in some human patients

Prognosis

- Approximately 50% of equine patients recover in 2 to 3 days with supportive therapy. Patients that do not recover often deteriorate rapidly over 6 to 12 hours.

Mycotoxic Encephalopathy

Known by many pseudonyms (moldy corn poisoning, blind staggers, leukoencephalomalacia, foraging disease), mycotoxic encephalopathy is caused by a toxin elaborated by the mold *Fusarium*, a common contaminant of corn. The clinical syndrome is highly variable and depends on the dose of toxin ingested, species of *Fusarium*, duration of the exposure, and individual susceptibility (see Chapter 34, p. 590).

History

- Highest occurrence is in late fall to early spring; incidence varies from year to year.
- Contaminated corn is part of the diet for several days.
- Multiple horses on the farm are often affected.
- Clinical signs generally begin 4 to 10 days after ingestion of the toxic mold.
- Death occurs within 1 to 3 days of onset of clinical signs.

Clinical Signs
Neurologic Syndrome
- Afebrile
- Behavioral changes (depression to mania)
- Ataxia and weakness that might progress to recumbency
- Blindness
- Asymmetric cranial nerve deficits
- Seizures
- Coma and death
- No consistent pattern of neurologic signs is seen because of the variability of the CNS lesion produced.

Hepatotoxic Syndrome
- Severe icterus
- Swelling of the muzzle and nose
- Difficulty breathing
- Coma and death
- Associated with high dose of the toxin

Cardiotoxic Syndrome
- No specific signs but decreased heart rate and increased cardiac enzyme activities are seen

Diagnosis
- Diagnosis includes history of feeding corn contaminated with *Fusarium* and multiple individuals affected with sudden onset of bizarre neurologic signs.
- Laboratory data usually are nonspecific: stress leukogram and normal to increased liver and cardiac enzyme activities.
- Results of CSF analysis might be normal or show neutrophilic pleocytosis with increased protein and xanthochromia.
- Diagnosis is confirmed postmortem with focal areas of liquefactive necrosis of cerebral white matter.
- Feed can be quantitatively analyzed for *Fusarium*.
- ***Practice Tip:*** *Feed can look grossly normal.*

Differential Diagnosis
- Hepatic encephalopathy
- Viral encephalopathy
- Trauma
- Equine protozoal myeloencephalitis
- Cerebral abscess
- Rabies
- Space-occupying mass
- Botulism
- Herpes myeloencephalopathy

●❯ WHAT TO DO

Moldy Corn Poisoning
- Remove the source of the toxicosis (the corn).
- Administer corticosteroids: dexamethasone, 0.1 to 0.2 mg/kg IV q24h for 1 to 2 days.
- Consider DMSO, 1 g/kg IV as a 10% solution in saline solution q24h for 5 days.
- Maintain hydration with intravenous fluids.
- Give broad-spectrum antibiotic therapy.
- Administer thiamine, 10 mg/kg in IV fluids q12h.
- Provide good nursing care.

Prognosis
- Prognosis is poor because of extensive CNS damage; few survive.

Viral Encephalitis
When any horse has an acute onset of behavior change and fever, viral encephalitis should be on the differential diagnosis list. In temperate regions, most cases occur in late summer and fall.

The absence of fever does not exclude viral encephalitis, especially WNV encephalitis (see p. 349).

Alphaviruses
The alphavirus subcategory of the family Togaviridae includes viruses that cause several diseases: eastern (EEE), western (WEE), and Venezuelan (VEE) equine encephalomyelitis. These diseases, clinically indistinguishable, manifest as an acute onset of fever and depression followed by diffuse CNS signs. Sporadic outbreaks occur in the eastern, Gulf Coast, and north central United States after excessive seasonal rainfall.

Signalment
- Disease can affect any age or breed and either sex. Encephalitis is not common among foals younger than 3 months of age.
- Disease occurs most commonly at the height of the vector (mosquito) season. In the southeastern United States, it can occur year-round.
- EEE and WEE: Usually one horse in a herd is affected. WEE not as common as EEE. WEE is almost always west of the Mississippi River, whereas EEE is predominantly east of the Mississippi River.
- VEE: Morbidity is as high as 50%. The last U.S. outbreak of VEE occurred in 1971, but the virus has since been found in Mexico, northern South America, and Trinidad. Monitoring of the viral encephalitides can be found at www.aphis.usda.gov/vs/nahss/equine/ee/.

Clinical Signs
- High fever
- Colic
- Anorexia
- Depression: might progress to somnolence
- Dementia: compulsive walking, excitability, aggressiveness
- Head-pressing
- Hyperesthesia
- Ataxia
- Blindness
- Circling
- Seizures
- Head tilt
- Recumbency
- Paralysis of pharynx, larynx, and tongue
- Irregular breathing
- Cardiac arrhythmias

Diagnosis
- IgM capture ELISA positive serology
  - Only the whole cell killed vaccine causes a positive IgM capture ELISA
- Fourfold increase in IgG serum titer over 2 to 3 weeks
- PCR or IHC analysis of brain tissue
- CSF analysis: leukocytosis, increased total protein value, xanthochromia. Most dramatic CSF changes are with EEE; changes are less dramatic with WEE and VEE. One might be able to isolate virus from the CSF. Early and mild cases have mononuclear pleocytosis; more severe cases have an equal or greater number of neutrophils, especially EEE.
- Histopathologic examination of the brain and spinal cord: No gross lesions are characteristic of the disease. Most pronounced microscopic lesions are in the cerebral cortex,

thalamus, and hypothalamus. Submit fresh or frozen brain specimen for virus isolation. Immunohistochemical analysis can be performed on fixed tissue.

Caution: Sufficient viral particles for human infection can be present in the CNS, especially with VEE. Use care at postmortem examination. *Do not* use power tools.

◉〉 WHAT TO DO

Viral Encephalitis

- No specific treatment is effective.
- Possibly administer DMSO, 1 g/kg IV as a 10% solution in saline or lactated Ringer's solution q24h for 5 days.
- Administer dexamethasone, 0.1 to 0.2 mg/kg IV q12 to 24h for 1 to 2 days for progressive cases.
- Administer NSAIDs: phenylbutazone, 2.2 mg/kg IV or PO q12h, or flunixin meglumine, 0.5 to 1 mg/kg IV or PO q12h.
- Administer anticonvulsants: diazepam, 0.1 to 0.4 mg/kg IV; phenobarbital, 5 to 10 mg/kg IV or to effect.
- Monitor hydration.
- Provide a laxative diet.
- Supply nutrients.
- Protect horse from self-induced trauma.

Prognosis

- EEE: Mortality is 75% to 100%; complete recovery is unusual. Many equine patients are recumbent for 3 to 4 days before dying.
- WEE: Mortality is 20% to 50%; persistent neurologic deficits are common.
- VEE: Mortality is 40% to 80%; viremia can be present for 3 weeks after recovery. Keep the patient isolated.

Report cases of EEE, WEE, or VEE to public health officials. The affected horse is not a source of WEE and EEE for human infection. *Note:* VEE can be readily transmitted to human beings directly or by mosquitoes.

Rabies

Because rabies is endemic in certain areas of the United States, serious consideration of this disease for cases with change in mentation, acute ataxia, and recumbency is imperative.

The antemortem diagnosis of rabies is difficult because of the wide spectrum of clinical signs and the absence of an accurate antemortem diagnostic test. Horses usually are infected by the bite of a rabid wild animal, but physical evidence of such a wound is seldom found. The incubation period can vary from 2 weeks to several months, but once clinical signs develop, typically a short course (average, 3 to 5 days) of progressive neurologic deterioration ends in death.

If rabies is considered a likely differential, barrier precautions should be used, including gloves and face shields.

Signalment

- The disease has no sex, breed, or age predilection.
- Young horses, being more curious, might be at increased risk.

Box 22-1	Clinical Signs of Rabies
Common	**Less Common**
Aggressiveness	Abnormal vocalizations
Anorexia	Blindness
Ataxia and paresis	Circling
Colic	Drooling
Convulsions	Head tilt
Depression	Paddling while recumbent
Fever	Pharyngeal paralysis
Hyperesthesia	Roaring
Lameness	Sweating
Loss of hind limb sensation	Teeth grinding
Loss of tail and anal tone	Tenesmus
Muscle tremors	
Paraphimosis	
Recumbency	

- Although vaccination is thought to be highly protective, consideration of rabies in any horse with an acute onset of neurologic signs is advised regardless of vaccination status.

Clinical Signs

- Signs are highly variable (Box 22-1).
- Rapid progression of clinical signs is a typical but not mandatory feature of equine rabies. Most patients are terminally recumbent within 3 to 5 days after the onset of clinical signs, although one patient is reported to have remained ambulatory for 9 days after the onset of clinical signs.

Diagnosis

- Complete blood count and serum biochemical testing provide little useful information. Severe hyperglycemia might occur as the result of stress.
- CSF can be normal or have mildly increased cellularity, with lymphocytes as the predominant cell type. Total protein level in the CSF might be normal or increased.
- No accurate antemortem test is available.

Caution: Any body fluid from a patient with suspected rabies must be handled with care. Label specimens properly, and inform laboratory personnel.

Precautions in Managing a Horse with Suspected Rabies

- Minimize human exposure, especially individuals with open wounds.
- Wear gloves and face shields.
- Wash hands thoroughly; the virus is relatively fragile and is killed by most detergents.
- Keep a list of all persons who come in contact with the horse suspected of having rabies. Petting the horse, touching the stall, or handling blood samples does not constitute exposure unless there are open wounds on the hand.

WHAT TO DO

Rabies

- Treatment might not be advisable if the findings are highly suggestive of rabies.
- Postmortem diagnosis is imperative because of zoonotic implications.
- Follow state public health guidelines if an unvaccinated horse is exposed to rabies.
  - Vaccination of horses after a bite has occurred might not be effective; however, a postexposure rabies prophylaxis protocol, developed and mandated in Texas, appears to be effective based on records from 72 horses.
  - This protocol involves immediate vaccination followed by a 90-day isolation period with booster vaccinations during the third and eighth weeks of isolation.

Submission of Rabies Material to the State Diagnostic Laboratory

- Brainstem and cerebellum are the brain samples of choice. Do not submit the entire head.
- Appropriate samples can be obtained with minimal contact through the foramen magnum. Wear latex gloves, surgical mask, and glasses during sample collection.
- Remove the head, and using a hacksaw, remove the back of the calvaria. *Do not* use power saws (including Stryker saws), which can aerosolize the virus. Scoop out cerebellum and some brainstem with a very large spoon.
- Refrigerate specimens before shipment. Do not fix tissues with chemical preservatives.
- Place specimens in at least two layers of separately sealed plastic bags with gel-type cold packs in a Styrofoam-insulated cardboard box.
- Test results are generally reported within 24 to 48 hours of laboratory receipt.
- Disinfect all instruments and surfaces with a 10% solution of household bleach in water.
- Veterinarians are encouraged to undergo rabies prophylaxis. With proper precautions, the risk of a human being acquiring rabies from a large animal is low. In the United States there have been no reported cases of human rabies transmitted from large animals, although a Brazilian veterinarian died from rabies after handling rabid cattle and goats.

Other Viruses

In Canada and the western United States, Bunyavirus encephalitis has been described. Recovery is possible. Other unidentified or identified (Cache Valley, snowshoe hare, St. Louis) viruses can also sporadically produce encephalitis with recovery. Horses with fever, lymphocytic pleocytosis in the CSF, and encephalitic signs can be tested (serologically) for these viruses if serum is sent to the Centers for Disease Control and Prevention. Japanese encephalitis virus affects horses in Japan, and Borna disease and African horse sickness (see Chapter 40, p. 667) can affect horses in Europe. Equine influenza virus has also been reported to cause nonsuppurative encephalitis in horses and mules. In Germany, a tick-borne virus (Flaviviridae) can cause encephalitis.

Verminous Encephalitis

Verminous encephalitis can cause acute ataxia and change in mentation. *Halicephalobus (Micronema) gingivalis (deletrix)* is the most common non-*Sarcocystis* parasite causing encephalitis.

Clinical Signs

- *Halicephalobus* encephalitis most often results in signs of cerebellar or vestibular ataxia (hypermetria, head tremors). Seizures might occur.
- Hematuria and signs of renal disease might be present along with the ataxia. Mandibular osteomyelitis, gingivitis, and head swelling might also be seen because the organism predominantly causes pathologic effects in bone and soft tissue of the head, kidneys, and CNS (most commonly in cerebellar/vestibular/upper cervical area).
- Optic neuritis or retinitis might be seen.

Diagnosis

- A confirmatory diagnosis antemortem is unlikely unless there is a lesion elsewhere in the body where a biopsy can be performed, such as gingiva, kidney, or bone.
- Urine should be examined for the presence of the parasite, although it is rarely if ever found in clinical cases.
- CSF pleocytosis suggests the presence of mixed inflammatory disease (lymphocytes, polymorphonuclear leukocytes), but this finding is nonspecific.

WHAT TO DO

Verminous Encephalitis Caused by *Halicephalobus gingivalis*

- Treatment can be attempted with fenbendazole, 10 to 50 mg/kg PO q24h for 5 days, and diethylcarbamazine, 50 mg/kg PO q24h for 5 days, given after meals.
- Administer corticosteroids: dexamethasone, 0.05 to 0.2 mg/kg IV q24h on days 1 and 2, with tapering dosage thereafter.
- Successful treatment is rare, but based on one recent report, might be possible. A single dose of ivermectin, 0.22 mg/kg PO, is controversial and might exacerbate neurologic signs.

Other Cause of Parasite-Mediated Encephalitis

Verminous encephalitis caused by *Strongylus vulgaris* is rare. Profound neurologic disease results from the migration of larvae within the brain or thrombosis of multiple small arteries to the brain. The thrombosis is caused by embolism of pieces of the verminous plaque, which can originate at the bifurcation of the brachycephalic trunk. The lesion is asymmetric and, in the case of thromboembolism, results in clinical signs that most closely resemble an intracarotid injection or acute, severe EPM. In one report, more than one horse on a farm was affected. Rare episodes of CNS migration by the cattle botfly *Hypoderma bovis* or *Hypoderma lineatum* and by *Setaria* organisms, filarial nematodes common in the peritoneal cavity, have been reported in horses. *Parela-phostrongylus tenuis* can migrate along the dorsal gray column of the cervical spinal cord in young horses, causing acute loss of sensation to one side of the neck and "C"-shaped scoliosis with the convexity on the same side as sensory loss.

●〉 WHAT TO DO

Verminous Encephalitis Caused by *Strongylus vulgaris*
- Corticosteroids and fenbendazole can be used as treatment, but efficacy is unproven. The CSF in affected horses might be normal.

Bacterial Meningitis
Signalment
- Bacterial meningitis is rare in equine medicine except in septic foals, following head injury, with immunodeficiency syndromes, or associated with THO. On rare occasions it can follow infection of a sinus or occur in growing foals without a predisposing cause although immunodeficiency in the foals should be ruled out.
- Adult horses with common variable immunodeficiency often have signs of meningitis (fever, fasciculations, stiffness, reluctance to move the neck freely, change in behavior, and hyperesthesia). These horses have B cell lymphopenia and hypogammaglobulinemia. *Staphylococcus aureus* is often cultured from the neutrophilic CSF.

●〉 WHAT TO DO

Bacterial Meningitis
- Antimicrobials with good penetration into the CSF and efficacy against gram-positive cocci should be the initial treatment in adult horses pending culture and sensitivity of the CSF. For foals, efficacy against gram-negative rods is imperative.
- Ideally, the antibiotics should be bactericidal.
- Enrofloxacin and/or a third- or fourth-generation cephalosporin is recommended (avoid enrofloxacin in foals).
- Ceftiofur could be used at the high dosage range (4 to 6 mg/kg q8h) or preferably ceftriaxone, ceftazidime, or cefotaxime, although these might be cost-prohibitive.
- Other choices include tetracycline or chloramphenicol, but both are bacteriostatic.
- Except in common variable immunodeficiency syndrome, anti-inflammatory therapy is extremely important.
- If the disease is rapidly progressive, a single dose of dexamethasone (0.06 to 0.2 mg/kg IV) and mannitol (0.5 to 1 g/kg IV) are recommended.
- For less severe cases, flunixin should be administered (0.5 to 1 mg/kg q12h), possibly in addition to DMSO (0.1 to 1 g/kg mixed in saline as a 10% solution).
- Horses with bacterial meningitis can make an apparent full recovery if appropriate therapy is provided early in the disease course.

Cerebral Abscess
Signalment
- Abscesses are most common in young foals.
- Often the horse has a history of strangles, pneumonia, or head trauma a few weeks before the onset of signs.

- The most common cause of brain abscess in older horses is infection following head trauma and fracture of the calvarium.

Clinical Signs
- Acute onset, might be febrile
- Depression progressing to stupor and narcolepsy-like signs
- Often episodes of violent behavior, head-pressing, or circling
- Hind limb or tetra-ataxia, falling, acute recumbency
- Unilateral or bilateral blindness
- Often multiple cranial nerves affected
- Head tilt and signs of neck pain common
- Seizures and coma
- Frequent waxing and waning of signs; affected horses might improve with treatment and then suddenly worsen despite treatment

Cause
- *S. equi* is the organism most frequently reported; *S. zooepidemicus* or *R. equi* rarely are reported.
- Access to CNS is through hematogenous spread from a suppurative lesion (bastard strangles), extension of suppuration from the sinus, nasal cavity, guttural pouch, or middle ear, or direct seeding of a variety of organisms from a penetrating wound or fracture.

Diagnosis
- History
- Clinical signs
- CSF sample (increased protein value and nucleated cell count, culture of spinal fluid); some cases have normal CSF
- Brain imaging (magnetic resonance imaging [MRI] or computed tomography [CT]) are best

Differential Diagnosis
- Neoplasia, rare even in adults
- Intracranial hematoma
- Cholesterol granuloma: most common in middle-aged, overweight adults
- EPM
- Rabies
- Hepatic encephalopathy
- Vestibular disease
- Encephalitis
- Idiopathic juvenile epilepsy in Arabian foals

●〉 WHAT TO DO

Cerebral Abscess
- Penicillin potassium, 22,000 IU/kg IV q6h or
- Trimethoprim-sulfamethoxazole, 30 mg/kg PO q12h
- +/– DMSO, 1g/kg IV as a 10% solution in saline solution or any isotonic fluid
- Flunixin meglumine, 0.5 to 1 mg/kg IV q12h

- Dexamethasone, 0.1 to 0.2 mg/kg IV, single dose, if necessary to reduce cerebral edema
- Phenobarbital to effect, 5 to 10 mg/kg IV as needed to control seizures
- Surgical drainage and catheter placement for administering cephalosporins into the abscess site

Prognosis

- Prognosis is poor to grave, although the rare adult horse has recovered. Excessive use of corticosteroids to control clinical signs might increase the risk of laminitis.

Moxidectin Coma

- Foals less than 4 months of age can develop coma following administration of moxidectin. This is a result of excessive gamma-aminobutyric acid production in the brain and occurs in young foals because of increased permeability of blood-brain barrier to the drug. The identical syndrome is reported in a premature foal administered ivermectin. Adult Quarter Horses rarely develop blindness, depression, and salivation following a standard ivermectin treatment.

●› WHAT TO DO

Moxidectin Coma
- Treatment is supportive care and administration of a single dose of sarmazenil (0.04 mg/kg IV).
- Intravenously administered lipids may also be used.

●› WHAT NOT TO DO

Moxidectin Coma
- Do not use moxidectin in young foals.

Fungal Meningitis

Cryptococcus is the most common fungal infection of the CNS. Affected horses can have predominantly cerebral or spinal cord signs. Fever usually is present. The CSF has considerable neutrophilic pleocytosis (generally greater than the clinical signs would indicate). The organism can be identified on close inspection of the CSF. On rare occasions, *Aspergillus* sp. can cause otitis media-interna and vestibular disease.

●› WHAT TO DO

Fungal Meningitis
- Administer itraconazole, 5 mg/kg PO q12 to 24h. This drug is highly protein-bound, so higher dosages may be needed to cross into the CSF.
- Or administer fluconazole, 14 mg/kg PO loading dose followed by 5 mg/kg daily. Although high CSF levels are obtained, *Aspergillus* sp. can be resistant.

Post–Endurance Race Cerebral Syndrome

Occasionally, a horse develops severe depression leading to recumbency and obtundation following an endurance race. This might be the result of the following:

- Hyperthermia
- Prolonged hypoxia
- Ischemia/reperfusion
- Free water consumption causing movement of water into damaged neurons, especially ones that have been chronically dehydrated from the race and have increased concentration of idiogenic osmoles

●› WHAT TO DO

Post–Endurance Race Cerebral Syndrome
- Horses that have signs of deranged cerebral function following an endurance race should be immediately placed on intranasal oxygen and treated for cerebral edema (see cerebral edema treatment, p. 369).
- Only oral and IV fluids containing sodium (at least 140 mEq/L) should be used.
- Once the horse becomes recumbent and obtunded, the prognosis is grave.

Equine Self-Mutilation Syndrome

Equine self-mutilation syndrome is a self-mutilating behavior described as biting at the flank area, tail, or lateral thoracic wall. The behavior often is precipitated by stress (anticipation of eating or interaction with others). Males are seven times more likely than females to develop the condition, which most often starts during the first 2 years of life. Heritable factors, inactivity or confinement, and stimulation of endogenous opioids might be involved in the development of the behavior.

●› WHAT TO DO

Equine Self-Mutilation Syndrome
- Castration, change in diet, stabling changes, and the use of opioid antagonists (nalmefene) have been used to manage the behavior with partial success.
- Imipramine, a tricyclic antidepressant drug, 1 mg/kg PO q12h, has been used successfully.
- Thorough diagnostic evaluation to investigate potential physical problems contributing to the behavior should be pursued.

Sudden Collapse

Examining a horse that has suddenly collapsed is an intimidating diagnostic and therapeutic challenge. Metabolic, respiratory, cardiovascular, and orthopedic causes of sudden collapse must be considered, as should the neurologic differential diagnosis list, sleep deprivation, narcolepsy/cataplexy, and polysaccharide storage myopathy. The prognosis for future use often is the determining factor in the owner's decision to pursue treatment. An accurate anatomic diagnosis is the first, and occasionally the most difficult, step. Always consider the possibility of rabies (see p. 364). Cataplexy can be a serious problem in some miniature horses and might require treatment in order for the horse to be functional and self-protective.

CNS

CNS

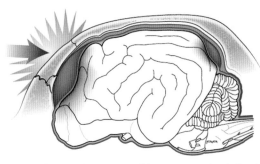

Figure 22-6   Schematic demonstrating blunt trauma to the skull and cortical injury at the site of the trauma (coup contusion—*arrow*) and the posterior cortical injury (contrecoup contusion) caused by rapid movement of the brain in the calvaria.

WHAT TO DO

Sudden Collapse

- Perform complete general physical, orthopedic, and neurologic examinations. Consider video-monitoring, possibly in conjunction with Holter monitoring, to capture episodes of collapse. The most common causes of collapse include sleep deprivation, seizures, and syncope. Video analysis should allow differentiation.
- Treatment is quite variable depending on etiology.

Cranial Trauma

Cerebral edema with hemorrhage is the most harmful and immediate pathologic result of cranial trauma, causing hypoxia and brain compression. Inflammation and oxidative injury begin soon after the injury and typically persist for at least 48 hours thereafter. Clinical signs are generally most severe within 12 hours, but uncontrolled cerebral edema and inflammation can result in progression of intracranial signs.

Causes

- Collisions, kicks
- Penetrating wounds
- Falls: over a jump; rearing and falling over backward (poll impact)
- Direct injury to neural parenchyma radiating from the point of impact and from the opposite margin of the brain (Fig. 22-6)
- Direct injury by displacement of basioccipital and basisphenoid bones into the overlying brain or brainstem

WHAT TO DO

Initial Clinical Management for Cranial Trauma

- Stabilize the medical condition.
- Maintain a patent airway. It is important to maintain Pa_{CO_2} at a low-normal value because elevations in Pa_{CO_2} increase cerebral blood flow and edema.
- Intubate if necessary and use an Ambu Bag. Supply oxygen if available.
- Control blood loss.
- Control seizures. Quiet the patient if the horse is having seizures or thrashing; use the lowest doses necessary of detomidine and butorphanol (2.5 mg of each, for example) or ideally diazepam, 0.1 to 0.4 mg/kg, to gain control of the horse. Then place a catheter and

give phenobarbital (which might decrease free radical injury, decrease cerebral metabolic rate, and decrease intracranial pressure, therefore improving perfusion) slowly IV to effect for more long-term seizure control.[11] The approximate IV dose is 5 to 10 mg/kg, which can be repeated (phenobarbital will not have full effect for several minutes). Another emergency option for immediate control of the recumbent horse having seizures is 5 to 10 mL of Fatal Plus (pentobarbital 390 mg/mL) mixed with 20 to 40 mL of saline; this should only be used when other treatments are unavailable.
- Obtain an accurate history.
- Perform as complete a physical examination as possible. Look for bleeding or leakage of CSF from wounds, ears, and nose; respiratory distress (abnormal respiratory patterns); and evidence of laryngeal injury.
- Perform an ophthalmic examination (fixed, dilated pupils are a poor prognostic finding). Retinal detachments can occur after head trauma, although optic nerve injury is more common. Palpate the skull carefully for fractures or crepitus, which often indicate that a fracture has occurred.

Neurologic Examination

- Assess mentation (alert, obtunded, stuporous, comatose).
- Assess visual response (menace); cortical injury often results in contralateral blindness.
- Perform a cranial nerve examination, especially pupil size; symmetry; pupillary light reflexes; menace response (a severely depressed horse might not menace, even though it is visual); and presence of nystagmus, strabismus, or dysphagia.
- Assess caudal brainstem function: respiratory pattern, swallowing, tongue tone, and vestibular signs.
- Evaluate voluntary limb movement and quality of the gait. Evaluate for concurrent spinal cord, orthopedic, soft tissue, thoracic, and abdominal injuries.
- Assess pain perception.
- Assess noxious perception by placing a finger in the patient's nose; this tests contralateral cortical response.
- Assess for abnormal body position or head tilt.
- Keep an accurate written record of all observations if possible; serial reassessment is crucial to evaluate progress and modify therapy.
- ***Practice Tip:*** *The presence of changes in pupil size from normal to miotic to dilated and fixed is a grave prognostic finding.*

Ancillary Procedures

- If possible, the following might prove valuable:
  - Skull radiographs, especially if palpable evidence of fracture or bleeding from ear or nose
  - CT or MRI
  - CSF collection and analysis: If the fluid is grossly contaminated with blood, and procedural contamination is unlikely, think fracture and a grave prognosis. ***Caution:*** Cisternocentesis and removal of a small volume of fluid should be done with caution because removal

---

[11]This treatment can also be used for seizures resulting from other causes, such as idiopathic, hypoxic/ischemic, and infectious causes.

of excessive fluid from a patient with severe cerebral edema can result in brain herniation. If there is an opportunity (gas anesthesia) to provide brief hyperventilation ($Paco_2 < 35$ mm Hg) before CSF collection, this should decrease the risk of herniation. CSF can be normal even with severe bleeding in the forebrain.

- Upper airway and guttural pouch endoscopy: Bleeding into the guttural pouches and from the nostrils can occur with fracture of basioccipital bones and ruptured rectus capitis muscle.

●〉 WHAT TO DO

Additional Treatment for Cranial Trauma

- *Administer polyionic crystalloids* with an osmolality slightly >300 mOsm/L at a maintenance rate to help support normal cerebral perfusion and provide electrolytes and buffers. Monitor systemic blood pressure with the goal of keeping mean arterial pressure >80 mm Hg. If needed, plasma expanders such as hetastarch or 25% albumin can be used. Approximately 100 mL of hypertonic saline should be added to each 5 L of balanced crystalloid fluid in an effort to maintain plasma osmolality at 310 to 320 mmol/L. This is believed to be effective in both decreasing cerebral edema and maintaining adequate cerebral perfusion. The initial treatment can be 7.5% hypertonic saline given at 1 to 2 mL/kg while the crystalloids are being set up or the horse is referred. If the patient is being referred any distance, 3.2% saline can be repeated a second time in 4 hours. Another treatment option to decrease brain swelling is mannitol,[12] 0.5 to 1 g/kg IV as a 20% mixture, repeated as needed at 4- to 8-hour intervals on the first day.
- Once the patient is hospitalized, the osmolality can be directly measured (necessary for mannitol), or if only saline is being used, it can be estimated as sodium concentration multiplied by 2.1 (if glucose and blood urea nitrogen are above normal range, the osmolality is further increased above the calculated value). The intravenous fluids should be refrigerated and administered cold unless the horse is already hypothermic.
- +/− DMSO, 0.1 to 1g/kg IV as a 10% to 20% solution in saline or other polyionic fluid q12 to 24h for up to 5 days.
- Vitamin E, 20,000 units PO q24h, for an adult, and coenzyme Q_{10}, 1000 mg or more per day PO and thiamine, 10 mg/kg diluted IV q24 h.
- Furosemide, 1 mg/kg IV q12h for 1 to 2 days. Furosemide is a potent diuretic; monitor for electrolyte imbalances and maintain hydration, especially when combined with mannitol.
- Keep the head elevated at 30 degrees if possible, and do not occlude the jugular veins.
- Dexamethasone, 0.1 to 0.2 mg/kg IV q6 to 8h, for the first 24 hours after injury and then q24h for 2 to 3 days (of questionable value for noninflammatory cerebral injury).
- Pentoxifylline, 8.4 to 10.0 mg/kg PO or IV q12h.
- Flunixin meglumine, 1 mg/kg q12h for 1 to 3 days; flunixin might not be effective in preventing brain-associated fever.
- Broad-spectrum antibiotics, especially if palpable fracture or evidence of bleeding is present.

[12]Do not use mannitol if bleeding in the cranial cavity has not been controlled (i.e., if there is bleeding from the nose or ears or a palpable skull fracture or a grossly bloody CSF sample). Mannitol treatment is controversial but might improve perfusion of the brain better than NaCl and has antioxidant properties. If a cerebral bleed is believed ongoing, aminocaproic acid, 10 mg/kg IV q6h can be administered.

- Magnesium sulfate, 15 to 30 mg/kg per hour IV (7.5 to 15 g/h in the 500-kg horse) if blood pressure is normal and plasma magnesium remains <4 mg/dL.
- Minocycline, 4 mg/kg PO q12h or doxycycline, 10 mg/kg PO q12h to inhibit metalloproteinase activity and apoptosis.
- Perform fracture repair if needed.
- Maintain blood glucose in normal range.
- Other treatments that have been used include:
  - 30% polyethylene glycol, 2 mg/kg IV
  - Progesterone
  - Vitamin C
- Give oxygen therapy if there is hypoventilation or pulmonary disease.
- Ventilate if needed.
- Omeprazole for gastric ulcer prophylaxis.
- Protect the patient from further injury by using a padded helmet and leg wraps and keeping the horse quiet and confined to a safe stall. Make sure the patient can urinate; disinfect the mouth with antiseptic flushes if dysphagic.
- CT, MRI, and exploratory craniotomy are available at some equine centers.

Monitoring

- Heart rate, respiratory rate and depth, and blood pressure should be maintained at near-normal values.
- Urine production should be adequate with the goal of 1 to 2 mL/kg/hr.
- Arterial oxygen should be 80 mm Hg or greater.
- Venous jugular oxygen saturation should be 60%. If it is not, attempt to increase perfusion and oxygen to the brain with IV fluids and supplemental oxygen.
- Maintain body temperature slightly lower than normal by administering chilled IV fluids and using other cooling methods (fans, ice packs, chilled enema, etc.).
- Assess pupil size and response.
- Monitor glucose (maintain normoglycemia).
- Monitor lactate.

●〉 WHAT NOT TO DO

Cranial Trauma

- Do *not* administer the following:
  - Glucose, unless the patient is confirmed hypoglycemic, which is rare except in foals
  - Calcium, unless the patient is confirmed hypocalcemic (low ionized calcium)
- Do *not* try to warm the patient too fast if hypothermia is present. Keep the head cool with ice bags, if possible.

Poor Prognostic Indicators

- Deterioration in vital signs
- Altered respiratory patterns (brainstem injury)
- Slow heart rate, decreasing blood pressure (medullary lesion)
- Unresponsive dilated pupils (midbrain lesion)
- Miotic pupils that become mydriatic (progressive midbrain edema or compression)
- Deterioration of mental status
- Tetraparesis or paraparesis progressing to recumbency
- Progressive loss of cranial nerve function (compression, hypoxia)

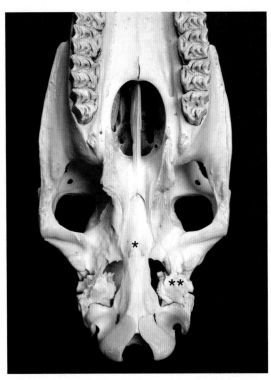

Figure 22-7   Ventral view of the equine skull. The basilar tubercles (*) are located between the basilar portion of the occipital and sphenoid bones. This is the site of attachment of the primary flexor of the head (rectus capitis muscle) and a common location for fracture when horses flip over and strike their poll on the ground. Signs may include seizure, coma, acute death, ataxia, and bleeding into guttural pouches, depending on degree and direction of fracture displacement. (**, Petrous bone.)

- Opisthotonos (cerebellum, brainstem)
- Fracture of the skull with severe CNS signs
- Intensifying seizures
- Gross hemorrhage into CSF

Basisphenoid and Basioccipital Fractures

Fractures of the basisphenoid or basioccipital bone, or both are particularly common among young adult horses that flip over backward (Fig. 22-7). Bleeding often is seen in the nose and sometimes the ear.

If the displacement is minimal, clinical signs might improve, and the individual recovers or is left with a mild residual head tilt. Minor displacement can be difficult to recognize on standard radiographs. If the displacement is severe, cerebral hemorrhage occurs, and the patient does not recover.

A bloody CSF sample might or might not be obtained with cerebral hemorrhage, depending on the location of the cerebral bleed.

Some horses that flip over backward rupture the muscles within the guttural pouch and sustain a fracture. Hemorrhage and a mild head tilt occur as a result of the muscle rupture. Check vision and pupillary light reflexes because many horses, especially foals, that experience severe backward flips have acute optic nerve injury and permanent blindness. Recovery is likely if the horse can stand, is not blind, and does not have a severe head tilt.

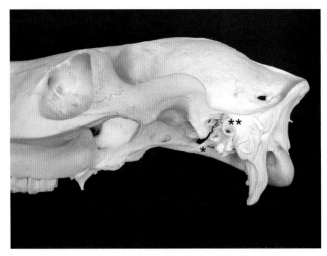

Figure 22-8   Petrous bone (**) is another common site for skull injury (fracture) in the horse that leads to acute neurologic deficits (mostly vestibular signs). Fractures of this bone may be hard to visualize on radiographs or computed tomography. (*, Basilar tubercles.)

➤➤ WHAT TO DO

Basisphenoid and Basioccipital Fractures
- Treat as for cerebral injury (see p. 368). Head tilt might be the only clinical sign.

Fractured Petrous Bone

A fractured petrous bone seems to be more common in weanlings and yearlings, once again associated with flipping over backward or falling on the side of the head (Fig. 22-8). Head tilt is a fairly consistent sign. Small fractures of this bone are difficult to confirm on radiographs or CT.

➤➤ WHAT TO DO

Petrous Bone Fractures
- Treatment is the same as for brain trauma (see 368). If the facial nerve is involved, remember to medicate the eye as a prophylaxis for exposure keratitis.

Frontal/Parietal Bone Trauma

Brain injury caused by trauma to the frontal and parietal bones is generally a result of a fracture with displacement or epidural hematoma. Variable degrees of stupor occur, and there can be blindness (with normal pupillary light reflexes) in the eye contralateral to the side of the head injury. Likewise, there might be loss of response to nasal stimulation on the contralateral side.

➤➤ WHAT TO DO

Frontal/Parietal Bone Trauma
- Treatments are similar to those for cerebral injury (p. 368). Antibiotics should always be administered if there is a fracture. Several horses have made remarkable recoveries in the first several days following the injury but have succumbed to a brain abscess later. If there is obvious fracture displacement, surgical reduction and stabilization are indicated.

Spinal Cord Trauma

Causes
- Falls, including over a jump and rearing over backward: Horses (especially timber horses) that land on their noses after falling often fracture/injure the caudal cervical/cranial thoracic area. Horses that flip directly over (poll impact) seem more commonly to have upper cervical injury. Less commonly, thoracolumbar fractures/injuries occur.
- Collision with a fixed object
- Pathologic fracture resulting from osteomyelitis (discospondylitis), especially *R. equi* or *S. equi* in 2- to 10-month-old foals

Clinical Signs
- Acute ataxia after an injury (or, in the case of discospondylitis, unassociated with a traumatic event). The ataxia can be para-ataxia, tetra-ataxia, or hemiataxia depending on the location of the lesion.
- Progression to severe ataxia or recumbency might be rapid.
- Perform a complete physical examination. The horse might be unmanageable because of pain.
- Remember that spinal cord trauma may or may not be associated with a fracture, and those cases without fracture often have rapid recovery from the ataxia.
- Acute concussion from flipping over can cause severe edema or hemorrhage in the cord, which can progress for 24 hours.

Emergency Stabilization of Medical Condition
- Support ventilation
- Control hemorrhage
- Manage shock with intravenously administered fluids (e.g., hypertonic saline solution)
- Assess and manage other injuries, such as orthopedic injuries

Neurologic Assessment of Spinal Cord Trauma
- If the horse is standing, evaluate attitude, posture, and gait. Look for ataxia: Are forelimbs involved or only hind limbs? Examine for palpable cervical abnormalities (swelling or crepitus) and neck pain.
- If the horse is recumbent, carefully assess whether the horse can become sternal, rise with assistance, or support weight. If the horse cannot become sternal, this supports a diagnosis of upper cervical injury.

Localizing the Lesion
- C1 to C3 lesion: horse might only lift head if recumbent or is tetraparetic/ataxia if standing
  - Hyperactive reflexes of all four limbs
  - Might prefer to lie on one side
- C4 to C6 lesion: horse can elevate head and neck if recumbent and is tetraparetic if standing
  - Hyperactive reflexes of all four limbs
- C6 to T2 lesion: tetraparesis or tetraparalysis

- Most severe signs in front legs
- Decreased spinal reflexes and tone in forelimbs
- Normal or hyperactive reflexes and tone in the pelvic limbs
- T3 to L3 lesion: horse might be able to dog sit and is paraparetic if standing
  - Thoracic limbs normal
  - Pelvic limb paresis to paralysis
  - With severe lesions, bladder paralysis
  - Might have patchy sweating along the trunk from damage to sympathetic nerves
- L4 to L6 lesion: horse might weakly dog sit
  - Pelvic limb paresis or paralysis
  - Loss of patellar reflex
- Sacral fracture: bladder paralysis with severe lesions
  - Pelvic limb gait deficit is possible
  - Pain found on rectal palpation and manipulation of the tail
  - Fecal retention and decreased anal and tail tone might be evident
  - Hyperesthesia of perineum, anus, and tail might be present
- Schiff-Sherrington syndrome: thoracolumbar trauma causes extensor rigidity of the thoracic limbs and hypotonic paralysis of the pelvic limbs
  - Rarely occurs in horses
- Horner syndrome (see p. 362)
  - Syndrome can result from a severe cervical spinal cord lesion, a T1 to T3 lesion, or perivascular jugular irritation involving sympathetic nerves. Signs are ipsilateral facial, neck, or truncal sweating, and include: miosis, ptosis, and third eyelid prominence on the side of the lesion.

Diagnosis
- Obtain radiographs.
- Perform a myelogram.
- Most CT and MRI units allow placement of only the proximal half of the neck of an adult horse in the gantry.
- Obtain a CSF sample if necessary.

●》 WHAT TO DO

Spinal Cord Trauma
- Provide stall rest for ambulatory patients.
- Dexamethasone, 0.1 to 0.2 mg/kg q12h IV for the first 1 to 2 days, for severely affected patients that are recumbent or grade 4 ataxic. Lower dosages can be used for less severely affected horses.
  OR
- Methylprednisolone sodium succinate, 10 to 30 mg/kg IV, within 1 hour of trauma (expensive).
- +/− DMSO, 0.1 to 1 g/kg IV as a 10% mixture in saline or lactated Ringer's solution.
- Broad-spectrum antibiotics if patient is recumbent, a fracture is diagnosed, or wounds are present.
- Maintain hydration and nutrition.
- Catheterize and drain bladder if necessary.
- Provide good nursing care.

- Vitamin E (aqueous), 2000 to 10,000 U/day PO per adult horse, and coenzyme Q₁₀, 1000 mg/day or more PO.
- Omeprazole for gastric ulcer prophylaxis (especially in foals and adults that have received high doses of steroids).
- Perform surgery for decompression or stabilization in selected cases. *Some horses with severe displacements of the upper cervical vertebral arches do well with only supportive treatment.*
- *Caution:* General anesthesia should be undertaken with care. Death can result from respiratory failure if the horse has severe cervical spinal cord lesions. Relaxation of muscle tone can cause displacement of fractures and can exacerbate neurologic injury.
- A sling can be useful in the care of some recumbent patients that have nondisplaced vertebral fractures.

Prognosis

Many weanlings or foals that fall over backward and have spinal cord signs recover completely within a few days. Adults seem to be more predisposed to fractures and therefore have a poorer prognosis. Fracture of the sacrum can result in cauda equina syndrome. Blindness is a common sequela among horses of all ages that flip over and have acute concussive injury to the head (see Chapter 23, p. 416).

- Obvious blood in CSF (not attributable to procedural contamination) indicates a poor prognosis.

Occipital or Atlantoaxial Injury or Malformations and Fracture of the Cranial Cervical Spine in Foals

Fracture of one or more of the occipital or atlantoaxial bones and subluxation are common problems in foals.

Clinical Signs

- Tetra-ataxia
- Tetraparesis
- Stiff neck
- Head or neck tilt
- Possible progression to recumbency

Diagnosis

- Crepitus on palpation
- Radiographs: sometimes can be difficult to image the lesion even when a fracture is present
- CT, MRI
- Fluoroscopy for those that have only dynamic compression

●〉 WHAT TO DO

For Injuries/Malformation of Cranial Cervical Spine in Foals

- *Fractures without ataxia and cord compression:* Provide stall rest, adapt feeding methods if needed, and administer ulcer prophylaxis.
- *Fractures with ataxia:* Consider administering DMSO, 1 g/kg IV q12-24h, and flunixin meglumine if pain is so severe that the foal does not move. If compression seems likely, perform myelography, CT, or MRI and then surgically stabilize or decompress the fracture.
- *Fractures or subluxation with head tilt, neck tilt:* Neck brace and stall confinement are generally the treatments of choice. The brace should be developed to help support the neck and maintain some

extension. The brace can make it difficult for the foal to rise and nurse and might predispose the foal to pneumonia, requiring antibiotics and significant nursing care.

Seizures

Seizures can be generalized or localized (focal seizures). Generalized seizures are characterized by tonic-clonic muscle activity, involuntary recumbency, and loss of consciousness. Postictal blindness and depression are common.

Focal seizures might not have obvious postictal signs or might have postictal localized clinical signs, such as facial or limb twitching, compulsive circling, self-mutilation of a particular area, and excessive chewing.

The diagnostic goal is to uncover a treatable underlying cause of the seizure, if one exists.

Causes

- Seizures can be classified as a manifestation of structural brain disease, metabolic/toxic disease, or an idiopathic condition.

Structural Brain Disease

- Neoplasia
- Abscess
- Parasitic (EPM; fairly common)
- Embolism caused by *Strongylus* spp.
- Pituitary adenoma, which can on rare occasions cause seizures or blindness
- Encephalitis (viral, bacterial, fungal)
- Meningitis
- Effect of trauma (bleeding, edema)
- Intracarotid injection
- Arterial air embolism
- Other intracranial masses: cholesterol granuloma
- Ischemic, hypoxic damage: mostly newborn foals (see Chapter 31, p. 545)
- Developmental causes, such as hydrocephalus and microencephaly
- If the lesion is in a quiet area of the brain, the affected individual is normal in an interictal period. If the lesion is in an active area of the brain, the individual shows signs of depression or a cranial nerve or proprioceptive deficit in the interictal period.
- *Practice Tip:* Do not misinterpret normal, vigorous rapid eye movement during sleep as seizure activity.

Metabolic/Toxic Disease

- Hyponatremia (common among foals with severe diarrhea or newborn foals with ruptured bladder, bilateral hydroureter, or inappropriate secretion of antidiuretic hormone)
- Hypoglycemia in foals and adults, which causes depression but rarely seizures
- *Neonatal encephalopathy* (also known as neonatal maladjustment syndrome, hypoxic-ischemic encephalopathy, and peripartum asphyxia syndrome): Foals have seizures, depression, or ataxia (see Chapter 31, p. 545).

- Hepatic encephalopathy: severe liver disease or portosystemic shunt
- Hyperammonemia without liver failure: 4- to 8-month-old Morgans and, infrequently, adults of any breed with colic (p. 362)
- Renal encephalopathy (rare)
- Hyperlipemia, hyperlipidemia
- Hyperkalemia (HYPP)
- Hyperthermia
- Kernicterus: Generally, this occurs in foals with neonatal isoerythrolysis with a bilirubin value in excess of 25 mg/dL. When bilirubin approaches this level, prevention of kernicterus includes plasma exchange or transfusion and small doses of phenobarbital or pentobarbital, 0.5 to 1 mg/kg IV q8h.
- Intoxication (see Chapter 34, p. 588)
  - Organophosphates
  - Propylene glycol
  - Mushroom toxicosis
  - Lead
  - Arsenic
  - Strychnine
- Hypocalcemia and hypomagnesemia (see p. 356)

◉ WHAT TO DO

Managing Severe Hyponatremia (<120 mEq/L)
- If severe hyponatremia is present, hypertonic saline solution can be administered until the serum sodium concentration is 125 mg/L and then further correction is made over several hours with isotonic crystalloids.
  - *Practice Tip:* As a rule, the more chronic the hyponatremia the slower it is corrected.
- Mannitol and thiamine can be administered while the serum sodium level is *slowly* corrected. Overly rapid correction can result in a permanent neurologic disorder.
- Hypernatremia generally causes depression rather than seizures. Sodium concentration should be returned to a normal value *slowly*. Do not use 5% dextrose alone for hypernatremia.

Idiopathic Epilepsy of Foals
- Onset usually at 3 to 9 months of age
- Generalized seizures with or without involuntary recumbency
- Hereditary in Egyptian Arabians

◉ WHAT TO DO

Idiopathic Epilepsy in Foals
- Respond well to anticonvulsants
- Usually outgrown after 3 months of anticonvulsant therapy

Lavender Foal Syndrome
- Lavender foal syndrome is a metabolic syndrome of newborn Egyptian Arabian foals with a "dilute" coat color. The foals are usually in opisthotonos immediately after birth and remain in lateral recumbency and paddle,

although they might be able to nurse and be aware of surroundings. The disorder is uniformly fatal.

Seizures During Estrus in Mares (Rare)
- Related to elevated estrogen level
- Occur during estrus only
- Underlying etiologic factor unknown
- This has rarely been reported in late-term pregnant mares that stop having seizures after delivery

◉ WHAT TO DO

Seizures During Estrus
- Control with progesterone or ovariectomy

Other Idiopathic Causes of Seizures
- Primary cerebrovascular disease (stroke) that is not related to an infection or a traumatic cause has been reported.
- On a rare occasion, acute and extensive (rostral) thrombosis of the jugular vein can cause seizures and circling.

Differential Diagnoses of Seizures
- Colic
- Exertional myopathy
- Sleep deprivation: some horses, when deprived of recumbent rest, begin collapsing during quiet times (in the stall, on cross-ties, in the field). The episodes of collapse are sometimes confused with seizures.
- Syncope: Cardiac problems such as severe bradycardia, prolonged Q-T syndrome, and obstruction of cerebral blood flow. Two types of noncardiac syncope are reported to exist.
- The presence of a mass in the lower thoracic region, such as *Corynebacterium pseudotuberculosis,* which can cause fainting when the horse lowers its head.
- Some individuals faint when the head is rapidly elevated.
  - Rapid recovery occurs when the head and neck are returned to a normal position in both the aforementioned conditions.
- Upper airway problems, such as laryngeal obstruction or acute pulmonary edema
- Narcolepsy, cataplexy: most common in miniature horses and Shetland ponies. Some respond to imipramine, 1 to 2.2 mg/kg PO q12h. Miniature foals often "outgrow" the problem.
- Tetanus
- A normal sleeping foal or horse can exhibit eyelid, lip, and limb movements that owners misinterpret as seizure activity.
- HYPP, hypocalcemia, and other tetanic disorders can have seizure-like signs.

Diagnosis
- Laboratory analysis (immediately after a seizure if possible) of glucose and electrolytes.
- Establish an accurate description of the seizure. If possible, place the horse under video surveillance to capture an episode.

- Interictal examination: Closely examine cranial nerves and look for evidence of proprioceptive deficits during a complete neurologic exam.
- Perform CSF sample and analysis.
- Obtain skull radiographs.
- Perform a fundic examination.
- Perform brain scan; CT or MRI.

●❯ WHAT TO DO

Seizures
To Stop a Seizure
- Diazepam, 5 to 20 mg IV for a foal; 0.1 to 0.4 mg/kg IV for an adult horse
- Midazolam, 0.04 to 0.2 mg/kg bolus followed by CRI of 0.01 to 0.04 mg/kg/hr
- Propofol, 4 mg/kg IV for uncontrolled seizures in foals (*not* ideal; attempt to control with benzodiazepines or phenobarbital)
- Pentobarbital (administer slowly to effect): approximately 3 to 10 mg/kg IV for immediate effect
- Phenobarbital (administer slowly to effect): approximately 5 to 15 mg/kg IV; requires 15 minutes for full effect. **Note:** Using dosages higher than 5 mg/kg might cause severe drowsiness and potentially respiratory depression, particularly in foals. Start with a low dose and increase if necessary for seizure control. Be prepared to administer ventilatory support if necessary. Doses higher than 15 mg/kg might be required in some cases.
- Potassium bromide, 50 to 120 mg/kg PO q24h × 5 days, can be added to treatments in individuals that do not respond to phenobarbital.
- Xylazine, 0.5 to 1 mg/kg IV, is not recommended as the first choice because it reduces cerebral blood flow after transiently increasing intracranial pressure, potentially exacerbating seizures. Xylazine or detomidine can be used as a last resort if only a small-volume injection is feasible because of uncontrollable seizure activity. *Also, see Cranial Trauma and Seizures (p. 368).*

Ancillary Treatments
- +/− DMSO, 1 g/kg IV as a 10% solution in saline or any other isotonic fluid once a day for 3 to 5 days
- Flunixin meglumine, 0.5 to 1 mg/kg IV q12 to 24h; potentially ulcerogenic in foals
- Antibiotics if a bacterial cause is suspected
- 10% dextrose IV for documented hypoglycemia, HYPP, and hepatic encephalopathy

Maintenance Therapy
- Phenobarbital, 5 to 10 mg/kg PO q12h (wide individual variation in dosage); might take 2 to 3 weeks to adapt to dosage and 10 to 14 days to reach steady-state. Reduce the dosage if patient is too sedated. Therapeutic range is considered 10 to 40 µg/mL, but some individuals seemingly respond to lower concentrations.
- Potassium bromide, 30 to 100 mg/kg PO q24h; takes several weeks to reach steady-state. Therapeutic range is considered 1 to 2 mg/mL.
- Pregabalin, 3 to 4 mg/kg PO q8h for seizure and pain control.

Prognosis
- Prognosis depends on the cause; i.e., whether there is a treatable intracranial or extracranial condition. Poor prognostic signs include increasing frequency of seizures, escalating intensity of seizures, and poor response to maintenance therapy.

Drug-Induced Hyperexcitability, Seizure, or Collapse
Drug-induced hyperexcitability, seizure, or collapse is caused by inadvertent intracarotid injection, penicillin procaine reaction, or drug-induced hypotension.

Inadvertent Intracarotid Injection
- Onset is during injection or a few seconds after injection.
- Acute seizure occurs with recumbency and paddling.
- Event might be preceded by facial twitching, head jerking with gradual raising of the head, and a wide-eyed appearance.
- Severity of signs depends on volume injected, properties of the drug, and individual sensitivity.
- *Caution:* It is difficult to differentiate arterial and venous (blood) puncture when a 20-gauge needle is used to administer intravenous medication.
- If drug is water soluble (xylazine, acepromazine), consider the following:
  - The affected individual can usually stand in 5 to 60 minutes.
  - The horse's condition usually is clinically normal in 1 to 7 days if no secondary injuries occur.
  - The following clinical signs can occur in addition to collapse: contralateral blindness, nasal septum hypalgesia, and subtle hemiparesis.
- Treatment might be unnecessary because most recover spontaneously.

●❯ WHAT TO DO

Intracarotid Injection
- Protect yourself and others first
- Dexamethasone, 0.1 to 0.2 mg/kg q12h for the first 24 hours IV
- +/− DMSO, 1 g/kg IV as a 10% solution in saline
- Diazepam, 0.1 mg/kg IV to quiet recovery or
- Phenobarbital to effect, 5 to 10 mg/kg IV q12h or q24h if seizures exist
- If drug administered into the carotid is insoluble or oil-based (e.g., phenylbutazone, penicillin procaine, or trimethoprim-sulfamethoxazole), consider the following:
  - Acute death often occurs
  - Recovery is usually unsatisfactory
  - Seizure is more severe
  - Persistent stupor or coma can occur
  - Humane destruction might be justified

Reaction to Intramuscular Procaine Penicillin Injection
- Reaction results from rapid intravenous absorption of procaine penicillin after intramuscular administration.
- Reaction might occur even with correct injection technique.
- Response is most common after several intramuscular injections have been given, causing the injection site to be more vascular.

- The "reaction" usually begins immediately after the injection or when it is nearly completed.
- Affected individuals act as if spooked, circle wildly, snort and/or bang around in their stall, or collapse and have behavior associated with a seizure.
- Keep the patient confined. Often the most serious consequence is self-inflicted injury, which can worsen if the patient is loose.
- Acute death can occur if a large volume is absorbed intravenously or the drug is mistakenly administered through an intravenous catheter.

●> WHAT TO DO

Reaction to Intramuscular Procaine Penicillin Injection
- Treatment usually is not possible. If the patient has collapsed and appears in a stupor, administer dexamethasone, 0.1 to 0.2 mg/kg IV.
- If treatment can be administered safely during the seizure, diazepam, 0.2 to 0.5 mg/kg IV, is the drug of choice.

●> WHAT NOT TO DO

Reaction to Intramuscular Procaine Penicillin Injection
- *Do not* administer phenytoin.

Drug-Induced Hypotension
- Usually occurs with intravenous administration of acepromazine
- Can also occur with xylazine or detomidine, especially in Draft and Warmblood horses
- Collapse is most common clinical sign

●> WHAT TO DO

Drug-Induced Hypotension
- Treat with intravenously administered fluids containing calcium, or administer a hypertonic saline solution.

Drug-Induced Hyperexcitability
- Butorphanol produces bizarre head tremors in some horses, especially when xylazine is not given several minutes before. No treatment is needed, although naloxone might reverse signs.
- Abnormally high plasma and CSF concentrations of aminophylline or lidocaine result in bizarre behavior, ataxia, tremors, and seizures.

●> WHAT TO DO

Drug-Induced Hyperexcitability
- Discontinue drug, give fluid therapy, and control any seizures.
- Lidocaine can cause CNS signs when used in individuals with cardiac dysfunction. *Note:* Lidocaine seldom causes a problem when treating ileus unless IV line/pump malfunction occurs and the horse is inadvertently administered a higher rate than anticipated.

- Many other causes exist, including fluphenazine decanoate or overdoses of pergolide or metoclopramide.

Venous Air Embolism Causing Seizure and/or Collapse
- If a fluid line becomes dislodged from a jugular catheter when the horse's head is elevated, air can be heard rushing into the venous system, and on rare occasion, the horse develops clinical signs associated with the air emboli. This can also occur when fluid bags are "internally" pressurized with air.
- Clinical signs include collapse, tachycardia, excitement, distress, pruritus, and even seizures if the air escapes to the left side of the heart. Auscultation of the heart might reveal an unusual "crepitus" or "sloshing" sound and a large amount of air bubbles can be seen on echocardiographic examination. Blindness of variable duration is occasionally seen.

●> WHAT TO DO

Venous Air Embolism
- Treatments include maintenance of blood pressure and adequate perfusion, sedation, or even general anesthesia with positive ventilation. Hyperbaric chamber or even catheterization of the right side of the heart and "vacuuming" the air (for right-sided air emboli) might be indicated. Experience is with supportive treatments; most horses recover.

Bizarre Behavior Associated with Fluphenazine Decanoate Administration
- Bizarre behavior might occur after treatment with the long-acting tranquilizer fluphenazine decanoate (Prolixin).
- The reaction appears to be idiosyncratic.

●> WHAT TO DO

Bizarre Behavior
- Administer benztropine mesylate, 0.018 to 0.04 mg/kg IV q12h.
- If benztropine mesylate is not available, antihistamines such as diphenhydramine, 0.5 to 2 mg/kg slowly IV or IM, might be beneficial, but phenobarbital or pentobarbital, 5 to 15 mg/kg IV, might also be needed to calm the patient. Phenobarbital, 5 to 15 mg/kg PO q12 to 24 h, might be needed for several days to keep the patient from injuring itself.
- Gross overdosing of piperazine can cause recumbency and dementia.
- Provide supportive care.

Dysphagia

Dysphagia (difficulty in swallowing) has many possible causes, such as oral irritation or injury, esophageal obstruction, a brainstem disease (nucleus ambiguus), diffuse neuromuscular disease (botulism), and peripheral damage to cranial nerve X (guttural pouch mycosis). Individuals with cerebral disease and severe depression also might have decreased tongue function; the tongue might remain extended or be slow to return to the mouth.

Causes

- Choke (see p. 177)
- Presence of an oral foreign body or irritation (see Salivation, p. 176): Look carefully for sticks or injury to and infection of the mouth and pharynx. This examination often necessitates sedation and use of a mouth speculum or general anesthesia and endoscopy through the mouth and the nose with manual examination of the mouth and pharynx. Wooden tongue–like infections do occur in horses; if there is no foreign body, these infections respond satisfactorily to penicillin and trimethoprim-sulfamethoxazole.
- EPM or other brainstem disease
- Guttural pouch disease: Mycotic plaques in the dorsomedial compartment, melanoma of the pouch, and flushing the pouch with an irritating substance can cause disease. Severe empyema can cause mechanical problems.
- Surgery involving the guttural pouch, such as removal of chondroids
- Botulism
- Yellow star thistle intoxication
- Viral encephalitis
- Cerebral abscess, mass or injury
- Pharyngeal swelling or obstruction
- Severe pharyngitis
- Rabies
- Organophosphate or lead intoxication
- Grass sickness (exotic; see Chapter 40, p. 664)
- Fractured mandible or stylohyoid bone

Specific Causes of Dysphagia in Foals

Most commonly presented for milk refluxing from the nose but might also have upper respiratory noise and often aspiration pneumonia.

- White muscle disease
- Botulism
- Neonatal maladjustment syndrome or soft palate dysfunction in foals (see Chapter 31, p. 545)
  - Soft palate dysfunction is a common cause and most foals recover with supportive treatments within a few days. Treatment should be directed for aspiration pneumonia.
- Cleft palate: Use endoscopy to carefully evaluate
- Pharyngeal collapse and/or persistent frenulum of the epiglottis
- Esophageal choke, which can occur in very young foals, especially miniature equines
- Fourth branchial arch defect can also cause milk to reflux from the proximal esophagus and nose
- Some foals with dysphagia at birth appear healthy otherwise and no cause is found. These foals may need to be raised by feeding from a bucket.

Fractured Jaw as a Cause of Dysphagia

- A fractured jaw can cause deliberate head tilt, tongue protrusion, and salivation.

- Diagnosis is made on physical examination, inability to properly align teeth, and radiographs.
- Consider surgical treatment if signs are severe.

Peripheral Nerve Disease

Suprascapular Nerve (Sweeny)

- Nerve injury is almost invariably caused by trauma:
  - Collision with a fixed stationary object or a kick
  - Ill-fitting driving collar on Draft horses
- Other possible causes are the following:
  - Peripheral nerve neoplasm or abscess compressing C6 area or suprascapular nerve
  - EPM
- Atrophy of supraspinatus and infraspinatus muscles results in an abnormal gait.
  - Initial stumbling, dragging of the toe
  - Abduction (lateral subluxation) of the shoulder on weight bearing
- If neuropraxia (nerve contusion) occurs, function returns in days to weeks.
- If the nerve has been severed, regrowth of the nerve along the fibrous framework occurs at a rate of 1 mm per day.
  - Most horses return to near normal function with stall rest after 3 to 18 months.
  - Surgery can be performed to decompress the nerve if there is no return of function within 3 months.
  - The suprascapular nerve is motor only, so loss of sensation in any part of the limb indicates damage to other nerves.
- Electromyograms can be useful 2 to 4 weeks after injury to detect involvement of other nerves.
- Anesthetic recovery can be physically difficult for any horse with nerve injury, muscle atrophy, or disuse of a limb.

●❯ WHAT TO DO

Peripheral Nerve Injury

For treatment of all peripheral nerve injury, see p. 378.

Musculocutaneous Nerve

- The musculocutaneous nerve originates from spinal cord segments C7-8.
- Musculocutaneous dysfunction causes the following:
  - Inability to flex the elbow, which results in an abnormally pronounced lifting of the shoulder to advance the limb
  - Dragging the limb when backing
- With severe lesions, there is loss of sensation on the dorsomedial aspect of the limb from the carpus to the fetlock.

Radial Nerve

- Radial nerve injury can accompany humeral fractures:
  - Evaluation before surgery can be difficult because there is no reliable autonomous zone for skin sensation. Examine the nerve at the time of surgical repair of the fractured humerus.

- Injury might be caused by prolonged lateral recumbency:
  - Most likely injury is a combination of ischemic myopathy and ischemic neuropraxia, most of which show considerable improvement within several hours. Some take a few days to improve, with the horse exhibiting severe pain and unwillingness to walk on the limb for 2 to 5 days.
- Direct trauma is less likely because of protection by surrounding muscle.
  - If trauma is the known etiologic factor, it is more likely the lesion is a contusion or avulsion of the brachial plexus (see the following section). Horses, especially young horses, occasionally are found in the pasture with radial nerve paresis/paralysis with no obvious trauma; it is assumed there has been some avulsion of the plexus in many of these cases, and recovery is generally slow or nonexistent.
- The affected individual is unable to bear weight because the radial nerve paralysis causes an inability to extend the elbow, carpus, and fetlock. The elbow drops during locomotion, and the toe drags; pectoral muscles might be able to advance the leg forward half-a-stride. When the patient is standing, the leg rests on the front of the toe, and the horse is able to paw with the limb.
- The limb must be supported with a splint or cast to avoid additional injury and muscle contracture.
- Recovery, in cases of neuropraxia, can take several weeks. If no improvement occurs in 6 to 8 weeks, the prognosis is poor but not hopeless. Radial nerve damage and separation combined with humeral fracture justify an extremely guarded prognosis.
- Rule-outs include septic arthritis of the elbow, fracture, EPM, rupture of the medial collateral ligament of the elbow, and focal myopathy.

Brachial Plexus Avulsion

Many cases of shoulder injury with signs of radial nerve paralysis are likely caused by damage to the roots of the brachial plexus.

- Limb carriage is almost identical to that described for radial nerve paralysis.
- Total avulsion results in flaccid paralysis of the entire limb and sensory loss distal to the elbow.
- Injury to the median and ulnar nerves, without radial nerve damage, results in a stiff, goose-stepping gait and hyperextension of the lower limb. Analgesia might be present over the lateral aspect of the cannon bone and pastern.
- The condition of patients that have sustained contusions progressively improves over 6 to 18 months. Physiotherapy (especially swimming) has been useful in returning the individual to function. Return to racing after brachial plexus injury has been reported.
- Neoplasia (nerve sheath) and EPM can have identical clinical signs.
- Prognosis in general is guarded to poor.

- The opposite limb should be bandaged for mechanical support.
- The affected limb should be bandaged or "lightly" casted in extension to protect the dorsal pastern area and to prevent tendon contracture.

Femoral Nerve

- The nerve is well-protected from external trauma but can be damaged by the following:
  - Penetrating wound of the caudal flank
  - Abscess, neoplasia
  - Aneurysm in the region of the external iliac arteries
  - Dystocia (hip or stifle lock) in a newborn foal
  - Femoral or pelvic fracture (rare)
  - Compression during anesthesia or complicated by myopathy (might be bilateral)
  - EPM
- The patient is unable to support its weight if femoral paralysis is present. The limb is advanced with difficulty. When the individual attempts to bear weight, the stifle collapses (flexes), and the hock and fetlock flex because of the reciprocal apparatus.
- At rest, all the joints are flexed.
- Atrophy of the quadriceps is evident in 2 to 4 weeks.
- Patellar reflex is depressed or absent.
- Hypalgesia might be evident over the medial thigh if the saphenous nerve or the femoral nerve, dorsal to the iliopsoas muscle, is involved.
- Prognosis is guarded regardless of the etiologic factor.

Sciatic Nerve

- In foals, sciatic nerve damage is often caused by *Salmonella, Rhodococcus,* or *Streptococcus* osteomyelitis of the sacrum and pelvis or, more commonly, an intramuscular injection into the caudal aspect of the thigh. Damage to the nerve occurs because of the following:
  - Needle puncture of the nerve
  - Irritation due to drug injection
  - Pressure from a hematoma
  - Scarring around the nerve
- In adults, damage to the sciatic nerve is caused by the following:
  - Pelvic fracture, especially the ischium
  - Coxofemoral luxation
  - Other injuries (kick), especially the peroneal branch of the sciatic nerve
  - Postfoaling, such as dystocia with delivery of a large foal
  - EPM: This should be considered when there are signs of focal lower motor neuron dysfunction.
- Gait and posture change occur as follows:
  - Patient can support its weight if the limb is positioned under the body.
  - At rest, the limb is held toward the rear, stifle and hock are extended, fetlock is flexed, and the front of the foot rolls forward.
  - The toe drags because limb flexion is poor.

CNS

- Hypalgesia exists over most of the limb, except the medial thigh.
- Postfoaling mares with sciatic damage might be unable to stand on the hind legs.

Peroneal Paralysis Versus Tibial Paralysis

Because the peroneal nerve is associated with sciatic nerve paralysis, the clinical findings are similar. In peroneal paralysis, hypalgesia might exist over the craniolateral gaskin, hock, and metatarsus. Paresis of the peroneal nerve is common after prolonged recumbency, and recovery generally occurs within 1 to 3 days; frequently, the individual is found standing on the fetlock. Tibial paralysis is less common than is peroneal nerve paralysis. The gait in tibial nerve paralysis resembles stringhalt. Flexion of the hock and extension of the digit are unopposed, so the individual overflexes the limb and raises the foot higher than normal. The hock is flexed (dropped hock), and the fetlock knuckles forward at rest. Sensation might be reduced in the caudal and medial coronet region.

Cranial Gluteal Nerve

Damage to the gluteal nerve results in profound atrophy of the gluteal muscles of the rump. There is little alteration in gait. This condition can be seen with a pelvic fracture or EPM involving the L6 ventral gray column. The condition can also occur following back injections with irritating drugs (iodine). The irritating substance is most likely injected adjacent to vertebra L4.

Lumbar, Sacral, and Caudal Roots

The lumbar, sacral, and caudal nerve roots are most commonly injured as the result of a vertebral fracture. Improvement or recovery can occur with supportive therapy. Radiographs and CT (in foals) might aid in recognizing a fracture or soft tissue swelling. Surgical decompression may be indicated. Ultrasonography in foals might identify an abscess.

- L6, L7, S1: Damage presents as sciatic nerve paralysis
- S1, S2, S3: Inability to close the anal sphincter, analgesia of anus and perineum, distention of bladder and rectum occur
- Caudal nerves: Analgesia of perineum and penis, but not prepuce, and inability to move tail occur
- Polyneuritis of the cauda equina can also affect the lumbar, sacral, and caudal roots; however, the onset of signs is insidious, and progression is slow

Facial Nerve

Facial nerve paresis or paralysis can result from THO, EPM, trauma, polyneuritis equi, or it can be idiopathic. If the facial nerve is affected at the nucleus (e.g., EPM) or as it courses through the middle and inner ear, all branches (auricular, palpebral, and buccal) are involved. With more distal injury, only one or two branches are usually affected (e.g., injury to the buccal branch caused by halter pressure during anesthesia). Horses might accumulate food in their cheeks with facial nerve dysfunction.

Injury to Buccal Branch of Facial Nerve: Clinical Signs

- Lower lip droop and decreased nostril diameter on affected side and deviation of nose to the contralateral side
- Cerebral disease may also cause decreased lip tone

Idiopathic Facial Paralysis

- Idiopathic paralysis often involves the buccal and the palpebral branches and usually is permanent.
- With any cause of facial paresis affecting the palpebral branch, monitor closely to prevent corneal ulceration.
- If no corneal ulcer is present at the first examination, apply ophthalmic ointment (Lacri-Lube) every 6 hours for 1 to 2 weeks.

⬤〉 WHAT TO DO

Facial Paralysis

- If a corneal ulcer is present, it should be treated immediately and intensively; a tarsorrhaphy might be required. Most affected individuals eventually compensate for the paresis and do not need further treatment.
- For corneal ulceration, see Chapter 23, p. 400.

⬤〉 WHAT TO DO

Management of Peripheral Nerve Disease

- Generally supportive, including bandaging of distal limbs to prevent abrasions of the front of the limb and support wraps and foot support on the opposite limb.
- Apply cold water hydrotherapy over the injured area.
- If an identifiable mass is compressing the nerve (e.g., hematoma or fracture), surgical decompression is indicated.
- NSAID or corticosteroid therapy: Corticosteroids (dexamethasone, 0.05 to 0.1 mg/kg) can be used for one to several days if there are no contraindications to corticosteroid therapy. Flunixin meglumine, 1 mg/kg q12 to 24h, can be given in place of corticosteroids. Treatment with vitamin E (10,000 units q24h for adult horses) and coenzyme Q_{10} can be considered.
- Gabapentin, 5 to 10 mg/kg PO q8 h or pregabalin, 2 to 4 mg/kg PO q8h can be used for anxiety and neurogenic pain.
- Treat postfoaling mares with sciatic nerve damage aggressively with anti-inflammatories (dexamethasone, 0.1 mg/kg IV q24h or flunixin, 0.5 to 1 mg/kg IV q12-24h) +/− 0.1 to 1 g/kg DMSO, as a 10% solution, and mild sedation if anxiety is a problem. Physical support (e.g., tail tie) for short periods is important to enable the mare to stand. If she continually tries to stand, she should be placed in a sling.
- Postfoaling mares that cannot stand are difficult to manage and often have severe myopathy due to recumbency. Dexamethasone (5 mg) epidural may benefit these mares.
- Injection of neurotropic growth factor as close to the damaged nerve as possible has been performed; however, the effectiveness is unknown.

References

References can be found on the companion website at www.equine-emergencies.com.

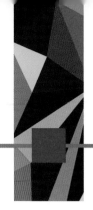

CHAPTER 23

Ophthalmology

Nita L. Irby

DIAGNOSTIC AND THERAPEUTIC PROCEDURES

Diagnostic and Therapeutic Aids to Treatment and Examination Basics

- All of the equipment necessary for field equine ophthalmology listed in Box 23-1 fits inside a small, three-tiered fishing tackle box and can travel with you wherever you go.
- *Practice Tip: Although they provide excellent general illumination, do not use any LED light source as a penlight for ocular illumination as they are painfully bright and leave a retinal after-image for many hours. Try one on yourself—if a light source is not comfortable when used on your own eye you should not use it on your patients.*

  Important! Every eye exam, in every species, should begin by asking the following questions, in this order:

  Question 1: Will I further injure this eye if I examine/manipulate it? If so, stop now and reassess.

  Question 2: Is this eye possibly dry? If so, be sure to do a Schirmer tear test now.

  Question 3: Do I need immunofluorescent samples for viral testing? If so, I should obtain them and some other culture samples now.
- Fluorescein dye tests should always be performed next, plus lissamine or rose bengal dye tests, if indicated.
- Intraocular pressure measurements should be obtained, followed by a complete anterior and posterior segment exam.

Schirmer Tear Tests

Dry eye, or keratoconjunctivitis sicca, is reported uncommonly in the equine patient, perhaps in part because it is underdiagnosed. Unless the patient has obvious epiphora, a Schirmer tear test should be performed in every equine patient and should absolutely be assessed in both eyes of all cases of:

- Chronic, recurring ulcerative or nonulcerative keratitis
- Partial to complete facial nerve paralysis
- Suspect temporohyoid osteoarthropathy (THO)
- Eosinophilic keratitis
- Facial fractures
- Any case where the eye(s) appears dry or has excess or tenacious mucoid discharge

The test should be performed as the first procedure in any eye exam, before any eye drops have been given and before patient handling causes reflex tearing.

Equipment

- Schirmer tear test strips[1]
- A 60-second timer or watch with a second hand

Procedure

- Bend the strip 90 degrees at the notch (the zero mark).
- Place the strip between the lower lid and third eyelid, approximately 1.5 cm from the medial canthus or one third the distance of the lower lid from the medial canthus.
- Begin timing immediately for 30 seconds or 1 minute (preferred) the distance that moisture has migrated along the filter paper strip.
- Read immediately and record value.
- Normal value: 15 to 30 mm wetting per minute or 15 to 20 mm wetting per 30 seconds

Corneal Culture and Cytologic Examination

Any breach in the corneal epithelium can result in secondary infections and subsequent ulcerative keratitis. The conjunctival sac normally contains predominately gram-positive bacteria, along with fungal organisms. These organisms may colonize disrupted tissue in horses with corneal ulcers or abrasions. Culturing of corneal lesions is always useful to better direct antimicrobial or antifungal therapy. This procedure is ideally performed at the beginning of the exam, if the patient permits, before administration of topical agents that may alter microbial yield. More aggressive corneal scraping should also be performed in order to aid in cytologic evaluation, an essential aid to diagnosing equine keratitis. Additional cultures of the deeper tissues should be obtained following scraping. It is always necessary to apply topical anesthetic before aggressive corneal scraping.

Important: This procedure should *not* be performed if the cornea is perforated and should be performed very carefully, or not at all, if a descemetocele is present.

Equipment

- Kimura platinum spatula or a sterile dulled scalpel blade (or the noncutting side or end of a scalpel blade also may be used; cytobrushes if available are excellent.)
- Culture swab plus transport media systems[2]

---

[1]Intervet, Inc., Rosewood, New Jersey.
[2]BBL Culture Media (Becton-Dickinson, Franklin Lakes, New Jersey).

Box 23-1	**Contents of Equine Ophthalmology Kit**

1. Welch-Allyn 3.5-V rechargeable halogen direct ophthalmoscope with Finoff transilluminator
2. Cobalt blue filter for transilluminator to enhance fluorescein stain fluorescence
3. 14-diopter or 2.2-D indirect ophthalmoscopy lens
4. 4× magnifying loupe
5. Waterproof white tape
6. Cyanoacrylate glue
7. Sterile cotton or polyester-tipped (preferred) applicators
8. Sterile gauze pads
9. Fluorescein stain strips, sterile
10. Lissamine green or rose bengal dye strips
11. Mosquito hemostats
12. Allis tissue forceps
13. Brown-Adson tissue forceps
14. Bishop-Harmon tissue forceps
15. Small Metzenbaum or Stevens tenotomy scissors
16. Small needle holder (Derf or large Castroviejo)
17. 2-0 nylon on a straight needle
18. 4-0 silk
19. 4-0, 5-0, and 6-0 polyglactin 910 (Vicryl) on small cutting needle
20. Schirmer tear test strips
21. Xylazine, detomidine, and butorphanol
22. Mepivacaine or lidocaine
23. 2% Lidocaine gel (for retrograde nasolacrimal lavage)
24. Tropicamide 1% ophthalmic drops (short-acting mydriatic to dilate pupils)
25. Atropine 1% ophthalmic drops (long-acting mydriatic and cycloplegic)
26. Proparacaine 0.5% (topical anesthetic)
27. 10% phenylephrine
28. Sterile eye collyrium, eye-irrigating solution in a spray bottle or sterile saline solution
29. 5% povidone-iodine solution
30. Alcohol swabs
31. Cyanoacrylate tissue adhesive
32. #11, #12, and #15 Bard-Parker scalpel blades (#12 works well for suture removal)
33. Glass slides (cleaned and in carriers)
34. Matches or lighter
35. 20-gauge intravenous catheters for normograde nasolacrimal cannulation; teat cannula, TomCat catheters, or 3.5F and 5F polypropylene canine urinary catheters and an equine nasolacrimal catheter for retrograde nasolacrimal lavage and cannulation
36. 30-, 25-, 20-, and 18-gauge disposable needles
37. 1-mL, 3-mL, 5-mL, 12-mL, and 2 20-mL syringes
38. Blood tubes, particularly red top (include one or two filled with formalin)
39. Synthetic culture swabs and transport media, preferably minitip
40. Port-a-Cul tubes for bacterial culture
41. Broth for bacterial culture
42. Mila eye lavage apparatus kit
43. TonoPen XL and tip covers

- Port-A-Cul tubes[3]
- Glass slides
- Gram stain and Wright-Giemsa stain, or alternatively, Diff-Quik stain
- Fungal staining agents (Grocott-Gomori methenamine silver, periodic acid–Schiff)

Procedure

- Do *not* use cotton swabs for sample collection because cotton is bacteriostatic.
- Samples can be inoculated directly onto blood and Sabouraud agar plates or placed into a small amount of blood culture broth; however, more routinely, commercial synthetic culture swab transport systems are used, with additional samples placed into anaerobic transport media. Viral culturing and certain fastidious organisms may require special media obtained from your laboratory.
- After confirming that the eye is *not* perforated and there is no descemetocele, premoisten the synthetic swab in the transport media and roll or rub the swab over the lesion(s). Repeat as needed and then return the swabs obtained to the appropriate transport media.
- Scrape the corneal lesion(s) or wound edges with the spatula or blade, obtaining several samples from the periphery of the lesion, and also from the center unless the ulcer is very deep. Roll each swab gently onto glass slides for cytologic examination. A minimum of 3 to

4 slides should be made to allow for multiple staining techniques.

- Keep culture samples at room temperature and process as soon as possible.
- Use Gram stain and a Wright-Giemsa stain or Diff-Quik stain to identify bacteria or fungal organisms in the cytologic smears and to analyze the cells present.
- Although many fungal organisms are seen on routine staining, special stains such as Grocott-Gomori methenamine silver and periodic acid–Schiff stain may be needed.
- If corneal scraping does not lead to the detection of microorganisms and the condition is unresponsive to treatment, a corneal biopsy may be needed.

Fluorescein Staining

Fluorescein staining is an important diagnostic aid to identify corneal epithelial disruption and to determine the patency of the nasolacrimal duct. The most common use of topical fluorescein is to localize corneal ulcers or abrasions. The hydrophilic corneal or conjunctival tissue beneath an epithelial defect such as an abrasion or ulcer absorbs the water-soluble fluorescein dye and stains the stroma bright green by conversion of absorbed light to fluorescent light. ***Practice Tip:*** *Fluorescein staining is indicated in every uncomfortable or painful eye, whenever a corneal ulcer is suspected, in all unexplained chronic ocular surface conditions, and whenever there is a history of direct trauma to the eye.* Samples for immunofluorescent assay should be collected *before* administration of fluorescein.

---

[3]BBL Media (Becton-Dickinson, Franklin Lakes, New Jersey).

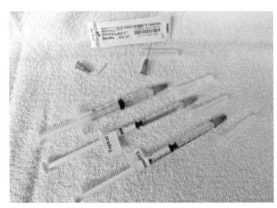

Figure 23-1 Topical medications for a routine eye exam. From *left:* fluorescein dye (strip has been placed in saline in a syringe), topical anesthetic, and a short-acting mydriatic. Needles are attached to each syringe *and the needles are broken from the hub* (25-*gauge* needles, shown at the *top*). The small-bore hub remains to ensure a fine spray of medication. ***Practice Tip:*** *Horses rarely notice when a small volume (0.05 to 0.1 mL) of room temperature solutions is sprayed gently on their corneas, but they notice immediately (and resent) when solutions are sprayed on their eyelids!*

Equipment

- Fluorescein strip[4]
- 0.5 to 1.0 mL sterile saline solution in a syringe or equivalent sterile collyrium (eye wash)
- Penlight, transilluminator, or ophthalmoscope. (Do *not* use LED lights; they are too bright.)

Procedure

- Moisten the fluorescein strip in the lacrimal lake (medially, between the nictitans and lower lid) or place the dry, sterile strip in a syringe with 0.5 to 1.0 mL sterile saline to create a fresh fluorescein solution that can be sprayed onto the cornea (Fig. 23-1). Gently close the lids 2 to 3 times to ensure the fluorescein is distributed throughout the tear film and covers the cornea. ***Practice Tip:*** *Direct contact of the impregnated fluorescein strip with the cornea causes stain uptake and discomfort and is to be avoided; the area of touch may be erroneously diagnosed as a corneal defect.*
- Gentle flushing with saline solution or collyrium removes any excess stain.
- Using a source of direct light, examine the entire eye for stain uptake. Very deep corneal ulcers (descemetocoeles) may take up stain only along their outermost borders.
- Ultraviolet, cobalt blue light, or a Wood's lamp excites fluorescein, facilitating detection of minute corneal epithelial defects.
- Patency of the nasolacrimal duct is verified if fluorescein dye appears at the nostril within 5 minutes, but this can take up to 20 minutes in a normal horse.

Lissamine Green and Rose Bengal Staining

Lissamine green (LG) and rose bengal (RB) stains:
- Can be used to identify dead or devitalized corneal or conjunctival epithelial cells

- Can be used to identify defects in the mucin layer of the tear film
- Can aid in diagnosing and assessing the extent of some neoplasias such as squamous cell carcinomas
- Can help detect the presence of minute foreign bodies
- Can aid in the diagnosis of some epithelial diseases such as viral keratitis and superficial fungal infections

LG and RB stain dead or damaged cells a teal-green or bright pink color, respectively. LG is less irritating to human patients than RB and is equally effective in evaluating the ocular surface and is recommended over RB. Interpretation is time- and concentration-dependent so repeatable dilution is important and interpretation of the stained eyes should be made at 1 to 2 minutes following application as the stains disappear at approximately 3 to 4 minutes. Excess concentrations of RB even stain healthy epithelial cells so judicious interpretation is warranted. Either dye should be used after the application of fluorescein dye.

Equipment

- RB[5] or LG[6] impregnated strips
- 0.5 to 1.0 mL sterile saline solution in a syringe or equivalent sterile collyrium (eye wash)
- Penlight, transilluminator, or ophthalmoscope. (Do *not* use LED lights; they are too bright.)

Procedure

- Moisten the strip with one drop of sterile saline or eye wash, shake off excess, and touch strip to the lacrimal lake and then proceed as described for Fluorescein staining or place the dry strip in a syringe with 0.5 to 1.0 ml sterile saline to create a fresh solution that can be sprayed onto the cornea.
- Gently close the lids 2 to 3 times to ensure stain is distributed throughout the tear film and over the cornea. As for fluorescein, direct contact of the impregnated strip with the cornea may cause stain uptake and discomfort and is to be avoided; the area of touch may be erroneously diagnosed as a corneal defect.
- Sponge the medial canthus gently to remove excess stain and examine immediately (no later than 1 to 2 minutes after staining).
- Using a source of direct light and magnification, examine the entire cornea and conjunctiva for stain uptake and note the pattern. For example, focal, vertically directed stain patterns suggest a conjunctival foreign body in the adjacent eyelid, and small serpiginous or punctate patterns may indicate herpetic or fungal keratitis. Consult veterinary ophthalmology texts for more details.

Topical Anesthesia

- Apply by means of gentle spray (see Fig. 23-1) from stock solution you have placed in a tuberculin or 3-mL syringe

[4]Ayerst Laboratories, Inc., New York.

[5]Rose Stone Enterprises, Alta Loma, California.
[6]HUB Pharmaceuticals, Rancho Cucamongo, California.

EYE

with a 25-gauge needle hub attached but *with the needle broken off flush with the hub.*

- Repeat administration of the topical anesthetic every 15 to 30 seconds for 1 to 2 minutes. If enhanced anesthesia is needed focally (such as before subconjunctival injection), an anesthetic-soaked cotton swab can be applied with gentle pressure to the area for 15 to 30 seconds.
- Proparacaine HCl[7] and other topical anesthetics cause vasodilation and hyperemia of the conjunctiva, as well as mild stinging on instillation. They also are somewhat toxic to the corneal epithelium. A faint, diffuse corneal epithelial "waviness" and faint, diffuse fluorescein uptake often occurs shortly after administration of a topical anesthetic.
- A complete external examination of the eye that includes fluorescein, RB, or LG staining always should be performed before instillation of an anesthetic.

Intraocular Pressure Measurements

- Intraocular pressure (IOP) measurements (via applanation tonometry) should be performed *on both eyes* of all equine patients presenting with:
  - An unexplained red, painful, or watery eye
  - Focal to diffuse corneal edema of no apparent cause
  - Any linear corneal opacity
  - A sluggish pupillary light reflex
  - A lens luxation in either eye
  - Suspected or previous glaucoma
  - A history of facial or ocular trauma
  - Uveitis cases
  - Any time there is an unexplained ocular complaint
- All prepurchase ocular exams should include an IOP assessment.
- IOP measurements are used to diagnose elevated pressure, but in the horse they are especially useful to document low intraocular pressures, a hallmark of uveitis. IOP readings in uveitis cases can help diagnose mild uveitis and help determine when uveitis is controlled.
- Sedation and lid akinesia are often needed to obtain IOP readings in the equine patient. If sedation is used, care must be taken to maintain the head position horizontal to slightly elevated at all times because a lowered head will falsely elevate IOP readings.

Equipment

- Sedative of choice and lid akinesia if needed
- Topical anesthetic eyedrops[8]
- Tono-Pen XL [9] or TonoVet[10]

Procedure

- Sedate the patient but maintain the head in a horizontal or slightly elevated position.
- Perform a motor nerve block (palpebral or supraorbital).

---

[7]0.5% (Akorn, Lake Forest, Illinois).
[8]0.5% Proparacaine (Akorn, Lake Forest, Illinois).
[9]TonoPenXL (Mentor Ophthalmics, 3000 Longwater Dr, Norwell, Massachusetts 02061-1672).
[10]ICare, Helsinki, Finland.

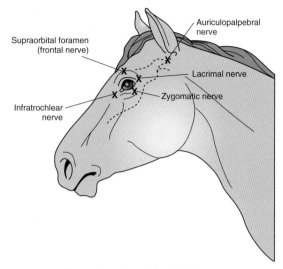

Figure 23-2   Nerve blocks of the eye.

- Open the lids *with your finger pressing on the bones of the orbit, not the globe!*
- Try to take readings between blinks because blinking may falsely elevate the IOP.
- IOP readings should be obtained from the central or most normal portion of the cornea because corneal edema and scarring can alter IOP readings.
- Perform readings according to the instrument used (i.e., gentle brushing or tapping the topically anesthetized cornea with the TonoPen or holding the TonoVet in front of the unanesthetized cornea as the plunger takes readings; see instructions accompanying your instrument).

Nerve Blocks (Akinesia) of the Eyelids
Anatomy Review

The facial nerve (cranial nerve VII) carries axons that provide motor control to all the muscles of the face. The palpebral nerve is the branch of cranial nerve VII that innervates the orbicularis oculi muscle and is responsible for eyelid closure. The trigeminal nerve (cranial nerve V) relays sensory information from the face via its three major branches: the maxillary, ophthalmic, and mandibular nerves. The maxillary nerve receives axons from the zygomatic nerve, carrying sensory innervation from the lateral lower eye. The frontal, lacrimal, and infratrochlear nerves contribute to the ophthalmic nerve and carry sensory innervation from, respectively, the central upper eyelid, lateral upper eyelid, and the medial canthus. Refer to Fig. 23-2.

Palpebral Nerve Block for Upper Lid Akinesia

- ***Practice Tip:*** *Never attempt to forcefully open a patient's closed eyelids without eyelid akinesia. This can result in rupture of a deep corneal ulcer or evisceration of a lacerated globe.*
- The sphincter muscle (orbicularis oculi) surrounding the equine eyelid is very powerful. To safely examine a painful, squinted eye, the orbicularis oculi muscle must be partially or completely paralyzed with a palpebral nerve block. This block should be performed to facilitate the examination of

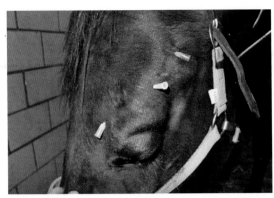

Figure 23-3 Needle placement for palpebral and frontal nerve blocks. Injecting 1 to 3 mL of local anesthetic immediately caudal to the most dorsal point of the zygomatic arch *(blue needle)* denervates most branches of the palpebral nerve *or* blocks a branch of the nerve as it crosses the zygomatic arch immediately caudal to the eye *(pink needle)*. Block the supraorbital branch of the frontal nerve by injecting 1 to 3 mL of local anesthetic subcutaneously over the palpable supraorbital foramen, dorsal to the medial canthus of the eye *(yellow needle)*.

every painful eye and in all cases in which the history is unknown and the eye is held shut. The palpebral nerve block affects motor function of the eyelid but does not desensitize the eyelid. A properly performed block results in akinesia (temporary paralysis) of the upper eyelid within 5 minutes and greatly facilitates a complete and safe examination of the eye.

- Branches of the palpebral nerve can be palpated in a number of sites as they cross the bones of the orbital rim dorsal and dorsolateral to the eye (Figs. 23-2 and 23-3). Cleanse one or more sites, and inject local anesthetic subcutaneously (1.5 to 2 mL per site) through a preplaced 25-gauge needle as described later.
- To anesthetize most of the palpebral nerve branches, fan 2 mL of local anesthetic subcutaneously immediately caudal to the most dorsal portion of the zygomatic arch. The nerve may not be palpable at this location (see Figs. 23-2 and 23-3).
- ***Practice Tip:*** *Sterile artificial tear ointment or other medication as indicated should be applied to the eye at the conclusion of the examination until the blink reflex returns to normal to prevent exposure keratitis.*

Equipment
- 25-gauge, $\frac{5}{8}$-inch (1.6-cm) needle, 5-mL syringe
- 2% mepivacaine (Carbocaine[11]), 2 to 3 mL

Procedure
- Palpate the area near the highest point on the zygomatic arch and the caudal border of the coronoid process of the mandible. A depression is felt caudal to the coronoid process. The nerve itself can often be palpated crossing the apex of the coronoid process in a horizontal direction (see Figs. 23-2 and 23-3).
- Cleanse the skin with 5% povidone-iodine solution (avoid alcohol and soapy scrubs).

[11]Pharmacia & Upjohn Co., Division of Pfizer, Inc., New York, New York.

- Insert the needle into the depression and direct the needle upward and caudal to the highest part of the arch or adjacent to the nerve if palpable.
- Aspirate first, and inject 2 mL of 2% mepivacaine hydrochloride (Carbocaine) SQ in a fanlike manner.
- Massage the injection site to disperse the drug along the nerve.

Anesthesia of the Eyelids

- The supraorbital, lacrimal, zygomatic, and infratrochlear nerves of the maxillary and ophthalmic branches of cranial nerve V carry sensory afferent fibers from the upper and lower lids.
- Each of these nerves can be blocked independently, as needed, for surgical or other procedures requiring uncomfortable eyelid manipulations or a line block along the orbit rim can be performed.
- ***Practice Tip:*** *The eye should be lubricated frequently after any sensory block until the blink reflex returns to normal because motor function is usually impaired as well.*

Supraorbital Nerve Block: Anesthesia of the Central Upper Eyelid

- The supraorbital (frontal) nerve block (a branch of ophthalmic V) provides analgesia to most of the upper eyelid and good, albeit partial, upper lid akinesia because instillation of local anesthetics in this area anesthetizes the frontal nerve and medial palpebral branches of the palpebral nerves.

  Note: The supraorbital or frontal nerve "block" is the preferred block for routine eye examination in a needle-shy or eye-shy horse because eyelid akinesia is good *and* the patient does not feel the manipulation of the central upper eyelid; a difficult patient is thus less resistant to the examination.

Equipment
- 25-gauge, $\frac{5}{8}$-inch (1.6-cm) needle, 5-mL syringe
- 2% mepivacaine (Carbocaine), 2 mL

Procedure
- Palpate the supraorbital foramen (located as the zygomatic process of the frontal bone widens, dorsal to the medial canthus of the eye) (see Figs. 23-2 and 23-3).
- Cleanse the skin with 5% povidone-iodine solution (avoid alcohol and soapy scrubs).
- Aspirate first, and instill 2 mL of 2% mepivacaine (Carbocaine) through a 1-inch (2.5-cm) needle placed subcutaneously, adjacent to the foramen. ***Note:*** It is not necessary to insert the needle into the foramen; a block so performed does not include motor blockade. A small artery and vein parallel this nerve. Reposition if blood is obtained.

Zygomatic Nerve Block: Anesthesia of the Lower Lateral Eyelid
Equipment
- 25-gauge, $\frac{5}{8}$-inch (1.6-cm) needle, 5-mL syringe
- 2% mepivacaine (Carbocaine), 2 to 3 mL

Procedure

- Place the index finger on ventral rim of the orbit at the lateral canthus of the eye, and firmly press against the supraorbital portion of the zygomatic arch.
- Cleanse the skin with 5% povidone-iodine solution (avoid alcohol and soapy scrubs).
- Inject medial to index finger along the rim of the orbit into the lower eyelid (see Fig. 23-2).

Lacrimal Nerve Block: Anesthesia of the Lateral Upper Eyelid

Equipment

- 25-gauge, ⅝-inch (1.6-cm) needle, 5-mL syringe
- 2% mepivacaine (Carbocaine), 2 to 3 mL

Procedure

- Cleanse the skin with 5% povidone-iodine solution (avoid alcohol and soapy scrubs).
- Inject in a line block medially along the dorsal rim of the orbit, medial to the lateral canthus (see Fig. 23-2).

Infratrochlear Nerve: Anesthesia of the Medial Canthus

Equipment

- 25-gauge, ⅝-inch (1.6-cm) needle, 5-mL syringe
- 2% mepivacaine (Carbocaine), 2 to 3 mL

Procedure

- Using firm pressure, palpate the irregularly shaped notch on the dorsal rim of the orbit near the medial canthus.
- Cleanse the skin with 5% povidone-iodine solution (avoid alcohol and soapy scrubs).
- Inject 2 to 3 mL of mepivacaine (Carbocaine) deeply and rostrally to the notch (see Fig. 23-2).

Nasolacrimal Duct Cannulation

- Cannulation of the nasolacrimal (NL) duct is indicated whenever obstruction of lacrimal drainage is suspected.
- Clinical signs seen with NL obstruction include epiphora (tearing), staining beneath the eye, and discharge at the medial canthus.
- The duct is cannulated retrograde from its rostral opening, where it emerges near the mucocutaneous junction on the ventrum of either nostril but can also be cannulated normograde. *Important:* Metal lacrimal cannulas are never recommended in the equine patient because they may cause significant trauma if the patient throws its head.
- Cannulation is also a procedure required for dacryocystorhinography (used to define a congenital obstruction or acquired inflammatory lesion of the nasolacrimal duct).
- Indwelling NL catheters placed retrograde can be used to deliver medications to the eye without having to manipulate the eye or eyelids when an eyelid lavage system (preferred) cannot be used.

Equipment

- Sedative of choice
- Penlight
- 4F to 6F polypropylene catheter[12] (French conversion: each French unit = 0.33-mm diameter) or equine-specific nasolacrimal catheters[13] (preferred) for retrograde flushing; 20-gauge IV catheter[14] for normograde flushing
- 20-mL syringe filled with warm sterile saline solution
- Gauze sponges
- Sterile topical anesthetic lubricant such as Lidocaine gel[15]

Procedure for Retrograde Cannulation

- Sedate the patient, but support the head in a horizontal or slightly elevated position, or nasal mucosal edema quickly develops, which impedes catheter passage.
- Reflect the lateral alar fold of the nostril and locate the puncta of the nasolacrimal duct; using a light source, it is easily located on the ventral aspect of the nasal meatus (Fig. 23-4, *A*), usually at the junction of the pink and colored mucosa. Some horses have two or more puncta in one nostril. *Practice Tip: The most proximal one is usually patent.*
- Swab the inside of the nostril clean of all debris. Lubricate the catheter with a small amount of topical anesthetic gel. While pulling rostrally on the nasal floor, slide the catheter into the duct at least 5 cm proximally (Fig. 23-4, *B*).
- To flush the duct, place a finger over the puncta to hold the catheter in place and to prevent the warm saline solution from refluxing normograde. *Practice Tip: If the saline is warm the patient objects less to the procedure. Attach the syringe and gently flush the duct retrograde, standing to the side as you do so because the patient usually sneezes. Patency has been achieved once the saline solution flows from the lacrimal puncta at the medial canthus.* Continue or repeat the flushing until the solution flows easily from the eye and is clear.
- The catheter can remain in the duct and its connector hub exited through a stab incision in the false nostril and sutured in place on the face with a butterfly taping technique for routine ophthalmic medication administration via the NL duct.

Procedure for Normograde Cannulation

- Normograde irrigation of the NL duct is easily and safely performed.

---

[12]Sovereign polypropylene catheter (Tyco Healthcare Kendall, Mansfield, Massachusetts) or MILA #NL 525 nasolacrimal catheters (MILA Intl, Erlanger, Kentucky) or #6 FR × 40-cm equine nasolacrimal catheter (Smiths Medical PM, Inc., Waukesha, WI 53186).
[13]Sovereign polypropylene catheter (Tyco Healthcare Kendall, Mansfield, Massachusetts) or MILA #NL 525 nasolacrimal catheters (MILA Intl, Erlanger, Kentucky) or #6 FR × 40-cm equine nasolacrimal catheter (Smiths Medical PM, Inc., Waukesha, WI 53186).
[14]Monoject Veterinary IV Catheter (Tyco Healthcare Group, LP, Mansfield, Massachusetts).
[15]Wedgewood Pharmacy, Swedesboro, New Jersey.

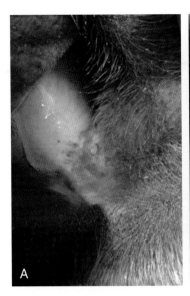
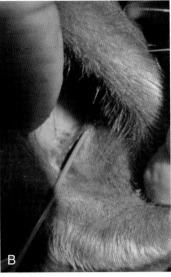

Figure 23-4   A, Nasolacrimal duct opening, ventrally in the nasal vestibule. **B,** A #6 French × 40-cm polytetrafluorethylene (PTFE) equine nasolacrimal catheter inserted into the distal nasolacrimal duct orifice.

EYE

- See the Equipment section for retrograde cannulation on p. 384.
- Sedate the patient if needed.
- Apply 1 to 2 drops of topical anesthetic to the eye.
- Remove the stylet from the catheter and insert the catheter into the NL punctal opening in the medial upper eyelid (Fig. 23-5) as you apply gentle upward traction on the lid. ***Practice Tip:*** *This is preferred to cannulating the lower lid puncta because the upper duct is less tortuous, but either can be used.* Attach a syringe filled with warm sterile saline and flush gently until fluid exits the opposite puncta in the medial canthus. Occlude that opposite puncta while maintaining a gentle flush until fluid exits the nose.

Subpalpebral Catheter Placement—Upper Eyelid

Uncooperative patients or ones that need frequent or long-term topical administration of an eye medication are candidates for subpalpebral or transpalpebral eye lavage catheters, placed from the conjunctival sac through the eyelid and secured to the face and down the neck; this allows delivery of medication(s) to the eye while standing at the patient's side. Silastic tubing systems are most highly recommended[16] (Fig. 23-6). If care is taken during placement, complications are extremely rare and the Silastic catheters can remain in place for many months (up to a year or more in some cases). They may be placed through the upper or lower eyelid; instructions below are for upper eyelid placement. Lower lid catheters are placed deep in the ventral conjunctival fornix, between the nictitans and medial lower eyelid.

Equipment
- Sedative (xylazine hydrochloride or other)
- Povidone-iodine swabs 10%[17]

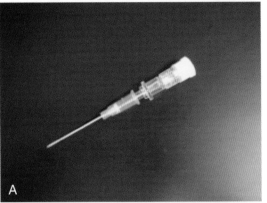
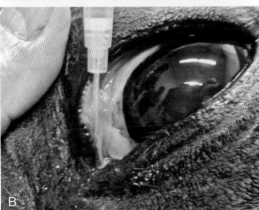

Figure 23-5   A, A 20-gauge IV catheter is shown on the *left.* **B,** With the stylet removed, the catheter passes easily into the upper nasolacrimal puncta as upward traction is applied to the eyelid for normograde nasolacrimal duct lavage.

- Povidone-iodine solution 5%[18]
- 2% local anesthetic with 25-gauge, ⅝-inch (1.6-cm) needle, 5-mL syringe
- Equine eye lavage kit with Silastic catheter[16]

---

[16]#6612 or #6613 Equine eye lavage kit (Mila International, Inc., Florence, Kentucky).
[17]Betadine Swabstick (Purdue Products, Stamford, Conneticut).

---

[18]Betadine 5% Sterile Ophthalmic Prep Solution (Alcon, Ft. Worth, Texas).

- Sterile surgical gloves
- Injection cap
- 5 mL of sterile saline in sterile syringe
- Waterproof tape
- 2-0 nonabsorbable suture on a straight needle
- Suture scissors
- Cyanoacrylate glue

Procedure for the Standing Horse

- Braid the forelock and at least 4 to 5 points in the mane.
- Sedate with xylazine (0.3 to 0.6 mg/kg IV), detomidine (0.02 to 0.04 mg/kg) or your preferred sedative.
- Anesthetize the palpebral and frontal nerves in the upper eyelid as described above (see Figs. 23-2 and 23-3) and, following cleansing with 5% to 10% povidone-iodine

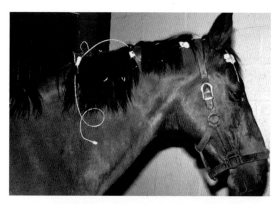

Figure 23-6   Equine eye lavage apparatus.

solution (*not* scrub), inject 1 to 2 mL of local anesthetic SQ in the dorsal eyelid at the intended exit point of the catheter, ideally just anterior to the bony orbit rim at the midpoint of the dorsal orbit. Prep the area with 5% to 10% povidone iodine *solution* (*not* scrub).

- If a marked amount of mucopurulent debris is present within the palpebral fissure, carefully rinse and sponge the debris from the eye. Rinsing with a 5% povidone-iodine solution and allowing the solution to remain in contact with the ocular surface for 2 to 3 minutes helps sanitize and cleanse the ocular surface and avoid carrying purulent debris through the eyelid during passage of the catheter.
- Open the kit. Ensure that the needle is securely attached to the tubing and that all materials are open and ready for use. Don sterile surgical gloves and rinse the insertion hand free of powder using sterile saline.
- Holding the needle as demonstrated (Fig. 23-7, *A*), grasp the eyelashes with a hemostat or the lid margins using a noncrushing instrument while inserting the finger and needle under the lid (Fig. 23-7, *B*); pull the lid firmly down and over the finger during insertion to prevent plication of the conjunctiva (i.e., do *not* hold the lid open during insertion). Maintain the lid as closed as possible as the needle and finger are directed into the dorsal conjunctival fornix (the index finger tip should be touching the ventral aspect of the dorsal orbit rim) (Fig. 23-7, *C*).
- When the fingertip is in position, approximately 1 mm anterior to the bony orbit rim, keep the finger in place against the bony orbit and between the point of the needle

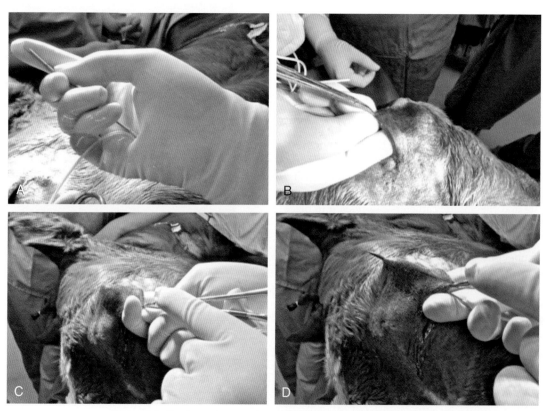

Figure 23-7   Tips for eye lavage catheter placement—see text for descriptions.

and the eye to protect the eye from the needle as you slide the needle off the fingertip (Fig. 23-7, *D*). If the needle is properly positioned in the palm, closing the palm of the hand or pushing with the palm drives the needle tip through the conjunctiva and skin in one smooth movement.

- The needle has penetrated the full thickness of the eyelid in the previous step. Remove finger from beneath eyelid and pull the needle and its attached catheter through the eyelid. When the footplate of the catheter is under the upper eyelid, close the upper lid and gently pull the footplate into position in the dorsal fornix. Palpate the fornix to ensure good positioning of the footplate, high in the fornix away from the cornea. ***Practice Tip:*** *If the eyelid opens significantly as you are seating the catheter footplate into the fornix, you may have penetrated the palpebral conjunctiva at some incorrect point, and the needle and catheter may require reinsertion (a small amount of eyelid movement is normal).*
- Using the needle, thread the catheter through the forelock and then through the underside of each neck braid. ***Practice Tip:*** *Placing the catheter on the underside of the braids, under and far dorsal in the mane, helps prevent the catheter from "catching" on objects in the stall.*
- Remove the needle from the Silastic tubing. Carefully insert the full length of the IV catheter provided in the kit into the Silastic tubing; retract the catheter stylet tip as you insert it to prevent penetration of the Silastic. Remove the stylet and attach the injection cap. Inject 3 to 5 mL of sterile saline into the line to ensure patency and note that the eyelid does not swell as you inject.
- Dry the portion of Silastic tubing over the face, attach two small pieces of waterproof tape and suture these in place as two white tape "butterflies" as shown (Fig. 23-6), one sutured near the eyelid and a second in the center of the forehead, *keeping the catheter taut between each butterfly and pressing the tape firmly against the dried tubing.* Avoid suturing the butterflies over the areas of motor nerves as you need access to these sites for future nerve blocks. Apply cyanoacrylate glue over the tape to further secure the Silastic tubing to the butterflies.
- The injection port and catheter should be "splinted" straight in some fashion (we do this by attaching it to a tongue depressor using waterproof tape and then to a braid in the mane). ***Practice Tip:*** *This is the "weak link" in this system; the catheter is subject to bending and subsequent leaking near the hub and should be replaced every 5 to 7 days as needed.*
- Administer eye medications through the injection cap while standing at the withers of the patient. Administer 0.2 mL of medication into the line followed by a slow flush of 3 cc of air until the patient blinks and moisture is seen spreading over the cornea to deliver the medication to the eye. Continuous administration of ophthalmic solutions or ulcer "cocktails" may be delivered via fluid pumps or discs attached to the Silastic and secured to the mane, halter, or a surcingle.

- Alternatively, a "homemade" SPL can be created very inexpensively using Silastic[19] or polyethylene (PE) tubing[20] (size 190-240). A customized flange is premade on the end of the PE tubing by heating the tubing over a flame and then pressing the softened tubing to a cool metal surface (***Caution:*** PE is very flammable!). A flange cut from a Silastic sheet must be glued onto the Silastic tubing. Either tubing can be attached to a wound drain insertion needle and inserted as described earlier, or a 12-gauge, 1½-inch needle with hub removed can be preplaced through the lid and the tubing threaded through it (pulling the needle through the eyelid while holding the tubing). Catheters fashioned from PE are usually removed at 2 to 3 weeks because of significantly more tissue reaction than occurs with Silastic.

Complications

- Regardless of whether catheters are placed through the upper or lower eyelids, complications can occur.
- Corneal ulceration can develop if the catheter is not sufficiently deep in the fornix or if it loosens and migrates adjacent to the cornea.
- If the patient is rubbing the eye excessively or an unexpected ulcer is noted, retract the eyelid and check the position of the catheter to ensure the catheter has not migrated near the cornea.
- If eyelid swelling or irritation develops, the catheter flange may have been pulled deep to the conjunctiva, and as a result, medications enter the subcutaneous tissues of the lid.
- Some patients rub their eyes because the catheter and ocular disease are irritating.
  - Hoods with hard plastic cups[21] over the eye help prevent trauma to the catheter and the eye; on rare occasion a cradle or cross-tying may be needed. ***Practice Tip:*** *Usually, if a horse is rubbing the eye lavage system, the catheter is malpositioned or leaking into the subcutaneous tissues.*
- The systems have been used with uniform success for more than 30 years and are rarely problematic.

OPHTHALMOLOGIC EMERGENCIES

Equine Ocular Emergencies

Many problems involving the equine eye are true emergencies, including:
- Blunt head trauma (see p. 388)
- Acute orbital cellulitis (see p. 396)
- Acute blepharitis (see p. 392)
- Eyelid lacerations (see p. 390)

[19]Silastic tubing (Bausch & Lomb Corporation, Midland, Michigan).
[20]Intramedic nonradiopaque polyethylene tubing (Clay Adams, Division of Becton-Dickinson and Co., Parsippany, New Jersey).
[21]EyeSaver Mask (Jorgensen Laboratories, Inc., 1540 N. Van Buren Ave., Loveland, Colorado 80538).

- Corneal ulcers or corneal stromal abscessation (see p. 399)
- Uveitis (see p. 412)
- Some cases of glaucoma (see p. 415)
- Acute blindness or visual disturbance (see p. 416)
- Traumatic injury to the eye (see pp. 388, 390)

These patients need to be examined immediately by a veterinarian or veterinary ophthalmologist because long-term prognosis for vision or retention of the globe may depend on immediate, accurate diagnosis and treatment.

Because many systemically administered drugs do not reach adequate ocular levels, owners or caregivers should be prepared to administer topical ocular medications as frequently as every 2 hours or more in acute conditions. In such cases, medication administration is greatly facilitated using an eye lavage apparatus[22] (see Figs. 23-6 and 23-7) placed through the conjunctival fornix of the upper (preferred) or lower eyelid. Referral to a facility providing 24-hour care may be necessary.

Acute Head Trauma with Eye Injuries

- Self-inflicted or induced traumatic injuries to the head, orbit, or globe, are common in horses because of the large size of the eye, the prominent lateral placement of the eye in the head, the nervous temperament of many horses, and the powerful reflex throwing of the head.
- Head, ocular, or orbital trauma is always an emergency.
- After injury, immediately restrain the patient's head to avoid self-induced injury that may occur from rubbing the eye and periocular area against objects, walls, or the forelimb.
- Avoid examination or manipulation of the ocular or periocular tissues until adequate restraint, tranquilization, and eyelid akinesia are completed.
- If you are on the phone with an owner, instruct them that they *do not* need to look at the eye and attempting to do so is likely to result in further damage.

Orbital and Periorbital Fractures

The dorsal (frontal bone) and temporozygomatic (temporal and zygomatic bones) regions of the orbit are most commonly injured.

Clinical Signs

- Edema, swelling, pain, blepharospasm, chemosis, and subconjunctival hemorrhage may or may not be accompanied by lacerations, contusions, or other injuries of the face or lids.
- Subcutaneous, subconjunctival, or orbital emphysema is common if the frontal or maxillary sinuses have been fractured (Fig. 23-8).
- Palpable disruption of the bones of the orbital rim may be felt if fracture fragments are displaced. Fractures generally appear more extensive on radiographs than on palpation.

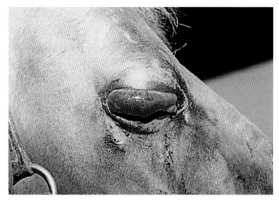

Figure 23-8 Eye of a 2-year-old Thoroughbred colt with severe subconjunctival emphysema resulting from dorsal orbital rim fracture involving the frontal sinus.

- Abnormal nasal or ocular discharge or reduced nasal airflow may be present.
- Strabismus or displacement of the globe is variable or absent.
- Globe may be enophthalmic, exophthalmic, or normally positioned.
- The nictitans may be protruded, recessed, or normal.
- Upper eyelid function may be impaired because of lid or conjunctival swelling or injury to the palpebral nerve.

Diagnosis

- Diagnosis is generally straightforward if a known traumatic event has occurred.
- Perform complete physical, ocular, and neurologic examinations; rule out orbital cellulitis (swelling, fever, leukocytosis, nictitans protrusion and supraorbital fossa swelling, +/-pain on opening mouth). Assess the ability of the injured eye to transmit a pupillary light reflex to the opposite eye. (A strong light is needed in horses to evaluate pupillary light response, but never use an LED light unless it does not hurt your own eye!)
- Be sure to examine and stain the cornea at presentation and again daily for several more days, even if the cornea is stain negative on day 1 because blunt corneal contusions may result in corneal epithelial sloughing that does not develop until several days later.
- Palpate the affected area and perform a gentle digital examination of the orbital rim from inside the palpebral fissure once the patient has been safely tranquilized and the eye topically anesthetized. Swelling and pain may prevent thorough palpation.
- Fully evaluate eye motility by moving the patient's head dorsally, ventrally, laterally, and in small circles while simultaneously observing for normal vestibular eye movements.
  - This evaluation may be difficult if significant periocular swelling is present.
  - Forced ductions of the eye may be needed for complete evaluation: after moderate sedation and topical anesthesia or under general anesthesia, grasp the limbal

conjunctiva with a small tissue forceps and "force" the globe through all planes of motion to ensure that it is not trapped in fractures.

- Computed tomography (CT) is recommended for diagnosis, but any combination of CT plus radiology, ultrasonography, and magnetic resonance imaging (MRI) may be needed for a complete diagnosis (see Ch. 14, p. 97).

●》 WHAT TO DO

Orbital Fractures
Symptomatic Treatment
- Administer cold compresses, analgesics, and anti-inflammatory agents.
- Systemic corticosteroids are *not* recommended because of concerns relative to a sinus or orbit infection.
  - ***Important:*** *If optic nerve damage is suspected, administration of systemic corticosteroids may be indicated.*
- Hot compresses may be used after the first 24 hours: Apply for 5 to 10 minutes every 2 hours.
- Systemic antibiotic therapy is necessary if open fractures, sinus fractures, or skin wounds are present or suspected.
- Frequent (8 times or more per day) application of topical eye lubricants is necessary if there is *any* impairment of eyelid function or integrity and a temporary tarsorrhaphy should be considered to protect the globe.
- ***Practice Tip:*** *Symptomatic treatment alone is* not *recommended if there is sinus compromise, significant displacement of fracture fragments, considerable facial deformity, displacement of the globe, or any impairment of normal eye movements. Fracture repair is urgently needed in cases of suspected optic nerve damage.*

Fracture Repair
- Repair is most easily accomplished in the first 24 to 48 hours as a general anesthetic procedure if the patient's physical condition is stable.
- Repair may be accomplished by digital manipulation and bony traction; however, most cases require moderate to extensive orthopedic manipulation, instrumentation, and fixation.

Blunt Trauma to the Head with Secondary Optic Neuropathy
- Blunt trauma is a common sequela to occipital trauma, rearing and striking the head, throwing the head and falling backward (especially common in youngsters).
- Trauma may result in sudden unilateral or bilateral visual impairment or blindness, resulting from partial or complete shearing or injury of the optic nerve fibers or from hemorrhage or fractures in the basisphenoid region.
- Complete cranial nerve examination including direct and consensual pupillary light reflexes, menace responses, obstacle course evaluation, and complete ophthalmic examination (including careful fundus and optic nerve examination) must be performed in all cases of blunt head trauma. Orbital ultrasound examination is sometimes helpful diagnostically. CT, MRI, or both, with or without a contrast agent, are highly recommended to establish a diagnosis and prognosis.
- Follow-up examination, even of a normal-appearing eye, should be performed at 6 to 8 weeks and again later after

trauma because post-traumatic demyelination and optic nerve atrophy may occur.

Immediate Findings
- Visual impairment: Horses with head trauma that are acutely blind will usually remain so forever. Occasionally, patients may be affected unilaterally or have a partially intact visual field in each eye.
- Blind patients have widely dilated and unresponsive pupils in each eye while partially sighted horses have variable pupillary responses.
- The fundus may be normal acutely, but optic nerve edema, hemorrhage, myelin loss, myelin extrusion, or other alterations may be present. These are rare findings because the most common site of injury is proximal on the optic nerves, quite a distance from the globes.

Chronic Cases (6 or More Weeks After Injury)
- Evaluate for optic nerve atrophy: Pallor, slight cupping, change in texture of the optic nerve head as scleral fibers (lamina cribrosa) become visible, and decreased diameter of the nerve head all may be observed.
- Retinal vasculature is decreased or absent.
- Peripapillary retinal or choroidal atrophy or pigment alteration may be present, often in a "butterfly wing" distribution.

●》 WHAT TO DO

Head Trauma with Blindness
- Partially sighted horses (with some intact optic nerve fibers) may improve with time and immediate, aggressive, appropriate management of central nervous system trauma (see Chapter 22, p. 368).
- Most patients are permanently visually impaired.
- Give an extremely guarded to grave prognosis in all cases. Vision loss may progress for the first few days after the injury.

Blunt Trauma to the Eye Without Laceration or Rupture
- Perform careful physical, neurologic, and ophthalmic examinations, including fundus examination and evaluation of direct and consensual pupillary light reflexes (as possible). The eye may appear normal or have any combination of injuries and degree of hyphema.
  - Indirect ophthalmoscopy is recommended because it is more useful for fundus examination through cloudy media than is direct ophthalmoscopy.
- Some patients may be normal; others may have mild to severe optic nerve edema or hyperemia with or without peripapillary retinal and choroidal edema.
- Check the sclera carefully (general examination, ophthalmoscopic exam, and with ultrasound) for occult ruptures, especially in the limbal and equatorial regions and in any areas of conjunctival hemorrhage. If not repaired, occult ruptures may result in phthisis bulbi (shrinkage of the eyeball). Ultrasound is invaluable but must be done cautiously, through the eyelids or supraorbital fossa or both

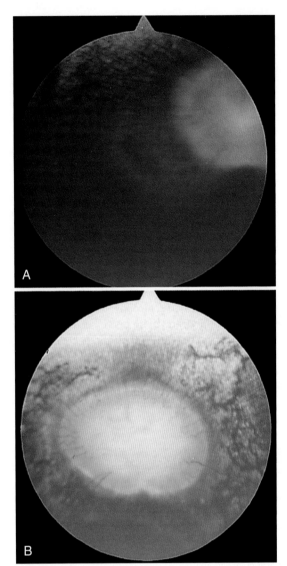

Figure 23- 9   A, Four weeks before this photograph was taken, a 3-year-old Warmblood stallion sustained iatrogenic blunt trauma to the eye. Resolving peripapillary retinal and choroidal edema are present; consolidating subretinal hemorrhage was also present not in this image. **B,** A photo obtained 1 year after injury shows a classic "butterfly" lesion (peripapillary choroidal atrophy and scarring with retinal pigment epithelium (RPE) hypertrophy).

but *with no pressure on the globe* or evisceration through an occult rupture can result.

- Perform repeat fundus examinations 1, 3, 6, and 12 months after injury because some patients develop "butterfly lesions" (areas of peripapillary choroidal and retinal pigment epithelial disturbance, or atrophy), possibly due to vascular disruption or as a result of compression of the posterior eye wall around the stalk of the optic nerve (Fig. 23-9). Visual disturbance has not been documented in these cases, and electroretinograms obtained in several cases were normal. Similar butterfly lesions occur from many causes, including equine recurrent uveitis (ERU); therefore, document all trauma-induced butterfly lesions to prevent any question of a diagnosis of ERU-associated unsoundness during future prepurchase examinations.

- Acute *hyphema* often is present.
  - If >50% of the anterior chamber is filled with blood or if spontaneous intraocular rebleeding occurs, the eye has a very poor prognosis, and phthisis bulbi often results.
  - See Acute Hyphema (p. 411).

●》 WHAT TO DO

Blunt Globe Trauma
- Monitor the cornea carefully for several days after any blunt traumatic injury. An initially normal cornea may slough its epithelium a few days later as a consequence of the contusion (Fig. 23-10).
- Monitor all subconjunctival regions for several days for swelling or pigment that may indicate an occult rupture.
- Administer systemic anti-inflammatory therapy as needed.

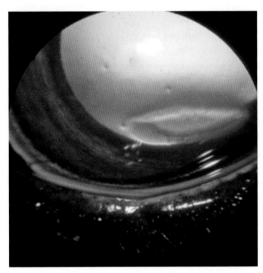

Figure 23-10   Corneal erosion in a 4-year-old Thoroughbred, 24 hours after blunt facial trauma. Note the loose epithelial edges and the absence of corneal edema. Normal-appearing eyes should be monitored closely for several days following trauma as corneal contusion may result in epithelial sloughing several days later.

Eyelid Emergencies
Eyelid Lacerations or Avulsions
- The classic equine eyelid laceration is usually an avulsion of the eyelid that occurs when the patient "catches" the upper or lower eyelid on a harness hook, nail, bucket handle, or other such object. The horse then pulls its head away forcefully, tearing through the thinnest part of the lid as it does so. The globe itself is usually surprisingly normal in these cases (Figs. 23-11 and 23-12)
- Lacerations that result from blunt compression or other direct trauma require careful ophthalmic exams because trauma to the globe is likely.
- Most eyelid lacerations or avulsions occur in the upper eyelid.

Diagnosis
- Usually the diagnosis is obvious.
- There may be a simple laceration perpendicular to the lid margin, a laceration that has removed the lid margin

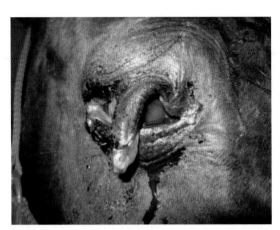

Figure 23-11 Acute eyelid injury. This 15-year-old Thoroughbred spooked while drinking from a bucket, caught its lateral canthus on the bucket handle and lifted the full bucket off of the ground before the eyelids tore. The globe was normal.

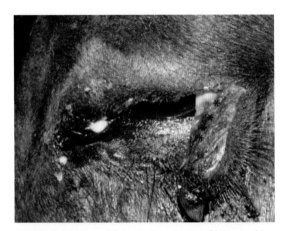

Figure 23-12 Subacute eyelid trauma in a 14-year-old Quarter horse, presented 16 hours after the injury. The *line of black asterisks* delineates the *tarsus* or *tarsal plate* layer, the connective tissue layer of the eyelid and the most important layer to surgically close. To the *left of the asterisks* is the smooth, moist conjunctival surface, which should *never* be sutured. To the *right of the asterisks* is the swollen orbicularis oculi muscle.

(uncommon), macerated tissue of any extent, or, most commonly, a flap of eyelid hanging from a pedicle (see Figs. 23-11 and 23-12).

- The wound usually is edematous and bloody, and swelling may be profound.
  - Blood, tears, and a mucoid to mucopurulent ocular discharge are seen on the lid and periocular area. The discharge is moist or dry, depending on the time since the injury. Tissues may be swollen 2 to 10 times normal.
- The individual usually is in mild to moderate pain and irritated by the tissue deformity.
- A fluorescein dye test *must* be performed to assess the integrity of the cornea. Manage any corneal injury appropriately.

⏺⏵ WHAT TO DO

Eyelid Lacerations

- Cleanse, if necessary, before complete examination using sterile saline or a 5% povidone-iodine *solution*. ***Important:*** *Never use alcohol, povidone-iodine scrub, or chlorhexidine anywhere near the eye.*

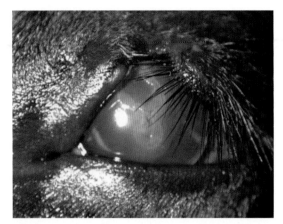

Figure 23-13 A 9-year-old Quarter horse mare with severe blepharospasm, chronic epiphora, and corneal ulceration secondary to severe trichiasis, resulting from an improper eyelid injury repair. (The skin was the only layer closed; the tarsal plate layer should be closed in *every* equine eyelid injury.)

- Perform a *complete ocular examination* including fluorescein staining and a careful examination of the adnexa and globe, including fundus and lens evaluation to assess occult injuries.
- Make sure the eye remains lubricated and protected from self-mutilation before, during, and after the examination.
- If the cause is unknown, skull radiographs may be indicated to rule out the presence of metallic foreign bodies and bony lesions.
- Explore wounds carefully before closing them.
- Administer tetanus prophylaxis.
- Administer systemic broad-spectrum antibiotics.
- Any periocular laceration that breaches the eyelid margin must be surgically repaired as soon as possible. ***Practice Tip:*** *Never excise any portion of torn eyelid margin.* The eyelid margin should be replaced and repaired in a minimum of two layers in every case.
- Eyelids are well vascularized and "forgiving" if properly repaired.
  - Tissue appearing hopelessly desiccated, inflamed, or infected can heal well if properly repaired and medicated.
- No other tissue in the body can substitute for lost eyelid margin. Preserve eyelid marginal tissue, *even when viability is in doubt.* Debride using a dry sponge or scrape with a blade; avoid cutting tissue away.
  - Removal or improper repair of an eyelid margin leads to chronic corneal irritation and ulceration from irritation by eyelid hairs (trichiasis, Fig. 23-13), exposure keratitis resulting from improper spreading of the tear film over the cornea, and chronic keratoconjunctivitis caused by an inability of the eye to properly cleanse itself.
- Preserve lid function or otherwise ensure that the lids can protect the globe during healing (e.g., performing a tarsorrhaphy is often a good idea).
- Prevent self-mutilation, possibly aided by an Eye Saver Mask.

Anesthesia and Wound Preparation

- Local anesthesia and heavy sedation are acceptable if the patient is cooperative. Use general anesthesia for all complicated repairs, repairs with fractures, or if the patient is difficult to manage.
- In either case, application of topical anesthesia is a useful adjunct to repair.
- Trim lashes and sensory hairs using petrolatum- or gel-coated scissors. Avoid clipping other lid hair around the wound because the small cut hairs are difficult to eliminate from the wound. Wounds that extend into the longer hair of the face may require clipping.
- Cleanse the wound thoroughly using sterile saline and a 5% povidone-iodine *solution*. ***Important:*** *Never use alcohol,*

povidone-iodine scrub or chlorhexidine anywhere near the eye. Avoid all detergent or scrub cleansers because they are highly toxic to ocular tissues; chlorhexidine in particular should never should be used in the periocular area.

- If the conjunctival surfaces are significantly contaminated, a commercial preparation of povidone-iodide[23] can be used to flush the ocular surface. Allow it to remain in contact with the cornea and conjunctiva for 2 minutes then rinse with sterile saline.
- Debride the wound margins with sterile gauze or scrape with a blade until the cut surfaces bleed freely. Minimize sharp debridement to preserve the maximum amount of eyelid tissue.

Acute Injuries (<12 Hours Old)

- Repair lacerations as soon as possible, cleansing and prepping as described above, but you may postpone repair for 24 hours or more to stabilize the patient's condition if other injuries are present.
- 5-0 absorbable suture material on a small needle is preferred.
- On all full-thickness lacerations, perform at minimum a two-layer closure. Some lacerations may require three layers.
- Examine the deeper layers of the cut eyelid until the white connective tissue layer of the eyelid (the *tarsus* or *tarsal plate*) is identified. It is immediately external to the conjunctiva, approximately three-fourths deep in the lid. ***Practice Tip:*** *This is the most important layer to close, and the layer in which to place deep sutures. Never suture conjunctiva nor allow any sutures to penetrate the conjunctiva at any point, or corneal irritation results* (see Figs. 23-11 and 23-12).
- The first suture placed (or preplaced) is critical: it should appose the eyelid margins perfectly, or chronic corneal irritation and poor cosmesis may result.
- A buried horizontal mattress, figure-of-eight, partially buried mattress, or cruciate suture that securely closes the eyelid margin, *with the knots completely buried or placed away from the eyelid margin and not penetrating the conjunctiva,* is recommended.
- If placement is not exact and a "step" develops in the lid margin as the suture is tightened, remove and replace the suture.
- This suture may be preplaced but not tied to facilitate placement of other tarsal sutures.
- Place additional sutures, as needed, completely closing the tarsus layer. Evert the lid as you go to confirm that these deep sutures do not penetrate the conjunctiva at any point and that the conjunctival margins are in gross apposition (precise conjunctival apposition not required).
- Tie any preplaced marginal suture(s), and perform routine skin closure.
- Place simple, interrupted sutures of 4-0 or 5-0 absorbable material in the subcuticular layers or skin with sutures 2 to 3 mm apart.
- Make *certain* that any cut suture ends cannot contact the cornea.
- Severe lacerations benefit by stenting the lacerated eyelid to the opposing eyelid by means of a simple tarsorrhaphy (split-thickness horizontal mattress sutures in the eyelid margins).
- If the eyelid injury is extensive or if the eyelids must be closed, plan ahead and place an eye lavage apparatus for administration of topical medications (if needed) before closure of the lids (see p. 385).

Postoperative Medical Management

- Avoid eyelid manipulations whenever possible and avoid placing excessive tension or stress on the eyelid during application of topical medications.

- Avoid topical corticosteroids.
- Administer topical broad-spectrum antibiotics q4h for 24 to 48 hours and then q6h for 7 to 10 days if tissue injury is excessive or if corneal integrity is in doubt; otherwise, antibiotics are unnecessary.
- If topical application is impossible, an eye lavage apparatus is recommended, or ophthalmic antibiotic solutions can be gently sprayed onto the cornea with a tuberculin syringe with the needle hub attached but with the needle broken off at the hub (see Fig. 23-1). This makes an effective, simple medication "squirt gun." ***Practice Tip:*** *Horses often strenuously resist sprays applied to the eyelids but rarely object to gentle spraying localized to the cornea.*
- If the cornea is injured, administer topical medications more frequently and judiciously.
- Administer systemic antibiotics for 5 to 7 days.
- Use of a systemic anti-inflammatory or antiprostaglandin agent is indicated depending on the degree of inflammation and discomfort. Minimally, administer phenylbutazone, 2.2 to 4.4 mg/kg q12h PO for 3 to 5 days.
- Ensure tetanus prophylaxis.
- Prevent self-trauma.
- Gently clean the periocular area as often as exudate and discharges accumulate. For excess swelling and to remove accumulated exudates, apply gentle warm compresses for 10 minutes every 2 to 3 hours.
- After cleansing and drying, coat the drainage area of the face beneath the eye with a film of petrolatum jelly to prevent hair loss from irritation by the eye secretions.
- Check daily to ensure normal eyelid function and absence of suture irritation.

Subacute to Chronic Lacerations (>12 Hours Old)

- See example in Fig. 23-12.
- Repair lacerations as soon as possible, cleansing and prepping as described earlier, but you may postpone repair for 24 hours or more to stabilize the patient's condition if other injuries are present.
- Provide topical and medical management as described previously.
- Restore the wound edges by means of sharp scarification with a #15 scalpel blade. *Take special care not to remove tissue but to instead restore a liberally bleeding surface* and repair as described above.

Acute Blepharitis

Blepharitis is an inflammation of the eyelids and can present as an acute or chronic condition. There are multiple causes for the inflammatory process, which can also affect the hair follicles and sebaceous gland openings of the eyelid margins. The changes can be seen as nonulcerative, ulcerative, or extensively necrotic lesions.

Etiology

Possible known causes include the following:
- Self-trauma
- Allergic reaction

---

[23]5% Betadine Ophthalmic Prep Solution (Alcon, Ft. Worth, Texas).

- Bacterial/fungal hypersensitivity
- Parasite infestation (e.g., *Demodex* or *Habronema*)
- Noxious chemical irritation or chemical sensitivity
- Exposure to noxious plants
- Insect stings or sprays (e.g., from bombardier beetles) or snake bite
- Immune-mediated purpura hemorrhagica and blood or vaccine reactions
- Orbital fat prolapse
- Cause unknown in most cases

Clinical Signs
- Lid and conjunctival swelling, edema, chemosis (may be profound)
- Blepharospasm
- Epiphora, mucoid to purulent discharge
- Exposure keratitis with or without ulceration resulting from poor lid-to-globe contact and poor tear film distribution

Diagnosis
- Take a careful history: Has this occurred before? To what chemicals, fertilizers, feed additives, soaps, cleansers, and plants has the patient been exposed?
- Perform careful examination of the head and eye, including all conjunctival surfaces of the lids, globe, and membrana nictitans.
  - Requires sedation, eyelid akinesia, and topical anesthesia
- Remove any foreign material present.
- Perform copious lavage with saline solution or ocular collyrium.
- Perform fluorescein staining (see p. 380).

⏺ WHAT TO DO

Acute Blepharitis
- Treat the cause, if found.
  - Cases with presumed bacterial blepharitis or inflammation of one or more eyelid glands ("styes") benefit from hot compress applications 2 or more times a day plus cleansing and good hygiene. Use a 1:10 solution of baby shampoo in water or a 5% povidone-iodine *solution; never use alcohol, povidone-iodine scrub, or chlorhexidine anywhere near the eye.*

⏺ WHAT TO DO

Facial Nerve Paralysis
- Rule out Horner's disease, which may have mild ptosis, but a blink reflex is intact with Horner's; ipsilateral facial sweating is always present with Horner's.
- Treat the patient for the primary disease (see Chapter 22, p. 350).
- Provide frequent (q2 to 4h) topical lubrication with artificial tear solution or ointment.
- Manage corneal ulceration if present (see p. 400).
- Perform temporary tarsorrhaphy:
  - Two horizontal mattress sutures placed split thickness in the eyelids may be adequate for 1 to 2 weeks. If these sutures are

- Most cases only require symptomatic therapy.
  - Administer systemic nonsteroidal anti-inflammatory drugs (NSAIDs).
  - Apply sterile ophthalmic lubrication with an agent such as Lacri-Lube (white petrolatum, mineral oil, and lanolin alcohol) or an antibiotic ointment, if indicated, until the lids have returned to normal contact with the cornea. Consider tarsorrhaphy if swelling is severe and blinking is severely compromised.
  - Monitor the cornea carefully for any exposure keratitis that may develop as the result of poor lid-to-globe contact and secondary poor tear film distribution.

Facial Nerve Paralysis
Facial nerve injury may result in the inability to close the eyelids, with exposure keratitis and corneal ulceration being common sequelae.

Etiology
- Trauma or compression of the facial nerve or any of its branches
- Equine protozoal myelitis (EPM)
- Temporohyoid osteoarthropathy (THO)
- Chronic, severe otitis media with or without THO
- Otitis interna
- Facial fractures
- Guttural pouch disease
- Vestibular syndrome
- Polyneuritis
- Other

Diagnosis
Obvious signs are usually the following:
- Ptosis
- Absent or reduced palpebral reflex. (Assess carefully! An apparent blink of the eyelids is often passive eyelid movement associated with globe retraction; however, this motion is insufficient to lubricate and protect the eye).
- Mucoid to mucopurulent ocular discharge caused by impaired lacrimal pump system
- Corneal epithelial thickening, erosion, or ulceration
- Positive rose bengal, lissamine green, or fluorescein stain uptake earlier, usually in a horizontal elliptical pattern just above the lower lid margin, slightly temporally (Figure 23-15, *A*).

left in place longer, chronic lid thickening, depigmentation, and necrosis occurs.
- The recommended suture is 4-0 silk.
- Sutures should be tightened to just appose the lids (no tighter or tissue necrosis can result).
- Sutures preplaced through rubber band stents and tied in a shoelacelike bow knot allow the lids to be easily opened for corneal examination.
- Perform a *reversible split-lid tarsorrhaphy* if facial nerve paralysis is from EPM, THO, or lasts longer than 2 weeks (Fig. 23-14).

EYE

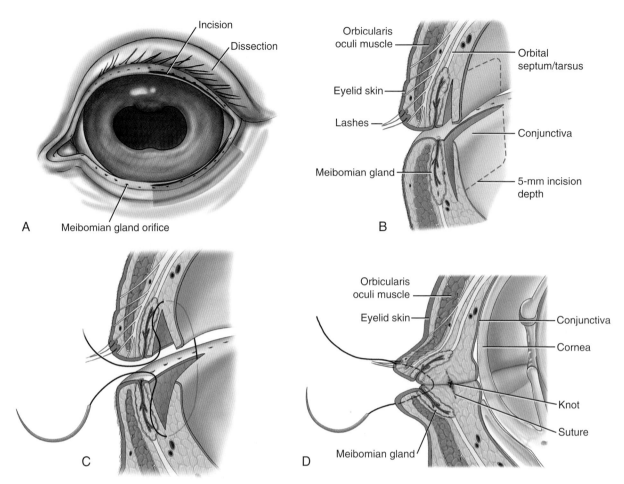

Figure 23-14   Split-lid tarsorrhaphy. The shaded areas in **A** and the incision in **B** indicate opposing 5- to 7-mm-deep incisions, made with care perpendicular to the lid margin and just caudal to the tarsal gland openings. The incisions must remain parallel, superficial to the conjunctival surface, and should be deep to and avoid the tarsal glands. Simple interrupted sutures are placed deep within the incision **(C);** when they are tightened, the wound margins will "pucker" together, burying the suture and providing a secure closure **(D).** (Modified from Divers TJ, Ducharme NG, de Lahunta A, Irby NL, et al: *Clin Tech Equine Pract* 5:23, 2006.)

- *Practice Tip: It is never indicated to remove eyelid margins to partially and permanently close the eyelids in cases of facial paralysis because most horses regain eyelid function in 6 to 18+ months. If the lid margins are completely excised the lids can never be reopened.*
- A simple, *reversible split-lid tarsorrhaphy* is recommended to close the temporal half of the palpebral fissure. It can be left in place for months to years and, if innervation and lid function return, the eyelids can be snipped open with return to normal appearance and function. While the split-lid tarsorrhaphy is in place, vision is possible from the open medial palpebral fissure and the nictitating membrane can provide protection to the medial aspect of the cornea.
  - The procedure can be performed with heavy sedation and local anesthetic blocks.
  - Cleanse the eyelid margins using a 5% povidone-iodine *solution* which is a completely safe product if it touches the ocular surfaces; *never use alcohol, povidone-iodine scrub, or chlorhexidine anywhere near the eye.*
  - Using a #15 scalpel blade, make a 10- to 15-mm-long incision, splitting to the eyelid margin as shown, following the tarsal (meibomian) gland openings but just caudal to them and incising to a depth of 4 to 6 mm. *The eyelid margins are not excised or otherwise destroyed; they are simply split into two layers* (see Fig. 23-14).

- Make a corresponding incision (same position, length, and depth) in the lower lid margin. The equine lower lid margin is thinner and the margin is less defined than the upper, so pay careful attention, ensuring that the lid is split properly into an outer skin–muscle-gland layer and a thinner, inner layer that includes conjunctiva and subconjunctival connective tissue. The inner layer (upper or lower lid) must not contain or invert *any* hairs, any hair follicles, or any cut hairs, which potentially regrow toward the cornea, possibly causing corneal ulceration.
- Using 5-0 absorbable suture, place one "bite" in the apex of the upper lid incision, parallel to the lid margin and then a corresponding bite in the trough of the lower lid incision. Repeat as needed (2 to 3 sutures usually suffice). When these sutures are tied, they bring the upper and lower eyelid wounds together, everting the inner conjunctival layer toward the cornea and everting the skin-muscle-gland layers outward. Preplacing the sutures before tying is recommended.
- Lastly, close the skin/lid margin with 2 to 3 horizontal mattress 5-0 absorbable sutures, split thickness in the everted marginal tissue as added wound security.
- Extreme care must be taken during closure to avoid causing trichiasis (hairs touching cornea as they regrow)
- The palpebral fissure appears overcorrected (over-closed) initially because of lid swelling.

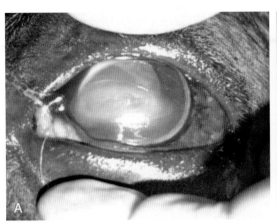 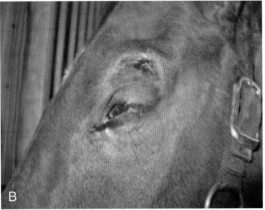

Figure 23-15 **A,** The left cornea of an 11-year-old Thoroughbred, showing a corneal ulcer secondary to facial nerve paralysis from THO before placement of a split-lid tarsorrhaphy. **B,** The same eye following removal of an eye lavage catheter, 4 months after the split-lid tarsorrhaphy was performed. When orbicularis oculi function returned 11 months later, the tarsorrhaphy was incised open by the home veterinarian, and the eye reportedly appeared normal.

- Medications can be applied through the open medial half of the palpebral fissure or through a preplaced eye lavage apparatus in fractious patients.
- Suture removal is unnecessary if absorbable sutures are used in the skin.
- Depending on the cause of the paralysis, normal eyelid function is very likely to return over 6 weeks to 3 years (in one reported case).

Ask the owner to regularly monitor the palpebral reflex. When the reflex returns, the tarsorrhaphy can be completely or gradually snipped opened using a small scissors or it can be left in place for life if nerve function does not return. Vision through the medial canthal opening is good (Fig. 23-15, *B*).

Prognosis
- Prognosis is guarded, but almost all patients have had partial to complete return of nerve function over a 6- to 36-month period.
- Cosmetic result after reversal of the procedure is excellent (eyelid aperture looks and functions normally).

Entropion
Entropion is inward rolling of one or more eyelid margins and can present as an acute or chronic condition. It is usually seen in newborn foals that have one or more medical conditions resulting in dehydration or excess recumbency.
- Entropion can occur secondary to corneal ulcer formation of any cause.
- Entropion can be the cause of corneal ulcer formation.

It is rare in adults except secondary to eyelid injury. In any case, entropion requires immediate correction to resolve the discomfort and disease that result from hairs rubbing the ocular surfaces.

Clinical Signs
- Lid and conjunctival swelling, edema, chemosis (may be profound)
- Blepharospasm
- Epiphora, mucoid to purulent discharge
- Keratitis with or without ulceration resulting from the eyelid hairs rubbing the cornea

Diagnosis
- History and clinical exam: The problem is readily apparent upon close inspection of the eyelid margins as one or more

eyelid margins are not visible because they are inverted toward the globe (Fig. 23-16, *A*).

● WHAT TO DO

Entropion
- Inspect the eye carefully for bedding or other foreign material and remove it. Liberally lavage the eye.
- Treat underlying cause, if found.
- The procedure requires topical anesthesia; use sedation as needed.
- Periocular instillation of local anesthetic may be necessary but this usually causes more irritation to the patient than three bites with the suture needle.
- ***Practice Tip:*** *As you suture, protect the cornea by closing the upper lid with your opposite thumb, gently placing your opposite thumbnail deep to the eyelid to be sutured.*
- The recommended suture is 4-0 silk, a nonreactive, soft material that is well tolerated by the periocular tissues.
- One or two horizontal mattress sutures placed centrally in the lid are sufficient (Fig. 23-16, *B*).
- The first suture bite is placed *perpendicular* to the lid margin; it should enter the skin half way between the lid margin and the orbit rim and should exit the skin approximately 0.5 to 1.0 cm from the lid margin. The second bite is placed *parallel* to the lid margin; it is a 5- to 7-mm bite, just at the hair line, approximately 3 mm from the lid margin, and paralleling the eyelid margin. The third bite reverses direction, again perpendicular to the margin and completes the mattress suture. If eversion is inadequate, place an additional suture bite near the orbital rim and tie to it. Ensure the trimmed suture ends do *not* touch the cornea (Fig. 23-16, *B*). ***Important:*** At *no* point should any suture bite penetrate the full thickness of the eyelid.

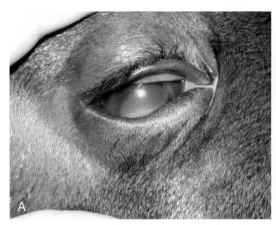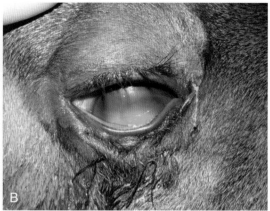

Figure 23-16   A, The right eye of a 2-day-old foal after the application of fluorescein dye. The upper eyelid margin is clearly seen and is normal; the lower eyelid margin is not visible as entropion is present. **B,** The same foal after placement of 2, 4-0 silk, horizontal mattress sutures that correct the entropion. The lower lid margin is now visible. Fluorescein, previously placed in the eye to delineate the corneal erosion (see part **A**) has now diffused into the corneal stroma, beyond the margins of the erosion.

Chemical Injuries to the Eye or Adnexa

◉› WHAT TO DO

Chemical Injuries

- Lavage, lavage, lavage.
  - A water hose is fine in an emergency. Owners should immediately and thoroughly wash the affected tissues and maintain continuous lavage for at least 45 to 60 minutes or until a veterinarian arrives. If the patient is to be transported, attempts should be made to maintain a lavage during transport if this can be done safely.
  - Under *no* circumstances instill any "product" into the injured eye in an attempt to neutralize the chemical agent; further tissue damage results!
- In general, alkali burns carry a much poorer prognosis than do acid injuries because alkaline substances progressively damage tissues for a considerable time after the insult. As a consequence of the tremendous tissue damage, severe, progressive keratomalacia occurs in most cases.
- Treat the patient as for complicated, melting ulcers (see p. 404).
- The prognosis is guarded to poor in all cases of alkaline corneal burn.

Emergencies Involving the Globe

Acute Exophthalmos

Acute exophthalmos is always an emergency.

Clinical Signs

- The eye protrudes any abnormal amount from the orbit and the supraorbital fossa may be distended.
- Assess the prominence of the cornea and also the eyelash angle compared to the normal side (it may be increased or decreased).
- The affected lids may be swollen and the conjunctiva (with chemosis, hemorrhage) may be protruding from the palpebral fissure; the nictitating membrane may be protruded or recessed from view.
- Fever is variable according to cause.

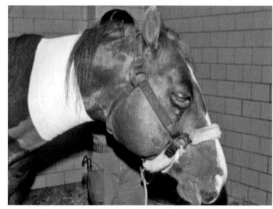

Figure 23-17   Exophthalmos and marked chemosis secondary to masticatory myopathy associated with selenium deficiency. The masseter muscle swelling is obvious in this image.

- Pain, redness, swelling, and discharge of serous to purulent material vary depending on the duration and cause.
- Bony alterations may be noted.
- Manual retropulsion of the eye into the orbit is reduced and may cause pain.

Differential Considerations

Orbital Inflammation, Infection, Cellulitis

- May be septic or nonseptic
- Possible causes:
  - Foreign body or traumatic perforation (wound may appear minor)
  - Extension of infection
    - Infected tooth root or sinus infection
    - Strangles
  - Result of a penetrating injury
  - Masticatory muscle nutritional myositis/selenium deficient myositis (Fig. 23-17)
  - Periorbital suture osteitis (Fig. 23-18, *A* and *B*).
  - Other

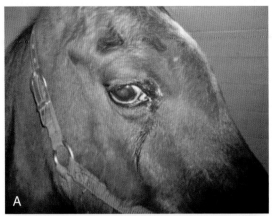

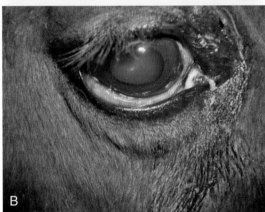

Figure 23-18   A, This 11-month-old Quarter horse presented with epiphora, a rapid onset of chemosis and a domed appearance of the forehead, and multifocal facial swellings. A crackling sound was noted in the eyelids of each eye (OU). Nasolacrimal duct obstruction was present OU. **B,** Subconjunctival emphysema was present with subcutaneous emphysema also noted elsewhere on the skull ("bubbles" are present in the conjunctiva, visible ventrally). Suture periostitis with air leakage from multiple sinuses was diagnosed.

- Fever, pain, reluctance to open mouth, and leukocytosis are present in some cases; nutritional myopathies may have markedly abnormal laboratory findings.

Glaucoma

- Glaucoma is rarely an acute problem causing exophthalmos in horses, but the condition may have gone unrecognized for long enough that a bulging eye is the first sign noticed by the owner.
- The eye usually has obvious abnormalities (see Glaucoma, p. 415), and the patient has no systemic signs.

Orbital Neoplasia

- Orbital neoplasia is rarely an acute problem but may present as one on some occasions.
- Numerous neoplasms can affect the equine orbit, primarily or as extensions from adjacent regions, including turbinates, sinuses, and the nasal cavity.
- Most equine patients have other clinical abnormalities (ipsilateral nasal discharge, altered airflow, abnormal sinus percussion, sinus or facial swelling, lymphadenopathy, neurologic abnormalities), depending on the location of the tumor.

Proptosis

- Proptosis is rare in the horse, often catastrophic, and carries a grave prognosis for vision.

- The eye should be enucleated if ruptured or if there is extensive extraocular muscle or optic nerve avulsion.
- Repair requires heavy sedation and an immediate lateral canthotomy, incising full-thickness the lateral eyelid commissure to relieve pressure on the globe and to allow its replacement.

Diagnosis

- Complete physical and ophthalmic examination including careful cranial nerve evaluation, percussion, and other assessment of sinuses and the caudal nasal cavity
- Complete blood cell count and chemistry profile
- Further diagnostic tests, including the following:
  - Radiography
  - Orbit ultrasonography
  - Endoscopy of the caudal nasal passage and pharynx, particularly of the periethmoidal area
  - CT or MRI or both
  - Anesthesia and exploration

●》 WHAT TO DO

Severe Exophthalmos

Immediate Therapy—First Steps

- Prevent self-mutilation; perform a lateral canthotomy as soon as possible to relieve pressure on the globe.
- Carefully cleanse the eye and periocular tissues with sterile saline solution or sterile eyewash. Contact lens solutions in squeeze bottles are readily available and easily used by owners.
- Perform fluorescein staining to rule out exposure keratitis and treat as needed.
- Consider placing a transpalpebral lavage apparatus (see p. 385) because the eyelids will be temporarily closed as part of the therapy.
- After cleaning, heavily lubricate the eye and any exposed periocular tissues with a sterile ophthalmic lubricant.
- Always perform a temporary tarsorrhaphy to keep the eyelids closed.
  - Use extreme care placing the tarsorrhaphy sutures so they do *not* rub the cornea and cause additional problems.
  - Protect the cornea as the sutures are tightened.

Further Therapy—Second Steps

- Therapy varies with the etiologic factor.
- In most acute cases and in cases of suture periostitis, initiate NSAID administration immediately.
- Aggressive antibiotic therapy is indicated if a septic process is suspected.
- Vitamin E and selenium plus careful medical management are indicated if nutritional myositis is suspected.
- Other treatments are directed at the specific cause as identified.

Nutritional Myositis

- Variable chemosis, nictitans prominence and mild to moderate orbit swelling and exophthalmos accompanied by difficulty chewing, temporal and masseter muscle swelling, and pain may be due to nutritional myopathy, which is a vitamin E and selenium deficiency associated with reduced access to fresh forage (see Fig. 23-17).

- The ocular signs are attributed in part to pterygoid muscle swelling; pain is noted on retropulsion of the globe; chemosis may be profound in some cases.
- The patient may have an anxious, uncomfortable attitude and trouble eating due to difficulty in opening the mouth.
- Muscle enzymes are elevated, and emergency medical and supportive care are warranted.
- Monitor corneal health via regular fluorescein staining. Ocular lubricants should be applied q2 to 4h until exophthalmos is resolved. A temporary tarsorrhaphy may be needed if severe corneal disease is present.

Lacerations and Ruptures of the Cornea and Sclera

- If there is any question that a laceration of the cornea or sclera has occurred, instruct the owner to prevent the patient from self-mutilating the eye and that the owner should *not* examine the eye or extrusion of intraocular contents may result (Fig. 23-19).
- Any examination of the eye or periocular area by the owner or veterinarian should await heavy sedation and akinesia of the lids.
- *Practice Tip:* *Failure to follow these guidelines can cause a simple full-thickness laceration to become a hopeless evisceration.*
- Also instruct the owner that nothing, particularly ointments, should be instilled into the eye.
- *Important:* At *no* time before or during the examination or during surgery should ophthalmic ointments be placed on an open eye—*use solutions only.*

Lacerations or Ruptures with a Poor Prognosis

- Prognosis is poor for any laceration associated with the following:
  - Hyphema of >50% of the anterior chamber
  - Lacerations of >24 hours' duration with flat anterior chamber
  - Lens rupture or dislocation

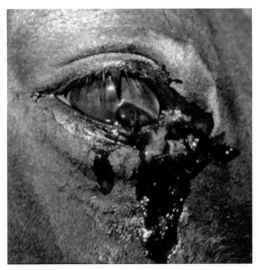

Figure 23-19 A simple corneal laceration, sealed by iris but with no iris prolapse, until the eyelids were forcefully opened.

- Blunt force rupture: the blunt force required to rupture an eye usually results in multiple, severe intraocular damage
- Extensive laceration with prolapse of intraocular contents other than aqueous or iris tissue (a partial evisceration)
  - If you believe there is vitreous prolapse, be sure (before you enucleate) that it is *not* just clotted aqueous humor, which carries a much better prognosis.
  - Globes with partial evisceration usually end as phthisis bulbi (a small, shrunken, and often painful or irritated eye). If the owner wants to preserve the appearance of an eye, an intraocular prosthesis can be placed through the wound after complete removal of the intraocular contents. Prognosis is variable because wound security and infection are unpredictable.
- Lacerations that extend across the limbus into the sclera have a poor prognosis if significant uveal tissue has prolapsed through the wound.
  - Uveal tissue in these cases usually includes the ciliary body.
  - Damage to the ciliary body results in decreased production of aqueous humor, hypotony, and phthisis bulbi.
  - Enucleation or prosthesis implantation may be indicated in these cases.

Lacerations with a Fair Prognosis

- Simple lacerations with minimal contamination and minimal iris prolapse
- Formed anterior chamber
- Small amount of hemorrhage or fibrin
- Iris may protrude through and close the wound but with minimal distortion of intraocular structures
  Transpalpebral or supraorbital fossa ultrasonography can be a useful prognostic tool to assess the posterior segment and lens but *only* if performed with extreme care, with no pressure on the eye, and only on a heavily sedated patient. Gel must *not* enter the palpebral fissure or eye.

Full-Thickness Lacerations

- All full-thickness lacerations of the equine eye necessitate immediate surgical repair under general anesthesia.
- Referral to a veterinary ophthalmologist is recommended for all but the simplest cases. Do *not* attempt surgery unless standard ophthalmic surgical instruments and appropriately sized suture material are available. *The surgery is usually more difficult than anticipated.*

Diagnosis

- Usually obvious
- Corneal or scleral defect, usually plugged with fibrin, iris, or other uveal tissue
- Decreased IOP
- Decreased depth or total collapse of the anterior chamber

- Fibrin, hypopyon, and hyphema may be present in the anterior chamber
- Fluorescein stain:
  - Usually stains corneal wound margins
  - May cause fluorescence of the aqueous humor if the wound has not sealed
  - Streaming of leaking aqueous humor may be visible in the stained precorneal tear film
- Assess dazzle and indirect/consensual pupillary light reflexes

●》 WHAT TO DO

Corneal and Scleral Lacerations
- Cases should be referred to a specialist whenever possible.
- Stereoscopic magnification should be used for repair.
- Muscle relaxants are helpful as part of the anesthesia protocol.
- A transpalpebral lavage device should be placed intraoperatively (see p. 385).
- Protect the eye during induction of anesthesia (hold head carefully to prevent further injury to the globe).
- Culture the wound and any excised tissue.
- Cleanse and prep the eye using sterile saline and a 5% povidone-iodine *solution; never use alcohol, povidone-iodine scrub, or chlorhexidine anywhere near the eye.*
- Gently lavage, cleanse, and carefully replace healthy-appearing prolapsed uveal tissue (usually iris) into the anterior chamber in acute injuries or excise if needed (prepare for bleeding). **Important Note:** Postoperative uveitis is proportional to the degree of uveal damage and handling. Keep it to a minimum.
- Irrigate and re-form the anterior chamber with balanced salt solution, lactated Ringer's solution, or viscoelastic substances. Viscoelastics are helpful to assist chamber formation and dissection of uveal tissue but should be removed if possible before complete wound closure.
- Wound apposition should be precise and water-tight.
  - Use 7-0 to 8-0 polyglactin 910 or other suitable ophthalmic absorbable suture material or nylon ophthalmic suture.
  - Sutures should be placed 1 to 2 mm apart, as deep as possible in the stroma, but *not* full thickness. Entry and exit points of the suture should be perpendicular to the corneal surface and wound edge, respectively.
- Re-form the chamber after wound closure.
- Apply fluorescein stain and mild external pressure to assess wound integrity.
- Unstable, irregular wounds or repairs should be reinforced with an overlying conjunctival flap.
- Consult ophthalmic textbooks for additional information. Refer whenever possible.

●》 WHAT NOT TO DO

Laceration Reconstruction
- The eye should *not* be covered by a membrana nictitans flap.
- Nictitans flaps frequently cause complications because they are often placed improperly.
- Nictitans flap placement can increase IOP, resulting in wound leakage.
- These flaps also prevent direct examination of the globe, which is important postoperatively.

Postoperative Management
- Examine the eye at least once daily for 7 to 10 days.
  - Severe secondary uveitis is common.
  - Endophthalmitis may develop.
- Treatment is facilitated by placement of a transpalpebral lavage apparatus (see p. 385) while the patient is under general anesthesia.
- Medications:
  - Topical 1% atropine *solution,* 4 times a day until pupil is dilated and then 1 to 2 times a day to facilitate pupillary dilation, for cycloplegia, and to stabilize the blood-aqueous barrier *(colic caution!)*
  - Topical broad-spectrum antibiotic *solutions,* q1 to 2h for 24 hours and then q2h for 3 to 4 days and finally q4 to 6h, depending on the condition of the eye
  - Systemic broad-spectrum antibiotics with a good gram-positive spectrum
  - A systemic NSAID until the wound is healed and any associated uveitis controlled; e.g., flunixin meglumine, 1.1 mg/kg q12h for 2 days and then q24h

Partial-Thickness Lacerations

●》 WHAT TO DO

Partial-Thickness Lacerations
- Wound margins separated by more than 2 to 3 mm necessitate surgical repair under general anesthesia.
- Manage superficial nonpenetrating lacerations as corneal ulcers, but perform a careful examination every 1 to 2 days to identify secondary infection, especially if the laceration is caused by plant material.
- Medications:
  - Topical 1% atropine, q8 to 12h or to effect, to maintain pupil dilation
  - Topical broad-spectrum antibiotics, q1 to 2h for 24 hours and then q2 to 6h, depending on the condition of the eye
  - Systemic NSAIDs until the wound is healed and any associated uveitis controlled
- Monitor the wound for enzyme activity (collagenase) as described in the ulcer section (see p. 400). Autologous serum should be added every 2 hours if there is doubt about enzyme activity.

●》 WHAT TO DO

Partial-Thickness Lacerations with Flap Formation
- Thin, superficial flap wounds should be treated as infected ulcers after the redundant tissue is trimmed.
- Deep flap wounds of varying thickness can be therapeutic dilemmas.
  - Ideally, repair flaps in the same manner as any laceration.
  - Carefully replace the cleansed flap over the cleansed wound bed, and press it firmly in place and secure the wound margins with sutures (7-0 to 8-0 ophthalmic suture); points of tissue adhesive may assist in the repair. A conjunctival flap may be needed to stabilize the wound.
  - For successful repair, the flaps should have minimal edema (not the usual presentation); otherwise, dehiscence is the more common sequela.

- If the flap detaches, excise it, but preserve corneal tissue whenever possible.
- Medications: Administer as for infected ulcers (see p. 403).

Corneal Abrasions and Bacterial Ulcers

- The cornea fills almost the entire interpalpebral space in the horse, prominently protrudes from the side of the face, and is easily and frequently traumatized.
- Corneal ulcers are self-induced or have numerous other causes.
- Any lesion that breaches the corneal epithelium is an emergency because of the following:
  - The patient experiences significant pain and discomfort and may cause additional self-trauma as a result.
  - The cornea is an avascular tissue, and corneal defense mechanisms are greatly reduced compared with those of well-vascularized parts of the eye or body.
  - A normal cornea is continually exposed to environmental contaminants, bacteria, and fungi.
  - *Practice Tip: The maximum thickness of the cornea is approximately 1 mm and a superficial infected ulcer in some cases can perforate the cornea in 24 hours.*

Important Note: All corneal ulcers, regardless of size or depth, should be considered emergencies, and the patient should receive prompt, aggressive treatment and follow-up care. All corneal ulcers should be considered infected until proven otherwise.

Corneal Abrasions vs. Superficial Erosions

Fig. 23-10 shows a *superficial corneal ulcer* with the surface epithelium lost but underlying basement membrane intact with minimal corneal edema.

- Eye is painful with significant blepharospasm. (Some cases with deep ulcers are less painful because the more abundant superficial nerve endings were lost to necrosis.)
- Lesion may or may not be visible to the naked eye.
- No change in contour of the cornea.
- Minimal or no corneal edema is present because the basement membrane and superficial stromal layers are intact, maintaining their barrier to corneal fluid imbibition.
- Fluorescein dye uptake is patchy to considerable, depending on the extent and depth of epithelial loss.

Corneal ulcers extend through epithelial basement membrane into the underlying stroma.

- Lesion is easily visualized.
- Corneal edema is obvious, adjacent to the ulcer bed and within it (except for *descemetoceles*).
- Intense fluorescein dye uptake.

Clinical Signs

- Pain is usually present, can be mild to severe.
  - Mild pain is indicated by a slightly dropped eyelash angle compared with the normal eye.
  - A severely painful equine eye cannot be opened manually.

- The severity of the problem and degree of pain are not directly proportional. A horse with a superficial corneal abrasion may exhibit more signs of pain than does a horse with a descemetocele or perforated ulcer.
- Blepharospasm, rubbing the eye, swelling of one or both eyelids, and redness and swelling of the conjunctiva are usually present.
- Epiphora and seromucoid, mucopurulent or purulent ocular discharge are usually present.
- Corneal clouding from edema or inflammatory cell infiltrate may be present or absent.
- Change in corneal contour may be present or absent. Examine the corneal surface from all oblique angles.

Practice Tip: Downer foals and all sick newborns should be examined carefully every day for any corneal disease and for entropion (see Fig. 23-16 and discussion on p. 395). The examination should include daily fluorescein staining. Young foals have decreased corneal and blink reflexes, particularly when they are neurologically or systemically compromised, and may have decreased tear production. Thick foam helmets can be used effectively in the care of recumbent foals to raise the down eye above the stall bedding. Artificial tear ointment every 6 hours is recommended prophylactically for the eyes of all downer foals, with ulcer treatment if needed.

Diagnostic Reminders

- The classic hallmark of corneal abrasions or ulcerations is the uptake of fluorescein stain by the corneal stroma. The examiner should be careful, however, because *dye uptake does not occur in all cases!* Intrastromal ulcerative processes can occur in the presence of an intact, overlying epithelium with active infection, stromal dissolution, and necrosis occurring in the absence of fluorescein stain uptake (Fig. 23-20). **Practice Tip:** *If the eye looks and is painful as if it has an ulcer, treat it for an ulcer even if it does not stain with fluorescein.*
- Deep ulcers that extend to Descemet's membrane retain stain only in the circumferentially adjacent stroma.

Diagnostic Steps

- Assess *tear production,* preferably as early as possible in the examination.
  - If the eye is painful and an ulcer is suspected, the patient should have obvious epiphora. If not, suspect decreased tear production as a cause of the ulcer. Dry eye is more common in horses than once thought.
- Assess *lid function, position, and corneal sensation.* Abnormal lid function and position (facial nerve dysfunction, decreased corneal sensation with resultant failure of reflex blinking, or entropion) cause corneal disease.
  - Assess the *palpebral reflex* before the lids are blocked.
  - Assess *corneal sensation* by a careful touch to the cornea of a sterile cotton swab *before applying topical anesthetic.*
- Tranquilize and restrain the patient as necessary, and establish eyelid akinesia.

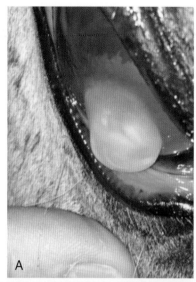

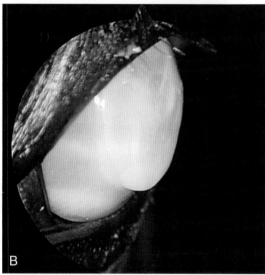

Figure 23-20 A, A 12-year-old gray Oldenburg stallion referred for an acute onset of pain and corneal edema. The cornea began to bulge less than 12 hours after onset. The cornea did not retain fluorescein stain. The diagnosis was keratomalacia and stromal ulceration, under an intact epithelium. **B,** Severe corneal stromal ulceration, with severe keratomalacia, hypopyon, and early corneal neovascularization. The cornea did not retain fluorescein stain before referral. A C-shaped tear in the loose corneal epithelium, evident dorsally, occurred during the examination.

- *Culture* the cornea with sterile, moistened swabs into aerobic and anaerobic transport media.
  - This step may be unnecessary for simple ulcers of known cause or when wound contamination is not expected. However, a culture specimen obtained at the start of the examination can be discarded if not needed.
- *Examine carefully* the cornea, conjunctiva, sclera, nictitating membrane, and eyelids, especially the palpebral conjunctival surface of the upper eyelid, *in the dark with a bright, focal light (but never with a bright LED).*
  - Perform a thorough examination, particularly if the etiologic factor is unknown.
  - Examine with magnification if possible, concentrating on the areas of the conjunctiva, nictitans, and eyelid

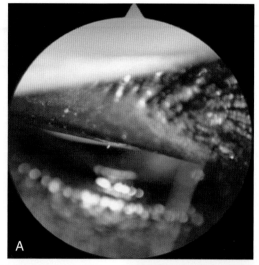

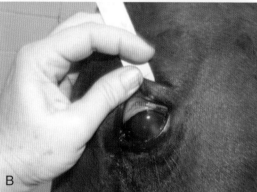

Figure 23-21 A, A plant foreign body (burdock pappus bristle), visible on the palpebral conjunctival surface of the upper eyelid of this horse, caused a corneal ulcer of 4 months' duration. **B,** A tongue depressor is used to "double evert" the upper eyelid to facilitate examination of the conjunctival surface.

that correspond to the position of the ulcer. Evert the corresponding area of the adjacent eyelid, looking across the tissue "horizon," rolled back over a finger or tongue depressor and examine the conjunctiva carefully for foreign bodies (Fig. 23-21). Careful examination of these areas in ulcer cases of unknown cause frequently discloses a foreign body (common), plant awn or spicule (common), or aberrant hair (very rare) as the cause of the problem.
- The bulbar aspect of the nictitating membrane should be examined in every corneal abrasion, especially in refractory cases (Fig. 23-22). A pocket-like fold of conjunctiva on the central aspect of the nictitans' bulbar surface may contain hairs or other foreign bodies that are difficult to see beneath this conjunctival fold. Knowing the location of this pocket, inspecting it for foreign material and sweeping it with a cotton swab (even when nothing is seen) is recommended (Figs. 23-23 and 23-24).
- Apply diagnostic stains to the eye.
  - *Fluorescein:* Ensure that stain covers the entire cornea. Lavage excess fluorescein from the eye, if necessary, and look for dye retention in the cornea (see p. 380).

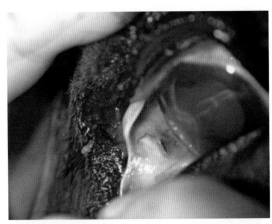

Figure 23-22   A plant foreign body is visible on the bulbar surface of the nictitating membrane of a 6-year-old horse (mosquito hemostat forceps are being used to retract the free margin of the nictitans). A corneal ulcer is present. The foreign body was imbedded in the nictitans pocket described in Fig. 23-23.

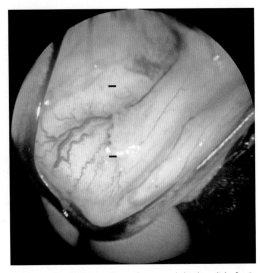

Figure 23-23   **A,** The bulbar surface of a normal third eyelid of a 9-year-old Thoroughbred showing the nictitans "pocket" present in most horses (free edge of nictitans is retracted on the *left*). A fold of conjunctiva is apparent between the *black lines* (note how the large, central nictitans venule "disappears" as the conjunctiva plicates over it—this venule is used to locate the pocket in most horses). This pocket is not present when lymphoid proliferation is present but otherwise should be routinely examined for small foreign bodies such as plant material in all horses with a complaint of keratitis (see Fig. 23-21) or hairs (see Fig. 23-24).

    ○ If dye retention is not obvious, use an ultraviolet light, Wood's lamp, illumination through a cobalt blue, or other blue filter (standard on many veterinary ophthalmoscopes) to enhance dye fluorescence.
- *Rose bengal* and *lissamine green* should be used next if fluorescein is inconclusive. Flood the cornea with stain and observe for pink or green staining of the corneal epithelium. Punctate uptake may be diagnostic of viral or fungal keratitis (complete diagnostic workup is needed for differential confirmation).

Important: Perform the corneal examination meticulously because failure to detect focal or punctate lesions has serious consequences, particularly if corticosteroids are prescribed to treat the eye.

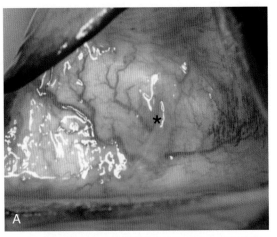

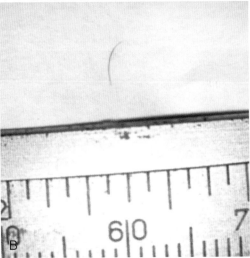

Figure 23-24   **A,** The bulbar surface of the third eyelid of an 11-year-old Thoroughbred with recurrent corneal ulceration in the left eye. Note the conjunctival hyperemia compared with normal nictitans above. The *asterisk* marks the nasal free margin of the nictitans pocket and a hair is immediately left of the asterisk (very difficult to see; hair removed in adjacent image). **B,** As seen in Figs. 23-21 and 23-22, note that the pocket is easily located by following the central nictitans venule.

- *Note and record* the size, shape, position, and depth of the corneal lesion(s), and document the amount of corneal edema present (the presence and extent of edema can help less experienced examiners assess the depth of a corneal lesion). Also note corneal clarity and infiltrate, depth and contents of the anterior chamber, and size, shape, and response of the pupils.
- *Apply a topical anesthetic* and obtain a *corneal cytologic sample* (see corneal scraping, p. 379) for interpretation and culture.
  - Two to four applications of topical anesthesia over a 2-minute period may maximize the depth of anesthesia.
  - The noncutting end of a sterile scalpel blade makes an excellent sampling instrument.
  - Remove surface debris before scraping (flush or gently swab).
  - Obtain three or four samples from stroma at the *wound margins* and smear them on four or five precleaned glass microscope slides.

- Cover the slides at once to prevent environmental contamination.
- Place final scrapings on sterile swabs that have been premoistened with transport medium for aerobic and anaerobic bacterial, fungal culture, *or* inoculate directly into broth or media.
- Stain cytologic samples with Giemsa-type stains for routine analysis and Gram's for classification of bacteria and for fungi. *All initial treatments of complicated or nonhealing ulcers should be based on this cytologic interpretation.*
  - Microorganisms invading the corneal stroma usually are resident conjunctival flora, most commonly streptococci, staphylococci, or *Pseudomonas,* but resident conjunctival flora and ulcer culture results vary with geographic location and housing. Anaerobic infections are also seen and should be considered in every severe or complicated ulcer, especially if gas bubbles are noted in the stroma.

  Note: Be sure to show the lesion(s) to the caretaker and instruct them of *signs that may indicate a worsening ulcer:*
- Any increase in edema
- Change in contour
- Originally clear cornea turning white (edema) or yellowish white (inflammatory cell infiltrate)
- Originally cloudy cornea turning color as follows:
  - More intensely white (increasing edema)
  - Yellow to white (inflammatory cells are increasing)
  - Clearing (may indicate that a descemetocele is developing)

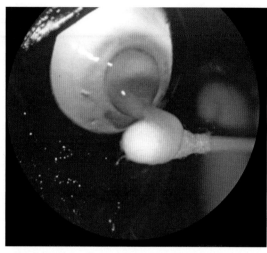

Figure 23-25 Eye of a 4-month-old Thoroughbred filly with a 9-mm-diameter superficial corneal ulcer of 3 days' duration at which time it became acutely more painful with increased edema, a bulging contour, and a mucoid "droopy" appearance, all indicating active keratomalacia. The cotton bud is elevating malacic stroma before excising it.

  - Developing a black spot (descemetocele or impending iris prolapse)
  - Pigment or blood, which may indicate focal perforation
- Decrease in the size of the pupil
- Purulent ocular discharge
- An ulcer beginning to develop a mucoid appearance may indicate that keratomalacia is occurring (see Figs. 23-20 and 23-25). *Important:* Keratomalacia can occur under intact epithelium.

●› WHAT TO DO

Corneal Abrasions and Ulcers in General

- Regardless of size, all ulcers necessitate aggressive management and careful follow-up care.
  - Remove, treat, or correct the cause, if known.
  - Control infection and microbial growth.
  - Control corneal enzymatic activity and secondary melting, if present.
  - Control inflammation and pain.
  - Place an eye lavage system if there is *any* concern with patient compliance.

- Maintain corneal hygiene.
- Maintain patient hygiene and comfort.
- *Never use* topical corticosteroids to manage an equine ulcer *or within 6 to 8 months after healing.* These agents *never* should be used to control pain, posthealing vascularization, or scarring in the horse.
  - Topical NSAIDs should also be avoided because corneal melting has been reported after their use.
- Tables 23-1 and 23-2 list common ophthalmic antibiotics and dosages.

Table 23-1	Commercially Available Ophthalmic Antibiotic Preparations		
Name of Drug	**Manufacturer**	**Concentration**	**Ophthalmic Preparations Available**
Azithromycin (AzaSite)*	Inspire	1%	S
Besifloxacin (Besivance)*	Bausch & Lomb	0.6%	S
Chloramphenicol	Various	0.16%-1.0%	O, S
Ciprofloxacin (Ciloxan)	Alcon and generic	0.3%	O, S, G
Erythromycin (Ilotycin)	Various	0.5%	O, G
Gatifloxacin (Zymar)*	Allergan	0.3%	S
Gentamicin	Various	0.3%	O, S, G
Levofloxacin (Iquix)*	Vistakon	1.5%	S
Moxifloxacin (Vigamox)*	Alcon	0.5%	S

Continued

Table 23-1	**Commercially Available Ophthalmic Antibiotic Preparations—cont'd**		
Name of Drug	**Manufacturer**	**Concentration**	**Ophthalmic Preparations Available**
Neomycin/polymyxin/ bacitracin	Various	Various	O, G
Neomycin/polymyxin/ gramicidin	Various	Various	S, G
Ofloxacin (Ocuflox)*	Allergan	0.3%	S, G
Tobramycin (Tobrex)	Alcon	0.3%	O, S

All drugs are commercially available in the United States. Some drugs are approved for human use only. *O*, Ointment; *S*, solution, *G*, Generic.
*These drugs should never be used prophylactically nor for any routine purposes. Please only use these drugs when indicated, for an appropriate duration and according to antibiotic susceptibility testing.

Table 23-2	**Antibiotics That Can Be Formulated for Ophthalmic Use**					
Name of Drug	**Topical Dose (mg/mL)**	**Subconjunctival Dose (mg)**		**Name of Drug**	**Topical Dose (mg/mL)**	**Subconjunctival Dose (mg)**
Amikacin	10	25-50		Erythromycin	50	100
Ampicillin (sodium)	50	50-100		Gentamicin sulfate	15-20	20-30
Carbenicillin disodium	5	100		Methicillin sodium	50	50-100
				Penicillin G	100,000 units/mL	0.5-1.0 million units
Cefazolin sodium	50-65	100		Ticarcillin disodium	6	100
Ceftazidime	NA	200		Tobramycin sulfate	15	20-30
Clindamycin	50	15-50				

Final dilutions in artificial tear solutions may enhance contact time. Consult package inserts for shelf life, which varies by drug from 3 to 30 or more days. *NA*, Not applicable.

●› WHAT TO DO

Simple, Noninfected Ulcers
- Manage simple ulcers *simply;* they should heal in 7 to 10 days.
  - Prevent infection with topical broad-spectrum antibiotics such as neomycin-polymyxin-bacitracin (or gramicidin), q4h for 24 to 48 hours, and then q6h as the lesion is resolving.
    - Fluoroquinolones should be reserved for confirmed infected ulcers and not used prophylactically.
  - Prevent or minimize reflex anterior uveitis with atropine.
    - Atropine stabilizes the blood-ocular barrier and decreases ciliary muscle spasm and its resultant pain.
    - Use 1% atropine solution (1 drop or 0.05 mL) or ointment (¼-inch strip); once or twice on the first day is usually sufficient to dilate the pupil in a noncomplicated, noninfected ulcer.
    - **Practice Tip:** *If atropine is needed more frequently, or if the once-dilated pupil becomes miotic, the ulcer may be worsening or may be infected.*
    - *Colic caution!* A 1% atropine concentration can be used safely every 6 hours if needed (rarely), *but the patient must be monitored carefully for decreased bowel sounds, prolonged gastrointestinal transit time, or bowel stasis* because atropine can cause idiosyncratic ileus and colic in certain horses. Instruct the owner to monitor gastrointestinal motility by observing bowel sounds and fecal output. If these diminish, discontinue atropine use until motility is normal, and monitor the individual carefully for signs of colic.
  - Prevent or minimize reflex anterior uveitis with NSAIDs.
    - Administer a systemic NSAID for 1 to 2 days in uncomplicated abrasion cases.
    - Use phenylbutazone, 2.2 to 4.4 mg/kg IV or PO q12h, *or* flunixin meglumine, 1.1 mg/kg IV or PO q12h.

●› WHAT TO DO

Complicated Ulcers
It is essential to recognize an infected, potentially melting, ulcer! (See Figs. 23-20 and 23-25.)
- The affected cornea swells, becomes blue-white, and swollen.
- Yellow-white areas may appear in the stroma (cellular infiltrates).
- If keratomalacia ("melting") develops, the affected area develops a swollen, gelatinous, mucoid appearance as the substances that "glue" corneal collagen fibrils together are "dissolved" (see Fig. 23-25).
- Corneal infection causes moderate to severe secondary uveitis with miosis, decreased IOP, and aqueous flare. Some patients have hypopyon because the inflamed anterior uveal tissue exudes inflammatory cells. The hypopyon does *not* usually mean that the eye is infected intraocularly (endophthalmitis) and has minimal correlation with prognosis.
  - Review additional signs noted under Diagnostic Steps, p. 400.

Melting Ulcers
Pseudomonas and beta-hemolytic *Streptococcus* are common causes of melting ulcers, but melting, or *keratomalacia,* can develop with any number of gram-positive or gram-negative bacterial infections, with fungal infections, or with corneal ulcers resulting from alkali injuries. Proteases and other tissue-toxic and tissue-digesting substances are released from certain bacteria and during corneal wound healing by rapidly dividing corneal epithelial cells, fibroblasts, corneal vascular ingrowth, and from white blood cells. An imbalance of normal enzyme production or presence of a corneal disease resulting in rapid, severe destruction or influx of neutrophils

can cause keratolysis, keratomalacia, and perforation of the globe within hours (see Fig. 23-25).

Melting Ulcers

- Melting ulcers require more aggressive treatment, and all cases benefit by eye lavage system placement (see p. 385).
- *Choose one drug from each of the following categories:*
  - *Antibiotics:* Drug choices are based on cytologic and Gram stain results whenever possible. Drugs may require fortification beyond the commercially available concentrations, but then stability cannot be assured.
    - The following is the recommended empirical regimen for topical use in suspected bacterial ulcers until the offending organism and sensitivities are identified. Alternate drugs every 1 to 2 hours or more often until there are *no* signs that the ulcer is progressing and then every 2 to 3 hours for 48 hours and then every 4 hours or as indicated:
    - Cefazolin, 50 mg/mL q1 to 2h *or* neomycin-polymixin-gram-icidin q1 to 2h, *or* chloramphenicol 0.5% *(prevent human exposure, e.g., wear gloves when handling medication)* plus
    - Ciprofloxacin 0.3%, ofloxacin 0.3%, *or* tobramycin, 10 to 15 mg/mL, *or* gentamicin, 10 to 20 mg/mL, *or* amikacin 10 mg/mL, q1h
    - Alter antibiotic treatment, if necessary, based on culture and sensitivity results.
    - Antibiotics may be administered through the eye lavage system (see p. 385) catheter 5 minutes apart. Each medication is followed with a gentle flush of 3 mL of air.
    - Subconjunctival antibiotics may be indicated for difficult patients and are indicated in some deep or rapidly deteriorating infections (cefazolin, 100 mg; gentamicin, 50 mg; penicillin, 10⁶ units; ticarcillin, 100 mg; tobramycin, 20 mg; vancomycin, 25 mg).
  - *Mydriatics, cycloplegics:*
    - 1% atropine topical ophthalmic solution, q12 to 24h, occasionally more often if the pupil does *not* dilate *(colic caution)*
    - See atropine discussion (p. 404).
  - *Topical antiproteases:* One of these should be used to control malacia.
    - Autologous serum:
      - Autologous serum is readily available, inexpensive, and beneficial.
        - Aseptic collection, aseptic storage, and aseptic administration are critical.
        - **Practice Tip:** *If the equine patient is receiving systemic antimicrobial therapy concurrently, harvesting serum at peak drug levels for autologous eye treatment makes good clinical sense.*
        - Refrigerate and replenish every 48 hours.
      - Apply a few drops, 0.2 mL via lavage catheter or small spray topically every 1 to 2 hours or more often, tapering as the ulcer stabilizes.
      - Serum can be used in combination with acetylcysteine.
    - Acetylcysteine 10% (Mucomyst), 1 to 2 drops or 0.2 mL via lavage catheter, q1 to 2h, more often in acute cases, tapering as the ulcer stabilizes and malacia decreases.
    - EDTA and topical tetracycline ophthalmics can also be used. **Practice Tip:** *Progressive keratomalacia is an indication that the ulcer must be reevaluated.*

- *Systemic NSAIDs:*
  - These drugs provide invaluable relief of the severe secondary uveitis that often develops in complicated ulcers.
  - Flunixin meglumine, 1.1 mg/kg IV or PO, is subjectively more effective than is phenylbutazone in these cases.
  - Use the lowest effective dose at the least frequency because NSAIDs decrease corneal angiogenesis, which is desirable in some infectious corneal diseases that affect horses.
  - Topical NSAIDs are *not* recommended with ulcers because they can worsen keratomalacia, delay wound healing, and suppress corneal neovascularization.
- *Systemic antibiotics* are recommended in most cases of severe corneal ulceration.
- Ensure stall rest.
- Control self-mutilation via eye cups or other means of ocular protection.
- Ensure protection of the periocular skin from ocular secretions via application of a thin coating of petrolatum once or twice daily.

Adjunctive and Supportive Therapy: Ulcer Debridement

- *Careful* debridement is beneficial in cases of melting ulcers (see Figs. 23-20 and 23-25).
  - Removes necrotic tissue bacterial load, and the quantity and activity of proteolytic enzymes
  - May enhance drug penetration
  - Helps maintain a more even corneal contour, which facilitates closure of the eyelids and the distribution of the tear film
- Perform debridement under tranquilization/sedation, lid block, and repeated administration of a topical anesthetic. Use a small, toothed forceps or dry cotton swab to pick up the malacic cornea and small corneal or eyelid scissors to excise it (Fig. 23-26). **Note:** The malacic cornea cannot be simply rubbed off or pulled off—the collagen fibrils are still attached peripherally. Gentle flushing with a commercial ophthalmic prep solution of 5% povidone-iodine may be beneficial.

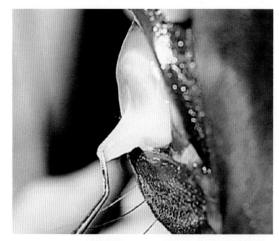

Figure 23-26 The right eye of a 12-year-old Thoroughbred gelding with a severe corneal ulcer of 8 days' duration. A toothed forceps is being used to elevate the malacic cornea for debridement with ophthalmic scissors.

- Complete debridement of all infected, necrotic tissue is beneficial but may be difficult to perform in the standing horse.

Ocular and Periocular Hygiene
- It cannot be overemphasized that it is important to enhance patient comfort and appearance and prevent periocular alopecia and dermatitis.
- Clean ocular exudates as often as possible.
- Apply a thin coat of petrolatum or A & D ointment to the tear drainage area ventral to the eye.

Surgical Intervention for Severe Corneal Ulcer Cases
- It may be necessary to perform a conjunctival flap.
  - This is a routine procedure that provides immediate blood supply to the ulcer to aid healing and acts as a source of fibrovascular tissue to reinforce the wound.
  - Use selectively for those ulcers located in the central cornea because the resulting scar is much more dense and permanent. This is of particular importance in the treatment of performance horses.
- Corneoscleral transposition, lamellar keratectomy, and superficial, posterior, or penetrating keratoplasty are also recommended as possible surgical aids to healing. These procedures require specialist referral for surgical expertise, instrumentation and operating microscopes.
- It is *not recommended* to use a third eyelid (membrana nictitans) flap or tarsorrhaphy in most cases of corneal ulceration. The resultant elevation in ocular surface temperature can increase the rate of bacterial growth. The inability to continuously monitor the eye covered by a flap and the possibility that the flap may cause additional problems completely preclude use of these techniques.

Antibiotic Comments
- Commercially available antibiotic preparations may have an insufficient antibiotic concentration to be clinically effective in deep, severe corneal infections. For example, commercially available gentamicin ophthalmic solution contains 3 mg/mL of drug while the clinically effective dose is considered to be 10 to 15 mg/mL. The commercial preparations can be "fortified" by adding to the ophthalmic solution an appropriate volume of the parenteral gentamicin to achieve the desired concentration.
- Selected antibiotics not available in ophthalmic formulations can be used if the parenteral medication is diluted in artificial tears to the topical dose concentrations listed in Table 23-2. Cefazolin, for example, a favorite drug when gram-positive cocci are found on cytologic examination, is made by diluting intravenous cefazolin to 500 mg/mL with sterile saline solution and then adding 1.5 mL (750 mg) of the intravenous solution to 13.5 mL of artificial tears. This makes a 55-mg/mL concentration for topical ophthalmic use. The preparation is refrigerated and replenished every 3 days.

Fungal Ulcers
Fungal ulcers rarely manifest as emergencies, occurring instead as mixed secondary infections of primary ulcers, as chronic stromal abscesses, or occasionally as superficial infections.

Diagnosis
- Corneal scraping (see p. 379) and routine cytologic examination are required procedures. Special stains, such as calcofluor white, acridine orange, periodic acid–Schiff, or Grocott-Gomori methenamine silver nitrate are necessary for diagnosis in some cases. Alert your laboratory if a fungal infection is suspected and submit sufficient cytologic samples to allow for special stains.
- Culture and sensitivity are of minimal clinical use because results often are not complete for several weeks. Polymerase chain reaction (PCR) testing is available at some research laboratories.

⊙❯ WHAT TO DO

Fungal Ulcers
- Prepare the owner for a long therapeutic course (4 to 10+ weeks).
- Referral for surgical excision of all apparently infected tissues is highly recommended.
- Perform daily ulcer debridement as described previously in addition to all of the following treatments:
  - Treat as an infected, melting ulcer (see p. 403) *plus*
  - Administer antifungal medications.
  - *Author's recommendation:* Minimize the frequency of topical antifungal medications for the first few days after diagnosis or acute keratomalacia and severe uveitis may result (begin every 6 to 8 hours, increasing slowly from this point to q2 to 4 h).
  - Natamycin (0.5%) is the only approved ophthalmic antifungal medication
  - Voriconazole (1%), 1% miconazole, and 1% itraconazole in 30% DMSO may be the best choices for stromal abscesses or cases with intact corneal epithelium.
  - Antifungals can be used systemically if not cost prohibitive (fluconazole 14 mg/kg PO once then 5 mg/kg PO q24h; voriconazole 3 mg/kg PO q12h).
  - Silver sulfadiazine may also be used topically for equine fungal keratitis. For a complete discussion of fungal keratitis, consult standard ophthalmology bibliography.

Eosinophilic Keratitis
Equine eosinophilic keratitis (EEK) usually manifests as an emergency because of its peracute onset and rapid progression. The etiology is unknown. It is a frustrating type of corneal ulcerative disease, usually seen in the summer and fall that can take months to resolve in some cases. Similar lesions have been attributed to ocular onchocerciasis, but this parasite has not been found in EEK cases. EEK may affect both eyes simultaneously and can recur in the same patient in one season or in subsequent years. Mini-outbreaks have occurred in some groups of horses. No cases of EEK have

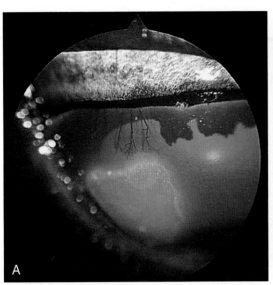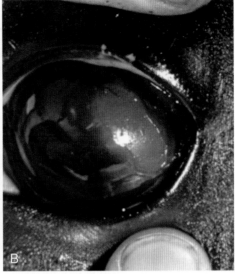

Figure 23-27   A, Right eye of a 12-year-old Thoroughbred mare with an 8-week history of refractory, bilateral, superficial corneal ulcers diagnosed as equine eosinophilic keratitis (EEK). This ulcer began in the ventrotemporal perilimbal cornea and gradually progressed centrally. **B,** The left eye of the same mare, showing a large, superficial, perilimbal ulcer with typical EEK appearance. The whitish membrane-like material on the ulcer surface OU debrided easily.

been seen in horses wearing fly masks all the time; therefore, it is highly recommended to use fly masks in affected geographic regions.

Clinical Findings

- Most cases have an acute, moderately severe conjunctivitis preceding the ulcerative EEK by 1 to 3 days. (Lid swelling, chemosis, epiphora, variable blepharospasm, and pruritus may be profound in some cases.)
- Some horses have acute, copious, caseous ocular discharge ("cake frosting" consistency).
- Corneal ulcers typically are acute in onset, rapidly increase in diameter (but not in depth), are often perilimbal in distribution initially (and often are adjacent to the nictitans), and may be unilateral or bilateral, with one unilateral lesion or multiple lesions in either eye, for example (Fig. 23-27). As the ulcers enlarge, they primarily parallel the limbus but may encroach on the central cornea as they increase in size. Some ulcers worsen due to self-trauma associated with pruritus.
- The presence of blepharospasm, epiphora, conjunctival hyperemia, and chemosis is variable after the first few days; some individuals are uncomfortable whereas others barely squint. Pain is typically minimal compared with non-EEK ulcers of like size.
- After the first day or so ulcers typically have a whitish, dry-appearing surface (see Fig. 23-27) or ulcer beds may be partially to completely filled with a firmly adherent, white, amorphous, caseous/necrotic exudate that may be thin and translucent or several millimeters thick and opaque, with accompanying granulation tissue (Fig. 23-28).
- Ulcers may or may not have associated neovascularization, depending on the duration of the disease. Vascularization

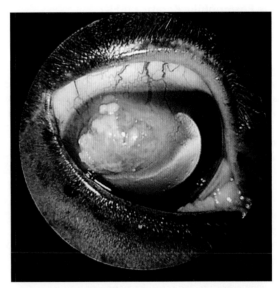

Figure 23-28   The right eye of a 9-month-old Thoroughbred filly with a 10-day history of corneal disease that began as a superficial erosion in the dorsotemporal perilimbal cornea. Photograph illustrates both the caseous, white surface exudate and extensive, rapid corneal neovascularization that develop in some EEK cases. The exudate contained a remarkable number of eosinophils and necrotic debris.

of the ulcer bed develops rapidly in some cases (see Fig. 23-28).
- Minimal corneal edema occurs beyond the ulcer bed, consistent with the depth of the lesions, but the ulcer bed often appears white, as noted previously.
- One or more small (1 to 2 mm diameter) to large (7 to 8 mm diameter) perilimbal or conjunctival granuloma-like lesions may be present in some cases.

EYE

Diagnosis

- History and clinical presentation are indicative.
- Fluorescein dye results may be difficult to interpret because of the large amount of surface debris and the white, pseudodiphtheritic membrane that develops in some cases. Remove all debris and repeat the stain.
- The classic findings on cytology are a very large number of intact and degranulated eosinophils with mast cells and neutrophils, a large amount of amorphous cellular debris, and degenerated to normal epithelial cells. Bacteria and fungi rarely are seen but may be present extracellularly, particularly if there is considerable amorphous debris and exudate. (**Note:** The normal equine eye typically shows a few eosinophils on cytology; there are hundreds in EEK cases.)
- Cultures should be performed after all surface debris is removed. The results usually are negative.
- Histologic examination of all excised lesions by a veterinary ophthalmic pathologist is highly recommended if a keratectomy is performed (because they may someday elucidate the cause).

▶▶ WHAT TO DO

Equine Eosinophilic Keratitis (EEK)

- Administer systemic NSAIDs and apply eye protection as soon as the diagnosis is made to control irritation and reduce self-trauma.
- Administer prophylactic topical triple antibiotic ophthalmic ointment every 6 to 12 hours.
- Cyclosporine (2%) 1 drop in each eye (OU) q12h is recommended.
- Antihistamines and mast cell stabilizers are recommended: the topical antihistamine, Zaditor[24] is available over-the-counter and can be used according to package insert instructions to provide symptomatic relief. Topical mast cell stabilizers (MCS) may be used q2h for 24 hours and then according to packaging (no veterinary products are available); *Alamast,*[25] *Alocril,*[26] *Alomide,*[27] and cromolyn sodium (inexpensive compared with others) have been used successfully. Other human prescription drugs that combine a MCS with an antihistamine, such as *Patanol*[28] or *Optivar,*[29] are sometimes helpful.
- Topical organophosphate-like drugs such as 0.125% echothiophate iodide may be beneficial but are usually unavailable.
- Systemic antihistamines are beneficial acutely.
- Deworm every affected case with ivermectin.
- Removal of the hyaline-like opalescent basement membrane/stromal surface is recommended to resolve these lesions. It may be beneficial to cleanse the ocular surfaces with a commercial ophthalmic prep solution (5% povidone-iodine *solution*), then use a scalpel blade to debride the lesion. The author has used a low-torque, 3.5-mm-diameter, round corneal diamond pterygium burr[30] with good success in all clinical cases treated. It is recommended to refer to a veterinary ophthalmologist for this treatment.

---

[24]Ketotifen 0.025% (Alcon Laboratories).
[25]Pemirolast (Santen).
[26]Nedocromil, Allergan.
[27]Lodoxamide tromethamine (Alcon Laboratories).
[28]Lopatadine (Alcon Laboratories).
[29]Azelastine (Bausch & Lomb).
[30]Algerbrush II (Alger, Inc.).

- If conjunctival or perilimbal granulomas are present, they should be completely excised whenever possible or, at a minimum, vigorously and sharply debrided.
- Consider surgical intervention via superficial keratectomy if there are many granulomas, if the ulcers are slow to resolve, or rapid return to use is indicated. Lamellar superficial keratectomy is recommended in chronic cases or in selected acute cases (performance horses) to speed disease resolution. (The cornea usually heals in 10 to 14 days postoperatively, which is a shorter course than medical treatment alone.)
- Referral to a veterinary ophthalmologist is recommended for all refractory cases.
- Control flies and always recommend fly masks during the warm-weather months!

Prognosis

- The ulcers may increase in diameter and number for the first several days after onset of the disease but ulcers rarely increase in depth (monitor the depth of the ulcer subjectively by noting the degree and extent of corneal edema adjacent to the ulcer).
- Neovascularization of the ulcer bed is variable. In some cases, neovascularization is very slow, whereas in others, it is rapid and extensive (see Fig. 23-28).
- Some cases heal in a few days to a few weeks while other cases remain unchanged for 6 weeks or longer than a year, despite aggressive therapy (or perhaps because of it?).
- Corneal pigmentation and scarring almost always occur, but the extent is unpredictable in all cases of EEK.

Corneal Foreign Bodies
Etiology

- Plant material is most common; superficial seed hulls are particularly tenacious.
- Metal, glass, gunshot, and many others have been reported.
- An eyelash can become a foreign body after a blunt traumatic injury to the periocular area; likewise, presumed fragments of tail hairs have been removed from some eyes.

Clinical Signs

- Signs are similar to those of corneal ulcer (see p. 400), but they vary with the size, location, nature, and extent of the injury and the type of foreign body.

Diagnosis

- Prevent self-trauma.
- Sedation, eyelid block, and topical anesthesia are necessary for diagnosis because most cases are painful with intense blepharospasm.
- Corneal foreign bodies may be readily seen or may be very small and difficult to see even with excellent lighting and magnification.
- Examine the iris and anterior chamber carefully for any change that may suggest penetration; slit lamp examination is often diagnostic.
  - Flare, fibrin, hyphema, and similar lesions can be subtle to obvious.

- Foreign body penetration into the anterior chamber has a guarded prognosis.
- Removing the foreign body with magnification and the patient under general anesthesia is highly recommended.

Caution: Small black bodies in the cornea that appear to be foreign bodies may be a piece of iris or corpora nigra sealing a corneal perforation. Approach these with care because disturbing such a lesion can result in aqueous humor leakage. Careful examination of the anterior chamber and iris should confirm the diagnosis.

●〉 WHAT TO DO

Corneal Foreign Bodies

- Regardless of the treatment used, it is critical to make sure that all foreign material is removed. This requires a very bright focal light source, excellent magnification, time, and patience.
- Patients with large, deep, or penetrating foreign bodies should be referred to a specialist trained in microsurgical technique and capable of managing a potential perforation.
- *Practice Tip:* After removal, send all foreign particles for bacterial and fungal culture and sensitivity.
- Medical management is as for complicated ulcers (see p. 404).

Superficial, Nonpenetrating Foreign Bodies

- Remove the foreign body using topical anesthesia, heavy sedation, and a lid block. Use a sharp stream of sterile saline solution directed tangentially at the foreign body.
- Removing the foreign body is facilitated by using a 25-gauge needle and small, toothed forceps (e.g., Bishop-Harmon 1 × 2).
- Use great care not to drive the foreign material deeper into the eye.

Deep, Nonpenetrating Foreign Bodies

- General anesthesia is usually needed for surgical removal and is much safer than local anesthesia and sedation in case the anterior chamber is entered during removal.

Penetrating Foreign Bodies

- Refer to a specialist as an emergency case.
- Prognosis is guarded, particularly if perforation by plant material or hair has occurred because of the high incidence of secondary endophthalmitis; however some plant material remains inert intraocularly.

Acute Corneal Edema Syndrome

Acute corneal edema can have many known causes, such as trauma, uveitis, and glaucoma, but a sudden onset of corneal edema with no apparent cause is a poorly understood syndrome among horses and may be a form of primary viral, bacterial (e.g., *Leptospira* spp.), or immune-mediated endotheliitis or endothelial degeneration. In most equine cases, the cause is never determined (Figs. 23-29 to 23-32).

Clinical Signs

- Any age, breed, and sex can be affected.
- Partial to complete corneal edema of mild to severe nature may occur. A 1-cm-wide vertical band of edema is a common acute presentation.
- Minimal pain is present in most acute cases. Pain may develop as the edema progresses and "water blisters" or vesicles form and then rupture, resulting in microerosions (see Fig. 23-30).

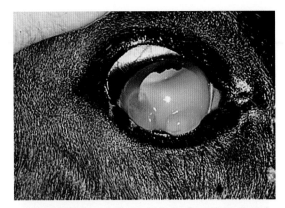

Figure 23-29 Severe corneal edema with bullae formation in the right eye of a weanling Thoroughbred filly. She was one of 18 Thoroughbred weanlings from a group outbreak of acute unilateral or bilateral corneal edema (mild to extremely severe); some cases developed concurrent retinal detachments. A cause was not conclusively determined.

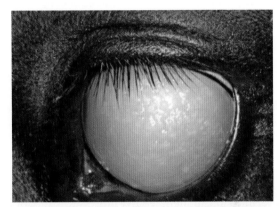

Figure 23-30 Acute, complete corneal edema of 3 days' duration in a 14-year-old Quarter horse. Numerous corneal vesicles or "water blisters" are evident. These rupture easily and cause recurrent microerosions and pain.

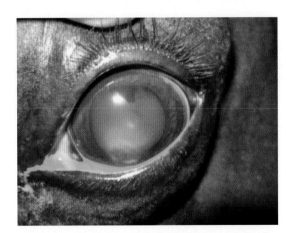

Figure 23-31 Focal, recurrent corneal edema with recurrent ulcer formation of weeks' duration in an 8-year-old Thoroughbred mare. Both eyes were symmetrically affected. A fine fibrinlike membrane was present on the endothelial surface with lightly pigmented keratic precipitates radiating centrifugally from the central, fibrinous area.

- One or both eyes may be affected.
- Affected cornea may have a considerable "bulge" or blisterlike appearance if the edema is intense (corneal hydrops) (see Fig. 23-29).
- Uveitis usually is mild to absent.

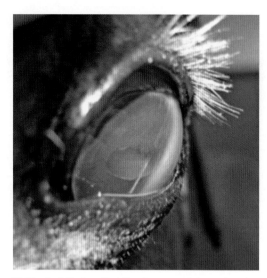

Figure 23-32 A distinct vertical line is apparent, traversing the anterior chamber of this 7-year-old Quarter horse gelding that presented with severe corneal edema of the entire temporal half of his cornea following blunt trauma to the eye 1 month earlier. Traumatic Descemet's membrane detachment and chronic, active uveitis were diagnosed.

Practice Tip: Corneal edema is common in cases of ERU. What differentiates this syndrome is the intense corneal edema with minimal intraocular pathologic changes.

Etiology

- Cause is usually unknown.
- Viral infection, immunoreactive processes, toxins, or toxic reaction may be the cause.
- Herd "outbreaks" have been reported in two groups of yearlings and weanlings; in 11% and 15%, respectively, of affected horses, some degree of retinal detachment occurred, acutely or over time; detachment was bilateral and complete in several horses (see Fig. 23-29).
- Horses, especially yearlings and weanlings, with unexplained corneal edema need repeated corneal and fundus examinations for 12 to 18 months.

Diagnosis

- Results of comprehensive ocular examination before and after complete mydriasis may indicate that referral to an ophthalmologist is appropriate.
- Perform a careful slit biomicroscopic examination.
  - A fine fibrinous weblike membrane with multiple, fine, golden-brown pigmented precipitates may be apparent on the endothelial surface of the affected area and small, pigmented keratic precipitates radiating from a point may be found in the affected area (see Fig. 23-31). This syndrome may be controlled with topical 2% cyclosporine.
  - A readily-apparent cause such as Descemet's membrane detachment may be evident (carries a grave prognosis for resolution of the edema; see Fig. 23-32).
  - Acute demarcation between edematous and normal cornea is usually evident (cellular precipitates and

keratic precipitates stop abruptly and distinctly at the edema margins; see Figs. 23-29 and 23-32).
  - Bullous keratopathy (subepithelial vesicles or "water blisters") or corneal hydrops may be present at the initial examination or may develop later in corneal edema cases from any cause. Corneal bullae or blisters form as the edema accumulates under the tight junctions of the epithelium (see Figs. 23-29 and 23-30).
  - Patients with chronic cases may have fibrosis of Descemet's membrane and endothelium.
- Peripheral indirect fundus examination is required to determine the condition of the retina and optic nerve.
- Use ocular ultrasonography, especially if the cornea is opaque, to assess health of the posterior segment.
- Perform a complete physical examination.
- Possibly submit serum and aqueous samples for equine herpesviruses (EHV), leptospirosis, Lyme disease, and equine viral arteritis (EVA) analysis. Vitreal sampling is recommended but carries more risks.
- If enucleation becomes necessary, aqueous and vitreal samples should be thoroughly analyzed and cultured and the eyes should be submitted to a veterinary ophthalmic pathologist for evaluation.

⏺➤ WHAT TO DO

Corneal Edema—Medical Management

- Management is generally extremely unrewarding if the edema is extensive and severe.
- Mild cases improve in 1 to 3 weeks.
- Use topical broad-spectrum antibiotics q6 to 8h because of the likelihood of epithelial slough or bullae rupture.
- Use topical 2% cyclosporine q12h.
- Topical hyperosmotic agents such as 5% NaCl q4h are always recommended but are of no apparent benefit in some cases except to reduce microbullae/vesicle formation.
- Administer systemic NSAIDs at standard dosages for 7 to 10 days.
- Topical NSAIDs every 8 to 12 hours may be beneficial acutely (diclofenac, ketorolac, flurbiprofen) but should *not* be used if ulcers are present.
- Topical corticosteroids are useful only if the corneal epithelium is intact and likely to remain so *(not so in most cases)*.
  - Administer 1% prednisolone acetate or 0.1% dexamethasone q6h, *not* hydrocortisone.
  - Discontinue immediately if pain increases or fluorescein dye retention is present.
- Systemic antihistamines may be beneficial in rare cases.

⏺➤ WHAT TO DO

Corneal Edema—Surgical Management

- Temporary or split-lid tarsorrhaphy (see p. 394) or a membrana nictitans flap may be indicated if sizable bullae develop in the cornea.
- Thermokeratoplasty: Meticulous multiple pinpoint thermal cauterizations of the affected superficial stroma may be beneficial in some cases but should be performed only by a specialist because corneal perforation can easily occur. The procedure induces adhesions between corneal collagen lamella that may provide stability, reduce lesion thickness, and decrease bullae formation.

- Surgical excision of a thin layer of superficial cornea followed by placement of a very thin conjunctival graft is recommended in some cases with intractable or chronic painful bullous keratopathy, termed keratoleptynsis. Although the procedure results in a permanent scar, the eye is usually comfortable with vision.

Prognosis

- Prognosis is guarded. Affected horses rarely return to normal but may improve slightly during the first 4 to 6 weeks.
- Fibrovascular ingrowth from the limbus develops in some cases, reinforces and reorganizes the swollen cornea, and may result in significant improvement.

Acute Hyphema

Etiology

- Hyphema can be caused by trauma, penetrating injuries, uveitis, glaucoma, intraocular neoplasia, retinal detachment, blood dyscrasia, congenital anomalies, tumors, surgery, and more.
- In human ophthalmology, hyphemas are graded according to the amount of blood in the anterior chamber (grade zero, a blood tinged aqueous humor, to grade 4, an anterior chamber completely filled with blood); prognosis is proportional to the hyphema grade.

Clinical Signs

- Signs are variable: from a small amount to the entire globe filled with blood.
- Clotted red blood usually is the result of recent trauma.
- Increased IOPs may be present with any degree of hyphema, particularly during the first 24 hours after injury.
- Rebleeding or apparent rebleeding as the clot retracts may occur.

Diagnosis

- Usually diagnosis is obvious. If cause is unknown, perform complete blood cell count (CBC), a chemistry profile, and a clotting profile.
- Perform a complete ophthalmic examination of both eyes.
- Perform a complete physical examination looking for other evidence of hemorrhage.
- Perform ocular ultrasonography and compare measurements to normal.

●》 WHAT TO DO

Hyphema

- How to manage these cases is controversial, at best.
- Manage the cause of the hyphema first, address any other systemic injuries, if present, and then worry about the blood in the eye(s).
- Keep the patient as quiet as possible to prevent self-trauma; tranquilize if necessary. The patient may be nervous as a result of blindness so caution is warranted.
- Feedstuffs should be raised to maintain an elevated head position as much as possible.
- Absolute stall rest is recommended unless this causes the patient to become agitated.

- Small hemorrhages (less than one fifth of the anterior chamber) can resolve without treatment.
- Measure IOP 2 to 3 times a day because secondary glaucoma is a common sequela.

Medical Management of Hyphema—Options

Mydriatics

- It is important to use them to prevent synechiae, but dilation may occlude the drainage angle.
- Usually mydriatics are contraindicated if IOPs are elevated.
- Use tropicamide q4 to 6h for 24h, then switch to 1% atropine q8 to 12h if IOP remains normal to decreased after 24 hours.

Miotics

- Not recommended as they greatly increase the risk of synechiae formation but have been recommended by some to facilitate drainage and expose a larger iris surface, which enhances fibrinolysis.

Anti-inflammatory Drugs

- Corticosteroids:
  - If fluorescein dye test is negative, use topical 0.1% dexamethasone or 1% prednisolone acetate, q4 to 6h, but not hydrocortisone.
  - Administer systemic corticosteroids at a standard anti-inflammatory dosage.
- Do not use aspirin or NSAIDs with antiplatelet effects because they predispose the patient to rebleeding.

Antiglaucoma Medications

- Timolol maleate plus dorzolamide (Cosopt) q8 to 12h
- Acetazolamide PO at standard doses

Other Treatments

- Administration of tissue plasminogen activator (tPA) into the anterior chamber can be used as an aid to clot dissolution but may have limited effect on large clots.
  - This is indicated when clot dissolution is slow (3 to 5 days with no significant change) or when IOPs are significantly elevated.
  - It may result in immediate bleeding or delayed rebleeding.
  - It is not recommended for the first 3 to 5 days after onset of hyphema.
- Lysine analogs such as oral or topical tranexamic acid and aminocaproic acid have shown promise in human studies but have not been evaluated in the horse.

Surgical Management of Hyphema

- Usually surgery is contraindicated and may cause additional damage as intraocular structures cannot be visualized during surgery.
- It can be considered in slow-resolving total hyphemas (grade 4) or when IOP remains elevated for more than 3 to 4 days despite glaucoma treatment.

Prognosis

- Prognosis varies depending on the amount of blood, the etiologic factor, and severity of any accompanying trauma, uveitis, glaucoma, secondary synechiae formation, retinal detachment.
- Nonclotted blood may be resorbed in 5 to 10 days, clotted blood in 15 to 30 days or more.
- ***Practice Tip:*** *Hyphema occupying more than one half the anterior chamber has a poor to grave prognosis.*
- Total hyphema with no change in 3 to 4 days carries a grave prognosis.

- Recurring hyphema has a poor prognosis.
- Possible sequelae include:
  - Synechiae
  - Cataracts
  - Blindness
  - Glaucoma
  - Phthisis bulbi

Anterior Lens Luxation

Anterior lens luxation is rarely a true emergency in horses because most cases result from anterior uveitis, but the condition may appear as an emergency to an alarmed owner. Luxated lenses may or may not be cataractous.

Etiology

- Secondary to chronic uveitis or glaucoma in the majority of cases
- Congenital, with or without multiple other anomalies
- Secondary to trauma

❱❱ WHAT TO DO

Lens Luxation

- Determine and treat the cause of the luxation, if possible.
- Anti-inflammatory medications should be used indefinitely in most cases.
- If anterior lens luxation is diagnosed in a small animal patient, immediate surgical removal via intracapsular lens extraction is recommended to prevent unwanted sequelae but *this is no longer the case in horses* as a multicenter, retrospective analysis showed a grave prognosis for both vision and retention of the globe (Brooks et al, 2009).
- Anterior positioned lenses can in some instances be manually displaced into the posterior chamber if the IOP is sufficiently low. Specialist referral is recommended.
- Posterior luxations should be treated with topical miotic ophthalmic agents to help maintain the lens in the posterior compartment.
- Currently, it is unclear in controlled studies what to recommend for sighted eyes when the anterior lens luxation cannot be manually reduced and maintained in the posterior compartment; small-incision phacoemusification of the lens with complete cortex and capsule removal through a small incision may be the best option. Specialist referral is recommended.
- If the eye is blind, enucleation or intraocular prosthesis is recommended.

Uveitis

- Along with corneal ulcers, anterior uveitis *(iridocyclitis)* is the most common ocular problem in horses and is the leading cause of blindness. The disorder usually presents as a nongranulomatous anterior uveitis with the inflammation confined to the iris, ciliary body, and the anterior and posterior chambers. Some individuals, however, may present with vitritis, chorioretinitis, and peripapillary inflammation.
- Uveitis can have many causes. Some causes are obvious, such as trauma. *Borrelia* sp. has recently been documented

in the eyes of two horses with uveitis (Priest et al, 2007). Most causes remain obscure, however, as is the case in any species. A specific uveitic syndrome in the horse known as equine recurrent uveitis (ERU, *moon blindness,* or *periodic ophthalmia*) has strong association with previous or current infection with one or more serotypes of *Leptospira interrogans.* A particularly difficult form of ERU, possibly a different syndrome altogether, is seen in Appaloosa horses.

- Uveitis most commonly occurs in middle-aged to older horses of either sex and may involve one or both eyes at the same or different times.
- Rarely is there any historical event more significant than something such as "eye irritation every so often caused by flies"
- Unfortunately, many cases of equine uveitis have subtle clinical signs and do not manifest as emergencies when they truly are. Rapid and prolonged treatment may prevent future recurrences and tragic long-term sequelae.
- The horse's uveal tissue has a profound ability to become inflamed after seemingly mild ocular insults. This fact, combined with the uveitic syndrome among horses that occurs after *Leptospira* infection and more commonly in some breeds, makes this group of diseases a diagnostic and therapeutic challenge.
- The risk of vision loss because of uveitis is very high. Sight is reduced in the acute period, and sight-threatening sequelae of inflammation are common. These sequelae include corneal decompensation and edema, glaucoma, cataracts, vitreal opacities and liquefaction, retinal detachments, and hemorrhage.
- In many cases, the eye being examined as an "emergency" has likely had subclinical disease for days to weeks; therefore, treatment results are usually poorer than expected.
- Most cases necessitate aggressive initial therapy (every 1 to 2 hours topically); therefore, use of an eye lavage system (see p. 385) may be beneficial.

Etiology

- The most common known causative agent is *Leptospira* infection; *Borrelia* sp. organisms have been documented intraocularly in two recent cases.
- Any number of bacterial agents that cause septicemia can cause uveitis (e.g., *Rhodococcus equi, Salmonella,* and *Escherichia coli*), as can intraocular parasites and some viruses (EHV, EVA, influenza).
  - Uveitis is common in septic foals or weanlings and usually is bilateral.
- Trauma
- Immune-mediated
- Lens induced
- Neoplasia, particularly lymphosarcoma

Clinical Signs

- It is important to examine both eyes.
- Complete examination often necessitates heavy sedation, eyelid akinesia, topical anesthesia, and pupil dilation.

Acute Signs

- Pain, lacrimation, blepharospasm, and photophobia may be mild to severe
- Hyperemia of the conjunctiva with scleral vascular engorgement
- Reduced IOP (<15 mm Hg)
- Corneal changes:
  - Edema: varies from none to mild and focal to severe and diffuse
  - Keratic precipitates may be present on the endothelial surface (whitish dots coalescing to greasy yellowish-white plaques)
  - May have corneal vascular ingrowth from the limbus
- Anterior chamber findings:
  - Aqueous flare is a hallmark of anterior uveitis
    - Flare results from the presence of protein and cells in the normally hypocellular and protein-poor aqueous humor. Flare usually is subtle and is easily assessed in a *very dark environment with a focal dot or slit of light directed into the eye at an angle from the examiner's line of view.*
  - More severe cases have fibrin, hypopyon, or hyphema in the anterior chamber
- Iris and pupil changes:
  - Miosis, a small pupil, is another hallmark of uveitis
    - Slow dilation, if at all, with 1% tropicamide
  - Iris:
    - Iris may be swollen with loss of the normal, finely detailed surface architecture
    - The iris color may be dulled, darker than normal to profoundly abnormal in light-colored irises (blue irises turn a yellowish green color)
    - Corpora nigra may be swollen and round, rather than with normal, spiculated contours
- IOP:
  - Decreased IOP is the third hallmark of uveitis
  - Pressures may be too low to record
- Fundus findings:
  - The fundus is often poorly seen because of anterior segment inflammation
  - Examination is facilitated by the use of indirect ophthalmoscopy, which is much more effective in penetrating hazy media
  - Vitreous humor may have cellular infiltrates, liquefaction, and "floaters"
  - Possible choroiditis, retinal edema, and focal to diffuse nonrhegmatogenous (without any tears or holes) retinal detachment
  - Peripapillary yellowish "rays" of subretinal exudate and retinal detachment are seen in many cases

Chronic Signs

- Corneal changes:
  - Diffuse edema and fibrosis
  - Fibrovascular ingrowth from the limbus, focal or diffuse
  - Focal to multifocal superficial erosions

- Corneal striae if glaucoma has occurred
- Calcific corneal deposits
- Iris changes:
  - Posterior synechiae: focal to diffuse with resultant dyscoria (abnormality of the shape of the pupil)
  - Loss of corpora nigra or loss of corpora nigra detail due to:
    - Preiridal fibrovascular membrane contraction (fine, whitish membrane most obvious at the pupil margin and on the corpora nigra and elsewhere)
    - Hyperpigmented iris (dark chocolate color; some patients have depigmented areas as well)
    - Abnormal surface neovascular changes (rubeosis iridis) in some instances
- Lens changes:
  - Cataract
  - Lens luxation
- Other possible findings:
  - Complete vitreal liquefaction
  - Secondary glaucoma
  - Retinal detachment with or without vitreous degeneration and traction bands
  - Retinal and optic nerve degeneration and atrophy
  - Blindness
  - Phthisis bulbi

Diagnosis

- CBC and chemistry profile
- Serologic assays with paired samples whenever possible
  - Leptospirosis titers: serovars *L. pomona, L. bratislava, L. autumnalis, L. grippotyphosa, L. hardjo, L. icterohaemorrhagiae, L. canicola,* and as many others as the laboratory can test.
    - Results may be difficult to interpret because many horses have positive titers and no clinical disease or may have negative serum antibodies but very high aqueous antibodies because of localized infection and intraocular antibody production.
  - Borreliosis
  - Brucellosis
  - Toxoplasmosis
- Conjunctival biopsy if *Onchocerca* infestation is suspected (extremely rare)
- Aqueous and vitreous sampling are recommended and may be of great value for cytologic analysis, serologic assay, PCR analysis, darkfield analysis, and culture (but should be performed by a specialist).
- ***Important:*** Perform a detailed examination of both eyes to determine primary versus secondary uveitis and ERU versus non-ERU causes of uveitis such as endophthalmitis, corneal stromal abscesses, foreign bodies, viral infections, etc.

●❯ WHAT TO DO

Equine Recurrent Uveitis (ERU)
- Aggressive, prolonged medical management of acute uveitis reduces the incidence of secondary complications. Place an eye

lavage apparatus if patient cooperation is difficult (see p. 385). *Treatment should not be discontinued prematurely (tell the owner!) but should continue on a tapering schedule for 4 to 6 weeks beyond the time when:*

- There is no evidence of aqueous flare
- The IOP is >12 to 15 mm Hg
- The eye looks normal

Note: *Lifelong treatment may be necessary*

- Chronically painful, blind eyes should be enucleated or an evisceration-intraocular implant procedure should be performed.
- Manage the cause, if known. The cause is often not discovered in cases of ERU, but leptospirosis and borreliosis should always be considered.

Medications

Use one from each category during acute flare-ups.

Corticosteroids

- Corticosteroids are the basis of therapy in most cases if no corneal ulcer is present (systemic corticosteroids may be used in the presence of a corneal ulcer).
- Topical 1% prednisolone acetate (*not* succinate) solution is the steroid of choice; 0.1% dexamethasone ointment is acceptable. Hydrocortisone is *neither* acceptable nor effective.
  - Administer every 2 to 4 hours in the acute period and taper slowly over weeks or months as signs diminish *if the corneal epithelium remains normal.*
  - Subconjunctival steroids (administered under the bulbar conjunctiva, not the palpebral conjunctiva) may be used in rare cases where topical treatment is impossible but only when the cornea is absolutely healthy. They do not substitute for topical agents but merely supplement them and are used with caution because of laminitis risk and because they cannot be removed once administered should a corneal ulcer develop.
- Systemic corticosteroids can be used at standard anti-inflammatory dosages but *not* in conjunction with systemic NSAIDs.

Mydriatic Agents

- Mydriatics must be used to dilate the pupil.
- Topical 1% atropine solution is the preferred mydriatic.
  - Administer 1 to 2 drops or a small spray every 6 to 8 hours to effect then as needed to maintain mydriasis.
  - Monitor for signs of colic (see p. 404).
- Phenylephrine (10%) can be added to atropine therapy if the pupil does not dilate with atropine; it is of questionable efficacy in equine patients.

Topical NSAIDs and Other Anti-inflammatory Immune Modulators

- Numerous ophthalmic NSAID preparations are available at any human pharmacy including flurbiprofen (0.03%), diclofenac (0.1%), Acular LS (ketorolac tromethamine ophthalmic solution) 0.4%[31]; Xibrom (bromfenac 0.09%[32]); and the prodrug nepafenac (Nevanac ophthalmic suspension 0.1%[33]).
  - The efficacy and side effects of most of these have not been studied in the equine eye.
  - These agents seem to be beneficial in some cases and of no apparent benefit in others.
  - NSAIDs may be the only anti-inflammatory option when the corneal integrity is in question, thus preclude the use of topical corticosteroids. NSAIDs should be used with caution because they can induce melting corneal ulcers.
  - NSAIDs may be used in combination with topical corticosteroids.
- Use of cyclosporine 2% q8 to 12h has been reported in some cases but intraocular penetration is very poor.

Systemic NSAIDs

- Phenylbutazone, 2.2 to 4.4 mg/kg *or*
- Flunixin meglumine, 0.5 to 1.1 mg/kg q12 to 24h, *not* for longer than 1 to 2 weeks (the drug of choice in all acute cases) *or*
- Dexamethasone, 0.05 to 0.1 mg/kg q24h
- Aspirin (10 to 25 mg/kg per day PO q24h) is an option for long-term maintenance in some cases but not for acute flare-ups.
- Continue all medications 10 to 14 days beyond the time when clinical signs have resolved and when the IOP has returned to normal range (>15 mm Hg). **Important:** *Only then begin a slow drug taper,* continuing topical corticosteroids q12h for 4 to 6 additional weeks. Before discontinuing, carefully examine the eye for signs of uveitis, recheck the IOP, and then reexamine weekly for 1 month. Advise the owner to examine the eye daily with a penlight for signs of inflammation (redness, mild cloudiness, miosis in dim light) and to request reexamination immediately if abnormalities develop. *Lifelong treatment may be necessary.*

Systemic Antibiotics

- Antibiotics should be administered in all cases of uveitis resulting from systemic disease and in any case suspected to be associated with *Leptospira* or *Borrelia* infection, although intraocular drug penetration is variable. Recommend systemic antibiotics in all acute ERU cases.
- Enrofloxacin (7.5 mg/kg PO or 5 mg/kg IV PO q24h) has been the preferred antibiotic.
- Gentamicin, 6.6 mg/kg IV q24h can be used.
- Beta-lactams are also very effective against *Leptospira.*
- Minocycline (4 mg/kg PO q24h) or doxycycline (10 mg/kg PO q12h) have potent anti-inflammatory effects and are very helpful in some cases. Minocycline was recently reported to have good aqueous humor

---

[31]Ketorolac tromethamine ophthalmic solution 0.4% (Allergan).
[32]Bromfenac 0.09% (Ista Pharmaceuticals, Inc., Irvine, California).
[33]Nevanac ophthalmic suspension 0.1% (Alcon Laboratories).

levels in noninflamed eyes (17.07% of corresponding plasma concentration) and excellent levels in mildly inflamed eyes (20.27% of corresponding plasma concentration).

Surgical and Other Treatments

- Surgically implanted slow-release cyclosporine (CSA) implants are beneficial for long-term management of uveitis in horses and are always recommended (80+% have less inflammation and fewer recurrent attacks). The suprachoroidal CSA implants have been reported to achieve therapeutic CSA levels intraocularly with few side effects and reduced incidence of disease flare-ups and complications (Gilger et al, 2006). **Practice Tip:** *Eyes with any active inflammation are* not *candidates for this surgery.*
- Intravitreal antibiotic injections *at doses proven safe for the retina* may reduce or eliminate disease flare-ups (seek consultation with a veterinary ophthalmologist for further recommendations).
- Any horse with ERU should routinely be pretreated with NSAIDs before any immune stimulus such as dewormings and annual vaccinations (Rx: 2 days before, day of, and 2 days after). Anecdotal reports say this prevents the post-vaccinal flare-ups that some horses experience.

Glaucoma

- Most cases of glaucoma are chronic, insidious sequelae of ERU (see Fig. 23-33, *A*). Glaucoma and ERU are most common among older horses and specifically Appaloosas.

Etiology

- Acute, primary glaucoma is uncommon among horses but it does occur.
- Secondary glaucoma is most common and is associated with the following:
  - Chronic ERU (anterior uveitis, moon blindness, iridocyclitis) possibly because of filtration angle obstruction by inflammatory debris, filtration angle fibrosis, filtration angle collapse (from iris bombé, chronic inflammation, and adhesions), postinflammatory fibrovascular pupil obstruction, obstruction of iris absorption of aqueous humor, or posterior synechiae
  - Trauma
  - Acute anterior displacement of a luxated lens (the usual cause of lens luxation is trauma or chronic uveitis)
  - Anterior vitreal prolapse
  - Tumors

Clinical Signs

- Elevated IOP is the hallmark of the disease.
- IOP should be assessed by means of applanation tonometry (Tonopen[34]) or rebound tonometry (TonoVet[35]). Normal values are approximately 15 to 28 mm Hg with the Tonopen. The examination should be performed

[34]Mentor Ophthalmics, Norwell, Massachusetts.
[35]ICare, Helsinki, Finland.

before sedation if possible and *not* with the head lower than the heart. See techniques section earlier (p. 382) and refer the case, if necessary, for IOP assessment.

- Signs of acute glaucoma are absent to subtle and easily missed.
  - Sight is variable. Horses can continue to see for a protracted period after the onset of elevated IOP, unlike dogs, which usually lose their sight shortly after elevated IOP.
  - Pain is variable. Some individuals seem normal, whereas others manifest exquisite pain.
  - Lacrimation, photophobia, blepharospasm, and small convulsive jerking movements of the head during rest may be present or absent.
  - Hyperemia of the conjunctiva and episcleral vein engorgement are occasionally present but not to the degree seen in canines.
  - Cornea:
    - Edema: mild and focal to severe and diffuse
    - Linear white lines or thin bands of mild to moderate edema traversing the cornea or branching in any direction: These striae (Haab's striae) or "stretch marks" are caused by breaks in Descemet's membrane with disruption of adjacent endothelial cell function (Fig. 23-33).
    - Focal to diffuse superficial ulcers if corneal edema is severe
  - Pupil:
    - Pupil is in midposition to slightly dilated but may be normal to small if uveitis is concurrent
    - Pupil is slowly responsive to unresponsive to bright light stimulus
    - Be sure to check direct and indirect responses to light
    - Pupil shape may be altered if synechiae are present
  - Iris:
    - Normal in an acute, primary case
    - Usually an abnormal dark chocolate brown or a darker color than normal for the eye (a change caused by uveitis)
    - Corpora nigra may be absent or abnormally smooth in contour because of previous bouts of inflammation and fibrosis
  - Lens:
    - If glaucoma results from anterior lens luxation, the lens (often cataractous) is seen in the anterior chamber. If corneal edema prevents examination of the anterior chamber, ultrasound examination is indicated.
    - Posterior lens luxation can occur
  - Fundus:
    - Optic and retinal atrophy may be present
    - Optic nerve cupping is unusual but may occur
  - Globe:
    - The eye may be slightly to grossly enlarged (buphthalmic, hydrophthalmic). This is a very chronic sign.

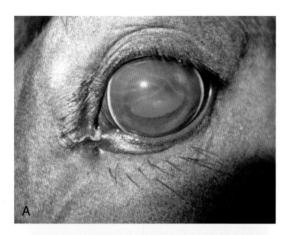

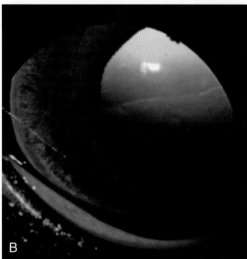

Figure 23-33   A, Numerous branching white lines of faint corneal edema are present in this 19-year-old Draft cross horse, consistent in appearance with classical Haab's striae, which are breaks or "stretch marks" in Descemet's membrane that occur secondary to glaucoma (the intraocular pressure in this eye was 58 mm Hg). **B,** In contrast are the corneal striae seen in this 11-year-old Dutch Warmblood import, with normal intraocular pressures on repeated exams (two faint parallel lines are evident traversing the pupil in this image). These striae lack the associated corneal edema seen in Haab's striae and are incidental findings in many Warmblood horses and some other breeds. Similar lesions can develop secondary to Descemet's fracture after blunt ocular trauma.

Diagnosis

- Measure the IOP as discussed in the techniques section, remembering to hold the eyelids open with pressure only on the bony rim. If the patient is tranquilized, the pressure should be obtained with the head above the level of the heart.
- Until tonometry can be performed, gross assessment of IOP can be made by gently rocking the index and middle fingers alternately back and forth on the dorsal portion of the globe, through the closed eyelid. Use the patient's other eye or the examiner's eye as a control. In these cases, immediate referral to a specialist for confirmation is recommended.

Glaucoma

- The insidious nature of glaucoma among horses means that some cases are hopeless from the outset and treatment is often unrewarding.
- The condition in some horses responds well to medical management, whereas others slowly progress despite medical treatment.
- Aggressive medical management should be reserved for eyes that still have vision.
- Individuals with acute to subacute disease, and some with chronic disease, may show improvement in the short term.
  - Administer combination ophthalmics: beta-adrenergic antagonists such as 0.5% timolol maleate, 1 to 2 drops q12h, in combination with the topical carbonic anhydrase inhibitor 2% dorzolamide (Cosopt) q8 to 12h.
  - Administer topical corticosteroids (0.1% dexamethasone or 1% prednisolone acetate, q4 to 6h). Ensure that the cornea appears healthy and is fluorescein negative before corticosteroid therapy.
  - Administer systemic NSAIDs at standard doses.
  - Consider adding oral carbonic inhibitors (acetazolamide 4.4 mg/kg PO q12h) if the foregoing treatments fail to effect adequate IOP control. Monitor serum K^+ level during treatment and supplement if needed. Efficacy in lowering IOP in the horse has not been assessed.
  - Consider administering 1% atropine q8 to 12h.
    - ○ **Practice Tip:** *Atropine is contraindicated in glaucoma in most species, but in the care of most horses, atropine may be a helpful and inexpensive glaucoma therapy.*
    - ○ Atropine is thought to enhance uveoscleral outflow of aqueous humor and is beneficial in some cases.
    - ○ It is critical to measure IOP every 6 to 12 hours in the first few days of atropine treatment because in the rare patient, pressure spikes are reported during atropine treatment and therefore the atropine treatment should be discontinued.
  - *Do not use* topical prostanoids such as 0.005% latanoprost. Though effective, they should be avoided because they cause uveitis and numerous side effects in the horse.
  - Hyperosmotic agents are of questionable efficacy in the horse and should be avoided because they cause diarrhea.
- Perform surgical management.
  - Referral to specialists for diode laser cyclophotoablation or cyclocryoablation can be considered but results are variable. Postoperative IOP spikes are common; operated cases require IOP monitoring several times a day. Either procedure works well in some cases and may provide good, long-term control of IOP. Cases that have dramatic postoperative elevations in IOP may lose any remaining vision.
- Blind eyes or eyes that are intractably painful should have an intraocular silicone prosthesis placed or should be enucleated. Chemical ablation of the eye, a less expensive option, can be used but with variable results and pain relief is questionable (50 mg gentamicin with 1 mg preservative-free dexamethasone, administered intravitreally—avoid the lens).

Acute Blindness

- An acutely blind horse is always an emergency.
- Most cases that appear acutely blind are, however, a more chronic problem such as uveitis that has gone unrecognized. This is especially true in Appaloosas.

- If the patient is truly acutely blind from a suspected neuro-ophthalmologic cause, the case must be worked up without delay. ***Practice Tip:*** *Compressive or traumatic optic nerve lesions (several listed below) should be treated urgently and referred immediately, if possible. There is a very short window of time, usually less than 24 hours, after the onset of a compressive optic nerve lesion until optic nerve function is permanently lost. Sphenopalatine (SP) sinus problems that receive emergency decompressive surgery may have a good outcome. The same may be true for some basilar skull fractures.*
- All acutely blind horses should have complete physical and neuro-ophthalmologic examinations performed, including menace response, assessment of palpebral reflexes, direct and indirect pupillary light reflex testing, an assessment of vestibular eye movements, and a detailed examination of the eye from cornea to retina, with particular attention paid to the optic nerves.
- A complete neurologic examination should be performed.
- If no cause for the blindness is found up to this point, upper airway endoscopy is recommended, with particular attention paid to the ethmoid region and to the drainage areas of the sphenopalatine sinuses if they can be reached in the patient in question.
- Differential considerations for an *acutely blind horse* that appears *otherwise healthy* but with an *abnormal ophthalmic examination* are many. The most common are:
  - Acute onset of bilateral cataracts
  - Acute severe bilateral uveitis
  - Bilateral retinal detachments
  - Bilateral optic neuritis
  - Bilateral exudative optic neuritis with or without hemorrhages
  - An SP sinus compressive lesion (fracture, tumor, blood clot, bony proliferative lesion, severe SP sinusitis)
- Differential considerations for an *acutely blind horse* that appears *otherwise healthy* but with a **normal** *ophthalmic examination* include:
  - Traumatic optic neuropathy secondary to basisphenoid fractures or other trauma
  - An SP sinus compressive lesion (tumor, blood clot, bony proliferative lesion, severe SP sinusitis)
  - Retrobulbar optic neuritis
  - Orbital, sinus, or ethmoid neoplasia affecting both orbits or that have extended to the optic chiasm
- An *acutely blind horse* that is also *systemically ill* may have any number of diseases including:
  - One of the viral encephalitides (EEE, WEE, VEE, West Nile)
  - Equine viral arteritis
  - African horse sickness
  - Thiamine deficiency
  - An acute blood loss neuroretinopathy

References

References can be found on the companion website at www.equine-emergencies.com.

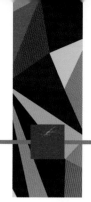

CHAPTER 24

Reproductive System

*Regina M. Turner, Tamara Dobbie, and
Dirk K. Vanderwall*

Physical Examination of the External Genitalia

- The normal stallion possesses two scrotal, ellipsoid testicles that are oriented with the long axis horizontal.
- It is normal for one testis to be slightly smaller or larger than the other; a large difference in size between the two testes is often indicative of a problem.
- The testes should be nonpainful and freely moveable within the scrotum and the testicular parenchyma resilient—not too hard, and not too soft—and nonpainful on palpation.
- Small amounts of peritoneal fluid (typically <5 mm measured ultrasonographically) are normally present within the vaginal cavity and can be visualized ultrasonographically with slightly deeper pockets of fluid imaged and possibly palpable around the epididymal tail. The height, width, and length of each testis and total scrotal width should be measured with calipers or ultrasonographically.
- The spermatic cord ascends from the craniodorsal aspect of the testis towards the external inguinal ring.
- The head of the epididymis is found near the base of the spermatic cord on the craniodorsolateral surface of the testis. The body runs dorsolaterally along the surface of the testis and the tail, the most readily palpable portion of the epididymis, is located on the caudal pole of the testis.
- The stallion has a musculocavernous penis consisting of a base (or root) connected by two crura to the ischial arch, a shaft that extends from the base to the glans, and a glans that is the enlarged free end of the penis.
- The urethra extends along the length of the penis.
- The cranial end of the glans penis has a deep depression called the fossa glandis.
- The urethral process (the termination of the penile urethra) extends outward from the fossa glandis.
- The fossa glandis contains two ventrolateral recesses and a large dorsal diverticulum called the urethral sinus. ***Practice Tip:*** *Smegma tends to accumulate in the urethral sinus and with time, aggregates into a clay-like mass referred to as a "bean." Remove the smegma using gentle massage and cleansing.*

- The penis is composed of three cavernous tissues:
  - The corpus cavernosus penis (CCP)
  - The corpus spongiosum penis (CSP)
  - The corpus spongiosum glandis (CSG)
- The CCP is the largest of the erectile spaces and extends along the length of the penile shaft dorsal to the urethra; it is crescent shaped and surrounded by the tunica albuginea.
- The CSP is a smaller area of erectile tissue extending along the penile shaft that surrounds the urethra:
  - It is directly continuous with and expands into the erectile tissue of the CSG that fills the glans penis.
- The cavernous tissues, in particular the CCP, become engorged with blood during sexual stimulation.
- The CSG expands immediately before and during ejaculation and is referred to as "belling" or "flowering" of the glans penis. The prepuce encloses and protects the flaccid penis and telescopes around the nonerect penis forming two distinct folds:
  - External prepuce (i.e., "sheath")
  - Internal prepuce
- The relationship between the various structural components of the entire prepuce and the erect penis is shown in Fig. 24-1.
- When examining the penis of a gelding, the horse can be sedated with xylazine or detomidine. A dosage that results in moderate sedation (+/− 0.5 mg/kg) causes the flaccid penis to descend.
- ***Practice Tip:*** *Do not sedate a stallion with acepromazine. Although infrequent, paraphimosis has been associated with the administration of phenothiazine tranquilizers. Any time the penis descends in response to administration of any drug, the horse should be monitored to ensure that the penis returns to its normal position in the prepuce within a reasonable period of time.*

Scrotal Enlargement

- There are many possible causes for scrotal enlargement, and many are extratesticular.
  - Scrotal fluid: hydrocele, hematocele, and pyocele
  - Inguinal and scrotal hernias
  - Spermatic cord torsion
  - Orchitis
  - Epididymitis
  - Sperm granuloma
  - Testicular abscess

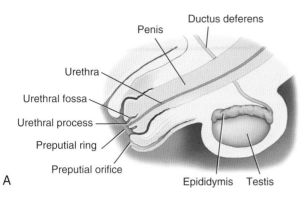

A

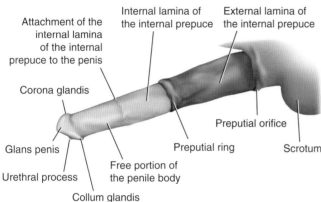

B

Figure 24-1 A, Schematic of normal penis and prepuce, showing the cavernous tissues, the urethra, the urethral fossa, and the location of the epididymis, testis, and ductus deferens. **B,** The internal preputial fold and external preputial fold (sheath).

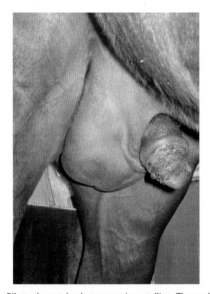

Figure 24-2   Bilateral scrotal enlargement in a stallion. The underlying cause cannot be determined by visual inspection of the scrotum alone.

- Testicular hematoma
- Testicular neoplasia
- ***Practice Tip:*** *Trauma, leading to hydrocele (fluid) and/or hematocele (blood), and systemic illness, leading to hydrocele, are the most common causes of scrotal enlargement in stallions.*
- Inguinal/scrotal hernias and spermatic cord torsion are seen occasionally.
- Identification of an enlarged scrotum is a nonspecific sign of any of the above conditions (Fig. 24-2). A detailed history usually combined with additional diagnostics is typically required to determine the underlying cause.

Clinical Signs: General
- Clinical signs are highly variable, depending on the underlying cause of the scrotal enlargement.

Diagnosis: General
- Careful physical examination combined with ultrasonographic examination is helpful in determining the cause of scrotal enlargement. It is recommended that an examination of the internal inguinal rings be performed per rectum to rule out the possibility of an inguinal hernia.

●》 WHAT TO DO

Scrotal Enlargement
- Specific treatment depends on the underlying cause.
- Sedation and analgesics are recommended in cases where the stallion is showing signs of pain associated with the enlarged scrotum.
  - Xylazine, 0.6 mg/kg IV *or*
  - Detomidine, 0.01 to 0.04 mg/kg IV
  - +/− Butorphanol tartrate, 0.02 mg/kg IV
- In the majority of cases, fine-needle aspiration of an enlarged scrotum is contraindicated; a diagnosis can usually be made without this information and the following risks are decreased:
  - Bowel perforation (in cases of inguinal hernia)
  - Disruption of a hematoma
  - Introduction or dissemination of infection
- Pyocele is a possible exception. Sampling the purulent fluid for culture and sensitivity testing may be indicated.

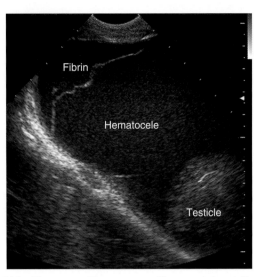

Figure 24-3 Ultrasonographic appearance of hematocele in a stallion. There is an excessive amount of slightly echogenic fluid surrounding the testicle, consistent with recent hemorrhage. Also note the presence of a fibrin strand within the fluid.

Scrotal Fluid: Hydrocele, Hematocele, and Pyocele

- The vaginal cavity is continuous with the peritoneal cavity, and increased amounts of anechoic fluid (hydrocele) in the vaginal cavity can result from systemic disease causing:
  - Increased production of peritoneal fluid
  - Decreased drainage of peritoneal fluid from the vaginal space
- Trauma, spermatic cord torsion, neoplasia, or systemic disease with dependent edema and/or pyrexia can cause a hydrocele.
- *Practice Tip: Hydrocele can also be seen congenitally, most often in Shire horses and ultrasonographically manifests as an increase in anechoic fluid within the vaginal cavity.*
- Hematocele can result from trauma or spermatic cord torsion with blood identified based on its ultrasonographic appearance within the scrotum (Fig. 24-3).
- *Practice Tip: Clotted blood has an appearance similar to a corpus hemorrhagicum on a mare's ovary (gray-black, mottled, irregular) and gradually increases in echogenicity as it organizes.*
- Pyocele can develop following a penetrating wound, secondary to rupture of an abscess, or as a result of peritonitis. Ultrasonographically, fluid appears relatively echogenic and often contains particulate debris.
- In cases of hematocele and pyocele, fibrin tags may form and be visible ultrasonographically as grayish structures floating or waving in the surrounding fluid.

◉› WHAT TO DO

Scrotal Fluid
- Manage the inciting cause, if possible.
- Cold water hydrotherapy

- Nonsteroidal anti-inflammatory drugs (NSAIDs):
  - Flunixin meglumine, 1.1 mg/kg IV q12 to 24h, *or*
  - Phenylbutazone, 2.2 mg/kg IV or PO q12h
- Prophylactic, broad-spectrum antimicrobial therapy is recommended for cases of hematocele to prevent secondary infection. Trimethoprim sulfa, 30 mg/kg PO q12h is a reasonable choice.
- Antimicrobial therapy is required for treatment of pyocele and is ideally based on culture and sensitivity. Pending culture and sensitivity results, a combination of potassium penicillin, 22,000 U/kg IV q6h, and gentamicin, 6.6 mg/kg IV q24h, is a reasonable choice. **Note:** Use gentamicin only if serum creatinine concentration is normal, the stallion is urinating, and hydration is ensured. An alternative antimicrobial choice pending culture and sensitivity is ceftiofur, 3 mg/kg IV or IM q12h.
- In severe cases of hematocele or pyocele resulting in permanent injury to the testicle, or unresponsive to treatment, unilateral orchiectomy should be considered.

Prognosis: Scrotal Fluid

- The prognosis for stallions with scrotal fluid depends largely on the underlying cause.
- Scrotal fluid can be expected to cause transient insulating effects on the testicle and a resultant lowering of semen quality.
- In cases of hydrocele in which the underlying cause is eliminated and the fluid resolves, semen quality is expected to improve in about one spermatogenic cycle, approximately 60 days.
- In cases of hematocele or pyocele with adhesions or fibrous tissue, the prognosis for normal function of the affected testicle(s) is more guarded and depends on the extent of the pathology; small adhesions may have little or no effect on future fertility, whereas extensive adhesions and fibrous tissue formation may interfere with the normal thermoregulation of the testicles and cause pressure necrosis and permanent damage to the testicular parenchyma. As long as one testicle is unaffected by the problem, that testicle would be expected to return to normal function once any insulating effects from the diseased testicle have resolved.

Inguinal and Scrotal Hernias

- An inguinal hernia occurs when a loop of bowel passes into the inguinal canal.
- A scrotal hernia is a progression of an inguinal hernia in which the bowel loop passes into the scrotum.
- Inguinal or scrotal hernias may be:
  - Congenital or acquired
  - Uncomplicated or complicated
- In cases of congenital hernias in foals, the problem typically resolves spontaneously within the first 12 months of age. Congenital hernias typically involve small intestine, the herniated piece is usually viable, and treatment is usually not necessary.
- Acquired inguinal and scrotal hernias can occur in geldings or in stallions and occur with a higher incidence in Standardbreds.
- Larger inguinal rings may predispose a horse to a hernia.

- In many cases, acquired inguinal and scrotal hernias are associated with exercise or trauma and involve the small intestine that is either strangulated or nonstrangulated.

Clinical Signs
- Most horses present for evaluation of an enlarged scrotum and/or colic.
- Some horses with nonstrangulating inguinal or scrotal hernias *do not* exhibit signs of discomfort.
- Moderate to severe hydrocele is often present in association with inguinal and scrotal hernias.

Diagnosis
- Examine the scrotum and its contents by palpation; scrotal edema and hydrocele often make palpation of the scrotal contents difficult.
- Ultrasonography should be used to examine the scrotum and the region around the external inguinal ring. Determine if loops of bowel are visible in the vaginal space and whether the bowel loops are viable.
  - Viable bowel: peristaltic waves, normal wall thickness
  - Nonviable bowel: reduced or absent peristaltic waves, thickened, edematous bowel wall
- If severe hydrocele is present, it may be difficult to find bowel loops. The testicle on the affected side may have increased echogenicity.
  - A 7.5 or 5.0 MHz linear array, microconvex or sector scanner transducer works well.
  - The type of bowel present in the hernia can also be determined using ultrasonography.
    - Small intestine is most common due to its small diameter and long mesentery
  - See Chapter 14, p. 86.
- If ultrasound diagnosis is not available or definitive, examine the internal inguinal rings by transrectal palpation. If a hernia is present, loops of bowel can be palpated passing through the affected inguinal ring into the inguinal canal.

●》 WHAT TO DO

Inguinal and Scrotal Hernias
- Treatment is *not* generally required for congenital hernias. In protracted cases, surgical correction may be needed.
- In cases of acquired hernia, treatment is indicated.
- In a few cases of uncomplicated acquired inguinal hernia, the hernia may be corrected manually by gentle transrectal traction on the herniated bowel.
- Bowel viability should be confirmed ultrasonographically before attempting to perform rectal taxis. *Practice Tip: Regardless of the condition of the bowel, rectal taxis carries a significant risk of rectal perforation and is not recommended in most cases.*
- Most often, surgical correction of the hernia is required. Any case involving strangulated bowel requires surgery for resection of the compromised tissue and reduction of the hernia.
- Generally, the testicle on the side of the hernia is removed at the time of surgery to prevent the recurrence of the hernia.
- In some cases, it may be possible to salvage the testicle, but the owner should be aware of the possibility of recurrence of the hernia.

- Sedatives, analgesics, and NSAIDs are recommended during transport to the surgical facility.

Prognosis: Inguinal/Scrotal Hernia
- The prognosis for congenital inguinal or scrotal hernia is very good and most resolve spontaneously with time.
- *Practice Tip: In cases of acquired hernia, the most important prognostic indicator is the duration of the hernia.*
- Regardless of whether or not the bowel is strangulated, prognosis is very good for cases in which the hernia is diagnosed and corrected early (<24 hours).
- Cases in which the hernia is left untreated for a long period of time are associated with a poorer prognosis.
- The prognosis for future fertility is good in most cases, if the contralateral testis was normal before the event.
- Even if a unilateral orchiectomy is performed as part of the surgical correction of the hernia, the remaining testicle typically returns to normal function once scrotal inflammation has resolved.

Testicular Enlargement
- Enlargement of the testicle is an uncommon cause for scrotal enlargement.
- Testicular enlargement can be caused by:
  - Orchitis
  - Vascular or lymphatic stasis within the testicle
  - Testicular abscess
  - Testicular hematoma
  - Testicular neoplasia

Clinical Signs
- Clinical signs vary, depending on the cause of testicular enlargement.

Orchitis
- Orchitis or inflammation of the testicular parenchyma is uncommon and can arise secondary to trauma, infection, parasites, or autoimmune disease.
- The affected testicle is typically enlarged, hot, and painful, and systemic signs such as fever, leukocytosis, and hyperfibrinogenemia may be present.
- If semen is collected and evaluated, large numbers of white blood cells are typically found and semen quality is often poor.

Vascular or Lymphatic Stasis
- Vascular or lymphatic stasis is most often associated with torsion of the spermatic cord.
- If testicular enlargement is caused by spermatic cord torsion, abnormalities of the spermatic cord should be evident on palpation and ultrasonographic examination (see later).
- The stallion is typically painful with pronounced scrotal edema and often hydrocele.

Testicular Abscess
- Testicular abscesses can arise as a result of:
  - Penetrating wound through the scrotum and testicle
  - Testicular biopsy
  - Progression of orchitis

- Descending infection from the bloodstream
- Descending infection from peritonitis
- Stallions typically present febrile with a unilaterally enlarged, warm, painful testicle; evidence of a previous wound or trauma to the scrotum may be found.

Hematoma

- Testicular hematomas usually result from testicular trauma.
- Small hematomas are often seen following testicular biopsy.
- Hematomas can form within the testicular parenchyma or on the surface of the testicle.
- Small intratesticular hematomas may *not* cause a noticeable scrotal enlargement and the stallion may be asymptomatic except for localized pain on palpation of the affected testicle.
- In the acute stages of a hematoma, the scrotum is enlarged, warm, and painful, and may be associated with scrotal edema and hydrocele.

Neoplasia

- Testicular neoplasia is uncommon in the stallion; the tumor is generally small, and the testicle is *not* noticeably enlarged.
- In many cases of testicular neoplasia, testicular degeneration is present and the affected testicle is actually reduced in size.
- Testicular tumors arise from either germinal or nongerminal cells; germinal tumors are more common. Histopathologic examination is needed for a definitive diagnosis.
- Tumors may be identified in fertile stallions during a routine testicular examination or in stallions with a history of declining fertility during a breeding soundness examination.
- Most, but not all, testicular tumors in the stallion are benign.

Diagnosis

- Palpation of the testicles should be attempted. In cases of traumatic injury, the scrotal contents may be painful and edematous, and a hydrocele may preclude a complete examination.
- Ultrasound examination is usually very informative.
- Ultrasonographic changes may be fairly subtle or quite apparent when comparing the normal testicle to the affected testicle.
- Ultrasonographic appearance varies with the underlying cause:
  - Orchitis: The testicle typically appears heterogeneous with hypoechoic or hyperechoic foci.
  - Vascular or lymphatic stasis: The testicular parenchyma usually maintains an overall homogeneous granular appearance and becomes hypoechoic with respect to its normal echogenicity.
  - Abscess: A well-defined pocket of purulent fluid is generally visible within the testicular parenchyma. Fibrin tags and adhesions may be seen around the testicle and hydrocele may be present; if the abscess ruptures,

pyocele may result. The ultrasonographic character of the surrounding testicular parenchyma may be altered because of pressure from the abscess.
  - Hematoma: Generally appears mottled, grayish black within the surrounding parenchyma (similar to a corpus hemorrhagicum on a mare's ovary). If bleeding is ongoing, large pockets of relatively hypoechoic unclotted blood may also be seen swirling within the scrotal sac. As the hematoma organizes, its ultrasonographic appearance becomes more echogenic, eventually appearing hyperechoic relative to the surrounding testicle. Fibrin tags and adhesions may also form in the affected area.
  - Neoplasia: Typically there is a localized heterogeneous appearance to the normally very homogeneous testicular parenchyma. The exact appearance is highly variable and most appear as localized, soft tissue densities within the surrounding parenchyma. Color Doppler ultrasonography can help confirm the presence of a vascular soft tissue structure within the testis.
- Cultures of ejaculated semen may aid in identification of the causative organism in cases of infectious orchitis.

WHAT TO DO

Testicular Enlargement
Orchitis
- Treatment should be initiated as soon as possible.
  - Broad-spectrum, systemic antimicrobial drugs can be used prophylactically in cases of traumatic orchitis and for treatment of infectious orchitis. The choice of antimicrobials for testicular infection should ideally be based on culture and sensitivity testing of the ejaculate. Potassium penicillin, 22,000 U/kg IV q6h and gentamicin, 6.6 mg/kg IV q24h are good initial choices. **Note:** Use gentamicin *only* if serum creatinine concentration is normal, the stallion is urinating, and hydration is maintained. An alternative antimicrobial selection pending culture and sensitivity is ceftiofur, 3 mg/kg IV or IM q12h.
  - NSAIDs: Flunixin meglumine, 1.1 mg/kg IV q12 to 24h or phenylbutazone, 2.2 mg/kg IV or PO q12h
  - Cold hydrotherapy
  - If the opposite testicle is normal, unilateral orchiectomy is a consideration

Abscess
- **Practice Tip:** *Unilateral orchiectomy before rupture of the abscess is the treatment of choice in most cases.*
- If the abscess ruptures, based on ultrasonographic appearance of the scrotal contents, the stallion should be treated as for infectious orchitis.
- Surgery may be indicated to remove the testicle and drain the scrotal contents to prevent an ascending peritonitis. Following surgical removal, the stallion should be placed on nonsteroidal antiinflammatory drugs and systemic antimicrobials based on culture and sensitivity results (see earlier for orchitis).
- If an attempt is made to salvage the testicle, nonsteroidal antiinflammatory drugs and systemic antimicrobials based on culture and sensitivity results from ejaculated semen are administered.

Hematoma
- If the hematoma is localized, anti-inflammatory drugs, cold hydrotherapy, and stall rest may be the *only* treatments needed.

- Prophylactic antimicrobials should be considered for large, diffuse hematomas.
- In cases of extremely large hematomas where bleeding is *not* controlled, unilateral orchiectomy should be considered.

Neoplasia
- Most testicular tumors are benign and small, and it may be best to refrain from treatment while continuing to monitor the lesion ultrasonographically for changes in tumor size and changes in the surrounding parenchyma. Sparing the affected testicle is usually justified because the unaffected parts of the testicle continue to function and contribute sperm to the ejaculate.
- If the tumor is unusually large, growing rapidly, or malignant, unilateral orchiectomy of the affected testicle is performed. Ultrasonographically guided testicular biopsy guides the decision to remove the affected testicle. Testis-sparing surgery for removal of testicular tumors has *not* been reported in the horse.

Prognosis: Testicular Enlargement
Orchitis
- Orchitis has a guarded prognosis for future fertility. In severe cases where both testicles are affected, inflammation and increases in local temperature result in fibrosis and degeneration of the testicular parenchyma.
- If *only* one testicle is affected, prognosis for return to normal fertility is greatly improved.

Abscess
- The prognosis for future fertility with a testicular abscess depends on the size, extent of resulting fibrous tissue formation, and pressure necrosis of the surrounding testicular parenchyma.
- Larger abscesses with extensive fibrous tissue decrease the likelihood that the testicle returns to normal function.
- If the opposite testicle is normal, the stallion may be fertile following successful treatment or removal of the abscess.
- Any disease process that causes pyrexia or insulates the testicle is expected to cause at least a temporary decrease in semen quality.

Hematoma
- The prognosis for future fertility of the affected testicle depends on the size of the hematoma and the degree of fibrous tissue formation.
- Small hematomas (<20 mm in diameter) cause *only* local changes in spermatogenesis.
- Large hematomas cause more severe effects on fertility.
- The degree of loss of testicular parenchyma depends on the amount of pressure necrosis and fibrous tissue formation. Once the hematoma consolidates and the testicular temperature is normal, the uninjured testicular parenchyma should contribute sperm to the ejaculate.
- ***Practice Tip:** If the contralateral testis is unaffected, the stallion should be fertile once the insulating effects have resolved.*

Neoplasia
- In the case of small, localized testicular tumors, it is likely that the unaffected parts of the testicle will continue to function and contribute sperm to the ejaculate; fertility is *not* noticeably affected.

- If the tumor grows or its presence results in degeneration to the surrounding parenchyma, a decline in semen quality is expected. If the contralateral testis is unaffected, the stallion should remain fertile.

Spermatic Cord Torsion
- Torsion of the spermatic cord can cause vascular compromise.
- Torsions of <180 degrees usually do *not* alter blood flow and *do not* cause clinical signs.
- Torsions of >180 degrees compromise blood flow to the testicle and/or cause lymphatic and venous stasis; clinical signs are typically apparent. Affected stallions present with signs of colic associated with:
  - Enlarged, painful testicle
  - Enlarged scrotum
  - Increased scrotal fluid
  - Scrotal edema
  - Enlarged spermatic cord

Diagnosis
- Because the stallion is usually painful, sedation and analgesics may be needed before examination.
- Palpate the spermatic cord and scrotum. The edema and hydrocele that often occur may preclude a complete physical examination.
- Attempt to identify the location of the tail of the epididymis:
  - In a normally oriented testis, the epididymal tail is pointing caudally.
  - In cases of 180-degree spermatic cord torsions, the tail is pointing cranially.
  - In cases of 360-degree torsion, the tail is pointing caudally and is often displaced dorsally, and changes in the spermatic cord are usually present.
- Ultrasonographic examination of the scrotal contents reveals abnormalities.
  - The spermatic cord vessel lumens are increased in diameter.
  - The testicular parenchyma may increase or decrease in echogenicity depending on the duration of vascular stasis (Fig. 24-4).
  - Hydrocele is often present. Evaluation of the testicular artery, arcuate arteries, central vein, and pampiniform plexus may allow the ultrasonographer to determine the presence or absence of blood flow to and from the testicle.
  - Vascular stasis may cause noticeable enlargement of any or all of these vessels.
  - If Doppler ultrasound equipment is available, it can provide additional information on the presence or absence of blood flow in the spermatic cord and testicle vessels.
- ***Practice Tip:** Many torsions of the spermatic cord are not pathologic. If vascular flow is not compromised, identification of a 180-degree spermatic cord torsion may be an incidental finding during routine examination of the testicles. In*

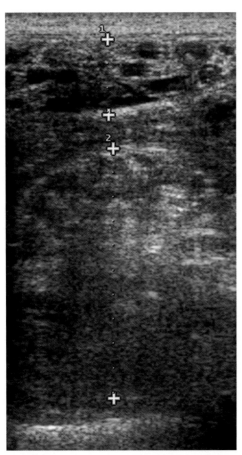

Figure 24-4   Ultrasonographic appearance of spermatic cord torsion in a stallion. Calipers marked "1" delineate the unaffected spermatic cord. Note the presence of numerous cross sections of the spermatic cord vessels. The lumens of the vessels appear as anechoic circular/elliptical structures. Calipers marked "2" delineate the affected cord. The spermatic cord torsion has resulted in a dramatic increase in size of the diameter of the affected cord. Additionally, the normal spermatic cord architecture is lost. The tissue appears more echodense, presumably due to chronic blood and lymphatic stasis. The normal, anechoic appearance of cross sections of the spermatic cord vessels is lost.

these cases, the stallion shows no clinical signs and the scrotal contents are nonpainful with no evidence of enlargement; however, the tail of the epididymis is displaced cranially. These torsions may be intermittent, and there is no evidence that their occurrence adversely affects semen quality.

●› WHAT TO DO

Spermatic Cord Torsion

- ***Practice Tip:*** *The usual treatment for spermatic cord torsion with vascular compromise is emergency castration of the affected testicle.*
- This surgery is generally performed at a referral hospital.
- In cases of spermatic cord torsion where the stallion is exhibiting signs of discomfort but the testicle is viable, surgical correction of the torsion and orchiopexy are possible to salvage the testicle.
- Before referral, the stallion should be treated as follows:
  - Administer sedation and analgesia before transport, depending on the degree of the stallion's physical comfort.
    - Xylazine, 0.6 mg/kg IV *or*
    - Detomidine, 0.01 to 0.04 mg/kg IV
    - +/− Butorphanol tartrate, 0.02 mg/kg IV

- NSAIDs:
  - Flunixin meglumine, 1.1 mg/kg IV q12 to 24h *or*
  - Phenylbutazone, 2.2 mg/kg IV or PO q12h
- Prophylactic broad-spectrum antimicrobial therapy is recommended because of the possible ischemic tissue and in preparation for surgery.
  - Potassium penicillin, 22,000 U/kg IV q6h *and*
  - Gentamicin, 6.6 mg/kg IV q24h
- ***Note:*** Use gentamicin *only* if serum creatinine concentration is normal, the stallion is urinating, and hydration is maintained. An alternative antimicrobial choice is ceftiofur, 3 mg/kg IV or IM q12h.

Prognosis: Spermatic Cord Torsion

- The prognosis for stallions with unilateral spermatic cord torsion and compromised blood flow is very good with prompt and appropriate treatment.
- If the contralateral testicle is normal before the torsion, the stallion should be fertile once normal thermoregulation is restored and following a complete spermatogenic cycle.
- ***Practice Tip:*** *Untreated, this condition can lead to tissue necrosis, endotoxemia, and death.*

Epididymitis

- Inflammation of the epididymis is uncommon and most often bacterial in origin.
- The problem rarely occurs primarily and is often a result of hematogenous spread or an extension of infection from the testes, bladder, or accessory sex glands.
- When epididymitis is suspected, the stallion should be carefully examined for another primary site of infection.
- Epididymitis can be unilateral or bilateral.
- *Streptococcus zooepidemicus* and *Proteus mirabilis* are reported as causative organisms.
- Besides scrotal enlargement, affected horses present with:
  - Signs of colic
  - Hind limb lameness
  - Lethargy
  - Pain associated with ejaculation
  - Poor semen quality
  - Neutrophils may be present in the ejaculate

Diagnosis

- Because the stallion is typically painful, sedation and analgesia are needed before examination.
- Palpation of the scrotal contents usually reveals an enlarged, painful epididymis.
- Ultrasonographic examination of the scrotum reveals changes in the affected epididymis. The specific appearance generally includes an increase in the number and size of hypoechoic regions in the epididymis believed to be associated with an accumulation of exudate and abscess formation. Scattered areas of increased echogenicity may be seen, and the epididymis may appear consolidated with loss of its fluid-filled lumen and concurrent hydrocele.
- If an ejaculate is obtained, evaluate cytologically for neutrophils; in chronic epididymitis, these may be absent. A

sample of the ejaculate that has been collected aseptically should be submitted for bacteriologic culture and sensitivity testing.

- ***Practice Tip:*** *Epididymal aspirates should be avoided because of the possibility of seeding the vaginal cavity or testicle with bacteria.*

◉〉 WHAT TO DO

Epididymitis
- In reported cases of epididymitis, the affected epididymides and testicles were removed by castration.
- In cases where the goal is to save the testicle and epididymis, systemic antimicrobial therapy based on culture and sensitivity testing of ejaculated semen, parenteral nonsteroidal anti-inflammatory drugs, and hydrotherapy are recommended.
- It is difficult to acheive adequate tissue concentration of antimicrobials in the epididymis. ***Practice Tip:*** *Antimicrobials with a high pKa and lipid solubility—trimethoprim sulfa and chloramphenicol—are the best choices.*
  - Duration of treatment is at least 3 to 4 weeks
  - NSAIDs:
    - Flunixin meglumine, 1.1 mg/kg IV q12 to 24h
    - Phenylbutazone, 2.2 mg/kg IV or PO q12h
  - Antimicrobials:
    - Trimethoprim sulfa, 30 mg/kg PO q12h
    - Chloramphenicol, 50 mg/kg PO q6h

Prognosis: Epididymitis
- Because the epididymis consists of a single, narrow, highly convoluted duct, there is a significant risk that the inflammation results in permanent obstruction of the lumen even if the infection is successfully treated.
- Even with hemicastration, bacterial organisms continue to be isolated from semen several months after surgery.
- Prognosis for future fertility is guarded in cases of unilateral epididymitis and is poor in cases of bilateral epididymitis.

Sperm Granuloma
- Sperm granuloma, uncommon in stallions, is the result of a severe inflammatory reaction to sperm extravasated from the epididymal lumen or seminiferous tubules.
- The condition is usually unilateral.
- Before modern anthelmintics, sperm granulomas were associated with parasitic migration of *Strongylus edentatus.*
- Trauma can also result in extravasation of sperm and subsequent granuloma formation.
- Clinical signs are similar to those seen with bacterial epididymitis:
  - Scrotal enlargement
  - Colic
  - Pain associated with ejaculation
  - Poor semen quality
  - Oligospermia
  - Neutrophils in the ejaculate

Diagnosis
- Because the stallion is typically painful, sedation and analgesia are required before examination.
- Palpation of the scrotum is performed and generally reveals an enlarged, painful epididymis.
- Ultrasonographic examination of the scrotum reveals epididymal abnormalities. ***Practice Tip:*** *Ultrasonographically, this condition frequently* cannot *be differentiated from bacterial epididymitis.*
- Semen analysis usually reveals the presence of neutrophils in the ejaculate. Submit a sample for culture and sensitivity testing; in contrast to bacterial epididymitis, it should produce no growth.
- Because of the similarities to bacterial epididymitis, a definitive diagnosis requires histopathologic examination of the affected epididymis after hemicastration. ***Note:*** Differentiation between the two conditions is important because the prognosis is different.

◉〉 WHAT TO DO

Sperm Granuloma
- Hemicastration is the most common treatment.
- If the goal is to preserve the affected testis, treatment should be directed as for bacterial epididymitis. The recommended treatment is the same.
  - Cold water hydrotherapy also may be beneficial.
- ***Note:*** Epididymal aspirates are *not* recommended in cases of epididymal pathology because of the risk of spreading infection in cases of bacterial epididymitis or the risk of introducing infection in a sperm granuloma.

◉〉 WHAT NOT TO DO

Sperm Granuloma
- *Do not* biopsy the epididymis.
- Because the epididymis is a single, highly convoluted duct, biopsy sampling may transect the epididymis.

Prognosis for Sperm Granuloma
- The affected testicle and epididymis are usually removed. Even if left in place, the outcome of an epididymal sperm granuloma is likely to be an impotent epididymis.
  - Therefore, the ipsilateral testicle no longer contributes sperm to the ejaculate.
- The contralateral testis should return to normal function once scrotal swelling resolves; the prognosis for fertility in stallions with unilateral epididymal pathology is good.
- ***Practice Tip:*** *If the condition is bilateral, the prognosis for future fertility is poor.*

Hemospermia
- Hemospermia is the presence of blood in the seminal fluid.
- The source of the blood can be from anywhere along the external genitalia—from the testicles to the external surface of the penis.

- Frequently bleeding originates from the skin or mucosal lesions of the urethra, urethral process, glans penis, or penile shaft.
- Other causes for hemospermia include:
  - Epididymitis
  - Blocked ampullae
  - Seminal vesiculitis
  - Cutaneous habronemiasis
  - Urethral strictures
  - Bacterial urethritis (most commonly associated with *Streptococcus* spp., *E. coli,* or *Pseudomonas aeruginosa*)
  - Urethral varicosities
  - Neoplasia
- ***Practice Tip:*** *Hemospermia can affect stallions of any age or breed; however, there is an increased incidence in Quarter Horses.*
- Blood may be present in all ejaculates or may be intermittent.
- Trauma causing bleeding from the penile skin or mucosa is a common cause of hemospermia.
  - The more common traumatic injuries include:
    - Kicks from a mare during breeding
    - Lacerations of the penis or urethral process from tail hairs of the mare during breeding
    - Urethral strictures or skin lesions caused by the use of stallion rings
- Iatrogenic hemospermia can occur following urinary bladder catheterization or urethroscopy.
- Idiopathic defects in the urethra communicating with the underlying corpus spongiosum penis are common causes of sometimes profuse hemospermia with many lesions found near the pelvic ischium.

Clinical Signs

- A diagnosis of hemospermia is usually based on seeing blood in the ejaculate.
- Affected stallions may exhibit pain with full erection or ejaculation.
- Stallions breeding by natural cover whose semen is *not* evaluated regularly may present for infertility because blood contamination of the ejaculate negatively affects pregnancy rates.
  - Additionally, blood may be seen around the vulva after breeding or in the dismount sample.

Diagnosis

- Gross examination of semen collected with an artificial vagina reveals hemospermia.
  - Gross appearance can range from pale pink (slight blood contamination) to bright red (significant blood contamination). Microscopic examination may be required to identify red blood cells in very mild cases.
    - If "round" cells are seen and you are unsure as to the type of "round" cell present, a smear of the ejaculate is prepared and stained with a Romanowsky-type stain. Red blood cells stain a pale pink and lack a nucleus.
- Bleeding can vary in severity among ejaculates and may be intermittent; collection of a single, blood-free ejaculate does *not* rule out the condition, particularly if the horse is at sexual rest.
- If the lesion communicates with the underlying cavernous tissue, bleeding can be impressive.
- Physical examination of the external surfaces of the penis, urethral fossa, and urethral process should be performed on the flaccid and erect penis to look for lesions.
  - Examination immediately following a blood-contaminated semen collection may facilitate identification of smaller lesions.
- Urethroscopy using a flexible fiber-optic endoscope should be performed to completely examine the penile and pelvic urethra and rule out the presence of urethritis or idiopathic mucosal lesions.
  - Performing the urethroscopic examination (see Chapter 12, p. 68) immediately following ejaculation may make the diagnosis more straightforward because blood may still be present in and around the lesion.
- Additional diagnostic techniques are employed to examine higher areas of the reproductive tract if indicated.
  - Palpation and ultrasonography of the scrotal contents may reveal abnormalities of the testes, epididymis, or spermatic cord.
  - Transrectal palpation and ultrasonography of the internal accessory glands may identify blocked ampullae or seminal vesiculitis.
- Retrograde infusion of contrast material into the urethra, followed by a series of radiographs, may help to identify strictures, masses, fistulas, and other similar urethral lesions. This technique is used less often when flexible endoscopy is readily available.

◆〉 WHAT TO DO

Hemospermia

- The treatment depends on the cause of the bleeding, so accurate identification of the bleeding source is important (i.e., a bleeding tumor involving the urethral process is different than bleeding from the seminal vesicles).
  - A minimum of several weeks, and often several months of sexual rest may be recommended when hemospermia is associated with traumatic lesions, urethritis, or idiopathic urethral lesions.
  - Hemospermia may recur once the stallion returns to an active breeding program, even with prolonged sexual rest; particularly if the source of the bleeding is an idiopathic urethral mucosal lesion.
- Surgery combined with sexual rest facilitates resolution of hemospermia from traumatic wounds or idiopathic mucosal lesions.
  - Suturing surface lacerations promotes first intention healing.
  - Laser ablation of the urethral mucosal lesions has mixed results.
  - In refractory cases of urethral mucosal lesions, a temporary (approximately 10 weeks' duration) subischial urethrotomy is performed to allow urine to bypass the distal urethra and potentially reduce pressure in the corpus spongiosum penis at the

end of urination. Side effects of this procedure include urethral strictures and fistulae.
- Primary closure of urethral mucosal lesions can be attempted if rest and subischial urethrotomy fail to resolve the problem.
- Depending on the degree of hemospermia, immediate extension of blood-contaminated ejaculates may be sufficient to allow pregnancies to occur.
  - In stallions breeding by natural cover, an extender can be placed in the mare's uterus before breeding, so the ejaculate mixes with the extender and blood contamination is diluted.
- Some horses may experience discomfort with ejaculation due to the underlying lesion. In these cases, anti-inflammatory medications are employed.
  - Flunixin meglumine, 1.1 mg/kg IV q12 to 24h *or*
  - Phenylbutazone, 2.2 mg/kg IV or PO q12h

WHAT NOT TO DO

Hemospermia
- *Do not* discourage normal spontaneous erections and penile movements/masturbation. These actions are physiologic, and it is well documented that aggressively discouraging spontaneous erection and masturbation can be harmful to the horse.

Prognosis
- The prognosis for recovery varies based on the cause of the hemospermia.
- Simple lacerations may heal with only rest.
- Puncture wounds are more difficult to manage and may require surgical intervention.
- For traumatic lesions, the prognosis for full recovery is good if the horse is given an appropriate period of rest and wound care.
- If rest alone is insufficient, or if the wound is large, surgical debridement and closure may be required.
- Idiopathic ulcerated or rentlike lesions of the urethra are more frustrating to treat.
- Surgical correction and/or laser ablation combined with sexual rest may be helpful initially, but recurrence is possible once the stallion is returned to active breeding.
- Temporary subischial urethrotomy increases the chances of a permanent resolution. Even when this treatment is used, recurrence is possible.

Acute Paraphimosis
- Paraphimosis is the inability to fully retract the penis into the preputial cavity (i.e., sheath; Fig. 24-5).
- This condition is most common in breeding stallions following a traumatic incident in the breeding shed; geldings can also be affected.
- Causes of acute paraphimosis include:
  - Penile trauma (see Penile Hematoma, p. 429)
  - Large lesions of the glans penis (e.g., squamous cell carcinoma)
  - Severe systemic disease, particularly those that cause extensive subcutaneous edema (i.e., purpura hemorrhagica)

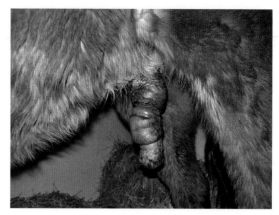

Figure 24-5   Acute paraphimosis in a stallion.

- Diseases that affect penile innervation such as EHV-1 or rabies
- Severe debilitation
- Severe exhaustion
- Penile paralysis associated with the use of phenothiazine-based tranquilizers (e.g., propriopromazine and acepromazine)
- Severe edema/swelling postcastration
- Under normal circumstances, the penis is held in the preputial cavity by the actions of the retractor penis muscles and smooth muscle within the cavernous spaces of the penis.
- Trauma or other factors can cause bleeding and/or edema in the loose connective tissue between the penis and internal preputial lamina.
- With the additional fluid weight, these muscles fatigue and the penis and internal preputial lamina protrude from the preputial cavity.
- This becomes a vicious cycle because the dependent penis further impairs venous and lymphatic drainage exacerbating the situation.
- The relatively inelastic preputial ring complicates the problem by serving as a constricting band. This ring impairs vascular and lymphatic drainage distal to the preputial ring.
- Once the penile and preputial skin is exposed, it rapidly thickens, excoriates and/or cracks, stimulating additional local inflammation.
- With prolonged protrusion, contusion, and stretching of the pudendal nerves across the ischial arch, a neuropathy results in penile paralysis.

Diagnosis
- Gently clean the penis and prepuce for complete inspection and physical examination to determine the extent of the injury or the extent of any secondary penile damage (e.g., edema, skin ulceration, tissue necrosis, etc.) in cases of traumatic paraphimosis.
- Ultrasonographic evaluation is useful to determine if penile enlargement is caused by swelling and edema or if other factors are present (e.g., hematoma/seroma or abscess).

●〉 WHAT TO DO

Acute Paraphimosis

- Treatment is directed at the inciting cause and managing:
  - Edema/inflammation
  - Maintaining the health of the penile and preputial skin while they are exposed
  - Returning the penis and associated preputial structures to the prepuce
- Reestablishing retention of the penis and prepuce in the preputial cavity:
  - Improves venous and lymphatic drainage
  - Minimizes pudendal nerve damage
  - Maintains health of the penile/preputial skin
- For acute trauma (see Penile Hematoma, p. 429), use cold hydrotherapy with a gentle stream of water for 20 to 30 minutes, several times a day.
- If large fluid pockets are seen ultrasonographically, drainage may be indicated before attempting to reduce the penile/preputial prolapse. The most dependent area is identified and drainage is established using a large-gauge needle (e.g., 14 gauge) or by sharp incision. Massage aids drainage of fluid and aseptic removal of blood/fibrin clots is performed with forceps. These procedures should be performed under aseptic conditions to prevent infection/abscess.
- An elastic compression (Esmarch[1]) bandage can be used to reduce penile swelling/edema and replacement of the penis within the sheath (Fig. 24-6). A tight bandage is placed beginning distally at the glans penis and moving proximally along the penis/prepuce. Remove the bandage after 10 to 15 minutes and attempt to reduce the penis/prepuce into the preputial cavity. The Esmarch wrap can be applied repeatedly in an effort to reduce the penis size for replacement into the prepuce.
- Once the penis and prepuce are reduced, an umbilical tape purse string suture is placed at the preputial ring or preputial orifice to prevent recurrent prolapse; leave enough of an opening for urination. The suture should be untied every 2 to 3 days for examination of the penis. If the penis cannot be retained within the prepuce, the penis should be cleaned and replaced into the sheath and the purse string retied for another 1 to 2 days. Alternatively, a sling can be fashioned out of porous, elastic material as an alternative to hold the penis in the sheath.
- External support is used if the condition of the penis prevents replacement or the purse string suture is *not* an option. The commercial supports are generally inadequate for proper support of the swollen penis. A better result can be achieved with the use of a hand-fashioned sling made out of "stretch lace." The fabric is cut to measure 0.5 × 3 m for most stallions. The stretch fabric is placed around the abdomen circumferentially and tied in a bow to the side of the dorsal midline. This arrangement holds the penis against the ventral abdomen, or the penis within the sheath (Fig. 24-7). The soft, nonlace side of the material should be adjacent to the skin to prevent ulceration. This fabric provides good support and allows the stallion to urinate.
- Before replacing the penis/prepuce or applying a support device, the tissues should be cleansed and lubricated with an emollient such as silver sulfadiazine cream[2] or a compounded product consisting of 80 mg dexamethasone and 3.88 g oxytetracycline per 1 pound lanolin base or a 1 : 1 mixture by volume of 2% testosterone cream[3] in emollient udder cream (i.e., Bag Balm[4]).
- ***Practice Tip:*** *The key to successful treatment of acute, traumatic paraphimosis centers around replacement and retention of the penis within the sheath. If the penis remains dependent or is inadequately supported, edema and swelling increase and the paraphimosis worsens, eventually resulting in penile paralysis. Complete replacement of the penis within the sheath is a major goal of treatment.*
- Ancillary treatments include:
  - Nonsteroidal anti-inflammatory drugs:
    ○ Flunixin meglumine, 1.1 mg/kg IV q12 to 24h *or*
    ○ Phenylbutazone, 2.2 mg/kg IV or PO q12h
  - Broad-spectrum systemic antimicrobial treatment is indicated if there is infection or cellulitis, or if surgical drainage is performed
- The duration of treatment varies, but it may take 7 to 10 days before the penis is spontaneously retained within the prepuce.
- If penile function is *not* regained, the penis is considered paralyzed. See Penile Paralysis, pp. 427 and 430.

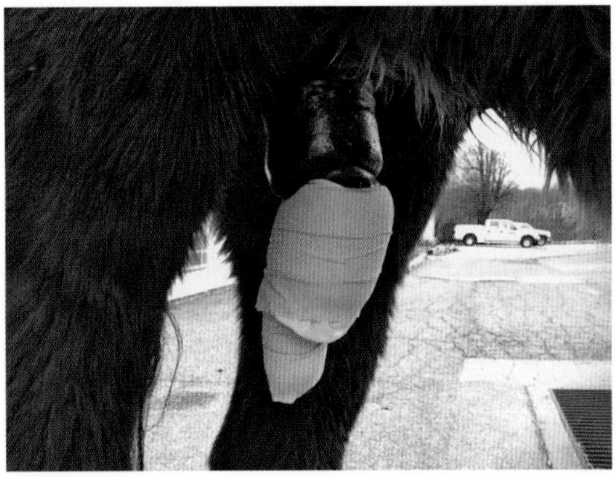

Figure 24-6   Application of a compression (Esmarch) bandage to the penis of a stallion affected with paraphimosis.

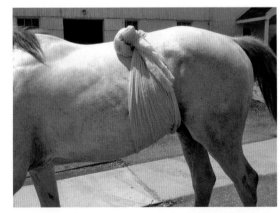

Figure 24-7   Application of a "stretch lace" support device to maintain the penis within the sheath.

[2]Silver sulfadiazine cream, SSD/Silvadene (Dr. Reddy's Laboratories, Bridgewater, New Jersey, 08807).

[3]First Testosterone MC (CutisPharma, Inc., Woburn, Massachusetts).

[4]Bag Balm (Dairy Association Co., Inc., Lyndonville, Vermont 05851)

[1]Esmarch bandage (Eickenmeyer Veterinary Equipment, Inc., Stony Plain, Canada; www.eickemeyerveterinary@telus.net).

Prognosis for Acute Paraphimosis

- With prompt and proper treatment, the prognosis is good for full recovery in cases of traumatic acute paraphimosis.
- Paraphimosis associated with large lesions of the glans penis is typically good if the lesion is removed and the penis is properly managed during the paraphimosis.
- Paraphimosis secondary to dependent edema and/or swelling is good if the edema/swelling resolves, and the penis is properly supported when extended.
- The prognosis for recovery of penile function is more guarded when penile innervation is affected (e.g., with EHV-1) and is poor when paraphimosis is associated with severe debilitation.
- ***Practice Tip:*** *Phenothiazine-associated paraphimosis has a guarded to fair prognosis if the penis is promptly replaced in the sheath and managed to avoid secondary complications.*

Penile Hematoma

- The most common cause of a penile hematoma is traumatic disruption of the vascular (primarily venous) network in the subcutaneous tissue located in the internal preputial fold on the dorsal aspect of the penis.
- Penile hematomas occur less commonly as a result of tearing of the fibrous tunica albuginea surrounding the CCP or disruption of the CSP (see Fig. 24-1).
- Traumatic disruption of the CCP or CSP is often referred to colloquially as a "fractured, broken, or ruptured" penis.
- Penile hematomas typically occur as a result of physical trauma to the erect penis such as:
  - A kick from a nonreceptive mare
  - Inadvertent forceful bending or stretching of the penis during vigorous attempts to gain intromission into the mare or artificial vagina
  - Awkwardly dismounting from the mare (or phantom)
- Trauma to the erect penis may occur outside of breeding activities (i.e., stallions that are used to determine estrous behavior in mares at a "teasing" rail may become injured with aggressive attempts to mount and/or hurdle the barrier).
- A stallion at pasture may be injured if he becomes sexually stimulated and tries to jump over a fence or other obstacle in an effort to reach a mare(s).

Clinical Signs

- Rapid, almost instantaneous, swelling of the superficial tissues of the penis and prepuce (Fig. 24-8)

⏺❯ **WHAT TO DO**

Penile Hematoma

- Treatment is directed at controlling the bleeding/swelling and minimizing edema.
  - Early and aggressive treatment is important to minimize the development of a chronic paraphimosis/penile paralysis.
  - Institute immediate cold hydrotherapy with a gentle stream of water from a hose for 15 to 20 minutes, repeated several times during the day.

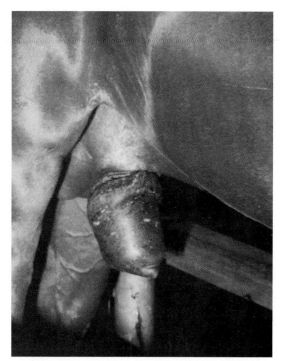

Figure 24-8 Direct trauma causing penile hematoma.

- Alternatively, the penis can be wrapped immediately with a compression bandage for 20 to 30 minutes; remove the bandage and repeat as needed several times a day.
- NSAIDs:
  - Flunixin meglumine, 1.1 mg/kg IV q12 to 24h *or*
  - Phenylbutazone, 2.2 mg/kg IV or PO q12h
- For uncomplicated cases, antimicrobial treatment is generally *not* necessary; if the penile/preputial skin is compromised as a result of trauma, systemic broad-spectrum antimicrobials are recommended.
- Supportive care:
  - Check and monitor the penis frequently.
  - Clean and apply an appropriate emollient ointment to the surface of the penis and prepuce to avoid drying/cracking (i.e., silver sulfadiazine [SSD] or "Bag Balm").
- Isolate the stallion for 1 week to avoid sexual stimulation, confine to a stall, and limit exercise. After 1 week of rest, sexual arousal may be beneficial to minimize adhesion formation. Similarly, light exercise can be resumed after 1 week in an effort to help resolve any residual edema/swelling.
- If the hematoma continues to enlarge in the acute phase in spite of the recommendations above, damage to the cavernous tissue(s) may have occurred, and additional diagnostics and treatment may be necessary. The tunica albuginea of the CCP can be examined ultrasonographically, radiographically using cavernosography, or surgically for a rent that extends into the corporeal tissue. If a rent is identified, surgical repair stops development of the hematoma and prevents formation of a shunt between the corporeal tissue and dorsal venous plexus that interferes with future erectile function.

⏺❯ **WHAT NOT TO DO**

Penile Hematoma

- *Do not* discourage normal spontaneous erections and penile movements/masturbation. These actions are physiologic, and it is well documented that discouraging spontaneous erections and masturbation can be harmful to the horse (e.g., with the use of stallion rings, shock collars, or other forms of physical punishment).

Prognosis

- With appropriate treatment, hematomas involving the dorsal penile subcutaneous vascular plexus generally resolve completely and *do not* result in any long-term disruption of reproductive function nor seem to predispose the stallion to a recurrence.
- If *not* repaired, hematomas associated with rupture of the tunica albuginea may result in impotence if a permanent vascular shunt occurs between the CCP and subcutaneous vascular plexus.
- A hematoma that remains confined to the CCP with an intact tunica albuginea may result in permanent deviation of the erect penis, presumably because of reduced blood flow through the cavernous tissue.
- Concurrent paraphimosis can complicate the situation. Please see Acute Paraphimosis, p. 427.

Chronic Paraphimosis/Penile Paralysis

- Penile paralysis occurs in stallions and geldings secondary to reduced retractor penis muscle tone/function which allows the penis and preputial tissue to passively prolapse.
- The dependent tissue becomes swollen and edematous, further exacerbating the problem. If uncorrected, venous and lymphatic drainage becomes impaired and secondary tissue damage occurs.
- Causes of penile paralysis include:
  - Severe exhaustion
  - Severe debilitation
  - Myelitis or spinal cord injury
  - Consequence of administration of phenothiazine-type tranquilizers (e.g., propriopromazine and acepromazine)
  - Chronic paraphimosis/paralysis can develop from acute paraphimosis if the condition is *not* treated promptly and appropriately (see Acute Paraphimosis, p. 427)

Diagnosis

- Diagnosis is similar as for acute paraphimosis.
- Gently clean the penis and prepuce for complete inspection and physical examination to determine the extent of penile damage (edema, skin ulceration, tissue necrosis, etc.).
- Ultrasonographic evaluation may help determine the extent of secondary damage to the penis. It may be possible to see thrombosis or fibrosis of the cavernous tissue spaces, which could affect prognosis and treatment.

●› WHAT TO DO

Chronic Paraphimosis/Penile Paralysis

- For protracted cases of penile paralysis, attempt to replace the penis within the sheath and maintain it in this position (see Acute

Paraphimosis, p. 427). This prevents secondary complications of dependent edema and may allow time for muscle function to be regained. The prognosis for return of penile function is guarded to poor in cases of chronic paraphimosis/penile paralysis.
- In the refractory case, the horse can be referred for permanent surgical retention procedures to avoid secondary complications associated with chronic dependency (i.e., tissue necrosis).
  - Phallopexy (Bolz procedure):
    ○ Stallions should be castrated with this procedure.
  - Posthetomy (circumcision) or a "reefing" procedure is used to remove all or part of the prepuce if fibrosis or stricture of the prepuce is present or a contributing problem.
  - Phallectomy is also to be considered.
- With good care, it is possible to maintain the health of a paralyzed penis and avoid the need for phallopexy or phallectomy.
  - Protect the horse from exposure to freezing temperatures.
  - Regularly monitor penile condition.
  - Regularly (3 to 4 times per day) apply emollients.
  - Apply external support (e.g., mesh lace slings; see Acute Paraphimosis, p. 427) to prevent dependent edema and trauma to the paralyzed penis.
  - Use penile massage 3 to 4 times per day to reduce edema if it develops.
- *Practice Tip: Some stallions with paralyzed penises are able to ejaculate into an artificial vagina with assistance and, in some situations, even return to natural service. Most stallions retain good sensation at the proximal end of the penis and respond in a positive manner with thrusting and ejaculation if sufficiently stimulated with hot compresses and manual pressure at the base of the penis.*

●› WHAT TO DO

Acute Paraphimosis

- *Practice Tip: Complications associated with sedative-induced penile prolapse/paralysis are avoided by monitoring the horse for the ability to completely withdraw the penis into the prepuce.*
- If the penis remains prolapsed for more than 30 minutes after the horse regains normal alertness after the administration of phenothiazines, then manually stimulate (i.e., squeeze with hemostats) the penis for a withdrawal response. If tactile stimulation does *not* result in withdrawal of the penis, then manually replace the penis in the prepuce and hold it in place by packing the preputial opening with rolled cotton.
- Remove the packing every 30 minutes to assess the ability of the penis to remain within the prepuce. Repeat cycles of penile replacement and packing are until normal spontaneous retention is restored.
- If the horse postures to urinate with the packing in place, remove the packing to allow urination to prevent urine scalding.

Prognosis for Chronic Paraphimosis/Penile Paralysis

- Horses with protracted cases of penile paralysis are *not* likely to regain the ability to retract the penis, or in the case of stallions, an erection.

Phimosis

- Phimosis is the inability of the penis to spontaneously protrude from the preputial cavity.

- It occurs in stallions and geldings and is generally due to trauma or disease of the tissues of the penis/prepuce and/or surrounding structures such as the scrotum.
- Phimosis can result in difficulty urinating and/or urinating within the preputial cavity, both of which can exacerbate the problem because of urine scalding of the penile/preputial tissues and local inflammation.
- ***Practice Tip:*** *Phimosis is normal in newborn colts. At birth, the internal lamina of the internal prepuce is fused with the free portion of the penis, and this mechanically prevents complete extension of the penis. These structures should spontaneously separate by the time the colt is 4 to 6 weeks of age, allowing the penis to fully extend.*
- Common causes of pathologic phimosis include:
  - Excessive swelling of the inguinal and preputial tissues following castration, particularly common in older horses
  - Penile/preputial and/or scrotal trauma after a breeding injury (e.g., kick from a mare or other injury to the area)
- Less common causes of pathologic phimosis include:
  - Large lesions on the penis that prevent penile extension (e.g., squamous cell carcinoma)
  - Severe systemic disease with severe dependent edema (e.g., purpura hemorrhagica)

●❯ WHAT TO DO

Phimosis
- For acute phimosis associated with a traumatic event (castration, etc.) treatment is directed at controlling local inflammation, edema, and hematoma formation.
  - Cold hydrotherapy with a gentle stream of water from a hose for 15 to 20 minutes, repeated several times a day
  - NSAIDs:
    ◦ Flunixin meglumine, 1.1 mg/kg IV q12 to 24h *or*
    ◦ Phenylbutazone, 2.2 mg/kg IV or PO q12h
  - Systemic broad-spectrum antimicrobials
  - Controlled exercise
  - Topical administration of appropriate antiseptic emollients (e.g., silver sulfadiazine [SSD], etc.) to the affected areas of skin
- Phimosis due to a space-occupying lesion of the penis or prepuce is effectively treated by surgical excision of the mass.
- Chronic phimosis with fibrotic stricture of the preputial fold is treated by:
  - Make a longitudinal incision through the preputial ring
  - Remove a wedge of tissue from the preputial ring and close the free edges with suture
  - For severe cases, remove the preputial ring by performing segmental posthetomy (i.e., "reefing" procedure)
- Chronic phimosis with a fibrotic stricture of the external preputial orifice is similarly treated by:
  - Make a longitudinal incision beginning at the preputial orifice and extend it caudally along the external preputial lamina
  - Excise a wedge of tissue as described earlier for the internal preputial fold/preputial ring

Prognosis for Phimosis
- The prognosis for acute phimosis is generally good following resolution of clinical signs.

- Stallions that develop phimosis following scrotal trauma and swelling may suffer a temporary or permanent reduction in semen quality, depending on the degree of injury to the testicles and scrotal tissues.
- The prognosis for chronic phimosis is generally good following elimination of the underlying problem causing the phimosis.
- Even after the reefing procedure, stallions can maintain breeding activity/function; radical excision of preputial tissue should be avoided to preserve reproductive function.

Priapism
- Priapism is the persistence of an erection without sexual arousal.
- Priapism occurs when arterial inflow or venous outflow to/from the CCP is pathologically changed; subsequently only the CCP is involved in the persistent erection (i.e., the CSP and CSG remain flaccid).
- Despite the fact that priapism shares similarities with penile paralysis, including the potential to occur after the use of phenothiazine-based tranquilizers, they are different syndromes (see Penile Paralysis, pp. 427 and 430).
- In cases of priapism, the penis is either fully or, more commonly, partially erect compared with the flaccid penis seen in penile paralysis.
- True priapism is uncommon; it has been reported to occur in both stallions and, less commonly, in geldings.
- Causes of priapism include:
  - Neurovascular trauma during breeding
  - Neuropathy
  - General anesthesia
  - Administration of phenothiazine-based tranquilizers such as acepromazine
- Priapism in the horse is referred to as low flow, or veno-occlusive, and occurs when alpha-adrenergic sympathetic neural impulses that cause detumescence are blocked; this is the mechanism by which phenothiazine-derived tranquilizers induce priapism in horses.
- The mechanism(s) by which other inciting factors cause low flow priapism are *not* known although they similarly impair detumescence of the penis.
- If unresolved, chronic priapism leads to fibrotic changes that subsequently impair the ability of the cavernous tissue to expand normally during erection.
- Should priapism persist, the penis ultimately loses its erectile function and tactile sensation, resulting in impotence.

Clinical Signs
- Persistent full or partial erection occurs in the absence of sexual stimulus.
- Regardless of whether the penis is fully or partially erect, manual examination reveals turgidity *only* within the corpus cavernosum penis. The corpus spongiosum penis and corpus spongiosum glandis remain flaccid.

●》 WHAT TO DO

Priapism

- Rapid recognition of the condition and instituting immediate treatment during the acute phase increase the likelihood of success and favorable outcomes, particularly in breeding stallions.
- Suppress parasympathetic "pro-erectile" activity by the immediate administration of an antagonist of acetylcholine.
  - Benztropine mesylate (16 µg/kg IV slowly)
- Local intracorporeal treatment is performed if medical treatment is unsuccessful, or in addition to medical treatment. Inject an alpha-adrenergic agent directly into the CCP to stimulate vascular and cavernosal smooth muscle contraction.
  - If administered in the acute phase, 10 mg of 1% phenylephrine injected directly into the erect CCP may be curative.
  - In chronic cases, this treatment may only provide a temporary (4 to 6 hours) resolution of clinical signs.
- If the erection does *not* resolve within a matter of hours after starting systemic and/or local medical treatment, more aggressive therapy includes flushing the CCP to remove stagnant blood.
  - This is best performed under general anesthesia in dorsal recumbency, but it can be performed as a standing procedure.
  - Irrigate the CCP with physiological saline containing 10 units heparin/mL.
  - Infuse, under pressure, through a 12- or 14-gauge needle inserted proximal to the glans penis.
  - Allow the effluent to escape by placing a similar-sized needle(s) caudally into the CCP at the level of the ischium.
  - Flush until fresh bleeding is evident in the effluent, which is indicative of functional arterial blood flow.
  - If fresh arterial blood does *not* appear at the end of the flushing process, it may indicate the arterial supply to the corpus cavernosum has been damaged making impotence more likely.
  - Instillation of 2 to 10 mg of 1% phenylephrine into the CCP at the end of the lavage may help maintain the flaccid state.
- If erection recurs after flushing the CCP, surgery may be needed. This involves shunting blood trapped in the CCP to the CSP by performing a side-to-side anastomosis between the two cavernous spaces. For a complete description of the procedure see Pauwels et al (2005) in the online references.
- Refractory cases of priapism in geldings or nonbreeding stallions are managed by permanently retaining the penis in the preputial cavity with the Bolz procedure (i.e., phallopexy, or partial penile amputation— phallectomy).
  - Castration is recommended before either of these procedures.

Prognosis for Priapism

- Although many treatments are described for this condition, most results are inconsistent or inadequate.
- The prognosis is poor for return to normal reproductive function.
- The prognosis improves if treatment is started in the acute phase.
- Future reproductive performance is often compromised by decreased penile sensation and/or poor erectile function (i.e., impotence).

- Some stallions with compromised penile function return to breeding with proper management (See Penile Paralysis, p. 427).

Postcastration Complications

- Complications can develop at the time of the procedure or within a few hours to days following the procedure.
- These include:
  - Excessive hemorrhage
  - Evisceration
  - Postoperative swelling
  - Peritonitis
- Other complications such as hydrocele and scirrhous cord may take weeks and months to occur and are *not* emergency conditions.

Excessive Hemorrhage

- Bleeding usually originates from the testicular artery; however, rupture or laceration of the branches of the external pudendal vein can also be a source of bleeding.
- Hemorrhage is generally the result of inadequate crushing of the vessels before transecting the spermatic cord with the emasculator.

Clinical Signs

- Continuous bleeding or streaming of blood from the castration site for more than 15 minutes is excessive; minor dripping of blood from the incision for 10 to 15 minutes is considered normal.

●》 WHAT TO DO

Post-castration Complications— Excessive Hemorrhage

- Examine the scrotum and the cut end of the spermatic cord for the source of the bleeding.
- If a scrotal vessel is bleeding, clamp and ligate it.
- If the horse was castrated standing, it may be possible to find the spermatic cord and re-emasculate the cord while still locally desensitized.
- If the horse was castrated while under general anesthesia, then the horse needs to be reanesthetized to examine the spermatic cord.
  - Find the spermatic cord using long forceps in the inguinal canal; emasculate or ligate the cord proximally, or leave the hemostat forceps in place for 12 to 24 hours.
- If the cord *cannot* be found, pack the scrotum with gauze and temporarily close the scrotum with sutures; remove the gauze and sutures in 24 hours.
- If the horse has lost a significant amount of blood and/or fluids, a blood transfusion may be required before anesthesia.
- Administer broad-spectrum antimicrobials, trimethoprim sulfa 30 mg/kg PO q12h, if prolonged exploration for the transected spermatic cord was necessary.

Evisceration

- Evisceration is an uncommon complication that can occur 4 hours to 6 days after castration surgery.

- Predisposing factors include:
  - Preexisting inguinal hernia
  - An increase in abdominal pressure after surgery
- *Practice Tip: Standardbreds are predisposed to congenital inguinal hernias, and it has been suggested that these horses should be examined for the presence of a preexisting inguinal hernia before castration.*

Clinical Signs

- Small intestine or omentum is seen protruding through the castration incision.

●〉 WHAT TO DO

Post-castration Complications—Evisceration

- Prevent further prolapse, contamination, and damage of the bowel.
- If a small piece of intestine has prolapsed, lavage and replace it in the scrotum and suture the scrotum closed.
- Begin broad-spectrum antimicrobials, procaine penicillin, 20,000 IU/kg IM q12h; *or* potassium penicillin, 22,000 IU/kg IV q6h; and gentamicin, 6.6 mg/kg IV or IM q24h; and NSAIDs, flunixin meglumine, 1.1 mg/kg IV or PO q12h.
- Refer to a surgical facility immediately; if surgery is *not* an option, attempt to retract the intestine into the abdomen by transrectal palpation and taxis; however, this generally is *not* successful.
- If a large piece of intestine has prolapsed and replacement into the scrotum is *not* possible, support and protect the intestines using a large moistened towel shaped into a sling.
- Begin IV fluids to prevent hypovolemic shock. Evisceration of omentum from the castration site is less serious than intestinal prolapse. The exposed omentum should be transected as proximally as possible using an emasculator in a standing or recumbent horse. The horse should be confined to a stall for 48 hours after the procedure to prevent further omental prolapse.
- *Practice Tip: Horses should be examined for evidence of inguinal herniation before castration, especially Standardbreds and horses with congenital inguinal hernias as foals. If inguinal herniation is suspected, perform an ultrasound examination of the inguinal rings/canals and scrotum before performing the castration.*

Postoperative Swelling

- Preputial and scrotal edema can be anticipated after any castration; it is most severe 3 to 6 days after surgery.
- Excessive swelling is a common complication when there is:
  - Infection
  - Inadequate wound drainage
  - Insufficient postoperative exercise
  - Excessive surgical trauma

Clinical Signs

- Excessive preputial and/or scrotal edema
- Surgical site may be painful and hot, and the horse may be reluctant to move.

Peritonitis

- Nonseptic peritonitis is common after routine castration due to the communication that exists between the vaginal and peritoneal cavities.

●〉 WHAT TO DO

Post-castration Complications—Swelling

- Administer NSAIDs such as flunixin meglumine, 1.1 mg/kg IV or PO q12h, for pain and inflammation.
- The patient should be exercised several times each day (i.e., ridden, lunged, etc.) and turned out in a paddock to encourage exercise.
- For an incision that closes prematurely, sedate the horse and reopen the incisions wearing sterile gloves. The incisions may need to be re-opened multiple times until the swelling resolves.
- If the surgical incisions are infected, begin antimicrobials, trimethoprim sulfa, 30 mg/kg PO q12h.
- Administer cold hydrotherapy several times a day to reduce edema and swelling.

- Blood and elevated nucleated cell counts (10 to 100 million cells/μL) are commonly found in the peritoneal cavity for at least 5 days after a castration, particularly an open castration.
- Septic peritonitis is a rare complication after castration.

Clinical Signs

- Fever
- Depression
- Colic
- Tachycardia
- Diarrhea
- Reluctance to move
- Weight loss

Diagnosis

- Abdominocentesis—elevated nucleated cell count (10 to 100 million cells/μL or greater) in addition to toxic or degenerate neutrophils and intracellular bacteria
- Culture and sensitivity of a peritoneal fluid sample

●〉 WHAT TO DO

Post-castration Complications—Peritonitis

- Immediately broad-spectrum antimicrobials: procaine penicillin, 20,000 IU/kg IM q12h; or potassium penicillin, 20,000 IU/kg IV q6h; and gentamicin 6.6 mg/kg IV q24h. Adjust if necessary based on the culture and sensitivity results.
- Administer NSAIDs: flunixin meglumine, 1.1 mg/kg IV or PO q12h; this acts as an antipyretic, analgesic, and decreases inflammation.
- Fluid therapy
- Peritoneal drainage and lavage
- Ensure adequate scrotal drainage.
- Remove the spermatic cord if infected.

MARE REPRODUCTIVE EMERGENCIES

Dirk K. Vanderwall, Tamara Dobbie, and Regina M. Turner

Abortion

- When a mare aborts, it is important to determine the cause both for the well-being of the individual mare and also to rule out a contagious infectious cause that would put other mares at risk of abortion.

REPRO

- Abortions prior to 4 months of gestation often go unnoticed because of the small amount of fetal material and vulvar discharge at this stage of pregnancy.
- Fetal tissue is often found when the abortion is after 4 months of gestation, usually along with other obvious external signs the mare has aborted.
- There are a variety of causes of abortion in the mare, both infectious and noninfectious.
- Diagnosing the cause for abortion requires a complete history and submission of samples from the fetus, fetal membranes, and the mare to a diagnostic laboratory in a timely fashion.

Clinical Signs

- After 4 months of gestation:
  - May find fetus and/or fetal membranes. The fetal membranes may be retained; therefore, perform a digital examination of the mare's uterus or an ultrasonographic evaluation of the uterus per rectum. If the fetal membranes are retained, see p. 443 on retained fetal membranes.
  - Generally, there is discharge from the mare's vulva or dried matter on the perineum, tail hairs, or the inside of the hind legs.
  - The mare may be systemically ill because of the abortion etiology (e.g., equine viral arteritis) or as a consequence of abortion (e.g., retained fetal membranes).

Diagnosis

- *Practice Tip: If within driving distance of a diagnostic laboratory, submit the entire aborted fetus and fetal membranes for a full necropsy and sampling; place aborted tissues in a leak-proof container and transport chilled.*
- Alternatively, perform the examination and sampling of aborted material on the farm and submit only the necessary samples to the diagnostic laboratory.
  - Contact the diagnostic laboratory because many provide an "abortion kit" that contains the list of samples to collect, various containers to transport the samples, and packing and shipping instructions together with submission and history forms.
- History:
  - Owner's name and address; veterinarian's name and address
  - Mare history:
    ○ Identification, breeding and foaling history, vaccinations, feeding program, pertinent medical history
  - Herd history:
    ○ Number of mares on the farm (pregnant and nonpregnant and resident and nonresident)
    ○ Number of other horses on the farm (i.e., stallions, pleasure horses, foals, etc.)
    ○ Other nonequine species on the farm
    ○ Number of previous abortions and the stage of gestation at which they occurred
    ○ Any foal illnesses/problems from previous foalings

- Fetal membranes—placenta:
  - Weigh the fetal membranes and check for completeness.
  - Measure the length of the umbilical cord.
  - Examine the membranes and record any abnormalities (photos of lesions/abnormal areas help the pathologist).
  - Collect tissue samples: <1 cm thickness for histopathology — cervical star, body, pregnant horn, nonpregnant horn, umbilical cord, amnion, and any gross lesions.
  - Label the samples and place in 10% buffered formalin.
  - Obtain 3 more samples (2 × 3 inches; 5 × 7.5 cm) from different parts of the placenta for bacteriology/virology and place in a labeled, sterile ziplock bag (include samples from abnormal areas).
- Fetus:
  - Weigh the fetus and measure the crown-rump length.
  - Examine the fetus for obvious congenital abnormalities and any internal lesions/abnormalities.
  - Collect the following fresh samples in labeled sterile ziplock bags for bacteriology/virology: lung, liver, spleen, thymus, adrenal (entire organ), kidney (entire organ), stomach contents (3 to 5 mL in a red-top blood collection tube), fetal heart blood (3 to 10 mL in a red-top blood collection tube).
  - Collect the following samples for histopathology and place in 10% buffered formalin: liver, lung, kidney, other adrenal gland, heart, thymus, spleen, small intestine, brain, and any other tissue believed important to the case based on the history and exam.
- Mare:
  - If mare shows systemic signs of illness, perform a complete physical examination and appropriate diagnostic evaluation (complete blood count [CBC], blood chemistry, etc.)
  - Collect a red-top and purple-top (ethylenediaminetetraacetic acid [EDTA]) blood collection tubes for assessment of antibody titers acute (time 0) and convalescent (2 weeks later).
  - Obtain an endometrial swab for aerobic culture.
- Ensure all specimens are sealed and double bagged to prevent content leakage.
- Fresh samples and blood collection tubes require ice packs for shipment.
- Send labeled samples via overnight shipping to the diagnostic laboratory with complete history and examination findings.

⦿〉 WHAT TO DO

Abortion
Treatment
- Mares with retained fetal membranes require prompt treatment (see p. 443) as do mares showing signs of systemic illness for other reasons related to the abortion.

- An "abortion" mare should be isolated from other pregnant mares until contagious causes of abortion have been ruled-out (i.e., EHV-1, EAV).
- Clean and disinfect the area where the abortion occurred.

Aftercare
- Once a diagnosis is made, steps to take:
  - Prevent an abortion storm (i.e., EHV-1); at-risk mares can receive booster vaccination.
  - Institute new protocols to prevent future abortions (i.e., vaccination for EHV-1 and EVA and careful ultrasonographic monitoring of mares with placentitis).
  - Consider assisted reproduction technologies—embryo transfer, oocyte transfer—to acquire pregnancies from mares that habitually abort (i.e., mares with placental insufficiency).
    - Ensure the selected "technology" is accepted for breed registry.

Vaginal Bleeding

- Vaginal bleeding is a fairly common problem in the mare.
- Vaginal bleeding can occur from a vaginal laceration or perforation following natural breeding.
- Mares may bleed from the vagina after foaling as a result of trauma to the reproductive tract.
- Older, multiparous mares often develop vaginal varicosities that bleed intermittently during late gestation.
  - Nonpregnant mares can occasionally develop varicosities.

Clinical Signs
- Mares with a vaginal laceration/perforation typically have a bloody discharge following natural service; mares can develop peritonitis and rarely vaginal or perirectal abscesses. Mares with perirectal and vaginal abscessation may strain to defecate or colic, respectively; mares with peritonitis are generally depressed and mildly uncomfortable.
- Vaginal varicosities can produce a small amount of blood infrequently to more significant amounts of blood persistently; blood clots can be found in the stall or dried blood may be attached to the tail hairs, perineum, or hind limbs.
- Rupture of vaginal vessels and tissue during foaling can cause minor to profuse bleeding.

Diagnosis
- Vaginal speculum examination:
  - Breeding lacerations are typically located in the vaginal fornix dorsal and lateral to the cervix.
  - Vaginal varicosities are generally located at the vestibulovaginal ring (on the cranial vestibular fold and the dorsal, caudal vaginal wall).
- Endoscopic examination:
  - Endoscopy may be required to see vaginal varicosities given their cranial and dorsal location; visualize the cervix and then retroflex the endoscope 180 degrees to view the cranial aspect of the vestibulovaginal ring.
  - Endoscopy may be helpful in identifying the source of postpartum hemorrhage.

- Digital vaginal examination:
  - Digital examination helps determine whether vaginal perforation has occurred following natural breeding.
- Abdominocentesis:
  - Recommended in cases of vaginal perforation
  - Septic peritonitis (see p. 219), or rarely, seminoperitoneum can occur
    - Seminoperitoneum refers to sperm in the peritoneal cavity; the reaction to the foreign protein (sperm) typically creates a nonseptic peritonitis; the sperm are found free in the peritoneal fluid or phagocytosed within leukocytes.

⊙❯ WHAT TO DO

Vaginal Bleeding
- Vaginal laceration/perforation:
  - Vaginal laceration without perforation:
    - Begin oral broad-spectrum antimicrobials, trimethoprim/sulfa, 30 mg/kg PO q12h.
    - Ensure mare is current on tetanus toxoid prophylaxis.
    - Do *not* rebreed the mare by natural cover during the current estrous cycle.
    - Use a "breeding roll" to avoid vaginal laceration/perforation.
    - Breeding rolls are recommended for:
      - A stallion with a long penis
      - Mares of small stature
      - An aggressive breeding stallion
  - Vaginal laceration with perforation:
    - These lacerations are rarely amenable to repair; therefore, allow to heal by second intention.
    - Begin broad-spectrum antimicrobials: potassium penicillin, 22,000 IU/kg IV q6h; or procaine penicillin, 22,000 IU/kg IM q12h with gentamicin, 6.6 mg/kg IV/IM q24h.
    - Start intravenous fluids if the clinical picture indicates their use is warranted.
    - Give flunixin meglumine (0.5 to 1 mg/kg IV/PO q12h) if the mare is straining or febrile.
    - If intestine has herniated through the vaginal perforation, rinse bowel with sterile saline and replace in the abdomen.
    - Place a Caslick's suture to prevent aspiration of air into the abdominal cavity.
    - If peritonitis is severe or bowel has entered the vagina, transfer to a referral center as quickly as possible for surgery and/or peritoneal lavage; if surgery is *not* an option or the peritonitis is *not* severe, the mare should be cross-tied for several days to reduce the risk of intestinal evisceration.
    - Mares should *not* be rebred until the following breeding season.
- Vaginal varicosity:
  - Often, *no* treatment is needed because the vessels regress and the bleeding stops once the mare foals.
  - If the bleeding is excessive or constant or the owners are concerned, the vessels can be ligated, cauterized, surgically resected, or hemorrhoid cream can be applied topically; transendoscopic laser photocoagulation is another option for the treatment of vaginal varicosities.
- Vaginal bleeding after foaling:
  - Most vaginal hemorrhage following foaling is *not* life threatening and seldom requires treatment.

- Profuse bleeding requires that the vessels be identified and ligated, if possible.
- If the source of bleeding cannot be identified, then the vaginal cavity can be packed with a large tampon made of rolled cotton, stockinette, and umbilical tape; cover the tampon with petroleum jelly and oily antibiotics, and leave in place for 24 to 48 hours.
- Minor vaginal lacerations heal by second intention.
- Significant lacerations should be sutured if possible.
- Mares with deep lacerations should be given broad-spectrum antimicrobials (trimethoprim/sulfa, 30 mg/kg PO q12h) and lavaged with dilute povidone-iodine solution (2%) to prevent abscess formation.
  - Mares with significant vaginal trauma may form vaginal adhesions; daily application of a topical antimicrobial ointment containing steroid (Animax[5]) may help prevent adhesion formation.
  - Large vaginal hematomas may form, making it difficult and painful for the mare to defecate; feed mares a laxative diet until the hematoma diminishes in size. Administer broad-spectrum antimicrobials (trimethoprim sulfa, 30 mg/kg PO q12h), NSAIDs (phenylbutazone, 2.2 mg/kg PO q12h or flunixin meglumine, 0.5 to 1.1 mg/kg PO/IV q12h) to alleviate pain, and tetanus toxoid prophylaxis.

Premature Placental Separation

- Normally, the chorioallantois separates from the uterus following the delivery of the fetus; however, occasionally the chorioallantois separates from uterus before the fetus is delivered.
- Premature placental separation occurs most commonly at birth; however, the condition is also seen in mid- to late gestation.
- There is a higher incidence of premature placental separation with induced deliveries and in mares suffering from mare reproductive loss syndrome (MRLS).
- Premature placental separation during delivery is an emergency situation because gas exchange is impaired between the dam and the fetus, so the fetus begins to suffer the effects of hypoxia.
- Similarly, large areas of separation between the placenta and uterus earlier in gestation also impair nutrient and oxygen exchange and often result in the birth of an abnormal foal.

Clinical Signs
- At birth:
  - The unruptured chorioallantoic membrane protrudes through the mare's vulvar lips; the cervical star is seen as a white shiny area, resembling a starburst in the center of the red, velvetlike surface of the chorion ("red bag").
- During gestation:
  - Signs may be similar to a mare with placentitis (i.e., premature udder development +/− premature lactation,

vulvar discharge); often mares present with hemorrhagic vulvar discharge only.
- Occasionally mares show no external signs of premature placental separation.

Diagnosis
- At birth:
  - Characteristic appearance of the unruptured chorioallantois; termed "red bag"
- During gestation:
  - Ultrasonographic evaluation of the uterus rectally and transabdominally:
    - Ultrasonographic examination reveals an area, or areas, of separation between the chorioallantois and uterus.
    - Often the chorioallantois takes on a "ribbon candy" appearance ultrasonographically.
    - Some of these mares may also have concurrent placentitis and the areas of separated chorioallantois may be thickened.

●› WHAT TO DO

Premature Placental Separation
Treatment
- At birth:
  - Immediately rupture the chorioallantois and deliver the fetus as quickly as possible.
  - The fetus is likely compromised, so resuscitation may be required to save the foal (see Chapter 29, p. 509).
- During gestation:
  - For premature placental separation without evidence of placentitis: Treat mare with 0.088 mg/kg altrenogest PO q24h; monitor pregnancy carefully for evidence of fetal death and discontinue altrenogest if fetal death occurs.
  - Premature placental separation with evidence of placentitis (see Chapter 27, p. 499, and Chapter 30, p. 522).

Outcome
- Foals born following premature placental separation often suffer from hypoxic-ischemic encephalopathy.

Hydrops of the Fetal Membranes
- *Definition:* Excessive accumulation of fluid (hydrops) in either the amniotic (hydramnios or hydrops amniosis) or allantoic (hydrallantois or hydrops allantois) cavity that occurs in late gestation (>7 months).
  - Hydrops allantois is generally the form that occurs in mares.
- If untreated, complications include:
  - Ventral rupture of the prepubic tendon and/or body wall
  - Uterine rupture

Clinical Signs
- Profound abdominal distention that leads to:
  - Difficulty walking and/or getting up/down
  - Dyspnea
  - Abdominal discomfort

---
[5]Dechra Veterinary Products, Overland Park, Kansas.

- Prolonged recumbency
- Ventral edema

Diagnosis

- Palpation per rectum reveals an enlarged/distended uterus that is typically "domed" dorsally, and inability to palpate/ballotté the fetus.
- Transrectal and/or transabdominal ultrasonography reveals excessive fluid accumulation around the fetus.

●❯ WHAT TO DO

Hydrops of the Fetal Membranes

- Plans should be made to induce abortion as soon as the diagnosis is confirmed because attempts to medically manage a mare with hydrops to the point that there is a chance of fetal viability may result in a catastrophic outcome, such as complete ventral or uterine rupture.
- If there is evidence of prepubic tendon/body wall compromise, a circumferential belly bandage should be applied to provide support.
- Before inducing abortion, place a large-bore IV catheter (ideally bilaterally) and begin fluid therapy in an effort to prevent cardiovascular collapse due to changing hemodynamics associated with removal of a very large volume of uterine fluid. Hypertonic saline 4 mL/kg should be administered IV if the mare develops cardiovascular shock!
- Procedure to induce abortion:
  - Wrap the tail, cleanse the perineum and then carefully manually dilate the cervix enough to allow passage of a 24F to 32F sharp thoracic trocar catheter through the cervix and puncture the chorioallantois.
  - If available, a balloon-tipped embryo transfer/uterine lavage catheter is passed into the chorioallantoic cavity after which the balloon is inflated, allowing it to remain in place without manual assistance (Fig. 24-9). If a balloon-tipped catheter is *not* available, an appropriately sized catheter/tubing can be introduced into the allantoic cavity and held in place manually.
  - Slowly drain the fluid over several hours thus allowing time for hemodynamic "adjustment" by the mare.

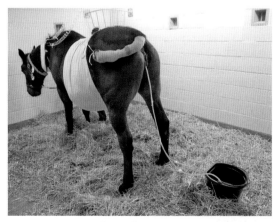

Figure 24-9 Mare with hydrops allantois being treated using a balloon-tipped embryo transfer/uterine lavage catheter passed transcervically into the chorioallantoic cavity allowing slow removal of the excessive fluid over the course of several hours (note tubing clamps that allow regulation of flow rate). If a balloon-tipped catheter is not available, a suitable catheter can be held in place manually.

- After the majority of the fluid is removed, manually dilate the cervix in preparation for assisted delivery of the fetus.
- Deliver the fetus using standard obstetrical procedures.
  - The fetus generally is alive, so be prepared for humane destruction of the fetus.
- Almost invariably, the fetal membranes are retained.
  - Since the uterus may *not* be responsive to oxytocin, cloprostenol (250 µg IM q6 to 12h) may be administered to stimulate uterine contractility in an effort to hasten passage of the fetal membranes.
- Monitor the mare closely for several days to assess passage of the fetal membranes, degree of uterine involution, accumulation of intrauterine fluid, development of metritis, etc.
  - If problems are identified, institute appropriate therapy.

Prognosis for Systemic Recovery

- Prognosis for complete recovery is generally good, particularly if no severe sequelae develop, such as ventral rupture or metritis/laminitis.

Prognosis for Future Fertility

- The prognosis for future fertility is influenced by the degree/completeness of uterine involution and/or whether any lasting damage to the reproductive tract has occurred (e.g., cervical trauma/tearing).
  - A complete breeding soundness examination is recommended before breeding.
- Mares in which ventral rupture has occurred may be at risk for recurrence of the problem in subsequent (normal) pregnancies, and accordingly, should be considered "high-risk" mares in the future.
  - If breed association rules allow embryo transfer, these mares can serve as embryo donors, obviating the need for them to carry a pregnancy to term.

Ventral Rupture

- Ventral rupture includes rupture of the prepubic tendon and/or abdominal muscles.
- These conditions can occur together, have the same predisposing causes, and have similar or identical clinical presentations.
- Ventral rupture tends to occur in older mares of any breed although draft breeds may be more predisposed.
  - Excessive uterine weight associated with hydrops and possibly twins is the most common predisposing factor; however, ventral rupture can occur in a seemingly normal pregnancy.

Clinical Signs

- Mares with ventral rupture are typically close to foaling and present with abdominal pain and reluctance to walk.
  - Mares with hydrops may develop signs any time between 7 months and term.
- A markedly thickened plaque of ventral edema is very sensitive to digital pressure in the area(s) of tissue trauma/damage.
- When the prepubic tendon ruptures, the tuber ischii become elevated and the udder moves cranially.

Diagnosis

- Transcutaneous ultrasonography is used to identify defects in the abdominal musculature and/or prepubic tendon.
  - Transabdominal ultrasonography is also used to assess if twin pregnancy is a contributing factor.
- Palpation and ultrasonography per rectum should be performed to determine whether hydrops of the fetal membranes is a contributing factor (see p. 437).

●› WHAT TO DO

Ventral Rupture

- Apply a circumferential belly bandage to provide abdominal support.
- If the mare is close to or at term, consider induction of parturition.
- Administer oxytocin, 20 to 40 IU IM, 2.5 to 10 IU IV, repeated q15 to 20min until delivery; or 40 to 80 IU IV in 1L of crystalloid over 30 to 60 min for 450 kg mare. (See p. 424 Edition 3 and companion website for complete details on Induction of Parturition.)
  - Be prepared to assist delivery of the fetus because the mare will not be able to develop normal intraabdominal pressure during delivery.
- If ventral rupture is associated with hydrops, termination of the pregnancy is indicated (see p. 437).

Prognosis for Systemic Recovery

- When recognized early and treated appropriately, ventral ruptures do *not* usually affect the life of the mare unless she is bred to carry a pregnancy to term again in the future, because of the risk of recurrence.
- Repair of ventral defects is described and is usually delayed for approximately 2 months after foaling to allow time for the edema to subside and the tissue margins of the defect to repair/remodel.

Prognosis for Future Fertility

- As noted above, because of the risk of recurrence in future pregnancies, if breed association rules allow embryo transfer, these mares should be considered for use as embryo donors, so they don't have to carry a pregnancy to term.
  - If that is *not* possible, these mares should be treated as "high-risk" mares in future pregnancies.

Uterine Torsion

- Uterine torsion generally occurs in the last trimester of gestation, 8 months to term; however, it can occur as early as 5 months of gestation.
- Degree of torsion can vary from 180 to 540 degrees in a clockwise or counterclockwise direction as viewed from the rear.
  - Clockwise = torsion to the "right"
  - Counterclockwise = torsion to the "left"
- There is no breed or age predilection.

Clinical Signs

- Low-grade, mild, or severe signs of colic are typically commensurate with the degree of rotation; more severe signs are associated with greater degree of rotation.

Diagnosis

- Definitive diagnosis is based on identification per rectum of asymmetrically taut broad ligaments with the broad ligament on the side of rotation "diving" ventrally under the uterus, while the contralateral broad ligament crosses tightly over the uterus in the direction of rotation.
  - Clockwise torsion: right broad ligament is drawn sharply ventrally under the uterus, while the left broad ligament is drawn tightly over the uterus from left to right.
  - Counterclockwise torsion: left broad ligament is drawn sharply ventrally under the uterus, while the right broad ligament is drawn tightly over the uterus from right to left.
- Uterine torsion in mares generally occurs cranial to the cervix, so a manual or vaginal speculum examination is generally unrewarding and is contraindicated in affected mares that are preterm in order to avoid contamination of the vagina/cervix.
  - However, a vaginal examination may be warranted in mares that are affected at term in order to assess the status of cervical opening and potentially correct the torsion as noted later.

●› WHAT TO DO

Uterine Torsion
Treatment

- When diagnosed at term, it may be possible to correct the torsion manually per vaginum by passing a hand/arm through the cervical canal and derotating the fetus.
  - This is only possible with torsions <270 degrees.
  - Keep the mare standing.
  - Use minimal sedation/tranquilization with epidural anesthesia (see p. 8) to minimize straining.
  - If the fetal membranes are intact, they should be ruptured to release fluid and reduce the size and weight of the uterus and its contents.
  - If possible, elevate the mare's hindquarters to help pull the uterus and gastrointestinal tract cranially.
  - Pass a hand/arm through the cervix and grasp a "substantial" part of the fetus (e.g., upper limb or trunk) and then rock the fetus back and forth to gain momentum and then with one concerted effort attempt to correct the torsion by swinging the fetus in the direction opposite to the torsion.
  - Depending upon the degree of initial rotation, a second attempt at correction may be necessary.
  - After correction, the mare should spontaneously begin second stage labor; however, labor may be delayed because of decreased uterine contractility caused by edema and/or vascular congestion.
  - If necessary, induce parturition with 10 to 20 IU oxytocin IM and repeat every 15 to 20 minutes as needed.
  - Approximately 80% of uterine torsions at term are corrected by this technique.
- Rolling with a "plank in the flank":
  - Rolling can be performed preterm, but avoid rolling at term because of the potential for greater risk of uterine rupture.
  - Induce general anesthesia (see Chapter 47) and place the mare in lateral recumbency on the side to which the torsion is directed.

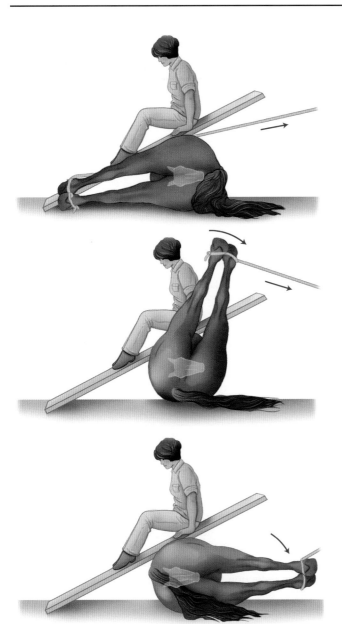

Figure 24-10   Rolling a mare with "a plank in the flank" to correct a uterine torsion.

- ◦ Clockwise = right side
- ◦ Counterclockwise = left side
- Place a board (3 to 4 meters long and 20 to 30 cm wide) across the mare's upper paralumbar fossa (Fig. 24-10).
- Have an assistant kneel on the board to stabilize it and exert pressure on the uterus/fetus.
- Roll the mare slowly (to avoid uterine rupture) to the opposite side.
- Assess progress after rolling with examination per rectum (may be difficult while mare is recumbent).
- Repeat as needed to fully correct torsion.
- Surgical correction via standing flank laparotomy (preterm):
  - Using standard procedures (see p. 217), prepare the mare for aseptic standing flank surgery on the side toward which the torsion has occurred.
    - ◦ Clockwise = right
    - ◦ Counterclockwise = left

- Once the abdomen has been entered, gently lift and rotate the gravid uterus back into normal position.
  - ◦ Depending on the degree of initial rotation, a second correction may be necessary.
- Although a uterine torsion can be corrected under general anesthesia using a ventral midline approach, it is *not* generally considered a "field" procedure.

Prognosis for Survival
- Mare survival—total = 84%
  - ≥320 days 65%
  - <320 days 97%
  - Method of correction does *not* affect mare survival.
- Foal survival—total = 56%
  - ≥320 days 32%
  - <320 days 72%
  - Method of correction does affect foal survival when the torsion occurs <320 days: Foal survival is significantly higher with standing flank laparotomy vs. ventral midline laparotomy.

Prognosis for Future Fertility
- The prognosis for the mare to successfully carry another pregnancy is good.
- Prognosis worsens with any of the following:
  - Cesarean section
  - Uterine rupture
  - More extreme degree of torsion and/or delay in diagnosis and management

Complications
- Premature placental separation resulting in fetal compromise (see p. 436).
- Necrosis and/or rupture of the uterine wall
- Peritonitis
- Endotoxic shock
- Recurrence of torsion, particularly if complete correction is *not* achieved

Terminal Cesarean Section
Indications
- A dystocia that cannot be relieved in which the foal is alive and more valuable than the mare (i.e., embryo recipient mare)
- A mare with an incurable illness that requires a C-section
- If humane destruction is imminent following the delivery of the foal
- In the case of a mare diagnosed with a surgical colic that is at or past her due date, if the owner is unable or unwilling to send the mare for surgery but is willing to try to save the foal.

How to Diagnose Fetal Viability
- Voluntary movement; withdrawal of a limb; corneal reflex; suckle reflex; anal reflex; pulses; heartbeat

REPRO

REPRO

Procedure

- Be prepared to resuscitate the foal after delivery.
- Place an intravenous catheter in the mare's jugular vein.
- Sedate the mare with xylazine, 1.1 mg/kg IV.
- Anesthetize the mare with ketamine, 2.2 mg/kg IV.
- Once the mare is in lateral recumbency, quickly enter the mare's abdomen through a low flank incision.
  - The surgical site does *not* require clipping or surgical preparation.
- Incise the uterus and quickly remove the fetus.
  - Be careful *not* to injure the fetus.
- Clamp the foal's umbilicus.
- Perform humane destruction of the mare.
- Resuscitate the foal (see Chapter 29, p. 509).

Uterine Prolapse/Uterine Horn Intussusception

- Uterine prolapse is an uncommon, life-threatening event that can occur following and/or in association with normal parturition, dystocia, retained fetal membranes, or mid- to late-term abortion. On very rare occasion prolapse of the cervix may occur.
- Uterine prolapse is a true emergency because continued prolapse may lead to permanent damage to the uterus and the potential rupture of uterine blood vessels.

Clinical Signs

- Protrusion of purplish to red (endometrial surface) mass of uterine tissue through the vulva
- Cases of partial prolapse or intussusception of the tip of a uterine horn may be more difficult to identify
  - In these cases, persistent tenesmus, restlessness, colic, and tachycardia may be present.

Diagnosis

- In cases of complete prolapse, the diagnosis is apparent on physical examination.
- In cases of partial prolapse and/or uterine horn intussusception, palpation per vaginum may provide a direct manual diagnosis, or transrectal palpation/ultrasonography may allow manual/visual identification of the intussuscepted uterine horn.

●❯ WHAT TO DO

Uterine Prolapse/Uterine Horn Intussusception

- Prompt resolution is important to minimize complications such as severe bleeding from the uterine blood vessels.
  - As soon as possible, the prolapsed tissue should be supported using any available material, such as a clean sheet or tray that is held at the level of the pelvic brim by two assistants.
- Epidural anesthesia (see Chapter 2, p. 8) combined with IV analgesia and sedation is administered to minimize straining before replacement is attempted.
- The everted tissue should be gently cleansed with sterile saline and/or dilute povidone solution, and it should be carefully palpated to determine if the bladder and/or portions of the gastrointestinal tract are present.

- Placement of a urinary catheter may be needed before replacement of a prolapsed bladder.
- The prolapsed uterus should be carefully examined for lacerations and to assess the overall condition of the tissue.
  - If lacerations are identified, they should be closed with absorbable suture.
- In cases where the fetal membranes are retained, it is common to find the retained portion of the membranes firmly attached to the area of the uterus that is prolapsing (i.e., the weight of the membranes likely contributes to the problem).
  - If membranes are present, gently attempt to remove them; however, if they cannot be removed, the membranes are trimmed before replacement of the uterus to reduce tension on the tissue.
- The uterus is replaced in its normal position using the flat of the hand beginning with the most caudal area and proceeding to the more cranial areas.
  - Care should be taken to ensure the uterine horns are completely everted, otherwise even small remaining intussusceptions result in renewed straining (after epidural anesthesia subsides) and the potential for re-prolapse of the uterus.
  - The rounded end of a sterile disposable vaginal speculum or glass bottle works well as an arm extension to ensure complete replacement of the tips of the horns.
- Once the uterus is completely replaced, oxytocin should be administered, 10 to 20 IU IV, to increase uterine tone.
- Broad-spectrum antibiotics and NSAIDs are generally administered, and additional supportive therapy is given if needed (e.g., IV fluids).
- Large-volume (3 to 12 liters total) sterile saline lavage is performed to aid removal of contaminants and fully expand the uterus to ensure all parts are returned to their normal positions.

Prognosis for Systemic Recovery

- The prognosis for survival is good if there are *no* tears in the uterus, and the uterine arteries have *not* been injured.
- Most mares that survive the initial prolapse and subsequent reduction of the prolapse have a normal recovery.
- Mares that die are almost exclusively those with tears of the uterine arteries.

Prognosis for Future Fertility

- Prognosis generally is very good, particularly in cases where replacement is rapid and trauma to the uterus is minimal.
- There are conflicting data on whether mares are or are not at greater risk for uterine prolapse in subsequent pregnancies.

Periparturient Hemorrhage

- Most cases of periparturient hemorrhage occur during or immediately after parturition; however, occasionally bleeding can occur in mid- to late gestation or several days after a delivery.
- Generally, the middle uterine artery ruptures and bleeds; however, other blood vessels including the external iliacs, utero-ovarian artery, pudendal artery, and vaginal artery can also rupture.
- Mares can bleed into the peritoneal cavity, broad ligament, serosal layer of the uterus, or lumen of the uterus.

- The outcome of a bleed is generally dependent on the site of bleeding, with bleeding into the peritoneal cavity carrying a poorer prognosis.
- Older, multiparous mares are predisposed to periparturient bleeds; however, mares of any age and parity can develop the condition.

Clinical Signs

- Lethargy, acute abdominal pain (pawing, rolling, discomfort), cold sweat, upward lip curl (i.e., Flehman response), tachycardia, tachypnea, pale mucous membranes, prolonged capillary refill time, muscle fasciculations, depression, weakness, ataxia, occasional vocalization, and +/− bloody vulvar discharge
- Some mares may show *no* signs of bleeding before peracute death.
- Clinical signs are more severe and physical findings are more abnormal when there is bleeding into the peritoneal cavity versus bleeding into a confined space such as the broad ligament.
- *Practice Tip: Mares with periparturient hemorrhage often have an upward lip curl, or Flehman response.*

Diagnosis

- Mares are painful and anxious; therefore, sedation and analgesics are generally necessary before proceeding with any diagnostics (Table 24-1)
- *Practice Tip: Avoid the use of acepromazine if the mare is believed to be hypotensive because of its potential to exacerbate the hypovolemia.*
- Physical examination:
  - Perform a complete physical examination paying particular attention to the color of the mucous membranes; capillary refill time; warmth of the ears; character of the pulse; evidence of a cold sweat over the lateral neck, dorsal thorax, or legs; auscultate the heart for rate, rhythm, and murmurs; evaluate the mare's temperature.

Table 24-1	Treatment Options for Analgesia and Sedation in Mares with Periparturient Hemorrhage	
	Dose	Method of Administration
Analgesics		
Flunixin meglumine	1.1 mg/kg	IV
Naloxone	8-32 mg	IV
Butorphanol tartrate	0.02 mg/kg (10 mg/500 kg)	IV
Sedatives		
Xylazine	0.25-1 mg/kg	IV or IM
Detomidine	0.01-0.04 mg/kg	IV or IM
Butorphanol tartrate	0.02 mg/kg (10 mg/500 kg)	IV

- Mucous membranes may be normal color in the acute phase.
- Clinical signs and physical examination findings are often highly suggestive of periparturient bleeding; therefore, a clinician may choose to begin treatment without pursuing a diagnostic workup.
- Mares with periparturient bleeding need to be stabilized immediately.
- Recommend an initial complete blood count and biochemistry profile to monitor the degree of anemia, hypoproteinemia, and azotemia.
- Diagnostic procedures may be stressful to the mare and may result in a rise in blood pressure and disruption of blood clot formation.
- Palpation/ultrasonography per rectum:
  - Perform with caution or avoid procedure altogether because it may dislodge a hematoma in the broad ligament and begin bleeding again.
  - In a recent retrospective study examining periparturient bleeding in mares, palpation per rectum was *not* significantly associated with an adverse outcome.
  - Palpation per rectum is useful in identifying the presence and size of a hematoma in the broad ligament or wall of the uterus; transrectal ultrasonography can confirm the diagnosis.
  - Transrectal ultrasonography can identify blood in the abdomen or within the lumen of the uterus.
  - Blood appears as hyperechoic particles swirling within anechoic fluid.
- Vaginal examination:
  - Vaginal speculum examination may identify uterine bleeding.
- Transabdominal ultrasonography:
  - Scan the ventral abdomen for evidence of blood within the peritoneal cavity.
  - Use a 3.5- to 5.0-mHz transducer.
  - Use liberal amounts of alcohol to obtain a diagnostic image; otherwise clip small areas of hair from the mare's ventral abdomen.
  - If the mare is quiet, comfortable, and cooperative, it is possible to visualize the uterus and broad ligaments from the ventral abdomen and diagnose broad ligament hematomas.
- Abdominocentesis:
  - Identify a fluid pocket in the ventral abdomen using ultrasonography and then obtain a sample of the fluid by abdominocentesis.
  - A fluid sample with the following characteristics is diagnostic of peritoneal hemorrhage: red fluid that does *not* clot; a packed cell volume (PCV) in the range of 8% to 20%; absence of platelets; +/− erythrophagocytosis.
- CBC and biochemistry profile:
  - Initially PCV and total protein (TP) are normal to mildly low or slightly elevated.
  - A drop in PCV and TP occurs over the next several days.

- Continue to monitor CBC and biochemistry to help direct treatment.
- Blood lactate should be closely monitored as a guide for a blood transfusion.

WHAT TO DO

Periparturient Hemorrhage
- Place the mare in a stall and keep her quiet and calm.
- Avoid removing the foal from the stall unless the mare is so violent that the foal is in danger of injury.
  - Separating the foal from the mare increases her anxiety and her blood pressure and may start bleeding and/or decrease clot formation.
- Control the mare's pain and anxiety.
  - Pain control can be achieved using flunixin meglumine, butorphanol tartrate, or naloxone.
  - Naloxone appears to provide analgesia; however, it does *not* appear to reverse hypotension in the actively bleeding mare.
  - Control the mare's anxiety with α_2-agonists (xylazine or detomidine) or butorphanol tartrate alone.
  - *Avoid acepromazine if the mare appears to be hypotensive.*
- Place an intravenous catheter.
- Begin hemostatic treatment:
  - Aminocaproic acid: Inhibits fibrinolysis and therefore stabilizes clot formation.
    - Initially give 20 g/500 kg (40 mg/kg) aminocaproic acid diluted in 1 L of isotonic fluids administered over 20 minutes intravenously.
    - A reduced dose of 5 to 10 g/500 kg (10 to 20 mg/kg) aminocaproic acid diluted in 1 L of saline can be repeated every 6 hours IV.
  - Yunnan Baiyou: A Chinese herb that has shown some efficacy in controlling hemorrhage in human patients.
    - Unsure of the exact mechanism of action, but it decreases template bleeding times and activated clotting times in anesthetized ponies.
    - Dissolve 16 capsules or 4 g (8 mg/kg) in 20 mL of lukewarm water and administer orally every 6 hours for 3 to 4 days.
  - Naloxone: A pure opioid antagonist
    - The drug has *not* improved hypotension during episodes of hemorrhagic shock in dogs.
    - Naloxone appears to relieve anxiety and provide analgesia to mares that are actively bleeding.
    - Administer 8 to 32 mg diluted in 500 mL of saline intravenously.
    - Mares should *not* receive naloxone following butorphanol tartrate administration because of the antagonistic actions of the two drugs.
  - Formalin: Used to treat severe bleeding in horses
    - Recent studies have been unable to show formalin is effective at improving hemostasis and therefore its use is questionable.
    - The dose currently recommended is 30 to 150 mL of 10% buffered formalin diluted in 1 L of isotonic fluids administered intravenously.
- Fluid therapy
  - Rapid volume expansion: If the mare's condition is deteriorating, then rapid volume expansion may be warranted; however, caution should be exercised.
    - A rapid rise in blood pressure could disrupt the clot and make the bleeding worse.
    - Hypertonic saline, 2 L/500 kg (2 to 4 mL/kg) IV bolus
    - Isotonic fluids, 10 to 20 L/500 kg bolused rapidly IV
  - Maintenance fluids: Fluid therapy may be warranted in large uterine artery bleeds in order to maintain adequate perfusion to the vital organs.
    - In less severe, contained bleeds, their use is *not* necessary provided the mare is eating and drinking.
    - Fluid amounts required to maintain perfusion: Isotonic fluids, 24 L/500 kg/day or 2 mL/kg/h
  - Blood products are reserved for those mares with severe, persistent hemorrhage with clinical and laboratory signs of deterioration.
    - Includes whole blood and plasma and best given in a hospital setting.
- ***Practice Tip:*** Do not *use hetastarch for volume expansion because of its negative effects on coagulation.*
- Corticosteroids: Consider corticosteroids if there is evidence of severe cardiovascular compromise.
- Antibiotics can be administered for large, contained hematomas to help prevent abscessation.
- Conjugated estrogen .05 to .1 mg/kg IV q4 to 8h may inhibit uterine hemorrhage.

Response to Treatment
- Mares that stabilize have a decrease in heart rate, stronger peripheral pulses, improvement in mucous membrane color, warming of the extremities, and become less anxious.
- Mares generally stabilize within 60 minutes of starting treatment.
- Mares that fail to respond to treatment may continue to deteriorate and may eventually die.
- Mares with uterine artery bleeding are best managed on the farm.
  - Moving mares may exacerbate the bleeding and worsen their prognosis.
  - Rapid and aggressive treatment should begin immediately on the farm.
  - Transfer to a referral center, if necessary, can occur once the mare is stabilized.

Aftercare
- Mares should be confined to a quiet stall for a minimum of 2 weeks.
- If the owner wants to rebreed the mare, perform a transrectal examination/ultrasonography at 30 days postpartum.

WHAT NOT TO DO

Periparturient Hemorrhage
- Do *not* rebreed the mare until the hematoma is well organized and consolidated.
  - Owners should consider giving the mare the entire breeding season off.

Future Reproductive Potential
- Mares remain fertile following uterine artery bleeds.
- A recent retrospective study found that 49% of mares produced a foal after recovery.

- Owners should be warned that mares who experience periparturient bleeding are at higher risk for subsequent bleeds during pregnancy.

Retained Fetal Membranes (RFM)

- Fetal membranes are defined as retained if they are not passed in their entirety within 3 hours of completion of second stage labor (i.e., delivery of the fetus).
  - The overall incidence of RFM is approximately 10%.
  - Incidence of RFM is increased after dystocia and some breeds (e.g., Friesian) seem to have a much higher incidence of RFM.
  - Fetal membranes are often retained after mid- to late-term abortion, particularly if elective abortion is performed.
- Complications arising from RFM include metritis, endotoxemia, and laminitis, which can be life-threatening.
  - ***Practice Tip:*** *The goal is to identify RFM early and begin therapy to both encourage passage of the membranes and prevent the development of secondary complications.*

Clinical Signs

- Initially, there are *no* clinical signs other than the presence of the membranes protruding from the vulva (when the membranes are retained in their entirety).
- With an increased duration of retention of fetal membranes, whether complete or partial, the likelihood of systemic signs of illness increases, which typically reflects evidence of endotoxemia:
  - Fever
  - Tachycardia/tachypnea
  - Dull/depressed attitude
  - Toxic/injected mucous membranes
  - Inappetence
  - Laminitis

Diagnosis

- If the fetal membranes are retained in their entirety, the diagnosis of RFM is readily apparent on physical examination, based on the presence of membranes protruding from the vulva.
- In contrast, if the fetal membranes have torn, smaller remnants of the membranes may be retained that are *not* evident externally.
  - To aid a presumptive diagnosis of partially retained membranes in a mare who has apparently passed the fetal membranes, gross examination of the membranes should be performed (if available) in order to determine if they were passed in their entirety.
    - ***Practice Tip:*** *The most common site of partial fetal membrane retention is the tip of the nonpregnant horn; therefore, lacerations or holes in this part of the tissue should heighten suspicion of potential partial membrane retention.*
- Palpation and ultrasonography of the reproductive tract per rectum may be helpful in identifying partially retained membranes.

- Palpation typically reveals a poorly involuted uterus.
- As the disease progresses, there often is an accumulation of intrauterine fluid although it may not be present initially.
- Ultrasonographically, retained membranes may appear as distinctive hyperechoic areas within the lumen of the uterus.
- Evaluation of the reproductive tract per vagina can also be helpful in arriving at a diagnosis, because it is often possible to palpate partially retained membranes.
- When a diagnosis of RFM is made, treatment should be initiated immediately, and the mare should be closely monitored for signs of complications including metritis, endotoxemia, and laminitis.

●❯ WHAT TO DO

Retained Fetal Membranes

- Administration of oxytocin is generally the most effective treatment for RFM, and many treatment protocols are used:
  - Administer 10 to 20 IU, IM or IV q1 to 2h.
  - Add 40 to 80 IU oxytocin to a 1-L bag of saline and administer IV slowly over 30 to 60 minutes.
  - If the mare begins to show signs of discomfort due to enhanced uterine contractile activity, the dose and/or frequency of oxytocin is reduced.
- For refractory cases, administration of calcium borogluconate in conjunction with oxytocin therapy may be effective.
  - Add 125 mL of 23% calcium borogluconate and 80 IU oxytocin to a 5-L bag of saline and administer slowly IV over the course of approximately 2 hours.
- Another option is to distend the chorioallantoic cavity with 10 to 12 L of warm saline (or water if necessary) through a sterile/disinfected large-bore nasogastric tube.
  - The chorioallantois is held tightly closed around the tube so the infused fluid distends the fetal membranes and uterus.
  - Distention of the uterus, cervix, and vagina stimulates endogenous oxytocin release and promotes separation of the chorionic microvilli from the endometrium.
- If the membranes are *not* passed in their entirety within 6 to 8 hours of foaling, then broad-spectrum antibiotic and anti-inflammatory treatment should be initiated.
  - Antibiotics: Potassium penicillin (22,000 IU/kg IV q6h) and gentamicin sulfate (6.6 mg/kg IV q24h)
  - NSAIDs: flunixin meglumine (1.1 mg/kg IV q12h) for its anti-inflammatory and anti-endotoxic effects
- Mares should be carefully monitored for signs of endotoxemia and laminitis and additional treatments (e.g., distal limb cryotherapy) may be added if signs of endotoxemia develop or the risk of endotoxemia is determined to be high.
- During the treatment period, gentle attempts at manual removal of the membranes may be performed using one of the following techniques:
  - Placement of gentle tension on the protruding membranes
  - Carefully sliding the hand between the chorion and endometrium
  - Twisting the exposed membranes to form a cord, which exerts gentle tension on the areas of membrane that are still attached.
  - The mare will likely need to be treated for septic metritis after RFM (see p. 444).

Prognosis for Systemic Recovery

- In uncomplicated cases of RFM in which the membranes are eventually passed without development of secondary complications, the prognosis for survival of the mare is excellent.
- If secondary complications arise, the prognosis is reduced commensurately.
- In the most severe cases of septic metritis, laminitis and death can occur.

Prognosis for Future Fertility

- If the mare survives and does *not* develop secondary problems, her prognosis for future fertility is very good.
  - Mares that have been treated for RFM are *not* good candidates for breeding on their foal heat.

Uterine Laceration/Rupture

- Laceration or rupture of the uterus generally occurs during second stage labor, often as a result of dystocia, although it can also occur during an apparent normal delivery.
  - Because lacerations can occur during a dystocia, manually evaluate the reproductive tract, per vaginum, after correcting a dystocia to identify any lacerations before secondary complications occur.
- During gestation, uterine rupture can result from violent intrapartum movement or as a sequela to hydrops or uterine torsion.

Clinical Signs

- In the acute stage, before abdominal contamination, there may not be any clinical signs.
  - The exception is with a visceral hernia (e.g., urinary bladder, small bowel, etc.) through a full-thickness tear. The herniated tissue is generally evident externally (visually) and/or internally (palpably) protruding into the caudal reproductive tract.
    - If abdominal viscera herniate, cleanse (i.e., rinse with sterile saline) and immediately replace into the abdominal cavity then initiate prophylactic antibiotic treatment for peritonitis.
- If *not* detected in the acute phase, signs of peritonitis are clinically evident in 24 to 48 hours after foaling and include:
  - Fever
  - Tachycardia/tachypnea
  - Dull/depressed attitude
  - Toxic/injected mucous membranes
  - Inappetence

Diagnosis

- Lacerations in the uterine body are often palpable, and identified during vaginal examination.
- Palpation per rectum usually reveals a toned uterus palpating smaller than normal for the time period after foaling.
- Abdominocentesis:
  - Immediately postpartum abdominocentesis may show minor or no changes.

- In contrast, if systemic illness is present secondary to the uterine laceration, peritoneal fluid findings support a diagnosis of peritonitis, with increased total protein and cellularity (see p. 219).

(see p. 219)

WHAT TO DO

Uterine Laceration/Rupture

- Medical and surgical treatment of uterine lacerations has been described; there are no evidence-based results to support one over the other.
  - Surgical correction is recommended for large lacerations, particularly those associated with severe dystocia and contamination of the abdomen.
  - Small lacerations sustained during an otherwise uneventful delivery generally do well with conservative treatment, especially lacerations located on the dorsal uterine wall.
- Surgical correction is usually performed under general anesthesia via a ventral midline approach.
- Medical management consists of systemic broad-spectrum antibiotics and anti-inflammatory treatment.
  - Potassium penicillin, 22,000 IU/kg IV q6h, and gentamicin sulfate, 6.6 mg/kg IV q24h
  - Flunixin meglumine, 1.1 mg/kg IV q12h, for its anti-inflammatory and anti-endotoxic effects
- Uterine lavage is contraindicated because the lavage solution could flush uterine contaminants and debris into the abdominal cavity.

Prognosis for Systemic Recovery

- The prognosis for complete recovery is good, although it depends on the degree of abdominal contamination that occurs.
- Whether treated surgically or medically, the survival rate of mares after a uterine laceration is 75%.

Prognosis for Future Fertility

- The uterus generally heals well with little evidence of the laceration.
- Foaling rates are very good for mares that recover, even breeding during the same year although they are *not* candidates for breeding on foal heat.
- Mares in which uterine adhesions form as a result of the laceration and peritonitis are exceptions to good fertility.
  - Mares with uterine adhesions may exhibit chronic and recurring signs of abdominal pain.
  - Or, uterine adhesions may interfere with normal uterine clearance mechanisms, predisposing mares to persistent "mating-induced" endometritis.

Postpartum Metritis

- Although postpartum metritis can vary in severity, it can be life-threatening with severe septicemia/endotoxemia and laminitis as sequelae.
- It is generally associated with dystocia and/or retained fetal membranes; however, it can occur after an apparently uneventful foaling.

Clinical Signs

- Signs are usually evident in 24 to 72 hours of foaling and are consistent with endotoxemia, including:
  - Fever
  - Tachycardia/tachypnea
  - Dull/depressed attitude
  - Toxic/injected mucous membranes
  - Inappetence
  - +/− Malodorous vaginal discharge

Diagnosis

- Rectal palpation and ultrasonography of the reproductive tract typically reveal an enlarged, atonic, poorly involuted uterus containing a large volume of echogenic fluid.
  - Retained fetal membranes may also be identified particularly if loose remnants are "floating" in the free fluid in the uterine lumen.
- Manual examination of the uterus may reveal remnants of fetal membranes, most commonly in the tip of the previously nongravid horn.

●〉 WHAT TO DO

Postpartum Metritis
Treatment
- Broad-spectrum antibiotics such as potassium penicillin, 22,000 IU/kg IV q6h, gentamicin sulfate, 6.6 mg/kg IV q24h, and metronidazole 15 to 25 mg/kg PO q8.
- Flunixin meglumine, 1.1 mg/kg IV q12h for its anti-inflammatory and anti-endotoxic benefits.
- Oxytocin therapy, 10 to 20 IU, IM q2 to 4h with large-volume sterile saline lavage to clear uterine fluid and debris; continue once or twice daily until signs resolve.
  - Uterine lavage can be performed with a sterile/disinfected large-bore stomach tube.
  - Two to 4 L of sterile saline are instilled at a time and then recovered by gravity flow.
  - A total of 10 to 12 L, or more, may be needed to completely evacuate the uterine lumen.
- Other treatments may include:
  - Polymyxin B, 1.5 million IU/550-kg horse diluted and administered slowly, IV q12h, for 3 days.
  - Pentoxifylline, 10 mg/kg PO q12h
- Affected mares should be monitored closely for the development of laminitis and treatments focused to prevent laminitis (see Chapter 43, p. 712).

Prognosis for Systemic Recovery

- If severe complications of metritis (e.g., laminitis) are avoided, the prognosis for systemic recovery is good.

Prognosis for Future Fertility

- After recovery, mares can be bred again and conceive with no increased risk of developing septic metritis after a future foaling.
  - Because metritis typically delays uterine involution, allowing the mare to have one estrous cycle (i.e., foal heat) without breeding is recommended.

- A complete breeding soundness examination before breeding is recommended.

Perineal Lacerations

- Most perineal injuries occur at the time of foaling, particularly unattended foaling, during stage II when the fetal forelimbs traumatize the structures of the caudal reproductive tract and rectum.
  - ***Practice Tip:*** *It is imperative that pregnant mares in which episioplasty, or Caslick's procedure, has been performed have the episioplasty opened before parturition in order to prevent a perineal laceration.*
- Perineal lacerations can also occur in pregnant or nonpregnant mares from fighting between mares.
  - When mares fight, they stand hind-end to hind-end and kick with both feet, which can result in perineal lacerations.
- *First-degree* lacerations involve only the mucosa of the vestibule and skin of the dorsal commissure of the vulva.
- *Second-degree* lacerations involve the mucosa and submucosa of the dorsal vestibule/vulva, and some of the musculature of the perineal body, in particular, the constrictor vulvae muscle.
- *Third-degree* lacerations result in tearing of the vestibular and possibly vaginal wall and disruption of the perineal body, anal sphincter, and rectum, causing a common "opening" between the rectum and caudal reproductive tract.

Clinical Signs

- *First-* and *second-degree* lacerations may only be evident on physical inspection of the caudal reproductive tract manually and/or with a vaginal speculum.
- *Third-degree* lacerations are apparent because of the loss of normal anatomy and fecal contamination of the vestibule/vagina.
  - These mares make a "windsucking" sound from air movement in and out of the abnormal orifice.

Diagnosis

- Manual palpation and/or a speculum examination are used to assess the severity of the laceration and injury.

●〉 WHAT TO DO

Perineal Lacerations
Treatment
- *First-degree* lacerations generally require *no* treatment other than local/topical application of an antiseptic ointment or cream.
- *Second-degree* lacerations may need an episioplasty and/or perineal body reconstruction.
  - If tissue damage has caused significant edema, inflammation, and infection, surgical correction may be postponed for 2 to 4 weeks.
    - Initially, systemic antibiotic and anti-inflammatory treatment is administered for the acute trauma.
- *Third-degree* lacerations are first treated with systemic antibiotics and anti-inflammatory drugs.

- Surgical correction is postponed for at least 4 weeks to allow second intention wound healing.
  - After surgical treatment, the mare should undergo a complete breeding soundness examination before breeding.

Prognosis for Systemic Recovery

- Perineal lacerations, including third-degree lacerations, do *not* adversely affect the health of a mare.

Prognosis for Future Fertility

- After treatment, future fertility should *not* be adversely affected; however, mares having had a third-degree laceration are at greater risk for recurrence, and therefore they should be closely monitored at the time of parturition in the future.

Foal Rejection

- Foal rejection consists of several abnormal maternal behaviors directed at the foal in the immediate postpartum period.
- The behaviors include:
  - Ambivalence towards the foal
  - Fear of the foal
  - Refusal to allow the foal to nurse
  - Aggression towards the foal
- The reason for these behaviors may include:
  - Inexperience of the mare—primiparous mares are most often affected
  - Disrupted bonding experience—human/animal commotion; early removal of fetal membranes/fluids
  - Abnormal/sick foal
  - Discomfort during nursing
  - Misdirected animal/human aggression
  - Breed—Arabians are more prone to foal rejection
- Foal rejection must be recognized and managed in order to maintain the health and well-being of the foal.

Clinical Signs

- Ambivalence towards the foal:
  - Mare shows little to no interest in the foal; no obvious protective or bonding behavior.
- Fear of the foal:
  - Mare moves away from the foal whenever it approaches.
- Refusal to allow the foal to nurse:
  - Mare does not stand still and allow the foal to nurse; mare kicks at the foal when it attempts to nurse.
- Maternal aggression towards the foal:
  - Mare aggressively attacks the foal by either biting or kicking; the biting is directed at the foal's neck, withers, or back. The foal is often lifted, shaken, tossed, and even stepped on; foals may be fatally injured or killed.

Diagnosis

- Foal rejection is diagnosed based on abnormal maternal behavior directed towards the foal.
- It is important *not* to confuse normal maternal behavior with foal rejection; mares often squeal when the foal first tries to nurse or mares nip at the foal when nursing becomes too aggressive.

●》 WHAT TO DO

Foal Rejection
Treatment
- Ambivalence towards the foal:
  - Keep mare and foal together with minimal disruption.
  - Reintroduce the fetal membranes for maternal bonding.
  - Examine the mare for evidence of pain/discomfort; treat the mare with flunixin meglumine,1.1 mg/kg IV, if it is believed there is an underlying cause.
  - Gently restrain the mare and assist the foal to nurse.
- Fear of the foal:
  - Densensitize the mare to the foal with positive reinforcement.
  - Tranquilize the mare with acepromazine or an α-adrenergic agonist (xylazine, detomidine); diazepam is helpful in reducing the fear response.
- Refusal to allow the foal to nurse:
  - For mares with painful, tender udders, treatment may include: oxytocin, 5 IU, IV/IM, to facilitate milk letdown; gentle hand milking to reduce udder distention; and flunixin meglumine, 0.5 to 1.1 mg/kg IV or PO, PRN for pain relief.
  - Gently restrain the mare while assisting the foal to nurse; two handlers are required. Reward the mare with grain when she permits the foal to nurse without adverse behavior.
  - Hand milk the mare and bottle-feed the foal in the mare's inguinal region; initially hand milking may be tolerated by the mare while nursing may not; eventually transfer the foal to the mare's teat.
  - Tranquilize the mare with acepromazine or an α-adrenergic agonist (xylazine, detomidine); the addition of butorphanol may be helpful in difficult mares.
- Maternal aggression towards the foal:
  - Tranquilize or restrain the mare; relapses are common.
  - Separate the mare and foal; find a nurse mare (see Lactation Induction Protocols, p. 448) to raise the foal or rear the foal on milk replacer, preferably with other orphan foals.

Prevention

- Allow the fetal fluids and fetal membranes to remain in the stall for several hours after delivery; examine the fetal membranes for completeness as soon as passed by the mare.
- Allow the mare and foal to interact undisturbed as much as possible after the delivery; avoid contact with other horses for several days.
- Desensitize the mare to udder and flank manipulation before foaling, especially in maiden mares; do *not* milk the teats before delivery.
- Mares with a history of foal rejection may benefit from hormonal treatment after delivery; the recommended regimen includes:
  - Administration of altrenogest, 0.044 mg/kg PO q12 to 24h
  - Estradiol benzoate, 10 mg IM q24h
  - Domperidone, 1.1 mg/kg PO q12 to 24h for 3 to 5 days after delivery
- Do *not* rebreed mares that have savaged their foals.

REPRO

Agalactia

- Agalactia is a failure of the mammary gland to produce milk or colostrum after parturition.
- The condition must be differentiated from the inability of the mare to "let milk down" after foaling or delayed lactation reported to occur in some mares.
- *Practice Tip: Agalactia is seen most commonly in mares with fescue toxicosis.*
- Occasionally lactating mares may develop agalactia due to inadequate nutrition, pain, or disease.
- *Practice Tip: Mares receiving pergolide mesylate for equine Cushing's disease should stop treatment 2 weeks before foaling for normal mammary development and lactation.*

Clinical Signs

- Mares with fescue toxicosis, fescue grass contaminated with the fungus *Neotyphodium coenophialum*, show minimal to no signs of impending foaling (i.e., increase in the size of the udder and teats, waxing, increases in calcium levels in mammary secretions).
- Less commonly, mares with fescue toxicosis have prolonged gestation, abortion, dystocia, dysmature or stillborn foals, thickened placenta, and retained fetal membranes.
- After delivery of the foal, mares have minimal udder development and minimal to complete absence of colostrum or milk production.

Diagnosis

- Agalactia due to fescue toxicosis is diagnosed based on clinical presentation, prolonged gestation with minimal udder development, and agalactia following parturition.
- A diagnosis can be made based on abnormalities in prolactin, progestagen, and relaxin concentrations during the last 30 days of pregnancy.
- Detection of urinary ergot alkaloids with enzyme-linked immunosorbent assay (ELISA) testing can confirm exposure to infected fescue.

● WHAT TO DO

Agalactia

- Mare:
  - Begin treatment with a dopamine antagonist: domperidone, 1.1 mg/kg PO q24h (preferred), sulpiride, 3.3 mg/kg PO q24h, or perphenazine, 0.3 to 0.5 mg/kg PO q12h or acepromazine, 20 mg IM q6h. Domperidone, unlike other dopamine antagonists, does *not* cross the blood-brain barrier and, therefore is less likely to induce extrapyramidal signs.
    - Alternatively, begin a lactation induction protocol.
- Foal:
  - Foals must receive 1 to 1.5 L of good quality colostrum, as evidenced by a sugar/BRIX refractometer[6] scale >23%, within the first 6 hours of life.

[6]Animal Reproduction Systems, Chino, California.

- Once adequate amounts of colostrum are consumed, begin bottle-feeding the foal with equine milk replacer. Start by feeding the foal 10% of its body weight divided into 6 to 12 feedings per day; for ongoing feeding of the foal, see Chapter 31, p. 556.
- Measure IgG levels at 12 hours; foals with levels ≤400 mg/dL can be administered additional high quality colostrum orally; otherwise administer 1 to 2 L of equine plasma IV.
- Foals that do *not* receive colostrum for several hours after delivery are started on a broad-spectrum antimicrobial, ceftiofur, 4.4 mg/kg IV q12h.
- Perform routine neonatal procedures:
  - Dip umbilicus using 1% chlorhexidine or 2% iodine.
  - Administer an enema if meconium is not passed soon after receiving colostrum.
  - Perform full routine neonatal examination.
- Foals can be bucket fed until the mare begins lactating; otherwise, a nurse mare is located (see Lactation Induction Protocols, see below), or the foal is raised in a group with other orphan foals.

Prevention

- Multiparous mares develop an udder several weeks before their expected due date.
- Maiden and miniature mares develop an udder very close to their due date or immediately after foaling.
- Mares that fail to develop an udder as foaling approaches should be closely scrutinized for fescue toxicosis.
  - If fescue toxicosis is suspected, remove the mare from infected pastures and hay 30 days before the foaling date.
  - Alternatively, domperidone, 1.1 mg/kg PO q24h, can be administered starting 10 to 14 days before the expected foaling date.
  - The domperidone dosage regimen needs to be adjusted if the mare begins dripping colostrum/milk prematurely.

Induction of Lactation

- Lactation induction in the barren mare is an alternative for raising:
  - An orphan foal
  - A foal whose dam must be shipped for breeding
  - Foals from mares that are "poor doers" or dams that have rejected their foals
- The protocol is also used in mares that suffer from agalactia after foaling.
- The prospective nurse mare should meet the following criteria for the induction and adoption protocol to be successful:
  - Has delivered and successfully nursed at least one foal
  - Has good body condition; is reproductively cycling; has a healthy, normal udder; is quiet with good maternal instincts
  - If the mare is in anestrus, it is important that the mare receive exogenous steroids, estrogen, and progesterone as part of the induction protocol.

◉〉 WHAT TO DO

Lactation Induction Protocols
- There are several protocols for lactation induction in the mare.
- The following protocols have been selected because of their ease of administration and the relatively rapid onset of lactation:

Protocol A
- The nurse mare and orphan foal should be housed in adjacent stalls.
- Day 1: Administer prostaglandin, 5 mg dinoprost IM; estradiol benzoate, 50 mg IM; altrenogest, 44 mg PO q24h; and domperidone, 1.1 mg/kg PO q12h.
- Day 2 to 15: Administer estradiol benzoate, 10 mg IM q24h; altrenogest, 44 mg, PO q24h; and domperidone, 1.1 mg/kg PO q12h.
  - Discontinue altrenogest on day 7 and domperidone/estradiol benzoate several days after adoption. *Important:* Do *not* use domperidone for more than 20 days total.
- Begin hand milking when the udder is enlarged and milk is present.
  - Milk the mare 5 times a day after administration of 5 IU of oxytocin IV.
  - The orphan foal should receive the milk from the mare.

Protocol B
- Day 1: Administer estradiol benzoate, 50 mg/500 kg IM; altrenogest, 22 mg/500 kg PO q24h; and sulpiride, 1 mg/kg IM q12h or domperidone, 1.1 mg/kg PO q12h.
- Day 2 and thereafter: Administer altrenogest, 22 mg/500 kg PO q24h; sulpiride, 1 mg/kg IM q12h or domperidone, 1.1 mg/kg PO q12h; recommend estradiol benzoate, 50 mg/500 kg IM q48 h if the mare is *not* cycling.
  - Discontinue altrenogest on day 7 and domperidone/estradiol benzoate several days after adoption. *Important:* Do *not* use domperidone for more than 20 days total.
- Begin hand milking on the fourth to seventh day of treatment (see Protocol A).

Adoption Procedure
- Adoption can begin once the mare is lactating, 3 to 5 L/day, and signs the mare is bonding with the foal (i.e., the mare paces and calls when the foal is removed from its stall).
- Initially the foal is brought to the mare's stall for short, supervised nursing sessions, and the mare is given oxytocin, 5 IU, IV, to facilitate milk "letdown."
- These sessions continue until the mare shows appropriate bonding behavior and anxiety when the foal leaves the stall, and the foal nurses without mare aggression.
- The final phase of the adoption procedure requires stimulation of maternal behavior by manual cervical massage. Massage the external cervical os for 2 minutes; repeat procedure in 10 minutes, or hormonally stimulate by using prostaglandin, 5 mg dinoprost IM, and oxytocin, 5 IU, IV.
  - The foal is held at the mare's head/shoulder during cervical stimulation and allowed to nurse after the procedure.
  - With the prostaglandin protocol, the foal is encouraged to nurse once the mare begins to show signs of abdominal discomfort.
- Once obvious maternal behavior—licking foal, following foal around the stall, calling to the foal—is seen, the mare and foal are allowed to interact freely in the stall.
- Some foals may require supplemental milk replacer in the first few weeks after adoption to give the nurse mare time to reach maximum milk production.

Outcome
- Foals may be slow to gain weight for several weeks after adoption; however, the weaning weight of these foals is not significantly different than "naturally" raised foals.
- In one report, the weaning weights differed between "naturally" raised and nurse mare foals when those mares did not receive exogenous steroids as part of the induction protocol. However as yearlings there was *no* difference between the two groups.

Mastitis
- The equine mammary gland is comprised of paired (left and right) glands, each with a glandular body and single teat.
  - The glandular part of each half is divided into two lobes (cranial and caudal), and each teat serves both the cranial and caudal lobes and therefore has two corresponding teat orifices.
- Mastitis occurs most commonly during lactation or in the postweaning period; it can also occur in maiden mares or mares that have not lactated for an extended period of time (i.e., years).
  - A higher incidence is described in the summer months. A higher incidence also occurs when the foal has to wear a muzzle.

Clinical Signs
- Warm, swollen, and painful udder
  - Generally unilateral involving a single lobe—cranial or caudal—although both lobes can be affected
- +/− Ventral edema
- +/− Systemic signs of illness:
  - Fever
  - Depression
  - Inappetence
- +/− Apparent lameness because of reluctance to move the hind leg on the affected side through its full, normal range of motion because of impingement on the mammary gland

Diagnosis
- Clinical signs are generally diagnostic; however, cytological, California mastitis testing (CMT), and/or bacteriological evaluation of mammary secretions is needed to confirm the diagnosis.
  - Cytology reveals large numbers of neutrophils.
  - The most common isolated organism is *Streptococcus zooepidemicus.*

‣ WHAT TO DO

Mastitis

- Manually milk frequently or use a milking device made from a 60-mL syringe:
  - Remove the plunger and cut the barrel of the syringe at the needle adapter, creating an open end.
  - Insert the plunger into the cut end of the barrel and place the smooth end of the syringe over the teat, withdrawing the plunger to create milk flow.
- Hot pack the affected gland several times a day.
- Administer systemic antibiotics; and/or infuse a bovine intramammary antibiotic preparation, daily to PRN. Ph bufferer Amikacin (500 mg) can be infused into each gland for gram-negative infections. A small cannula is needed to infuse the gland.

- Flunixin meglumine, 1.1 mg/kg IV q12h, for its analgesic and anti-inflammatory effects.

Prognosis

- With treatment, signs usually resolve within a few days to 1 week.
- Recurrence is unlikely.

References

References can be found on the companion website at www.equine-emergencies.com.

REPRO

CHAPTER 25

Respiratory System

DIAGNOSTIC AND THERAPEUTIC PROCEDURES

Barbara Dallap Schaer and James A. Orsini

Nasotracheal and Orotracheal Tube Placement

It is critical to establish an airway in a patient exhibiting respiratory distress (cyanotic mucous membranes, respiratory stridor, apnea). Intubation is the most rapid and least invasive method and is performed through the nose or mouth. Alternatively, a tracheostomy is used in patients with obstruction of the upper airway. Nasotracheal intubation is preferred to orotracheal intubation because it can be performed on a conscious horse, and the tube can be left in place until the respiratory crisis has resolved. General anesthesia is required for orotracheal intubation. For an anesthetized or severely obtunded patient, orotracheal intubation is preferred because a larger endotracheal tube can be used for oxygen supplementation or assisted ventilation (see p. 454).

Nasotracheal Intubation

Equipment
- Sedatives (xylazine hydrochloride and butorphanol tartrate)
- Appropriately sized nasotracheal tube
  - Adults, 11- to 14-mm internal diameter[1]
  - Foals, 7- to 12-mm internal diameter[2]
- Lubricating jelly[3] or warm water
- White tape
- 20-mL syringe, not Luer-Lok

Procedure
- Sedation may be required for an adult. Sedation is generally unnecessary for foals. Suggested adult (physiologically stable) dose is 0.3 to 0.5 mg/kg xylazine and 0.01 to 0.02 mg/kg butorphanol IV.
  Caution: Sedation or tranquilization of a dyspneic patient may lead to cardiopulmonary depression, increased upper airway resistance, and apnea.

- Lubricate the tube sparingly or place it in warm water.
- Reflect the alar fold of the nostril and insert the tube medially along the ventral nasal meatus.
- Extend and elevate the head to allow easier access to the trachea and to prevent the tube from being swallowed.
- Advance the tube into the pharynx. *Do not* use force. If resistance is encountered, rotate and advance. If still meeting resistance, use a smaller-diameter tube.
- Confirm that air is flowing through the tube, which indicates correct placement.
- Use an air-filled syringe to inflate the cuff to the point at which air cannot escape around the tube.
  Caution: Do not inflate the cuff past the point where resistance is first encountered.
- Secure the tube by placing tape around the tube end and tying it to the horse's halter.

Orotracheal Intubation

Equipment
- Drugs for general anesthesia (xylazine hydrochloride and ketamine for adults; diazepam and ketamine for physiologically stable foals)
- Appropriately sized orotracheal tube with inflatable cuff[4]
  - Adults, 18- to 28-mm internal diameter
  - Foals, 8- to 11-mm internal diameter
- Oral speculum made of polyvinyl chloride pipe, 5-cm diameter, 4 to 5 cm long, wrapped with white tape
- Lubricating jelly[5]
- 20- or 30-mL syringe, not Luer-Lok

Procedure
- General anesthesia should be used if the patient is fully conscious. The recommended dose for adults is 0.3 to 1.1 mg/kg xylazine IV for sedation followed by 2.2 mg/kg ketamine IV. Diazepam and guaifenesin are additional considerations as part of the preanesthetic and induction drugs. The recommended dose for foals is 0.1 mg/kg diazepam IV administered slowly for sedation, followed by 1 mg/kg ketamine IV administered slowly.
  Caution: Intubate as soon as the patient is anesthetized. Equipment for cardiopulmonary resuscitation should be available.

---

[1]Cuffed endotracheal tubes (Advanced Anesthesia Specialists, LLC, Prescott, Arizona, Seaforth, Australia).
[2]Cuffed nasotracheal tubes for foals (MedVet International, Mettawa, Illinois).
[3]Priority Care sterile lubricating jelly (VetDepot, Encinitas, California).

[4]Cuffed endotracheal tubes (MedVet International, Mettawa, Illinois).
[5]Priority Care sterile lubricating jelly (VetDepot).

450

- Dorsiflex the head and pull the tongue out through the interdental space.
- Place the speculum between the upper and lower incisors.
- Sparingly lubricate the endotracheal tube.
- Advance the tube through the center of the speculum. If resistance is encountered, rotate and advance the tube gently. If the patient repeatedly swallows, administer 0.1-mg/kg doses of ketamine IV until swallowing stops; allow 2 to 3 minutes for effect after each dose.
- The endotracheal tube placement is confirmed by demonstrating air moving through the tube. The tube should not be palpable in the proximal cervical area.
- Use a 20-mL syringe to inflate the cuff until resistance is encountered.
- Maintain general anesthesia while the orotracheal tube is in place.

Complications

- Overinflation of the endotracheal tube cuff can cause pressure necrosis of the tracheal mucosa and sloughing. In the most severe cases, tracheal stenosis may result. *Do not inflate the cuff beyond the point where resistance is first met.*
- An excessively long tube may end in a main stem bronchus with ventilation of only a portion of the pulmonary tree.
- Bleeding from injury to nasal mucosa occurs commonly during nasotracheal intubation. Generally, this is not clinically significant.

Transtracheal Aspiration and Bronchoalveolar Lavage

Transtracheal Aspiration

- Transtracheal aspiration is a simple, commonly used technique for assessing disease in the lower respiratory tract. The fluid obtained from aspiration is a mixture of secretions and cellular material that has collected in the distal trachea.
- Results of cytologic examination of the aspirate determine the type and severity of inflammation and may give some indication as to the bacteria involved in an infectious process.
- The upper respiratory tract is host to a large bacterial population, and culture results of specimens from the nares or guttural pouch are difficult to interpret when not seeking a particular pathogen.
  - Transtracheal aspiration bypasses the upper respiratory tract and is the best method for obtaining a representative sample for bacterial culture of the lower respiratory tract.
- Tracheal aspirates also can be retrieved through a flexible, fiber-optic endoscope biopsy channel; a sterile endoscopic catheter is available for sampling via the endoscope.[6]

- Results of cultures are not as reliable when sampling via the biopsy channel, but using an endoscope allows the clinician to see the area being sampled and avoids complications from tracheal puncture.

Equipment
- Twitch
- Sedation may be necessary if patient is young, difficult to restrain, or coughs excessively during the procedure; xylazine hydrochloride, 0.3 to 0.5 mg/kg, with butorphanol tartrate, 0.01 to 0.02 mg/kg IV, is recommended for restraint and as a cough suppressant
- Clippers
- Material for aseptic preparation
- Sterile gloves
- 2% mepivacaine (Carbocaine) for local anesthetic
- 16-gauge through-the-needle catheter[7] with or without a 7-inch (17.5-cm) extension set[8]
- An alternative is a 12-gauge nondisposable needle and 5F polyethylene tubing or one of several commercial TTW kits available.
- 60-mL syringe (sterile)
- 100-mL sterile 0.9% saline solution without bacteriostatic agent
- Plain and ethylenediaminetetraacetic acid (EDTA) Vacutainer tubes[9]
- Port-a-Cul culture system[10]

Procedure
- Appropriately retrain and/or sedate the patient as needed.
- Clip and sterilely prepare a 10-cm area on the ventral midline of the middle third of the trachea.
- Aseptically block the intended aspiration site with local anesthetic.
- Palpate the trachea with sterile gloves, and stabilize it with one hand.
- ***Practice Tip***: *A small skin incision using a #15 blade facilitates cannula or needle passage through the skin.*
- Position the cannula bevel downward, and place the catheter through the skin and between tracheal rings into the tracheal lumen (Fig. 25-1).
- Stabilizing the cannula or needle with one hand, feed the catheter down the trachea to the thoracic inlet. Coughing may cause the catheter to retroflex into the pharynx and become contaminated.
- Attach the syringe and rapidly inject 20 to 30 mL of sterile saline solution.
- Aspirate the fluid injected into the sampling syringe; only a portion of the fluid instilled is retrievable.

---

[6]Endoscopic Microbiology Aspiration Catheter (Mila International, Inc., Florence, Kentucky).

[7]Intracath intravenous catheter placement unit (Deseret Medical, Inc., Becton, Dickinson and Company, Sandy, Utah).
[8]Seven inch (17.5 cm) or 30-inch (75 cm) extension set (Abbott Laboratories, North Chicago, Illinois).
[9]Vacutainer (Becton-Dickinson Vacutainer Systems, Rutherford, New Jersey).
[10]Port-a-Cul (Becton-Dickinson Microbiology Systems, Cockeysville, Maryland).

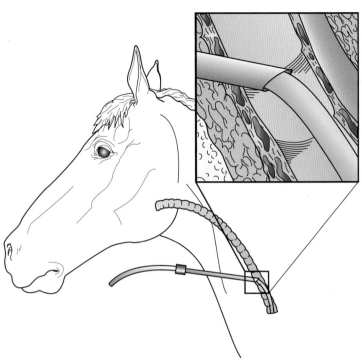

Figure 25-1   Technique for transtracheal aspiration and washing. Through-the-needle catheter is placed between tracheal rings.

- Inject another aliquot of fluid through the catheter if the sample collected is inadequate. *Do not* inject more than 100 mL total volume. Reposition or slowly withdraw the catheter to assist aspiration of the sample.
- Carefully withdraw the catheter after obtaining the sample; if there is resistance, remove the needle before withdrawing the catheter.
- If the sample contains any purulent debris, an antibiotic can be administered systemically or be infiltrated subcutaneously at the puncture site.

Complications

- Catheter laceration and loss into the airway can occur. The catheter almost always is coughed out within 30 minutes.
- Subcutaneous abscess or cellulitis can occur at the site of needle puncture. In severe cases, infection may extend to the mediastinum. In these cases, administer systemic antimicrobial therapy. Apply a hot pack, topical diclofenac or dimethyl sulfoxide (DMSO) over the infected site. If needed, incise for drainage.
- Mild subcutaneous emphysema around the trachea is common and can result in pneumomediastinum. Emphysema is rarely a problem unless the patient is in respiratory distress.

    Practice Tip: *Performing a transtracheal wash (TTW) in horses with severe heaves and respiratory distress can lead to severe pneumomediastinum.*
- Damage to the tracheal rings can result in chondritis or chondroma formation. Stenosis of the tracheal lumen would be the most severe sequela.

Bronchoalveolar Lavage

- Bronchoalveolar lavage (BAL) is used to sample the terminal airway and associated alveoli.
- BAL is an excellent method for examining pathologic changes in the most distal portion of the respiratory tract.
- BAL should be performed for the diagnosis of noninfectious lower airways (heaves, inflammatory airway disease [IAD], neoplasia) because only a limited section of the lung can be evaluated and the sample is generally not as suitable for culture as is tracheal aspirate, diseases, or EHV-5 infection.
- BAL may be performed blindly or with endoscopic guidance.

Equipment

- Sedatives (xylazine hydrochloride and butorphanol tartrate)
- 3-m BAL catheter[11] or 2- to 3-m, 9-mm-diameter flexible fiber-optic endoscope[12]
- 2% mepivacaine (Carbocaine) hydrochloride or 2% lidocaine (xylocaine)
- 3-5 sterile 60-mL syringes
- 180- to 300-mL sterile 0.9% saline solution without bacteriostatic agent, warmed to body temperature
- Plain and EDTA Vacutainer tubes

---

[11]240- to 300-cm (2.4- to 3-m) BAL Catheter (Advanced Anesthesia Specialists, LLC, Prescott, Arizona).
[12]GIF 130 gastroscope (2- or 3-m long, 9.8-mm outer diameter (Olympus America, Inc., Center Valley, Pennsylvania).

Procedure

- Sedation usually is required. Recommended doses are 0.4 to 0.6 mg/kg xylazine with 0.01 to 0.02 mg/kg butorphanol IV.
- If using a BAL catheter, extend the horse's head and gently pass the catheter through the nose and into a terminal airway. Wedge the catheter into the bronchus of a lower lung lobe. The main disadvantage to this procedure is that the location of the catheter is unknown.
- Pass the endoscope, if using an endoscope, clean the biopsy channel or catheter starting in the endoscope with antiseptic solution and rinse with sterile water. Pass the endoscope, and inject 35 mL of lidocaine (2.0%) through the biopsy channel starting in the distal trachea to minimize excessive coughing. Gently "wedge" it into the smallest-possible diameter bronchus, inflate the balloon at the catheter tip, and inject the remaining 10 mL of lidocaine. Infuse up to 300 mL (60 mL for a foal) using 60 mL aliquots sequentially injected and then aspirated.
- If excessive coughing occurs, consider increasing the sedation and/or infuse 5 mL of dilute mepivacaine.
- Keep sample on ice if cytologic analysis is completed within a few hours or place sample in an EDTA Vacutainer tube (purple top) if delayed examination is expected.

Complications

- Complications are rare, focal pneumonia at the point of the lavage is uncommon.
    - Temperature should be monitored for 3 to 5 days after BAL.

Respiratory Fluid Analysis

- A direct smear of the fluid can be made if the sample appears cellular; otherwise, the sample is centrifuged, and the centrifugate is placed on a glass slide. (See Chapter 11, p. 38.)
- The slide prep may be air dried and stained with Wright stain.
- Cytologic examination should include a differential cell count, degenerative status of the cells, and an assessment of the bacterial component.
    - Total cell counts are not meaningful because the density of the cell population varies with the amount of saline solution retrieved.
    - The differential cell count should be determined, although the aspiration reflects only a small segment of the pulmonary tree in transtracheal aspiration and BAL.
    - Normal results of BAL, in particular, do not rule out lung disease, because a normal section of lung can accidentally be lavaged.
    - Cell populations may vary in normal horses based on their environment (e.g., housed in a stable or housed outdoors).
- Normal TTW aspirate contains strands of mucus.

- Columnar epithelial cells and pulmonary alveolar macrophages are the predominant cell types in TTW. Lymphocytes and macrophages account for most of the cell population in a BAL sample.
- Neutrophils and eosinophils are normally less than 5% of the BAL differential cell count.
- Increased numbers of nondegenerate neutrophils (>25%) are common in recurrent obstructive pulmonary disease (recurrent airway obstruction [RAO], heaves, formerly chronic obstructive pulmonary disease [COPD]).
- Increased numbers of neutrophils (>5%), mast cells (≥2%), or eosinophils (≥1%) are suggestive of IAD.
- An infectious process is supported by the presence of intracellular bacteria.
- The presence of squamous epithelial cells as part of the TTW sample, usually in rafts or rolled into a cigar shape, indicates pharyngeal contamination or metaplasia in the lower respiratory tract from chronic irritation or inflammation.
- Curschmann spirals are coiled mucous plugs from terminal airways that are indicative of chronic inflammation, most commonly RAO.
- Pulmonary hemorrhage is detected by means of finding hemosiderin-laden alveolar macrophages.
- Free bacteria and fungal elements (especially in stabled horses with heaves) are common in normal TTW samples.
- For a morphologic description of cell types and their role in disease processes, see p. 54.
- The transtracheal aspirate should be submitted for aerobic and anaerobic culture for adult horses and aerobic culture for foals.
    - Gram stain is useful in determining initial antibiotic therapy while awaiting culture results.
    - The significance of the results should be interpreted in conjunction with cytologic findings because contamination is always a possibility, and the normal trachea can contain bacteria.

Nasal Oxygen Insufflation

- Oxygen administration is more frequently used to treat neonatal foals than it is to treat adults but is therapeutic for both.
- Supplementation of oxygen should be based on clinical signs and results of blood gas analysis.
    - Hypoxia is suspected in patients with pneumonia, pulmonary edema, hemolytic anemia, considerable blood loss, obstructive pulmonary disease, hypoventilation, and recumbency-associated or neonatal ventilation/perfusion mismatch.
- Nasal oxygen insufflation is beneficial to all patients undergoing general anesthesia.
- Increasing the concentration of oxygen in the inspired air increases blood Pao_2 levels.
- Patients with severe parenchymal disease or right to left shunts may not respond clinically to nasal oxygen administration.

RESP

Equipment

- Oxygen source (high-pressure oxygen cylinder[13])
- Oxygen flowmeter/humidifier (humidifier should be filled with sterile water)
- Oxygen tubing (2 to 4 m) to extend from the flowmeter to the patient
- Nasal catheter[14]
- 1-inch (2.5 cm) white tape, or in neonates, half of wooden tongue depressor
- Examination gloves
- 2-0 nonabsorbable suture on a straight needle

Procedure

- Attach the humidifier to the flowmeter on the oxygen source.
- Connect the nasal catheter to the oxygen tubing and then connect the oxygen tubing to the humidifier. *Practice Tip: Humidified air should be used for all oxygen administration >30 minutes.*
- Using the nasal catheter, measure the distance between the nostril and the medial canthus. This is the approximate distance to the nasopharynx.
- Reflect open one nostril and place the catheter along the ventral meatus (the most ventral and medial portion of the nasal passage) and into the nasopharynx.
- Place a butterfly square of tape around the tubing (approximately 6 cm from the nostril), and then curve the tubing around and suture the tape to the nostril. Gloves are optional but are recommended for handling suture material. Tubing may have to be sutured in several places. Alternatively, in neonates, the nasal catheter can be curved around half of a wooden tongue depressor, placed alongside the nostril and face, and secured in place with white tape.
- Set the flow of oxygen between 5 and 15 L/min, depending on the size and needs of the patient.
- Check the setup frequently (every 2 hours) to ensure tube patency. Replace the nasal catheter daily.
- *Note:* This procedure may have variable effect on FiO_2.
  - Use of two catheters and two lines may result in a further increase in FiO_2. In healthy neonatal foals, a single intranasal catheter with an oxygen flow rate of 50 mL/kg (2.5 L/min) increases FiO_2 from 21% (room air) to 23% to 26%; bilateral catheters at this flow rate increase FiO_2 to 31% to 34%.
  - A flow rate of 200 mL/kg(10 mL/min) O_2 via a single catheter has a FiO_2 of 52%, and bilateral catheters at this flow rate have a FiO_2 as high as 75%.
  - A slightly lower FiO_2 is expected in adult horses, and in some cases, intratracheal oxygen is needed to substantially increase FiO_2.

- Healthy adult horses administered 5 L/min, 10 L/min or 15 L/min oxygen via single catheter had reported FiO_2 values of 29%, 41%, and 49%, respectfully; FiO_2 values are reported lower in RAO horses supplemented with the same oxygen flow rates.
- If the catheter is positioned in the trachea, the FiO_2 is higher but coughing is generally moderate to severe.
- Monitoring of arterial blood gases for efficacy is useful.
- An occasional complication of oxygen supplementation can be increased Pa_{CO_2}, possibly altering the patient's acid-base status.
- *Practice Tip: There is no concern of oxygen toxicity with intranasal oxygen.*

Assisted Ventilation

- Assisted ventilation is used in the care of patients with apnea, hypoventilation, persistent fetal circulation, or respiratory distress not corrected by oxygen supplementation.
- Clinical disorders in which mechanical ventilation might be necessary include foal maladjustment syndromes (neonatal encephalopathy), respiratory disease resulting in decompensation, thoracic injury or disease, and botulism.
- Persistent cyanotic mucous membranes and dyspnea or hypoventilation with an arterial P_{CO_2} greater than 60 mm Hg are strong clinical indicators of hypoventilation and tissue hypoxia.
- Short-term ventilation is relatively easy, whereas long-term ventilation is expensive and labor intensive, requiring 24-hour nursing care and sophisticated equipment.
- *Note:* Unless the patient is semiconscious or unconscious or has diffuse neuromuscular weakness (i.e., botulism), a neuromuscular blocking agent is needed before assisted ventilation.
- Assisted ventilation can be performed in a standing patient but is not well tolerated. Endotracheal intubation (or tracheostomy) must be performed before an attempt is made to ventilate.
- Placement of a cuffed, wide-diameter orotracheal tube may be advantageous in an adult, but nasotracheal intubation is more commonly used in neonates requiring assisted ventilation (p. 450).

Equipment

- Oxygen cylinder[15] with a regulator[16] that has a flowmeter and a diameter index safety system (DISS) fitting for a demand valve (the small "E" cylinder is portable)
- Regulator for E cylinder with a flowmeter giving 1, 2, 4, 6, 10, 15, and 25 L/min and a DISS connection for a demand valve

---

[13]High-pressure oxygen cylinder (size E is small and portable). Oxygen supply service is available through local health care companies. Reusable oxygen cylinders are provided.
[14]Nasal catheter "Levin tubes" 235200-160 (Rusch, Inc., 1-800-514-7234, csrusch@teleflexmedical.com).

---

[15]Oxygen supply service is available through local health care companies. Reusable oxygen cylinders are provided.
[16]LSPO2 Regulator 270-020 (Allied Healthcare Products, St. Louis, Missouri).

- One of the following methods for delivering positive-pressure ventilation:
  - Oxygen demand valve[17]
  - Ambu Bag with an adapter for oxygen insufflations

Procedure

- Intubate the patient and inflate the cuff of the endotracheal tube (see p. 450).

Ventilation with a Demand Valve

- Attach the demand valve to the oxygen cylinder.
- Open the tank by turning the valve on the tank regulator counterclockwise.
- Attach the demand valve directly to the endotracheal or tracheostomy tube.
- Ventilation is achieved by pressing the button on the demand valve. The demand valve delivers oxygen at 160 L/min. Monitor the chest expansion and then release; exhalation occurs passively. (Check to be certain the release/pop-off valve is open!)
- *Practice Tip: Generally, allow 2 to 3 seconds to deliver one breath to an adult; to a foal, allow significantly less time. It is safest to watch the chest rise and end inspiration as soon as the chest nears full expansion.*
  Caution: Do not overinflate the lungs; overinflation causes barotrauma and can decrease cardiac output. This can readily occur in foals when a demand valve is used. Therefore, an Ambu Bag with appropriate pop-off valve is preferred for foal resuscitation.
- If the chest does not rise, check for leaks and tube placement. Confirm that the esophagus has not been accidentally intubated. This can be established by seeing and/or palpating the tube or by use of a capnograph to monitor exhaled carbon dioxide (if the tube is in the esophagus there is no reading for CO_2).
- For an adult, deliver 10 to 12 breaths per minute; for a foal, deliver 15 to 20 breaths per minute.
- The demand valve can be used to assist ventilation if the patient breathes independently. The demand valve triggers automatically when inspiration begins and shuts off when exhalation begins. This method increases airway resistance and the work of breathing and should be discontinued as soon as the patient is able to breathe room air.
- A full E oxygen cylinder contains $\approx$ 600 L of O_2 and lasts only 15 to 20 minutes in resuscitation of an adult (see Chapter 47, p. 736).

Ventilation with an Ambu Bag in Foals

- Attach the Ambu Bag to the endotracheal or tracheotomy tube.
- Place the oxygen insufflation tube into the reservoir of the Ambu Bag to increase inspired O_2 concentration.
- Open the oxygen tank, and turn the flowmeter to 15 L/min.

- Compress the Ambu Bag until full expansion of the lungs is achieved.
- Exhalation is passive through a valve on the Ambu Bag.
- Administer approximately 20 breaths per minute.
  - Foal resuscitator may be used if intubation is not possible. There are at least two commercial resuscitators[18,19] sold for use in foals through distributors worldwide.

Ventilation with a Nasotracheal Tube and Demand Valve

- Intubate the patient with a clean, lubricated nasotracheal tube (see intubation procedure, p. 450). Do not advance beyond the midcervical area of the trachea.
- Attach the free end of the tube to the oxygen cylinder regulator.
- Open the regulator on the tank to a maximal flow rate.
- Occlude both nares and watch the chest rise to full inflation, which can take as long as 8 seconds in an adult, depending on lung compliance. *Do not* overinflate the lungs.
- Once the lungs are inflated, open the nostrils to allow passive exhalation.
- Deliver 10 to 12 breaths per minute to an adult and 15 to 20 breaths per minute to a foal.
- The E oxygen cylinder lasts only 10 to 15 minutes at maximal flow.

Complications

- Overinflation of the lungs results in barotrauma and injury to the alveoli, and possibly, pulmonary emphysema.

Nebulization

- Nebulizers that aerosolize particles 0.5 to 2 μm are required.
- Ultrasonic nebulizers are preferred because they have high aerosol output and are much faster than other forms of nebulization; nebulization of 30 to 50 mL of solution can usually be accomplished in 15 to 20 minutes; The Nouvag-Altraneb nebulizer[20] works well.
- Antibiotics, ideally preservative free, although not mandatory, *mixed with a bronchodilator* (most commonly albuterol, 3 to 5 mL of a 0.5% commercial solution; q.s. to 30 mL with sterile water [for ceftiofur] or preferably 0.45% sterile saline for other drugs) are a combination commonly used for bacterial infection of the lower airways and lung.
  - Gentamicin, 2.2 mg/kg as a 50 mg/mL solution, q24h (it is a concentration-dependent drug) and ceftiofur, 1 mg/kg as a 25 mg/mL solution q12h (it is a time-dependent drug) are the most frequently nebulized antibiotics.

---

[17]LSP Demand Valve (with 6-foot [1.8-m] hose and female DISS fitting) 063-03; must specify 160 LPM when ordering (Allied Healthcare Products).

[18]Resuscitator (Animal Reproduction Systems, Chino, CA 91710).
[19]Resuscitator (McCulloch Products in Auckland New Zealand).
[20]Nouvag-Altraneb nebulizer (Susquehanna Micro, Windsor, Pennsylvania).

- Amikacin at 6.6 mg/kg can be used in place of gentamicin.
- Aminoglycosides are poorly absorbed after nebulization; the nebulization dose is one third the systemic dose.
- If systemic treatment with aminoglycosides is also being performed, the systemic dose can be decreased by 10%.
- All nebulized antibiotics should be either mixed with a bronchodilator (i.e., albuterol) or a bronchodilator should be nebulized just before the antibiotic.
- One to 2.5 mL of 10% acetylcysteine may be added to the mixture if there is a large amount of exudate in the airways or in neonatal foals with acute respiratory distress because acetylcysteine may have antioxidant properties.
- In addition, surfactant may be nebulized, although intratracheal administration is preferred; 30-mL nebulizations require approximately 20 minutes and can be repeated q4 to 8h.
- The mask should be fitted so that CO_2 can be adequately exhaled.
- All tubing should be kept clean, away from barn dust, and replaced every 1 to 2 days.
- Steroids (preferably budesonide, 0.5 to 2 mg, or dexamethasone, 1 to 2 mg, sodium phosphate–preservative free) may be added to the solution for aspiration pneumonia.
- Metered dose inhalers are also available and can be used for bronchodilatory therapy.
- The Equine Haler[21] and the AeroHippus[22] are comparable in efficacy and can be used to administer the following in the adult horse:
- Albuterol, 360-900 µg
- Salbutamol, 500-1000 µg
- Ipratropium, 100-200 µg
- Combivent is a combination of albuterol and ipratropium.
- Corticosteroids such as:
  - Fluticasone, 2000 to 3000 µg
  - Beclomethasone, 1500 to 3500 µg

Metered dose inhalers are best used for maintenance therapy, whereas nebulization and systemic therapy are better for more acute respiratory diseases.

Temporary Tracheostomy

Janik C. Gasiorowski and James A. Orsini

- The terms tracheotomy and "temporary" tracheostomy are frequently used interchangeably; temporary tracheostomy is preferred when an indwelling tracheal cannula is placed in the tracheal lumen as part of the surgical procedure.
- Tracheotomy is performed on an emergency basis when acute respiratory obstruction occurs. This procedure establishes an airway that bypasses the larynx and nasal passages and can be lifesaving if there is an obstruction of the upper respiratory tract.

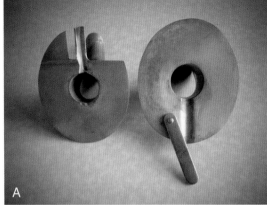

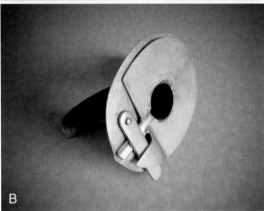

Figure 25-2   Metal tracheostomy device. **A,** Device as two pieces. **B,** Device assembled.

- A temporary tracheostomy provides a direct route for manual ventilation or even inhalant anesthesia regardless of the cause of upper respiratory obstruction. This procedure does not help in cases of lower respiratory problems resulting in respiratory compromise.
- Tracheostomy occasionally is indicated before operations on the larynx or nasal passage when upper respiratory obstruction is anticipated (i.e., debridement of necrotic laryngitis) or in which orotracheal intubation would preclude surgical access (i.e., arytenoidectomy).

Equipment

- Clippers
- Material for sterile scrub
- 2% local anesthetic, 5- to 10-mL syringe, and 22-gauge, $\frac{1}{2}$-inch (1.25-cm) needle
- Sterile gloves
- #10 scalpel blade and handle
- Appropriately sized tracheotomy tube[23]
  - ***Practice Tip:*** *For those inexperienced in performing tracheostomy, a two part metal tracheotomy tube[24] is easier to use! See Fig. 25-2.*
- Size 0 nonabsorbable suture on a straight needle (optional)

---

[21]Equine Haler (Jorgensen Labs, Loveland, Colorado, 800-525-5614).
[22]AeroHippus (Trudell, 866-761-6578).

[23]Tracheostomy tube, 18-mm or 28-mm internal diameter (Jorgensen Laboratories, Inc., Loveland, Colorado).
[24]Two part metal tracheostomy tube (Jorgensen Labs, Loveland, Colorado).

Procedure

- Sedate patient if circumstances allow/neccesitate.
  Landmarks: The trachea is easily palpated directly on the ventral midline of the neck. Isolate a section of the trachea between the upper and middle third of the neck in a horse and middle of the neck in a pony.
- Clip the surgical area and prepare with a sterile scrub.
- Inject 5 to 10 mL of local anesthetic into the subcutaneous tissue over the trachea. The bleb should be 5 to 7 cm long on the midline.
- With sterile gloved hands, grasp the trachea and make a vertical 5-cm incision through the skin and subcutaneous tissue parallel to the length of the trachea with a scalpel blade.
- Bluntly separate the underlying muscle bellies (paired sternothyrohyoideus) on the midline raphe; retract each belly laterally until the trachea is located on the midline (Fig. 25-3).
- Incise the tracheal annular ligament between two cartilage rings. The incision should be parallel to the cartilage rings and thus perpendicular to the skin incision. The incision should be only long enough to allow passage of the tracheal tube and should not exceed more than a third to one-half of the circumference of the trachea (see Fig. 25-3).
- Insert the tracheal tube through the incision (suture in place if necessary).
- Suction and clean or replace the tracheostomy tube daily because it can become easily obstructed with secretions. It may need to be cleaned more frequently.
- The tracheostomy tube should be large enough to fill the tracheostomy site and must not extend beyond the bifurcation of the trachea to ensure that all lung fields are ventilated.
- **Important:** Sedation may not be necessary, and often contraindicated, for a horse that is in upper respiratory distress but still tractable. Attempting to sedate a horse that is flailing from acute, complete upper airway obstruction is extremely dangerous. In may be safer to perform the procedure quickly immediately after the horse loses consciousness. In a life-threatening emergency, sterile technique is abandoned, any sharp object is used to incise in the described procedure, and any tube available (stomach tube, garden hose, and so on) may be used to initially establish an airway.

Complications

- Wound infection can occur, particularly if sterile technique is not used. The airway is a contaminated environment. The tracheostomy site should be allowed to heal by second intention after removal of the tube and cleaned several times daily during this period.
- Subcutaneous emphysema is likely if air can move around the outside of the tube. The air is a problem only if it carries infectious agents with it or if it dissects along tissue planes, leading to pneumomediastinum, pneumothorax, or both.
- Tracheal stricture is possible as the tracheal mucosa contracts during healing. Granulation tissue is produced intraluminally and can contribute to luminal narrowing if excessive.
- If tracheal rings are damaged in the process, cartilaginous deformity and luminal narrowing may result.

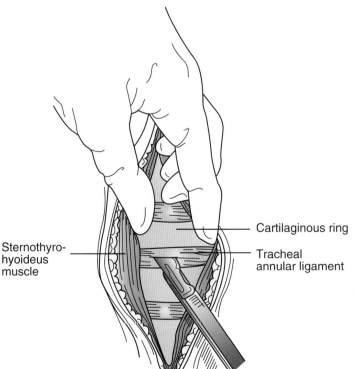

Sternothyro-hyoideus muscle

Cartilaginous ring

Tracheal annular ligament

Figure 25-3 Surgical technique for tracheostomy. Make a vertical midline incision in the skin, divide the sternothyrohyoideus muscle, and horizontally incise an annular ligament to allow passage of the tracheotomy tube.

Paranasal Sinus Trephination

- Sinus trephination, or creating a hole in the bone overlying the paranasal sinuses for access to the sinus cavity, is a procedure used for diagnosis and treatment of paranasal sinus disease.
- Clinical signs suggestive of sinus disease (nasal discharge, facial asymmetry) are frequently supported by abnormal findings on radiography that help localize the disease to a particular sinus.
- If findings on radiography are normal or inconclusive, exploratory sinoscopy of the frontal and caudal maxillary sinuses can be performed through a small trephination site.
- If a bacterial infection is suspected, sinocentesis provides a laboratory sample suitable for cytologic examination and culture and sensitivity determinations.
- Trephination with sinus lavage is the treatment of choice for patients with chronic sinusitis and associated empyema that are refractory to systemic antimicrobial therapy.
- The frontal sinus is dorsal and medial to the orbit. The left and right frontal sinuses are separated by a median septum. The frontal sinus communicates with the caudal maxillary sinus through the frontal maxillary opening.
  - Sinoscopy of the frontal and caudal maxillary sinuses is most easily performed by means of trephination of the frontal sinus.
- The maxillary sinus is paired and is rostral and ventral to the orbit. The sinus is divided into rostral and caudal compartments by an incomplete oblique septum. Both compartments communicate with the ventral nasal meatus through the nasomaxillary opening.
  - Because of its more ventral location, the maxillary sinus is usually the site of greatest fluid accumulation in sinusitis.
  - Ideally, both compartments should be cultured and lavaged, but lavage of the rostral compartment only can provide satisfactory results.

Equipment

- Sedative (xylazine hydrochloride or detomidine)
- Clippers
- 2% local anesthetic, 25-gauge, $\frac{5}{8}$-inch (1.6-cm) needle, 3-mL syringe
- Material for a sterile scrub
- Sterile gloves
- #15 scalpel blade with handle
- The trephine used depends on availability and the size of the hole required
  - For sinus lavage: 2.5-, 3.2-, or 4.5-mm ($\frac{3}{16}$ to $\frac{1}{4}$ inch) drill bit and drill or 2.0- to 4.5-mm ($\frac{5}{32}$, $\frac{3}{16}$, or $\frac{1}{4}$ inch) Steinmann pin[25] with Jacobs chuck[26]
  - For passage of a 4-mm endoscope: 6.34-mm Steinmann pin with Jacobs chuck

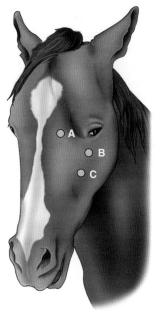

Figure 25-4   Sites for paranasal sinus trephination in an adult. ***A,*** *Frontal sinus.* Draw a horizontal line from midline to the medial canthus and trephine at a location 1 cm lateral to the midpoint of this line. ***B,*** *Caudal maxillary sinus.* Trephine at a location 3 cm rostral from the medial canthus and 3 cm dorsal from the facial crest. ***C,*** *Rostral maxillary sinus.* Trephine at a location half the distance along a line drawn from the medial canthus to the rostral end of the facial crest.

- For sinocentesis and sinus lavage: Intravenous catheter[27] (14-gauge, 2-inch [5 cm] long): Remove stylet and cut end so that the catheter is only $\frac{3}{4}$ inch (1.9 cm) long, or alternatively, a 1-inch teat cannula can be used.
- 2-0 nonabsorbable suture
- 5-mL syringe
- EDTA (purple top) Vacutainer tube[28] for cytologic examination
- Culturette[29] or Port-a-Cul[30] culture system or both
- 1 L saline solution with 0.5% to 1% povidone-iodine (Betadine) and a 30-inch (75-cm) extension set[31] for sinus lavage

Procedure

- Procedure may be done on a standing, sedated patient or with general anesthesia. For sedation, administer 0.01 to 0.02 mg/kg detomidine IV or 0.4 to 0.7 mg/kg xylazine IV.
- See Fig. 25-4 for trephination sites for each paranasal sinus.
- Choose a trephination site clip a 5-cm area, and perform a sterile scrub.
- Infiltrate 2 mL of 2% local anesthetic subcutaneously to the level of the periosteum.

---

[25]Steinmann pin (size 2.5, 3.2, 4.5, or 6.34 mm; Synthes [USA] Paoli, Pennsylvania).
[26]Jacobs chuck (A.J. Buck and Son, Inc., Owings Mills, Maryland).
[27]Abbocath-T radiopaque FEP Teflon IV catheter, 14-gauge, 2-inch long (Abbott Laboratories, Inc., Abbott Park, Illinois).
[28]Vacutainer tubes (Becton-Dickinson Vacutainer Systems).
[29]Culturette collection and transport system (Becton-Dickinson Microbiology Systems).
[30]Port-a-Cul tube (Becton-Dickinson Microbiology Systems).
[31]30-inch extension set (Abbott Laboratories, Inc.).

RESP

- Maintaining aseptic technique, make a 0.5- to 1.5-cm stab incision (depending on the portal size required) through the skin down to the periosteum.
- Using a $\frac{1}{8}$- to $\frac{1}{4}$-inch (0.3- to 0.6-cm) Steinmann pin or a 3.2-mm drill bit, drill a hole in the bone overlying the sinus perpendicular to the bone surface.
- **Note:** Review anatomy of overlying soft tissue and intrasinus structures is recommended before performing the procedure to minimize post-operative complications.

  Practice Tip: Be careful not to overdrill the bone and traumatize the sinus cavity. The bone is only a few millimeters thick, and drilling should stop as soon as there is loss of resistance. When a drill bit is used, there is a greater chance of breaking the drill bit if the patient moves.

For Sinocentesis and Sinus Lavage

- Insert the catheter, and attempt to seat the injection portal into the bone.
- Attach a 5-mL syringe to the catheter, and aspirate any fluid within the sinus. If no fluid is obtained, inject 30 mL of warm sterile saline solution before reaspirating. A sample for culture and cytologic examination should be collected at this time.
- Once a sample is obtained, attach the extension set to the catheter, and flush the dilute povidone-iodine solution into the sinus. The saline solution and any purulent exudate are lavaged from the sinus through the nasal passages if the nasomaxillary opening is patent.
- If repeated lavage is needed, suture the catheter to the skin. If not, remove the catheter and place several interrupted sutures in the skin. If purulent material has exited from the trephination site, clean the area and place topical antibiotics in the wound before suture placement.

Complications

- Wound infection or abscess formation can occur at the trephination site. Incise and drain the abscess or remove the sutures, and allow the area to drain and heal by secondary intention. Clean aseptically and apply topical antibiotics until the area is healed.
- Epistaxis occurs if the sinus mucosa is excessively traumatized during trephination or catheter placement.

Thoracocentesis and Chest Tube Placement

- Thoracocentesis is the aspiration of fluid from the thoracic cavity and serves both diagnostic and therapeutic functions.
- The procedure is easily performed on a standing horse and may be indicated when pleural effusion is suspected on the basis of findings on auscultation of the chest, radiography, or ultrasonographic evaluation.
- Pleural effusion most often accompanies pleuropneumonia, formation of a pleural abscess, and neoplasia. Pleural effusion may also occur as a result of hemothorax in foals with fractured ribs and rarely in exercising horses or older horses receiving phenylephrine.

- Analysis of pleural fluid differentiates these problems and can be lifesaving if the effusion compromises respiratory function.

Equipment

- Clippers
- Material for sterile scrub
- Local anesthetic
- 5-mL syringe and 25-gauge, $\frac{5}{8}$-inch (1.6-cm) needle
- Sterile scalpel blade (#12) and handle (#3)
- Sterile metal teat cannula ($2\frac{1}{2}$ to 4 inches [6.2 to 10 cm] long)[32] or metal bitch urinary catheter ($10\frac{1}{2}$ inches [26.2 cm] long)[33]: Blunt-tipped cannulas are less likely to lacerate the lung.
- Three-way stopcock[34] or extension set tubing[35]
- 60-mL syringe
- Nonabsorbable size 0 suture
- Chest tube[36] 20 to 24 French with or without Heimlich one-way valve[37] for repeated drainage
- Plain and EDTA Vacutainer tubes[38]
- Port-a-Cul (aerobic/anaerobic) culture system[39]

Procedure

- Sedation may be necessary, depending on the disposition and degree of illness of the patient. Recommended dosage is 0.3 to 0.5 mg/kg xylazine with 0.01 to 0.025 mg/kg butorphanol IV.

Thoracocentesis

- Choose a site for thoracocentesis based on results of auscultation of dull lung fields, or preferably, by ultrasound examination. Fluid usually collects ventrally. A common site for thoracocentesis is the lower third of the thorax between the seventh and eighth intercostal spaces. Both sides of the chest should be aspirated if bilateral effusion is suspected because most horses with pleuritis have an intact mediastinum.

  Caution: Avoid the heart when placing the needle or chest tube ventrally! Ultrasound guidance is recommended for precise placement.
- Clip and prepare the site aseptically.
- Inject 5 to 10 mL of local anesthetic subcutaneously and into the intercostal muscle. Perform final skin preparation.

---

[32]Ideal udder infusion cannula (Butler Animal Health Supply, Dublin, Ohio).
[33]Metal bitch urinary catheter (Jorgensen Laboratories, Inc.).
[34]Pharmaseal K75 3-way stopcock (Baxter Healthcare Corp., Deerfield Illinois).
[35]Extension set, 7 or 30 inch (Abbott Laboratories, Inc.).
[36]Thal-Quick chest drainage catheter set (24F to 36F, 41-cm long; Advanced Anesthesia Specialists, LLC, Prescott, Arizona).
[37]Heimlich chest drainage valve (Advanced Anesthesia Specialists, LLC, Prescott, Arizona).
[38]Vacutainer (Becton-Dickinson Vacutainer Systems).
[39]Port-a-Cul (Becton-Dickinson Microbiology Systems).

- Make a stab incision through the skin and fascia at the cranial aspect of the rib to avoid the intercostal vessels and nerves, which are located on the caudal border. Also look for and avoid the lateral thoracic vein.
  - ***Practice Tip:*** *Extension of the stab incision into the intercostal muscle makes passage of the teat cannula or thoracic trocar easier. If there is considerable resistance when passing the teat cannula, it can break! It is also important to inject lidocaine close to the parietal pleura because of the sensitivity of the pleura.*
- Maintaining aseptic technique, hold the cannula and attach a three-way stopcock or tubing with the end clamped to prevent pneumothorax if negative pressure exists in the thoracic cavity. Alternatively, a cannula can be inserted with sterile syringe attached.
- Insert the cannula into the skin incision and push through the intercostal muscle. A sudden loss of resistance is felt as the pleural space is entered. If there is not a large quantity of pleural effusion, it is important not to advance the cannula any further at this point so as to avoid lacerating the lung.
- Attach a 60-mL syringe to the stopcock or tubing. Aspiration should yield fluid if an effusion is present. Rotation or gentle redirection of the cannula often is needed. If fluid is freely flowing, which is normal in these cases, it can be siphoned off into a bucket.
- Keep the tubing or stopcock closed when not removing fluid to prevent aspiration of air and iatrogenic pneumothorax.
- Once fluid is no longer retrievable, place a purse-string suture around the cannula and tighten the suture as the cannula is removed. If septic fluid is removed, antimicrobials can be infiltrated around the incision. Apply an antiseptic or antibiotic ointment, and bandage the wound.

Chest Tube Placement

Repeated drainage often is necessary, particularly when large volumes of fluid are present or infection is suspected. For these patients, an indwelling human chest tube is required.

- Choose the smallest-size tube that allows fibrinous material to drain.
- Follow the instructions for chest tube placement that accompany the product. A one-way valve can be used to maintain negative pressure.
- Use a purse-string suture or Chinese finger knot to attach the tube to the skin; tie the free suture ends around the tube several times in a locking pattern, or use rapid-curing glue.
- The chest tube can be clamped when it is not being used; however, this is not necessary if the Heimlich valve or "condom," acting as a one-way valve, is sufficiently adhered to the tube. An open condom (closed end cut) can be placed around the outside of the tube and tightly taped to the tube to prevent air entering the thorax in lieu of a commercially available Heimlich valve.
- The chest tube may be left in place for up to 1 month. It can be changed as needed if debris occludes the

lumen. Lavage of the pleural space with pH-balanced polyionic fluid may be helpful. Sinus tracts that form around the tube often heal spontaneously after tube removal.

- ***Practice Tip:*** *Use of tissue plasminogen activator (tPA), 4 to 12 mg infused into the pleural space, early in the treatment of pleuritis can be helpful in preventing the formation of fibrinous pockets.*

Pleural Fluid Analysis

- Only 1 to 2 mL of straw-colored fluid is retrieved from a normal pleural cavity.
- Color, opacity, volume, and odor are useful parameters.
  - Yellow, opaque fluid with fibrinous clots suggests a septic exudate.
  - The presence of foul-smelling effusion correlates well with the presence of anaerobic bacterial colonization.
  - A relatively clear to serosanguineous exudate occasionally is seen in neoplastic processes.
- Cytologic examination (with a total cell count and differential) and measurement of total protein should be performed to classify the effusion definitively.
  - The normal total protein level is less than 2.5 g/dL, and the total nucleated cell count is typically less than 8000 cells/µL.
  - Neoplastic disease often has a significant inflammatory component and can mimic an infectious process. Often neoplastic cells are shed into the pleural fluid and can be identified at cytologic examination.
- Specimens for anaerobic and aerobic cultures should be submitted to the laboratory if infection is suspected. ***Practice Tip:*** *If the presence of sepsis is unclear from the clinical signs and cytology, comparison of glucose and lactate between the pleural fluid and plasma may be helpful in determining the existence of sepsis.*

Complications

- Pneumothorax can occur when air enters the pleural cavity if the cannula is placed too dorsally during thoracocentesis. The thorax normally has negative pressure, and when fluid has been removed, the thorax should return to negative pressure. To correct pneumothorax, aspirate air dorsally with a 4-inch cannula, catheter, or chest tube in the same manner that fluid is aspirated (see Chapter 46, p. 730).
- Hemothorax can occur if a large vein or artery is punctured during insertion of a cannula. Avoid the lateral thoracic vein (in the ventral third of the thorax) and *always enter along the cranial margin of a rib.*
- If the heart is accidentally punctured during cannula placement, fatal cardiac arrhythmia can result. Avoid the cranial/ventral aspect of the thorax and use ultrasound guidance to place a chest tube.
- Hypovolemia is rare as a result of pleural fluid removal even when large volumes (10 to 20 L) are removed by means of thoracocentesis; however, fluid therapy should be instituted to replace the volume lost.

RESPIRATORY TRACT EMERGENCIES

*Jean-Pierre Lavoie, Thomas J. Divers,
and Fairfield T. Bain*

Emergencies of the respiratory system are generally conditions causing respiratory distress; however, in some cases the disease can be life-threatening without producing distress, such as pleuropneumonia, and therefore is treated as an emergency.

- The initial diagnostic goal when evaluating a patient with respiratory distress is to determine whether the problem is:
  - Upper respiratory disorder (obstruction)
  - Lower respiratory problem (e.g., pulmonary edema, bronchoconstriction, or pneumothorax)
- The presence of upper respiratory disease, including tracheitis, usually can be determined on the basis of the noise (stridor) the patient is making when breathing, especially on inspiration.
- The presence of lower respiratory disease causing respiratory distress usually can be determined by means of auscultation of the thorax.
- *Practice Tip: Inspiratory dyspnea often is more pronounced than expiratory dyspnea with upper airway obstruction, whereas the reverse is true with lower airway obstruction, such as heaves (RAO).*
- The presence of life-threatening respiratory infection without respiratory distress that necessitates emergency care, such as pleuropneumonia or aspiration pneumonia, usually can be determined with the history, auscultation of the thorax, and routine diagnostic procedures, such as ultrasonography and tracheal aspiration.

Respiratory Distress with Respiratory Noise: Upper Airway Obstruction

- Labored breathing due to upper airway obstruction usually produces noise.
- The list of differential diagnoses is long, so perform a complete physical examination with ancillary diagnostic equipment (e.g., endoscopy and radiography) to identify clinical features that narrow the possible causes.
- Remember that acute respiratory obstruction often is rapidly progressive for three reasons:
  - The primary disease process, such as edema, often is progressive.
  - Constant turbulence of airflow against the compromised airway leads to increased edema.
  - Increased negative pleural pressure caused by increased respiratory effort against an obstructed airway may lead to pulmonary edema.
- Consider any acute respiratory noise an emergency.

Nasal Obstruction

For respiratory distress to occur, both nares must be compromised. The most common causes of acute, bilateral nasal obstruction are the following:

- Trauma, including foreign bodies
- Atresia of the choanae
- Anaphylaxis
- Bee sting
- Snake bite (see Chapter 45, p. 724)
- Facial clostridial myonecrosis
- Acute obstruction of one or more commonly both jugular veins, along with low head carriage (depression or tranquilization)
- Some chronic diseases of the nasal cavity, such as neoplasia, granuloma, or ethmoid hematoma, can occasionally cause acute onset of respiratory distress
- Postanesthetic period when the head has remained in a dependent position during prolonged surgeries (nasal hyperemia and edema)
- Expansive disorders of the sinuses such as primary empyema, sinus cysts, and neoplasia causing compression of the nasal meatuses; rarely do these require emergency treatment
- Horner syndrome in addition to tranquilization and prolonged lowering of the head, which may cause nasal edema and obstruction

Trauma to the Nasal Cavity

- Trauma to the nasal cavity can occur when a horse:
  - Runs into a fixed object in the field
  - Is kicked
  - Engages in continuous head pressing with cerebral disease
- Trauma also occurs in severely depressed individuals that keep their heads lowered and frequently have a nasogastric tube inserted. Trauma may result in nasal septum fracture/deviations with exuberant callus formation and subsequent persistent nasal obstruction.

◉ WHAT TO DO

Management of Blunt Nasal Trauma

- Keep affected individual as quiet as possible. Apply ice packs to the external nasal surface.
- Spray lidocaine with epinephrine 2% (25 mL in each nostril for an adult) into the nasal cavity. Phenylephrine spray (0.1%, 20 to 30 mL total per adult-sized horse) also can be used.
- If progressive nasal swelling is expected, secure a small intranasal tube (9- to 15-mm diameter, 4- to 8-cm length) by suturing to the nostril to help maintain a patent nasal airway. This is easier than performing a tracheotomy; however, nasal mucosal necrosis can result from the pressure of the tube. A nasotracheal tube can also be used.
- Tracheotomy may be needed in some cases.
- Try to keep the head elevated to at least the level of the shoulder. If the affected individual safely tolerates it, the head should be tied or supported in an elevated position.
- Maintain complete patency of jugular veins.
- Begin administration of appropriate antibiotics.
- Suture any wounds.
- Administer tetanus toxoid (or antitoxin, if indicated) if no previous vaccination.

• Always consider the possibility of serious head trauma and its sequelae.

WHAT NOT TO DO

Management of Blunt Trauma (Injury to the Nose)
• *Do not* use xylazine or any tranquilizer that causes lowering of the head or an increase in upper airway resistance.

WHAT TO DO

Atresia of the Choanae
• Can be unilateral or bilateral
• When bilateral, atresia of the choanae is life-threatening and detectable at birth; emergency temporary tracheostomy is required to maintain airway patency

Thrombosis of Jugular Veins
• Bilateral thrombosis of the jugular veins can occur in severely ill patients receiving intravenous medications, especially hypertonic fluids or acidic or alkaline drugs, through the jugular vein.
• Unfortunately, many of these patients are depressed and hold their heads lower than normal because of the primary disease, and progressive nasal edema can result.
• Tracheostomy can be avoided with medical treatment if the patient can maintain its head in a normal position.
• Critically ill horses with acute thrombosis of one jugular vein should ideally have medication and fluids administered in the lateral thoracic vein (see Chapter 1, p. 3), and blood samples should be collected from the catheter or facial sinus (see p. 2) to prevent injury to the remaining jugular vein. Avoid large-volume fluid administration to minimize phlebitis and thrombosis.

WHAT TO DO

Acute Jugular Vein Thrombosis
• Avoid traumatic manipulation of the veins; if one jugular vein is still patent and must be used, aseptic technique for introduction of a "low" thrombogenic catheter is recommended, and if possible, dilute high or low pH drugs with a normal pH fluid before administration.
• Maintain the head at the level of the shoulder or elevated if possible. Feed horses with a hay net placed at normal head position. If the affected individual tolerates it, the head should be tied in an elevated position or supported, but the patient must be closely monitored to prevent self-induced injury.
• Administer antiedema therapy (e.g., furosemide, 1 mg/kg IV slowly) if edema of the head is severe.
• If one jugular vein is patent with a catheter in place, remove the catheter and place it in the lateral thoracic vein or cephalic vein if possible.
• Begin aspirin, 10 to 20 mg/kg or 4.5 to 9 g/450-kg adult PO q48h. Give aspirin every 2 to 3 days for its antiplatelet effect. Pentoxifylline does not inhibit platelet aggregation in the horse, but it may make red blood cells more deformable. Clopidogrel (Plavix), 2 to 3 mg/kg PO q24h, inhibits platelets better than aspirin in the horse.

• Low-molecular-weight heparin, 50 U/kg, or regular heparin, 50 to 80 IU/kg, administered subcutaneously may be helpful in decreasing progressive thrombosis.
• If the thrombosis is acute, tPA can be injected with a 25-gauge needle just proximal to the thrombosis in hopes of lysing the clot. This carries a risk of pulmonary thromboembolism.
• If hypoproteinemia is compounding the problem, administer plasma (2 to 10 L), fresh or fresh frozen, or hetastarch (2 to 10 mL/kg). Consider cost and expected benefit.

Bee Sting
Bee stings or vaccine reactions can produce acute severe nasal edema.

WHAT TO DO

Bee Sting or Fire Ant Bite on Nose
• Apply cold compresses
• Administer antihistamines:
  • Diphenhydramine (Benadryl), 1 mg/kg IM or slowly IV
  • Doxylamine succinate, 0.5 mg/kg slowly IV (unusual behavior may occur when administered rapidly)
• Consider examethasone if the edema is progressive and severe: 0.1 to 0.2 mg/kg IV q24h
• Administer epinephrine, 3 to 5 mL of 1:1000 solution IV to a 450-kg adult, if the swelling is rapidly progressive or if there are signs of systemic hypotension (tachycardia, poor pulse quality)
• Consider whether a tracheotomy is indicated (see p. 438)
• Keep the head level or elevated.

Snake Bite
• Venomous snakes may bite horses and cause severe tissue necrosis (see Chapter 45, p. 724).
• The nose is a common site for a bite, and severe swelling results.
  • Swelling is considerable with rattlesnake bites.

Clinical Signs and Diagnosis
• The swelling is initially warm and then becomes cool as the skin becomes necrotic.
• It may be necessary to shave the area to identify the fang marks. Bite marks may help differentiate the snake species.
• Severe cellulitis often is associated with infections with *Clostridium* organisms.
• Hemolytic anemia occurs infrequently.
• Gastrointestinal signs (colic, diarrhea) may be present.
• Tachycardia can result from pain, relative hypovolemia, or myocarditis.
• Severe systemic effects from the venom are not common in adults.
• In foals, systemic effects include hypotension and shock.

WHAT TO DO

Snake Bite on Nose
• If the airway becomes obstructed, perform tracheostomy (also see p. 456).
• If the nose is bitten and airway obstruction has not developed, keep the head level or elevated to minimize severe swelling. Pass a

nasotracheal tube, shortened stomach tube, or syringe case, and leave it in place to prevent airway obstruction.
- Administer flunixin meglumine to decrease inflammation and diminish systemic effects caused by proinflammatory prostanoids. It has little effect on platelet function.
- Administer penicillin in all cases, 22,000 to 44,000 U/kg IV (preferably q6h), or 22,000 U/kg IM q12h.
- Administer metronidazole, 15 to 25 mg/kg PO q8h, and gentamicin, 6.6 mg/kg IV q24h. Substitute ceftiofur, 3.0 mg/kg IV or IM q12h, for gentamicin if hydration and renal function are a concern.
- Administer tetanus toxoid for adults or toxoid and antitoxin to foals or if vaccination status is unknown or deficient.
- If hypotensive therapy is needed, give fluids including hypertonic saline solution, plasma, and finally pressor drugs if the fluids do not correct the hypotension (see Systemic Shock, Chapter 32, p. 565). *Caution:* Dehydration must be avoided if gentamicin is used!
- Antivenin (equine origin) is recommended if it can be administered within the first 24 hours of the bite. Antivenin may also benefit foals bitten by coral snakes.
- Foals should be managed appropriately with:
  - Intravenous fluids
  - Inotropic or pressor drugs (e.g., dopamine, 5 to 10 µg/kg per minute; or dobutamine, 5 to 15 µg/kg per minute; or norepinephrine, 0.02 to 0.1 µg/kg per minute)
  - Fluids
  - Drugs
- **Practice Tip:** *Remember that foals do* not *have as dramatic an increase in blood pressure in response to pressor drugs as do adults.* Change in heart rate should be monitored in foals receiving beta- and alpha-agonist combination drugs. More than a 40% increase in heart rate is a signal to slow the rate of drug administration.
- Antivenom[40] is available and can be administered.

Laryngeal/Pharyngeal Obstruction

WHAT TO DO

Airway and Breathing
- Nasotracheal intubation can be difficult to perform on a distressed patient.
- In most cases, tracheotomy is preferred.
- If the instruments to perform the tracheotomy are not readily available, attempt nasotracheal intubation.
- If the patient collapses, perform nasotracheal intubation because it is faster.
- Secondary pulmonary edema is a common occurrence with acute severe upper airway obstruction; routinely administer furosemide in these cases.

Laryngeal Edema Associated with Anaphylaxis
- The cause often is unknown, but it can be an anaphylactic reaction to vaccine antigens or can accompany purpura hemorrhagica.

Diagnosis
- Endoscopic examination is the best diagnostic tool. Edema and collapse of the tissues around the larynx are seen. Avoid tranquilization if possible.

[40]Antivenom (Lake Immunogenics, Ontario, New York: 800-648-9990; Red Rock Biologies, Woodland, California; 866-897-7625).

- Administer acepromazine, 0.02 to 0.04 mg/kg IV, and butorphanol, 0.01 to 0.02 mg/kg IV, for sedation if necessary to better examine the larynx endoscopically.

WHAT TO DO

Laryngeal Edema Associated with Anaphylaxis
- If laryngeal edema is caused by an anaphylactic reaction, administer epinephrine, 3 to 7 mL/450-kg adult (1:1000 as packaged) slowly intravenously. If time permits, dilute in 20 to 30 mL of 0.9% saline solution. Similar doses of epinephrine may be administered intramuscularly or subcutaneously in less severe cases.
- If respiratory stridor is present, which suggests 80% or more compromise of the airflow, pass a nasotracheal tube to prevent further obstruction and the need for tracheotomy. Caution: The tube might increase the edema via mechanical irritation.
- If laryngeal edema is severe, perform tracheotomy (see p. 455).
- If pulmonary edema has developed (crackles on auscultation or froth at the nostril), begin furosemide therapy, 1 mg/kg IV, and see p. 472.
- Dexamethasone, 0.1 to 0.2 mg/kg IV bolus; DMSO, 1 g/kg IV in 3 L of 0.9% saline solution; or dextrose 5% may also be administered.
- For systemic anaphylaxis, administer crystalloid and colloid fluids because affected individuals may be hypotensive except for those that have received large doses of epinephrine.
- Provide intranasal or intratracheal oxygen delivery.

WHAT NOT TO DO

Laryngeal Edema
- *Do not* administer acepromazine if systemic anaphylaxis and hypotension are a possibility.
- *Do not* use α_2-agonists, such as xylazine and detomidine, because they increase upper airway resistance.

Prognosis
- Prognosis is generally good, but the condition may persist for several days or recur.

Epiglottitis
- When acute, epiglottitis may cause a respiratory noise, and on rare occasions, produce respiratory distress similar to croup in human beings.
- Epiglottitis is more common in racehorses.
- Examine the underside of the epiglottis to determine the full extent of the inflammation; slowly instill topical 2% lidocaine (30 mL) around the pharynx through the endoscope to facilitate epiglottic elevation.

WHAT TO DO

Epiglottitis
- Provide rest.
- Throat spray (colloidal silver or a dexamethasone/[nitrofurazone {Furacin} spray, DMSO]) and nonsteroidal anti-inflammatory drugs (NSAIDs) are recommended.
- Administer oral antibiotics such as:
  - Trimethoprim-sulfamethoxazole, 20 to 30 mg/kg PO q12h
  - Ceftiofur, 3 mg/kg IV q12h

- Metronidazole, 15 to 30 mg/kg per rectum q8h, should be added if the breath smell is fetid. Metronidazole may be irritating to the oral and esophageal mucosa if they are already injured.
- Replace hay with less abrasive feeds such as grass hay, wetted pelleted or cubed hay, or hay silage.
- Tracheotomy is rarely needed for epiglottitis.

Subepiglottic Cysts
- Patient has history of exercise respiratory noise, coughing, and dysphagia. In rare instances a subepiglottic cyst may completely obstruct the upper airway and cause respiratory distress.
- Perform tracheotomy before the surgical removal of the cyst if labored breathing is present.

Arytenoid Chondropathy
- In most cases, the chondrosis has been present for an extended period, though the obstruction may be acute.
- ***Practice Tip:*** *If noise is apparent at rest, there is generally an 80% or more compromise of the airway. Once noise and labored breathing are clinically noticeable, the progression towards complete obstruction can be rapid!*

Diagnosis
- Endoscopic examination

◉▸ WHAT TO DO

Arytenoid Chondropathy
- Perform a tracheostomy (see p. 455 for procedure).
- Throat spray (dexamethasone, nitrofurazone [Furacin], DMSO), systemic antibiotics, and NSAIDs are recommended.
- Surgical removal (arytenoidectomy) of the diseased cartilage is required if medical treatment fails.

Pharyngeal Dysfunction in Neonatal Foals
- Pharyngeal dysfunction may cause oronasal reflux after nursing in the newborn foal.
- Secondary aspiration pneumonia is common.
- Pharyngeal endoscopy rarely reveals dorsal displacement of the soft palate; a cause for the dysfunction is rarely seen.
- The cause is often unproven but may be due to:
  - Neonatal encephalopathy
  - Selenium deficiency
  - Dysmaturity of pharyngeal function
- Many foals recover sufficient function to nurse without aspiration while others are fed by bucket.
- Fourth branchial arch defects may also cause milk to drain from the esophagus into the nose.
- A small number of affected foals may not regain the full respiratory function needed for racing.

◉▸ WHAT TO DO

Pharyngeal Dysfunction: Neonatal Foal
- Feed the foal by nasogastric tube.
- Administer selenium if serum concentration is low.
- Treat aspiration pneumonia if present.

- If a neonatal foal is unable to nurse by 5 to 7 days of age, it is recommended to bucket feed with the bucket at ground level to minimize aspiration.

Laryngeal Paresis/Paralysis
Postanesthetic Laryngeal Spasms
Postanesthetic laryngeal spasm is an anesthetic complication and therefore a problem at referral centers that perform general anesthesia. Most commonly spasm occurs after removal of the endotracheal tube during anesthetic recovery and only rarely occurs following nasogastric intubation. Pulmonary edema quickly follows the obstruction thus it must be immediately managed.

◉▸ WHAT TO DO

Postanesthetic Laryngeal Spasms
- Tracheostomy (see p. 455) or nasotracheal intubation
- Provide oxygen supplementation (10 L/min) through the tracheotomy or nasotracheal tube
- Furosemide 1 mg/kg IV
- DMSO, 1 g/kg IV in 3 L of 0.9% saline solution, plus dexamethasone, 0.1 to 0.2 mg/kg, in cases of pulmonary edema

Hypocalcemia
Hypocalcemic patients can develop laryngeal paresis and consequently laryngeal obstruction.
Diagnosis
- History is important, such as lactation in a mare; however, idiopathic cases have occurred not associated with lactation.
- Other clinical signs are trismus of facial muscles, thumps, and trembling.
- Confirm all presumptive cases by measuring serum calcium levels. Serum calcium concentration usually is less than 6.5 mg/dL (<1.0 mmol/L ionized Ca^{++}) in adults with severe clinical signs. Profuse sweating, hypochloremia, and resultant alkalosis further exacerbate hypocalcemia.

◉▸ WHAT TO DO

Airway Obstruction Due to Hypocalcemia
- Administer calcium borogluconate, 11 g slowly IV over 20 minutes, to an adult (450 kg) while monitoring heart rate and rhythm. ***Note:*** Calcium borogluconate is safer than calcium chloride.
- If clinical signs do *not* resolve, a second treatment may be required. Give additional calcium diluted with polyionic fluids at a slower rate.

◉▸ WHAT NOT TO DO

Calcium Administration
- *Do not* administer calcium borogluconate subcutaneously.

Idiopathic Laryngeal Paralysis in Foals and Adult Horses
History
- A young foal with stertorous breathing with no other physical abnormalities
- Adult horses may also have this condition

Diagnosis

- Perform endoscopy.
- Rule out other known causes in young foals:
  - Hyperkalemic periodic paralysis (HYPP) in Quarter Horses with "Impressive" breeding homozygous for the defective gene: There should be laryngeal and pharyngeal collapse with HYPP, and HYPP is often associated with dysphagia. HYPP does *not* usually cause clinical signs in newborn foals.
  - Transient displacement of the soft palate in newborn foals: Milk reflux is more of a problem than respiratory obstruction, although affected foals may make a noise when handled.
  - ***Practice Tip:*** *Selenium deficiency also can cause collapse of the airways and respiratory noise with distress in very young foals. Consider this in areas (primarily northern United States and Canada) known to be selenium-deficient.*
  - Retropharyngeal strangles lymphadenopathy (see p. 467).

●》 WHAT TO DO

Idiopathic Laryngeal Paralysis

- Perform a tracheostomy for immediate relief (see p. 456).
- Administer selenium intramuscularly (*not* intravenously) if a deficiency is suspected.

Prognosis

- Prognosis is very poor for idiopathic cases and severe selenium deficiency; most cases have little improvement.
- For other differential diagnoses, prognosis is good.

Liver Failure

Acute bilateral laryngeal paralysis may occur in cases of pyrrolizidine alkaloid poisoning and other causes of hepatic encephalopathy. Clinical and biochemical evidence of liver disease is present.

●》 WHAT TO DO

Laryngeal Paralysis /Liver Failure

- Tracheostomy relieves respiratory distress; the prognosis is poor with liver failure.

Bilateral Laryngeal Hemiplegia

- Idiopathic/traumatic
  - Rare
  - Traumatic: right laryngeal hemiplegia (periphlebitis following intravenous injections, neck trauma) in a horse with preexisting left laryngeal hemiplegia
  - Idiopathic: foal laryngeal paralysis (see previous text) and on rare occasion may occur in adults
- Organophosphate poisoning (see Chapter 34, p. 586)

Guttural Pouch Tympany

- In foals, guttural pouch tympany can cause a respiratory noise and predispose the foal to pneumonia; however, it rarely causes respiratory distress.

- Diagnosis is based on obvious distention of the retropharyngeal areas (easily compressible). The condition may be confirmed using lateral radiographs of the head and neck (the guttural pouch extends beyond the second cervical vertebra), or by the decompression of the pouch by applying manual pressure on both sides of the retropharyngeal area or inserting a catheter in the affected pouch.
- Temporary relief of airway obstruction is achieved by applying manual pressure on both sides of the retropharyngeal area or inserting an indwelling catheter in the affected pouch via the nasopharyngeal opening. Avoid transcutaneous decompression of the pouches using a needle because it may cause severe bleeding by inadvertent puncture of a vessel(s) within the guttural pouch and lead to secondary guttural pouch empyema.
- Tracheostomy is usually *not* required.
- Treat aspiration pneumonia, which is almost always present.

Strangles: Diagnostic Approach and Management
Fairfield T. Bain

- Strangles is an infection caused by the gram-positive bacteria *Streptococcus equi* subspecies *equi.*
- It is typically characterized by infection of the upper respiratory tract and associated lymph nodes but can also be seen as a source of internal abscessation and immune reactions within the skin and internal organs.
- The disease more commonly affects young horses and is common worldwide.
- Most outbreaks are associated with introduction of a new horse that is shedding the organism to a group of susceptible horses.
- The organism is maintained within groups of horses by asymptomatic carriers.

Etiopathogenesis

- *Streptococcus equi* subspecies *equi* is commonly known as *Streptococcus equi.* The organism enters the horse either through the oral cavity or nasal passages and subsequently invades the tonsillar epithelium.
- Transfer from the tonsils to the regional lymph nodes may occur within hours. Abscess formation occurs within 3 to 5 days, depending on a variety of factors including infective dose and individual immunity.
- Mandibular lymph adenopathy and node abscessation is considered characteristic with this disease; however, it may affect the retropharyngeal and other lymph nodes of the head. ***Practice Tip:*** *Abscess formation is the hallmark of the disease with rupture and drainage being the eventual path to resolution.*
  - Endoscopy of the guttural pouches is important to identify enlargement of the retropharyngeal lymph nodes protruding into the floor of the medial compartment of the guttural pouches.

RESP

Clinical Signs

- Strangles may infect susceptible horses of all ages, but is much more common in younger animals (<5 years).
- The earliest detectable clinical sign is fever (up to 103° F/39° C or higher), which may coincide with early suppurative inflammation within the regional lymph nodes—mandibular or retropharyngeal—often before detectable lymph node enlargement.
- There may be an initial serous nasal discharge that progresses to mucopurulent discharge within a few days.
- The amount of clinically detectable discharge may be a reflection of the individual's immunity against the organism. ***Practice Tip:*** *Enlargement of the retropharyngeal lymph nodes may compress the dorsal pharyngeal walls and result in some degree of airway obstruction. The external retropharyngeal area may not clinically appear enlarged; however, affected horses may extend their head and neck to compensate for the compromised upper airway.*
- In addition to airway obstruction, pharyngitis and retropharyngeal lymphadenitis may result in painful or difficult swallowing and some degree of inappetence or dysphagia.
- The retropharyngeal lymph nodes may also protrude into the floor of the medial guttural pouch compartment resulting in impairment of nerve function and control of swallowing.
- Lymphadenitis may initially present as painful enlargement of affected lymph nodes, followed by exudation of serum through the overlying skin and eventual rupture and drainage of the affected lymph node.
- Rupture of the retropharyngeal lymph nodes may take several days and result in empyema of the guttural pouches with compression of the pharynx. ***Practice Tip:*** *The more "classically" described appearance of mandibular lymph node enlargement may be absent in many outbreaks, resulting in a delay in diagnosis and additional spread between in-contact horses.*
- Other lymph nodes may also be affected, such as parotid lymph nodes; cervical lymph nodes; or more rarely, internal lymph nodes such as mesenteric lymph nodes.
- Abscesses in the deep cervical or cranial mediastinal lymph nodes can occasionally result in tracheal compression and dyspnea in the absence of upper airway involvement.
- Complications associated with strangles are estimated to occur in up to 20% of cases.
  These complications include:
  - Spread to other sites within the body
  - Internal abscesses
  - Pneumonia
  - Pleuropneumonia
  - Immune reactions
- Pneumonia is reported to be the most common cause of death as a complication of strangles.
- Purpura hemorrhagica is an immune-complex deposition vasculitis associated with exposure to the strangles organism and development of an anamnestic immune response, usually in older horses.

- This complication can result in clinical signs of fever together with painful swelling and serum exudation.
- There is the potential for skin necrosis in severe cases, usually involving the skin of the lower limbs and ventrum.
- Petechiae and variably-sized ecchymotic hemorrhages can occur within the mucosa of the nasal passages.
- ***Practice Tip:*** *Some forms of purpura hemorrhagica can result in acute and rapidly progressive immune-mediated myositis or infarctive lesions within the skeletal muscles (see Chapter 35, p. 615).*
- Clinical signs may appear similar to myositis of other causes and may be severe enough to result in the breakdown of musculotendinous support of the affected limbs.
- A preexisting high serum antibody titer to antigens of *S. equi* (e.g., strep M protein) may be involved in the development of purpura hemorrhagica following either infection or immunization.
- In addition to the classic skin lesions, similar patterns of vasculitis and tissue necrosis can occur within the skeletal musculature and internal organs (i.e., lung and intestine).
- The resulting clinical signs depend on the particular organ system involved:
  - Myopathy
  - Respiratory difficulty
  - Colic

Diagnosis

- Clinical suspicion of strangles infection should be considered in outbreaks of febrile respiratory disease with nasal discharge and lymph node enlargement in groups of young horses.
- ***Practice Tip:*** *Because of the high proportion of horses without external lymph node enlargement, it is important to consider guttural pouch endoscopy in outbreaks of fever within groups of horses.*
- Diagnosis is made by demonstration of the specific etiologic agent *Streptococcus equi* subspecies *equi* by:
  - Bacterial culture:
    - Nasal swabs
    - Purulent exudate from draining lymph nodes
    - Nasopharyngeal or guttural pouch washes
  - Polymerase chain reaction (PCR) of nasopharyngeal or guttural pouch washes
- ***Practice Tip:*** *In some outbreaks, a higher percentage of isolation of the organism may come from the guttural pouches rather than the nasopharynx.*
- The technique for nasopharyngeal wash uses a 20-cm, 10F polypropylene catheter to rinse the nasal passages with 60 mL of sterile saline; this is collected in a sterile collection container as it drains from the nares.
- Endoscopic evaluation of the guttural pouch permits direct visualization of the floor of the medial compartment to look for enlargement of the retropharyngeal lymph nodes, presence of empyema, and chondroids. Direct

lavage of the guttural pouch may be performed using a sterile transendoscopic catheter.[41]

- Initial evaluation of the nasopharynx in affected horses using only a twitch for restraint is recommended to determine the degree of airway compromise before sedation with α_2-agonists because these drugs may result in relaxation of pharyngeal musculature and further compromise airway diameter.
- In certain cases, the use of serology may be useful in obtaining a diagnosis.
  - These may include diagnosis of an internal abscess where obtaining a culture is not possible cases demonstrating immune reactions in the absence of classic infection.
  - Serum antibodies to the streptococcal M-protein (SeM) can be measured by enzyme-linked immunosorbent assay (ELISA). Several laboratories perform this assay including IDvet in Europe and IDEXX laboratories in the United States and Canada. An ELISA detecting antibodies against other streptococcal proteins is also available in the United Kingdom and is used to screen for early infection or carriers.

⊙ WHAT TO DO

Strangles
- Treatment of a horse with strangles depends on the stage of the infection.
- Many young horses progress to rupture and drainage of affected lymph nodes.
- Most affected horses recover with rest and provision of easily accessible feed and water.
- Some horses may require short-term anti-inflammatory treatment to reduce the pain associated with pharyngitis and physical lymph node enlargement; skin care may be necessary at the abscess sites.
- Some horses present with more severe complications such as *airway obstruction or dysphagia.*
- It is important to evaluate the affected horse with airway obstruction via endoscopy to determine the degree of compromise and determine if tracheostomy is indicated to relieve respiratory distress.
- Tracheostomy is often more easily performed as an elective procedure rather than after the development of severe respiratory distress and collapse (see p. 456). Cuffed tracheostomy tubes may be used in dysphagic horses to prevent the potential for aspiration pneumonia.
- In cases of guttural pouch empyema, after rupture and drainage of retropharyngeal lymph nodes, repeated lavage may be needed to reduce compression of the nasopharynx, to speed resolution of the infection, and to reduce persistent purulent exudate that could result in chondroids and establishment of a carrier state.
  - The usual course of treatment is repeated lavage with 500 mL to 1 L of crystalloid solution, followed by instillation of penicillin gel once the purulent exudate has been removed. ***Practice Tip:*** *Prepare the penicillin gel by heating gelatin (2 g) with 20 to 30 mL physiologic buffered saline (PBS) or sterile water*

(enough PBS to make a suspension) and then adding 5 million units aqueous penicillin. This can be stored as a gel and infused by a pipette or Chambers catheter into the guttural pouch. After infusion of the guttural pouch, the horse's head should be maintained in a neutral or slightly elevated position for 20 minutes if possible. Commercial bovine mastitis suspensions are also used in the guttural pouch; however, these preparations seem to increase the risk of intestinal dysbiosis.
  - In cases where there is a persistent thick purulent exudate, 10 mL of 10% to 20% acetylcysteine solution can be instilled following lavage to help facilitate removal by breaking down the disulfide bonds in the exudate.
  - Once the majority of the purulent exudate is removed, penicillin gel can be instilled for a residual effect and aid in "clearing" the infection.
  - The goal is to achieve a negative culture from the guttural pouch before releasing the horse into the general population.
- The use of antimicrobial agents for strangles is controversial.
- There is no evidence to support the belief that antimicrobial use increases the likelihood of internal abscess formation with strangles.
- If administered during the early phase of the disease—at the initial fever, and before palpable lymphadenopathy—immediate treatment with antimicrobial therapy for 3 to 5 days may on rare occasion resolve the infection and prevent abscess formation.
  - This protocol may be useful in a racing or performance stable situation.
  - While curative, this may prevent development of protective immunity; treated horses may therefore be susceptible to future infection.
  - These individuals should be isolated from clinically infected horses to prevent reinfection. *Once lymphadenopathy develops, antimicrobial therapy is considered contraindicated in most uncomplicated cases.*
  - The belief is that antimicrobial therapy may only temporarily improve fever and lethargy, and when discontinued before complete resolution of the infection enlargement and rupture of the lymph node abscess may occur or that the infection may later reemerge.
- Antimicrobial therapy is indicated in complicated cases with retropharyngeal lymph node enlargement that results in airway obstruction or dyspnea requiring tracheostomy. Antimicrobial therapy helps to allow for reduce the size of the abscessed lymph node and addresses secondary complications associated with dysphagia and tracheostomy.
  - Penicillin remains the antimicrobial drug of choice; isolates are consistently sensitive to penicillin.
  - Other drug classes, such as cephalosporins, macrolides, or trimethoprim-sulfa combinations, may be used depending on antimicrobial sensitivity testing. ***Practice Tip:*** *Trimethoprim-sulfa may produce a clinical response but is not expected to "sterilize" infected lymph nodes and is inactivated in the presence of purulent material.*
- Treatment of clinical signs associated with purpura hemorrhagica generally involves antimicrobials with concurrent dexamethasone (0.05 to 0.2 mg/kg IV or PO q24h) to suppress the inflammation associated with vasculitis.
  - The length of time for steroid therapy can be prolonged, and most often, tapering the dose is recommended.
  - When to discontinue the steroid therapy remains a decision based on clinical signs and recurrence when the drug is stopped.

[41]Endoscopic Microbial Aspiration Catheter (Mila International, Inc., 12 Price Avenue, Erlanger, KY 41018).

- Elevation in serum total protein and globulins may indicate the potential for immune complex deposition and the development of purpura hemorrhagica.
- In addition to steroid therapy, nonsteroidal anti-inflammatory drugs may be useful in addition to supportive care of affected skin (bandages, hydrotherapy).
- In those patients with an active infection concurrent with clinical signs of purpura hemorrhagica, antimicrobial therapy is also indicated.

Prevention

- Prevention of strangles remains a challenge.
- Vaccination is an imperfect process due to:
  - Adverse reactions
  - Vaccine failure
  - Immune reactions reported to occur with most vaccines
- Newer vaccines are currently being evaluated.
- It is critical to educate clients on principles of biosecurity, especially in racing and performance horse populations.
- Recent efforts at screening new additions to groups of horses by guttural pouch endoscopy and testing (culture or PCR) have helped reduce the incidence on premises with historic problems with strangles.
- Remember to consider a common water source as a mode of transmission. ***Practice Tip:*** *Restricting this route of spread is important in prevention.*

Strangles with Involvement of the Retropharyngeal Lymph Nodes

Obstruction usually is caused by septic lymphadenopathy. In most cases, there is *not* a "mature" abscess to be drained. These cases are difficult to manage, although the prognosis for survival is good. Dysphagia may be a presenting sign.

Diagnosis

- Obtain a history and observe clinical signs.
- Radiographs and/or ultrasound examination of the head/pharynx may be needed in absence of discernible abscess.

●❯ WHAT TO DO

Laryngeal Obstruction/Strangles

- Tracheostomy (see p. 456); endoscopy may need to be delayed until a tracheostomy is performed, to allow for improved airflow.
  Note: Expect a purulent discharge from the tracheotomy site with soft tissue reaction around the area that resolves after the tracheotomy tube is removed; healing is by second intention.
- Drain the lymph node if an abscess is present. Ultrasound examination may be helpful in determining whether there is an abscessed lymph node. Often a well-developed abscess, "ripe for draining," is not present. Endoscopy of the guttural pouches may reveal a "bulging" abscess on the floor of the guttural pouch. If this is the clinical finding, the abscess can be incised and drained using a surgical laser with endoscopic guidance. Because the anatomy is complicated, and the vagus nerve must be avoided when incising the abscess.

- Transcutaneous ultrasound examination may allow imagining of the abscess after incising so that a 12-gauge teat cannula can be inserted into the diseased lymph node.
  Note: With or without drainage, laryngeal paralysis or dysfunction often is seen at endoscopic examination months later.
- Administer penicillin. Clinical improvement may take 1 week or more. Penicillin, 22,000 to 44,000 U/kg IV q6h, is preferred in the initial stages of treatment to speed the recovery. If a tracheostomy is performed, place the intravenous catheter as far from the tracheotomy site as possible. If aspiration occurs, broader-spectrum antibiotics are indicated.
- See also the previous What To Do box on Strangles in general, on the previous page.

Acute Guttural Pouch Empyema

- Often associated with *Streptococcus equi* ssp. *equi* or ssp. *zooepidemicus* infection
- Rarely causes respiratory distress

Diagnosis

- Perform endoscopic examination of pharynx, larynx, and guttural pouch
- Perform ultrasound examination and identify fluid within guttural pouch
- Radiographic findings include a fluid line in the guttural pouches
- Nasal discharge is likely present
- Swelling and pain behind ramus of mandible may be present clinically

●❯ WHAT TO DO

Guttural Pouch Empyema with Airway Obstruction

- Tracheotomy is rarely needed.
- Appropriate antibiotic (penicillin) administered systematically and through an indwelling catheter in the guttural pouch which also serves to improve drainage.
- Pass a Chambers catheter, appropriate-sized stomach or nasotracheal tube, into the guttural pouch for drainage, and lavage with 1 L of nonirritating polyionic fluid (warm saline solution alone or with penicillin potassium). If sedation is needed, administer acepromazine, 0.02 mg/kg IV, and butorphanol, 0.01 mg/kg IV. If the respiratory obstruction is not severe, substitute xylazine for the acepromazine to lower the head during the flushing procedure and improve drainage. Feeding hay at ground level during flushing may help keep the head low and reduce aspiration of lavage fluid.
- Note: This procedure will likely need to be repeated.
- See also the previous What To Do box on Strangles in general, p. 467.

Proximal Esophageal Obstruction

On rare occasions, proximal esophageal obstruction can cause respiratory distress if the obstruction is in the proximal esophagus.

Diagnosis

- A dorsally collapsed larynx may be visible on endoscopic examination
- Feed material is seen at the esophageal opening or immediately on entering the esophagus via endoscopy

●〉 WHAT TO DO

Proximal Esophageal Obstruction with Laryngeal Obstruction

- Discontinue oral feeding and drinking.
- Tranquilize the horse with xylazine or detomidine if patient's condition permits.
- Pass a nasogastric tube to relieve the esophageal obstruction. If intubation is unsuccessful, perform tracheostomy.
- Administer antimicrobials to prevent/treat aspiration pneumonia and provide anti-inflammatory therapy.

Pharyngeal Trauma

Lacerations, puncture wounds, foreign bodies, and blunt trauma (including insertion of a nasogastric tube) may cause trauma to the pharynx. Clinical signs may include dysphagia, labored breathing, and respiratory noise.

Diagnosis

- Endoscopy of the pharynx may show the lesion.
- Radiography is best to identify metallic foreign body.

●〉 WHAT TO DO

Pharyngeal Trauma

- Throat spray (colloidal silver, or dexamethasone/nitrofurazone [Furacin], DMSO), systemic antibiotics, and NSAIDs are recommended.
- Replace hay feeding with less abrasive feed such as grass, wet pelleted or cubed hay, or hay silage.
- Temporary tracheostomy rarely is required.
- Administer antibiotics such as trimethoprim-sulfadiazine (TMP-S) and metronidazole or potassium or sodium penicillin with gentamicin and metronidazole.

Hyperkalemic Periodic Paralysis

Airway obstruction occurs in homozygously affected foals. A loud fluttering sound may be made during episodes, and a persistent noise may be made after treatment. Most cases do not necessitate tracheostomy and can be managed medically. Stressful events such as weaning or excitement may precipitate onset or worsening of clinical signs.

Diagnosis

- Young Quarter Horse foals (<5 months) are most commonly affected.
- Endoscopically, there is collapse of the soft palate, pharynx, and larynx. Do not use xylazine for sedation because doing so increases upper airway resistance.
- Delayed eyelid opening occurs after manual closing in homozygotes.
- Patient is direct descendant of Impressive on both sides of lineage.
- Confirm homozygous status for the defective gene by DNA means of evaluation:
  - Collect one EDTA tube (5 to 10 mL) of blood labeled with the patient's name. Do not freeze or separate. The diagnosis can also be performed on hair samples from the mane or the tail.

- Send to Veterinary Genetic Laboratory/HYPP Test, School of Veterinary Medicine, University of California, Davis, CA 95616-8744 or other approved testing laboratory. See Chapter 31, p. 71.

Clinical Chemistry Findings

- Serum potassium value often is normal; slight elevations are found in some foals. Some patients have an elevated creatine kinase value, but this finding is not uniform.

●〉 WHAT TO DO

Pharyngeal Collapse with HYPP

- Administer 50 to 250 mL of 50% dextrose IV if hyperkalemia is present. Do not use if the patient has collapsed and is believed to have suffered hypoxic brain damage. The high concentration of dextrose can aggravate central nervous system (CNS) intracellular acidosis because dextrose is metabolized anaerobically to lactic acid. The benefit of glucose is to stimulate insulin release and move potassium intracellularly. Insulin level is elevated within 5 minutes after glucose infusion and causes an immediate intracellular potassium shift.
- Give calcium gluconate, 0.2 to 0.4 mL/kg IV of a 23% solution diluted in 1 L of 5% glucose to stabilize cell membranes.
- Give 1 mEq/kg of 7.5% or 8.4% $NaHCO_3$ IV over 5 to 10 minutes to shift potassium intracellularly. Dextrose may be preferred in place of $NaHCO_3$ because $NaHCO_3$ decreases the level of ionized calcium, which has "cellular protective" activity against hyperkalemia. $NaHCO_3$ may also contribute to respiratory acidosis. Paradoxical CNS acidosis may be caused by the administration of $NaHCO_3$ although evidence of this phenomenon is not strong in the horse.
- Give acetazolamide, 2.2 mg/kg PO q12h.
- Remove alfalfa hay, molasses, and electrolyte supplements.

Selenium Deficiency

Selenium deficiency can cause a variety of signs in foals and adults. In young (sometimes newborn) foals, pharyngeal and laryngeal paresis result in respiratory noise or milk reflux.

Diagnosis

- Diagnosis is based on geographic location and clinical signs (there may be involvement of the skeletal muscles resulting in weakness and abnormal gait).
- Serum creatine kinase values are variable but if elevated should arouse suspicion. Collect blood for measurement of selenium (<10 mg/dL supports the diagnosis).

●〉 WHAT TO DO

Selenium Deficient Myopathy

- Administer intramuscular injection of selenium (not intravenous). Repeat in 3 days. Do not expect rapid improvement in the foal's condition because selenium takes a few days to be incorporated in enzymes and tissues. Oral supplementation with selenium, 0.002 to 0.006 mg/kg of body weight, is recommended in selenium deficient areas.
- Supportive therapy is required for the survival of severely affected cases.
- Prognosis is poor in recumbent weanlings and newborn foals with severe leg edema.

RESP

Selenium Deficiency
- *Never* administer selenium by the *intravenous* route!

Tracheal Obstruction
Tracheal Collapse
- Tracheal collapse may be caused by trauma or a progressively enlarging mass (e.g., hematoma, thyroid cyst, abscess) dorsal to the trachea.
- Collapse in absence of the previously listed causes is most common in adults, miniature horses, and Shetland ponies.
- The collapse generally occurs throughout the cervical and thoracic area.
- *S. equi* or *Rhodococcus equi* abscesses also can collapse the trachea at the thoracic inlet in individuals 6 months to 1 year of age, and *Corynebacterium pseudotuberculosis* may rarely cause a similar problem in adults in the western states of the United States.
- Rarely, chondrodysplasia of tracheal cartilage due to trauma (e.g., previous tracheostomy), or the idiopathic syndrome in ponies, may cause airway obstruction.

Clinical Signs
- Respiratory noise (stridor)
- Inspiratory distress if the collapse is extrathoracic and expiratory distress if intrathoracic
- Cyanosis

Diagnosis
- Diagnosis is confirmed at endoscopic examination of the upper airway and trachea. Provide oxygen intranasally during the endoscopic examination.
- The edges of the flattened trachea may be palpated in the jugular furrow in some cases of tracheal collapse.
- Radiography or ultrasonography is useful in cases resulting from an impinging mass, especially a mass at the thoracic inlet.

⬤〉 **WHAT TO DO**

Tracheal Collapse
- The extent of the collapse in miniature horses and Shetland ponies makes repair difficult. If the collapse is in only a single area of the neck, extraluminal prosthetic devices can be implanted to increase tracheal diameter. If possible, surgically drain or incise the compressing masses using ultrasound guidance.
- Intraluminal stents may be placed in miniature horses.
- A rare cause of tracheal collapse is a mediastinal abscess or tumor (e.g., *S. equi* abscess) or severe pneumomediastinum. The diagnosis is based on radiographic, endoscopic, or ultrasonographic examination. Treatment requires tracheostomy and placement of an endotracheal tube through the tracheostomy site and passed beyond the site of the obstruction. Drainage of a cranial thoracic abscess can be performed with ultrasound guidance. It may be necessary to anesthetize the foal with a short-acting anesthetic to move the leg far enough forward to place the drainage tube.
- Tracheal collapse associated with pneumonia may respond to antimicrobial administration.

Tracheal or Bronchial Foreign Body
In rare instances, horses inhale foreign bodies such as sticks or twigs and the foreign body lodges in a primary bronchus. This results in acute onset of coughing with variable respiratory distress. Small objects, such as a broken indwelling catheter used for transtracheal wash, are usually expelled spontaneously with coughing.

Diagnosis
- Endoscopic examination

⬤〉 **WHAT TO DO**

Tracheal/Bronchial Foreign Body
- Removal by means of endoscopy is difficult depending on the size and location of the foreign body.
- Referral and a surgical approach for removal of the foreign body may be required.

Additional Causes of Respiratory Distress Leading to Upper Airway Obstruction
- Intralaryngeal granulation tissue
- Neoplasia

Respiratory Distress Without Noise
Pneumothorax
- Pneumothorax may be due to a lesion in the lung parenchyma (closed pneumothorax) or in the thoracic wall (open pneumothorax). (See Chapter 46, p. 729, on thoracic injury.)
- Severity depends largely on the inciting cause and the completeness of the mediastinum.
- Horses with tension pneumothorax (ingress of air into the pleural space, but without egress) may rapidly develop life-threatening hypoxemia because the significant increase in the intrapleural pressure on the affected side compromises the opposite side.
- Idiopathic pneumothorax (no evidence of infection or trauma but probable lung rupture) often is bilateral.
- Inflammatory causes, such as pleuropneumonia, rarely result in bilateral pneumothorax, whereas traumatic pneumothorax can be unilateral or bilateral.

Diagnosis
- The patient exhibits signs of respiratory distress (flared nostrils and increased respiratory rate).
- Auscultation reveals little or no dorsal movement of air (bilaterally or unilaterally).
- Confirm findings with radiographs (the dorsal lung margin can be seen) or ultrasonography (air echo that does not move with respiration; see Chapter 14, p. 95). In horses with respiratory diseases causing air trapping into the peripheral lung tissue (heaves or severe pneumonia), radiographs and ultrasonography may underestimate the severity of the pneumothorax.
- Perform diagnostic aspiration with a paracentesis catheter (blunt) or a $3\frac{1}{2}$-inch (8.8-cm) needle or catheter with stylet. ***Practice Tip:*** *Attach a short extension tube to the needle or catheter, place 3 to 5 mL of sterile saline solution into the tube,*

●> WHAT TO DO

Pneumothorax

- Administer oxygen intranasally, 10 to 20 mL/kg per minute through a nasopharyngeal tube. Even with unilateral pneumothorax, the opposite side of the lung can be physically compromised because of the positive pressure on the mediastinum with tension pneumothorax.
- Cover any wounds with an occlusive dressing (cellophane wrap works well) and suture as soon as possible unless internal tension pneumothorax is also suspected.
- After routine sterile preparation and local analgesia, sterilely place a 3½-inch (8.8-cm), 16-gauge IV catheter high in the thirteenth intercostal space. As soon as the chest is entered, pull the stylet back ¼ inch (0.6 cm). Using a 60-mL syringe and three-way stopcock or vacuum pump (make certain the pump is set on suction), aspirate the air. For continuous leaks, passive evacuation of air within the pleural space can also be achieved using a chest valve (Heimlich valve or a perforated condom; Fig. 25-5). Rarely, continuous aspiration using a suction pump is needed.
- Start broad-spectrum antibiotic therapy for all forms of externally induced pneumothorax: penicillin potassium or sodium, 22,000 to 44,000 U/kg IV q6h, and gentamicin, 6.6 mg/kg IV q24h, or ceftiofur, 3.0 mg/kg IV q12h.
- Analgesics (NSAIDs) may improve depth of ventilation and may reduce likelihood of atelectasis, secondary bacterial pneumonia, and adhesions.

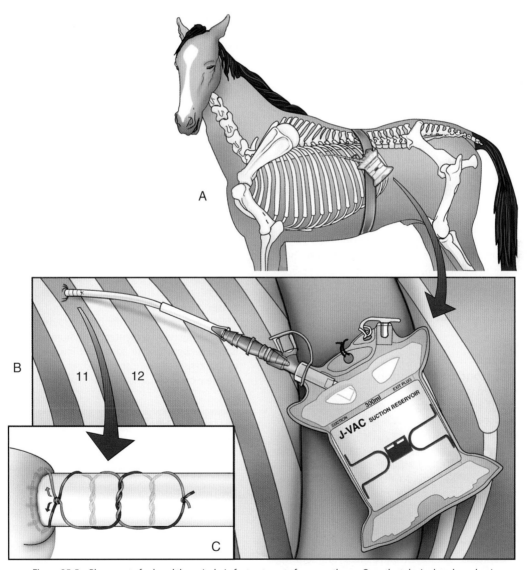

Figure 25-5 Placement of a dorsal thoracic drain for treatment of pneumothorax. Once the tube is placed, mechanical suction can be applied to the chest or a Heimlich valve can be attached. After most of the air is removed, a J-VAC can be attached to provide *short-term positive suction*. The Chinese locking pattern used to suture thoracic tubes in place is shown in part **C**.

and hold the tube proximally as the needle is sterilely advanced into the dorsal thorax (usual depth is 2 inches [5 cm]) after routine sterile preparation and appropriate local analgesia and systemic restraint. If pneumothorax is present, the saline "bubbles" back up as the thorax is entered and the air is forced out. If negative pressure is still present, the saline solution is sucked into the thorax.

Traumatic Pneumothorax
- Caused by:
  - Thoracic wall and lung injuries (see Chapter 46, p. 728)
  - Small axillary wounds
  - Tracheal trauma
  - Transtracheal washes
  - Thoracoscopy
  - Bone marrow aspiration (sternum or ribs)
- If the mediastinum is complete, the pneumothorax is unilateral. The patient has a rapid respiratory rate, but its condition remains stable.
- If pneumothorax is bilateral, signs are more severe and respiratory distress is progressive.

Pneumothorax Secondary to Pleuropneumonia
- Generally, pneumothorax is unilateral because the mediastinum usually is complete with inflammatory disease.
- Alveoli may rupture in severe pneumonia, or air leaks into one side of the chest from a chest drain, resulting in bronchopleural fistula and pneumothorax.
- Unilateral pneumothorax in patients with pleuropneumonia can cause severe respiratory distress because the pneumothorax is compounded by bilateral lung disease, and the pressure of the tension pneumothorax forces the mediastinum to the opposite side.
- Pneumothorax associated with pleuropneumonia has a guarded to poor prognosis.

●》 WHAT TO DO

Pneumothorax Secondary to Pleuropneumonia
- Replace leaking chest valve if a problem.
- Place a 3½-inch (8.8-cm), 16-gauge IV catheter high in the thirteenth intercostal space after routine sterile preparation. As soon as the chest is entered, pull the stylet back ¼ inch (0.6 cm). Using a 60-mL syringe and three-way stopcock or vacuum pump (make certain the pump is set on suction), aspirate the air.
- If the pneumothorax persists, consider thoracoscopy to diagnose and assist closure of the bronchopleural fistula if visualized.

Idiopathic Pneumothorax
Affected individuals have no evidence of external trauma, nor do they have pneumonia. They often have bilateral pneumothorax or bilateral compromise, are in severe respiratory distress, and may die acutely. Tension pneumothorax is suspected in these cases.

●》 WHAT TO DO

Idiopathic Pneumothorax
- Bilateral: With severe respiratory distress, decompress the thorax as described, and place an indwelling one-way chest tube and a Heimlich valve (or perforated condom as an alternative) high on the chest wall. This must be done quickly. Affected patients have tension pneumothorax; therefore, an incision into the thorax may reduce internal thoracic pressure.
- Unilateral: If the patient's condition is stable, there is no need to place suction in the thoracic cavity unless pressure in the hemithorax is compromising the opposite side of the thorax.

Pneumomediastinum
- Pneumomediastinum is commonly found radiographically after transtracheal aspiration but rarely necessitates treatment.
- An exception to this would be a horse with respiratory distress (most commonly heaves) that continually coughs and develops a severe pneumomediastinum following a transtracheal aspirate.
- Tracheal perforation (most often from kicks or severe axillary wounds) occasionally results in pressure pneumomediastinum, which can severely affect preload (venous return) to the heart and cause life-threatening hypotension with respiratory distress.
- Less commonly, gas originates from the lungs, the esophagus, or the abdominal cavity.
- The diagnosis is confirmed radiographically and endoscopically.
- Rupture of the esophagus results in sepsis and pneumomediastinum; the prognosis is poor (see Chapter 18, p. 181).

●》 WHAT TO DO

Pneumomediastinum
- *Tracheal perforation:* Endoscopic examination of the trachea reveals the point of perforation. Repair surgically through a ventral cervical incision in the standing patient.
- *Axillary wound:* Cross-tie the patient to decrease movement, and pack the wound to prevent more air from entering the wound.
- It may be beneficial to administer intravenous fluids to improve venous return and cardiac preload.
- In severe cases of tracheal perforation, surgery is needed.

●》 WHAT NOT TO DO

Pneumomediastinum
- *Do not* close the skin incision!

Pulmonary Edema
- Acute pulmonary edema frequently arises from conditions that increase pulmonary vascular pressure, such as left-sided heart failure (e.g., ruptured chordae tendineae), or that alter the permeability of the pulmonary vascular endothelium, such as endotoxic shock, purpura hemorrhagica, adverse drug reactions, or anaphylaxis.
- Other causes of pulmonary edema include the following:
  - Smoke inhalation (see p. 475)
  - Neurogenic pulmonary edema that may accompany head trauma
  - Iatrogenic overzealous administration of intravenous fluids in recumbent neonates, adults with anuric acute

renal failure or severe hypoproteinemia, or patients with increased vascular permeability

- Traumatic acute pulmonary edema, a common cause of mortality in horses sustaining a fracture while in training or racing
- Severe upper airway obstruction (See sections on nasal, laryngeal, and pharyngeal obstruction)
- Viral infections including:
  - Influenza virus
  - Equine herpes virus
  - Equine arteritis virus
  - Equine Hendra virus (*Morbillivirus*)
  - African horse sickness (endemic to the African continent; see Chapter 40, p. 674).
- Pulmonary edema results in a reduction in lung volume and elasticity and causes hypoxemia. Edema usually occurs with acute problems and rarely is observed in hypoproteinemic patients with glomerulopathy or protein-losing enteropathy despite the presence of severe subcutaneous edema.

Diagnosis

- Diagnosis is by physical examination and the presence of a preexisting disease such as acute heart failure, endotoxic shock, or anaphylaxis.
- Frothy blood-tinged nasal discharge may be present with inflammatory diseases.
- Ultrasound examination (see Chapter 14, p. 96)

●⟩ WHAT TO DO

Pulmonary Edema

- Manage the primary disease.
- Administer furosemide, 1 mg/kg IV.
- Administer oxygen intranasally, 10 to 20 mL/kg per minute (5 to 10 L/min per 500-kg adult) until adequate ventilation is restored.
- Inhaled bronchodilators may be helpful via bronchodilation and improved fluid clearance. Nebulization with combination bronchodilators and surfactant may be attempted for cases with severe froth.
- If fluid therapy is needed because of hypotension, a colloid (e.g., 25% human albumin) and hypertonic saline should be administered.

  Note: If anxious, sedate with diazepam, 0.05 to 0.2 mg/kg IV, or acepromazine, 0.02 to 0.04 mg/kg IV.

Pulmonary Edema Resulting from Heart Failure
(See Chapter 17, p. 146)

●⟩ WHAT TO DO

Pulmonary Edema from Heart Failure

- Digoxin, 1 mg IV/450-kg adult
- Furosemide, 1 to 2 mg/kg IV followed by 0.5 to 1.0 mg/kg PO q12h or 0.12 mg/kg/h as a continuous rate infusion (CRI)
- Intranasal oxygen delivery, 10 to 20 mL/kg per minute (5 to 10 L/min per 500-kg adult)
- Arterial vasodilator to decrease afterload (see Chapter 17, p. 148)

Pulmonary Edema Resulting from Anaphylaxis
(Adverse Drug Reaction)

●⟩ WHAT TO DO

Pulmonary Edema from Anaphylaxis

- Epinephrine, 3 to 5 mL (1:1000 dilution) for adults, diluted in 20 to 30 mL of saline solution and administered slowly IV or in less severe cases, IM or SQ
- Dexamethasone, 0.1 to 0.2 mg/kg IV bolus
- Furosemide, 1 mg/kg IV
- Intranasal oxygen delivery, 10 to 20 mL/kg per minute (5 to 10 L/min per 450-kg adult)
- Intravenously administered plasma or synthetic colloid (hetastarch)

Purpura Hemorrhagica

- Rarely causes acute pulmonary edema

●⟩ WHAT TO DO

Pulmonary Edema Purpura

- Dexamethasone, 0.1 to 0.2 mg/kg IV
- Furosemide, 1 mg/kg IV q24h
- Intranasal oxygen delivery, 10 to 20 mL/kg per minute (5 to 10 L/min per 450-kg adult)

Pulmonary Edema Resulting from Endotoxic Shock/ Systemic Inflammatory Response Syndrome

- *Definition:* A shock-like syndrome similar to endotoxic shock that can be initiated by any inflammatory disorder.
- Rare cause of pulmonary edema.

●⟩ WHAT TO DO

Pulmonary Edema from Systemic Inflammatory Response

- Administer low-dose flunixin meglumine, 0.25 mg/kg IV; DMSO, 1 g/kg IV diluted in 3 L of 0.9% saline solution or 5% dextrose; and dexamethasone, 0.25 mg/kg IV bolus. The use of corticosteroids is controversial.
- Give furosemide, 1 mg/kg IV (monitor systemic blood pressure because it can lower cardiac output).
- Administer oxygen intranasally, 10 to 20 mL/kg per minute (5 to 10 L/min per 450-kg adult).
- Cardiac output usually is low; manage with plasma/albumin or hetastarch and dobutamine, 2 to 10 μg/kg per minute.
- Hypertonic saline solution is the fluid of choice when intravenous fluids are needed in the initial management of pulmonary edema and hypotension.

Fluid Therapy in Patients at High Risk of Development of Pulmonary Edema

- High-risk patients include the following:
  - Septic foals
  - Recumbent foals
  - Patients with increased vascular permeability (endotoxic shock, systemic inflammatory response syndrome, smoke inhalation, and others)

- Patients with generalized anaphylactic diseases causing rapid protein loss
- Patients with increased hydrostatic pressure (oliguric renal failure, heart failure)
- Fluid therapy for hypovolemia is required for many of these patients, and central venous pressure should be monitored when possible.

●〉 WHAT TO DO

Hypovolemic Patients at Risk of Pulmonary Edema
- Administer hypertonic saline solution initially, 4 to 8 mL/kg, to improve cardiac output and blood pressure, and to decrease pulmonary arterial pressures.
- Oncotic plasma expanders (e.g., equine plasma, 25% human albumin, vetstarch, or hetastarch) may decrease lung fluid volume and are recommended, but these agents are expensive.

Acute Lung Injury/Acute Respiratory Distress Syndrome: Foals and Adults
- There are *no* strict criteria established to define acute lung injury (ALI) and acute respiratory distress syndromes (ARDS) in horses.
- These terms are loosely used to describe conditions associated with severe respiratory dysfunction and refractory hypoxemia associated with diffuse pulmonary infiltrates and interstitial pattern on thoracic radiographs.
- ALI may be triggered by a systemic inflammatory response, aspiration, or viral infection. If triggered by a systemic inflammatory response, treatment with corticosteroids, NSAIDs, pentoxifylline, furosemide CRI, hypertonic saline, and colloids followed by maintenance crystalloid therapy, may be successful.

Aspiration Pneumonia
- Aspiration pneumonia is common among horses.
- Chronic aspiration caused by a mechanical or neurologic condition of the pharynx or larynx is generally *not* an emergency.
- Acute aspiration results from esophageal choke, iatrogenic causes, or meconium aspiration in foals.
- In rare instances, horses spontaneously reflux gastric contents because of anterior enteritis, small-bowel obstruction, or gastric dilatation.
- Occasionally, horses have severe respiratory distress after aspirating a large volume of foreign material.
- ***Practice Tip:*** *Severe respiratory distress may be caused by misdirected nasogastric tubes and meconium aspiration in foals.* THIS IS AN EMERGENCY!

Diagnosis of Iatrogenic Aspiration Pneumonia
- History of coughing and distress after tubing
- Auscultation of the trachea and lungs reveals a loud fluttering sound with crackles and wheezes hours later; ingesta is seen at the nostrils
- Tracheal endoscopic examination
- After 12 to 48 hours, the following may be seen:
  - Hemorrhagic, often foul smelling, nasal discharge
  - Cranio/caudo ventral opacities on thoracic radiographs

- Lung consolidation and pleural effusion may be present on ultrasonographic examination.
- Development of secondary septic pleuritis (see p. 480)

●〉 WHAT TO DO

Aspiration Pneumonia
- Broad-spectrum antibiotics:
  - Penicillin potassium or sodium, 44,000 U/kg IV q6h; and gentamicin, 6.6 mg/kg IV q24h; and metronidazole, 15 to 25 mg/kg PO q6 to 8h
  Caution: Monitor renal function and provide intravenous fluids if needed.
  - or Ceftiofur, 2.2 to 3.0 mg/kg IV q12h, and metronidazole, 15 to 25 mg/kg PO q6 to 8h
- Corticosteroids: dexamethasone, 0.1 to 0.2 mg/kg q24h on day 1 and 0.05 to 0.1 mg/kg on day 2
  Note: Corticosteroids are for chemical aspiration *only!*
- Adjunct Supportive Treatment
  - Intranasal oxygen delivery: 10 to 20 mL/kg per minute (5 to 10 L/min per 450-kg adult) continuously. Place a soft rubber tube in the nasopharynx, suture it to the false nostril, and administer humidified oxygen from a portable tank or a portable oxygen concentrator. Adjust rate of administration based on arterial blood gas values or pulse oximeter when possible.
  - Flunixin meglumine, 0.25 to 1.1 mg/kg or phenylbutazone, 2.2 to 4.4 mg/kg IV or PO, after discontinuing any corticosteroid therapy.
  - ***Practice Tip:*** *Aspirate the lower airway by suction if aspiration occurred within a "window" of 30 minutes after the insult or if foreign material is easily seen on endoscopic examination of the trachea. If the suction is forceful using a pump, it should be for brief periods of <15 seconds, with simultaneously administered oxygen.*
  - Nebulize with antibiotics, gentamicin or amikacin, 50 mg/mL in 0.45% saline or ceftiofur, 25 mg/mL in sterile water and 5 mL of 0.5% albuterol for inhalation. Total volume is generally 30 to 40 mL.
  - ***Practice Tip:*** *In rare instances, distress occurs after proper nasogastric tube procedures or administration of oral medication. These episodes of reflux esophageal spasm or esophageal or gastric irritation are alarming because the immediate concern is aspiration pneumonia or gastric rupture; however, within 30 to 60 minutes, the patient is normal.*
  - ***Important:*** *Almost all adults with choke have some aspiration pneumonia. Ultrasound examination of the chest 24 to 48 hours after the onset of choke generally reveals moderate to significant pleural changes. In most cases, recovery is excellent regardless of these findings.*

Viral (or Postviral) Respiratory Distress Syndrome
- The condition is most often seen in young adults, and rarely, foals exposed to viral infections of the upper respiratory tract. The incidence of respiratory distress among horses with viral upper respiratory infections is low.
- Affected individuals initially have a fever (often as high as 41.4° C [106° F]) associated with the viral infection and experience severe tachypnea with labored breathing within 1 to 3 days.
- The pathophysiologic mechanism of the syndrome is undetermined but is believed to result from hyperreactivity

of the airways triggered by the virus or irritant. This syndrome is distinctly different from pleuropneumonia (see p. 480), which results in severe weight loss and significant ventral ultrasonographic and/or radiographic abnormalities.

- Equine multinodular pulmonary fibrosis (EMNPF) is a chronic disease of horses that has been associated with equine herpesvirus 5 (EHV-5). It can cause respiratory distress at rest and is a fatal disease in the majority of cases.
- Mules exposed to influenza virus may have respiratory distress and die.

Diagnosis

- History includes recent arrival from a sale barn or recent exposure (e.g., a show) to a large group of young horses.
- Fever may be as high as 41.4° C (106.5° F).
- Auscultation: Wheezes and crackles are heard but are less dramatic than the clinical signs; lung sounds are quiet for the effort expended in breathing.
- During the acute phase, transtracheal aspirate usually is nonseptic, although bacteria (such as *Streptococci* and *Pasteurella/Actinobacillus* organisms) and fungi (such as *Aspergillus*) are occasionally cultured. Secondary bacterial colonizations/infections are common during the recovery phase.
- Most individuals affected are not toxic, and they have a normal appetite but labored breathing.
- Affected individuals may look like patients with heaves, but the age (foals and young adults) and history are different.
- Radiographs and ultrasonography show abnormalities (e.g., interstitial pattern or alveolar edema and roughening of the pleura), but the abnormalities are generally not severe.
- EMNPF: Horses often have lymphopenia, neutrophilia, and increased fibrinogen and may clinically look similar to horses with heaves, except there is often more weight loss and less cough and nasal discharge, and fever may be present. Ultrasound and radiographs demonstrate diffuse multinodular areas of consolidation (fibrosis) (see p. 96). BAL findings support an inflammatory process and PCR for EHV-5 is usually positive on BAL (though may be negative on TTW). Lung biopsy with histopathology and PCR testing is definitive.

●》 WHAT TO DO

Viral (or Postviral) Respiratory Distress Syndrome

- Provide stall rest in a cool environment.
- Administer NSAIDs if fever >40° C (104° F) or if there is severe depression or complete anorexia.
- Administer bronchodilators:
  - Inhaled bronchodilators:
    - Albuterol, 1 to 2 µg/kg q1h in metered-dose inhaler (MDI)[42]; rapid onset (<5 minutes) but short-acting (30 minutes to 3 hours)

[42]MDI; Equine Aeromask, EquineHaler, AeroHippus.

- Ipratropium bromide, 0.5 to 1 µg/kg q6h in MDI; onset within 15 minutes, lasts 4 to 6 hours
  - Clenbuterol, 0.8 to 3.2 µg/kg PO q12h for 2 to 3 days
- Administer intranasal oxygen, 10 to 20 mL/kg per minute (5 to 10 L/min per 450-kg adult) continuously.
- Antimicrobial therapy for secondary bacterial infections:
  - Penicillin procaine, 22,000 U/kg IM q12h or
  - Ceftiofur, 3.0 mg/kg IV, IM q6 to 12h, especially when *Pasteurella* spp. (*Actinobacillus* spp.) organisms are cultured
- After viral infection, some cases may be difficult to control without corticosteroid administration (dexamethasone, 0.5 to 1.0 mg/kg IV q24h, 1 to 2 doses).
- If referral is considered:
  - Avoid shipping during daytime if ambient temperature is high.
  - Control fever before shipping.
- Treatment for EMNPF includes valacyclovir, 25 mg/kg PO q12h; and corticosteroids: dexamethasone, 0.05 to 0.1 mg/kg IV q24h; or colchicine, 0.03 mg/kg PO q12h, along with supportive care.

Prognosis

- Despite respiratory distress for 3 to 6 days, the prognosis is generally good.
- In rare cases, such as when a horse has not been vaccinated or a mule has not been previously exposed to influenza, rapid progression to death may result from the influenza virus infection.
- Prognosis for EMNPF is poor.

Smoke Inhalation (and Other Noxious Fumes)

- Horses may be seriously affected or die of smoke inhalation in a barn fire.
- They can die in the absence of skin burns.
- Three pulmonary consequences can occur in association with smoke inhalation:
  - Carbon monoxide poisoning: immediate
  - Edema of the upper airways and lungs: hours later
  - Pneumonia: hours to days later
- *Practice Tip: Smoke inhalation, causing carbon monoxide poisoning and pulmonary edema, are the immediate primary concerns when affected individuals are examined after a fire.*

Clinical Findings

- Respiratory signs following smoke exposure:
  - Coughing
  - Labored breathing
  - Polypnea
  - Frothy nasal or oral exudate
- Other clinical findings:
  - Tachycardia
  - Widespread wheezes and crackles
  - Cyanosis

●》 WHAT TO DO

Smoke Inhalation

- Manage pulmonary, laryngeal, or pharyngeal edema and prevent proteinaceous cast formation in the airways.

- There is *no* specific treatment for carbon monoxide (CO) poisoning. The half-life of CO can be decreased by providing oxygen therapy.
  - If the horse can be treated with a hyperbaric oxygen chamber within 5 hours of exposure, this may rapidly reduce the CO.
- Prevent airway obstruction from fibrin debris: Suctioning through an endoscope is preferred. (Suction should be performed in multiple, brief [<15-second] pulses because prolonged, continual suction causes hypoxemia.)
- Perform tracheotomy only if life-threatening laryngeal edema is occurring. Tracheotomy prevents the patient from removing necrotic casts from the lower airway by coughing.
- Provide oxygen therapy: humidified, 10 to 15 L/min for adults, administered intranasally or through a tracheotomy; continue oxygen during suctioning.
- Alleviate bronchoconstriction:
  - Inhaled bronchodilators:
    - Albuterol, 1 to 2 µg/kg q1h in MDI (Equine Aeromask, EquineHaler, AeroHippus); rapid onset (<5 minutes), but short acting (30 minutes to 3 hours)
    - Ipratropium bromide, 0.5 to 1 µg/kg q6h in MDI; onset within 15 minutes, lasts 4 to 6 hours
  - Clenbuterol, 0.8 to 3.2 mg/kg IV or PO q12h (may be nebulized: 10 mL containing 0.03 mg/mL)
- Nebulization with bronchodilators, saline, surfactant acetylcysteine and continual oxygen therapy may reduce cast formation.
- Provide prophylactic therapy for shock. Despite the presence of pulmonary edema, fluid therapy is needed to maintain tissue perfusion. Fluid therapy is essential for patients receiving furosemide to manage pulmonary edema.
  - Administer polyionic fluids to prevent shock: maintenance rate, 1 to 2 L/h (adult). Add KCl (20 to 40 mEq/L) if renal function is normal and if serum potassium value is normal or low.
- Vitamin B_{12} may be administered as a slow bolus (generally 20 to 30 mL of multi-B complex) to bind cyanide to form the rapidly excreted product, cyanocobalamin. Carbon monoxide should be considered in all smoke inhalation patients and cyanide poisoning should also be considered in those exposed to the combustion products of nitrogen- and carbon-containing substances, including wool, silk, cotton and paper, as well as synthetic substances, such as plastics and other polymers.
- Vitamin C (30 mg/kg) may be administered IV to treat oxidative injury.
- Plasma: a larger volume in severe cases or synthetic colloids such as hetastarch.
- NSAIDs: flunixin meglumine, 0.25 mg/kg IV q8h or ketoprofen, 1 mg/kg IV q12h.
- Therapy for sepsis. Administer broad-spectrum bactericidal antibiotics to patients believed to be in a septic state (fever or the presence of intracellular bacteria on examination of tracheal sputum). Bacterial airway colonization may not peak for 2 to 4 days after smoke inhalation. If deep burns exist on the body or if tracheotomy is performed, administer antibiotics:
  - Ceftiofur, 3 mg/kg IV q12h *or*
  - Penicillin, 22,000 IU/kg IV q6h; and gentamicin, 6.6 mg/kg IV q24h; or amikacin, 15 to 25 mg/kg IV q24h; or enrofloxacin, 7.5 mg/kg PO q24h or 5 mg/kg IV q24h; and metronidazole, 15 to 25 mg/kg PO q8h.

Acute Lung Injury (ALI)/Acute Respiratory Distress Syndrome (ARDS): Foal-Specific Information

- ALI or ARDS may occur because of:
  - Severe birth asphyxia
  - Prematurity
  - Meconium aspiration
  - Fractured ribs
  - Sepsis
- Management and treatment are often complex, and the specifics are presented below.

WHAT TO DO

Acute Lung Injury in Neonatal Foal
- Begin intranasal oxygen immediately if available! Portable oxygen concentrators provide flow rates adequate for foals (up to 6 L/min).
- If oxygen treatment stabilizes the foal but the foal remains hypoxic and has typical prematurity heart murmurs, then nitric oxide may be mixed in the oxygen line at a ratio of 5 to 10 L O_2:1 L NO (special value needed for NO tank) in hopes of decreasing pulmonary hypertension.
- Premature foals with respiratory distress that does not respond to intranasal oxygen may need to be ventilated. Intubate and use Ambu bag with 100% oxygen at 20 breaths/min if the foal is cyanotic or stops breathing. If Ambu bag and intubation are *not* possible, the foal aspirator and resuscitator[43] may be used.
- If the foal is premature, administer thyrotropin-releasing factor, 1 mg slowly IV, or give thyroxine (T_4), 1 mg PO daily, and liothyronine (T_3), 1 to 2 µg/kg/day.
- If available and financially possible, surfactant should be administered for prematurity or meconium aspiration–induced respiratory distress. Commercially available surfactant is expensive, but it can be collected from healthy cows/horses via BAL (use 50 mL sterile saline for BAL and take top 5 mL of collection to use for surfactant harvest). This can be administered intratracheally.
- Surgically repair any fractured or displaced ribs; remove hemothorax and pneumothorax.
- Administer vitamin E and selenium (1 mL IM).
- Maintain hydration but do *not* overhydrate!
- A single dose of corticosteroids, dexamethasone, 10 mg IV, can be given. If there is dramatic improvement, this may be continued in a tapering fashion over 3 days. This treatment appears to be most important with aspiration of meconium (see later).
- If parenchymal disease is suspected, nebulize with 0.5% albuterol, 5 mL, and 5 to 10 mL of acetylcysteine (10% or 20%) in addition to aminophylline, 5 mg/kg for first treatment followed by 2 mg/kg IV q12h in a CRI.
- Antibiotic treatment should be given for most cases even if sepsis is not believed to be present at the time. Third-generation cephalosporins are preferred. Aminoglycosides may decrease respiratory muscle strength.

Meconium Aspiration in Foals
Diagnosis
- Diagnosis is based primarily on the history.
- Aspiration is commonly seen with fetal (in utero) diarrhea and stress associated with a colicky mare.

---

[43]Foal aspirator and resuscitator (McCulloch Medical).

- Affected foals typically are born with brown-stained amniotic fluid or amnion.
- Foals with this history should be presumed to have aspirated meconium and generally show respiratory distress in the first few days of life.

●》 WHAT TO DO

Meconium Aspiration
- Administer corticosteroids: dexamethasone, 0.1 to 0.2 mg/kg IV q24h on day 1, 0.05 to 0.1 mg/kg on day 2. Use of corticosteroids is controversial, but in the newborn, immediate anti-inflammatory treatment may be needed to decrease the pulmonary inflammatory response to prevent hypoxia and reversion to fetal circulation due to pulmonary hypertension.
- Administer broad-spectrum antibiotics:
  - Penicillin, 44,000 U/kg IV q6h, and amikacin, 18 mg/kg IV q24h
  - Ceftiofur, 3.0 mg/kg IV q12h, and amikacin, as an alternative
- If aspiration is severe, administer oxygen intranasally at 5 to 10 L/min (see Nasal Oxygen Insufflation, p. 453).
- Perform tracheal suction if the foal has labored breathing and a fluttering sound is heard on auscultation of the trachea. Pass a catheter down the trachea, infuse 10 mL of saline solution, and aspirate using a 60-mL syringe. Repeat several times if aspirated material is retrieved. *Oxygen should be administered simultaneously and aspiration is brief (10-second bouts) to prevent further oxygen debt.*

Rib Fractures
- Rib fractures are common in newborn foals.
- Rib fractures may lead to respiratory distress because of:
  - Lung lacerations
  - Pneumothorax
  - Hemothorax
  - Ventilation impairment if flailed chest
- Rib fractures have also been associated with cardiac lacerations and diaphragmatic hernia.
- The fractures generally occur at the costochondral junction or immediately above it.

Diagnosis
- Depression at, or near, the costochondral junction best seen when the foal is in dorsal recumbency
- Subcutaneous crepitations, edema, and pain occasionally present on palpation
- Thoracic radiographs and ultrasound examination to confirm the diagnosis

●》 WHAT TO DO

Rib Fractures
- Most foals with thoracic trauma are asymptomatic.
- Handle foals with care to avoid secondary thoracic trauma.
- Blood transfusion, intranasal oxygen insufflation, and antimicrobials may be indicated with severe lung lacerations.
- Give NSAIDs to decrease pain and increase ventilation if *no* hemothorax is present.
- If flail chest or severe lung laceration is present, internal stabilization of selected rib fractures may be indicated.

Bronchointerstitial Pneumonia in Nursing/Weanling Foals
- Bronchointerstitial pneumonia can present clinically like *R. equi* infection and affects the same age or older foals; it is of unknown cause.
- Bronchointerstitial pneumonia causes severe respiratory distress with a high fever, usually affecting one horse per farm.
- Consider this disease when a patient with suspected *R. equi* infection has negative culture results for *R. equi* on tracheal aspiration.
- The prognosis for these foals is fair to poor with corticosteroid treatment. If not treated with corticosteroids, most of the affected individuals have respiratory distress for 3 to 5 days before dying.
- Less severely affected foals with slowly progressive chronic pulmonary interstitial disease have a favorable prognosis with corticosteroid treatment.
- The cause of the syndrome is unknown; it may be toxic, immunologic, or a nonbacterial infection.

Diagnosis
- Clinical presentation
  - 1 to 9 months of age
  - Respiratory distress: tachypnea and cyanosis
  - Frequently bright, alert, and nursing
  - High fever: 38.9° to 41.7° C (102° to 107° F)
  - Variable inflammatory changes on leukogram (normal to severe neutrophilia and hyperfibrinogenemia)
- Tracheal washes:
  - Not always possible because of severe respiratory distress
  - Suppurative inflammation
  - *R. equi* negative
  - Bacterial growth common
  - No intracellular bacteria

Ultrasound Findings
- Diffuse roughening of pleura, without abscessation, and rarely obvious consolidation: The ultrasound findings generally do not look as bad as the foal clinically appears.

Radiographic Findings
- Diffuse bronchointerstitial pattern, usually focal to coalescent alveolar opacities
- No pulmonary abscesses

●》 WHAT TO DO

Acute Bronchointerstitial Pneumonia in Nursing/Weanling Foals
- Administer *corticosteroids* (*only* if *R. equi* infection is believed to be unlikely): dexamethasone, 0.1 to 0.4 mg/kg IV or IM q12h for 3 to 6 days, followed by a tapering dosage. Inhaled corticosteroids (beclomethasone, 8 µg/kg q12h, or fluticasone, 4 µg/kg q12h, using Aeromask, EquineHaler or AeroHippus may be considered in less severely affected foals.
- Improvement should be seen within 48 hours after corticosteroids are started.
- Administer oxygen intranasally: 5 L/min continuously.
  Caution: Small oxygen tanks may last for 1 to 2 hours only.

RESP

- Give antibiotics: ceftiofur, 3.0 mg/kg IV q12h
- Administer bronchodilators:
  - Inhaled bronchodilators:
    - Albuterol, 1 to 2 µg/kg q1h in MDI (Equine Aeromask, EquineHaler, or AeroHippus); rapid onset (<5 minutes), but short acting (30 minutes to 3 hours)
    - Ipratropium bromide, 0.5 to 1 µg/kg q6h in MDI; onset within 15 minutes, lasts 4 to 6 hours
  - Clenbuterol, 0.8 to 1.6 µg/kg PO q12h
  - Aminophylline, 3 to 5 mg/kg slow IV infusion over 3 hours or PO q12h, may have some anti-inflammatory effects and strengthen diaphragmatic muscles in foals with severe and prolonged respiratory distress, but plasma levels may need to be monitored to prevent toxicity.
  - Nebulization is preferred over MDI if equipment and adequate personnel are available.
- Balanced polyionic fluids to maintain hydration. *Do not* administer sodium bicarbonate because this may increase the respiratory rate and even decrease blood pH if there are severe alveolar ventilation-perfusion abnormalities.
- Administer ulcer prophylaxis medication:
  - Omeprazole, 4 mg/kg PO q24h, or ranitidine, 6.6 mg/kg PO q8h or 1.5 mg/kg IV q8h
- Provide thermoregulatory control:
  - Alcohol or cold water bath and fan
  - NSAIDs if needed: dipyrone, 5 to 10 mL q6 to 12h, is preferred when available
- If referral is considered:
  - Avoid shipping during daytime if ambient temperature is high.
  - Control fever before shipping.

ARDS from Pneumonia in Foals Caused by *Rhodococcus Equi*

- ARDS generally affects foals between 2 weeks and 3 months of age and rarely horses older than 4 months.
- ARDS may manifest as acute respiratory distress. *R. equi* infection must be differentiated from bronchointerstitial pneumonia of viral or unknown causation (see previous section) because it also results in respiratory distress in this age group of foals.

Diagnosis

- The age of the foal (2 weeks to 4 months)
- A history of previous *R. equi* infection on the farm
- Swollen joints without severe lameness are common; uveitis may also occur
- Geographic location (increased prevalence in some areas of the country, such as dry, dusty, warm areas)
- Season: most commonly affects foals in the late spring
- Clinical presentation:
  - Labored breathing
  - High fever
  - Often minimal cough or nasal discharge
- Auscultation:
  - Harsh lung sounds are heard diffusely, except for the caudal tip, which is generally loud but normal.
  - Lung sounds often are less musical than with other bacterial infections.
- Tracheal aspiration: Use the least traumatic method of collection: percutaneous TTW with an Intracath or similar

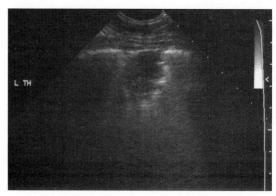

Figure 25-6   Sonogram of a foal thorax with *Rhodococcus equi* and pulmonary abscessation (*dark area*).

catheter (see p. 451). Insertion of an Intracath does not require local anesthesia or an incision and therefore is less stressful. If sedation is needed, use diazepam, 5 mg IV, or xylazine, 0.02 to 0.05 mg/kg IV.

Note: This method of tracheal aspiration is more expensive than other diagnostic methods. Culture and Gram stain the aspirate. ***Practice Tip:*** R. equi *organisms are small, pleomorphic, gram-positive rods (see Chapter 11, p. 57).*

- Affected foals often have very high neutrophil counts and high fibrinogen concentrations.

Ultrasound Findings

Peripheral lung abscesses typical of *R. equi* can be seen (Fig. 25-6) in most cases when labored breathing is present.

Radiographic Findings

- Radiography may have a similar sensitivity as ultrasound but is not as easily performed on the farm. Use standard units and a 400-speed film or screen combination, and 80 kV(p) at 20 mA 0.2 to 0.3 second, nongrid.
- *R. equi* infection often produces a "white out" of the lungs, except for the caudal tips of the diaphragmatic lung lobes, which remain black. Discrete pulmonary abscesses may also be seen.

●》 WHAT TO DO

Rhodococcus Pneumonia

- Administer antibiotics:
  - Clarithromycin, 7.5 mg/kg PO q12h and rifampin, 5 mg/kg PO q12h. (For the first 5 days of treatment the administration of these drugs should be separated by at least 1 hour to improve absorption of the macrolide.) Clarithromycin is preferred for initial treatment of severe cases; or
  - Azithromycin, 10 mg/kg PO q24h for 5 days and then 10 mg/kg PO q48h, and rifampin, 5 mg/kg PO q12h; or
  - Erythromycin, 25 mg/kg PO q6 to 8h, and rifampin, 5 mg/kg PO q12h
  - *Important:* When foals are medicated with macrolides, make an effort to do the following:
    - Administer the oral antibiotics away from feed buckets, hay, and water, and wipe the mouth after administration to lower the risk of the mare ingesting the macrolide.
    - Manure should be removed from the stall frequently, and hay should be fed in a rack to lower the risk of the mare consuming the gut-passed macrolide in the foal's manure.

Note: Compliance by owners is important to ensure that the entire dosage is swallowed especially when foals are in respiratory distress.

- Erythromycin, 5 mg/kg IV q8h, could be administered intravenously to foals that cannot be properly medicated via the oral route, but this is very expensive.
  - As a last option, when *R. equi* is resistant to all other antibiotics, use vancomycin, 5 to 7.5 mg/kg diluted and administered slowly IV, q8 to 12h.
- Trimethoprim-sulfamethoxazole, 20 mg/kg PO q12h, should be added if *Pneumocystis carinii* infection is suspected. This organism is only rarely seen on TTW, but ground-glass appearance of lung parenchyma around the focal abscesses may be seen on radiographs and may raise suspicion of dual infection with *Pneumocystis.*
- If additional aerobic bacteria are observed on Gram stain, ceftiofur, ninocycline, or gentamicin can be added to the *Rhodococcus* therapy until antimicrobial susceptibility is available. The importance for the additional treatment is not evidence based.
- Administer oxygen intranasally, 10 to 20 mL/kg per minute continuously (see p. 453).
- Administer intravenous fluid therapy. Polyionic fluids may be required at a maintenance rate of 40 mL/kg IV over 24 hours if dehydration is present and foals are unable to nurse.
- Bronchodilators often have limited efficacy in these foals.
  - Clenbuterol, 1.6 µg/kg PO q12h, also has mucokinetic properties.
  - **Important:** *Do not* use aminophylline unless plasma levels are monitored; there is risk of drug interaction with macrolides, and toxic levels of aminophylline can cause seizures in foals. The drug may have some anti-inflammatory effects and strengthen diaphragmatic muscles in foals with severe and prolonged respiratory distress.
  - Provide ulcer prophylaxis: omeprazole, 1 to 4 mg/kg PO q24h, or ranitidine, 6.6 mg/kg PO q8h. *Do not* combine or administer sucralfate simultaneously with orally administered antibiotics, bronchodilators, or H₂/proton pump blockers.

Practice Tip: *On hot days, some foals receiving macrolides experience high fevers (41.1° to 43.4° C [106° to 110° F]). Cool with alcohol or cold water bath and fans, provide shade, and administer dipyrone, 10 mL IV. Keep indoors on hot days.*

ARDS from Pneumonia in Foals Caused by Bacteria Other Than *Rhodococcus Equi*

- This is most common in neonatal foals with sepsis and less common in older foals.
- Fever and respiratory distress in a nursing foal with radiographic cranioventral pattern of disease or pleural effusion (uncommon) are compatible with bacterial pneumonia.
- Age, tracheal wash, and farm history are important in ruling out *R. equi* infection in 2-week-old to 4-month-old foals.

Clinical Findings and Diagnosis

- Auscultation of the chest varies; crackles and wheezes or a "consolidated bronchial tone sound" are frequently heard cranioventrally. Quiet bronchial sounds due to pleural effusion are occasionally heard ventrally on auscultation.
- Clinical pathology: Results of a leukogram generally support sepsis: *toxic neutrophils with a left shift and elevated fibrinogen value.*

- Tracheal wash: Perform TTW for aerobic and anaerobic culture and Gram stain. The most frequent organisms are gram-positive cocci such as *S. equi* ssp. *zooepidemicus*; gram-negative rods such as *Pasteurella/Actinobacillus* organisms; *Escherichia coli* are most common in growing foals. Anaerobic infection of the lung in foals is unusual. In neonatal foals gram-negative organisms are most common.
- Thoracic ultrasound: consolidated lung with or without pleural fluid. However, pleuropneumonia is uncommon in foals.
- Thoracocentesis: *only* if ultrasound findings indicate pleural effusion and the fluid is believed to contribute to respiratory distress or when an etiologic agent is not isolated with TTW. Butorphanol, 0.025 mg/kg IM, or diazepam, 5 mg IV, can be administered before the procedure.
- Radiography: to rule out diffuse bronchointerstitial pneumonitis. Radiographic findings may be similar to those found with *R. equi* infection.
  - A radiographic pattern suggesting abscesses and diffuse involvement of the lung, with multiple joint swellings (usually nonpainful), significant neutrophilia, and thrombocytosis is indicative of the presence of *R. equi* infection.
- Acute interstitial pneumonia, viral or idiopathic, should be ruled out and may sometimes differ from severe bacterial pneumonia with:
  - Lower fibrinogen value
  - Less responsive leukogram
  - More diffuse disease pattern at clinical and radiographic examination
  - No peripheral abscess or ventral consolidation observed on ultrasound examination
  - Absence of pathogenic bacteria in tracheal aspirate

●▶ WHAT TO DO

Severe Bacterial Pneumonia Foals Other Than *R. Equi*

- Broad-spectrum antibiotics:
  - Penicillin potassium or sodium, 22,000 to 44,000 U/kg IV q6h or
  - Ceftiofur, 3 to 5 mg/kg IV q8 to 12h and
  - Amikacin, 18 to 25 mg/kg IV q24h, should be added for the synergistic benefit and improved gram-negative spectrum if renal function is normal and the foal is receiving fluids intravenously
  - Metronidazole, 15 mg/kg PO q12h for foals younger than 3 weeks and q8h for older foals, *only* if anaerobic-like organisms appear on cytology or if *E. coli* or *Enterobacter* organisms are cultured. The latter finding may indicate increased risk of an anaerobic organism also being present. Metronidazole is not part of the routine treatment regimen for severe foal bacterial pneumonia.
- Intranasal oxygen delivery, 10 to 20 mL/kg per minute
- Consider antiulcer prophylaxis:
  - Omeprazole, 4 mg/kg PO or
  - Ranitidine, 6.6 mg/kg PO q8h or 1.5 mg/kg IV q8h, or other H₂ blocker

RESP

- If indicated, remove pleural fluid using diazepam (Valium) for sedation and adequate restraint; use a teat cannula and 60-mL syringe with a three-way stopcock. The fluid is often bright red in color in the neonatal foal with a generalized sepsis and severe pneumonia.
- Nebulization with antibiotics and bronchodilators may be helpful.

Acute Respiratory Distress in Foals After Anthelmintic Treatment

- Although this complication is rare, nursing or weanling foals may develop respiratory distress 1 to 3 days after administration of an anthelmintic.
- This is believed to be a result of the death of a large number of ascarid or strongyle larvae in the lungs.

Diagnosis

- History of receiving an anthelmintic, often for the first time
- Signs of respiratory distress within 48 hours after anthelmintic treatment

Clinical Signs

- Labored breathing
- Tachypnea
- Coughing
- Nasal discharge
- Fever possibly present
- Auscultation:
  - Wheezes heard over lung fields bilaterally
- TTW:
  - Usually nonseptic
  - Cellular reaction that may be a mixture of neutrophils and eosinophils

◉〉 WHAT TO DO

Respiratory Distress After Anthelmintic Treatment

- Corticosteroids, single dose only: dexamethasone, 0.1 mg/kg; usually considerable improvement is seen
- Antibiotics:
  - Trimethoprim-sulfamethoxazole, 20 mg/kg PO q12h and/or
  - Penicillin procaine, 22,000 U/kg IM q12h or
  - Ceftiofur alone, 3.0 mg/kg IV q12h
  - Nebulization with antibiotic, bronchodilator, and steroid might be helpful.

Prognosis

- Prognosis is good.

Pleuropneumonia and Septic Pleuritis

- Although the disease process may have been present for several days, consider pleuropneumonia an emergency!
- *Practice Tip: Unlike most forms of pneumonia in foals, pleuropneumonia in an adult is commonly complicated by anaerobic infection, which is associated with a greater risk of necrosis and infarction of the lung.*
- Pleuropneumonia is the most common cause of infectious pleural effusion in the horse (Table 25-1).

Table 25-1	Signs and Physical Findings of Pleuropneumonia	
	Clinical Signs	**Auscultation Findings**
Acute	Respiratory distress, cough (usually soft), red to dark brown exudate at nostril, severe depression	Crackles and in some areas wheezes, increased ventral bronchial sounds if effusion is minimal
Subacute to chronic	Weight loss, soft cough, poor performance, normal to increased respiratory rate	Pleural effusion, no ventral lung sounds, normal to loud dorsal sounds, radiating heart sounds

Clinical Signs

- Lesions usually are most severe in the midventral right lung, and abnormal lung sounds commonly are more prominent in this area.
- Clinical signs include:
  - Forelimb or sternal edema
  - Low-grade colic
  - Pleurodynia (often confused with, but rarely laminitis)
  - Fever
  - Anorexia

Diagnosis

- The odor of the sample obtained by means of TTW or thoracocentesis can be important in management. A fetid odor indicates the presence of anaerobic bacteria, worsens the prognosis, and increases the cost of treatment. Air echoes within the pleural fluid may also indicate the presence of anaerobic infection or bronchopleural fistula. (See also p. 94.) Discuss this finding with the owner.
- Transtracheal aspiration: Use a BBL Vacutainer, Columbia broth with sodium polystyrene sulfonate (SPS) and increased cysteine.[44] *Submit for aerobic and anaerobic culture.*
- Thoracocentesis is indicated if there is the suspicion of pleural effusion (decreased ventral lung sounds and radiating heart sounds). Ultrasonographic findings confirm the presence of fluid. *Submit for cytology and aerobic and anaerobic culture.*
- *Practice Tip: Quick method (for culture only) for thoracocentesis: Procedure requires 18-gauge, $1\frac{1}{2}$- to $3\frac{1}{2}$-inch (3.75- to 8.9-cm) needle for pleurocentesis. Use aerobic-anaerobic culture medium (BBL Vacutainer, Columbia broth with SPS and increased cysteine[44]).*
- Indwelling chest drain: Procedure is indicated if a large volume of fluid is present or if the effusion is septic (the same site as the thoracocentesis is preferred if the site is ventral enough to provide adequate drainage).
- Requires a blunt-tipped 24F trocar catheter[45]; one-way valve (it is possible to make a latex condom into a one-way

---

[44]Becton-Dickinson, Cockeysville, Maryland.
[45]Trocar catheter (Deknatel, Howmedica, Inc., Floral Park, New York).

valve by opening the closed end and attaching the other end to the catheter with tape).

Protocol for Thoracocentesis

- See p. 459.
- Pass the blunt-tipped 24F trocar catheter 4 to 6 cm through a stab incision. (**Note:** The intercostal blood vessels run caudal to the ribs.).
- Remove the trocar and manipulate the catheter to obtain the best flow rate; suture to skin using Chinese finger trap pattern (see Fig. 25-5, *C*).
- Attach the one-way valve (Heimlich valve or perforated condom) to the catheter to prevent pneumothorax. Tape the condom over the end of the tube with the cut end distal and place a purse-string suture around the catheter to hold it in place.
- Determine the site for the thoracocatheter using ultrasound examination. (**Important:** Avoid the lateral thoracic vein and associated vessels. Place the catheter at a distant site from the heart.)
- In a low number of cases, both sides may drain with one catheter.

●▷ WHAT TO DO

Pleuropneumonia

- Manage all cases of adult pleuropneumonia aggressively.
- Start broad-spectrum antibiotics immediately.

Option 1

- Penicillin, 44,000 U/kg IV q6h
  and
  - Gentamicin, 6.6 mg/kg IV q24h
  and
  - Metronidazole, 15 to 25 mg/kg PO q6 to 8h

Option 2

- If decreased renal function is a concern or if cost of option 1 is prohibitive:
  - Ceftiofur, 3 mg/kg q12h IV or IM, and enrofloxacin, 7.5 mg/kg IV or PO q24h (depending on culture results). Important: Enrofloxacin is generally not highly effective against *Streptococcus equi ssp. zooepidemicus!*
  and
  - Metronidazole, 15 to 25 mg/kg PO q6 to 8h
- Serum creatinine concentration must be monitored during treatment. If azotemia is present, administer fluids or use option 2. Monitoring peak and trough gentamicin levels is the best method to reach therapeutic levels and prevent renal toxicity associated with aminoglycoside usage. Dosages higher than 6.6 mg/kg may be needed and appropriate for some cases.
- NSAID treatment to control fever and pain: NSAIDs may potentiate the nephrotoxicity associated with aminoglycoside administration.
- Recombinant tPA (4 to 12 mg) placed in the thoracic cavity immediately after drainage may reduce fibrin accumulation.
- Clopidogrel (Plavix), 4 mg/kg PO as a loading dose, followed by 2 mg/kg, q24h and/or aspirin, 20 mg/kg PO or per rectum, may be used in horses with hemorrhagic or fetid-smelling pulmonary exudate with the goal of decreasing pulmonary thrombosis.

Supportive Therapy for Concurrent Toxemia

- For adults with abnormal mucous membrane color, toxic-appearing neutrophils or bands, and tachycardia:
  - Intravenous therapy with polyionic fluid
  - Flunixin meglumine, 0.25 mg/kg IV or PO q8h, rather than phenylbutazone if toxemia is present
  - J5 hyperimmune plasma, 2 L IV
  - Pentoxifylline, 10 mg/kg IV or PO q12h
  - Other possible treatments: polymixin B 6000 U/kg if there is evidence of severe toxemia and normal renal values
  - Low-molecular-weight heparin, 50 mg/kg SC q24h, with the goal of preventing thrombosis
  - Intranasal oxygen delivery if respiratory rate is elevated
  - Cryotherapy—feet

Prognosis

- Prognosis for survival is generally good in acute cases unless severe tachypnea, severe polypnea, toxemia, and hemorrhagic-fetid nasal exudate or pleural fluid are present.
- These findings support the presence of infarction and a poorer prognosis.
- In patients with pulmonary infarction, rib resection ultimately may be needed to improve recovery.
- Note: Complications such as laminitis, renal disease, and bronchopleural fistula worsen the prognosis.

Heaves/Recurrent Airway Obstruction (Formerly COPD)/Summer Pasture-Associated Obstructive Pulmonary Disease

- Horses with heaves often experience respiratory distress after exposure to allergens and dust.
- Airways of affected patients appear to be hyperactive to particulate matter (e.g., dust, mold spores, noxious fumes, and even high humidity), predisposing the individual to respiratory crises, sometimes despite good management.
- Increased mucus production and decreased lung function provide the ideal environment for secondary infections, which may trigger episodes of respiratory distress.
- Fever of 39.5° to 40° C (103° to 104° F) in horses with heaves suggests secondary bacterial bronchitis or bronchiectasis.

History

- Cough and exercise intolerance of >3 months' duration in an adult horse (usually >7 years old) that is otherwise normal
- Period of labored breathing at rest with a more pronounced expiratory effort and generally no fever
- Respiratory signs that may wax and wane, even when horse is kept in the same conditions

Clinical Findings

- Findings include increased respiratory rate, extended neck and head, flared nostrils, and double expiratory effort.

RESP

- A "heave line" caused by hypertrophy of the external abdominal oblique muscles may develop.
- Weight loss is common if respiratory distress is prolonged—weeks to months.
- Horses may appear normal when at pasture although in the southeastern United States horses may develop acute onset of respiratory difficulty caused by some component of the pasture such as mold.
- Auscultation: Fine crackles and wheezes usually are heard over most lung fields. The lungs sometimes are abnormally quiet (especially ventrally) in severe episodes. This sign is confused with ventral consolidation (pneumonia) or pleural effusion, but horses with pleuropneumonia infrequently have respiratory distress, and when they do, they usually have signs of sepsis (injected, discolored mucous membranes; severe depression; and commonly a hemorrhagic or fetid discharge from the nostrils).
- Response to treatment (see the following) is a useful diagnostic test if heaves is thought to be the problem. Multiple diagnostic tests are generally unnecessary; if it looks like heaves, then it probably is.
- A significant response to a single injection of atropine (7 to 10 mg/450 kg slowly IV) supports the diagnosis but is seldom indicated unless the horse is in respiratory distress. Atropine administration causes tachycardia and, less commonly, colic. An alternative is N-butylscopolammonium bromide, 0.3 mg/kg IV, a potent bronchodilator, which reaches maximum effect 10 minutes after intravenous administration, and causes fewer side effects than using atropine.
- Increased neutrophil percentages (>25%) in BAL (see Chapter 11, p. 58) on cytologic examination helps confirm the diagnosis but is usually not required/indicated when respiratory distress is present.
- Sedation for the BAL procedure: xylazine, 0.3 to 0.5 mg/kg IV, and butorphanol, 0.01 mg/kg IV. Try to keep the head at the level of the shoulder or elevated to decrease airway resistance.
- Bacterial culture of TTW if there is clinical (fever) and hematologic evidence of secondary bacterial infection (leukocytosis, increased fibrinogen).

Important: If the patient is in severe respiratory distress, do *not* perform a TTW because severe pneumomediastinum can occur. Tracheal aspirate via an endoscope may be used. An endoscopic microbiology aspiration catheter (Mila International) can be used if culture is needed. A sterile polyethylene #205 tubing with an adapter[46]) also works well for sample collection for cytologic examination and culture.

⯈⯈ WHAT TO DO

Severe Heaves
- Corticosteroids:
  - Dexamethasone, 0.04 to 0.06 mg/kg PO or parenterally q24h, for 7 to 14 days. A clinical response is expected within 3 days. Except

for cases that can be removed from the "allergen," such as pasture-associated heaves, systemically administered steroids are required if there is obvious distress.
- Inhaled corticosteroids: beclomethasone dipropionate, 7 µg/kg q12h, or fluticasone, 4 to 6 µg/kg q12h (via MDI, e.g., Aeromask, EquineHaler, or AeroHippus). The mask may be poorly tolerated in horses with labored breathing. If the facemask is not initially well-tolerated, begin with dexamethasone treatment and then continue with inhaled corticosteroids.
  - When using MDI: (1) warm, (2) shake for 30 seconds, (3) keep vertical, and (4) fire into spacer at end of expiration/beginning of inspiration.
- Bronchodilators:
  - Albuterol, 1 µg/kg q1h in MDI (Equine Aeromask, EquineHaler, AeroHippus); rapid onset (<5 minutes), but short acting (30 minutes to 3 hours). This β1-agonist not only provides bronchodilation but improves ciliary clearance and production of surfactant.
  - Ipratropium bromide, 0.5 to 1 µg/kg q6h in MDI (Equine Aeromask, EquineHaler, AeroHippus); onset within 15 minutes, lasts 4 to 6 hours.
  - Clenbuterol, 0.8 to 1.6 mg/kg IV or PO q12h; limited efficacy in horses with labored breathing.
  - Atropine, 0.014 to 0.02 mg/kg (7 to 10 mg IV/450-kg adult one dose), for immediate relief in severe cases unless significant tachycardia (>80 beats/min) is present. Or N-butylscopolammonium bromide, 0.3mg/kg IV or IM, and reaches maximum effect 10 minutes after intravenous administration; the clinical effect wanes within 1 hour after drug administration, more rapidly than does atropine.

Note: Response to inhaled bronchodilators is often less dramatic than with atropine or with N-butylscopolammonium bromide in horses experiencing respiratory distress.

Note: Atropine decreases intestinal motility, so advise owners to monitor for signs of colic, although colic is unusual when this dosage is used once. Be careful when administering bronchodilators to patients with severe tachycardia.
- Antibiotics: If there is a fever or if bacterial bronchitis is suspected, administer penicillin procaine, 22,000 U/kg IM q12h, or ceftiofur, 3 mg/kg IV or IM q12h.
- Intranasal oxygen delivery: 10 to 15 L/min through a nasopharyngeal catheter sutured at the nostril. Humidify the oxygen through warm water if possible.
- Maintain adequate hydration because dehydration thickens the mucous plugs in the airways. Provide fresh, clean water and electrolytes. In some cases it may be necessary to administer fluids through a nasogastric tube or intravenously.

Prognosis
- Prognosis is good in most cases. However, satisfactory clinical improvement may require 3 to 5 days. *Do not* expect improvement in horses with heaves and concurrent bacterial bronchitis until corticosteroid therapy is added to the antimicrobial therapy.
- Some older patients with a prolonged history of heaves with severe parenchymal disease may not respond to this treatment; this is a rare occurrence.
- Radiographs are recommended because bronchiectasis may be present.

---

[46]Intramedic sterile polyethylene #205 tubing and Intramedic Luer Stud Adapter (Becton-Dickinson, Parsippany, New Jersey).

Management

- Management of heaves involves minimizing contact with allergens by changing feeds. Remove exposure to hay and straw; pasture is generally preferred.
- Alternatively, use a pelleted or cubed hay, hay silage, or hydroponic hay, and a low-dust bedding (newspaper or low-dust shavings can be used).
- Most affected individuals should be kept outside 24 hours a day if possible. If not, it is best to move them to the end of the barn (or an area with the best ventilation) and outside at haying time and during bedding change.
- In the southeastern United States, some individuals exhibit respiratory signs of heaves while at pasture (summer pasture–associated obstructive pulmonary disease) and may improve within 24 hours if they are simply housed in a barn.

Note: On rare occasion, a 3- to 6-month-old foal recovering from "typical" foal pneumonia develops "heavy" signs. A transtracheal aspirate may reveal *Aspergillus* sp. and no bacteria. Treatment with bronchodilators and occasionally corticosteroids is recommended.

Pulmonary Infiltrative Diseases

- Pulmonary infiltrative diseases are uncommon causes of respiratory distress in horses.
- They more commonly cause chronic respiratory signs often resembling those observed in heaves.
- Affected horses fail to respond to conventional therapy for heaves.
- Anorexia, weight loss, and evidence of multisystemic involvement are often present.
- In suspected cases, the diagnosis is based on lesions found on thoracic radiographs and in lung biopsies.
- Conditions associated with pulmonary infiltrative diseases in horses are as follows:
  - Idiopathic granulomatous pneumonia
  - Multisystemic eosinophilic epitheliotropic diseases
  - Neoplasia
  - Silicosis
  - Fungal infection
  - Equine multinodular pulmonary fibrosis (see p. 475)

Additional Causes of Respiratory Distress without Noise

- Compromised ventilation can result from the following:
  - Botulism
  - Tetanus
  - Increased intraabdominal volume/pressure preventing normal lung expansion
  - Diaphragmatic hernia
- Tachypnea associated with severe metabolic acidosis or tissue hypoxia (hemolysis, intoxication)
- Pain
- Idiopathic tachypnea in young foals; more common in Draft foals; hyperthermia also common in these foals
- Hepatoencephalopathy or other cerebral/brainstem disorders

Epistaxis

- Epistaxis caused by head trauma rarely necessitates emergency treatment unless the nares are obstructed; tracheotomy is then required.
- Conditions causing epistaxis that can be life-threatening and necessitate emergency evaluation and therapy are:
  - Guttural pouch mycosis
  - Epistaxis caused by thrombocytopenia
  - Rupture of the longus capitis muscle

Guttural Pouch Mycosis

- Bleeding may be the only clinical sign in adults with guttural pouch mycosis; or bleeding and neurologic signs may occur simultaneously.
- In some cases, yellow exudate is seen at the nostril before bleeding is observed.
- Middle-aged or older pastured horses are most commonly affected.
- Owners report finding blood on the stall wall or on the nose before the major bleed occurs.
- The bleeding is generally unilateral unless severe hemorrhage happens, in which case blood may be draining from both nostrils.

Diagnosis

- Mycosis is rarely seen in hot and dry climates.
- A tentative diagnosis is based on history; endoscopic examination is needed for a definitive diagnosis.
- Endoscopic examination: Unless there is evidence of hypotension, elevated heart rate, pale mucous membranes, or slow capillary refill time, light sedation facilitates the passage of the endoscope. Use of a guidewire passed through the biopsy channel assists in entering the pouch. An alternative is to pass a Chambers catheter in the opposite nostril to elevate the guttural pouch flap. The lesion, often a yellowish green, diphtheritic membrane with clot formation, is most commonly found dorsally in the medial or lateral compartment.

▶ WHAT TO DO

Guttural Pouch Mycosis/Epistaxis

- Once the diagnosis is confirmed, surgery is needed as soon as possible.
- If blood loss is severe, blood transfusion (see Chapter 20, p. 287) and polyionic fluids are needed to stabilize the patient's condition. Hypertonic saline usually is not administered unless hypovolemic shock is clinically evident.
- If sedation is needed to transport the patient, use diazepam, 0.05 mg/kg IV.
- If the bleeding is uncontrollable and life-threatening, ligation of the common carotid artery on the affected side is useful even though some bleeding continues.

Important: Ligation of the common carotid artery can result in severe neurologic signs and blindness.

Epistaxis Caused by Thrombocytopenia

Epistaxis can be an emergency requiring specific treatments. Please see discussion of thrombocytopenia and blood transfusion in Chapter 20, p. 287.

Rupture of the Longus Capitis Muscle

- Rupture can mimic severe guttural pouch hemorrhage and is differentiated at endoscopic examination.
- Treatment is symptomatic:
  - Keep the affected individual quiet.
  - Administer fluids and blood transfusion.
  - Maintain a patent airway.

Ethmoid Hematoma

- The initial clinical sign usually is a unilateral blood-tinged nasal discharge.
- With progression of the hematoma, respiratory noise develops due to partial airway obstruction.

Diagnosis

- Endoscopic examination usually reveals a dark reddish-black or even greenish discolored mass in the ethmoid turbinate region. Radiographs are helpful in identifying masses in the paranasal sinuses.

● WHAT TO DO

Ethmoid Hematoma

- Laser surgery or cryosurgery is generally recommended for large lesions, although intralesion injections with 4% formalin via endoscope can be effective for smaller lesions.

- Rarely, an adverse event, including acute death, may occur immediately after the formalin injection. If the cribriform plate is necrotic, the formalin may enter the calvaria and brain.
- Computed tomography can be used before the injection to determine whether the cribriform plate is intact.
- Large ethmoid hematomas require excision of the mass via paranasal sinus surgery.
- Autologous blood transfusion (collection in blood bag containing citrate-phosphate-dextrose solution 10 days before surgery) should be considered.

Exercise-Induced Pulmonary Hemorrhage

- Rarely is the bleeding so severe that it results in respiratory distress and death.
- In some cases of acute death, bleeding is within the thoracic cavity.

Nasal Masses

- Rarely are nasal masses (e.g., tumor and granuloma) a cause for emergency treatment; however, they are some of the most common causes of epistaxis and upper respiratory noise and obstruction.

References

References can be found on the companion website at www.equine-emergencies.com.

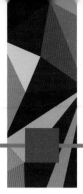

CHAPTER 26

Urinary System

DIAGNOSTIC AND THERAPEUTIC PROCEDURES

Barbara Dallap Schaer and James A. Orsini

Urinary Tract Catheterization

Urinary tract catheterization ensures an accurate, uncontaminated urine sample obtained in a convenient manner. A midstream, free-catch urine sample is adequate for urinalysis but is not appropriate for culture. The same technique is used for passage of the fiber-optic or videoendoscope in performing cystoscopy or urethroscopy.

Equipment
- Sedative or tranquilizer (xylazine hydrochloride or detomidine hydrochloride with butorphanol tartrate and acepromazine)
- Smooth muscle relaxant (N-butylscopolammonium bromide, Buscopan)—sometimes useful in males (foals and adults)
- Tail tie for mares
- Sterile gloves
- Sterile lubricating jelly
- Appropriate urinary catheter (sterile)
  - Stallions and geldings: 9-mm outer diameter urinary catheter
  - Mares: 11-mm outer diameter urinary catheter
- 60-mL catheter-tip syringe (sterile)
- Three sterile vials for urinalysis, cytologic examination, and culture specimens

Procedure
Male Catheterization
- Stallions and geldings usually need sedation and tranquilization for restraint and penile extension. (Recommended dosage is 0.3 to 0.5 mg/kg xylazine and 0.01 to 0.02 mg/kg butorphanol, combined with 0.02 mg/kg acepromazine IV—for geldings only.)
  - Although the risk of acepromazine causing paraphimosis in stallions is inconclusive, avoid its use in stallions if at all possible.
- Clean the penis with a dilute antiseptic solution (povidone-iodine or chlorhexidine) and rinse with water.
- Wear sterile gloves while minimally lubricating the catheter.
- Stabilize the penis with one hand and gently advance the catheter through the urethral opening.

- Advance the catheter. The catheter should glide through the urethra easily until the urethral sphincter is reached. Injection of 60 mL of air and/or 10 mL of lidocaine into the urethra may aid passage through the sphincter. Excessive force in inserting the catheter can cause bleeding and retroflexion of the catheter, which further inhibits passage into the bladder.
  - In some cases it is difficult to pass the catheter through the urethral sphincter. In the adult horse, rectal palpation and gentle manual pressure on the bladder may be needed to facilitate passage of the catheter into the bladder. Administration of Buscopan can be used to relax the urethral sphincter.
- If urine does not flow freely when the catheter has reached the bladder, gently aspirate with a 60-mL syringe.
- Place samples directly into the sterile vials for urinalysis, cytologic examination, and culture and colony count.

Female Catheterization
- Sedation is generally not needed, although use of a twitch is recommended.
- Wrap the tail and pull it to the side.
- Scrub the perineum with a dilute antiseptic solution (povidone-iodine or chlorhexidine) and rinse with water.
- Wearing sterile gloves, minimally lubricate the catheter.
- Place a hand within the vagina and locate the urethral opening on the floor of the vagina. Insert one finger into the urethra and gently guide the catheter with the opposite hand.
  - Many times the procedure is done "blindly" without a hand in the vagina.
- Advance the catheter approximately 5 to 10 cm. If urine does not flow freely, aspirate with a 60-mL syringe.
- Place samples in appropriate containers.

Complications
- Infection of the lower urinary tract can occur if sterile technique is not maintained, particularly if the bladder is atonic.
- Injecting large volumes of air into an inflamed urethra should be avoided because of the possibility of a potentially fatal air embolism, although a small probability.

Urinalysis
- Urinalysis is useful in the diagnosis of lower and upper urinary tract disorders. Each sample should be submitted

for a complete urinalysis, cytologic examination, and bacterial culture with colony count.

- A urine sample should be examined within 20 minutes of collection or be refrigerated immediately.
- Gross examination of equine urine is difficult because of the high mucous content.
  - Pigmenturia is easily seen but must be differentiated as either hematuria, hemoglobinuria, bilirubinuria, or myoglobinuria by means of clinical exam, plasma color, serum creatine kinase, and direct bilirubin measurement along with urine dipstick and microscopic examination.
- A urine dipstick is routinely used to determine pH, protein content, glucose, bilirubin, and the presence of pigments. ***Practice Tip:*** *Hemoglobin, myoglobin, and hematuria all cause occult blood to be positive.*
- A refractometer is used to determine specific gravity.
  - The specific gravity of the urine of adults is normally between 1.008 and 1.045; the urine of foals is between 1.001 and 1.025.
  - Highly concentrated urine is often caused by decreased water intake.
  - If urinary specific gravity remains isosthenuric (equal to blood specific gravity of approximately 1.010) despite changes in water intake or a water deprivation test, significant renal disease should be suspected.
- Normal urine should not contain protein, glucose, or bilirubin.
  - If a dipstick is used, protein may be falsely elevated to "trace" if the urine is highly concentrated or very alkaline.
  - Protein is detected if there is pigmenturia or inflammation or infection in the urinary tract.
  - Absolute (true) proteinuria should be quantitated with analytical measurement followed by calculation of urine protein : urine creatinine ratio with high ratios >3 : 1 seen with glomerulonephritis.
  - Glucosuria occurs in hyperglycemia with normal renal function. If the blood glucose level is normal, glucosuria is highly suggestive of renal tubular disease.
  - Normal equine urine is alkaline; adult urinary pH is 7.5 to 8.5, foal urinary pH is 5.5 to 8.0. Increased acidity occurs with strenuous exercise, metabolic acidosis, and anorexia or starvation.
- Cytologic examination of the urine is important in differentiating urinary tract inflammation and infection. Slides should be made from the sample centrifugate, air dried, and stained with Wright or Diff-Quik stain.
  - Five red blood cells (RBCs) and 5 white blood cells (WBCs) per high-power field (100×) are normal. More than 10 RBCs per field suggests bleeding, and more than 10 WBCs per field suggests inflammation.
  - If inflammation is present, a Gram stain should be performed to look for bacteria. Bacteria should not be detected in normal urine if the sample is collected using aseptic technique. Assessment of bacterial morphology

helps in instituting antibiotic therapy before culture results are obtained.
- Casts (cellular debris shed from the renal tubules) indicate renal tubular damage.
- Calcium carbonate crystals are common and are considered within normal limits unless clinical signs suggest the presence of urinary calculi.

URINARY TRACT EMERGENCIES

Thomas J. Divers

Primary urinary tract emergencies in the horse are uncommon; however, when they do occur, the disease can be life-threatening if not properly diagnosed and treated. The most common urinary system emergencies are the following:
- Acute renal failure
- Discolored urine
- Lower urinary tract obstruction
- Ruptured bladder in the foal and occasionally in the adult

Acute Renal Failure

Acute renal failure (ARF) usually results from nephrotoxic causes or vasomotor nephropathy (e.g., ischemic causes). The most common pathologic finding is acute tubular necrosis.

Nephrotoxic Causes

- Consider aminoglycoside nephrotoxicity if a patient becomes depressed while being treated with aminoglycosides or a few days after therapy is discontinued. Depression and anorexia are the most common clinical signs of uremia in the equine.
- Aminoglycoside-induced renal failure usually results in polyuric renal failure and is typically responsive to treatment if diagnosed and treated early.
- Tetracycline-induced renal failure may occur if 20 mg/kg per day or greater is administered or lower doses are administered for several days to a dehydrated horse.
- Euvolemic foals appear more resistant to toxic effects of oxytetracycline, but they may sporadically develop signs of ARF 3 to 4 days after 1 or 2 doses of 3 g oxytetracycline are administered for treatment for contracted tendons. Foals that are treated with large doses of oxytetracycline for contracted tendons should:
  - Be euvolemic (well hydrated)—this may not be the situation in the severe tendon contracture when the foal has difficulty rising and nursing.
  - Have serum creatinine measured if there is a report of change in clinical behavior (i.e., depressed 2 to 4 days after the oxytetracycline treatment).
- On rare occasion a horse may develop signs of renal failure 3 days after receiving intravenous tiludronic acid, caco copper, or vitamin preparations; cause and effect remain unproven.

Diagnosis

- History, physical examination, laboratory findings

Laboratory Findings

- Findings include azotemia, isosthenuria, hyponatremia, and hypochloremia.
- Azotemia in the horse is best determined by measurement of serum creatinine.
  - In some cases of ARF, especially those with diarrhea, the blood urea nitrogen (BUN) value may be only mildly elevated, but the creatinine value is greatly elevated; believed to be due to dialysis of urea into colon fluid.
  - The presence of prerenal azotemia is best determined by clinical examination, urinalysis, and time required for serum creatinine concentration to return to normal after fluid therapy is started (most prerenal azotemia is corrected within 36 hours after initiation of fluid therapy). The upper range for creatinine from prerenal azotemia may be as high as 7 to 8 mg/dL. A BUN-to-creatinine ratio >20 suggests a prerenal component.
  - Suspect renal azotemia if the BUN-to-creatinine ratio is <10, serum potassium concentration is elevated, urine specific gravity is 1.006 to 1.012 despite large volumes of intravenous fluid therapy, and creatinine concentration does not decline or declines slowly over several days after fluid therapy is started.
  - Newborn foals sporadically may have a serum creatinine concentration in the 5- to 8-mg/dL range (and sometimes higher) without other evidence of renal dysfunction. This is most common in foals born to mares with placental dysfunction. The creatinine concentration generally returns to normal in these patients within 2 days. Some adult Quarter Horses and rarely Warmbloods have a normal serum creatinine concentration of up to 2.4 mg/dL.
- Serum potassium and calcium values typically are normal and low, respectively, with ARF, but the potassium and calcium concentration may be high if the renal failure is oliguric. The finding of hyperkalemia in a patient with ARF suggests a more guarded prognosis because it often indicates oliguric or anuric renal failure.
- Blood ammonia may be elevated if neurologic signs are present (uremic encephalopathy).

Pigment Nephropathy

- Pigment nephropathy is most common after a severe episode of myopathy. Some mild to moderately severe cases may not receive intravenous fluid therapy, providing an explanation for the ARF in these cases. Grossly discolored urine is not a prerequisite for myositis-induced ARF.
  - ***Practice Tip:*** *Not every horse that "ties up" requires fluid therapy; if urine is discolored or the clinical signs are severe, fluids should be given and/or creatinine checked 2 to 3 days after resolution of clinical signs and discolored urine.*
- Hemolysis is less likely to result in renal failure than is myopathy, although individuals with hemolysis and disseminated intravascular coagulation are at risk of ARF, especially red maple poisoning.

- Depression caused by uremia occurs 3 to 7 days after the tying-up episode or hemolytic crisis.
- Aspartate aminotransferase (AST) measurement helps confirm previous myopathy in horses with an unknown cause of ARF.

Vasomotor Nephropathy

- There are no published numbers on the incidence of ARF in horses with sepsis, but it is common. Renal failure may well be the most common organ failure following sepsis in the horse. Any condition predisposing to hypotension or release of endogenous pressor agents has the potential of causing hemodynamic-mediated ARF.
- Causes include acute blood loss, severe intravascular volume deficits, septic shock, thrombotic episodes, coagulopathy, and acute heart failure, including pericarditis.
- Vasomotor nephropathy can cause severe renal failure without accompanying histologic findings. Alternatively, diffuse renal, cortical, or medullary necrosis occasionally occurs.
- Acute glomerulopathy is rare in horses but can occur with purpura hemorrhagica or other systemic vascular diseases.

Diagnosis

- History, physical examination, clinical signs

Laboratory Findings

- Findings include elevated serum creatinine value with concurrent low urine specific gravity (<1.020), hematuria, hypochloremia, and hyponatremia.
- The rare case of acute glomerulopathy may cause gross hematuria and significant proteinuria.
- Hyperkalemia suggests primary intrinsic renal failure as opposed to prerenal azotemia. This seems to be especially true in horses with colitis.

General Treatment Principles for Acute Renal Failure—Acute Tubular Nephrosis

Treatment of Acute Renal Failure

- General treatment (Fig. 26-1): With nephrotoxic-induced ARF, the creatinine may not decrease for 2 to 3 days after treatment is started. If the patient is polyuric the prognosis is usually good, and the creatinine slowly returns to normal.
- Specific treatment (rarely needed): Peritoneal or pleural dialysis may be useful in reducing toxic agents, but the results are variable. This procedure is rarely used unless there is a need to remove a nephrotoxin still present in the blood.
- Peritoneal dialysis protocol for oliguric or anuric ARF:
  - Monitor electrolyte status, especially sodium and potassium.
  - Administer warm lactated Ringer's solution with 1.5% dextrose for peritoneal dialysis; heparin (1000 units/L) can be added in hopes of decreasing adhesions.

URN

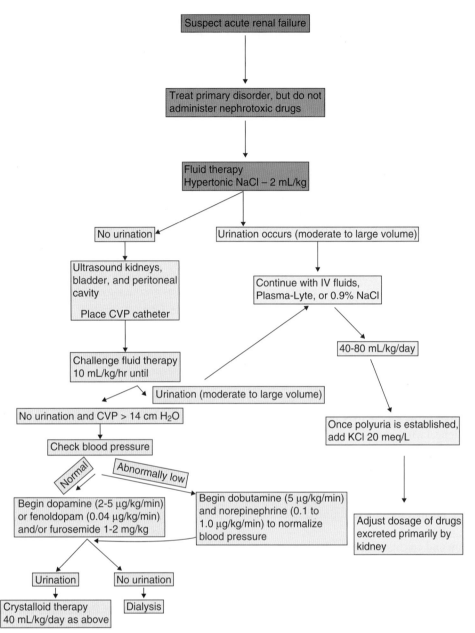

Figure 26-1   General treatment principles for acute renal failure. *CVP,* Central venous pressure.

Peritoneal catheters can be obtained from Cook Critical Care in Bloomington, Indiana, or a mushroom catheter or human thoracic catheter (28F) can be used to drain the urine. These catheters should be placed in the ventral abdomen for drainage of the dialysate fluid. Fluid can be administered via these catheters, although it is better to administer the dialysate fluid via another smaller catheter placed into the abdomen at the left paralumbar fossa (*Note:* Make sure it is not in the retroperitoneum and that it is caudal to the spleen!) Ultrasound examination should be performed following catheter placement to ensure that catheters are placed within the peritoneal cavity.

• If no cardiopulmonary abnormalities are identified, dialysis may be administered at 40 mL/kg. After 30 to 60 minutes, drain most of the fluid, leaving enough in

the abdomen to keep the omentum from "plugging" the drainage catheter opening (this can be determined by ultrasound, or discontinue drainage when the flow slows). If the horse is euvolemic, nearly 60% of the fluid should be recovered in order to continue with the dialysis. With repeated dialysis, nearly 80% of the previous dialysate fluid volume should be retrieved, and the horse's body weight should be essentially unchanged. If dialysis is to be continued for a few days, cytologic examination and WBC counts should be performed on the collected fluid for monitoring of peritonitis. If WBC counts become elevated, continuous flow and drainage may be indicated.

• In foals, the omentum often interferes with this procedure, making peritoneal dialysis more difficult in the recumbent foal.

- Hemodialysis is performed at a small number of critical care facilities.
- *Note:* The jugular veins must be patent and in good health for hemodialysis

●› WHAT TO DO

Acute Renal Failure—Acute Tubular Nephrosis
See Fig. 26-1.

- Treat predisposing condition.
- Provide fluid replacement for volume deficits and electrolyte and acid-base correction. Hypertonic saline solution (2 mL/kg) followed by 0.9% saline or Plasma-Lyte solution is the preferred initial fluid therapy in most cases. Potassium (20 mEq/L) is added after it is confirmed that the patient is polyuric.
- Monitor serum sodium, chloride, calcium, and potassium levels, and correct any abnormalities. Although high-sodium fluids are not generally recommended in neonatal foals, foals with polyuric ARF can be treated with high-sodium fluids because of their enhanced urinary sodium loss associated with the renal failure.
- Assess the character of ARF: polyuric (excessive excretion of urine) versus oliguric (diminished urine excretion). Determine whether the patient has oliguric or polyuric renal failure. If oliguric renal failure is suspected, monitor the packed cell volume (PCV), plasma protein concentration, jugular vein distention, peripheral edema, blood pressure, and central venous pressure (CVP).
  - To measure CVP, insert a 24-inch (60-cm) Intracath[1] catheter into the jugular vein and into the anterior vena cava of the adult horse. Use a manometer with a baseline positioned at the level of the right atrium. Normal CVP is <8 to 10 cm H_2O with the horse's head held at a normal height or slightly higher. When the CVP catheter is properly positioned there is a 1- to 2-cm change in CVP associated with breathing. Although the measurement is not precise, if the CVP measurement is performed exactly the same (i.e., same height related to a 0 position on the manometer using the point of the horse's shoulder and maintaining a similar head position), monitoring the trend during treatment can be very helpful in determining the correct volume of intravenous fluids to be administered. In foals, measurement can be done with a 20-cm Mila catheter.[2] Determination of CVP in a recumbent foal is difficult and probably inaccurate; however, accuracy is improved by placing the foal in sternal recumbency for the measurement.
  - Monitor blood pressure to help assess adequacy of volume replacement in conjunction with cardiac output and vascular tone. If blood pressure remains low despite adequate volume replacement, administer dobutamine and/or dopamine (both can be given at approximately 5 µg/kg/min) with the goal of restoring cardiac output, blood pressure, and adequate glomerular filtration pressure. The systolic arterial pressure must be at least 90 mm Hg and ideally 110 mm Hg with the horse's head held in normal position. This can be monitored with a Critikon Dinamap,[3] Cardell[4] or other monitoring device. The measurements may be only an estimate of the true blood pressure. The cuff (bladder) width should be 40% or more of the tail circumference for the most accurate mean measurement.

- Once volume deficits are corrected and systemic blood pressure is restored, do the following for oliguric or anuric ARF:
  - Manage oliguric renal failure with dopamine, 3 to 7 µg/kg/min IV continuously, and furosemide, 1 to 2 mg/kg IV q2h, for 4 treatments. Blood pressure should not rise above normal values (mean value, 110 to 120 mm Hg) during the infusion. Dobutamine, 5 µg/kg/min, may be administered if the CVP is normal and blood pressure is low normal. Controversy exists among clinicians regarding the efficacy of dopamine in the treatment of ARF in humans and some other species. Its use is recommended in the care of horses with oliguric or anuric ARF; some horses with ARF have an increase in urine production after dopamine administration. Dopamine (2.5 to 5.0 µg/kg/min) has been shown to increase renal blood flow and urine production in healthy horses. If dopamine treatment does not increase urine production within 2 to 4 hours, its continuation is probably futile. A dose of fenoldopam (0.04 µg/kg/min) has been shown to be effective for foals but its advantage over dopamine is unproven in the horse, and it is more expensive.
  - Discontinue dopamine administration within 24 to 48 hours and furosemide immediately if therapy is successful in converting oliguria to polyuria.
  - Continue to monitor urine output. If oliguria reoccurs, repeat dopamine and furosemide treatment.
  - Some consider furosemide therapy alone to be contraindicated in the management of rhabdomyolysis-induced or aminoglycoside-induced renal failure in other species, but it can be used alone *following volume replacement* as treatment for other causes of ARF.
  - Mannitol, 0.5 to 1.0 g/kg IV, may be used in acute oliguric renal failure caused by rhabdomyolysis after correction of volume deficits with intravenously administered fluids.
  - Do *not* use mannitol if the patient is anuric.
  - Administer aminophylline, 0.5 mg/kg over 30 minutes, in an attempt to improve glomerular filtration rate in premature or septic foals with respiratory distress and renal failure. If there is improvement, this can be repeated 2 to 3 times daily.
  - Refractory hypotension, defined as an adequate fluid therapy and high CVP but low arterial pressure and anuria in foals, should be managed with norepinephrine, 0.1 to 1.0 µg/kg/min, and 1 to 2 days' treatment with low-dose corticosteroids (0.5 to 2 mg/kg hydrocortisone IV q6h). Norepinephrine may have positive effects on renal and cardiac hemodynamics. If this is unsuccessful, vasopressin (0.01 to 0.04 units/kg/h) can be used for 1 hour with the goal of initiating urine production. The expectation of vasopressin use is to constrict efferent vessels more than afferent vessels.
- For polyuric ARF, do the following:
  - Administer 60 to 80 mL/kg per day polyionic fluids (usually 0.9% saline solution with 20 mEq/L potassium chloride) IV until a precipitous drop in serum creatinine concentration occurs.
  - Continue with intravenous fluids at 40 to 60 mL/kg a day for the next several days until creatinine concentration has returned to normal or has plateaued.
  - Furosemide and dopamine should *not* be used in polyuric states.
  - If sedation is required, use small doses of xylazine because it can increase urine production.
- If the patient is anorectic, add 50 to 100 g of dextrose/L to the intravenous fluids for calories.
- Acute glomerulopathy, a rare condition in the horse, is managed as described before with treatment for the systemic condition (i.e., steroids for vasculitis).

---

[1]Becton-Dickinson, Franklin Lakes, New Jersey.
[2]Mila, 12 Price Avenue, Erlanger, KY 41018.
[3]Absolute Medical Equipment, 55 West Railroad Ave, Garnerville, NY 10923.
[4]Midmark Corporation, 60 Vista Drive, PO Box 286, Versailles, Ohio.

- Omeprazole or an appropriate H₂-blocker and/or sucralfate are administered to diminish the incidence of gastric ulceration.

Acute Septic Nephritis

- Acute septic nephritis is rare in horses other than *Actinobacillus equuli* nephritis in foals. These foals usually are younger than 7 days (most are 2 to 4 days old), and many are found dead in the pasture without obvious clinical signs.
  - Overwhelming bacteremia and endotoxemia are the primary concerns with *A. equuli* rather than renal failure. Most infected foals have a low serum immunoglobulin G concentration.
- Gram-negative enteric bacteria, even *Actinobacillus,* and gram-positive *Streptococcus zooepidemicus* may occasionally cause acute bilateral septic nephritis in adults.
  - Treatment should include intravenously administered fluids and antibiotics.
  - Initial antibiotic therapy, pending microbiology results of urine culture and sensitivity, is ceftiofur, 4 mg/kg IV q12h, or trimethoprim-sulfamethoxazole, 20 mg/kg PO q12h.
- *Leptospira interrogans* serogroup *Pomona* (most likely *kennewicki*) can cause ARF and hematuria in horses. Although not common, the organism may rarely affect multiple horses simultaneously (more commonly weanlings and yearlings) causing fever and acute renal failure.
  - Fever, leukocytosis, and pyuria without microscopically detectable bacteriuria should raise the index of suspicion for *L. pomona kennewicki.*
  - Serum titers are very high for *L. pomona* and other cross-reacting serotypes at the onset of disease. With acute infection there is usually more than one serovar with a very high titer.
  - Treatment includes intravenously administered fluids as recommended for other causes of ARF. Also administer penicillin, 22,000 U/kg IV q6h, or enrofloxacin, 5 to 7.5 mg/kg IV q24h.
  - Prognosis is fair to good with appropriate treatment.

Renal Tubular Acidosis

- Type I renal tubular acidosis (RTA) may occasionally cause acute and severe depression in horses related to unusually low blood pH.
- This type of RTA occurs usually, although intermittently, in adults and may be preceded by drug therapy for another condition or renal injury, or there may be no predisposing cause.
- Genetic predisposition is unproven but possible and recurrence may occur.

Diagnosis

- The diagnosis is based on the presence of a severe metabolic acidosis and hyperchloremia with a neutral to alkaline urine pH.

⊙› WHAT TO DO

Renal Tubular Acidosis

- Administer sodium bicarbonate, intravenously (severe RTA) and orally (up to 100 g PO q12h added to 4 to 8 L of water for oral administration and 8 L of sterile water for IV administration), with supplemental potassium chloride (40 meq/L IV or 20 g PO. Most cases of RTA are transient and the patient recovers with treatment and time. Some horses require intermittent or persistent therapy.
- The amount of bicarbonate to correct the deficit is more precisely determined by the formula: mEq deficit per L plasma × 0.3 to calculate extracellular fluid deficit in mEq. To determine grams of sodium bicarbonate needed, divide the mEq value by 12 (there are 12 mEq/g of sodium bicarbonate per gram). To make an isotonic solution (approximately 300 mmol/L) for IV administration there are 24 mmol of sodium bicarbonate/g or 12.5 g/L. ***Practice Tip:** Administering a large and hypertonic dose of sodium bicarbonate orally may cause diarrhea!*

Discolored Urine

Discolored urine results from bilirubinuria, hemoglobinuria, myoglobinuria, pyuria, hematuria, or drug discoloration (Table 26-1). The color and consistency of normal adult urine vary widely because of the amount of mucus in the urine. The urine of some horses normally contains pigments that cause a reddish-brown discoloration best seen in urine-stained snow or shavings. The most common drugs to cause urine discoloration are rifampicin and phenazopyridine.

Hematuria

Hematuria is recognized as blood clots or uniform red discolored urine without blood clots.

Causes

The most frequent causes are the following:
- Urethral hemorrhage: habronemiasis, calculi, idiopathic (proximal dorsal urethral hemorrhage in males), urethritis, neoplasia (squamous cell carcinoma most common)
- Bladder: calculi, cystitis, neoplasia, amorphous debris, bleeding diathesis (warfarin toxicity), blister beetle toxicity, cystic hematomas in newborn foals, rupture of an infected umbilical artery and bleeding into the bladder in newborn foals, rarely NSAID administration
- Ureter: Occasionally one or both ureters are torn near the entrance to the bladder, causing uroperitoneum and sometimes hematuria. This is most common in newborn foals; it is unknown if there is a tear or a congenital defect in the foal's ureter(s). Clinical signs are generally seen at day 3 of age and urine may accumulate in either the retroperitoneal space or peritoneum. The swelling in retroperitoneal space can be seen via ultrasonography. The defect may sometimes heal without surgery.
- Kidney: calculi, trauma, nephritis, vascular anomaly, idiopathic, parasite migration (*Strongylus* or *Halicephalobus deletrix*), neoplasia, glomerulopathy, papillary necrosis, NSAID administration, blister beetle toxicosis, and leptospirosis (though most do not have hematuria)

Table 26-1   Differential Diagnosis of Discolored Urine

	Hematuria	Hemoglobinuria	Drugs	Bilirubinuria	Myoglobinuria
Urine color*	Red, bright, or dark	Pink (also red or dark red)	Any color (e.g., orange), rifampin, phenazopyridine	Dark brown (green foam when shaken in a tube)	Brown to red to black
Consistency	Occasional clumps of blood are seen, and the discoloration is not uniform	Consistent discoloration	Consistent discoloration	Consistent discoloration	Consistent discoloration
Plasma color	Normal	Usually pink	Variable	Icteric	Usually normal unless anuric
Urine dipstick blood result	Almost always positive for both hemolyzed and nonhemolyzed blood	Consistently strongly positive for hemolyzed blood	Negative	Negative unless secondary renal disease with hemolysis or hematuria	Consistently strongly positive for hemolyzed blood
Sediment and cytologic features of urine	RBCs and ghost cells	Pigment casts and some secondary RBCs due to tubular disease	Normal	Normal to few RBCs if renal disease	Pigment casts, RBCs due to tubular disease
Laboratory tests	Variable PCV and protein; MCV may be increased; creatinine is increased if both kidneys sufficiently diseased	Low PCV; normal to high protein; MCV may be increased; increased unconjugated bilirubin	No change	Increased liver enzymes and bilirubin (both conjugated and unconjugated)	Increased creatine kinase; any increase in serum creatinine is a reflection of decreased glomerular filtration rate

MCV, Mean corpuscular volume; *PCV*, packed cell volume; *RBCs*, red blood cells.
*Never use this alone for diagnosis because color can vary.

Diagnosis

- Signalment, age, duration of hematuria, and the time during urination when hematuria is most pronounced are helpful. Examples include:
  - Hematuria after exercise suggests cystic calculi.
  - Hematuria only at the beginning of urination indicates a distal urethral lesion.
  - Hematuria uniformly throughout urination implies a bladder lesion or more likely bleeding from the kidney.
  - Hematuria only at the end of urination suggests bladder hemorrhage or proximal urethral syndrome in adult males.
- If discolored urine is recognized but clots are not seen, hemoglobinuria, bilirubinuria, or myoglobinuria must be ruled out (see Table 26-1).
  - Differentiate using urine dipstick evaluation, PCV, plasma protein, color of plasma, color of mucous membranes, serum chemistry (e.g., creatine kinase, AST, γ-glutamyltransferase, conjugated bilirubin), and urine sediment examination (presence of RBCs). A few patients with normal urine produce reddish-brown spots in snow or on shavings after urination. This is believed to be caused by metabolized plant pigment.
- Confirm the origin of hematuria with a physical examination. Examine the urethra (after tranquilization in males) and bladder via endoscopic and/or ultrasonographic exam; palpate the urethra, bladder, ureters, and left kidney. Also a 1-m endoscope may be long enough to examine the bladder except in large geldings or stallions although a 2-m scope is preferred and may be required for larger horses.
  - After disinfecting the instrument, tranquilize the patient for penile relaxation, and gently pass the scope retrograde by way of the urethra after lightly lubricating the outside of the scope with sterile K-Y jelly or similar lubricant (see Chapter 12, p. 68). The mucous membrane of the urethra is generally pale white to pink, although a few small red foci are normal. Minimal dilation with air is needed in some cases to move the mucosa away from the tip of the scope. Excessive use of air causes the patient to strain, and the urethral mucosa becomes very hyperemic. ***Note: In rare cases after prolonged inflation, fatal air embolism occurs.***
  - The presence of a mucosal defect or hyperemia and tortuous vessels in the urethra near the opening of the accessory sex glands is evidence to confirm the diagnosis of idiopathic urethral hemorrhage in adult males (Fig. 26-2). This occurs in otherwise healthy geldings, or rarely, stallions that discharge dark blood immediately after urination. This syndrome seems to be more common in Quarter Horses. Hyperemia throughout the urethra is more consistent with urethritis or endoscopy irritation. Once the endoscope is in the bladder, the ureteral openings can be seen by retroflexing the endoscope. Evaluation of urine draining from each ureter, as well as complete bladder evaluation, can

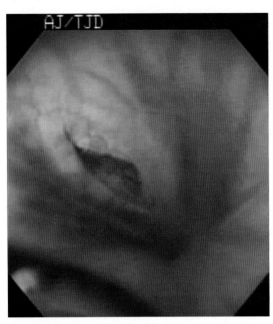

Figure 26-2 Endoscopic examination of urethra of a 9-year-old gelding with hematuria at the end of urination. The defect in the urethra is dorsal and just distal to the accessory sex gland openings.

further distinguish the source of the hematuria. During the examination, urethral hyperemia rapidly occurs, even in a normal horse.

>> WHAT TO DO

Discolored Urine

- Emergency treatment is rarely required unless clots are causing urinary obstruction or rupture of the kidney has occurred, resulting in life-threatening bleeding or colic.
- Management of life-threatening hemoglobinuria, myoglobinuria, and bilirubinuria is discussed with hemolytic anemia, rhabdomyolysis, and liver failure.
- If bleeding from the urinary tract is believed to be life-threatening, conjugated estrogens (0.05 to 0.1 mg/kg slowly IV) can be given.
- If there is straining caused by catheterization of the bladder or cystitis, phenazopyridine can be administered.

Obstruction of the Lower Urinary Tract

Clinical Signs

- Hematuria, pollakiuria (frequent urination), dysuria (painful or difficult urination), and tenesmus (ineffectual and painful straining in urinating) are common.
- Dribbling of small amounts of urine and signs of colic, agitation, and sweating also occur.
- Stranguria (slow and painful discharge of urine) is most commonly a result of lower urinary tract obstruction and may also be caused by acute lower urinary tract infections or neurologic disorders, such as herpes myelitis.

General Information

- Obstruction is usually caused by urethral calculi or calculi at the trigone of the bladder that prevent normal urine voiding.
- Obstruction is rarely caused by blood clots.

- Urethral obstruction is more common in males and rarely occurs in individuals <1 year.
- Urethral obstruction can be caused by severe preputial trauma or cellulitis.

Diagnosis

- Rectal examination:
  - The bladder is enlarged and tense (patients with abdominal or intestinal pain also may have bladder distention but the bladder is not tense).
  - Cystic calculi can generally be palpated during rectal examination and/or be seen during rectal ultrasound examination (7.5-MHz rectal probe).
  - *Practice Tip: Most cystic calculi are easily felt with only the hand and wrist in the rectum.*
  - In males, urethral calculi are frequently palpated percutaneously a few inches below the anus in the perineum.
  - In males, the urethra seems painful to palpation, and pulsations or swelling of the urethra is detected.
  - Passing a urethral catheter (stallion catheter) after tranquilization is helpful, but it may be difficult to transverse the urethral sphincter in some normal horses, which should not be confused with obstruction.
  - Ultrasonography of the perineal region and urethra with a 7.5-MHz scanner can depict calculi and urethral swelling.
  - Urethral endoscopy can be used, although it generally is not necessary.

Laboratory Findings

- Unless bladder rupture is suspected (see the next section below), laboratory tests are unnecessary.

>> WHAT TO DO

Obstruction of Lower Urinary Tract

- Surgical removal of the urethral or bladder stone: In mares with bladder stone, removal can often be performed manually with epidural (lidocaine and xylazine) anesthesia, a small hand, and patience. Many mares with calculi, and all males with calculi, need to be referred for emergency surgery.
- In some cases of urethral calculi in males, the stone can be accidentally forced back into the bladder during urethral catheterization.
- Follow-up examination of the urinary tract is important to determine:
  - Bladder function (via rectal examination)
  - Presence of other stones (via ultrasound examination of the entire urinary tract)
  - Urinary tract infection (via culture and urinalysis)
  - Renal function (via measurement of serum creatinine)
- Some horses with cystic calculi in the trigone area develop bladder scarring in this area leading to chronic partial obstruction of both ureters and chronic renal failure.

Ruptured Bladder

- Most cases of ruptured bladder occur in young male foals at birth and signs are observed within the first few days of

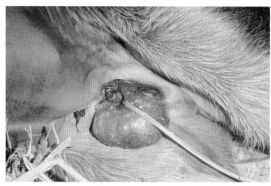

Figure 26-3 Subcutaneous and preputial edema caused by urachal leakage of urine into the subcutaneous space.

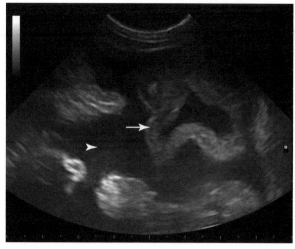

Figure 26-4 Ultrasound photo of uroperitoneum in a foal (*arrow,* bladder; *arrowhead,* uroperitoneum). (Courtesy Nora Grenager, VMD).

life (average, 4 days), although it can occur in older sick foals and also in adults as a result of urinary calculi, or in foaling mares.

- Rupture of the bladder or urachus, causing uroperitoneum, occurs in neonatal or older foals with:
  - Urachal abscess
  - Ischemia of the apex of the bladder
  - Recumbent foals (e.g., premature or septic foals)
  - Botulism
  - Central nervous system (CNS) disturbances
  - Abdominal trauma
- If the urachus ruptures outside the abdominal cavity and in the subcutaneous space, a large accumulation of urine causes severe stranguria, subcutaneous swelling, colic, and distress (Fig. 26-3). Differentiate the subcutaneous swelling from hematoma or septic cellulitis by means of ultrasound aspiration with cytologic examination of the edema fluid. If urine is confirmed and the swelling continues to enlarge, prompt surgical removal of the urachus is required.
- Some newborn foals apparently have some leakage of urine subcutaneously without urachal rupture, causing stranguria and noticeable swelling of the prepuce. Unless the swelling is enlarging, these can be treated medically with:
  - Sedation, flunixin meglumine 0.5 mg/kg, 1 or 2 treatments
  - Sedation, diazepam 0.1 mg/kg IV
  - Appropriate antiulcer medication
  - Local cold packing of the area
  - Systemic antibiotics
  - If the prepuce is swollen, an indwelling Cook male urinary catheter[5] may be needed.

Ruptured Bladder in Foals

Clinical Signs

- Ruptured bladder is usually diagnosed within the first 2 to 3 days of life in otherwise healthy foals and is most common in males. In these cases, the rupture most likely occurs during delivery. The most common site of bladder rupture in foals is the dorsal or dorsocranial region. Urachal rupture occurs within the peritoneal cavity or subcutaneously as described previously.

- Rupture may also occur anytime during the first 2 weeks in septic and specifically recumbent foals. Recumbent neonatal foals, especially those receiving intravenous fluids, should have an indwelling urinary catheter placed to monitor urine output and prevent bladder rupture. Catheterization of fillies is difficult; however, it is most easily achieved with a Cook 8F or 10F catheter,[5] or a 12F 55-cm Foley catheter.[6]
- In recumbent foals, rupture of the urachus may also occur.
- There is no sex predilection in this group of sick, recumbent foals.
- Stranguria, dysuria, depression, and bilaterally symmetric ventral abdominal distention are the most common signs in 1- to 4-day-old foals with ruptured bladder that occurs at birth.
- Stranguria and dysuria are often misinterpreted as rectal tenesmus. With tenesmus, the pelvic limbs are positioned farther under the body than in stranguria or dysuria. After a foal with ruptured bladder has received a couple of enemas for the mistaken diagnosis of meconium impaction, the foal may develop a straining response to the rectal irritation rather than the uroperitoneal irritation.

Diagnosis

- History: generally occurs in young males but can occur in females
- Clinical signs: depression, stranguria, abdominal distention (ventral and symmetric)
- Ultrasound examination of the abdomen (Fig 26-4): uroperitoneum in foals creates hypoechoic fluid, accentuates small intestine imaging, and with a ruptured bladder often an "inverted bladder" is seen.
- Laboratory findings: hyponatremia, hypochloremia, hyperkalemia, and azotemia. ***Practice Tip:*** *These classic*

---

[5]Cook Australia, Queensland, Australia.
[6]MILA International, Inc. 12 Price Avenue, Erlanger, KY, 41018.

laboratory abnormalities are often not as pronounced in sick neonatal foals on IV fluids.

- The ratio of peritoneal fluid creatinine concentration to serum creatinine concentration >2:1 confirms the diagnosis of uroperitoneum. With large amounts of peritoneal fluid, as in uroperitoneum, it is preferable to perform abdominocentesis with an 18-gauge needle. A teat cannula creates a large defect in the abdominal wall, and if surgery is not performed within a few hours, urine leaks through the abdominal wall defect into the subcutaneous tissues. The history, clinical, ultrasound, and serum laboratory findings are so characteristic that peritoneal fluid evaluation generally is not necessary. Accuracy of peritoneal fluid creatinine determinations using point of care equipment such as I-Stat is unproven; it is reported to be reliable.

●❱ WHAT TO DO

Ruptured Bladder

- Begin to correct acid-base and electrolyte abnormalities before surgery.
- Administer 0.9% saline solution with 5% to 10% glucose IV.
- Avoid exogenous insulin therapy (to drive potassium into cells) for hyperkalemia. If significant electrocardiographic (ECG) abnormalities (QRS complexes without P waves) are recognized, administer 50 mL of 50% dextrose with 0.5 g calcium borogluconate (22 mL of 23% calcium borogluconate) to increase the endogenous insulin level and protect the myocardium respectively. Another option for decreasing plasma potassium that many prefer is to give 1 mEq/kg of sodium bicarbonate intravenously.
- If severe hyperkalemia with associated ECG abnormalities and significant abdominal distention are present, remove abdominal fluid before general anesthesia. Make sure the foal is on IV fluids when this is performed to decrease the risk of systemic hypovolemia and hypotension. If drainage is performed several hours before surgery, subcutaneous leakage of abdominal fluid and prolapse of omentum occurs if the intraperitoneal catheter is removed. If omental prolapse occurs, simply disinfect the area and resect the omentum flush with the skin and apply an abdominal bandage. If the peritoneal catheter is left in the abdomen, frequent walking of the foal may improve drainage because the omentum has a tendency to plug the catheter openings.

Surgery

- Surgery is usually successful if performed within the first 5 days of life. Ruptured bladder is not a surgical emergency if electrolyte abnormalities are corrected, and in some cases, such as severe distention or hyperkalemia, the abdominal fluid can be drained before surgery. Occasionally, there is translocation of a portion of the abdominal fluid into the thoracic cavity compromising respiratory function. Drainage of the abdominal fluid allows resolution of the thoracic effusion.
- Induction of general anesthesia is best performed by mask induction using isoflurane, sevoflurane, or desflurane (expensive) as agents of choice.
- A two-layer surgical closure of the bladder tear after debridement of the torn edges is recommended.

- A second procedure is sometimes, albeit rarely, needed if urine continues to leak from the bladder.
  - It is often advantageous to place an indwelling urethral catheter at surgery for the first 24 to 48 hours postoperatively, particularly in male foals that may have had chronic bladder distention before rupture because of other problems (maladjustment syndrome, prematurity, and sepsis). If straining is a problem following surgery or in catheterized foals, phenazopyridine (4 to 10 mg/kg PO q12h) should be administered.

Ruptured Bladder In Older Nursing Foals

- Ruptured bladder rarely occurs without warning in 4- to 10-week-old foals. The apex of the bladder is necrotic, resulting in rupture.
- Affected foals are depressed, have abdominal distention, and may or may not have the classic electrolyte abnormalities of *hyponatremia, hypochloremia, and hyperkalemia* that occur in younger individuals.
- Diagnosis is confirmed with ultrasound examination and comparison of urine to blood creatinine concentrations.
- Treatment is similar to that of younger patients, except the urachus and apex of the bladder are removed.
- Ruptured bladder may also occasionally occur in growing foals that have severe external trauma.

Ruptured Bladder in Adults

- Rupture is unusual in the adult from causes other than urethral calculi or occasionally after foaling in mares.
- Rupture can occur from abdominal trauma or in recumbent males.

Clinical Signs

- Ruptured bladder is difficult to diagnose from clinical signs alone since the abdominal distention commonly seen in foals may not be apparent. Depression and anorexia 2 days after rupture may be the only signs seen. Stranguria may be present.

Diagnosis

- Peripheral blood sample:
  - Azotemia
  - Hyponatremia
  - Hypochloremia
- Abdominal ultrasonography: large volume of slightly echogenic fluid (more echogenic in adults than in foals)
- Abdominocentesis:
  - Peritoneal fluid creatinine: plasma creatinine ratio >2:1
  - Identification of calcium carbonate crystals. **Practice Tip:** *This is unique to the adult horse and is not seen in foals with uroperitoneum.*
- Endoscopy of the bladder can be used to determine the location and extent of the tear. The endoscope should be properly disinfected and the urethral opening or vaginal area appropriately cleaned before the procedure! Antibiotics should be administered if endoscopy is performed.

●❯ WHAT TO DO

Ruptured Bladder in Adults

- Surgical repair: Not always needed immediately but generally is recommended.
  - Small dorsal tears may not require surgery.
- Drainage of peritoneal fluid: Use an indwelling mushroom catheter.
- If chronic distention of the bladder preceded the rupture (e.g., urethral calculi), a urinary catheter should be left in place after surgical repair and treatment with bethanechol 0.25 mg/kg SQ q8h may be required.

Rule-Outs for Stranguria in Foals

- Ruptured bladder: Older foals with bladder apex necrosis may not have stranguria
- Meconium impaction. **_Practice Tip:_** *Tenesmus can look like stranguria or it can be the result of an irritating treatment for suspected meconium impaction.*
- Hematoma in bladder seen on ultrasound
- Ruptured urachus
- Neonatal encephalopathy (hypoxic-ischemic encephalopathy/*dummy bladder*):
  - This appears to be a variant of the neonatal encephalopathy syndrome that interferes with normal micturition and causes a persistently distended bladder with severe straining.
  - Affected foals, usually males, should have an indwelling catheter placed in the bladder and be treated for neonatal encephalopathy in addition to antimicrobials.
  - Most foals recover within a few days.
  - Some show no others signs of neonatal encephalopathy.
  - Some have electrolyte abnormalities suggestive of uroperitoneum but *no* rupture.
  - Phenazopyridine should be administered.
- Urachal abscess in 2- to 6-month-old foals
- Ureteral tear occurs in newborn foals and may be bilateral. The urine may accumulate in the retroperitoneal space or in the abdomen.

Intraperitoneal Drain Placement for Continuous Urine Removal

- Place the catheter at the ventral-most aspect of the abdomen, 1 cm off midline (preferably to the right to avoid the spleen).
- Clip and aseptically prepare the catheter site after local anesthesia is administered.
- Make a stab incision with a #20 blade through the skin and the external sheath of the rectus abdominis muscle
- Introduce a 4-inch (10-cm) cannula, if needed, to confirm the presence of fluid.
- Use a bitch catheter to help direct the mushroom catheter in the opening made by the cannula. Alternatively, a 16F to 20F thoracic catheter may be positioned in the abdomen to allow fluid removal.
- Suture the skin around the mushroom catheter after removing the bitch catheter. Apply antiseptic cream and keep the catheter end clean when it is not draining; use a small syringe to prevent ascending contamination or allow continual drainage with an open or cut condom taped to the end of the catheter.
- Intravenous fluids: administer polyionic fluids at maintenance or *slightly* higher rate when needed.
- Antimicrobial therapy: Trimethoprim-sulfamethoxazole, 20 mg/kg PO q12 to 24h, or for adults, enrofloxacin, 5 mg/kg IV q24h or 7.5 mg/kg PO q24h, and metronidazole, 15 to 25 mg/kg PO q8h, should be added if endoscopy or catheterization is performed.

Prolapse of the Bladder

- Prolapse of the bladder can occur as eversion of the bladder or in association with a prolapsed or torn vagina.
- Eversion of the bladder through the urethra occurs in females with severe straining, e.g., with a dystocia.
- The mucosal surface of the bladder is obvious, and the ureteral opening may be seen. The ureters may still be patent.
- Eversion of the bladder from the umbilicus is reported and surgically repaired.

●❯ WHAT TO DO

Prolapse of the Bladder

- Perform epidural anesthesia. For a 450-kg mare, administer 5 to 7 mL of 2% lidocaine and/or 80 mg of xylazine diluted with 8 mL of sterile saline using an 18-gauge, 1½-inch (3.8-cm) needle (see Caudal Epidural Catheterization, p. 8). The xylazine may also be mixed in the lidocaine without using saline.
- Clean the bladder with sterile saline solution, and examine surrounding tissue to rule out intestinal involvement in the herniated bladder. If a part of the bladder is necrotic, debride and suture it. Make sure to avoid the ureteral openings.
- Use gentle, consistent pressure on the bladder to return the everted bladder to the abdomen with or without sphincterotomy. This is generally difficult because of bladder swelling; general anesthesia and abdominal laparotomy may be required.
- If necessary, refer the horse for laparotomy and sphincterotomy to return the bladder to its normal position.
  - Use the ligaments of the bladder as a guide for inverting the bladder through the urethra.
  - Infuse 1 L of warm saline solution into the bladder to ensure repositioning and to check for tears.
  - Leave a Foley catheter with the cuff inflated with saline solution in the bladder for 24 hours, and administer antibiotics prophylactically.
- To replace a bladder that has prolapsed through a vaginal tear, it may be necessary to remove the urine by aspirating before the bladder is returned.

Ruptured Ureter(s)

- Rupture of one or both ureters may uncommonly occur in newborn foals and even more uncommonly in postfoaling mares.
- In foals (males and females), signs may not be seen for 3 to 5 days.

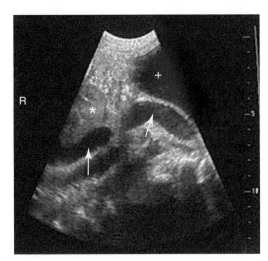

Figure 26-5 Ultrasound photo of dilated ureter *(arrows)*, kidney *(*)*, and bladder *(+)* in a 4-day-old foal with hydroureters and hyponatremic encephalopathy. (Photo courtesy of F.T. Bain.)

- Serum creatinine is elevated, and electrolyte abnormalities, similar to those seen with a ruptured bladder, may occur.
- Ultrasound examination of the abdomen, including the retroperitoneal space, and radiographic contrast studies may be needed to confirm the diagnosis.
- Surgical repair with temporary placement of ureteral catheter(s) is the treatment of choice in most cases.

Hydroureters in Foals
- Foals affected by hydroureter most often are first examined at 3 to 7 days for signs of acute cerebral dysfunction (seizure, head pressing, obtunded mentation).
- The CNS signs are a result of the hyponatremia caused by:
  - Insufficient ureteral emptying
  - Hydronephrosis
  - Presumed tubular dysfunction
  - The foals are also hypochloremic and azotemic.
  - Ultrasound examination reveals distended ureters (almost always bilateral) (Fig. 26-5).
  - Recumbent foals receiving large-volume IV fluids normally have some ureteral distention.
- The CNS signs usually resolve with *gradual* sodium replacement (see treatment for hyponatremia, Chapter 22, p. 373).
- Unfortunately, the ureteral dysfunction seems to be permanent in most foals.
- Surgical transpostion of the ureters to another location in the bladder may be attempted; low-dose alpha-agonist treatment that enhances ureteral motility can also be tried.
- Foals, especially recumbent foals, receiving intravenous fluids frequently have the ultrasound appearance of ureteral and renal pelvis distention; this does not appear to cause a significant problem.

Acute Urinary Incontinence in Mares Associated with Foaling
- Acute urinary incontinence can be caused by damage to the bladder muscle or, more commonly, damage to the urethral sphincter during foaling.

●》 WHAT TO DO

Acute Urinary Incontinence
- If the urethral sphincter is lacerated, suture it after a Foley catheter is placed in the bladder.
- If the sphincter is injured but not lacerated, treatment includes the following:
  - Phenylpropanolamine, 1 to 2 mg/kg PO q12h, to improve sphincter tone if the mare is dribbling urine and the bladder is small
  - Systemic antimicrobials, such as trimethoprim-sulfamethoxazole
- If the bladder wall (detrusor muscle) is damaged and the bladder is enlarged with no physical obstruction of the urethra:
  - Bethanechol, 0.03 to 0.05 mg/kg SQ q8h or 0.16 mg/kg PO q8h, to enhance detrusor activity
  - Phenoxybenzamine, 0.4 mg/kg PO q6h, to relax the sphincter; unfortunately this drug is expensive. Low doses of acepromazine, 0.02 mg/kg q6h IV or IM, can be used.
  - Place an indwelling urinary catheter
  - Some affected mares may have fever and peritonitis

Acute-Onset Polyuria/Polydipsia
- Acute-onset polyuria/polydipsia may occur as a result of:
  - Acute renal failure
  - Other nephrogenic causes including drug administration and nephrogenic diabetes insipidus
  - Psychogenic causes following management, feed, or temperature changes
  - Central diabetes insipidus (i.e., following acute or chronic brain/brainstem disease)
- Central and, less commonly, nephrogenic diabetes insipidus can be an emergency because severe hypernatremia may develop in only a few hours if water consumption is inadequate.

●》 WHAT TO DO

Acute-Onset Polyuria and Polydipsia Not Caused by Renal Failure
- Rehydrate with one-half to normal sodium-containing fluids and limited free water if there is severe hyponatremia until the serum sodium is normal.
- Administer antidiuretic hormone (ADH) (vasopressin) 0.25 U/kg IM or SQ.

References
References can be found on the companion website at www.equine-emergencies.com.

CHAPTER 27

Monitoring the Pregnant Mare

Tamara Dobbie

- Health problems in a pregnant mare at any time in gestation can adversely affect the pregnancy.
- Minor illnesses that last for short periods are less troublesome than those conditions that occur later in gestation and/or persist for longer periods.
- Some disorders that affect late gestation mares may severely compromise:
  - Uterus
  - Placenta
  - Fetus
  - Combination of ALL three
- Pregnancies with compromise of the above organs and tissues are at higher risk of loss or poor neonatal survival.
- High-risk pregnancies can be broken down into two categories:
  - Past or recurrent problems during pregnancy
  - Newly diagnosed conditions that increase the risk of pregnancy loss
- The following are some of the conditions that define a pregnancy as "high risk":
  - Past or recurrent problems:
    - Placentitis
    - Premature placental separation (red bag delivery)
    - Dystocia
    - Late-term abortion
    - Premature foals
    - Peripartum hemorrhage
  - Newly diagnosed conditions:
    - Uterine torsion
    - Hydrops allantois or amnion
    - Endotoxemia
    - Gastrointestinal colic
    - Colitis
    - Laminitis
    - Abdominal wall hernia
    - Prepubic tendon rupture
    - Twins
    - Placentitis
- It is critically important to accurately evaluate high risk pregnancies in order to establish a prognosis and formulate a treatment plan.
- Fetoplacental well-being is most accurately assessed ultrasonographically.
- Several hormone profiles are available that assess fetoplacental well-being; each has its own merits and pitfalls.
- High-risk mares need to be monitored closely for signs of foaling and have trained personnel in attendance when foaling occurs.
- A plan should be in place for all high-risk mares so that decisions can be made quickly, especially in the event of a complication.

Ultrasonography

- Ultrasonographic evaluation of the fetus and placenta is a valuable method of assessing fetoplacental well-being in the high-risk mare.
- Transabdominal and transrectal examinations are performed in the initial examination of the high-risk mare and then are repeated weekly, or as deemed necessary, to continue monitoring the health of the fetus and placenta.

●》 WHAT TO DO

Fetal Evaluation

- Any clinical problem that affects the health of the pregnant mare can adversely affect the developing fetus.
- Monitoring the fetus is vitally important in the high-risk mare.
- ***Practice Tip:*** *The fetus can be imaged transabdominally after 70 days of gestation; however, detailed assessment is not possible until 4 months of pregnancy.*
- The fetus can be viewed transabdominally using a 3.5 to 5 MHz probe early in pregnancy and a 2 to 2.5 MHz probe later in gestation or for heavier horse breeds.
- The mare's entire ventral abdomen needs to be scanned (udder to xiphoid and laterally).

- It is often helpful to divide the ventral abdomen into 4 quadrants—right cranial, right caudal, left cranial, left caudal—to ensure all parts of the uterus are evaluated.
- Initially it is important to determine fetal numbers and fetal orientation; there should be one fetus in the uterus.
  - If twins are identified, reduction to a singleton is possible before 150 days of gestation. The orientation of the fetus varies depending on the stage of pregnancy; however, after 9 months of gestation, the fetus should be in an anterior longitudinal, dorsopubic orientation.
- Fetal heart rate and rhythm and breathing movements are important indicators of fetal well-being.
- Fetal heart rate and rhythm can be determined using M-mode ultrasonography or by using a stopwatch and counting beats in B-mode ultrasonography.
  - It is important to take several measurements at rest and following periods of activity.
  - Fetal heart rates correlate with the age of the fetus and fetal activity.
  - The resting fetal heart rate decreases with increasing gestational age.
  - Accelerations in heart rate are expected with fetal activity and are a sign of fetal well-being in the equine fetus.
  - *Practice Tip: During the last weeks of pregnancy, the equine fetus usually has a baseline heart rate between 60 to 75 beats/min, a low heart rate range of 40 to 75 beats/min, and a high heart rate range of 83 to 250 beats/min.*
  - *Practice Tip: Low fetal heart rates and those that lack heart rate variation may indicate fetal hypoxia. Prolonged low heart rates are abnormal and may indicate impending death.*
  - Sustained elevated heart rates are equally concerning and generally indicate fetal distress.
  - *Practice Tip: Transient low (<60 beats/min) or high(>120 beats/min) fetal heart rates are common. If fetal heart rates are consistently too low or high (<60 beats/min or >120 beats/min) during the observational period, perform another ultrasound examination within 24 hours.*
  - The fetus is monitored continually throughout the ultrasound examination for breathing, body movements, and fetal tone.
  - Breathing movements may be difficult to see; however, the equine fetus should move several times throughout the examination.
  - A fetus is usually quiet for less than 10 minutes in late gestation although periods of 30 to 60 minutes are reported.
  - A lack of movement and absence of fetal tone are indicators of fetal distress and potentially poor outcome.
- *Practice Tip: The size of the fetus is determined from the aortic and thoracic measurements.*
  - The diameter of the aorta is measured in long axis as close to the heart as possible.
  - The thoracic diameter is measured from the fetal spine to the sternum in the caudal thorax.
  - Normal indices for aortic and thoracic diameter indicate normal fetal size for gestational age and a healthy uterine environment.
  - Fetuses larger than expected for gestational age may be at risk for dystocia. The normal fetal and maternal parameters in late gestation are in Table 27-1.

Table 27-1   Normal Fetal and Maternal Measurements in Late Gestation

Fetal and Maternal Measurement	Mean +/− SD	Range
Fetal Heart Rate (HR)		
Low HR <330 days (beats/min)	70.1 +/− 6.8	61-85
Low HR >329 days (beats/min)	66.4 +/− 8.7	52-81
High HR (beats/min)	92.9 +/− 11.0	56-118
HR range (beats/min)	16.7 +/− 10.0	1-40
Mean HR (beats/min)	74.6 +/− 7.4	53.8-87.8
Aortic Diameter		
Ascending aorta (mm)	22.8 +/− 2.2	18-27
Thoracic Width		
At diaphragm (cm)	18.4 +/− 1.2	16.2-21.3
Fetal Breathing		
Presence and rhythm	Present and rhythmic	
Fetal Activity*		
(0-3)	1.6 +/− 0.6	1-3
FETAL TONE		
Presence	Present	
Fetal Fluids		
Allantoic Fluid		
Maximum depth (cm)	13.4 +/− 4.4	5.5-22.7
Quality (0-3)	1.41 +/− 0.7	0-3
Amniotic Fluid		
Maximum depth (cm)	7.9 +/− 3.5	2-14.3
Quality (0-3)	1.6 +/− 0.6	1-3
Uteroplacental Thickness		
Maximal thickness (mm)	11.5 +/− 2.4	6-16
Minimal thickness (mm)	7.1 +/− 1.6	4-11
Uteroplacental Contact		
Vessels	Small uterine and placental vessels imaged	
Continuity	Rare small areas of discontinuity	

SD, Standard deviation.
From Reef VB: *Equine diagnostic ultrasound*, Philadelphia, 1998, WB Saunders, p. 431.
*See page 500 for description of fetal activity and fetal fluid scale.

●> WHAT TO DO

Placental Evaluation

- The health of the placenta is most accurately assessed using ultrasonography.
- The placenta of the high-risk mare should be evaluated both transrectally and transabdominally.

Transrectal Placental Evaluation

- Transrectal ultrasonography is performed using a 5 to 7.5 MHz linear array transducer.

Evaluation of Uteroplacental Unit

- ***Practice Tip:*** *The combined thickness of the uterus and placenta (CTUP) is an important measurement that needs to be assessed in all high-risk mares.*
- The position for the measurement is slightly lateral of midline and approximately 5 to 7 cm cranioventral to the cervical star. The tissue dorsal to the uterine blood vessel in longitudinal section is the uteroplacental unit (Fig. 27-1); several measurements should be taken and then averaged. ***Important:*** It is key to accurate CTUP evaluation not to include the amnion in the measurement because this falsely increases thickness; the normal values for the combined thickness of the uterus and placenta during gestation are in Table 27-2.
- Because the CTUP is generally thicker dorsally than ventrally, perform the measurement in the cranioventral location. Caution is recommended when interpreting CTUP values in the high-risk mare.
- Often the position of the fetus in the maternal pelvis or lack thereof can alter the measurements.

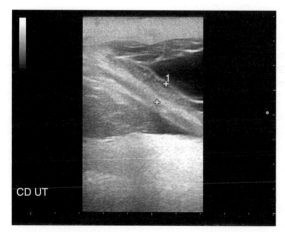

CD UT

Figure 27-1   Transrectal sonogram from a late-gestation pregnant mare. Note the location for obtaining the measurement of the combined thickness of the uterus and placenta *(plus signs)*.

Table 27-2	Normal Values for the Combined Thickness of the Uterus and the Placenta (CTUP) at Various Stages of Gestation

Days of Gestation	Normal CTUP (mm)
<270	7
271-300	8
301-330	10
>330	12

- Additionally, the cervical pole can become edematous during the last month of gestation. ***Practice Tip:*** *For these reasons, a diagnosis of placentitis is rarely made based only on an increased CTUP; the diagnosis is contingent on a combination of consistently increased CTUP values for the stage of gestation together with the presence of other clinical signs (i.e., vulvar discharge, premature udder development).*
- The fetal orbit is often imaged during a transrectal examination.
- ***Practice Tip:*** *Identification of the fetal orbit after 9 months of gestation signifies the fetus is in the correct presentation.*
- Orbital dimensions provide a rough estimate of fetal growth.
- The fetal fluids should be evaluated during transrectal examination.
  - Allantoic fluid is generally anechoic with some echogenic particles, whereas amniotic fluid tends to be slightly more hyperechoic.
  - Any significant increase in echogenicity in either chamber—allantoic and amniotic—may indicate placental infection or fetal stress.
- When palpating the late-gestation, high-risk mare per rectum, the uterus should have adequate tone and the fetus should be palpable.
- ***Practice Tip:*** *If the examination reveals a uterus that bulges above the brim of the pelvis and a fetus that is* not *palpable or seen ultrasonographically, then hydrops allantois or hydrops amnion should be suspected.*
- When abnormalities of the fetal fluids are suspected on transrectal ultrasonographic evaluation, a follow-up transabdominal evaluation is strongly recommended.
- The transrectal window, although important, covers a relatively small area of the entire fetoplacental unit and therefore can be prone to isolated atypical measurements.
- The larger window visualized transabdominally is often necessary to confirm difficult and somewhat subjective diagnoses like hydrops.

Transabdominal Placental Evaluation

- Transabdominal ultrasonography of the uteroplacental unit is best performed using a 10-MHz microconvex linear array transducer.
- The uteroplacental unit is comprised of two layers: the uterus and chorioallantois.
  - The outer layer, the uterus, is slightly more echogenic than the inner layer, the chorioallantois, which tends to be more hypoechoic.
- Normally the uteroplacental unit measures 1.15 +/− 0.24 to 1.38 +/− 0.23 cm in the pregnant horn during late gestation.
- ***Practice Tip:*** *Increased thickness of the uteroplacental unit >2 cm in the fetal horn is abnormal and suggestive of placentitis (Fig. 27-2) or another placental problem (i.e., placental edema, premature placental separation) and is generally associated with an unfavorable outcome.*
  - Ultrasonographically, premature placental separation (Fig. 27-3) and placentitis creates a ribbon candy appearance of the uteroplacental unit in the fetal horn.
  - It is important to recognize these conditions and monitor them carefully.
  - If there are large areas where the placenta does not contact the uterus, the outcome is generally unfavorable.
- The significance of a uteroplacental unit that is too thin (<0.7 cm) is unclear.

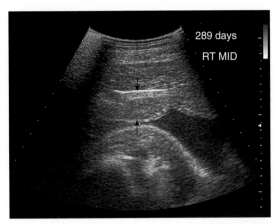

Figure 27-2   Transabdominal sonogram from a late-gestation mare with placentitis. Note the increased thickness of the uterus and placenta *(arrows)*.

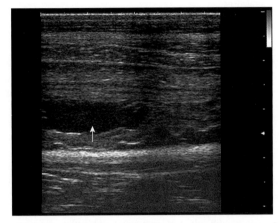

Figure 27-3   Transabdominal sonogram from a mare with premature placental separation. Note the area of placental detachment from the uterus *(arrow)*.

- Foals born from these pregnancies are sometimes abnormal at birth. Fluid accumulation between the chorioallantois and the uterus can also occur and is abnormal.
- Allantoic and amniotic fluids are assessed during the examination.
- Fluid compartments are best evaluated using an ultrasound probe with deeper penetration (2 to 3.5 MHz).
- The maximal fetal fluid depths for both allantoic and amniotic fluids are measured in all four quadrants—right cranial, right caudal, left cranial, and left caudal—perpendicular to the uteroplacental surface.
- *Practice Tip: The amount of fetal fluid present is an indicator of fetal and maternal well-being.*
- **Important:** Decreased fetal fluids (maximum amniotic fluid depth <0.8 cm and maximum allantoic fluid depth <4.7 cm) are considered abnormal and are indicative of fetal stress and an unfavorable outcome. Conversely, excessive fetal fluids (amniotic fluid depth >14.9 cm and allantoic fluid depth >22.1 cm) are also abnormal and indicative of hydrops allantois or hydrops amnion.
- The character of the fetal fluids are graded on a scale from 0 to 3; 0 = anechoic fluid with no particles, 3 = echogenic fluid with many particles.
- Fetal fluids are normally anechoic until late gestation.
  - Echogenic particles in the fetal fluids increase as the pregnancy progresses.
  - The presence of echogenic particles in the fetal fluids in early gestation is abnormal.
  - Allantoic fluid generally contains more echogenic particles than amniotic fluid.
  - Transporting the pregnant mare may mix the particulate debris in the allantois and increase the echogenicity of the fluid.
  - The amniotic fluid often appears more echogenic than the allantoic fluid because fetal activity mixes the particulate debris in the amniotic compartment.
  - *Practice Tip: Significant increases in the echogenicity of fetal fluids in early or late gestation are indicative of fetal distress.*
- Normal placental parameters for the late-gestation mare are in Table 27-1.

◉❯ WHAT TO DO

Hormone Profiles for Assessing and Monitoring Fetoplacental Well-being

- Hormone profiles can be used in conjunction with ultrasonography to evaluate and monitor fetoplacental well-being in the high-risk mare. Each profile has its own merits and pitfalls, which limit the practicality and use of them.

Progestins

- Progesterone and its related progestins are required to maintain pregnancy in the mare.
- During the first trimester, progesterone is produced by the primary and accessory corpora luteii (CL) of the ovaries.
- Following the regression of the CL and the decline of the ovarian progesterone, the fetoplacental unit becomes the primary source of progestins for the remainder of the pregnancy.
- Maternal progestins rise slowly over the second and third trimesters; during the last 2 to 3 weeks of pregnancy, progestin levels rise rapidly, peak 2 to 3 days before parturition, and then dramatically decline the last day, or often hours, before delivery.
- *Practice Tip: Fetal adrenal glands are involved in the production of progestins and therefore measurement of maternal progestins indirectly assesses fetal stress.*

- There is no commercial radioimmunoassay or enzyme-linked immunosorbent assay (ELISA) that measure progestins specifically. The commercial assays available for measuring progesterone cross-react with one or more of the progestins in the mare's plasma in late gestation and can be used for measuring progestin levels.
- Measurement of maternal plasma progestins in late gestation are useful for:
  - Monitoring placental function and fetal health
  - Identifying impending abortion
  - Anticipating premature delivery and fetal outcome
- Three abnormal progestin profiles can be observed in the late-gestation mare.
  - The *first* is the rapid fall of progestin levels associated with acute conditions (i.e., colic, uterine torsion, maternal stress) where the fetus is dead or soon to be.
  - The *second* is the accelerated rise in progestins weeks before delivery. This rise is generally associated with placental pathology (i.e., placentitis) and often results in the birth of a live foal, even those born before the anticipated birth date. This occurs because of the activation of the fetal hypothalamo-pituitary-adrenal axis stimulates precocious fetal maturation.

- The *third* involves a failure of the progestins to peak before parturition; this pattern is found almost exclusively in mares suffering from fescue toxicosis.
- Progestin levels in late-gestation mares remain constant between 2 and 12 ng/mL until the last 3 weeks of pregnancy, at which time the levels rise dramatically.
- When monitoring the high-risk mare, several blood samples are needed to determine whether there is an increasing or decreasing trend in the progestin profile.
- Some advocate 3 samples a day, while others recommend sampling every 2 to 3 days until a total of 3 samples are collected; once the initial trend has been identified, regular sampling should continue to monitor fetoplacental health.
- **Practice Tip:** *The initial profile helps formulate a prognosis and direct therapy.*
  - Progestin levels that are elevated (>50% of the laboratory high normal) and/or continue to increase are indicative of ongoing fetal stress (i.e., placentitis) and should be treated appropriately and monitored carefully.
  - Progestin levels that are decreased (<50% of the laboratory low normal) and/or continue to decline are indicative of a dead or severely compromised fetus.
- **Important:** After 305 days of gestation, progestin concentrations should be interpreted with caution because levels begin to rise as part of the normal sequence of events before parturition.

Estrogens
- There are four estrogens produced by the pregnant mare:
  - Estrone
  - Estradiol 17-beta
  - Equilin
  - Equilenin
- Estrogens, like progestogens, are produced by the fetoplacental unit and therefore can provide an assessment of fetal viability and placental health.

- Total estrogen concentrations decline slowly over the last several months of pregnancy and reach basal levels after delivery.
- Estrone sulfate concentrations accurately determine pregnancy and fetal viability in early gestation (after 60 days); however, in late gestation, estrone sulfate concentrations alone are *not* an accurate indicator of fetal well-being.
- A single plasma sample measuring total estrogens, estradiol 17-beta and its metabolites, can be used to monitor fetal health in mid to late gestation.
- **Practice Tip:** *Between 150 to 280 days of gestation, total estrogen concentrations should be >1000 ng/mL.*
  - Concentrations <500 ng/mL are associated with a dead or severely compromised fetus.
  - Concentrations <1000 ng/mL are abnormal and associated with fetal stress and compromise.

Relaxin
- Relaxin is produced by the mare's placenta.
- Relaxin can be detected after 80 days of gestation; concentrations peak during midgestation and then remain elevated until parturition, after which time they drop rapidly.
- **Practice Tip:** *Because relaxin is produced by the placenta, it has the potential to be a marker for monitoring placental health and identifying mares at risk for placental dysfunction.*
- Mares with a variety of placental disorders including placentitis, premature placental separation, and hydrops have demonstrated decreased relaxin concentrations.
- Unfortunately, there is no commercial assay currently available for measuring relaxin levels in the mare.
- The assay has also failed to show reliable correlation between the clinical response to treatment of affected pregnancies and improved relaxin concentrations, thereby limiting its usefulness.

●❯ WHAT TO DO

Monitoring the Mare for Readiness of Foaling
- High-risk mares need to be monitored carefully for foaling to ensure someone trained and knowledgeable is in attendance when foaling occurs.
- Milk electrolytes and careful observation of the external physical signs are techniques of determining impending parturition in the mare.
- Unfortunately, neither method is very accurate in the high-risk pregnant mare.

Milk Electrolytes
- In the normal late-gestation mare, monitoring mammary electrolytes (calcium, potassium, and sodium) can provide useful information about impending parturition and fetal readiness for birth.
- **Practice Tip:** *Typically, mammary calcium concentrations reach peak levels of 400 ppm (equivalent to 40 mg/dL or 10 nmol/L) or greater the day of, or a few days before, foaling.*
- Potassium and sodium concentrations also invert in the last few days before foaling with potassium concentrations greater than sodium concentrations.
- Once these changes are seen, the fetus is mature, foaling is generally imminent, and parturition can be induced should this be necessary.

- Mares with placental abnormalities, such as placentitis or twins, often have precocious udder development in addition to a premature rise in milk calcium concentrations.
  - It has also been suggested that an elevation in milk calcium concentrations before 310 days of gestation may be indicative of an abnormal pregnancy.
  - Therefore, mammary calcium concentrations are generally unreliable in high-risk mares and should *not* be used alone for determining impending parturition or predicting fetal maturity.

External Genitalia
- As parturition approaches, the external genitalia and musculature of the normal pregnant mare begin to change:
  - The sacrosciatic ligaments on either side of the mare's tail relax, causing the tail head to appear more prominent.
  - The vulva lengthens and softens and the mare's udder increases in size.
  - The teats become distended and eventually a small amount of waxy residue is visible on the end of each teat.
- Unfortunately, it is highly variable as to exactly when these changes occur in relation to foaling.
- In the high-risk pregnant mare, the physical changes indicative of parturition are even less reliable.

- Mares with placentitis and twins often have premature udder development and some mares with placentitis may lactate and/or "wax" for many weeks before foaling.
- Mares with ventral abdominal wall herniation or prepubic tendon rupture may have a significant amount of ventral edema that may complicate monitoring of udder development.
- Mares with hydrops are often placed in belly support wraps, which tends to create edema in the area of the udder, making mammary gland monitoring difficult.

Attended Foaling

- Attended foalings are important in all mares.
- *Practice Tip: Stage II labor is very short in the horse compared with our other domestic species and any complication that prolongs delivery or prevents progression of the delivery can result in severe and even fatal consequences for the mare, foal, or both.*
- The high-risk mare is more likely to:
  - Lose a pregnancy
  - Have a dystocia
  - Deliver a foal that is nonviable
- Mares need to be monitored carefully for the remainder of the pregnancy once they are identified as high-risk.

- With routine assessment of the fetus and placenta using ultrasonography and/or hormone profiles, it is possible to monitor the health and well-being of the pregnancy and determine whether there is imminent danger of pregnancy loss or fetal death.
- *Practice Tip: Mares close to foaling or those in danger of aborting should be checked every 15 to 20 minutes by a trained foaling attendant, or have video monitoring in place.*
- Other monitoring options include:
  - Halter monitors that activate alarms when the mare lies in lateral recumbency
  - Foalert[1] that is activated when the vulvar lips separate during labor
- Whatever system is used, a trained assistant needs to be in attendance when the mare begins to foal.
- If complications arise, a veterinarian should be contacted immediately.
- A plan should be in place for all high-risk mares, detailing the importance of the mare and foal and the extent to which the owner is willing to go to save either one.
- Having a plan in place allows quick decisions without jeopardizing the future well-being of the mare or foal.

▶ WHAT TO DO

The High-Risk Mare

- Once a high-risk pregnancy has been identified and a fetoplacental evaluation has occurred, it is important to develop a treatment protocol that creates a healthy uterine environment to sustain the pregnancy for as long as possible.
- Various drugs/therapies are used to accomplish this:
  - **Progestogens** promote uterine quiescence and inhibit prostaglandin-mediated abortion.
    - They are important to use in any condition where there could be prostaglandin release (i.e., colic, endotoxemia, laminitis) or an increase in uterine myoelectric activity (i.e., placentitis).
    - Preparations available:
      - Altrenogest (Regu-Mate[2])
      - Daily progesterone in oil, 300 mg/day
      - Long-acting progesterone formulation (BioRelease P4 LA 150[3]; 150 mg progesterone/mL)
    - Altrenogest (Regu-Mate) is typically administered at a dose of 0.044 mg/kg PO q24h in early gestation, and higher doses, 0.088 mg/kg PO q24h, are recommended whenever prostaglandin release is a concern.
    - Progesterone in oil (daily formulation) is administered at a dose of 300 mg/day intramuscularly (IM).
    - Long-acting progesterone formulation (BioRelease P4 LA 150) is administered at a dose of 10 mL IM q7days.
    - No studies have been published using the long-acting progesterone formulation (BioRelease P4 LA 150) in mares carrying high-risk pregnancies. However, studies performed in normal pregnant mares indicate that these formulations can support normal pregnancies.
    - Progesterone daily formulation (300 mg/day IM) and altrenogest (44 mg/day PO) have been used successfully in

preventing pregnancy loss in cloprostenol-induced abortion in mares.
    - Mares can foal while receiving altrenogest although a study reported that these foals were slower to adapt to extrauterine life; discontinuing altrenogest therapy at 320 days of gestation alleviates neonatal adaptation problems.
    - Mares on progestogen therapy should be monitored frequently by ultrasonography to ensure fetal viability.
    - *Practice Tip: Never discontinue progestogen therapy abruptly; always taper the dose gradually over several days!*
  - **Nonsteroidal anti-inflammatories** are used to reduce placental and uterine inflammation and inhibit prostaglandin production.
    - Phenylbutazone or flunixin meglumine are the two most common nonsteroidal anti-inflammatories used.
    - Flunixin meglumine is known to completely inhibit endotoxin-induced prostaglandin-F2 alpha ($PGF_{2\alpha}$) secretion, but appears to be ineffective in the prevention of pregnancy loss associated with cloprostenol-induced abortion.
    - Phenylbutazone is administered at a dose of 2.2 mg/kg IV or PO q12 to 24h.
    - Flunixin meglumine is administered at a dose of 1.1 mg/kg IV or PO q12 to 24h; Long-term treatment generally uses a lower dose of 0.25 mg/kg IV or PO q8h.
  - **Antimicrobials** are used to treat bacterial infections.
    - A variety of antimicrobials are used to treat mares with placentitis:
      - Trimethoprim-sulfamethoxazole, 15 to 30 mg/kg PO q12h
      - Procaine penicillin, 22,000 IU/kg IM q12h
      - Potassium penicillin, 22,000 IU/kg IV q6h

[1]Foalert (Acworth, Georgia).
[2]Regu-Mate (Intervet, Inc., Millsboro, Delaware).
[3]BioRelease P4 LA 150, 150 mg progesterone/mL (BETPHARM, Lexington, Kentucky).

- Gentamicin, 6.6 mg/kg IV q24h
- Cefazolin, 20 mg/kg IV q6h
- Ceftiofur, 2.2 mg/kg IV/IM q12h
○ Potassium penicillin, gentamicin, and trimethoprim sulfa-methoxazole all concentrate in the allantois of the pregnant mare. Procaine penicillin, cefazolin, and ceftiofur have not been critically evaluated to determine whether they concentrate in allantoic fluid.
○ Antimicrobials to avoid in the pregnant mare:
- Enrofloxacin: It has the potential to cause cartilage abnormalities and other arthropathies in the fetus, but these are mostly a problem when administered after birth.
- Doxycycline: Tetracyclines can delay skeletal development and discolor deciduous teeth; use only in the last half of pregnancy provided the risk can be substantiated.
- Chloramphenicol: It may affect protein synthesis, particularly in the fetal bone marrow; use only if benefits outweigh the risks.
- **Pentoxifylline** improves peripheral blood flow, reduces inflammation, and can aid in the treatment of endotoxemia.
  ○ Used predominantly in the treatment of placentitis
  ○ Administered at a dose of 10 mg/kg PO q12h
- **Tocolytics** are used to relax the uterus.
  ○ Tocolytics are used in the high-risk mare to promote uterine quiescence and prolong pregnancy.
  ○ Clenbuterol and isoxsuprine are tocolytics.
  ○ Studies using clenbuterol have not clearly demonstrated its ability to delay parturition or abortion in the normal or high-risk late-gestation pregnant mare, respectively; therefore, its use is questionable.
  ○ Isoxsuprine has poor bioavailability following oral administration and therefore its ability to affect uterine relaxation is doubtful.

○ Clenbuterol is administered at a dose of 0.8 μg/kg PO PRN (as circumstances may require).
○ Isoxsuprine is administered at a dose of 0.4 to 0.6 mg/kg PO q12h.
- **Vitamin E** is an antioxidant.
  ○ Vitamin E is used in high-risk mares with uteroplacental dysfunction/compromise.
  ○ High doses of vitamin E prepartum are protective against hypoxia-induced injury in newborn rats.
  ○ No evidence-based studies support high doses of vitamin E prepartum; however vitamin E reduces the incidence of hypoxia-related problems in foals.
  ○ Vitamin E is administered at a dose of 6000 to 10,000 IU PO q24h.
- **Oxygen:** Supplemental oxygen can be given to mares with reduced oxygen saturation (i.e., pneumonia) or mares with placental dysfunction.
  ○ The objective of the treatment is to improve oxygen delivery to the fetus and reduce the risk of peripartum fetal hypoxia.
  ○ Intranasal oxygen flow rate is 10 to 15 L/min.
- **Nutrition:** Preventing hypoglycemia in the late gestation, high-risk mare is very important to avoid premature delivery of nonviable foals.
  ○ Equine placenta is sensitive to poor nutrition and rapidly produces prostaglandins in response to hypoglycemia and hyperlipemia.
  ○ Late-gestation mares that need to be held off feed (i.e., post-colic) should be maintained on intravenous infusions of dextrose, 2.5% or 5% dextrose in 0.45% saline, administered at a rate of 1 to 2 mg/kg/min.
  ○ Anorectic late-gestation mares should receive supplemental nutrition (i.e., partial parenteral nutrition or nasogastric intubation) to prevent hypoglycemia and hyperlipemia (see Chapter 51, p. 775).

References

References can be found on the companion website at www.equine-emergencies.com.

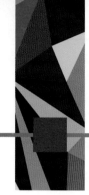

CHAPTER 28

Emergency Foaling

Tamara Dobbie and Regina M. Turner

Dystocia

- Dystocia is an abnormal or difficult delivery.
- Generally caused by abnormal fetal:
  - Presentation
  - Position
  - Posture

  Note: Disproportionate fetal oversize is rare in the mare.
- Every dystocia is different and *no* single management option is right for all circumstances.
- The decision on how to manage the dystocia is based on:
  - Experience of the practitioner
  - Value of the foal/mare
  - Wishes of the owner
  - Viability of the foal
  - Availability/affordability of a referral hospital

●〉 WHAT TO DO

Dystocia

Identification of a Problem

- Stage II labor begins with the rupture of the chorioallantois (or water breaking) and ends with the delivery of the foal.
  - Normal duration is 30 minutes or less.
  - Signs of a potential problem include:
    - Upside down hooves
    - Abnormal combination of extremities at the vulva
    - Absence of strong contractions
    - No progression of the delivery within 10 minutes of the water breaking
    - Failure of the fetal extremities or amnion to appear at the vulva within 5 minutes of the water breaking

Examination of the Mare

- Obtain a brief history: age, previous number of foals, expected due date, time since the rupture of the chorioallantois, any attempts to relieve dystocia/deliver foal, any fetal movement observed.
- Perform a brief physical exam: color of mucous membranes, capillary refill time (CRT), appearance of the perineum.
- Restraint is used, if needed, to perform a safe and comprehensive vaginal examination or to minimize mare straining (see vaginal delivery):
  - Physical restraint: chain shank, twitch, gum chain
  - Sedation: xylazine, detomidine, acepromazine, +/− butorphanol
- Some recommend performing an abdominocentesis to rule out a uterine tear before the infusion of large volumes of lubricant into the uterus; however, abdominocentesis:
  - Can cause delays with delivery of the foal
  - May *not* be necessary in the majority of cases of dystocia
  - Is unlikely to be realistic in practice

Examination of the Fetus

- Prepare the mare for a vaginal examination:
  - Wrap tail and secure off to one side.
  - The tail can be tied with a long rope to the mare's neck or held by an assistant.
  - Clean perineum with disinfectant scrub and water.
  - Dry perineum.
  - Apply generous amounts of lubricant to clean arms or obstetric sleeves.
- To determine if the fetus is viable, assess for:
  - Withdrawal reflex
  - Corneal reflex
  - Suckle reflex (anterior presentation)
  - Anal reflex (posterior presentation)
  - Peripheral pulses or umbilical pulse
  - Heartbeat
- **Practice Tip:** *A positive response to any of the listed tests confirms that the fetus is alive, although possibly compromised. A negative response to all of the above tests does not mean the fetus is dead. It can be difficult to determine if a fetus is dead.*
- Do take the time to make an accurate diagnosis of the cause of the dystocia. This is the most important component of the examination. Without an accurate diagnosis, the chances of resolving the dystocia are greatly reduced.
- Carefully examine the fetus to determine:
  - Presentation: Anterior longitudinal is normal. However, a fetus can also be delivered in posterior longitudinal presentation.
  - Position: Dorsosacral is normal
  - Posture: Head, neck, and forelimbs extended is normal
  - Any obvious fetal abnormalities, contracted tendons, wry neck
  - Any obvious uterine, cervical, or vaginal abnormalities
- Choice of treatment option depends on:
  - Viability of the fetus
  - Value of the fetus
  - Value of mare
  - Experience of veterinarian
  - Proximity to a referral center
- **Practice Tip:** *There are only 3 ways to deliver a foal.*
  - Vaginal delivery:
    - Assisted vaginal delivery
    - Controlled vaginal delivery: The mare is under general anesthesia with hindquarters elevated
  - Cesarean section (C-section):
    - If a cesarean section is an option, make the decision for referral quickly in order to maximize the chances of delivering a healthy, viable foal
  - Fetotomy is considered an option *only* if the fetus is dead.

⟫ WHAT TO DO

Assisted Vaginal Delivery

- ***Important:*** *Do* have a bystander keep track of time; if *no* progress is made after 15 minutes an alternative approach should be considered (i.e., fetotomy, controlled vaginal delivery, or cesarean section).
- Minimize mare straining:
  - Sedation—xylazine, detomidine, acepromazine +/− butorphanol. ***Note:*** Monitor the effects of the sedation on a live fetus.
  - Tocolytics—clenbuterol, 10 mL Ventipulmin orally; 30 minutes for full effect
- Lubricate the reproductive tract:
  - Use *large volumes* of lubricant administered via a stomach pump and sterile nasogastric tube.
  - Use carboxymethylcellulose/propylene glycol formulations.
    - *Avoid* polyethylene polymer powder (J-Lube, Jorgensen Laboratories) because of its potential to produce peritonitis and death in the case of peritoneal contamination.

Perform Fetal Mutations

- Fetal mutations are manipulations that return the fetus to normal presentation, position, and posture. They include the following:
  - Repulsion—always the first mutation!
    - Push the fetus back into the uterus.
    - Be careful *not* to rupture the uterus.
    - Use large volumes of lubricant; tocolytics, e.g., clenbuterol, 10 mL Ventipulmin syrup orally, may prevent uterine rupture.
  - Rotation: Rotate the fetus on its longitudinal axis.
  - Version: Rotate the fetus on its transverse axis; this is difficult to perform in a term fetus.
  - Extension of head/neck and limbs may be necessary.

Forced Extraction

- Apply obstetric chains (Box 28-1) to the limbs. ***Important:*** Position the chain one loop above and a half hitch below the fetlock; the chain between the two loops should lie along the dorsum of the limb.
- An obstetric chain or snare can be applied to the head to keep the neck in extension.
- Apply traction during abdominal straining.
- Allow periods of rest between periods of traction.
- Initially pull dorsally to engage the fetus into the pelvic canal.
- Once the fetus is in the pelvic canal, traction should be directed ventrally towards the hocks to allow the fetus to follow the normal direction of the mare's caudal reproductive tract.

Box 28-1 | **Standard Obstetric Equipment**

- Clean/sterile obstetric chains/straps and handles
- Sterile nasogastric tube and clean stomach pump designated for dystocias only!
- Sterile lubricant: Carboxymethylcellulose is strongly preferred.
  - ***Note:*** Polyethylene polymer powder (PEP)–based lubricants are reported to cause severe peritonitis and even death if they leak into the abdominal cavity. Therefore, PEP-based lubricants (i.e., J-Lube, Jorgenson Laboratories) should be avoided if there is any risk of a uterine laceration or if cesarean section is an option.
- Clean buckets for water and lubricant
- Disinfectant scrub
- Rectal sleeves (optional)
- Tail wrap

Dystocia in Cranial Presentation

- Carpal flexion:
  - Repel fetus.
  - Rotate carpus dorsolaterally while bringing the fetlock and foot medially and caudally into the pelvic canal; cup the hoof to protect the uterus.
- Incomplete elbow extension:
  - Position of the foal's muzzle is at the same level as the fetlocks.
  - Repel fetus.
  - Extend flexed limbs with traction.
- Foot-nape posture:
  - One or both of the forelimbs is positioned over top of the foal's extended head.
  - Repel the fetus and reposition the legs under the head and neck.
  - ***Practice Tip:*** *There is the potential for a rectovaginal fistula or third-degree perineal laceration with this malpresentation.*
- Poll presentation:
  - This is a ventral deviation of the head.
  - Repel the fetus, grasp the foal's muzzle, and rotate the head laterally in an arc.
  - Lift the muzzle up and over the brim of the pelvis.
  - A head snare is recommended to maintain the neck in an extended posture.
- Ventral deviation of the neck:
  - The neck is ventrally deviated between the forelimbs, bringing the foal's mandible to lie next to the ventral thorax.
  - Repel the fetus deeply into the uterus and locate the head.
  - Rotate the head laterally in an arc, and attempt to pull the muzzle caudally and medially.
  - It may be necessary to push the forelimbs into carpal flexion and return them to the uterus in order to manipulate the head.
  - A cesarean section or fetotomy is often indicated with this malpresentation.
  - If successfully corrected, a head snare is recommended to maintain the neck in an extended posture.
- Neck flexion:
  - Neck is flexed laterally such that the foal's head is located beside the thorax.
  - Repel the fetus and bring head and neck into extension.
  - The length of the foal's neck can often make it impossible to reach the foal's head to perform this maneuver.
  - Consider the possibility of wry neck for those cases where the malpresentation *cannot* be corrected.
  - Fetotomy with neck amputation may be the best option for a dead fetus.
  - If successfully corrected, a head snare is recommended to maintain the neck in an extended posture.
- Shoulder flexion:
  - Repel the head and neck back into the uterus.
  - Locate the retained leg and work down the limb until the distal radius is identified.
  - Pull the leg cranially and medially into a carpal flexion while repelling the fetus further into the uterus.
  - Rotate the carpus dorsolaterally while bringing the fetlock and foot medially and caudally.
  - Cup the hoof to protect the uterus.
  - Cesarean section may be the best option if the foal is alive, given the difficulty in performing this mutation.
  - Fetotomy should be considered if the fetus is dead.

NEO

Dystocia in Posterior Presentation
- Hock flexion:
  - Locate the metatarsus and repel the fetus forward into the uterus.
  - Rotate the hock dorsolaterally while at the same time directing the fetlock and foot medially and caudally.
  - Cup the hoof to protect the uterus.
  - ***Practice Tip:*** *This malpresentation can be extremely difficult to correct!*
- Hip flexion:
  - *Breech* is the term used to describe a bilateral hip flexion.
  - ***Practice Tip:*** *This malpresentation is very challenging to correct, and a cesarean section is often the best alternative for obtaining a viable foal and a reproductively healthy mare.*
  - Correction requires converting the hip flexion into a hock flexion by pulling the distal tibia caudodorsally.
  - Once the hock is flexed, see correction above.
  - Fetotomy with amputation of the distal limb (at the level of the tarsus) may be the best option if cesarean section is *not* feasible and the foal is dead.

Dystocia in Transverse Presentation
- Ventral: All four limbs and the ventral abdomen are presented toward the birth canal.
- Dorsal: The spine/back of the fetus is presented toward the birth canal.
- ***Practice Tip:*** *Transverse presentation is a very difficult malpresentation to correct and generally requires a cesarean section.*
- Fetotomy is challenging in true transverse presentations.
- ***Practice Tip:*** *It may be possible to convert a ventral transverse presentation into a caudal presentation by repulsion of the head and forelimbs of the fetus forward into the uterus while at the same time extending the hindlimbs into the birth canal.*
- **Note:** Often fetuses in transverse presentation have congenital malformations due to their restricted space and activity in utero.

▶▶ WHAT TO DO

Fetotomy
- Reserved *only* for situations in which the fetus is dead.
- Many malpresentations can be corrected by fetotomy, partial or complete.
  - Partial fetotomy requires a minimum of one to three cuts to deliver the fetus vaginally.
    - A partial fetotomy carefully performed by a skilled veterinarian should *not* negatively impact the mare's reproductive potential.
    - Partial fetotomy is an excellent alternative for:
      - A dead fetus with carpal flexion
      - Deviation of the head and neck
      - Shoulder flexion
      - Hock flexion
  - Complete fetotomy (six cuts in anterior presentation) is sometimes used in bovine dystocias to reduce the mass of a large fetus.
  - ***Practice Tip:*** *Because fetal oversize is rare in mares, complete fetotomies are rarely performed in the horse and may carry more risk than in the cow.*
  - Fetotomy should *not* be attempted if the practitioner is unfamiliar with the procedure, and instead a cesarean section or terminal C-section should be performed as the alternative.

Box 28-2   Fetotomy Equipment

- Fetotome
- Wire threader
- Fetotomy wire
- Wire cutters
- Wire saw handles
- Wire introducer
- Krey hook
- Fetotomy knife
- Routine obstetric equipment (see Box 28-1)

- Equipment required, see Box 28-2
- Restraint of the mare:
  - Physical restraint—chain shank over the nose, lip chain, twitch; *no stocks*
  - Tranquilization—xylazine, detomidine, acepromazine, +/− butorphanol
  - Epidural anesthesia does *not* eliminate uterine contractions or abdominal press but decreases the reflex straining associated with vaginal manipulations
    - 1 to 1.25 mL 2% lidocaine per 100 kg or
    - 35 mg xylazine/500 kg plus 2.6 mL 2% mepivacaine added to 0.9% sterile saline for a final volume of 7 mL. ***Practice Tip:*** *Drug combination reduces the risk of ataxia and hindlimb paresis, but the full effect may take up to 30 minutes.*
  - General anesthesia: xylazine, 1.1 mg/kg IV, followed by ketamine, 2.2 mg/kg IV. **Note:** Elevation of the mare's hindquarters is required.

General Guidelines for Fetotomy
- Use large volumes of lubricant to protect the reproductive tract and to provide additional space between the uterus and the fetus.
- Tocolytics: Clenbuterol, 10 mL Ventipulmin syrup, may help relax the uterus and provide additional space.
- Hold the fetotome with two hands, one hand on the head of the fetotome to ensure the correct position is maintained and the other hand on the base to stabilize the instrument during cutting.
- Check the fetotomy wire following placement to make certain the wire has *not* become kinked or crossed and that there is *no* direct contact between the wire and the mare's reproductive tract.
- Perform the minimum number of cuts.
- ***Practice Tip:*** *Avoid repeated in-and-out arm movements because this leads to vaginal and cervical abrasion and subsequent adhesion formation.*

▶▶ WHAT NOT TO DO

Dystocia
- *Do not* use stocks for restraint during examination of a mare in labor. Often, these mares lie down unexpectedly and this can be very dangerous for the veterinarian and the mare.
- *Do not* tie the tail to a fixed object. It is common for a standing mare to lie down suddenly when vaginal manipulations are performed.
  - *Do not use* polyethylene polymer powder (J-Lube, Jorgensen Laboratories) if peritoneal contamination is possible because of the risk of a uterine laceration or if a cesarean section is an option. The powder can cause peritonitis and even death.

Aftercare

- Mares are at an increased risk for a retained placenta following a dystocia and/or fetotomy. Follow the protocol outlined for a retained placenta, see Chapter 24, p. 443.
- Cervical lacerations are possible following a dystocia and/or fetotomy. It is generally *not* possible to determine the extent of the cervical injury after dystocia/fetotomy, and therefore the cervix should be reevaluated when under the influence of progesterone (i.e., a week following the foal heat ovulation).
- Vaginal and cervical adhesions may occur if there has been significant mucosal trauma. A topical antimicrobial and steroid preparation (Animax[1]) is applied to the damaged tissue daily to prevent adhesion formation.

Outcome

- Mare survival rates following:
  - Cesarean section, uncomplicated: 90% to 100%
  - Controlled vaginal delivery (CVD): 90% to 100%
  - Fetotomy: Fifty-six to 96%; survival is likely related to the experience of the obstetrician
  - Assisted vaginal delivery:
    - One study reported better mare survival following assisted vaginal deliveries compared with controlled vaginal deliveries. This is probably because mares undergoing CVD had more severe and more protracted dystocias.
- Mare fertility following:
  - Cesarean section:
    - 60% foaling rate in mares bred the same year as C-section
    - 72% foaling rate in mares bred the year following C-section
    - Breed the mare the same year for C-sections performed early in the season and without complications; breed the mare the following year for C-sections performed later in the season or those with complications.
  - Controlled vaginal delivery:
    - 58% pregnancy rate for mares bred the same year as the controlled vaginal delivery
  - Fetotomy
    - 80% pregnancy rate for mares bred the same year as partial fetotomy when the fetotomy is performed by a skilled veterinarian
- Foal survival:
  Practice Tip: The length of stage II labor is the single most important determinant for the outcome of the foal, whether the foal is delivered vaginally or by cesarean section.
  - Foal survival following vaginal delivery:
    - For every 10-minute increase in stage II labor beyond 30 minutes, there is a 10% increased risk of a dead foal and a 16% increased risk of the fetus *not* surviving.
  - Foal survival following cesarean section:
    - 11% to 42% chance of delivering a live foal
    - 5% to 31% chance of the foal surviving to discharge
    - The wide range in foal survival consistently depends on the duration of stage II labor; therefore, *refer early!*

Premature Separation of the Chorioallantois: Red Bag Delivery

- At the beginning of normal, stage II labor:
  - The chorioallantois generally ruptures at the cervical star, releasing the allantoic fluid or "breaking of the water."
  - This allows the chorioallantois to remain intimately attached to the endometrium, thus allowing ongoing transfer of oxygen and nutrients from the dam's circulation to the fetal circulation through the umbilical cord.
  - The intact amnion containing the foal should progress through the opening in the chorioallantois.
  - *Practice Tip: The first fluid-filled "bag" seen at the vulva should be the pearly white, translucent amnion.*
- In a red bag delivery, the chorioallantois does *not* rupture and delivery progresses:
  - The entire fetoplacental unit (intact chorioallantois with the intact allantoic cavity containing the amnion and the foal) separates from the endometrium and passes through the birth canal.
  - If this occurs, then the connection of the foal to the mare's oxygen supply via the chorionic villi becomes severely compromised.
  - Since the foal *cannot* breathe during passage through the birth canal, the foal becomes hypoxic if the condition is *not* corrected.
  - *Practice Tip: The first sign of a problem is the appearance of the thick, velvety, intact chorioallantois at the vulva, rather than the pearly white amnion, thus the use of the term* red bag delivery.
  - *Important Note: A red bag delivery is an extremely time-sensitive emergency that must be corrected immediately to avoid fetal hypoxia and death.*

●〉 WHAT TO DO

Red Bag Delivery

- Foaling attendants should be aware of the signs of a red bag delivery *in advance of foaling* and know to contact a veterinarian *immediately* if a red bag delivery occurs.
- The chorioallantois should be immediately manually ruptured and an assisted vaginal delivery performed as soon as possible.
- Judicious traction should be applied to the foal to facilitate delivery in an attempt to minimize the duration of the hypoxic insult.
- If veterinary assistance is some distance away, an experienced foaling attendant is instructed to rupture the chorioallantois and deliver the foal.

---

[1]Dechra Veterinary Products, Overland Park, Kansas.

Practice Tip: *"Blunt" dissection of the chorioallantois is strongly recommended. However, in some cases of red bag delivery, the chorioallantois is abnormally thickened and* cannot *be ruptured using your hands. In these cases, sharp incision may be required.*

- Less common possibilities for a protruding structure at the vulvar opening include:
  - Vaginal prolapse
  - Evisceration
- After delivery, the foal should be treated for a possible hypoxic insult.
- The cause of most red bag deliveries is *not* known. However, in some instances, the chorioallantois is obviously thickened as a result of disease such as ascending placentitis or fescue toxicosis. Samples of the chorioallantois are obtained and submitted for histologic analysis if more information is desired.

⬤〉 WHAT NOT TO DO

Red Bag Delivery

- *Always confirm* that the anatomic structure at the vulvar opening is the chorioallantois before rupturing. Do *not* proceed without confirmation!
- ***Important Note:*** Vaginal prolapse and intestinal evisceration emergencies are not managed like red bag delivery. Know the difference!
- Do *not* incise prolapsed vaginal or intestinal tissue; this is contraindicated.

References

References can be found on the companion website at www.equine-emergencies.com.

CHAPTER 29

Foal Resuscitation

Kevin T. Corley

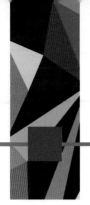

Neonatal foals deteriorate rapidly with disease and debilitation. This rapid deterioration demands early identification and treatment of compromised foals. This chapter outlines emergency resuscitation in the foal, including:

- Cardiopulmonary cerebral resuscitation
- Rapid restoration of circulating volume with emergency fluid therapy
- Respiratory support with oxygen therapy
- Nutritional support with glucose supplementation

Cardiopulmonary Cerebral Resuscitation (CPCR) of the Foal

Anticipate

Cardiopulmonary arrest is a sudden event, and requires immediate treatment. Predicting which foals are likely to require resuscitation can speed up the institution of appropriate resuscitation.

- Risk factors for newborn foals include factors affecting the mare during pregnancy:
  - Vaginal discharge during pregnancy
  - Placental thickening identified by ultrasonography
  - Illness of the dam during pregnancy
  - Dystocia
  - Delivery by cesarean section (C-section)
- Risk factors for foals undergoing hospital treatment include:
  - Worsening respiratory compromise
  - Septic shock
  - Severe metabolic disorders

Prepare

- It is not possible to successfully resuscitate a foal without an ordered plan. CPCR is a high intensity activity, and having a plan allows the resuscitator to prioritize and focus on lifesaving measures.
- Elements of the plan that can be prepared in advance are the general order of resuscitation and which attendant takes the lead role in resuscitation.
  - If a veterinarian is present, they should direct resuscitation.
- Equipment must be available, ready to use, and in an easily accessible place. The basic list of equipment is given in Box 29-1.
  - The equipment for CPCR should be placed in a dedicated, single, easily movable container. All CPCR equipment should be thoroughly checked before the foaling season.

Recognize Early

- Early identification of foals that will require resuscitation is critical. This is particularly important for resuscitation at birth, because the foal may have arrested during parturition and therefore may have a prolonged period of arrest. Familiarization with the normal sequence of events during parturition is essential for successful resuscitation.
- Second Stage of Labor: Expulsion of the Foal
  - Expulsion of the foal should take no more than 20 minutes.
  - The foal takes a few gasps initially.
  - Foal should be breathing spontaneously within 30 seconds of birth.
  - Heart rate averages 70 beats/min immediately after birth and should be regular.
  - A few normal foals may have arrhythmias for up to 15 minutes following birth, including:
    - Atrial fibrillation
    - Wandering pacemaker
    - Atrial premature contraction
    - Ventricular premature contractions
  - ***Practice Tip:*** *These dysrhythmias do not require specific treatment.*
  - Foals have pain and sensory awareness at birth and develop a righting reflex within 5 minutes and a suck reflex within 2 to 20 minutes.
- Respiratory arrest almost always precedes cardiac arrest in the newborn foal. The arrest is usually a result of asphyxia, itself caused by:
  - Premature placental separation
  - Early severance or twisting of the umbilical cord
  - Prolonged dystocia
  - Airway obstruction by fetal membranes
- **Note:** Some foals do not start spontaneously breathing even without any apparent birthing misadventure.
- Foals that are deprived of oxygen undergo a sequence of changes:
  - They begin with a brief period of rapid breathing.
  - As the asphyxia continues, the heart rate begins to drop, respiratory movements stop, and the foal enters *primary apnea.*

NEO

Box 29-1	**Equipment for CPCR**

Basic Equipment
8-mm and 10-mm internal diameter 55-cm-long nasotracheal tubes*
5-mL syringe (to inflate the cuff of the nasotracheal tube)
Self-inflating resuscitation bag[†]
Small flashlight (pen torch)
Epinephrine (adrenaline) bottle[‡]
Five 2-mL sterile syringes
20-gauge 1-inch needles

Additional Equipment for Newborn Foals
Bulb syringe
Clean towels

Equipment That Should Be Available If Possible
Oxygen cylinder and flow valve
Steel 14-gauge 1- to 1.5-inch needles
Four 1-L bags of lactated Ringer's solution
Fluid administration set
14-gauge IV catheter
End-tidal carbon dioxide monitor
Electrical defibrillator

For Studfarms Without Resident Veterinarians
Suitable facemask together with a resuscitation bag or pump[§]

*For example, V-PFN-8 and V-PFN-10 (Cook Veterinary Products, Bloomington, Indiana).
[†]For example, Laerdal "The Bag" Disposable Resuscitator Adult 840043 (Wappingers Falls, New York).
[‡]For example, Epinephrine injection 1:1000 (Butler, Dublin, Ohio).
[§]C.D. Foal Resuscitator (McCulloch Medical Products, Glenfield, New Zealand).

- In some foals in primary apnea, spontaneous breathing may be induced by tactile stimulation.
- The next stage is irregular gasps, which become weaker until the foal enters *secondary apnea.*
- There are no further respiratory efforts and the heart rate continues to drop until it stops.
- Part or all of this sequence may occur in utero and during delivery, and a foal may already be in secondary apnea by the time it is born.
- *Practice Tip: Primary apnea cannot be differentiated from secondary apnea on clinical grounds alone.*
- Newborn foals requiring resuscitation are:
  - Those that gasp for longer than 30 seconds
  - Foals with absent respiratory movements or heartbeat
  - Those with a heart rate less than 50 beats/min and falling
  - Foals with obvious dyspnea
- In the hospitalized foal, similar parameters apply.
  - Foals (<7 days old) with a heart rate that is below 50 beats/min and falling and those with apnea require resuscitation.
  - For foals with failing respiratory systems, intubation and positive pressure ventilation with a self-inflating resuscitation bag may be a prelude to mechanical ventilation.
  - Decreases in venous oxygen saturation, end-tidal carbon dioxide, and muscle tone may all be early signs of arrest or impending arrest.

Select

- Not all foals are suitable candidates for resuscitation. Foals with obvious congenital defects at birth should probably not be resuscitated.
- It is not uncommon for foals with congenital defects (i.e., severe arthrogryposis, hydrocephalus, etc.) to present as a dystocia and for the foal to arrest during the birthing process.
- Although it is technically possible to successfully restore spontaneous circulation in hospitalized foals that arrest, the long-term outcome in severely ill foals is very poor.
  - Many of these foals arrest again within a short period of time and become increasingly difficult to successfully resuscitate.
  - The welfare and financial implications of resuscitation should always be considered and used to determine the degree of effort to resuscitate the foal.
  - *Practice Tip: In contrast to the severely sick foal, the prognosis for the relatively healthy foal that arrests during anesthesia is relatively good.*

The First 20 Seconds

- The first thing to do is to decide whether CPCR is appropriate for the foal, as outlined previously.
- Thereafter, the effort is directed in preparing the foal for CPCR.
- The foal should be placed in lateral recumbency on a hard flat surface.
- If any of the ribs are fractured, the side with the broken ribs should be placed against the ground.
- If ribs are fractured on both sides, the side with more of the cranial ribs (3, 4, and 5) fractured should be placed on the ground.
- The head should be extended, so that the nose is in a straight line with the trachea.
- In the newborn foal, the nares and mouth should be cleared of fetal membranes before proceeding.
- Vigorous towel drying should also be started, which acts as a strong tactile stimulus for the foal to begin breathing.
- In a foal that is born with meconium staining, the first 20 seconds should be devoted to suctioning and clearing the airway.
- Airway suctioning should ideally start as soon as the meconium-stained head appears at the vulva, before the foal takes its first breath. This early suctioning is not always possible.
- If the foal is covered in thick meconium, suctioning of the trachea should also be attempted.
- *Practice Tip: Suctioning of the oropharynx can induce bradycardia or even cardiac arrest via vagal reflexes, and for this reason, suctioning with a bulb syringe may be safer than using a mechanical suction unit.*
- Mechanical suction should not be applied for longer than 5 to 10 seconds at a time. An aspiration mask for clearing the airways is included as part of a commercially available

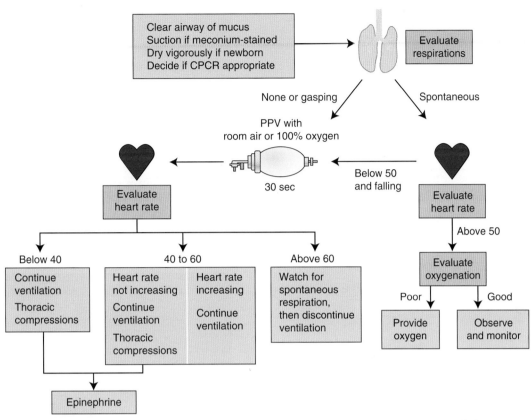

Figure 29-1   Flow chart for cardiopulmonary cerebral resuscitation (CPCR). *PPV,* Positive pressure ventilation.

pump-and-mask system[1] and may be especially appropriate for suction by nonveterinarians.

CPCR
Cardiopulmonary cerebral resuscitation (CPCR) (Fig. 29-1) includes 3 critical steps:
- **A**irway
- **B**reathing
- **C**irculation

Airway
- The best way to ensure an adequate airway is to intubate the foal.
  - *Practice Tip: Nasal intubation is generally preferred to oral intubation because there is less risk of the tube being damaged as the foal regains consciousness.*
- If two brief attempts at nasotracheal intubation are unsuccessful, oral intubation should be used.
- The internal diameter of the tube should be matched to the size of the foal.
- As a rough guide, term Thoroughbred foals (45 to 60 kg) require a 9- to 10-mm internal diameter tube for nasotracheal intubation and a 10- to 12-mm internal diameter tube for orotracheal intubation.
- It may be necessary to use a tube with a 7- to 9-mm internal diameter in smaller breeds of foals (20 to 35 kg) and premature Thoroughbred foals.

- Smaller tubes are easier to pass, but create more resistance to airflow.
- For intubation, the foal can be in lateral or sternal recumbency.
- The head should be in a straight line with the neck.
- To pass a tube nasally, one hand is used to direct the tip of the tube medially and ventrally into the ventral meatus. The other hand is used to advance the tube.
- To pass a tube orally, the tongue should be gently pulled forward and to the side with one hand to stabilize the larynx. The tube is advanced over the tongue in a midline position.
- In both intubation techniques, rotation of the tube, 90 to 180 degrees when the tube end is in the pharynx, is helpful.
- Once the tube is in place, the cuff should be gently inflated to provide a "seal" for assisted ventilation.
- It is important to check that the endotracheal tube has successfully passed into the trachea by:
  - Compressing the thorax and simultaneously feeling expired air at the exposed tube end.
  - The thoracic wall should also be seen to rise when the first breath is given.
  - If the tube has entered the esophagus, it is often felt in the cranial neck just left and dorsal to the larynx or proximal trachea.
  - It is also possible to check the tube position with an end-tidal carbon dioxide monitor or a colorimetric carbon dioxide indicator. For these devices, the

---
[1]Foal Resuscitator (McCulloch Medical, Glenfield, New Zealand).

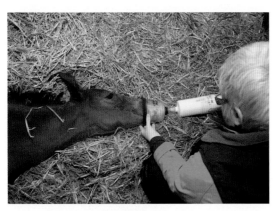

Figure 29-2 Using a pump and mask to provide breaths during CPCR. The rate should be 10 to 20 breaths per minute. (Copyright Veterinary Advances Ltd., 2012. From the iOS App "Equine Techniques." Used with permission.)

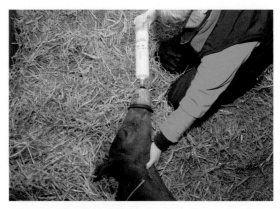

Figure 29-3 Gently occluding the esophagus during pump-and-mask CPCR to prevent aerophagia. (Copyright Veterinary Advances Ltd., 2012. From the iOS App "Equine Techniques." Used with permission.)

presence of carbon dioxide on exhalation confirms that the tube is in the airway.

Breathing

- The optimum rate of ventilation is unknown, but experience suggests rates between 10 and 20 breaths per minute are appropriate.
  - Higher rates may be associated with impaired blood flow in the heart muscle.
- Oxygen is not necessary during resuscitation but is helpful immediately postresuscitation.
- The best method of providing artificial respiration is a self-inflating resuscitation bag connected to a nasotracheal or endotracheal tube. This allows controlled ventilation and avoids the risk of aerophagia or driving foreign material, meconium, or mucus into the lower airways.
  - Aerophagia fills the stomach with gas and limits the lungs' ability to fully expand.
  - When using a resuscitation bag, the optimum method is to place the bag on the floor and to kneel next to the bag with the shoulders over the bag. The hands should be placed flat and together, on the bag. This allows controlled use of body weight to help compress the bag.
- An alternative to a self-inflating resuscitation bag is a resuscitation pump. The commercially available model[2] delivers a tidal volume of 780 mL and can be connected to a nasotracheal tube or a mask.
- Anesthetic machines with a minimum reserve bag of 1 L and oxygen demand valves may also be used for resuscitation, but carry a significant risk of volutrauma.
- ***Practice Tip:*** *Masks, rather than endotracheal tubes, probably represent the best option for CPCR by nonprofessionals (Fig. 29-2).*
- If possible, the proximal esophagus should be gently occluded to prevent air from being forced into the stomach, which hinders movement of the diaphragm (Fig. 29-3).
  - The esophagus is best occluded just dorsal to the trachea (which can be felt as a tube with semirigid rings of

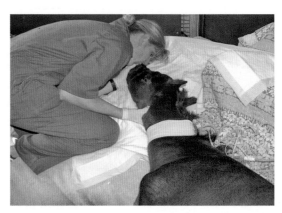

Figure 29-4 Mouth to nose resuscitation, with occlusion of the esophagus to prevent aerophagia. (Copyright Kevin Corley and Jane Axon, 2004. From the iOS App "Equine Techniques." Used with permission.)

cartilage), cranially and ventrally on the neck, just caudal to the larynx. For people with medium to large hands, the fingers can be used on one side of the neck, and the thumb of the same hand on the other side of the neck. The fingers and thumb are gently pressed together so that the tissue just dorsal to the trachea gently occludes the esophagus. People with smaller hands may need to use a hand on either side of the neck.

- If neither an endotracheal tube nor a pump and mask are available, it is possible to perform mouth-to-nose resuscitation (Fig. 29-4).
  - One hand should be used to cup the chin and occlude the down nostril. The other hand should gently occlude the proximal esophagus, as described earlier. The head should be dorsiflexed as far as possible to straighten the airway, but the head should not be lifted. The resuscitator should check that the thorax rises as an assistant blows into the foal's nostril.
- Doxapram is a highly controversial treatment for stimulating respiration at birth.
  - The drug clearly has a role for increasing ventilatory rate in hemodynamically stable foals with perinatal asphyxia syndrome and neonatal encephalopathy.

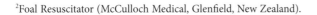

[2]Foal Resuscitator (McCulloch Medical, Glenfield, New Zealand).

- However, doxapram reduces cerebral blood flow, especially at higher doses in foals. It also increases myocardial oxygen demands in experimental animals.
- It is these effects, together with the evidence that this class of drugs is ineffective in secondary apnea, that have led to the recommendation that doxapram *not* be used in acute cardiopulmonary resuscitation.
- The drug may have a role if no other elements of cardiopulmonary resuscitation are possible but should *not* be substituted for the other steps outlined in this chapter.

Circulation

- Thirty seconds after beginning ventilation, the foal should be assessed to determine whether circulatory support is required.
- ***Practice Tip:*** *Thoracic compressions should be started if the heartbeat is absent, <40 beats/min, or <60 beats/min and not increasing.*
- The optimum rate for thoracic compressions in the foal is unknown. In adult horses, a rate of 80 compressions per minute (cpm) has been shown to result in significantly better circulation than 40 or 60 cpm.
- Rates between 80 and 120 cpm are therefore likely appropriate for foals. However, rates of 80 to 120 cpm rapidly fatigue the resuscitator. Therefore, switch the personnel performing thoracic compressions every 2 to 5 minutes.
- Ventilation must continue during thoracic compressions. The recommended ratio is 2 breaths per 15 thoracic compressions. Thoracic compressions should not be stopped during breaths.
- The foal should be in lateral recumbency.
- The foal should be placed on a firm dry surface.
- The person doing the thoracic compressions should kneel by the foal's spine, and place their hands on top of each other, just caudal to the foal's triceps, in the highest point of the thorax (Fig. 29-5).

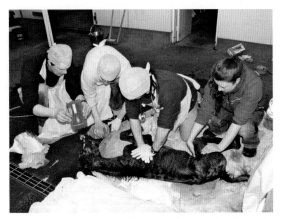

Figure 29-5   CPCR of a foal after C-section, showing resuscitation bag and nasotracheal tube, thoracic compressions, checking for pulse in the femoral artery, and checking for pupillary light response. (Copyright Veterinary Advances Ltd., 2012.)

- The resuscitator should have their shoulders directly above their hands, enabling them to use their body weight to help compress the thorax. This helps reduce resuscitator fatigue.

Drugs

- *Epinephrine* (adrenaline) is the major drug for foal resuscitation. It should be given if the heart rate remains very low (<40 beats/min) or absent after 2 minutes of full CPCR with thoracic compressions and breathing.
  - The dose is 0.01 to 0.02 mg/kg IV or 0.5 to 1 mL per 50 kg body weight, using the standard 1 mg/mL (1 : 1000) epinephrine.
  - This dose should be repeated every 3 to 5 minutes until a regular heart rate returns, or it is determined that CPCR is unsuccessful.
  - If venous access is not possible, epinephrine can be injected into the trachea below the cuff of the endotracheal tube, if present.
  - The intratracheal epinephrine dose is 0.1 to 0.2 mg/kg or 5 to 10 mL per 50 kg body weight.
  - ***Important:*** Intracardiac injection should be avoided. Epinephrine was not found to improve outcomes in human patients undergoing out-of-hospital CPCR.
- Other drugs play a minor role in CPCR of foals and are rarely used in acute resuscitation.
- Fluid therapy (bolus of 10 mL/kg crystalloids) may be helpful in restoring the circulation (see Emergency Fluid Resuscitation, p. 514).
- ***Important:*** The following drugs—atropine, calcium, and doxapram—are ineffective or dangerous in resuscitation of the newborn foal.

Defibrillation

- If a defibrillator is available, it should only be used for foals in ventricular fibrillation (recognized by rapidly undulating electrical activity with no discernable complexes).
- Electrical defibrillation may be tried on a foal in asystole that does not respond to thoracic compressions and epinephrine injection.
- The defibrillation setting is 2 to 4 J/kg or 100 to 200 J per 50 kg, increasing the energy by 50% with each defibrillation attempt.

Monitoring the Effectiveness of CPCR

- During CPCR, monitoring the effectiveness of the resuscitative efforts helps adjust the technique for each patient. For example, the rate of ventilation and the rate and pressure of thoracic compressions can vary.
- The pulse, if palpable, is the best way to monitor thoracic compressions (see Fig. 29-5).
- The progress of CPCR can be monitored by the heartbeat, if present, and used to decide when to stop thoracic compressions.
- Although an ECG is useful for monitoring heart rhythm, it is not adequate for monitoring CPCR because electrical

NEO

activity in the heart can continue without effective contractions (pulseless electrical activity).

- CPCR can also be monitored by the pupillary light reflex (see Fig. 29-5). If the people doing thoracic compressions keep a flashlight in their mouth, they can lean across and assess the pupil response and size without interrupting the resuscitation efforts.
  - **Practice Tip:** *The pupil is widely dilated and fixed with inadequate resuscitation, whereas effective circulation results in a more normal pupil that responds to light.*
- If the equipment is available, an end-tidal carbon dioxide monitor (capnograph) is extremely useful to assess the effectiveness of CPCR. The greater the expired carbon dioxide tension, the more effective the resuscitation efforts because more carbon dioxide is being transported to the lungs and expelled.
  - End-tidal carbon dioxide tensions >15 mm Hg indicate good perfusion and portend a good prognosis, whereas tensions persistently <10 mm Hg indicate ineffective CPCR and a poor prognosis.

When to Stop CPCR

- Ventilation should be stopped when the heart rate is >60 beats/min and spontaneous breathing is established.
  - This can be tested by stopping ventilation and disconnecting the bag or pump for 30 seconds and checking for a respiratory rate >16 beats/min, a regular respiratory pattern, and normal respiratory effort.
  - The first few breaths may be a gasping pattern, and should be followed by a normal respiratory rate and pattern.
  - **Practice Tip:** *Premature withdrawal of ventilation is reported to be the most common mistake in human neonatal CPCR.*
- If started, thoracic compressions should be continued until a regular heartbeat of >60 beats/min has been established.
  - There should be no lag period between the cessation of support and the onset of a spontaneous heartbeat.
  - Therefore, CPCR should not be stopped for longer than 10 seconds to assess the circulation.
  - Clinical experience suggests that if spontaneous circulation and respiration are not present after 10 minutes, then survival is unlikely.

Care for Foals After Resuscitation

- Foals that have been resuscitated continue to require support, and should be intensively monitored for at least 30 minutes.
  - Supplemental oxygen should be provided by either facemask or nasal cannula.
  - A careful physical examination should be performed, and if equipment is available, the heart rhythm should be monitored with an electrocardiogram.
- The consequences of a period of asphyxia during arrest and resuscitation are serious and may not be apparent for 24 to 48 hours after the arrest.

- Asphyxia can result in a syndrome of:
  - Altered neurologic status
  - Seizures
  - Impaired gastrointestinal and cardiovascular function
- There is no way to prevent the effects of asphyxia. Vitamin E, Vitamin C, selenium, corticosteroids, mannitol, acetylcysteine, and dimethyl sulfoxide might possibly reduce oxidative damage.
- A decision whether to refer a foal for intensive care is based on several factors, including:
  - Availability
  - Costs versus the economic worth of the foal
  - Success rates are variable and generally are 70% to 80% for most referral centers
  - Foals that have been successfully resuscitated are at high risk of complications, and referral should be strongly considered if circumstances permit.
- Whether or not referral is undertaken, it is important *not* to immediately warm foals after CPCR. Extensive research in human patients indicates that hypothermia for 12 to 24 hours after CPCR results in remarkably better neurologic outcomes.
  - **Practice Tip:** *Although it is difficult to replicate the clinically induced hypothermia in the veterinary setting, foals should not be deliberately warmed-up to "normal" body temperature in the period immediately after CPCR.*

◖❯ WHAT TO DO

Cardiopulmonary Resuscitation of the Foal
- Place the foal in lateral recumbency and extend the head.

Airway/Breathing
- Clear the nostril of mucus and debris to open airways and stimulate breathing.
  - If meconium stained, attempt suction of trachea for 5 to 10 sec
- Intubate if needed (usually a 9- to 10-mm tube), make sure "pop-off" valve is open.
- Ventilate at 10 to 20 breaths/min

Circulation
- If the heart rate is absent or low (<40 beats/min), begin thoracic compression at 80 cpm.
- Continue simultaneous ventilation—2 breaths/15 thoracic compressions.
- If there is no response in heart rate in 2 minutes, give 0.5 to 1 mL epinephrine IV for a 50-kg foal.
  - Repeat every 3 to 5 minutes until heartbeat returns.
- Ventricular fibrillation: Defibrillate with 100 to 200 J/50 kg.

Stop Resuscitation
- When heart rate is >60 beats/min and spontaneous breathing is well established
- If *no* response occurs after 10 minutes of continuous CPCR

Aftercare
- Supplemental intranasal or intratracheal oxygen at 5 to 10 L/min
- Monitor function of all body organs

WHAT NOT TO DO

Cardiopulmonary Resuscitation of the Foal

- Stop thoracic compressions to perform assisted ventilation
- Mistakenly intubate the esophagus
- Perform thoracic compressions on the fractured rib side of the foal if the other side has no obvious fractures
- Give doxapram if any other alternatives for ventilation are available
- Give sodium bicarbonate to a nonventilating foal

Emergency Fluid Resuscitation

Prompt, adequate fluid therapy is one of the easiest and most effective ways to maximize a foal's chance of survival. However, determining which foals require emergency fluids can be difficult.

Recognition of Hypovolemia in Foals

- Many of the clinical signs of hypovolemia (inadequate circulating volume) that are familiar in adult horses are inconsistently present in the foal.
- The clinical signs of hypovolemia in adults are:
  - Tachycardia
  - Weak pulses
  - Poor filling of the jugular vein
  - Tachypnea
  - Cold extremities
- When any of these clinical signs occur in the foal, hypovolemia should be suspected.
- Hypovolemic foals may have heart rates above, below, or within the normal range.
- Because the clinical signs of hypovolemia are vague in the foal, more reliance must be placed on the history than in adult horses.
- *Practice Tip: Foals become dehydrated very rapidly when they do not nurse. Hypovolemia should be suspected in any foal that has not nursed for the previous 4 hours.*
- Foals that are born by C-section may be clinically hypovolemic immediately after birth.
  - This may be due to lack of transfer of blood from the placenta during the birthing process, or in the case of foals taken from mares undergoing colic surgery, due to the effects of endotoxemia.
- Blood lactate concentrations may also be useful to detect hypovolemia in foals.
  - Lactate is an end product of anaerobic metabolism, and it accumulates in the tissues when there is insufficient oxygen for aerobic respiration.
  - Increased blood lactate concentrations (>2.5 mmol/L) in foals primarily reflect inadequate tissue perfusion, which occurs with hypovolemia.
  - However, lactate has also been reported to be increased in sepsis, the systemic inflammatory response syndrome (SIRS), trauma, after seizures, and during periods of increased circulating catecholamines.

- As for all laboratory information, lactate concentrations should be assessed in context of the entire clinical picture.
- Handheld lactate monitors[3] are available and not prohibitively expensive and therefore are suitable for field use. These monitors have good accuracy in the horse, especially when lactate is measured in plasma rather than whole blood. The Lactate-Pro[4] accurately measures L-lactate in whole blood, plasma, or peritoneal fluid.
- It is important to remember that prognostically, the lactate concentration before resuscitation is *not* as important as the trend following resuscitation!
- In hospitalized foals, blood pressure can also be used to determine hypovolemia.
- In adults, increased creatinine concentrations reflect inadequate perfusion to the kidney in the absence of nephropathy or postrenal problems such as ruptured bladders.
  - The most common cause for inadequate perfusion to the kidneys is hypovolemia.
  - In foals during the first 36 hours of life, increased creatinine concentrations may reflect compromised placental function in utero, and therefore are *not* a reliable marker for hypovolemia.
  - Foals with a ruptured bladder may also have increased plasma creatinine concentrations.
- Urine specific gravity can be used as an indicator of hydration in the foal without renal disease. The specific gravity should be <1.012; higher values indicate hypovolemia.
- *Practice Tip: Packed cell volume (PCV) is a poor indicator of circulatory status in the neonatal foal.*
  - It is uncommon to find an increase in PCV in the severely hypovolemic foal in contrast to adults.
  - The normal range for PCV in foals during the first week of life (28% to 46%) is slightly lower than in adults.
  - It is common for critically ill foals to have PCVs of 22% to 26%, possibly as a result of a combination of fluid therapy and bone marrow suppression with illness.
- Total solids concentration (measured by a refractometer) provides an estimate of total plasma protein and is also an unreliable indicator of hypovolemia in foals.
  - Total solids may be decreased by failure of passive transfer or by loss of protein through the gastrointestinal tract or kidney.
  - There is no correlation between total solids concentration and PCV or other signs of circulatory status such as lactate concentration in the foal.
  - The normal range for total solids is quite variable in the foal (4.3 to 8.1 g/dL; 43 to 81 g/L); total solids are usually lower than the adult.

---

[3]Accutrend Lactate Monitor (Roche Diagnostics, Switzerland).
[4]Lactate-Pro (Biomedical Labs, Queen Creek, Arizona).

Fluid Choices for Hypovolemia

- Balanced electrolyte solutions designed for resuscitation (i.e., Hartmann's solution,[5] lactated Ringer's solution,[6] or Normosol-R[7]) are the best fluids to use for treating hypovolemia.
- These fluids approximate the concentration of electrolytes in blood. They are therefore the safest fluids to use if electrolytes cannot be measured.
- *Practice Tip:* It is not recommended to attempt major electrolyte replacement before restoring a circulating volume.
- *Important:* Exceptions to this rule are *hyperkalemia, hyponatremia,* and *hypochloremia,* which are seen in ruptured bladder cases. These foals require 0.9% or 1.8% sodium chloride solution for resuscitation.
- Sodium chloride has traditionally been used as a resuscitation fluid in human medicine.
  - Sodium chloride is an acidifying fluid and therefore may *not* be the best choice for acute resuscitation in foals because most of these foals are acidotic because of lactic acidosis.
- *Practice Tip:* Hypertonic saline (7% to 7.5% sodium chloride) has no role in resuscitation of neonates.
- Hypertonic saline may cause a rapid change in plasma osmolarity, resulting in:
  - Brain shrinkage and subsequent vascular rupture with cerebral bleeding
  - Subarachnoid hemorrhage
  - Permanent neurologic deficit or death, to which neonates are particularly susceptible
- The change in plasma osmolarity is more severe in patients with renal insufficiency, a common finding in critically ill foals.
- Colloids are solutions that contain large protein or starch molecules, as opposed to crystalloids, which contain only electrolytes and water or glucose and water.
  - The role of colloid solutions such as modified gelatins (Haemaccel[8] and Gelofusine[9]) and hydroxyethyl starches (tetrastarch, pentastarch, VetStarch, and hetastarch) for acute resuscitation of the foal is unclear.
  - The theoretic advantage is that they expand the plasma volume by a greater amount than the balanced electrolyte formulas and persist in the circulation longer, prolonging their positive effect.
  - They also increase the plasma oncotic pressure, in contrast to crystalloids, which decrease it.
  - There are no clear-cut benefits of colloids for neonatal foals in clinical practice.
  - The total daily dose of hydroxyethyl starches should not exceed 15 mL/kg. At higher doses, these starches may interfere with coagulation and may cause clinical bleeding.

- Hydroxyethyl starches might be indicated for resuscitation in foals with a plasma total solids concentration of <3.5 g/dL (<35 g/L).
- There is evidence in humans that tetrastarch has fewer negative effects on coagulation and the kidneys than does hetastarch.
- The initial plasma expansion is greater with lower-molecular-weight colloids, and higher-molecular-weight colloids persist longer in the circulation.
- The average molecular weight of modified gelatins is small (30 to 35 kD) when compared with albumin (69 kD), pentastarch (200 kD), and hetastarch (450 kD).
- Modified gelatin solutions are therefore preferred for initial resuscitation of markedly hypovolemic foals, and hydroxyethyl starches may be better for long-term maintenance of plasma colloidal oncotic pressure.
- Plasma is a colloid solution often used for supplementing passive immunity in foals.
  - Plasma needs to be defrosted (if stored) or collected from a donor, and is therefore rarely available for acute fluid resuscitation.
  - Furthermore, because some foals may have anaphylactoid reactions or transfusion-related acute lung injury with plasma transfusions, it is good practice to infuse plasma slowly and monitor for a reaction.
  - This patient complication detracts from the use of plasma for fluid resuscitation.

Rate of Fluid Administration

- There are two ways to approach the treatment of hypovolemia—the shock dose and fluid boluses; both result in similar treatment patterns.
- Hypovolemic foals typically require 20 to 80 mL/kg of crystalloid fluids immediately.

Shock Dose

- The *shock dose* concept is borrowed from small animal medicine, and therefore is a concept familiar to many.
- The shock dose for a neonatal foal is 50 to 80 mL/kg of crystalloid fluids.
- Depending on the perceived degree of hypovolemia, one fourth to one half of the shock dose is given as fast as possible (in <20 minutes), and the foal is reassessed.
- If the foal requires additional fluid, another one fourth of the shock dose is given, and the foal is again reassessed.
- The final one fourth of the shock dose is only given to severely hypovolemic foals.

Fluid Boluses

- The incremental *fluid bolus* concept is borrowed from human medicine and is a much more practical method. The caveat is that it assumes a similar bodyweight among all patients, and therefore has not been adopted in small animal medicine.

---

[5]Baxter Healthcare Corporation, Deerfield, Illinois.
[6]Dechra Veterinary Products, Shrewsbury, Shropshire, UK.
[7]Abbott Laboratories, North Chicago, Illinois.
[8]Haemaccel (Intervet, Cambridge, UK).
[9]Gelofusine (B. Braun Medical Ltd, Sheffield, UK).

- The bolus method is simple:
  - Give a bolus of 1 L of crystalloids (i.e., approximately 20 mL/kg for a 50-kg foal), and reassess.
  - Up to 3 additional boluses may be given, reassessing the foal after each.
  - Most hypovolemic foals require at least 2 boluses.
- In foals where the body weight varies from 50 kg, the method needs to be adjusted so that the bolus is approximately 20 mL/kg.
- In pony foals and very premature Thoroughbred foals, boluses of 500 mL are usually appropriate. In large draft foals, the first bolus should be 2 L.
- Whether using the *shock-dose* method or the *fluid-bolus* method, the foal is reassessed during acute fluid therapy to determine if more fluids are needed.
- Foals with a strong pulse and improved mentation and that are urinating probably do not require any further fluid resuscitation.
- These foals are likely to still require fluids to correct dehydration and electrolyte imbalances, and for maintenance and ongoing losses.
- Foals with continued weak pulses (or low blood pressure), depressed mentation, and who have *not* urinated may require more rapid fluid administration, up to the maximum of 80 mL/kg or 4 L unless there is jugular vein distention, indicating increased CVP.

Possible Complications

- It is recommended to auscultate the lungs and trachea before and during rapid fluid therapy because pulmonary edema is an important theoretic complication.
- Pulmonary edema appears to be extremely rare in critically ill foals aggressively resuscitated with crystalloids.
- *Practice Tip: Crackles, classically associated with pulmonary edema, are more likely to represent opening and closing of collapsed alveoli rather than edema in foals.*
- Severe pulmonary edema results in wet sounds in the trachea, and a frothy pink fluid from the nares or mouth.
- If edema does occur, albuterol/salbutamol (50 μg for a 50-kg/110-lb foal) should be administered by metered dose inhaler and further fluid therapy carefully titrated, preferably by means of evaluating central venous or pulmonary pressures.
- *Practice Tip: Treatment of hypovolemia takes precedence over any concerns about possible cerebral edema and thus worsening perinatal asphyxia syndrome.*
  - Inadequate cerebral perfusion, due to hypovolemia, prolongs the ischemic event and is extremely detrimental in these foals. This is far more important than concerns about cerebral edema.
- Foals with neonatal isoerythrolysis are generally *not* hypovolemic, unless they become so debilitated that they stop nursing for 4 hours or more.
  - In foals with isoerythrolysis and hypovolemia, aggressive fluid therapy is not contraindicated as long as the PCV is 8% or greater.

- Although fluid therapy decreases the hematocrit, it does *not* decrease the number of circulating erythrocytes and may improve their distribution to the tissues unless the blood viscosity becomes extremely low.
- However, in foals with low PCVs, restoring blood oxygen-carrying capacity is a priority, and donor blood, washed mare's blood, or hemoglobin substitutes should be given as soon as possible.

Important Exception to Aggressive Fluid Therapy

- Aggressive fluid therapy should be avoided in uncontrolled bleeding because it may increase bleeding.
- This is uncommon in neonatal foals, but may occur with rib fractures, trauma resulting in internal bleeding, or rupture of an inaccessible vessel.
- In humans and experimental animals, aggressive fluid therapy in uncontrolled bleeding has been shown to increase mortality.
- If blood pressure can be measured, fluid therapy should be titrated to maintain the mean arterial pressure as close to 60 mm Hg as possible without increasing the systolic pressure over 90 mm Hg.
- If blood pressure cannot be measured, then a fluid rate of 2 to 3 mL/kg/h should be used until bleeding is stopped.
- In uncontrolled hemorrhage, the use of vasopressors (i.e., norepinephrine, vasopressin, or terlipressin) in addition to low fluid rate could be considered. There is *no* evidence in foals to guide doses of vasopressors in this clinical situation.

Emergency Glucose Support

- *Practice Tip: Intravenous glucose therapy is often part of emergency treatment in foals.*
- This is because the glycogen stores at birth are only sufficient to meet 2 hours of energy requirements in the unfed foal; fat stores are also very low at birth.
- Therefore, foals that are not nursing are at risk for hypoglycemia.
- Septicemia may also result in hypoglycemia, possibly as a result of lack of glycogen reserves and poor nursing in septic foals.
- Foals may also be hyperglycemic, presumably as part of the physiological response to cortisol release or associated with unregulated glucose metabolism with disease processes.
- Both hypoglycemia and hyperglycemia are harmful.
- Severe hypoglycemia is associated with seizure activity, coma, and death.
- Following cerebral hypoperfusion, a feature of hypovolemia and of perinatal asphyxia syndrome, hyperglycemia may be more detrimental than hypoglycemia.
- For this reason, it is advisable to monitor the blood glucose frequently in foals.
- Hypoglycemia is treated with glucose-containing fluids or parenteral nutrition.

NEO

NEO

- Hyperglycemia is treated with infusions of normal insulin (0.05 to 1 U/kg/h) starting at the bottom of this dose range.

Measuring Blood Glucose

- Blood glucose concentrations are easy to measure.
- A small volume of blood can be obtained from a venous stick or from capillary ooze from a small cut.
- Handheld monitors are the most convenient way to measure blood glucose, because the results are available very quickly, allowing accurate titration of treatments.
- There are many inexpensive handheld monitors available, designed for monitoring of humans with diabetes mellitus. However, the accuracy of these monitors is controversial, and generally these monitors are better at detecting hypoglycemia than hyperglycemia.
- *Practice Tip: One monitor, AlphaTRAK,*[10] *has been validated for use in horses and foals with blood glucose greater than 20 mg/dL and hematocrit range of 15% to 65% (see Chapter 15, p. 110).*

Fluids for Supporting Blood Glucose Concentrations

5% Glucose Solution

- One liter of 5% glucose provides approximately 190 kcal (796 kJ), and 1 L of 5% dextrose contains 170 kcal (712 kJ).
- These fluids are not a great source of energy for the foal.
- To meet resting energy requirement (44 kcal/kg/day [184 kJ/kg/day]) for a 50-kg foal, 11.5 to 13 L per day would need to be given. This is more than double the foal's maintenance fluid requirements and causes important electrolyte derangements.
- Five percent glucose has been recommended as a resuscitation fluid for foals because it:
  - Provides both volume and energy, but
  - However, it is not a good fluid for treating hypovolemia.
  - Only 10% of the volume administered remains in the circulation after 20 minutes; each liter of 5% glucose is expected to drop the plasma sodium concentration by 4 to 5 mmol/L (4 to 5 mEq/L) in a 50-kg foal.

50% Glucose Solutions

- These fluids are preferable to the 5% solutions. Each milliliter of 50% glucose is equivalent to 1.9 kcal (8 kJ), and 50% dextrose provides 1.7 kcal (7.1 kJ) per mL.
- It may be used in 2 ways:
  - In the hospital setting, the solution should be administered via an electronic pump, separately from the resuscitation fluids.
    - The starting rate depends on the degree of hypoglycemia.
    - A rule-of-thumb is to start at 20 mL/h for mild hypoglycemia (50 to 70 mg/dL; 2.8 to 4 mmol/L)

and 50 mL/h for severe hypoglycemia (<50 mg/dL; <2.8 mmol/L).

- In the field, it is probably best to add the 50% glucose solution to the resuscitation fluids.
  - In this situation, 10 to 20 mL of the 50% solution should be added per liter of resuscitation fluid.
  - If blood glucose can be measured, the amount of 50% solution added to the resuscitation fluids should be varied, based on measured blood glucose, to deliver approximately 20 mL/h for mild hypoglycemia and 50 mL/h for severe hypoglycemia.

Practice Tip: Glucose is not suitable for long-term nutritional support for foals. If enteral feeding is not possible or desirable after the first 12 to 24 hours of treatment, parenteral nutrition solutions containing dextrose or glucose; amino acids; vitamins and trace minerals; and in many foals, lipids, should be instituted.

●》 WHAT TO DO

Fluid Resuscitation of the Hypovolemic Foal

- Place a 14- to 16-gauge jugular catheter.
- Administer 2 L of a "balanced" crystalloid to a 50-kg foal (30 to 40 mL/kg).
- Reassess the foal and administer an additional 15 to 40 mL/kg crystalloid treatment.
  - Clinical assessment should include:
    - Mentation changes
    - Pulse pressure
    - Speed of jugular vein distention when held off
    - Urine production
    - Heart and respiratory rates
    - Mucous membrane color
    - Capillary refill time (CRT)
- Check and monitor blood glucose.
  - Add 10 to 20 mL of 50% dextrose to each liter as needed.
- Continue maintenance therapy (100 mL/kg/day) and replace ongoing fluid losses
  - Monitor "fluid in" and "fluid out" balance plus:
    - Serum electrolytes
    - Creatinine
    - Urea
    - PCV
    - Total solids
    - Body weight

◐》 WHAT NOT TO DO

Fluid Resuscitation of the Hypovolemic Foal

- Do not use 5% dextrose as a volume resuscitation fluid if a balanced crystalloid is available.
- *Do not* use 7.5% hypertonic saline in foals.

Emergency Oxygen Therapy

- Oxygen therapy is extremely useful for support of foals. It should be considered in all foals following resuscitation and dystocia.

---

[10]AlphaTRAK (Abbott Animal Health, Abbott Laboratories, North Chicago, Illinois).

- Other foals that are likely to benefit from oxygen are those that are:
  - Dyspneic
  - Cyanotic
  - Meconium stained after birth
  - Recumbent
- In the hospital setting, oxygen therapy should be based on the oxygen tension (Pao_2) in an arterial blood sample.
  - Oxygen should be supplemented if the arterial tension is <60 to 65 mm Hg (8.0 to 8.7 kPa).
  - The most convenient places for sampling arterial blood in the foal are the dorsal metatarsal artery and the brachia artery (see Chapter 31, p. 531).
- Small-bore flexible rubber feeding tubes are useful as oxygen cannulas for intranasal oxygen therapy in the foal.
  - The length to be inserted into the nares should be measured by the distance from the nares to the medial canthus of the eye.
  - The tube is then inserted into the ventral meatus of the nose.
  - There are a variety of ways of fixing the tube in place.
    - One method is to attach the tube to a tongue depressor, which has been previously wrapped in tape. The oxygen tube is taped along one edge of the tongue depressor, and then curled around one end, so that it heads back in the direction it is coming from. It is not taped to the bottom edge of the tongue depressor. The tube and depressor are then attached to the foal's muzzle using tape or Elastikon (Elastoplast[11]), taking care not to prevent the foal from opening its mouth (Fig. 29-6).
    - An alternative method is to stitch the cannula to the foal's skin at the point it enters the nares.
    - Oxygen may also be delivered in the short-term by facemask.
- ***Practice Tip:*** *Oxygen should be humidified before delivery to the foal if given for >1 hour.*
  - The simplest way to achieve this is to bubble O_2 through sterile water.
  - Easily sterilized bottles, designed for humidification, are available commercially.
- Oxygen therapy should be started at 9 to 10 L/min and titrated according to the response of the patient and, if available, measured arterial oxygen tensions.

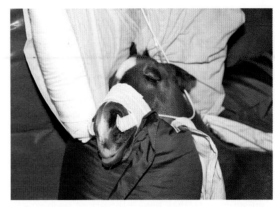

Figure 29-6 Intranasal oxygen in a foal. The oxygen tubing is measured to the medial canthus of the eye and then taped to a tongue depressor. The tongue depressor is attached to the foal using Elastoplast. (Copyright Veterinary Advances Ltd., 2012. From the iOS App "Foal Techniques." Used with permission.)

- If measuring arterial oxygen tension, the oxygen flow rate should be decreased if the tension is >120 mm Hg (16 kPa).
- Oxygen is not a completely benign therapy.
  - Inspired oxygen fractions of >60%, for more than 48 hours can result in pulmonary pathology causing tracheobronchitis, leading to acute respiratory distress syndrome (ARDS) and subsequently to pulmonary interstitial fibrosis.
  - This is believed to be mediated through oxygen free-radical formation; increased free-radical formation with increased inspired oxygen overwhelms scavenging capabilities. There may also be non–free-radical mediated injury through cellular metabolic alteration or by enzyme inhibition.
- ***Practice Tip:*** *It is very difficult to generate inspired oxygen fractions of >60% with intranasal oxygen therapy. Healthy foals receiving 10 L oxygen/min by nasal cannula have a Fio_2 of approximately 52%.*

Conclusion

Early recognition of foals needing emergency support is key to success. This is achieved through a review of the history to anticipate which foals are likely to require intervention, rapid clinical assessment of foals, and a high index of suspicion. CPCR, fluid resuscitation, and glucose and oxygen supplementation, applied judiciously, can reduce mortality and morbidity.

References

References can be found on the companion website at www.equine-emergencies.com.

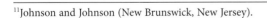

[11]Johnson and Johnson (New Brunswick, New Jersey).

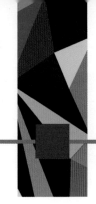

CHAPTER 30

Perinatology and the High-Risk Pregnant Mare

*Pamela A. Wilkins**

Important: Pregnant mares are considered at high-risk of a poor outcome when they have a history of problems during past pregnancies or have a new problem during the current pregnancy. As such, these cases can be classified as recurrent, historical, reemergent, or new problems resulting in a pregnancy being classified as high-risk.

High-Risk Pregnancy Classification

- Determination of current or recurrent threats to pregnancy aids in assessment and the development of a plan for that pregnancy.
- It is important that the team that manages the pregnancy, parturition, and postparturient care of the dam and foal are in place early and that the desires of the owner are clear. It is *not* unusual for the owner of the dam to plainly value one over the other, and knowledge of any preference for survival of the dam or foal by the owner is important to help direct any decisions made regarding management.
- A "decision maker" for the equine patient needs to be identified, along with reliable contact information for this person. This information should be clearly marked and readily available in the record.

Historical or Recurrent Problems

- Placentitis
- Premature placental separation
- Recurrent dystocia
- Recurrent abnormal foals
- Premature termination of pregnancy
- Abortion
- Premature birth
- Prolonged pregnancies
- Uterine artery hemorrhage

Current Problems

- Precocious udder development
- Placentitis
- Twin pregnancy
- Premature placental separation
- Over-term relative to past gestations

- Musculoskeletal problems:
  - Fractures
  - Laminitis
  - Lameness
- Endotoxemia:
  - Colic
  - Colitis
- Recent hypotension, hypoxemia
- Recent abdominal surgical incisions
- Recent anesthesia—mid-term is safest
- Uterine torsion—especially if >320 days pregnancy
- Development of body wall hernia
- Previous fractured pelvis
- Neurologic disease:
  - Ataxia
  - Weakness
  - Seizures
- Hydrops allantois, hydrops amnion
- Pituitary hyperplasia
  - ***Practice Tip:*** *Recommend discontinuing pergolide 1 to 2 weeks before foaling to allow adequate colostral production.*
- Chronic inflammatory diseases
- Lymphosarcoma or other neoplasia
- Melanoma in the pelvic canal
- Hypoparathyroidism
- Recent hemorrhage
- Small volumes of clinical bleeding from the vagina in older mares is generally considered benign
- Innumerable other problems
- Any critical illness in the dam, including organ failure

Threats to Fetal Well-Being

- Any problems exhibited by the mare should be viewed in terms of how it threatens *not* only the dam but also fetal or neonatal well-being. After understanding the risks to both, develop an action plan to minimize or eliminate the risks and execute the plan.
  - For example, critical illness in the dam puts the fetus at great risk, and the converse may also be true because a compromised or dead fetus may complicate the clinical course of a critically ill dam.
- Important physiological changes occur with pregnancy, primarily associated with the cardiovascular system and the respiratory system.

*With acknowledgment to Jonathan E. Palmer, who authored this chapter in the second edition.

- Late-term pregnant mares have a reduced functional residual capacity (FRC) in their lungs accompanied by an increase in minute volume, resulting in increased respiratory rates at rest that when combined with increased alveolar ventilation produce chronic respiratory alkalosis.
- The enlarged uterus limits lung expansion, contributing to the reduction in FRC and ventilation-perfusion mismatching.
- The reduction in oxygen reserve and higher rate of oxygen consumption (20% to 25% increase compared with not being pregnant) result in intolerance of apnea and a propensity for hypoxemia.
- Cardiac output during pregnancy increases 30% to 50% and is associated with higher resting heart rates and stroke volumes. Fifty percent of this increased output goes to the uterus, and the rest goes to the skin, gastrointestinal tract, and kidneys to compensate for the increased demands of pregnancy.
- During the last trimester, blood flow to the placenta increases tremendously in parallel with fetal growth because the late-term fetus has a much higher oxygen demand needed to support growth.
- *Practice Tip: A high rate of placental perfusion must occur for the fetus to receive enough oxygen, resulting in pregnant mares being at greater risk for severe complications should blood loss or hypovolemia occur.*
- Late-term pregnant mares have an increased plasma volume and a relative (physiological) anemia.
- Uterine blood flow is *not* autoregulated and is directly proportional to the mean perfusion pressure and inversely proportional to uterine vascular resistance.
- Blood gas transport is largely independent of diffusion distance in the equine placenta, particularly in late gestation, and is more dependent on blood flow.
- Information from other species cannot be extrapolated to the equine placenta because of its diffuse epitheliochorial nature and the arrangement of the maternal and fetal blood vessels within the microcotyledons.
  - For example, umbilical venous Po_2 is 50 to 54 mm Hg in the equine fetus, compared with 30 to 34 mm Hg in the sheep, whereas the maternal uterine vein to umbilical vein Po_2 difference is near zero. Also unlike the sheep, mare umbilical venous Po_2 values decrease 5 to 10 mm Hg in response to maternal hypoxemia and increase in response to maternal hyperoxia.
- The mare has total control of the fetal environment.
  - The fetus must receive everything from the dam.
  - There is *no* physiologic feedback for the fetus to communicate its changing needs to the mare.
  - The fetus can compensate for some changes brought about because of disturbances in maternal homeostasis but always at some cost to the fetus.
  - Threats to fetal well-being include the following:
    - Lack of placental perfusion
    - Lack of oxygen delivery

- Nutritional threats
- Placentitis, placental dysfunction
- Loss of fetal-maternal coordination of maturation
- Interaction with other fetuses, multiple pregnancy
- Iatrogenic factors
  - Drugs or other substances given to the dam
  - Early termination of pregnancy (e.g., induction)

Lack of Placental Perfusion
- *Practice Tip: Poor placental perfusion can be compensated for only in the short-term through redistribution of fetal blood flow, and the margin of safety in late pregnancy is small.*
- Whenever maternal perfusion is compromised, placental circulation and oxygen delivery may also be compromised; the result is a significant threat to the fetus.

Lack of Oxygen Delivery to the Fetus
- Causes of reduced oxygen delivery are as follows:
  - Decreased placental perfusion
  - Maternal anemia
  - Maternal hypoxemia
- In the horse, alignment of fetal and maternal vessels results in a countercurrent flow pattern.
  - The vessels are parallel to each other and the flows are opposite.
  - The venous side of the fetal capillary bed is aligned with the arterial side of the maternal capillary bed so that the gradient of oxygen and other nutrients is the highest possible.
  - This is the most efficient pattern for transfer of oxygen and nutrients and removal of waste products.
- Consequences of countercurrent flow pattern in the horse are the following:
  - Changes in maternal Pao_2 significantly change fetal Po_2.
  - Maternal hypoxia or hypoxemia may have a profound effect on the fetus.
  - Hypoxia and hypoxemia may predispose the foal to hypoxic-ischemic asphyxia disease and/or neonatal encephalopathy syndrome.
  - When maternal Pao_2 is increased with inhaled oxygen, umbilical Po_2 increases significantly, and the driving force increases, allowing more efficient transport of dissolved oxygen to the fetus.

➤➤ WHAT TO DO

Placental Hypovolemia/Hypoxemia
- Maternal hypovolemia must be managed aggressively.
  - Supplement the mare with intranasally administered humidified oxygen (10 to 15 L/min) (Fig. 30-1).
  - Increased oxygen delivery to the fetus may help with fetal hypoxia.
- *Practice Tip: Serious consideration should be given to blood transfusion therapy in the treatment of anemic mares to prevent fetal hypoxia. Loss of red cell mass impacts oxygen content of blood much more than does hypoxemia!*

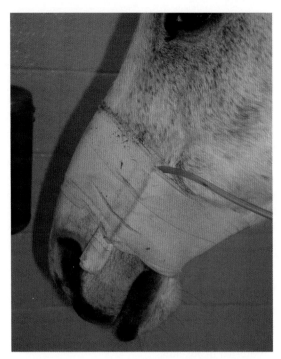

Figure 30-1   Intranasal oxygen insufflation in a mare.

Caution: Giving blood transfusions to a broodmare may predispose the mare to producing antibodies against foreign blood groups and puts successive foals at risk for neonatal isoerythrolysis (NI). This should be included in any discharge instructions so subsequent decision makers are aware of the increased risk.

Poor Maternal Nutritional State

- Chronic maternal malnutrition can be due to:
  - Lack of intake (because of lack of opportunity)
  - Malabsorption
  - Tumor cachexia
  - Organ failure
  - Acute fasting
  - Elective surgical procedures
  - Colic
  - The capricious appetite of the late-gestational mare
- *Practice Tip:* *Thirty to 48 hours of complete fasting in the late-term mare decreases glucose delivery to the fetus and increases circulating plasma free fatty acids, resulting in an increase in prostaglandin production in the maternal and fetal placenta.*
- Maternal and fetal placenta and fetal fluids contain a complex mix of prostaglandins that are believed important in maintaining pregnancy and may have a role in initiation of parturition.
- The risk of preterm delivery increases within 1 week of an anorectic episode; the foal often appears premature and *not* ready for delivery.

◉❯ WHAT TO DO

Maternal Malnutrition: Negative Energy Balance
- Support the mare's nutritional needs at the end of gestation.
  - Provide nutritional supplementation.
  - Encourage the mare to stay on a high plane of nutrition.

- Avoid acute fasting.
  - If the mare is fasted or becomes completely anorectic, start by administering glucose supplementation, 0.5 to 1 mg/kg IV per minute. Further parenteral nutrition may be required if the mare remains anorectic for >72 hours.
  - This negates the changes in prostaglandins and greatly decreases the risk of early delivery.
- When periodically anorectic mares are refractory to being encouraged to eat:
  - Treat with flunixin meglumine, 0.25 mg/kg IV q8h.

Placentitis/Placental Dysfunction

- *Practice Tip:* *The percentage of placenta affected is not a predictor of the outcome of the pregnancy; a foal born with widespread placental lesions may be better off than a foal with a focal placental lesion.*
- The presence of placentitis, no matter how extensive, is predictive of a serious problem because 80% of foals born from mares with placentitis are abnormal in some clinically detectable way.
- Placentitis is a common cause of late-term abortion in mares and perhaps the most common cause of a mare displaying high-risk pregnancy clinical signs of:
  - Precocious udder development
  - Premature lactation
  - Cervical softening
  - Vaginal discharge
- The cause is generally considered to be an ascending infection that enters the uterus via the cervix, although hematogenous spread of some bacterial and viral agents, equine herpesvirus-1 and equine viral arteritis in particular, is possible.
- Mares at increased risk of placentitis include those with:
  - Poor perineal conformation
  - Abnormal cervical anatomy, sometimes resulting from a previous birth trauma
  - Lower urinary tract disorders
  - History of vaginal/cervical examination performed late in pregnancy
  - History of being placed in dorsal recumbency while anesthetized and pregnant
- Common bacteria that have been isolated in equine placentitis/abortions include:
  - *Streptococcus equi* (subspecies *zooepidemicus*)
  - *Escherichia coli*
  - *Pseudomonas aeruginosa*
  - *Klebsiella pneumoniae*
  - *Nocardioform* species
- Fetal loss and premature delivery resulting from placentitis is not fully understood. Recent studies, however, suggest that infection of the chorioallantois results in increased expression of inflammatory mediators that, in addition to other local effects, alters myometrial contractility. Combined, these observations suggest that fetal loss can occur because of a compromised fetus, increased myometrial contractility, or both.

- Ultrasonographic evaluation of the uterus and conceptus per rectum and transabdominally can provide valuable information, particularly regarding placental thickness if placentitis is a concern (Figs. 30-2 and 30-3). (See Chapter 27 for more details on placental and fetal evaluation.)
- **Practice Tip:** *Fetal fluids can be evaluated and fetal size can be estimated from the size of the eye later in gestation.*
- Placental diseases that occur in late-term pregnancy include the following:
  - Premature placental separation
  - Placental infection/infectious placentitis
    - ○ Ascending pathogens:
      - Bacteria
      - Fungi
    - ○ Hematogenous spread of pathogens
      - Viruses
      - Bacteria
      - *Ehrlichia*
      - Fungi
  - Noninfectious inflammation
  - Placental degeneration
  - Placental edema
  - Hydrops allantois, hydrops amnion

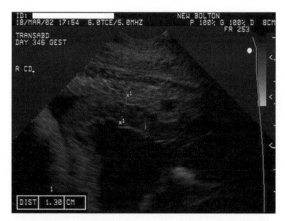

Figure 30-2   Transrectal ultrasonographic view of thickened placenta consistent with placentitis.

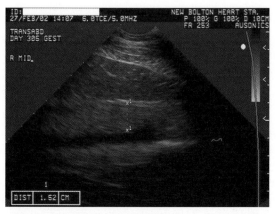

Figure 30-3   Transabdominal ultrasonographic view of thickened placenta consistent with placentitis.

Placental Insufficiency

- Treat all cases of suspected or proven bacterial placentitis/placental dysfunction.
- All cases of premature onset of lactation should be managed as such until proved otherwise.
- **Important:** Recognize early signs of placental dysfunction (i.e., premature udder development in placentitis, etc.) and if needed, measure acute phase proteins such as serum amyloid A (SAA) when placentitis is suspected. Early treatment for placentitis is important.
- Treatment consists of the following (see Table 30-1):
  - Administer broad-spectrum antimicrobial agents. Trimethoprim-sulfa drugs appear to cross the placental/uterine barrier, and recently, using microdialysis, gentamicin and penicillin were found in the allantoic fluid after administration to mares. If culture and sensitivity results are available from uterine discharge, directed therapy should be instituted toward the specific organism.
  - Nonsteroidal anti-inflammatory agents, such as flunixin meglumine, are used in an effort to combat alterations in prostaglandin balance that may be associated with infection and inflammation.
  - Pentoxifylline has been used for its rheologic effect, potentially improving blood flow within the placenta, and also for its general anti-inflammatory effect. **Note:** Absorption of orally administered pentoxifylline is reportedly quite variable in horses.
  - Tocolytic agents and agents that promote uterine quiescence have been used and include:
    - ○ Altrenogest (Regu-mate) is most commonly used.
    - ○ Isoxsuprine's efficacy is unproven and its bioavailability is variable and often poor.
    - ○ Clenbuterol is most indicated in managing dystocia and in preparation for assisted delivery or cesarean section; intravenously, it decreases uterine tone for up to 120 minutes.

Table 30-1	Drugs Used to Treat High-Risk Pregnancy Mares	
Drug	**Dose/Frequency/ Route**	**Indication**
Trimethoprim-sulfonamide	25-30 mg/kg q12h PO	Antimicrobial
Flunixin meglumine	0.25 mg/kg q8h PO/IV	Anti-inflammatory
Altrenogest*	0.044-0.088 mg/kg q24h PO	Tocolytic
Isoxsuprine	0.4-0.6 mg/kg q12h PO	Tocolytic; poor absorption
Clenbuterol	0.8 μg/kg as needed PO or slowly IV	Tocolytic; minimal clinical effect
Pentoxifylline	4-6 g/500 kg q12h PO or IV	Anti-inflammatory
Vitamin E–water soluble	5000 IU/d PO	Antioxidant

*Injectable progesterone in oil may also be obtained from compounding companies—0.8 mg/kg IM is recommended (see Chapter 27, p. 502); swelling at the injection site may occur.

- Three additional strategies can be used in managing high-risk pregnancy patients:
  - Provide intranasal oxygen supplementation (insufflation) to the mare with the goal of improving oxygen delivery to the fetus: 10 to 15 L/min.
  - Vitamin E (tocopherol) is administered orally to some high-risk mares as an antioxidant for placental/uterine inflammation and as a neuroprotectant strategy for the fetus. Recent evidence suggests that large (>5000 IU/day) vitamin E doses do *not* increase maternal vitamin E concentration more than smaller (1000 IU/day) doses.
  - Many high-risk mares are anorectic or held off feed because of their medical condition. These mares are at increased risk for fetal loss because of their lack of feed intake, which alters prostaglandin metabolism. Therefore, intravenously administered dextrose, 2.5% to 5% in 0.45% saline or water (5% dextrose), at fluid rates providing 1 to 2 mg/kg per minute dextrose should be given to these patients.
- ***Note:*** Few of the strategies just described are specifically aimed at the fetus, but rather in maintaining the pregnancy.
- ***Practice Tip:*** *Even if the pregnancy* cannot *be maintained to term, prolonging the pregnancy speeds development of the premature fetus and may improve survival.*
- Immediately following delivery, the foal should be treated for sepsis although treatment of the mare with antibiotics may prevent sepsis in the foal. Many foals born to mares with bacterial placentitis are not infected.
- In a compromised pregnancy in which clinical signs of early delivery do *not* regress with treatment, this therapy, with or without exogenous corticosteroid therapy, may be considered to increase the chances of fetal survival.
- Recently, evidence was reported that prenatal administration of adrenocorticotropic hormone and large doses of dexamethasone (0.2 mg/kg IV/IM q24h for 3 days) may be beneficial in advancing the maturity of the fetus.

Loss of Fetal/Maternal Coordination of Readiness for Birth

- Normal timing of parturition is decided cooperatively by:
  - Maternal events
  - Fetal events
  - Placental events
  - Dynamic interaction among these three distinct forces
- Loss of coordination results in the following:
  - A premature foal
  - A dysmature foal
  - A postmature foal

Iatrogenic Causes

- A major cause is poor timing of induction of delivery; in other words, *"open no womb before its time."*
  - Timed based on the calendar and convenience
  - Timed based on emergency considerations for the mare
- Maternal drug therapy
  - Drugs affect the fetus in a variety of ways.
  - Tranquilizers and analgesics (e.g., detomidine and butorphanol) have immediate (<30 seconds) and profound effects on the fetal cardiovascular system.

- Although drugs clearly indicated for the mare should be administered, the effect on the foal and possible alternative agents should be considered.

Twinning

- The mare is unique in being generally unable to support multiple fetuses.
- The reason for this is not entirely clear.
- Twins compete in ways detrimental to both mare and foal.
- One twin suffering from fetal distress may initiate early parturition.
- Twins increase the risk of dystocia.
- The presence or absence of twins can be readily determined in the late-term pregnant mare by transabdominal ultrasound.

Ventral Body Wall Tears and Hydrops Allantois/Hydrops Amnion

- ***Practice Tip:*** *Any late-pregnant mare that has a rapidly enlarging abdomen and an area of painful flank edema that progresses to the ventral body wall could be suffering from rupture of the abdominal musculature, the rectus abdominis muscle, or the prepubic tendon.*
  - These conditions occur together or separately in pregnant mares. Together, these defects are referred to as ventral ruptures and "body wall tears."
- Other clinical conditions with similar presentations include the following:
  - Hematoma: subcutaneous or intramuscular
  - Hydrops allantois/hydrops amnion as a primary cause leading to the rupture
- There may *not* be an obvious predisposing cause for these conditions. Some predisposing factors include the following:
  - Severe edema associated with the advanced pregnancy sometimes caused by increased uterine weight such as hydrops or twin pregnancy
  - Trauma in late pregnancy—appears to be more common in older, unfit mares believed to occur because of their size and Draft breeds. Affected mares are generally close to term.
- ***Important:*** Mares with hydrops conditions are more susceptible to developing ventral body wall tears.
- ***Note:*** Hydrops allantois is an emergency condition requiring attention in a short time interval to ensure the health of the mare.
- Secondary complications associated with intraabdominal hypertension may develop, leading to abdominal compartment syndrome, including:
  - Respiratory compromise
  - Hypovolemic shock at delivery
  - Body wall hernia
- Abdominal compartment syndrome is often noticed by the owner as a sudden onset of abdominal distention, with progressive lethargy and anorexia, and possibly dyspnea. Diagnosis is made by rectal palpation revealing an enlarged fluid-filled uterus; hydrops is confirmed by sonographic

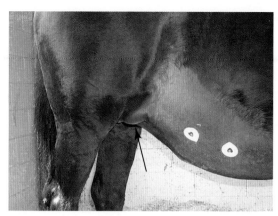

Figure 30-4 Mare with flank edema as an early sign of ventral body wall tear/rupture. Edema is highlighted by *black arrow*. Note fetal electrocardiogram leads on body wall as part of monitoring fetal well-being.

examination per rectum showing a large amount of allantoic or amniotic fluid.

- Body wall hernias and prepubic tendon rupture are usually detected by the owner as an abrupt change in the contour of the abdominal wall and lethargy and anorexia in the mare.
  - Mares with ventral ruptures may have ventral edema from the udder to the xiphoid cartilage of the sternum or only in the flank region initially (Fig. 30-4).
    ○ Some mares develop marked ventral edema without a known cause; in these cases, foaling is usually uneventful.
  - Mares with ventral ruptures have signs of distress and intermittent colic. If the pain is severe, there is an increase in heart rate and respiratory rate. These mares are generally reluctant to move or lay down.
  - Ventral body wall defects may easily lead to rupture of the blood supply to the mammary gland, disrupting its attachment to the body wall and causing bleeding of the adjacent musculature; blood may be detectable in the milk.
  - The udder may be displaced cranially and ventrally because of loss of its caudal attachment to the pelvis. The plaque of edema can almost obliterate the outline of the mammary gland.
- Ultrasonographic examination of the posterior aspect of the ventral abdomen and flank regions may be useful to detect the presence of tears or a hernia. Any defect in the abdominal musculature may be complicated by bowel incarceration.
  - All examinations are generally less than satisfactory because of the fetus and edema of the body wall.

◉› WHAT TO DO

Body Wall Rupture

- Initial treatment for ventral ruptures is aimed at stabilizing the horse by restricting activity. *Box stall confinement is mandatory.*
- Examine the mare for hydrops if the abdomen is rapidly enlarging in size.

- It is important to closely monitor for signs of blood loss, which can be significant.
- Monitor fecal production—generally decreased
- Continued discomfort suggesting progression of the tear
- Anti-inflammatory drugs, such as phenylbutazone or flunixin meglumine, may help relieve discomfort.
- Use of a suitable bandage (ReWrap BOA[1]) or CM Heal hernia Belt[2] around the abdominal wall, acting as an abdominal sling, may provide support for the ventral abdominal wall. Any abdominal bandage must be well padded to avoid pressure necrosis along the top!
- The possibility of bowel entrapment and strangulation should be evaluated, and surgical correction may be necessary if bowel strangulation has occurred. Repeated ultrasonographic examination of any entrapped bowel may be needed (see Chapter 14, p. 86).
- In a few cases, because of rapidly changing clinical parameters, the mare gains little from supportive treatment, and induction of parturition (or termination of the pregnancy in mares earlier in gestation) must be performed.
- *Practice Tip: If it is apparent that the mare cannot be maintained until term and the foal is >314 days of gestation, the administration of dexamethasone (0.2 mg/kg IV/IM q24h for 3 days) stimulates precocious fetal maturation and foal survival.*
- Pregnancy termination may be desirable in some mares with hydrops conditions or twins that present well before their anticipated parturition date even if ventral body wall tears have not yet occurred.
- Induction of parturition or cesarean section, *not* required to save the life of the dam, has been associated with poorer outcomes for the fetus because of lack of readiness for birth. *Practice Tip: The best outcomes for the fetus seem to be achieved with conservative management and assistance at the time of parturition.*
- *Practice Tip: The clinician should anticipate that assistance with parturition may be needed because the mare may be reluctant to lie down and/or may experience difficulty developing sufficient abdominal pressure during active labor.*
- Equipment needed for assistance with parturition and resuscitation of the delivered foal should be available.
- Clear communication with the owner should be established regarding whether the mare or the fetus is the priority because this crucial decision may determine the decisions made as the case progresses.
- Edema usually resolves quickly after foaling, and the mare can suckle the foal normally.
- Supplementation with colostrum or plasma is likely in cases in which the mare has leaked colostrum before delivery!

Idiopathic Factors

- Many foals born with hypoxic-ischemic asphyxial disease or neonatal encephalopathy syndrome have *no* history of known abnormalities occurring during gestation or parturition.
- Although it is easy to blame problems in the neonatal foal on complications occurring during parturition, most problems occur during the antepartum period.

NEO

NEO

Fetal Monitoring

Fetal Monitoring

- A biophysical profile of the fetus can be generated from fetal monitoring in the late-term fetus, making it easy to determine that the fetus is alive.
- Viability cannot be determined by itself because we are unable to determine if the fetus is ready to transition to neonatal life using current techniques.
- Obtaining a good image of the fetal heart requires:
  - Meticulous preparation of the skin
  - A 2.5 to 3.5 MHz transducer at 25 to 30 cm depth (see Chapter 14, p. 92)
  - Patience
- Currently, there is not enough evidence from large prospective trials to evaluate the use of a biophysical profile as a test of fetal well-being in high-risk pregnancies in human beings or horses.
- In human beings, a normal biophysical profile performed close to the time of parturition confers a large probability of perinatal survival and lack of acidosis.
- However, a normal biophysical profile does *not* guarantee a normal foal, nor does an abnormal profile always accurately predict an abnormal foal.
- The presence or absence of twins is also easily determined in the late-term pregnant mare by transabdominal ultrasound.
- The sonogram is performed through the acoustic window present from the udder to the xiphoid ventrally and laterally to the skinfolds of the flank.
- *Practice Tip:* *Imaging of the fetus usually requires a low-frequency (3.5-MHz) probe, whereas examination of the placenta and endometrium usually requires a higher-frequency (7.5-MHz) probe. Imaging the fetal heart generally requires a 2.5-MHz probe and depth of at least 30 cm. Transrectal ultrasound examinations are also necessary to determine uteroplacental integrity.*
- Locate the thorax of the fetus by the recognizable "striped" pattern caused by shadowing of the transverse processes of the vertebrae and the ribs. The heart is imaged as you move the probe away from the liver and toward the cranial thorax. The fetal heart is visualized within the fetal thorax and is generally the only beating object observed. If the heart is *not* beating, careful examination, ensuring that the entire fetal thorax has been seen, is usually needed to be positive of in utero fetal death.
- A complete description of this examination is beyond the scope of this chapter. (See Chapter 14, p. 92.)
- The value of this type of examination lies in its repeatability and low risk to the dam and fetus. Sequential examinations over time allow the clinician to follow the pregnancy and identify changes as they occur.

Comments on the Biophysical Profile

- Lacks sensitivity:
  - Fetus with normal profile may have a life-threatening problem
- Lacks specificity:
  - Extreme values are found in normal fetuses
- Information gathered about the placenta in conjunction with other critical information can be valuable.

Fetal Heart Rate Monitoring

- Ultrasound technique:
  - The monitor measures the rate only by calculating the difference between two beats; therefore, the results can be inaccurate.
  - Long-term measurements are *not* generally recorded, and the results may be misleading.
- Fetal electrocardiography (ECG):
  - Any ECG machine with recording capabilities works
- The fetal ECG is a companion to transabdominal ultrasonography.
- One can record fetal ECGs continuously using telemetry or more conventional techniques at planned intervals throughout the day.
- Electrodes are placed on the skin of the mare in locations aimed at maximizing the magnitude of the fetal ECG, but because the fetus frequently changes position, multiple sites may be needed in any 24-hour period (Fig. 30-5).
- Begin with an electrode placed dorsally in the area of the sacral prominence and two electrodes placed bilaterally in a transverse plane in the region of the flank.
- The fetal ECG maximal amplitude is low, usually 0.05 to 0.1 mV, and can be lost in artifact or background noise, so it is common to move electrodes to new positions to maximize the appearance of the fetal ECG (Fig. 30-6).
- *Practice Tip:* *The normal fetal heart rate has a wide distribution during the last months of gestation ranging from 65 to 115 beats/min. However, the range of heart rates of an individual fetus can be narrow.*

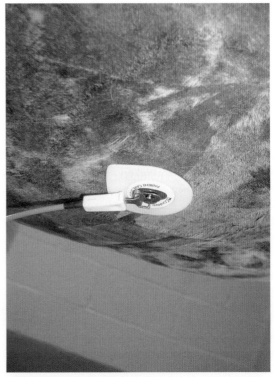

Figure 30-5 Fetal electrocardiogram lead placed on ventral abdomen of mare.

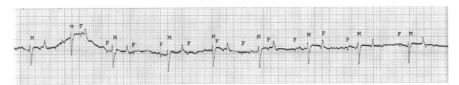

Figure 30-6 Fetal electrocardiogram tracing. Fetal beats are marked with *F,* whereas maternal beats are marked with *M.* Note the difference in amplitude and rate between fetal and maternal tracings. The fetal rate is ~2 times the maternal rate.

- If conventional techniques are used, recordings should ideally be made during a 10- to 20-minute period and repeated several times a day.
- If telemetry is used, paper recordings should be obtained at approximately 2-hour intervals to allow for calculation of fetal heart rate and observation of rhythm.
- ***Practice Tip:*** *Bradycardia in the fetus is an adaptation to in utero stress, most usually thought to be hypoxia. By slowing the heart rate, the fetus prolongs exposure of fetal blood to maternal blood, increasing the time for equilibration of dissolved gas across the placenta and improving the oxygen content of the fetal blood.*
- The fetus also alters the distribution of its cardiac output in response to hypoxia, centralizing blood distribution.
- Tachycardia in the fetus can be associated with fetal movement, and brief periods of tachycardia should occur in the fetus in any 24-hour period. ***Practice Tip:*** *Persistent tachycardia is a sign of fetal distress and represents more severe fetal compromise than bradycardia. Tachycardia, followed by severe bradycardia, can be observed terminally in some fetuses.*
- Dysrhythmias have been recognized in the challenged fetus, most commonly believed to be atrial fibrillation, but runs of ventricular tachycardia also are apparent.
- During the last weeks of pregnancy, fetal foals usually have the following:
  - All have a baseline heart rate between 60 and 75 beats/min; a low heart rate is in the range of 40 to 75 beats/min, and the high fetal heart rate (FHR) is in the range of 83 to 250 beats/min.

- Eighty percent have a low fetal heart rate <70 beats/min: 55%, low FHR <60 beats/min; and 14%, low FHR <50 beats/min.
- Eighty-six percent have a high fetal heart rate >100 beats/min: 50%, high FHR >120 beats/min; and 20%, high FHR >200 beats/min.

Important: Transient low heart rates <60 beats/min are common and should *not* be considered ominous unless they are consistent with *no* accelerations. Also, FHR transiently may be >200 beats/min. Transient FHR >120 beats/min is *not* threatening unless it is persistent and does not return to baseline levels.

●〉 WHAT TO DO

Abnormal Fetal Heart Rate

- Whenever FHRs are <60 or >120 beats/min throughout an observation period, repeat assessment within 24 hours or less is indicated.
- Beat-to-beat variability generally ranges from 0.5 to 4 mm, with most in the range of 1 mm. This beat-to-beat variability requires an intact central nervous system and functioning sympathetic and parasympathetic systems. When measuring the variation, periods when the heart rate is *not* accelerating or decelerating should be used for an accurate observation.
- The finding of *no* beat-to-beat variation in the absence of maternal drug therapy, which may sedate the fetus, is an indication of loss of fetal central nervous system input into cardiac function; repeat observations are indicated.

References

References can be found on the companion website at www.equine-emergencies.com.

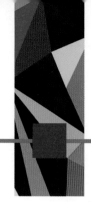

CHAPTER 31

Neonatology

K. Gary Magdesian

Physical Examination of the Newborn Foal

- Physical examination is fundamental to the workup of the critically ill foal. To fully understand the subtle changes associated with disease, one must be familiar with the physical examination findings and behavior of the healthy foal. Healthy, term foals are precocious neonates that can stand and nurse from the udder within 2 hours of delivery.

  Practice Tip: An easy rule of thumb is the "1,2,3" rule: most foals should stand by 1 hour, they should nurse by 2 hours, and the placenta should be passed by the mare within 3 hours postpartum. Normal vital signs change dramatically within the first 24 hours of life (Table 31-1).

- At 1 minute of age, the foal should have a heart rate and respiratory rate >60. By 1 to 2 hours after birth, the heart rate should be 80 to 120 beats/min, and the respiratory rate should be 30 to 40 breaths/min.

- At 10 minutes of age, a normal, healthy foal has an effective suckle reflex, can sit sternally without assistance, and attempts to rise within 20 minutes.

- A finger inserted in the ear or nostril results in a head shake and a grimace reflex.

- Thoracolumbar stimulation performed by briskly running the thumb and forefinger down either side of the foal's thoracolumbar spine elicits attempts to rise characterized by throwing the front legs forward, lifting the head and neck upward, and trying to push off with the hind limbs.

- The foal's heart rate at this age approaches 100 beats/min, and the respiratory rate averages between 40 and 60 breaths/min.

- A newborn foal that displays generalized hypotonia and an inability to rise, sit sternally, or suckle may be suffering from the following:
  - Peripartum hypoxia/asphyxia or other adverse peripartum challenge
  - In utero–acquired sepsis
  - Prematurity or dysmaturity

- A thorough history of peripartum events and careful examination of the foal and placenta help differentiate among these conditions.

- Scleral injection and mucosal hemorrhages (petechiae) are consistent with sepsis in the neonate, and these findings warrant consideration of sepsis until proven otherwise.

- Signs of hypovolemic shock in the neonatal foal include:
  - Cold extremities
  - Sunken eyes
  - Obtundation
  - Poor pulse quality
  - Pale mucous membranes
  - Unlike the adult horse, heart rate may *not* reflect hypovolemia in the form of tachycardia.

- At birth, the normal foal is relatively tachypneic and tachycardic, but this should resolve with time as the neonate transitions to extrauterine life. Increased respiratory rate and effort can be clinical signs of pulmonary or cardiac disease.

- *Practice Tip: Of the two signs, increased or abnormal respiratory effort and pattern may be the most reliable indicators of respiratory difficulty because foals with central respiratory depression due to hypoxia, hypothermia, hypoglycemia, or hypocalcemia may* not *have an appropriate increase in respiratory rate in response to hypoxemia or hypercapnia.*

Placenta

- *Practice Tip: A history of premature separation of placental membranes, prolonged delivery or dystocia, and meconium staining of the foal or placenta are periparturient events associated with acute or chronic hypoxia/asphyxia.*

- A maternal history of prepartum purulent vaginal discharge, precocious udder development and lactation, or evidence of abnormal discoloration of the placenta, particularly in the area of the cervical star, increases the index of suspicion for placentitis and in utero sepsis or fetal inflammatory response syndrome (FIRS) associated with abnormal cytokine release.

- *Note: A normal placenta weighs approximately 10% to 11% of the foal's birth weight. Evaluate unusually heavy (or light) placentas by means of gross and light microscopic examination.*

- Peracute cases of placentitis may produce only generalized edema without obvious areas of infection.

- Small placentas with large areas of abnormal villus formation have been associated with neonatal dysmaturity.

- Therefore, histopathologic examination of the placenta is strongly recommended if a neonate shows early abnormalities.

- *Practice Tip: Foals born with high serum creatinine concentration, especially when blood urea nitrogen (BUN) is normal, should be suspected of having had abnormal placental function in utero with "spurious hypercreatinemia." These foals should be evaluated and monitored closely for 3 days for signs of neonatal encephalopathy and sepsis.*

	Age		
Parameter	**<10 Minutes**	**≤12 Hours**	**24 Hours**
Heart rate (beats/min)	<60	100-200	80-100
Respiratory rate (breaths/min)	40-60	20-40	20-40
Body temperature (°F/°C)	99-102/37-39	99-102/37-39	99-102/37-39

Table 31-1   Neonatal Vital Signs During the First 24 Hours After Foaling

- The possibility of kidney injury in utero, although rare, is evaluated by urinalysis and renal and urinary tract ultrasonography.
- The serum or plasma creatinine in foals with spurious increases should rapidly decrease.

Prematurity

- *Definition:* Prematurity is a relative term indicating that the gestational length was inadequate for an individual mare.
- The gestational length in mares can vary widely (320 to 365 days); however, the individual mare has a relatively consistent gestational length from year to year.
  - Therefore, a foal born to a 320-day gestational length may be normal for one mare, while premature for another.
- Foals from abnormally long gestations can also exhibit signs of prematurity. The term *dysmaturity* rather than *prematurity* may be more appropriate in these cases.
  - These foals may be the result of intrauterine growth retardation, often the result of placental insufficiency.
  - Abnormally large foals occur in mares with prolonged gestation, often as a result of fescue toxicity; these foals are generally healthy in utero but may have an increased mortality as a result of high incidence of dystocia.
- Unusually short (<320 days) or abnormally long (>360 days) gestation has been associated with the birth of foals with signs of prematurity, including the following:
- Small body size
- Fine, silky hair coat
- Generalized weakness; hypotonia
- Increased passive range of limb motion
- Flexor tendon and periarticular ligament laxity
- Incomplete cuboidal bone ossification, usually in premature foals
- Domed forehead
- Floppy ears
- Inability to regulate body temperature
- Many premature foals have inverted neutrophil to lymphocyte ratios, with a neutrophil/lymphocyte ratio <1:1, unless they have experienced subacute to chronic intrauterine stress, in which case the neutrophil/lymphocyte ratio is normal to high.

- This is a better prognostic indicator for the premature foal than is the inverted neutrophil:lymphocyte ratio.
- *Practice Tip: Hypoglycemia is common in premature foals.*
- Some foals born after a prolonged gestation have slightly different clinical features, characterized by a large frame size with poor muscle development, erupted incisors, and long hair coats.
  - The physiological findings may be similar to those of dysmature foals, but these foals are considered "postmature."

Mucous Membranes and Sclera

- At birth and during delivery, it is normal for mucous membranes of foals to appear cyanotic; however, this should resolve rapidly as the neonate makes the transition to extrauterine life. The mucous membranes of a healthy neonate quickly become pale pink with a capillary refill time (CRT) of 1 to 2 seconds. Pale mucous membranes suggest anemia or hypovolemia, whereas pale yellow mucous membranes are consistent with the presence of icterus, as occurs with neonatal isoerythrolysis; hepatopathy; and occasionally, sepsis.
- Gray or slightly blue mucous membranes indicate shock, poor peripheral perfusion, or hypoxemia. Cyanosis appears only if the Pa_{O_2} is <35 to 45 mm Hg and only when the packed cell volume (PCV) is within the normal range. Tissue or organ damage may begin when Pa_{O_2} is <60 mm Hg.
- *Practice Tip: Do not rely on mucous membrane color to diagnose hypoxemia.*
- Hyperemic, injected mucous membranes and hyperemic coronary bands may indicate sepsis, systemic inflammatory response syndrome (SIRS), or fetal inflammatory response syndrome (FIRS). Petechiae on oral mucous membranes or inside the pinnae also are associated with sepsis and SIRS. Icteric mucous membranes may be observed with hemolysis, sepsis, hepatic disease or dysfunction, equine herpesvirus-1 (EHV-1) infection, and meconium retention.
- *Practice Tip: It is important to differentiate large- and small-vessel injection. Small-vessel injection imparts a generalized or diffuse, bright red appearance to the mucous membranes and suggests more severe disease.*
- The sclera should be white with only faint vessels apparent. Significant injection is indicative of sepsis/SIRS. Prominent scleral hemorrhages can also be observed after birth trauma, but this should rapidly improve over the first 2 to 3 days of life.
- Differential diagnoses for icterus in the neonatal foal include the following:
  - Liver or biliary disease: Examples are hepatic dysfunction as part of multiple organ failure resulting from sepsis, hepatitis/cholangitis (bacterial or viral, especially equine herpes virus, or congenital malformations), biliary atresia or dysfunction, glycogen branching

enzyme deficiency (GBED), Tyzzer's disease, and toxic or drug-induced hepatopathy.

- Neonatal herpes viremia
- Neonatal isoerythrolysis or other hemolysis
- Meconium retention (meconium is rich in bilirubin): Intestinal reabsorption of unconjugated bilirubin occurs and contributes to neonatal icterus.
- Septic foals may sporadically have increases in both conjugated and unconjugated bilirubin without evidence of liver dysfunction.

Cardiovascular System

- The cardiac rhythm of a neonate should be regular. However, nonpathologic sinus arrhythmia may be present for a few hours postpartum.
- Up to 15 minutes postpartum, normal foals may exhibit wandering pacemaker, atrial premature contraction, atrial fibrillation, ventricular premature contraction, partial atrioventricular block, and tachycardias.
  - However, the duration should be short (5 minutes) and should disappear within 15 minutes of birth.
- Heart rate averages between 70 and 110 beats/min during the first week of life.

Bradycardia

Bradycardia is associated with hypoglycemia, hypothermia, hyperkalemia, and tissue hypoxia.

●› WHAT TO DO

Hypoglycemia
- Hypoglycemia: Use a stall-side dextrometer or glucometer, available in most human pharmacies, to monitor or measure blood glucose (see Chapter 15, p. 111). The AlphaTRAK[1] has been validated for use in foals. Stall-side dextrometers may be inaccurate under conditions of high humidity or extremes of temperature.
- Avoid the temptation to administer a bolus dose of 50% dextrose.
- Introduce 5% dextrose as a constant rate infusion beginning at 4 mg/kg/min equaling a rate of 4.8 mL/kg/h of 5% dextrose.
- Increase the rate or concentration up to 8 mg/kg/min (no more than 15% dextrose) as needed to reach a target glucose concentration in the foal between 60 and 180 mg/dL.

●› WHAT TO DO

Hypothermia
- Carefully rewarm the foal.
- Unless bradycardia is present, the rewarming should occur slowly during initiation of other therapies in order to avoid rapid increase in metabolic rate; target approximately 1°F per hour.
- Heating pads, covers, heat lamps, and IV fluid warmers can also be used but should frequently be reassessed to avoid thermal damage or overheating.
  - Be careful of direct heat application in the form of warming pads because they may "thermally" damage the skin.

[1]Abbott Animal Health, Abbott Park, Illinois; www.abbott.us.

●› WHAT TO DO

Hyperkalemia
- Hyperkalemia is most common with anuric renal failure or uroperitoneum (ruptured bladder) but also occurs with massive tissue damage resulting from severe shock (sick cell syndrome, hypoxia/asphyxia) or muscular diseases such as white muscle disease. Hyperkalemic periodic paralysis and adrenal dysfunction are other differential diagnoses.
- Treatment of hyperkalemia is with potassium-free fluids (such as 0.9% saline or isotonic sodium bicarbonate); calcium (do *not* mix with bicarbonate; dose depends on ionized calcium laboratory results), add 0.2 to 1.0 mL/kg of 23% calcium gluconate diluted in saline once (no more than 50 mL 23% calcium gluconate per liter of saline or as guided by ionized calcium concentrations); dextrose (4 to 8 mg/kg/min), insulin (0.005 to 0.01, up to 0.1 U/kg/h of regular insulin); and sodium bicarbonate (1 to 2 mEq/kg diluted in fluids over ≥15 minutes; do *not* mix with calcium).

●› WHAT TO DO

Tissue Hypoxia
- The most common cause of bradycardia is hypoxemia or severe anemia leading to tissue (myocardial) hypoxia.
- Many foals respond readily to increased oxygen in the inspired air administered by means of a mask, intranasal insufflation, flow-by oxygen, or nasotracheal intubation and ventilation.
- In cases of severe anemia, as with neonatal isoerythrolysis, blood transfusion is indicated.

Tachycardia

- Tachycardia occurs with the following:
  - Sepsis or SIRS: Fever often is absent at examination in the neonate. Hypothermia is more common.
  - Hypovolemia, hypotension
  - Hypoxemia
  - Anemia
  - Pain: abdominal or musculoskeletal
  - Stress
  - Cardiac failure or congenital cardiac anomalies
  - Hyperthermia
  - Hypocalcemia: occurs with severe asphyxia

Murmurs

- Many foals have physiological flow murmurs that may persist for several days after birth.
- Soft, blowing murmurs usually are associated with turbulent blood flow and are exacerbated by anemia or alterations in hemodynamics.
  - These are typically grade III/VI or less in intensity.
- The typical patent ductus arteriosus (PDA) murmur is a continuous machinery murmur or a holosystolic murmur (most common) loudest over the left side of the base of the heart.
- *Practice Tip: Persistent or loud (>grade II/VI) murmurs; murmurs present for more than 5 to 7 days after birth that do not resolve or diminish in intensity; or murmurs associated with exercise intolerance, persistent tachycardia, or*

hypoxemia may be caused by persistent PDA, patent foramen ovale, ventricular septal defect (VSD), or another congenital heart anomaly and should be investigated further. Murmurs that are due to right-to-left shunts, such as a right-to-left flow through a VSD with tetralogy of Fallot, are seen in cases with severe hypoxemia that is oxygen unresponsive.

- Normal foals should have a 5:1 ratio for PaO_2: Inspired O_2% (FiO_2). Nasal oxygen at 5 L/min can increase FiO_2 to nearly 30%, which means the PaO_2 should be 150 or greater.

Peripheral Pulses

- Peripheral pulses should be easy to palpate.
- ***Practice Tip:*** *The metatarsal artery is the easiest site to access; other sites include the digital, caudal auricular, facial, transverse facial, and brachial arteries. Bounding, hyperkinetic pulses are associated with early stages of compensated sepsis/SIRS. Weak, thready pulses indicate cardiovascular collapse and shock.*

Respiratory System

- The resting respiratory rate of a newborn foal averages between 20 and 40 breaths/min; immediately after birth, the respiratory rate should be >60 breaths/min.
- Because foals have a thin chest wall and a relatively rapid respiratory rate, thoracic auscultation often reveals air movement throughout the chest and absence of crackles and wheezes even when there is lung pathology, especially diffuse interstitial disease.
- Moist end-expiratory crackles and "fluid" (large airway) sounds are commonly auscultated immediately after birth as the normal foal expands its lungs.
- Unusually quiet adventitial lung sounds associated with large airway sounds auscultated immediately after birth can be compatible with incomplete alveolar inflation and lung atelectasis.
- Significant areas of ventral dullness on auscultation and percussion indicate:
  - Areas of consolidation
  - Atelectasis
  - Pleural effusion
- Breathing effort should be minimal once the pulmonary liquid has been reabsorbed, which takes several hours.
- Areas of dorsal dullness when the foal is in sternal recumbency suggest the presence of pneumothorax.
- Neonatal foals rarely have significant pleural effusion, but this should be ruled out in cases of ventral dullness.
  - Pleural fluid may occur in the neonatal foal with:
    - Hemothorax; often secondary to fractured ribs
    - Bacterial pneumonia
    - Necrotizing pleuropneumonia
    - Chylous effusion
    - Cardiac failure
    - Uroperitoneum

Respiratory Distress

- Respiratory distress is exacerbated by recumbency and characterized by the following:
  - Nostril flare
  - Expiratory grunting
  - Rib retraction
  - Increased abdominal effort
- In paradoxical respiration, the chest wall collapses during inspiration. This is referred to as a *flail chest* and is a life-threatening medical condition that occurs most commonly when multiple (usually 3 or more) adjacent ribs are broken in multiple places. The flail segment moves in the opposite direction as the rest of the chest wall during respiration.
- In some cases, respiratory distress is associated with congenital upper airway abnormalities such as choanal atresia and subepiglottic cysts, warranting endoscopic examination.
- Rule out rib fractures (gentle palpation, ultrasonographic evaluation of ribs) in all foals showing respiratory distress or abnormal respiratory function. This is done early in the examination and before the foal is forcefully restrained.

Apnea

- Apneic episodes, slow respiratory rates, or irregular respiratory patterns such as apnea interspersed with tachypnea (e.g., "cluster breathing," ataxic respiratory patterns), are abnormal and are associated with the following:
  - Central respiratory depression resulting from asphyxia or extrauterine maladaptation—generally the most common cause in neonatal intensive care units
  - Hypoglycemia
  - Hypothermia
  - Prematurity

Diagnostic Tests

- Thoracic radiography and ultrasonography aid in identifying:
  - Rib fractures
  - Hemothorax
  - Pneumothorax
  - Pulmonary consolidation
  - Abscessation
  - Pleural effusion
- Arterial blood gas analysis is the most accurate assessment of pulmonary function. Samples are most easily collected from the dorsal metatarsal artery or the brachial artery (Fig. 31-1). The artery can be used for repeat sampling. A small, subcutaneous or intradermal bleb of 2% lidocaine (without epinephrine) just proximal to the sampling site makes collection easier for foals sensitive to arterial puncture. Special blood collection syringes for arterial blood also makes sampling easier (see Chapter 1, p. 4).
- If frequent monitoring is needed, rectal pulse oximetry can be used. ***Note:*** When using rectal pulse oximetry, be sure the recorded heart rate is accurate; if *not*, the oxygen saturation may be inaccurate.

NEO

NEO

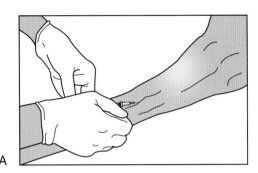

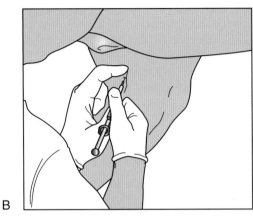

Figure 31-1   Arterial blood gas samples are most easily collected from **(A)** the dorsal metatarsal artery (located between MtIII and MtIV), or **(B)** the brachial artery (crosses the elbow cranial to the medial collateral ligament where it can be palpated).

- Upper airway endoscopy is valuable in assessment for congenital anomalies and laryngeal dysfunction.

Abdominal Cavity

- Absence of manure passage can be associated with the following:
  - Atresia coli: Suggested by lack of fecal-staining in enema fluid and the absence of fecal colored material in the rectum; white mucus may be present.
  - Meconium retention/impaction
  - Ileus
  - Intestinal obstruction
  - Ileocecocolic aganglionosis in white homozygous frame overo foals, the homozygous state of lethal white overo syndrome (see Chapter 13, p. 70).
- Because of the foal's thin body wall, distention of the small or large intestine results in visible, generalized abdominal enlargement.
- Simultaneous auscultation or percussion of tympany indicates the presence of a gas-distended viscus.
- **Practice Tip:** *Tight, tympanic, dorsally distributed distention is compatible with gas accumulation in the GI tract. Turgid, ventrally distributed, pendulous distention can be seen with uroperitoneum and peritoneal effusion.*
- Abdominal distention can contribute to cardiorespiratory failure by increasing intrathoracic pressure and reducing venous return to the heart, a phenomenon known as thoracic tamponade associated with intraabdominal hypertension and abdominal compartment syndrome.

Abdominal Auscultation

- Auscultation should demonstrate bilateral borborygmi. Ingestion of colostrum and the act of sucking itself enhance gastrointestinal (GI) motility and the passage of meconium and feces.

Meconium

- The first manure a foal passes, meconium, is composed of cellular debris, intestinal secretions, bilirubin, and amniotic fluid ingested by the fetus.
- Meconium is a dark, blackish brown color and is firm, pelletlike, or pasty.
- **Practice Tip:** *All meconium should be passed within 24 hours of birth and is followed by a softer, yellow/orange to tan "milk feces."*

Causes of Colic: With or Without Abdominal Distention

- Meconium or fecal impaction: Aboral or distal impactions usually can be found by means of careful and well-lubricated digital rectal examination, although abdominal radiography or ultrasonography may be needed to find more proximal (orad) impactions.
  - Many foals allow abdominal palpation. In these cases, if abdominal distention is *not* severe, meconium may sometimes be palpated.
  - Some foals have meconium retention without colic, particularly when they are obtunded or weak as with prematurity or hypoxic-ischemic injury. In these cases, passage of meconium/feces is delayed because of primary GI dysfunction, but it does *not* necessarily result in colic and is common in foals with peripartum asphyxia or sepsis. Such foals may be less tolerant of enteral feeding because of this meconium retention and remain so until the meconium impaction is resolved.
  - Foals with true meconium impaction may become uncomfortable because of proximal (orad) gas distention.
  - **Practice Tip:** *Meconium impaction is most common in colts that do* not *receive adequate volume of colostrum.*
- Enteritis (see Chapter 18, p. 220) is a cause of colic in foals, particularly in the early stages before development of diarrhea.
  - Fever and leukopenia are other clinical findings suggestive of enteritis.
  - Ultrasonographic evidence of thickened, fluid-filled small intestine with some motility is a diagnostic finding.
- Ileus can develop secondary to hypoxic-ischemic or asphyxial injury, sepsis, hypovolemia, prematurity, or shock.
- Intussusception may be found with ultrasound (target lesion sign) (see Chapter 14, p. 88).
- Gastroduodenal ulceration: Classic signs of this problem in older foals include rolling onto the back, sialorrhea or ptyalism, and odontoprisis (grinding teeth). The foals often have poor body condition.
  - Ulcers can be clinically silent in the neonatal foal.

- Peritonitis: Differential diagnoses include:
  - Ruptured duodenal or gastric ulcer
  - Other GI luminal breach
  - Enteritis
  - Urachal abscess or other internal umbilical infection
  - Chyloperitonitis, or peritonitis secondary to the presence of chylous effusion (typically mild or transient colic)
- Intestinal volvulus: Severe pain can progress to depression; abdominal distention, usually considerable, and reflux are common.
- Uroperitoneum: Increased amount of free fluid visible on sonogram.
  - Diagnosis is by measurement of concurrent peritoneal and serum creatinine concentrations. Peritoneal creatinine concentration is at least two times the serum or plasma creatinine concentration is diagnostic of uroperitoneum.
  - Most commonly, uroperitoneum results from rents in the bladder; urachal structures necrotic secondary to infections; and rents/tears in the ureters, kidneys, or proximal urethra.
- Pancreatitis is a rare cause of colic, diarrhea, and peritonitis in neonatal foals.

Diagnostic Aids
Nasogastric Intubation
- Perform nasogastric intubation to check for gastroduodenal reflux in foals with colic.
- Reflux can be associated with ileus caused by:
  - Ischemic-hypoxic intestinal damage, neonatal gastroenteropathy/neonatal necrotizing enterocolitis
  - SIRS
  - Peritonitis
  - Enteritis
  - Obstruction due to intussusception, impaction, volvulus, or duodenal stricture
- The presence of occult blood–positive reflux may be associated with:
  - Neonatal gastroenteropathy/neonatal necrotizing enterocolitis
  - Gastric ulceration
  - Enteritis caused by clostridial organisms or occasionally salmonellosis
- If severe gastric distention is present, passage of the tube beyond the cardia may be difficult. Lidocaine applied to the nasogastric tube or injected down the tube (monitor volume used to avoid lidocaine toxicity) helps relax the cardiac sphincter and facilitate entry into the stomach.
- Use the largest diameter tube that can be safely passed in cases in which the presence of reflux is suspected, but *no* fluid was obtained with routine tube passage.

Abdominal Radiography
- Abdominal radiography can be used to determine the location and the severity, but *not* necessarily the cause, of gas or fluid distention.

- Gas distention of the small intestine characterized by gas–fluid interfaces within the lumen can be found in foals with ileus caused by enteritis, peritonitis, neonatal gastroenteropathy, neonatal necrotizing enterocolitis, and small-intestinal obstruction (see Chapter 18, p. 191).
- Concurrent large-bowel distention is frequently associated with ileus caused by neonatal gastroenteropathy, neonatal necrotizing enterocolitis, or enteritis.
- Primary large-bowel distention occurs with obstruction caused by meconium impaction/retention, volvulus, or displacement. Sand or dirt accumulation can also be detected in foals with pica. Meconium can be seen in some cases of meconium impaction.
- Radiographic settings on portable and stationary machines vary a great deal and depend on the model and brand of the unit, cassettes, film-screen combinations, and focal distance. Consultation with a radiologist or radiologic technician is recommended for guidelines.

Contrast Studies
- Barium enema radiographic examination (barium mixed with warm water and administered by gravity flow through a cuffed Foley catheter inserted in the rectum) helps identify meconium impaction and may aid in the diagnosis of atresia coli.
- White foals born of frame overo heritage, or to two known carriers of the overo lethal white syndrome mutation, retain the barium with no or little expulsion from the anus. The diameter of the small colon is often reduced as compared with normal foals.
- Upper GI contrast radiography is used to document delayed gastric emptying and prolonged transit time that occur with ileus, obstruction, and gastroduodenal ulcer disease. This is particularly helpful in foals with gastric outflow obstruction/dysfunction due to ulcers or strictures in the duodenum.
- Contrast radiography of the upper GI tract is performed by administering 5 mL/kg barium sulfate suspension through a nasogastric tube. Serial radiographs are obtained 10, 20, 30, and 60 minutes, and 2 and 4 hours after administration of the contrast agent. Contrast radiography is used to find GI obstruction, ulceration, and delayed transit time. Normal findings are as follows:
  - Barium begins leaving the stomach immediately and is gone after $1\frac{1}{2}$ to 2 hours.
  - The cecum fills by 2 hours.
  - The transverse colon fills by 3 hours.

Transabdominal Ultrasonography
- Ultrasonography allows evaluation of the following:
  - Small-intestinal motility
  - Bowel wall thickness
  - Degree of gastric and small- or large-intestinal distention
  - Volume and character of peritoneal fluid
  - Assessment of urinary and umbilical structures
- Healthy foals have flaccid, motile, and apparently empty or mildly fluid-filled loops of small intestine. The wall

thickness should be <3 mm and there should be a minimal amount of peritoneal fluid.

- Round, fluid-distended loops of bowel can be seen with ileus, enteritis, and small-bowel obstructive disease.
- Enteritis results in a generalized increase in bowel wall thickness and edema, and there is usually at least some motility, although often nonprogressive.
- Severe neonatal gastroenteropathy or neonatal necrotizing enterocolitis bowel diseases can produce focal increases in bowel wall thickness with or without intramural gas accumulation (i.e., pneumatosis intestinalis).
- Small-intestinal intussusception has a doughnut-shaped pattern ("target lesion") caused by the telescoping of one segment of bowel into another; the intussusceptum invaginates into the intussuscipiens (see Chapter 14, p. 88).
- The presence of an excessive volume of clear, nonechogenic peritoneal fluid is compatible with uroperitoneum; however, comparison of abdominal to serum creatinine concentration needs to be evaluated for a definitive diagnosis.
  - Other differential diagnoses include effusions associated with intestinal diseases and cardiac failure.
- An increase in peritoneal fluid echogenicity is associated with increased cellularity with:
  - Peritonitis, possibly associated with uroperitoneum if caused by ruptured urachal abscess
  - Hemoperitoneum
  - Chylous effusion or chyloperitoneum
  - Ruptured abdominal viscus

Abdominocentesis

- Abdominocentesis is used to obtain peritoneal fluid for analysis and cytologic examination. It is indicated in foals when peritoneal effusion is present.
- The procedure is best performed by means of sterile technique and ultrasound guidance with a 20-gauge needle or a teat cannula/bitch catheter.
- *Practice Tip: Use care in performing abdominocentesis in foals using a teat cannula: omental herniation can result. An opening created by the procedure is sometimes closed with a cruciate suture after the cannula is withdrawn to prevent the potential for omental herniation. Needles can penetrate the intestine and should be used cautiously in foals. Perforation of the intestine can cause life-threatening septic peritonitis.*
- The finding of peritoneal fluid with an increased nucleated cell count and total protein concentration is consistent with peritonitis.
- Peritoneal fluid with a creatinine concentration greater than twice the serum creatinine concentration establishes a diagnosis of uroperitoneum.
- If there is distended intestine, abdominocentesis can result in bowel perforation and peritonitis; ultrasound-guided abdominocentesis is recommended in performing the procedure.
- Any peritoneal fluid collected may be tested for:
  - Creatinine concentration
  - Nucleated cell count
  - Total protein concentration

- Culture and sensitivity
- Cytologic analysis
- Sanguineous fluid should be measured for PCV to evaluate for the relative amount of hemorrhage.
- Peritoneal lactate and glucose concentrations may be useful in assessing peritonitis and bowel ischemia when compared with plasma concentrations.
- *Practice Tip: Amylase and lipase should be measured if pancreatitis is suspected.*
- Opaque peritoneal fluid is consistent with chylous effusion. Ultrasonographically it appears as an echoic effusion. The common presenting clinical sign is colic.
  - *Practice Tip: To confirm the presence of a chylous effusion, measure triglyceride concentrations. Chylous effusions have a high triglyceride peritoneal concentration compared with serum concentrations and a low cholesterol concentration.*
  - The leukocyte and total protein concentrations vary widely in chylous effusions. Typically, they are normal to mildly increased; however, in some foals chylous peritonitis is present with increased white blood cell counts.
  - In a minority of cases, the presence of chyle appears to be inflammatory.
- The differential diagnoses of chylous effusions or chyloperitonitis include:
  - Idiopathic causes—most cases recover with supportive treatment
  - Lymphangiectasia
  - Abdominal trauma
  - GI disease
  - Pancreatitis
  - Congenital malformation of lymphatics

Gastroscopy

- See Gastric Ulcers, Chapter 18, p. 181.
- Gastroscopy is used to document gastric and duodenal ulceration. *Practice Tip: Withhold food and water for at least 3 to 6 hours before gastroscopy to ensure adequate gastric emptying.*
- It is important that the stomach of the foal *not* be excessively filled with air during the examination because this can lead to or exacerbate colic. Insufflated air should be evacuated before removing the gastroscope. Resist performing gastroscopy without a clear indication (just to "have a look") because many normal foals exhibit signs of colic after the procedure because of the air introduced into the GI tract during the examination.

Urogenital System

- Palpate the umbilicus, inguinal region, and scrotum (in colts) for congenital hernias. The testes may *not* be descended at birth or may move back and forth through the inguinal canal.

Urination

- *Practice Tip: Time to first urination is generally 6 to 12 hours; fillies take longer than colts to void for the first time.*

- Because of a persistent frenulum, many colts do *not* drop the penis to urinate for the first week or more after birth: this is normal. Resist the urge to exteriorize the penis because this is uncomfortable for the foal, can cause penile or preputial trauma, and is *not* necessary.
- The specific gravity of the first urine produced usually is >1.035 because of fetal (in utero) urine. Within 24 hours the urine should be hyposthenuric <1.010 although it can occasionally be higher.
- Observe for urination closely to be certain the foal does *not* have a patent urachus, in which case urine "drips" from the umbilicus.
- Colts urinating in their prepuce may appear to have a patent urachus because the urine runs down the ventral abdomen and drops off the external umbilical remnant or may create one because of the umbilical stump being constantly urine soaked.
- Healthy, well-hydrated foals urinate frequently, often after nursing. Urine specific gravity is low in nursing foals (often 1.001 to 1.010) because of the high-volume liquid diet in the form of milk.
- Foals with peripartum asphyxia may have oliguria because of decreased renal blood flow and urine production (neonatal nephropathy) which warrants close monitoring of urine output.
- Dysuria or stranguria can be observed in foals with:
  - Uroperitoneum
  - Urachitis, patent urachus
  - Cystitis
  - Cystic blood clots resulting from umbilical bleeding
  - Urachal diverticulum
- Occasionally, foals with hypoxic-ischemic injury (peripartum asphyxia) cannot urinate despite greatly distended bladders. Such foals have stranguria and require indwelling urinary catheterization for 1 or more days until the micturition reflex normalizes in order to prevent bladder rupture.
  - Soft infant feeding tubes, Foley or Cook catheters (5F to 8F) can be used as urinary catheters.
  - Closed systems with sterile urinary bags are optimal. ***Practice Tip:*** *"One way valves," such as a condom with the end cut off, can be used on the end of urinary catheters in ambulatory foals where a closed system is impractical.*
- ***Note:*** A lack of urine production due to oliguria, anuria, uroperitoneum, or abnormal micturition reflexes is considered an emergency, and the cause is pursued when a euvolemic neonatal foal has *not* urinated for 2 hours or more. Foals receiving IV fluid therapy urinate at least hourly.
- Uroperitoneum associated with a urachal or bladder defect at the site of urachal attachment most likely occurs in the postpartum period in association with:
  - Infection
  - Shock
  - Internal umbilical remnant trauma

- Tissue hypoxia associated with poor blood flow
- Adverse peripartum events
- Urachal defects, or those occurring at the junction of the urachus and bladder, are commonly associated with urachal infections. Bladder rents can occur either during parturition or in the postpartum period.
- Signs of uroperitoneum include the following:
  - Decreased urination
  - Straining to urinate
  - Pendulous, fluid-filled abdominal distention
  - Varying degrees of lethargy and anorexia
- Large amounts of free fluid on a sonogram are consistent with uroperitoneum. Confirmation requires measurement of peritoneal and serum creatinine concurrently.
- ***Practice Tip:*** *Peritoneal fluid creatinine concentration at least 2 times the serum creatinine concentration is diagnostic for uroperitoneum. Measurement of abdominal electrolytes and cytologic analysis is supportive, but these are* not *as specific a diagnostic tool as measurement of creatinine concentration.*
- Rupture of a ureter or urachus (subcutaneous or intraabdominal) causes postrenal azotemia and may cause perineal or periumbilical edema, respectively. Ultrasonographic examination is also useful in these cases.
  - Ureteral rents demonstrate retroperitoneal fluid accumulation before abdominal effusion if recognized early.
- An unexplained syndrome of unilateral or bilateral hydroureter occurs in neonatal foals. Affected foals often present between days 3 to 7 of age with encephalopathic signs associated with severe hyponatremia.
  - Pseudohypoaldosterone was blamed as the cause in one case while several other cases have dramatically improved by catheterizing the bladder and ureter(s).
  - Transposing the ureteral(s) opening into the bladder at a location away from the trigone may be useful if a ureteral flap is the cause.

Umbilicus

- Examine the umbilical stump for signs of infection characterized by thickening or abnormal discharge. Many foals allow abdominal palpation and examination of the internal umbilical remnant by palpation.
- Transabdominal ultrasonography is used to measure internal umbilical remnants. Normal diameter in light breed foals 3 to 7 days of age is as follows:
  - Umbilical vein at external stump, <1 cm
  - Umbilical vein at liver, <1 cm
  - Umbilical artery at bladder, <1 cm
  - Umbilical arteries and urachus combined; transverse view toward stump, <2.5 cm

Omphalitis/Omphalophlebitis/Omphaloarteritis

- The microorganisms associated with umbilical infections include those associated with sepsis in neonatal foals. Gram-negative enteric and nonenteric bacteria, *Streptococcus* sp., *Enterococcus,* and occasionally anaerobes can be involved.

- Therefore, broad-spectrum antimicrobials, such as beta-lactam drugs (ampicillin, penicillin, ceftiofur, cefazolin, combined with amikacin), should be instituted before culture results are known if renal function is normal; serum creatinine should be serially monitored in foals on amikacin.
  - Ampicillin may have some advantage over the other previously mentioned beta-lactams because of better efficacy against many isolates of the genus *Enterococcus.*
  - Penicillin and ampicillin have increased activity over anaerobes as compared with the cephalosporins.
  - If renal function is abnormal, or the foal is experiencing hypoperfusion, ceftiofur or another third-generation cephalosporin is used. Adjustments in the dosing interval may be required for cephalosporins used in azotemic foals.
  - If anaerobes are suspected based on odor or the presence of significant gas shadows on ultrasonography, metronidazole is indicated.
- Treatment of umbilical infections consists of long-term use of systemic antimicrobials. Duration of antimicrobial therapy is dictated by resolution of clinical signs (fever, umbilical size, resolution of discharge if present) ultrasonographic findings, hematologic results, resolution of leukocytosis, and change in acute phase reactants such as fibrinogen (if it was increased).
- If the foal's clinical status deteriorates during medical management, or the ultrasonographic appearance of infected structures worsens or fails to improve with time, surgical resection is indicated.
- Surgical intervention is rarely needed with early and targeted antimicrobial therapy.
  - The exception is the walled-off abscesses that may be difficult to treat with antimicrobials alone.
  - Even if surgery is planned, 24 to 48 hours of antimicrobial treatment during the preoperative period aids in surgical resection by "reducing" the inflammation and periumbilical swelling.

Visual System

- A pupillary light response should be present, though is more sluggish in foals than in adult horses.
- A consistent menace response often is not present until 2 to 3 weeks of age.
- Newborn foals have decreased corneal sensation and may not appear painful with corneal ulceration.
- Some foals have decreased tear production and red conjunctiva associated with the "dry eyes"—keratoconjunctivitis sicca (KCS).
  - KCS should be treated with artificial tears and/or an antibiotic ophthalmic ointment.
- Mild, ventral medial strabismus is common.
- Examine the foal's eyes for corneal cloudiness, congenital cataracts, microphthalmia, or entropion. Foals with a silver hair coat color, particularly the Rocky Mountain Horse, Kentucky Mountain Saddle Horse, Icelandic, and pony breeds, should be closely examined for multiple congenital ocular anomalies (MCOA), including:
  - Ciliary or peripheral retinal cysts in heterozygotes
  - Iris hypoplasia
  - Enlarged corneas
  - Uveal cysts
  - Lens subluxation
  - Cataracts in homozygous individuals
- *Practice Tip: Ophthalmic examination may show a persistent hyaloid artery remnant coursing from the optic disc and spreading to the posterior lens capsule, often resembling a spider's web. This is* not *an abnormality and should disappear with time. Suture lines frequently are seen in the center of the lens.*
- Examine the retina for signs of detachment and hemorrhage, especially in cases of head trauma. Scleral hemorrhage can be associated with sepsis, disseminated intravascular coagulation (DIC), or birth trauma.
- The optic disc is round in foals compared with the elliptical shape in adults.
- Corneal ulcers are common in recumbent and weak foals. *Important:* All septic and peripartum asphyxia foals should be evaluated for the presence of ulcers with fluorescein stain.
- Entropion is common in premature and dysmature foals. Most of these cases are transient and respond to temporary sutures for a few to 20 days.
  - After local anesthesia, two to three single vertical mattress sutures are placed in the affected eyelid using 4.0 silk or nylon. Skin staples may also be used.
- Congenital cataracts can be removed surgically if determined to be congenital and *not* resulting from inflammation.
  - Phacoemulsification of the lens is highly successful and best performed in foals under 6 months of age.

Neurologic System

- Healthy foals are bright, alert, and responsive to touch and sound.
- While being restrained in a standing position, normal foals often alternate between periods of hyperactivity and struggling and episodes of sudden, complete relaxation (flopping).
- Foals should stand with an erect, angular head and neck carriage and a base wide stance in front.
- Their gait is exaggerated and appears hypermetric compared with adults, just as limb reflexes are increased compared with adult horses.
- When recumbent, foals have strong resting extensor tone and a crossed extensor reflex that persists for as long as 1 month of age.
- *Practice Tip: Foals normally spend approximately 50% of their time sleeping. When "sound" asleep, normal foals can be extremely difficult to arouse; this is especially common in miniature horse foals. Foals in "deep" sleep can also exhibit rapid eye movement, limb twitching, irregular breathing*

patterns, and vocalizing. To the untrained eye, this activity can be confused with seizure activity.

Neurologic Disease

- The most common cause of neurologic disease among newborn foals is peripartum asphyxia injury (hypoxia/ischemia) associated with:
  - Dystocia
  - Prolonged delivery or cesarean section
  - Damage resulting from cytokine release associated with placental inflammation/infection or neonatal sepsis
- These perinatal injuries (neonatal encephalopathy) can produce the following clinical signs:
  - Loss of menace response, central blindness
  - Fixed, dilated pupils
  - Nystagmus
  - Hypertonic, hyperresponsiveness ("jittery" behavior)
  - Seizure activity ranging from grand mal clonic seizures to tonic posturing, extensor rigidity, and focal seizures
  - Obtunded, stuporous mentation, even coma
  - Hypotonia
  - Abnormal respiratory patterns including cluster breathing and ataxic respiration
  - Failure to locate udder, loss of ability to recognize the dam
  - Barking noise or other abnormal vocalizations
  - Dysphagia
  - Dysuria
  - Wandering

Causes of Neonatal Seizures

- The most common cause is peripartum asphyxia (see below)
- Metabolic causes include:
  - Hyponatremia
  - Hypernatremia
  - Hypoglycemia: Foals often simply show obtundation and hypotonia
  - See specific disorders below in this section
- Hepatoencephalopathy: rare in neonatal foals
- Congenital malformations are rare (e.g., Dandy-Walker syndrome and hydrocephalus)
- Genetic/congenital causes:
  - Juvenile epilepsy
  - Lavender foal syndrome of Egyptian Arabians (see Chapter 13, p. 70)
  - Glycogen storage disease IV (glycogen branching enzyme deficiency) in Quarter Horses and related breeds (see Chapter 13, p. 72)
  - Epilepsy in miniature horse foals, ponies, and other breeds
- Meningitis: Antimicrobial and other supportive therapies are indicated. Pharmacology of antimicrobials should be considered, especially regarding blood-brain barrier penetrability. Third-generation cephalosporins (cefotaxime, ceftazidime, or ceftriaxone) are advantageous in terms of spectrum of activity and central nervous system (CNS)

penetrability. *Halicephalobus gingivalis* nematode infection (older nomenclature: *Halicephalobus deletrix, Micronema deletrix*) has been documented as a cause of CNS disease in foals younger than 3 weeks.
- Toxin- or drug-induced seizures: Aminophylline, theophylline, cimetidine, imipenem, and doxapram, for example, can cause seizures.
- Idiopathic epilepsy is treated long-term with phenobarbital or potassium bromide. Acute seizures are usually abolished with diazepam or midazolam.

Head Trauma

- If associated with neurologic signs such as obtundation to coma, medical treatment is instituted to restore adequate cerebral perfusion pressure and decrease intracranial pressure by ensuring the foal is well hydrated and normovolemic with good tissue perfusion.
- Adequate perfusion is ascertained before using osmotic agents.
- Oxygenation and ventilation are assessed using arterial blood gases. While hypoxemia is promptly treated, *hyperoxemia* is avoided.
- To reduce increased intracranial pressure, treat with mannitol (0.25 to 1.0 mg/kg as a 20% solution), unless there is severe, active bleeding, as suggested by CSF fluid or the presence of ongoing bilateral nasal bleeding and a nasal/sinus/guttural pouch source of hemorrhage has been ruled out.
- *Practice Tip: Plasma osmolarity is ideally monitored when mannitol or other hyperosmolar therapy is used to avoid persistent and severe hyperosmolarity.*
- *Practice Tip: Hypertonic saline should* not *be used in neonatal foals unless serum sodium concentrations are monitored closely. Neonatal foals have difficulty regulating high sodium fluids.*
- Dexamethasone is controversial and is currently contraindicated in the treatment of acute head trauma in humans.
- Dimethyl sulfoxide (DMSO), 1 g/kg IV diluted in 1 L of lactated Ringer's solution q12 to 24h, is used by some, although its use and popularity are dwindling. ***Practice Tip: Neonatal foals may*** not *eliminate DMSO as rapidly as adult horses; therefore, it can cause undesirable, persistent hyperosmolarity. DMSO solutions can cause hemolysis (rare in foals) and should be administered at no greater than 10% strength.*
- If multiple hyperosmotic agents (mannitol, hypertonic saline, or DMSO) are administered to the head trauma patient, they should *not* be administered concurrently because of concerns in causing excessive hyperosmolarity.
- Foals with head trauma or encephalopathy should have their heads positioned above the heart to avoid cerebral venous congestion.

⏺⟩ WHAT TO DO

Neonatal Encephalopathy

- Primary treatments include:
  - Supportive therapy: Maintain normal blood pressure and cardiac output with the goal of providing adequate cerebral perfusion.

- Physiologic homeostasis is the goal using vital signs and blood pressure as one indicator of clinical trends.
- Control seizures (see What to Do box).
- Begin early treatment with intranasal oxygen. Hypoxemia should be prevented and treated; severe *hyperoxemia* is best avoided in order to minimize potential oxidant damage. **Note:** Oxygen insufflation rates should be dictated by arterial blood gases.
- Other treatments include:
  - Balanced, polyionic crystalloids: Normosol R, Plasma-Lyte A, or lactated Ringer's solution (LRS)
  - Colloids: plasma
  - Dextrose in water, 5% to 15% to provide 4 mg/kg per minute of dextrose
  - Positive inopressor (inotropic) drugs:
    - Dobutamine: 2 to 10 µg/kg per minute (if fluids fail to normalize blood pressure and perfusion)
    - Norepinephrine: 0.01 to 3.0 µg/kg per minute (if dobutamine fails to normalize blood pressure and perfusion) to normalize arterial pressure with hypoxia or head trauma
  - Magnesium may have some benefit in reducing secondary or reperfusion injury, although its administration in *supraphysiological* doses (20 to 50 mg/kg infused over one hour followed by 10 to 25 mg/kg/hr as a continuous rate infusion/CRI) is controversial.
  - Vitamin C (see Equine Emergency Drugs; Appendix 9, p. 859) and thiamine (10 mg/kg slowly IV) may provide some antioxidant and positive energy metabolism effects, respectively.
  - Respiratory stimulants—Caffeine (10 mg/kg PO) or doxapram (0.5 mg/kg IV then 0.04 mg/kg/min for 20 minutes) for encephalopathic foals with hypoventilation and respiratory acidosis. Doxapram may increase heart and brain oxygen demand. These treatments are used when there is hypoventilation and severe respiratory acidosis, and mechanical ventilation is not practical.
  - High blood ammonia, secondary to constipation, can exacerbate neurologic signs; enemas and laxatives are indicated.

Hypoglycemia
See previous discussion and pp. 529-530.

Hypocalcemia
- Administer 10% calcium borogluconate, 1 to 2 mL/kg (Ca^{2+}, 9 to 18 mg/kg), slowly IV over 5 to 10 minutes diluted in crystalloids. Alternatively, administer 0.5 mL/kg of 23% calcium slowly and diluted in crystalloid fluids.
- Slow or stop infusion if bradycardia develops.
- Follow with a maintenance infusion of calcium: 10% calcium borogluconate, 2.3 to 5 mL/kg/day, or 23% calcium borogluconate, 1 to 2 mL/kg/day, diluted and administered slowly.

Hyponatremia
- Cortical (central) blindness is a common finding with severe hyponatremia ($[Na^+] \leq 105$ to 110 mEq/L).
- The seizures associated with hyponatremia are often focal in nature and facial only in clinical presentation. Jaw drop, or inability to raise the mandible or close the jaw, is very common.
- In more severe cases, the seizures may be generalized and blindness occurs.

- ***Practice Tip:*** *Hyponatremia should be corrected slowly to avoid central pontine myelinolysis.*
- In human patients, it is recommended that the plasma sodium concentration *not* be increased by more than 0.5 mEq/h, or 10 mEq/day.
- However, an exception is when hyponatremic seizures are present.
  - In these cases, the plasma sodium concentration should be increased by 2 to 5 mEq/L rapidly, to abolish the seizures.
  - Once the seizures abate, a slow correction (0.5 mEq/L) regimen is instituted.
- To raise the plasma sodium a few mEq/L quickly, commercial replacement fluids are administered. Plasma-Lyte A ($[Na^+] = 148$) or Normosol R ($[Na^+] = 140$ mEq/L) are preferred over LRS ($[Na^+] = 130$ mEq/L).
  - Physiological to hypertonic saline can also be used if these balanced commercial fluids do *not* increase the sodium concentrations fast enough to stop seizures.
- Once seizures stop, the rate of sodium correction should be slowed to 0.5 mEq/L per hour once plasma sodium is 116 to 120 mEq/L or greater.
- ***Practice Tip:*** *The more chronic the hyponatremia, the more important it is to slowly raise the serum sodium.*
- Sodium concentration in other cases of hyponatremia (longer duration or *no* seizure activity present) should only be increased at a rate of 0.5 mEq/L per hour.

●) WHAT TO DO

Seizures
- Immediately control seizures by administering benzodiazepines.
  - Diazepam: 0.04 to 0.2 mg/kg IV, up to 0.4 mg/kg if needed IV *or*
  - Midazolam: 0.04 to 0.1 mg/kg IV, up to 0.2 mg/kg IV
- An exception to the recommendation for benzodiazepine use is in foals with hepatic encephalopathy, where endogenous benzodiazepines are believed to contribute to encephalopathy.

Musculoskeletal System
- Examine the musculoskeletal system, including mandible, limbs, and ribs, for fractures resulting from birth trauma.
- Fractured ribs often are difficult to detect but frequently produce a clicking sound on auscultation, heard in synchrony with respiration.
  - Displaced fractures or those associated with hematomas or edema can be palpated.
  - Nondisplaced or minimally displaced fractures are detected using ultrasound.
  - Foals with fractured ribs should be kept quiet.
  - Foals with multiple or medially displaced rib fractures may be candidates for surgical repair, particularly if there is any evidence of internal thoracic trauma (hemothorax, pneumothorax) or if the rib fractures are located directly over the heart.
- Foals normally have an initial and transient, mild carpal and fetlock valgus conformation in the thoracic limbs.

Examine limbs for more severe angular and flexural deformities that may require surgical intervention.
- Palpate joints and physes for signs of swelling, edema, and heat (see Chapter 21, p. 301).
- Lameness should be thoroughly evaluated in the neonatal foal because septic arthritis, physitis, or osteomyelitis may be the etiology.

Dysmaturity, Prematurity
- Musculoskeletal signs:
  - Increased passive range of joint motion
  - Periarticular ligament and flexor tendon laxity
  - Incomplete cuboidal bone ossification (see Chapter 21, p. 309; detectable only on radiographs) of carpus and tarsus. The navicular bone and epiphyses of long bones should also be evaluated in very premature foals.
- Foals with incomplete ossification of the cuboidal bones, epiphyses, or navicular bones should *not* be allowed to exercise without some support of their body weight during physical therapy.
  - Severely affected foals are often maintained in a recumbent position in a small foal box, with frequent body position changes, rotating every 2 hours. They are allowed to stand for a few minutes every 1 to 2 hours, initially only with assistance (supported under the sternum and tuber ischii) in order to reduce the compressive forces on their limbs and to prevent crushing of the ossifying bones.
  - Tube casts and splinting are generally not recommended for these cases because they contribute to laxity of the supporting structures and may be associated with increased morbidity from cast sores; if used, change them frequently.
  - Casts can be made to end just above the fetlock to minimize development of the ligament and tendon laxity.
- Angular limb deformities should be corrected early in affected foals to avoid abnormal compression of the immature cartilaginous bones. Standing on slippery floors is to be avoided!

Severe Flexor Tendon Laxity
- Treatment includes the following:
  - Controlled exercise
  - Shoes with heel extensions
  - "Light" protective wraps if weight bearing results in trauma to heel bulbs and fetlock, but keep in mind that wraps can compound laxity

Limb Contracture/Congenital Flexural Deformity
- Contracture and deformity can involve proximal (carpus, tarsus) or more distal (fetlocks, pasterns) joints.
- Tendon contracture is associated with:
  - In utero malpositioning
  - Toxins such as Sudan pasture
  - Genetic causes (Norwegian Fjord horses)
  - Neonatal hypothyroidism

Limb Contracture/Congenital Flexural Deformity
- Mild cases of contracture often respond to stall confinement and support wraps.
- Additional treatments for contracted tendons include physical therapy, systemic analgesics, Robert Jones wraps, and controlled (limited) exercise to prevent worsening of contracture and extensor tendon rupture.
- Moderate to severe cases include the use of toe extensions (for distal limb contracture) and splints along with the bandages.
- Severely affected cases may benefit from the administration of supra-antimicrobial doses of oxytetracycline (1 to 3 g, or 20 to 60 mg/kg IV q24 to 36h for a maximum of 3 doses) in addition to the previously mentioned treatments. *Practice Tip: Oxytetracycline should be administered as a dilute solution in fluids. Measuring serum creatinine concentration before and after each treatment is ideal and should be done if repeated doses are needed.*
- *Caution:* Acute anuric-to-oliguric renal failure is occasionally reported to occur after treatment with this higher dose oxytetracycline. Concurrent intravenous administration of fluids is recommended if there are any concerns about concurrent dehydration.
- Casting and splinting are associated with exacerbation of lateral laxity, may promote the development of rubs and pressure sores, and should be used with great attention to monitoring skin and limb integrity.
- Rupture of the common digital extensor tendon (CDET) may occur with significant carpal contracture and has been reported associated with hypothyroidism, forelimb contracture, and mandibular prognathism.
  - Serum thyroid hormone concentrations should be measured in affected foals.
  - Treatment for rupture of the CDET consists of stall confinement and the use of support wraps. A firm fetlock bandage extends the digit and assists the foal in foot placement.
  - Splints may be needed for foals that are unable to advance or extend the limb or that frequently knuckle over at the fetlock.
  - The ruptured tendon ends heal, presumably with fibrosis, and the foals generally have an excellent prognosis for soundness. Early and aggressive treatment is recommended to minimize the possible sequelae of fetlock subluxation.
- Rupture of the gastrocnemius muscle may occur in neonatal foals causing inability to stand and swelling (hematoma) at the proximal insertion of the tendon at the caudal thigh. Some of the foals have a history of a dystocia delivery.
  - There is disruption of the reciprocal mechanism on flexing the stifle and hock.
  - For mild gastrocnemius injury, exercise restriction by forced recumbency, with minimal or *no* bandaging, may be sufficient treatment.
  - For more severe disruption of the muscle, limb stabilization by splinting and intensive nursing and monitoring are needed.
  - As the hematoma resolves and healing of the tendon insertion begins, some physical therapy is recommended for a normal range of motion after healing.

Septic Arthritis
- Lameness is usually present, although septic arthritis/physitis can be difficult to identify in weak or recumbent foals. Careful, frequent palpation and visual assessment of

all joints and growth plate regions are warranted in such foals.

- ***Practice Tip:*** *If a neonatal foal becomes acutely lame, septic arthritis should be the top differential diagnosis unless another cause is positively identified; too often an overly optimistic diagnosis of "the foal might have been stepped on by the mare" is made, and early and important treatment of septic arthritis is delayed.*
- Fever is variable.
- Painful, warm joint effusion is frequently accompanied by significant leukocytosis and hyperfibrinogenemia. Osteomyelitis commonly is associated with marked hyperfibrinogenemia (>800 mg/dL).
- Radiographs of affected joints are indicated to evaluate for concurrent septic physitis or osteomyelitis. Ultrasonography, computed tomography, or magnetic resonance imaging can aid in diagnosis of bone infections when equivocal results are obtained radiographically.
- Arthrocentesis reveals a neutrophilic pleocytosis and increased total protein concentration.
  - Neonatal foals with septic arthritis may *not* develop as great an elevation in white blood cell count as adult horses. Synovial fluid leukocyte counts of ≥10,000 cells/µL are indicative of sepsis in the foal.
  - Synovial fluid lactate, glucose concentrations, and pH are helpful adjuncts in evaluating for sepsis; lactate increases, whereas glucose and pH decrease relative to serum/plasma concentrations of these analytes.

WHAT TO DO

Treatment of Septic Arthritis

- Treatment of septic arthritis is with systemic antimicrobial therapy and joint lavage using balanced electrolyte solutions with 10 g DMSO added per 1 L.
  - Small volumes of an antimicrobial (amikacin, 250 mg per joint) can be instilled in the joint after lavage, but the total dose should be monitored.
  - Arthroscopic examination and lavage is indicated in joints where fibrin deposition or osteomyelitis is suspected.
  - ***Note:*** Regional limb perfusion, using one third the calculated total systemic dose of aminoglycoside, is indicated in some cases (see Chapter 5, p. 16).
  - ***Practice Tip:*** *The total daily dose of amikacin should not exceed 25 mg/kg for either intraarticular injection or regional limb perfusion. The balance of the dose can be administered simultaneously with the release of the tourniquet after regional limb perfusion has been completed.*
  - Ideally, amikacin therapy is guided by therapeutic drug (i.e., peak and trough concentrations) and renal function monitoring (i.e., serial creatinine and BUN) in affected foals.
  - Some severe osteomyelitis cases may benefit from debridement of affected bone or other more invasive procedures.
  - Intraosseous and intraphyseal perfusion, especially if there is a septic physis, is an alternative route when intravenous perfusion is *not* possible.
- Continuous intrasynovial antimicrobial infusion has been studied recently for use in equine septic joints and appears to be an effective adjunct.

Septic Osteomyelitis

- Foals present with variable lameness.
- Fever is inconsistent (intermittent).
- There may be painful swelling/edema over the physis, epiphysis proximal to the joint, or at site of bone infection with or without secondary sympathetic joint effusion. If joint effusion cannot be readily palpated, consider less commonly affected joints (distal interphalangeal or scapulohumeral).
- Radiographic evidence of periosteal osteolytic and proliferative changes is often present.
- Leukocytosis and hyperfibrinogenemia (often >800 mg/dL) usually accompany the clinical condition.

WHAT TO DO

Prognosis

- Treat with long-term antimicrobial therapy; aspirate physis for culture and sensitivity if septic physitis is present. Antimicrobials can be injected directly into the septic physis.
- Use nonsteroidal anti-inflammatory drugs conservatively to provide analgesia and decrease inflammation. Ketoprofen (1 to 2 mg/kg IV q24h) and flunixin meglumine may be associated with reduced risk of adverse effects, including gastrointestinal and renal toxicity, as compared with phenylbutazone. Carprofen (0.7 to 1.4 mg/kg IV or PO q24h) is another option, but it requires study in foals. Recently, firocoxib has been studied in the neonatal foal and is an alternative, particularly in those foals with renal compromise.
- Regional limb perfusion, using one third the calculated total dose of aminoglycoside, is indicated in many cases. The total daily dose of amikacin should *not* exceed 25 mg/kg, and is optimally guided by therapeutic drug monitoring. The balance of the dose is administered at the time of tourniquet release. Renal function (creatinine and BUN) is monitored closely in foals receiving amikacin.
- Some severe cases of osteomyelitis may benefit from surgical debridement of affected bone. Support of the unaffected limbs with support wraps is recommended to prevent limb deformities when a severe lameness is present in another limb.
- The need for long-term analgesia with nonsteroidal anti-inflammatory drugs should prompt prophylaxis for gastric and duodenal ulcer disease in the care of these patients (see Chapter 18, p. 181).
- A recent study (Neil KM et al, 2010) reported the prognosis for survival of foals with septic osteomyelitis to be favorable (80.6% discharge from hospital). In addition, 65.8% of those discharged (48% of those treated) ultimately raced. Multiple septic joints, but *not* multiple bone involvement, had an unfavorable prognosis for racing; however, both led to a decreased discharge from the hospital.

Nursing Behavior

- A healthy foal consumes upward of 15% to 25% of its body weight in milk daily with an average daily weight gain of 1 to 3 lb (0.45 to 1.35 kg).
- Foals nurse, on average, seven times per hour during the first week of life. As they age, the nursing frequency decreases. At 24 weeks of age, the nursing frequency is once per hour.
- ***Practice Tip:*** *Udder distention and milk streaming in the mare are some of the earliest signs of a "fading foal" that is no longer nursing effectively.*

- Milk dripping from a foal's nose after nursing may be the result of the following:
  - Cleft palate: Although it has to be ruled out, cleft palate is one of the least common causes of dysphagia among foals. Upper airway endoscopy is an excellent diagnostic method to rule out a cleft palate.
  - Subepiglottic cyst
  - Persistent or restricted epiglottic frenulum
  - Dorsal displacement of the soft palate
  - Generalized weakness caused by sepsis/SIRS/FIRS or dysmaturity is common
  - Dysphagia associated with perinatal asphyxial syndrome is common
  - White muscle disease is common in certain geographic regions
  - Esophageal pooling of milk (megaesophagus or branchial arch defect)
  - Transient pharyngeal paresis (idiopathic) may resolve in a few to several days or persist, requiring the foal to be bucket fed. This condition is common in some regions and breeds.
  - Congenital fourth branchial arch defects may cause milk to reflux from the esophagus. Diagnosis is made by endoscopy and observing the pharyngeal arch "hanging" over the right dorsal arytenoid. A physical defect in the area just dorsal to the right larynx is palpable externally.

Nutrition

- The caloric requirements of the healthy, active foal are approximately 120 to 150 kcal/kg per day.
- **Practice Tip:** *Sick neonates, such as foals with sepsis or peripartum asphyxia injury, often have reduced caloric needs because of inactivity and recumbency.*
- Feeding excessive calories is potentially harmful in septic human patients because these calories can be used to drive the inflammatory response. **Note:** Preliminary investigations using indirect calorimetry suggest that sick and nonexercising (orphan) foals have reduced resting energy requirements, as low as 40 to 55 kcal/kg per day.
- **Practice Tip:** *Mare's milk is the optimal food source for foals. Mare's milk has approximately 500 kcal/L of milk. To provide 50 kcal/kg per day to a critically ill foal, a total of 2500 kcal is needed for a 50-kg foal, equaling 5 L of milk. This is equivalent to 10% of body weight in milk.* If the foal does *not* gain weight on this volume of milk and the GI tract is normal, a larger volume of milk is fed.
- Alternatives for orphan foals include:
  - Commercial milk replacers
  - Goat's milk
- Goat's milk alone may predispose the foal to constipation and metabolic acidosis. A 1 : 1 mixture of foal milk replacer and goat's milk is preferred.
- Foals should be fed small amounts frequently because milk serves as a buffer for gastric pH, and increased frequency of small volume feedings are particularly necessary in foals with subnormal GI motility.

- It is optimal to divide the daily requirement into small feedings every 2 hours or more frequently. Please see section on nutritional support and parenteral nutrition for more information (see Chapter 51, p. 548).

Catheterization and Blood Sampling

- The jugular vein is the most common site for venipuncture in an awake, active foal.
- In more depressed foals, the saphenous and cephalic veins are used.
- Sites for arterial blood gas sampling include the dorsal metatarsal (first choice); brachial; transverse facial; facial; and less frequently, the brachial or caudal auricular arteries (Fig. 31-1, p. 532).

Triage of the Critically Ill Foal: Emergency Stabilization

●❯ WHAT TO DO

Emergency Stabilization

- **Practice Tip:** *Refer to this list as the "5 Hypo's" for ease of memory. Regardless of cause or underlying disease, the following guidelines are applied to most weak, recumbent foals.*
- **#1**—Hypoxemia: Defined as Pao_2 <70 mm Hg in lateral recumbency, <80 mm Hg in sternal recumbency on room air (pulse oximeter reading <95%)
  - Administer oxygen insufflation via nasal cannula at 5 to 10 L/min for an average-sized foal, 100 to 200 mL/kg/min.
  - Keep the foal sternal.
  - The nasal cannula is placed at the level of the medial canthus.
  - Mechanical ventilation is performed if these interventions are inadequate or if the foal is fatigued from respiratory distress.
  - The most common causes of hypoxemia in the neonatal foal include ventilation-perfusion mismatch and hypoventilation.
  - Right-to-left cardiac or pulmonary shunt should be suspected with poor response to increasing inspired oxygen concentration through nasal insufflation.
  - See Chapter 25, pp. 454-455, for more information on ventilatory support.
- **#2**—*Hypercapnia:* Defined as $Paco_2$ >55 mm Hg and pH ≤7.25 or central narcosis
  - Keep foal in sternal recumbency; provide chemical stimulation of ventilation with caffeine or doxapram for central origin hypoventilation (neurogenic).
  - Provide manual or mechanical ventilation if foal is in respiratory failure (muscle fatigue, neuromuscular disease, severe respiratory disease).
  - Causes of hypoventilation include rib fractures, neurologic disorders (peripartum asphyxia), neuromuscular disease (botulism, which occurs most commonly in foals nearly 4 weeks of age), muscular disorders (white muscle disease or HYPP), airway obstruction, severe pulmonary disease, and pleural disorders (pneumothorax, effusion).
- **#3**—*Hypovolemia:* Clinical findings of hypovolemia in neonatal foals include obtundation/depression, cold extremities, poor pulse quality, prolonged CRT, pale mucous membranes, and delayed jugular fill.
  - Monitoring tools that indicate hypovolemia include low arterial blood pressure, low central venous pressure, and decreased urine output.

- Laboratory indicators include hyperlactatemia, high PCV, metabolic acidemia with high anion gap, and increased oxygen extraction ratio (decreased venous oxygen saturation).
- Treatment is with the "fluid challenge" technique:
  ○ Administer 10 to 20 mL/kg of isotonic crystalloid such as lactated Ringer's solution, Plasma-Lyte A or 148, Normosol R, or isotonic saline 0.9%, and then reassess. Monitor sodium if high [Na⁺] fluids are administered.
  ○ *Practice Tip: If hyperkalemia is suspected (uroperitoneum, hyperkalemic periodic paralysis [HYPP], acute renal failure, severe rhabdomyolysis, or adrenal insufficiency) potassium-free fluids, saline, or isotonic sodium bicarbonate are optimal fluid replacements.*
  ○ Reassessment of perfusion parameters, both clinical and laboratory, and serial monitoring, dictates the need for more fluid volume.
  ○ Each subsequent bolus is administered at a slower rate than the preceding.
  ○ Though central venous pressure (CVP) is *not* an accurate goal of fluid therapy (i.e., normal CVP does *not* necessarily mean euvolemia) it is a reasonable ceiling or limit to fluid therapy.
  ○ Reaching a CVP of 10 to 12 cm H_2O (7.4 to 8.8 mm Hg) should guide discontinuation of bolus fluid administration.
- If hypoproteinemia or failure of passive transfer is present, plasma should also be administered (3 to 20 mL/kg) depending on IgG status. Plasma should be administered slowly, especially initially, to monitor for adverse effects, including fasciculations, tachypnea, tachycardia, fever, or colic.
- Monitor colloid osmotic pressure and coagulation parameters.
- **#4**—Hypoglycemia:
  - Administer 4 mg/kg/min dextrose (or up to 8 mg/kg/min if severe hypoglycemia is present) by fluid pump as constant rate infusion (CRI), or spike fluids to a percentage that provides 4 mg/kg/min with the volume infused.
  - *Practice Tip: If a 20-mL/kg crystalloid bolus is being administered over 30 minutes, then the dextrose percentage can be 0.6% to 12% depending upon blood glucose values. Spiking bolus fluids with 5% dextrose often results in hyperglycemia; therefore a lesser percent than 5% is recommended for a maintenance rate of fluid administration.*
- **#5**—Hypothermia:
  - Provide slow warming of body temperature, while hypovolemia and hypoglycemia are corrected.
  - Mild hypothermia is protective of cerebral function and against reperfusion injury in other species.
  - Strive for a rate of increase of body temperature to be 1°F per hour, unless considerable hypothermia is present (associated with bradycardia), in which case faster rewarming is indicated.

Generalized Weakness, Loss of Suckle

The most common causes of weakness and reluctance to suckle among newborn foals are the following:

- FIRS
- Sepsis/ SIRS
- Peripartum asphyxia
- Prematurity, dysmaturity
- There are several additional causes, including enteritis, uroperitoneum, myositis, renal or liver disease, and colic

Fetal Inflammatory Response Syndrome (FIRS)

- FIRS was described in human perinatology and is applicable to foals, characterized by a condition of systemic inflammation in the fetus and an increase in fetal plasma inflammatory cytokines.
- In humans, FIRS is characterized specifically by an increase in fetal plasma interleukin-6. It has been observed in fetuses with:
  - Preterm labor and intact placental membranes
  - Premature rupture of fetal membranes
  - Fetal viral infections such as cytomegalovirus in humans
- In horses, FIRS likely is present in foal fetuses with:
  - Premature placental separation
  - Placentitis, EHV-1, or equine viral arteritis infection
  - Prematurity
- In human pediatrics, FIRS is a risk factor for short-term mortality and long-term sequelae such as bronchopulmonary dysplasia and even brain injury. Short-term morbidity of FIRS in human infants, which can also contribute to mortality, includes:
  - Pneumonia
  - Intraventricular hemorrhage
  - Necrotizing enterocolitis
  - Respiratory distress
  - Neonatal sepsis
- Foals may be born septic or weak and demonstrate signs of maladjustment or unreadiness for birth. If placental disease is recognized early and believed associated with bacterial sepsis, early treatment of the mare with antibiotics (e.g., trimethoprim-sulfamethoxazole) is indicated along with anti-inflammatory therapy for placentitis (flunixin meglumine, pentoxifylline, vitamin E, and altrenogest).

Sepsis/Systemic Inflammatory Response Syndrome (SIRS)

- *Practice Tip: Sepsis/SIRS are the leading causes of neonatal foal morbidity and mortality.*
- The clinical criteria for SIRS in human medicine apply to foals and include two or more of the following:
  - Tachycardia
  - Tachypnea or hypoventilation
  - Fever or hypothermia
  - Leukocytosis
  - Leukopenia
  - >10% band neutrophils
- The conditions are most commonly associated with gram-negative bacterial infections and endotoxemia, although gram-positive microbes often are present concurrently.
- The clinical signs associated with sepsis are the result of an unbalanced stimulation of the immune system after exposure to microbial toxins.
- During sepsis, release of endogenous proinflammatory and anti-inflammatory mediators (e.g., tumor necrosis factor and interleukins -1, -2, and -6) precipitate a cascade of metabolic and hemodynamic changes that result in multiple organ system failure if left unchecked.

- As septic shock progresses, the patient succumbs to a combination of:
  - Cardiopulmonary failure
  - Generalized coagulopathy
  - Disruption of metabolic pathways
  - Loss of vascular endothelial integrity
- The definitions of *sepsis, severe sepsis,* and *septic shock* apply to the neonatal foal.
  - *Sepsis* is the presence of infection with concurrent SIRS.
  - *Severe sepsis* is sepsis with fluid-responsive hypotension or signs of organ dysfunction such as azotemia, hyperbilirubinemia, hypoxemia, or coagulopathy.
  - *Septic shock* is sepsis in which the hypotension is fluid refractory and vasopressor dependent.
- The microorganisms most commonly associated with neonatal foal sepsis include:
  - *Escherichia coli*
  - *Actinobacillus*
  - *Pasteurella*
  - *Klebsiella*
  - *Salmonella*
  - Other enteric microbes
  - *Streptococcus*
  - *Enterococcus* is increasing in prevalence and is a common cause of sepsis in foals with diarrhea.
  - Other gram-positive microbes or anaerobes are occasionally isolated from blood cultures.
  - Viral pathogens such as EHV-1 and equine arteritis virus also can produce sepsis-like syndromes (or SIRS), as can tissue damage associated with adverse peripartum events or severe tissue hypoxia.

Clinical Signs and Diagnosis

- The clinical signs observed with sepsis depend on the integrity of the foal's immune system, the duration of illness, and severity of the insult.

Signs During Early Hyperdynamic Phases of Sepsis/SIRS
- Lethargy
- Loss of suckle ("milk face")
- Hyperemic, injected mucous membranes and sclera
- Hyperemic coronary bands
- Petechiae inside pinnae and on oral mucosa
- Decreased CRT
- Tachycardia, increased cardiac output, hyperkinetic bounding pulses
- Tachypnea
- Variable body temperature
- Extremities that often remain warm to the touch
- The foal remains responsive

Signs During Advanced Uncompensated (Hypodynamic) Septic Shock
- Depression, lethargy
- Profound weakness, recumbency
- Dehydration, hypovolemia
- Hypotension unresponsive to fluid support (shock)
- Decreased cardiac output, tachycardia, cold extremities, thready peripheral pulses

- Prolonged CRT
- Oliguria
- Hypothermia
- Respiratory compromise: tachypnea, increased respiratory effort, hypoxemia, cyanosis

Localized Sites of Infection: Specific Signs
- Pneumonia, pleuritis: tachypnea, respiratory distress, fever, abnormal lung sounds, ventral dullness with pleural effusion, friction rubs with pleuritis
- Meningitis: seizures, stupor, opisthotonos. Other clinical signs include hyperesthesia, rigidity, cranial nerve abnormalities, nystagmus, and obtundation. Definitive diagnosis is through CSF analysis, which demonstrates neutrophilic pleocytosis, and occasionally bacteria are observed. CSF should also be cultured.
- Hepatitis: icterus and encephalopathic signs
- Nephritis: variable urine production, proteinuria, hematuria
- Peritonitis, enteritis: colic, ileus, diarrhea, abdominal distention
- Synovitis: painful, warm joint distention, lameness, fever
- Physeal, epiphyseal osteomyelitis: variable joint distention, localized pain over epiphysis or physis, lameness, fever, edema over affected areas
- Uveitis: blepharospasm, miosis, hypopyon, epiphora, fibrin accumulation in the anterior chamber
- Omphalitis: variable enlargement of umbilical remnant, umbilical discharge, fever, periumbilical edema. (See Omphalitis on p. 535.)

Clinical Pathologic Findings

- Leukopenia, neutropenia (white blood cell [WBC] count, <5000 cells/μL; neutrophils, <3400 cells/μL), increased band neutrophil count (bands, >50 cells/μL). Neutrophils may show toxic changes. Leukocytosis (white blood cell count >12,000 cells/μL) with neutrophilia is sometimes present.
- *Practice Tip:* If the total WBC count is <1200 (low neutrophils and lymphocytes) and the foal appears septic based on clinical examination; consider EHV-1! Some of the EHV-1 foals have toxic changes and left shift in neutrophils.
- Plasma fibrinogen concentration may be normal with acute sepsis: Fibrinogen increases in response to inflammation over 12 to 24 hours. *Practice Tip: Hyperfibrinogenemia in a newborn foal indicates some degree of chronicity and suggests the presence of in utero infection associated with placentitis. A failure to increase fibrinogen concentration in the face of sepsis/SIRS may indicate presence of coagulopathies such as DIC.*
- Hemoconcentration caused by hypovolemia is often present.
- Hypoglycemia (glucose, <60 mg/dL): Depletion of reserves or loss of control over glucose homeostasis may occur. Occasionally, and sometimes early in sepsis, hyperglycemia may be present.
- Hypogammaglobulinemia may result from failure to absorb colostral antibodies or increased protein

catabolism associated with sepsis. ***Practice Tip:*** *Foals with adequate passive transfer of colostral antibodies have a serum or whole blood immunoglobulin G (IgG) concentration >800 mg/dL. In partial failure of passive transfer (FPT), IgG is between 200 and 800 mg/dL, and in complete FPT, IgG is <200 mg/dL.*

- Hyperbilirubinemia is caused by a combination of sepsis-associated hemolysis or increased red cell turnover, anorexia, and hepatic dysfunction. Meconium retention can also contribute to hyperbilirubinemia.

- Lipemia resulting in opalescent serum is due to impaired lipid clearance associated with the cytokine upregulation in sepsis.

- Azotemia: increased creatinine or BUN concentration can be associated with dehydration/hypovolemia or hypotension, poor glomerular filtration rate resulting from any cause, and direct renal damage from ischemia, cytokine release, or coagulopathy.

- Hypoxemia: Pao_2 <60 mm Hg is associated with pulmonary pathology, ventilation-perfusion mismatching, pulmonary hypertension, or hypoventilation. These may occur in combination with respiratory acidosis.

- Metabolic acidosis: Defined as arterial pH <7.35, HCO_3 <24 mEq/L, due to poor peripheral perfusion and anaerobic metabolism. An increase in lactate concentration in these cases often contributes to the observed acidemia.

- Lactate concentration in neonates is higher than adults in the first 24 hours of life. Lactate is highest in the immediate postpartum period (2.3 ± 0.9; 4.9 ± 1.0; 3 ± 0.4 mmol/L in different studies) then declines to 1.2 ± 0.3 by 24 hours of age. Sick neonates with high lactate concentrations may clear part of the lactate concentration rapidly with resuscitation; persistently increased lactate (>2.5) concentrations without any decrease may carry a poorer prognosis!
  - ***Note:*** Lactate concentrations decrease in sick foals with initial fluid therapy but may *not* normalize. In these cases, it is hypothesized that some of the hyperlactatemia is due to sepsis and inflammatory mediators directly, rather than hypoperfusion.
  - ***Clinical Example:*** Pyruvate dehydrogenase activity is often reduced during cytokinemia, which occurs during sepsis.

Cultures for Diagnosis
- Culture blood, synovial fluid, CSF, peritoneal fluid, and/or urine, depending on which body system(s) are affected.
- Tracheal aspiration, although useful in the evaluation of foals with pneumonia, is too stressful to perform on septic neonates with severe respiratory distress; it is another useful diagnostic sample only if it can be rapidly and expertly performed.
- All samples obtained should be submitted for bacterial (aerobic and anaerobic) culture and susceptibility testing.
- Fungal culture and viral isolation or polymerase chain reaction (PCR) are additional tests to be considered in select cases where these pathogens are suspected and are especially important in foals with severe lymphopenia and neutropenia when EHV-1 is a possible cause.

Radiographs
- Obtain thoracic radiographs with the foal in lateral recumbency or standing. Take thoracic radiographs with the foal standing when possible to reduce effects of recumbency-induced atelectasis. Radiographs of the thorax with the forelegs pulled forward improves evaluation of the cranioventral lung fields.
- It is optimal to image both sides of the thorax.
- *Bacterial bronchopneumonia* is commonly associated with an alveolar pattern and air bronchograms in the cranioventral and caudoventral lung fields (Fig. 31-2). Pulmonary consolidation with loss of air bronchograms may be present with severe disease. Acute bacterial pneumonia can also present as diffuse interstitial disease.
- Both alveolar and interstitial patterns can be seen in acute lung injury and acute respiratory distress syndrome.
- *Viral pneumonia* is characterized by a diffuse interstitial pattern (Fig. 31-3).
- *Aspiration pneumonia,* including meconium aspiration, is associated with caudoventral and cranioventral infiltrates.
- *Surfactant deficiency* and *hyaline membrane formation* produce a diffuse, ground-glass appearance of the lung with prominent air bronchograms. This radiographic appearance also has been seen in foals with respiratory distress associated with viral pneumonia (Fig. 31-4). The ground-glass appearance can be mimicked in lateral thoracic radiographs of foals with pulmonary hemorrhage or hemothorax.
- Serial radiographs of swollen, painful joints or physes are recommended to detect signs of articular damage and osteomyelitis. These radiographs should be repeated in 2 to 5 days if swelling or pain persists.

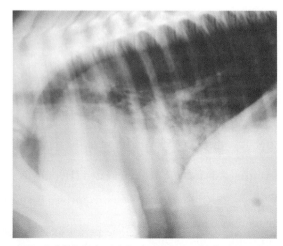

Figure 31-2 Recumbent lateral thoracic radiograph of a foal with bacterial pneumonia. The radiograph shows significant alveolar infiltrate involving the caudal and ventral lung fields. This finding is compatible with consolidation resulting from bronchopneumonia.

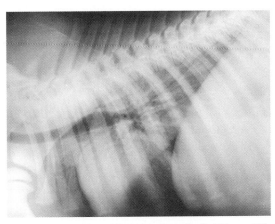

Figure 31-3 Recumbent lateral thoracic radiograph of a 24-hour-old foal. The pregnancy was complicated by septic placentitis. Radiograph shows an interstitial pattern most pronounced in the caudodorsal lung fields.

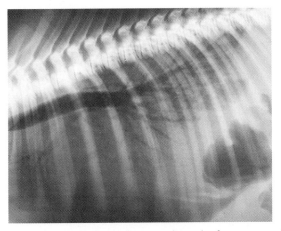

Figure 31-4 Recumbent lateral thoracic radiograph of a premature foal. Cesarean section was performed at 322 days of gestation. A diffuse alveolar pattern in all lung fields is compatible with diffuse pulmonary atelectasis.

- Plain abdominal radiographs can identify the location of gas distention. Ileus associated with enteritis or peritonitis is associated with generalized mild to moderate distention of the small and large intestines. Radiographs can demonstrate meconium in foals with impactions or retention.

Shock

- Shock is a pathophysiologic state of inadequate energy production for cellular function.
- Categories of *shock* include the following:
  - *Cardiogenic:* Examples include myocardial failure and white muscle disease (selenium deficiency).
  - *Distributive:* Examples include septic shock and anaphylactic shock in which vasomotor tone is lost.
  - *Hypovolemic:* Examples include hypovolemia and hemorrhagic shock.
  - *Obstructive:* Examples include pericardial tamponade or pulmonary arterial thromboembolism.
  - *Hypoxic:* Examples include severe hypoxemia, severe anemia, and mitochondrial dysfunction.

Peripartum Hypoxic/Ischemic/Asphyxia Syndrome: Neonatal Maladjustment Syndrome or Neonatal Encephalopathy

- This syndrome can result from any periparturient event that impairs or disrupts uteroplacental perfusion or umbilical blood flow often causing focal areas of cerebral injury due to ischemia/hypoxia or hemorrhage.
- Hypoxic/ischemic/asphyxia syndrome produces multiple organ system damage in addition to the more commonly recognized behavioral and neurologic deficits.
- This syndrome may also be associated with abnormal cytokine release in utero, a phenomenon currently being investigated.
- The following are periparturient events associated with this syndrome:
  - Dystocia
  - Induced delivery: Cervical dilation is a prerequisite for induction to reduce the risk of dystocia. Induction is rarely used because it increases the risk of dystocia and fetal morbidity.
  - Cesarean section
  - Premature placental separation
  - Placentitis: indicated by fetal membranes >11% of foal's body weight
  - Severe placental edema: indicated by uteroplacental thickness >2 cm
  - In utero meconium passage with or without postpartum meconium aspiration
  - Twinning
  - Severe maternal illness, especially with hypoxia/hypoxemia
  - Abnormally prolonged gestation
  - Pregnancy complicated by reduced fetal fluid volume increases risk of umbilical cord compression during labor and suggests the presence of chronic placental dysfunction

Diagnosis

- The syndrome produces a wide range of clinical signs.
- Asphyxia induces a critical redistribution of cardiac output.
- The result is preferential blood flow to the heart, brain, and adrenal glands and decreased perfusion of the lungs, GI tract, spleen, liver, kidneys, skin, and muscles.
- Diagnosis is based primarily on clinical signs.

Signs Associated with Specific Organ Injury

- Hypoxic-ischemic encephalopathy (neonatal encephalopathy): loss of suckle, loss of dam recognition, apnea, irregular respiratory patterns (inappropriate tachypnea, ataxic or cluster breathing), hypotonia, anisocoria, sluggish pupillary light reflex, dilated pupils, depression, tonic posturing (preference for lying in extensor posture with occasional pedaling limb movements), hyperesthesia, focal or grand mal seizures, and coma
- Renal tubular necrosis (neonatal nephropathy): oliguria, anuria, and generalized edema with fluid or sodium overload associated with the oliguria or anuria

NEO

- Ischemic enterocolitis (neonatal gastroenteropathy): colic, ileus, abdominal distention, gastric reflux, diarrhea (possibly bloody), necrotizing enterocolitis, and feeding intolerance
- Pulmonary dysfunction: meconium aspiration, pulmonary hypertension, or surfactant dysfunction—respiratory distress, tachypnea, increased respiratory effort, rib retractions, apnea
- Cardiac dysfunction caused by myocardial infarction or ischemia/hypoxia and persistent fetal circulation: arrhythmia, tachycardia or bradycardia, murmurs, generalized edema, hypotension, dysrhythmias
- Hepatocellular necrosis, biliary stasis: icterus, increased liver enzymes
- Adrenal gland necrosis: weakness, hypotension, hyponatremia, hypochloremia, hyperkalemia, and hypoglycemia
- Parathyroid necrosis: lipemia, seizures, hypocalcemia

Clinicopathologic Abnormalities
- Vary widely depending on the severity of specific organ injury
  - *CNS:* increased blood-brain barrier permeability, increased CSF protein
  - *Renal:* proteinuria, increased urinary concentration of gamma-glutamyl transferase (GGT), azotemia, hyponatremia, hypochloremia, increased fractional sodium excretion
  - *GI:* occult blood–positive reflux
  - *Respiratory:* hypoxemia, hypercapnia, respiratory acidosis
  - *Cardiac:* hypoxemia, increased values of myocardial enzymes (creatine kinase MB) and cardiac troponin I, decreased cardiac output
  - *Hepatic:* increased values of hepatocellular and biliary enzymes, hyperbilirubinemia
  - *Endocrine:* absolute or relative hypocortisolemia, hypocalcemia, hypoinsulinemia, or peripheral insulin resistance resulting in poor control of blood glucose

Other Diagnostic Aids
- Abdominal ultrasonography or radiography (recommended technique: 85 kV(p)/20 mA-s) to assess for signs of necrotizing enterocolitis, such as intramural gas accumulation (pneumatosis intestinalis), generalized intestinal distention, thickening of bowel wall. Consider performing a horizontal beam view with the foal in lateral recumbency to better assess for gas pneumatosis intestinalis.
- Thoracic radiographs (65 to 75 kV(p)/5 to 8 mA-s) to detect diffuse lung atelectasis as evidenced by a pulmonary vascular pattern with distention of pulmonary arteries resulting from pulmonary hypertension and persistent pulmonary hypertension of the neonate (PPHN). Normal findings on thoracic radiographs do *not* exclude the presence of respiratory abnormalities.
- Echocardiography to assess for patent foramen ovale, patient ductus arteriosus, and pulmonary hypertension associated with persistent fetal circulation; assessment of contractility (fractional shortening) and cardiac output (Bullet method)

- Cardiac output measurement: lithium dilution or Bullet method through echocardiography:
  - The Bullet method is as follows:

$$CO = SV \times HR;$$
$$SV = (\tfrac{5}{6} \times LVAd \times LVLd) - (\tfrac{5}{6} \times LVAs \times LVLs)$$

where
CO = cardiac output
SV = stroke volume
HR = heart rate
LVAd = left ventricular area in diastole (in short axis)
LVLd = left ventricular length in diastole (in long axis)
LVAs = left ventricular area in systole (in short axis)
LVLs = left ventricular length in systole (in long axis)

Prognosis
- Between 60% and 80% of foals suffering from peripartum asphyxia recover fully and mature into neurologically normal adults.
- A poor outcome is associated with severe, recurrent seizures that persist for >5 days postpartum, severe hypotonia that progresses to coma, and severe multiorgan system damage that includes unresponsive renal failure or hypotension. These foals should be monitored closely for development of concurrent septicemia.
- Dysmature and premature foals exposed to severe acute peripartum asphyxia have a poorer outcome than do term foals.

Prematurity and Dysmaturity
- *Prematurity* is defined as the condition of a foal born before a gestational period of <320 days, although foals born with longer gestational ages can be considered premature if born to dams with historically longer gestational periods.
- *Dysmaturity* is defined as the condition of a foal born after a normal or prolonged gestation period in which there are signs of underdevelopment. Dysmaturity is associated with abnormal uteroplacental function, which can result in delayed fetal growth and maturation when chronic, and in varying degrees of fetal asphyxia when acute.
- *Postmaturity* is the term some clinicians apply to the foal born after a prolonged gestation with signs of dysmaturity, yet they have large frame size, poor body condition, and long hair coats.

Clinical Signs
In addition to generalized weakness and hypotonia, the following signs are characteristic of dysmaturity and prematurity:
- Low birth weight; thin body condition
- Short, silky hair coat
- Floppy ears, soft muzzle, flexor tendon laxity, periarticular laxity
- Increased range of passive limb motion
- Domed forehead

- Absent or diminished suckle reflex, ineffective swallow reflex
- Time to nurse and stand delayed >3 to 4 hours postpartum
- Hypothermia caused by poor thermoregulation
- Intolerance of enteral feeding, colic, abdominal distention, diarrhea, reflux
- Respiratory distress caused by lung immaturity or surfactant dysfunction
- Visceral wasting, "gaunt" abdomen

Laboratory Findings

- Leukopenia: white blood cell count, $<6.0 \times 10^3$ cells/μL; neutropenia with neutrophil to lymphocyte ratio <1.0
- Hypoglycemia caused by lack of nursing and insulin response that contributes to abnormal glucose homeostasis
- Hypocortisolemia and poor cortisol response to stress and exogenous corticotropin (adrenal insufficiency) in some cases
- Hypoxemia, variable hypercapnia, and respiratory acidosis because of lung immaturity
- Hyponatremia and hypochloremia associated with renal immaturity or dysfunction

●> WHAT TO DO

Central Nervous System Disturbances

Neonatal Encephalopathy

- Supply supplemental oxygen to the mare using an IN cannula or nasotracheal tube. This raises the maternal PaO_2 and aids in reducing fetal hypoxia.
- Seizure control:
  - Administer diazepam, 0.04 to 0.44 mg/kg IV, for immediate seizure control; effect is short lived; repetitive doses contribute to respiratory depression.
  - Midazolam, 0.04 to 0.1, up to 0.2 mg/kg, can also be used and results in less accumulation than diazepam with repetitive doses.
  - For severe, recurrent (>2 episodes), or persistent seizure activity, use phenobarbital, 2 to 3 mg/kg IV q8 to 12h, up to 5 mg/kg q12h; monitor serum values (15 to 40 μg/mL). Higher doses can produce respiratory depression and hypotension.
  - Midazolam can be used as a CRI at 2 to 5 mg/h for 45-kg foals or 0.04 to 0.1 mg/kg/h for intermediate-term seizure control during hospitalization, with others using higher hourly rates if needed.
  - **Practice Tip:** *Monitor for respiratory depression whether using benzodiazepines or barbiturates.*
  - If using phenobarbital, serum concentrations can be measured; target concentrations in other species range from 14 to 40 μg/mL.
  - Potassium bromide can be used for longer-term seizure control in the newborn. Doses of 60 to 90 mg/kg once a day orally have been determined for adult horses and used in neonatal foals. Bromide is *not* an immediate control for seizures because it has a long half-life. Therapeutic drug monitoring of bromide in other species targets serum concentrations of 700 to 2400 μg/mL.
- The use of magnesium in hypoxic-ischemic encephalopathy (HIE) is controversial. Magnesium is believed to play a role in ameliorating secondary neuronal cell death after hypoxic-ischemic insults to the CNS, although this is equivocal in the natural setting. Magnesium has effects on calcium channels, N-methyl-D-aspartate receptors, and vascular reactivity. The loading dose is 50 mg/kg over 1 hour and is followed by 25 mg/kg per hour.
  - Using sterile technique, remove 20 mL from a 100-mL bag of 0.9% saline solution or 0.45% saline with 2.5% dextrose. Replace that volume with 20 mL 50% magnesium sulfate. For the average 50-kg foal, begin CRI at 25 mL/h for 1 hour, and then decrease to 12.5 mL/h. **Important:** Monitor for CNS and respiratory depression and muscle weakness; monitor plasma magnesium concentrations.
- **Practice Tip:** *Avoid xylazine for sedation unless it is the only drug available. Xylazine causes transient hypertension, which may exacerbate existing CNS bleeding and contribute to respiratory and cardiovascular depression (bradycardia) and reduced GI motility.*
- Avoid acepromazine because it may lower seizure threshold and produce significant hypotension.
- The use of osmotic agents for HIE is controversial. Osmotics are beneficial for interstitial edema; however, whether interstitial or intracellular edema is present in most cases of HIE requires further study. If the foal is hydrated, a mannitol trial is attempted and evaluated for a response in terms of mentation, since intracranial pressure is *not* routinely measured. Mannitol can be administered at 0.25 to 1.0 g/kg IV as 20% solution over 10 to 20 minutes as an osmotic diuretic. The duration of action of mannitol may be 5 hours or less; therefore, repeated dosing (3 to 4 times) may be required. If improvement is *not* seen in the first 24 hours, treatment is often suspended.
  - Mannitol may theoretically exacerbate active, ongoing cerebral hemorrhage. Questions remain as to the location of any edema that develops in neonatal encephalopathy. If edema has a role in the pathophysiology of this syndrome, most current evidence, in other species, suggests that it is intracellular (cytotoxic, not interstitial or vasogenic); therefore, the use of osmotic diuretics may be unwarranted in many cases. Some clinicians never use DMSO or mannitol in the management of cerebral edema and report *no* change in outcome. Others suggest that the antioxidant properties, with or without anti-edema properties, of mannitol are of clinical benefit.
  - Some clinicians continue to use DMSO at 0.5 to 1.0 g/kg given as *no* more than a 10% solution IV over 30 to 50 minutes.
  - **Practice Tip:** *Neonatal foals do* not *appear to eliminate DMSO as effectively as adult horses and can remain hyperosmolar for several days. Hemolysis is rarely observed in neonatal foals after DMSO administration unless administered at concentrations greater than 10%.*
  - Optimally plasma osmolarity should be monitored during osmolar therapy to ensure that persistent hyperosmolarity does *not* exist. The osmolarity should decrease into the normal range before the next dose.
- Protect the foal from self-trauma: Wrap legs, apply a soft head helmet (Velcro foam leg wraps and helmet available; 702-851-1217), pad walls and provide soft bedding, and apply ocular lubricant to reduce risk of traumatic corneal ulceration.
- Keep the patient's head low during resuscitation (CPR) to aid cerebral blood flow. However, after successful resuscitation and during other times, the head should be kept level to elevated 30 degrees when the patient is in lateral recumbency if cerebral injury is suspected. *The goal is to minimize intracranial pressure.*
- Do *not* overhydrate, but aim to maintain appropriate cerebral perfusion, with a normal mean arterial pressure: Cerebral Perfusion Pressure = Mean Arterial Pressure – Intracranial Pressure.

NEO

NEO

Renal Failure

- Hypovolemia should be corrected as soon as possible.
- Lack of urine production should be considered an emergency. It could be due to prerenal or renal oliguria or anuria, or a lack of urine voiding may be due to an inability to micturate. Prerenal oliguria should be rapidly addressed in order to prevent progression to renal disease. Inability to micturate associated with an enlarged, hypotonic bladder can lead to a ruptured bladder if *not* addressed.
- Monitor fluid balance (fluid input and urine output) to evaluate renal function. This ensures adequate hydration while avoiding overhydration.
- If hypotension occurs despite IV fluid administration: Dobutamine (2 to 15 µg/kg/min) can be administered as an inotropic agent. Use dobutamine if cardiac dysfunction and secondary hypotension are contributing to poor renal perfusion; discontinue or reduce dosage if tachycardia develops. Norepinephrine (range: 0.01 to 3.0 µg/kg/min) causes an increase in systemic vascular resistance and therefore elevates arterial blood pressure. Using 0.3 µg/kg/min (with or without fenoldopam) increases urine output and creatinine clearance; this regimen may be useful in treating hypotension with concurrent oliguria (Hollis et al, 2008).
- If correction of hypovolemia and hypotension does *not* result in correction of anuria, then anuric renal failure is a concern, particularly if concurrent azotemia is present and creatinine is increasing over time. If nonresponsive anuria or marked oliguria is present, despite adequate hydration, blood pressure, and fluid balance, and dialysis is *not* an option, then medical therapy geared to increasing urine output can be tried.
  - Furosemide: Administer small boluses (0.12 to 0.5 mg/kg IV q30 to 60min, up to 1 to 2 mg/kg total dose) to enhance diuresis, or begin or follow with continuous infusion (0.12 mg/kg per hour after a loading dose of 0.12 mg/kg). Monitor for development of hypochloremic metabolic alkalosis and additional electrolyte abnormalities such as hypokalemia.
  - Mannitol: Administer 0.5 to 1.0 g/kg IV as 20% solution over 15 to 30 minutes or 75 to 100 mg/kg/h CRI (osmotic diuretic). Do *not* repeat the bolus if anuria persists.
  - Dopamine infusion: Administer 2 to 3 µg/kg/min if anuria or oliguria is present.
    - *Lower* doses stimulate dopaminergic receptors and enhance urine output by natriuresis.
    - *Medium* doses recruit beta-receptors and support cardiac function, which may further improve renal perfusion.
    - *High* doses stimulate alpha-receptors and result in decreased splanchnic blood flow, renal blood flow, and urine production.
    - Titrate the dose to the individual patient. In one report, a dose of 0.04 µg/kg/min fenoldopam, a dopamine-1 receptor agonist, increased urine output in foals; however, creatinine clearance did not change (Hollis et al, 2006).
    - Recommend bladder catheterization to allow accurate assessment of urine production.
    - *Note:* The use of dopamine in renal failure is controversial as to benefit in human patients and is *no* longer commonly recommended. However, in cases of oliguria or anuria in foals, it may be worth trying because hemodialysis (or possibly peritoneal dialysis) is the only alternative when medical therapy fails.

Renal Failure

- ***Caution:*** Furosemide is *incompatible* with many medications. If administering furosemide through the same intravenous line as dopamine, avoid prolonged mixing of solutions in the line by administering dopamine or furosemide solution as close to the catheter port as possible.
- Protect furosemide CRI solutions from light by wrapping the line in paper or foil.
- Although furosemide administration can result in diuresis, prolonged use is associated with electrolyte and acid-base disturbances.
- The use of dopamine or furosemide in the management of oliguric renal failure does *not* correct the underlying problem. Judicious use of intravenous fluids, and "protecting" from dehydration, is indicated in these cases where oliguria or anuria is present.
- Close attention to matching "ins and outs" is important.

Colic, Reflux, Abdominal Distention

- Perform nasogastric decompression to check for reflux. Discontinue feeding if significant reflux is present. Reduce the volume or frequency of enteral feeding if there is a low volume of residual feed present on subsequent nasogastric intubation.
- If abdominal distention is severe and life-threatening and causing significant respiratory compromise, and abdominal exploration is *not* an option or is delayed, then percutaneous large-bowel trocarization can be performed (see Chapter 18, p. 160). Use a 16-gauge, $3\frac{1}{2}$-inch (8.75-cm) catheter-over-stylet attached to a 30-inch (75-cm) extension set. Sedate the foal if needed to keep it quiet in lateral recumbency. Clip and surgically prepare a site over the right paralumbar fossae at the point of maximal bowel distention. Infuse a small bleb of lidocaine at the puncture site. Using sterile technique, advance the catheter and stylet through the skin and body wall into distended viscus. Remove the stylet and connect the extension set. Place the free end of the extension set into a small beaker of sterile water to monitor gas-bubble production. Once bubbling stops, a small volume of antimicrobial (e.g., amikacin diluted 50:50 with sterile water) can be infused as the catheter is withdrawn. Broad-spectrum systemic antimicrobial therapy is recommended for 3 to 5 days after trocarization. ***Important:*** There is a risk of septic peritonitis, and the procedure should only be performed if distention is severe and life-threatening.
- Prokinetic drugs: In general, the cause of ileus should be addressed rather than resorting to prokinetic drugs. Hypoperfusion, hypoxemia, hypoglycemia, and meconium retention should be addressed as possible contributors to ileus. Ileus due to gut injury associated with hypoxic-ischemic damage or sepsis/SIRS needs time to heal, and parenteral nutrition may be indicated. When prolonged ileus is noted, but *no* mechanical obstruction is present, prokinetic drugs may be indicated. These drugs are *not* recommended for routine use because they can cause additional GI problems, such as possibly predisposing to intussusception, worsening colic, or neurologic complications. They may be indicated in foals with postoperative ileus.
  - Metoclopramide, 0.02 to 0.04 mg/kg/h as a CRI; can also be used as 0.25 to 0.5 mg/kg as slow IV infusion or per rectum q6h; observe for extrapyramidal adverse effects (CNS excitation, motor restlessness, muscle spasms). Metoclopramide stimulates

gastroduodenal motility and thus may be useful in the management of delayed gastric emptying associated with gastroduodenal ulceration in older foals.

- Cisapride, 0.2 to 0.4 mg/kg PO q4 to 8h, stimulates small- and large-intestinal motility. Motility is not necessarily coordinated or progressive, and signs of colic may worsen. Cisapride is currently *not* available as an FDA approved drug in the United States because of concerns of dysrhythmias in human patients.
- Lidocaine: The adult horse dose is 1 to 1.3 mg/kg slowly (over 15 minutes) IV, followed by 0.05 mg/kg per minute. The pharmacokinetics of this drug have *not* been studied in neonates; neonates are more susceptible than older horses to toxicity and may require a lower dose because of possible reduced liver metabolism and also a lower plasma protein concentration (lidocaine is highly protein bound), thereby increasing free drug concentrations. Discontinue if the following signs of toxicity develop:
  - Collapse
  - Muscle fasciculations
  - Ataxia
  - Excitation
- ***Important:*** Use lidocaine with caution. It may have several advantages with respect to analgesic and anti-endotoxic effects, but it also has anti-inflammatory effects that have unknown influences on natural protection against infection.
- Neostigmine, 0.005 to 0.01 mg/kg SQ q4h has been used successfully to evacuate "gas" (distended large intestine) but *not* a displacement or obstruction. Neostigmine reduces gastric emptying and jejunal motility in healthy adult horses; therefore, its use in foals with reduced gastric emptying is *not* recommended.
- Bethanechol, 0.03 to 0.04 mg/kg SQ or IV q6 to 8h: This drug increases gastric emptying and stimulates small-intestinal and pelvic flexure smooth muscle contraction. It may therefore improve gastric emptying in foals with duodenal and pyloric ulcers.
- Gastroprotectants (see Gastric Ulcers, Chapter 18, p. 181): Foals with hypoxic or ischemic GI damage are at increased risk of GI ulcers because of poor GI perfusion and the primary disease process. Acid production is not necessarily the cause of the ulcers, and the gastric milieu is likely more alkaline in sick foals from duodenal reflux than it is in normal foals. Therefore, H_2-antagonists and proton pump inhibitors may not be needed. In addition, the neonatal foal has a blunted response to H_2-antagonists. A recent retrospective (Furr M et al, 2012) study suggested that the use of antacid medications in foals predisposed foals to diarrhea. Antiulcer medications used in foals are:
  - Ranitidine, 6.6 mg/kg PO q8h or 1.5 to 2 mg/kg slow IV q8 to 12h; ranitidine also has some motility-enhancing effects
  - Famotidine, 2.8 mg/kg PO q12h or 0.3 mg/kg IV q12h
  - Sucralfate, 20 mg/kg PO q6h
  - Omeprazole, 4 mg/kg PO q24h
  - Pantoprazole, 1.5 mg/kg slow, dilute IV q24h
  - Antacids, such as Maalox or Di-Gel: 30 to 60 mL q3 to 4h. Most antacids have a short half-life, produce minimal change in gastric pH, but may provide transient pain relief.
- Administer broad-spectrum, bactericidal antimicrobials to reduce the risk of sepsis from translocation of luminal bacteria across a compromised GI mucosa. Sucralfate may also decrease bacterial translocation.
- PN: With mild GI compromise, reduce the volume or frequency of enteral feeding and support the foal with PN. In cases of severe asphyxia accompanied by hypothermia, hypotension, shock, or advanced prematurity, recommend delaying all enteral feeds and providing PN until GI function returns (as evidenced by passage of meconium, borborygmi present).
- Foals with colic: Withhold feeding or nursing until the signs of colic or distention resolve.
- Glucose supplementation: 4 mg/kg/min is used for the first 24 hours in foals with an adequate body condition score; however, after 24 hours of withholding enteral feeding, PN is instituted.

⦿〉 WHAT TO DO

Persistent Pulmonary Hypertension of the Neonate (PPHN) and Pulmonary Vasoconstriction

- Control of hypoxemia in the neonate is vital because it is a consistent stimulus for pulmonary vasoconstriction. Control is accomplished by providing a high concentration of oxygen of up to 100% delivered during nasal insufflation with high flow rates, or mechanical ventilation if necessary.
  - Administer oxygen intranasally, 5 to 10 L/min for an average-sized foal—100 to 200 mL/kg/min. The FiO_2 achieved with IN oxygen cannot be accurately predicted but can be high in the neonatal foal especially if two nasal catheters and oxygen lines are used. The use of oxygen insufflation with two nasal catheters at a rate of 100 to 200 mL/kg/min in healthy foals yields an FiO_2 of 48% to 75% oxygen (Wong et al, 2010).
- Acidosis accentuates hypoxic pulmonary vasoconstriction. Acid-base imbalances should be corrected. The goal is to achieve a pH of 7.4. Use of sodium bicarbonate to correct acidosis cannot be recommended if $PaCO_2$ is increased and the foal does *not* improve with mechanical ventilation with appropriate minute volumes.
- Consider pulmonary vasodilators if other techniques (i.e., oxygen therapy) fail to reverse pulmonary hypertension:
  - Tolazoline: infant dose, 1 to 2 mg/kg IV over 10 minutes; if there is a good clinical response with an increase in PaO_2, follow with intravenous infusion at 0.2 mg/kg/h for each 1-mg/kg pulse-dose administered.
  - Tolazoline causes adrenergic blockade, peripheral vasodilation, GI stimulation, and cardiac stimulation.
  - ***Important:*** Tolazoline therapy frequently results in severe tachycardia and hypotension because of the nonselective vasodilation produced, and it is *not* considered a first-choice approach. There is a report of fatalities associated with tolazoline and yohimbine use in horses, including in a 4-month-old foal that had been administered tolazoline.
- Nitric oxide (NO) is an important modulator of vascular tone needed to achieve neonatal circulatory patterns. Ventilation with NO in 100% oxygen reduces pulmonary vascular resistance. Inhalation of 5 to 40 ppm NO has been effective in reversing hypoxic pulmonary vasoconstriction in foals. Use approximately 5:1 to 9:1 ratio of O_2:NO. ***Note:*** A special regulator/flow valve is needed to attach to the NO tank.
- Future directions for management of PPHN include endothelin-1 receptor antagonists and specific phosphodiesterase inhibitors. Inhaled or nebulized prostacyclin is gaining favor in the human neonatal intensive care field.
- Monitor blood pressure. Support cardiac function with dobutamine if indicated.
- Correct hyperthermia if present: Remove covers and heating pads.

WHAT TO DO

Respiratory Compromise

- For mild hypoxemia, Pao$_2$ 60 to 70 mm Hg; Sao$_2$, 90% to 94%: Increase periods that the foal spends in sternal or standing position; turn every 2 hours if recumbent; stimulate periodic deep breathing to reinflate atelectic lungs; administer humidified IN oxygen, 2 to 10 L/min for average-sized foal – 40 to 200 mL/kg/min.
- For moderate to severe hypoxemia, Pao$_2$ <60 mm Hg, Sao$_2$ <90%, accompanied by hypercapnia, Paco$_2$, >70 mm Hg: Initially try oxygen insufflation, sternal positioning, and doxapram if hypoventilation is neurogenic in origin (i.e., HIE). If neurogenic in origin and *not* improved by treatment with a respiratory stimulant (e.g., doxapram or caffeine), or if respiratory acidosis is causing pH <7.25, and is *not* associated with metabolic alkalosis and therefore *not* compensatory, provide positive pressure ventilation (PPV). Respiratory muscle fatigue (in premature foals), severe lung disease, botulism, and muscular diseases should also be treated with PPV. Intubate nasotracheally, using a 7- to 10-mm-diameter, 55-cm long, cuffed, silicone nasotracheal tube.[2]
  - If respiratory muscle fatigue is a concern and mechanical ventilation is not an option:
    - Aminophylline (5 mg/kg mixed in a small volume of crystalloid fluid) can be administered IV over 30 minutes q12h to help maintain strength of diaphragm muscle contractions.
    - Aminoglycoside administration may be switched from IV to IM with the goal of decreasing the neuromuscular blocking effect of the drug.

Mechanical Ventilation

- Ventilator modes:
  - *Controlled mandatory ventilation:* All breaths are machine-triggered, and depth/timing are determined by machine settings.
  - *Assist/control ventilation:* In this mode, the breaths can be patient-triggered, machine delivered or both. The patient may trigger the breath depending on the level of sensitivity, which can be varied. However, whether the breath is patient or ventilator derived, the tidal volume, inspiratory time, and flow rate are machine determined (based on settings) and fixed.
  - *Synchronized intermittent mandatory ventilation (SIMV):* This is an assist-control mode in which a minimum number of machine-delivered breaths are guaranteed, while the patient can trigger its own breaths in addition to the set number. The tidal volume, inspiratory time, and flow rate are determined by the patient with spontaneous breaths (i.e., under complete control of the patient), whereas machine-triggered breaths are ventilator controlled. Pressure support ventilation can be combined with SIMV so that patient-triggered breaths are supported.
  - *Pressure support ventilation:* This is a "supported" or assisted means of ventilation for spontaneous breaths only. The inspiratory tidal volume and time are augmented by the machine, which decreases the work of breathing, but the control of tidal volume and inspiratory time are under patient control. The patient controls all parts of the breath, including triggering, respiratory rate and tidal volume, except for the pressure limit. The patient initiates each breath, and the ventilator assists by delivering support with a present pressure value. Pressure support may be combined with SIMV mode, in which the spontaneous breaths are supported.

- *Continuous positive airway pressure (CPAP):* This is a spontaneous breathing mode in which there is maintenance of positive airway pressures during inspiration, exhalation, and in between breaths. This mode results in increased functional residual capacity and improves ventilation-perfusion ratios. CPAP can be combined with pressure support ventilation.

WHAT TO DO

How to Do Mechanical Ventilation and Airway Support

- Typical settings: Begin PPV with initial tidal volume of 6 to 10 mL/kg and PEEP of 4 to 6 cm H$_2$O. Low tidal volumes (6 mL/kg) are associated with protective lung strategies in human critical care.
- A starting point for breath rate is 20 to 30 breaths/min, which should be adjusted using capnography and arterial blood gas analysis. The inspiratory/expiratory ratio should be set at 1:2.
- Providing pressure support (PS) without mandatory machine breaths may be sufficient for many foals. PS should start at 8 to 12 cm H$_2$O. In this mode, foals generate each breath and determine the depth, volume, and duration of the breath but are assisted by machine-generated pressure throughout each inspiration. CPAP is a weaning mode and may be useful for foals with milder respiratory compromise.
- Use a Fio$_2$ of 60% to 100% initially and reevaluate arterial blood gas values within 30 minutes of initiating PPV. Adjust inspired oxygen concentration accordingly with the goal of rapidly reducing Fio$_2$ to <50% to 60% to minimize the risk of oxygen toxicity.
- Attempt to maintain peak airway pressures below 30 to 40 cm H$_2$O to reduce barotrauma.
- Breath rate is determined by Paco$_2$ and the foal's initial breathing rate; some increase in Paco$_2$ is permissible and may be necessary to prevent barotrauma. Some foals respond best to pressure support ventilation only, with no mandatory machine-driven breaths. Foals tolerate SIMV/PS modes well.

Other Means of Improving Ventilation

- If meconium aspiration has occurred, attempt to treat the foal with IN oxygen alone. PPV can predispose to alveolar rupture and pneumothorax in these cases. Suctioning of the airways is attempted, but do *not* perform prolonged suction without oxygen administration.
- Intratracheal surfactant instillation may be beneficial if surfactant dysfunction is suspected because of severe asphyxia, pulmonary hypoperfusion, sepsis, or meconium aspiration.
  - Commercial products are expensive; surfactant can be collected from healthy donors (cows or horses) after bronchoalveolar lavage (BAL) using the top "frothy/foamy" layer.
- Apnea and irregular respiration may be caused by hypoxic-ischemic damage to the central respiratory center, maladaptation to extrauterine life, hypocalcemia, hypoglycemia, or hypothermia. Check body temperature and correct hypothermia if present. Correct hypoglycemia and/or hypocalcemia. If central respiratory depression is suspected, consider respiratory stimulants:
  - Doxapram CRI, 0.01 to 0.05 mg/kg/min; begin at the low end of the dose range and titrate. Doxapram may increase myocardial oxygen consumption; therefore, this agent should be used in the hemodynamically stable foal. Monitor the foal for hyperarousal or excitability, and reduce the dose if these occur.
  - Caffeine: Caffeine is *not* as effective as doxapram at improving hypoventilation in foals in two published studies. If used, begin with a loading dose of 10 mg/kg PO initially and then a

[2]Bivona, Inc., Gary, Indiana.

maintenance dose of 2.5 to 3 mg/kg PO q24h. Therapeutic range for caffeine is 5 to 20 µg/L; toxic concentration is >40 mg/L.

- If apnea persists, PPV may be needed.
- If PaO_2 does *not* have a significant increase with 100% oxygen, on ventilator, or high volume nasal oxygen flow after 3 to 4 hours of treatment, suspect the presence of a shunt or primary cardiac anomaly (a poor prognostic indicator). Rule out persistent pulmonary hypertension (PPHN) by a trial with NO in the inspired gas. The ratio of PaO_2 to inhaled oxygen % should be 5:1.

Secondary Infection

- Evaluate serum IgG. If IgG is <800 mg/dL and the foal is <18 hours of age and has a functional GI tract, administer good-quality colostrum (specific gravity, >1.060) enterally, or administer IV plasma transfusion, or both. If the foal is >18 hours of age or has compromised GI function, administer plasma. Serum IgG should remain >800 mg/dL. Provide broad-spectrum antibiotics if GI compromise is suspected, if the foal has signs of sepsis, or serum IgG is <800 mg/dL.

⦿》 WHAT TO DO

Prematurity/Dysmaturity

- Attempt to establish the cause of prematurity or dysmaturity. Examine the placenta. If evidence of placentitis is present, initiate broad-spectrum, bactericidal antibiotic therapy. Be watchful for preterm deliveries associated with EHV-1 infection.
- Observe closely for signs of respiratory distress and progressive respiratory fatigue. Therapy depends on the degree of respiratory dysfunction:
  - PaO_2, <60 mm Hg; $PaCO_2$, >60 mm Hg: Initiate IN oxygen therapy, 3 to 10 L/min for an average-sized foal—60 to 200 mL/kg; increase time spent in sternal recumbency; monitor arterial blood gas values.
  - PaO_2 <60 mm Hg, $PaCO_2$ >65 to 70 mm Hg with respiratory acidosis: Begin PPV with PEEP. Use PPV with tidal volumes of 6 to 10 mL/kg. Attempt to keep peak airway pressure <30 to 40 cm H_2O and inspired oxygen concentration <50% to reduce risk of barotrauma and oxygen toxicity, and keep PEEP at 4 to 8 cm H_2O. Excessive PEEP reduces cardiac output and necessitates CRI of dobutamine. Insufficient PEEP may *not* increase functional residual volume as desired.
- If a foal shows signs of advanced prematurity and signs of severe respiratory distress immediately postpartum, consider intratracheal instillation of surfactant in addition to PPV. **Important:** This is uncommon: most foals, unless born before 280 days of gestation, do *not* have primary surfactant deficiency.

Hypothermia

- Maintain carefully controlled environmental temperature if foal shows poor thermoregulation.
- Provide external warmth using warm water pads, radiant heaters, forced warm air blankets, warmed intravenous fluids, and insulated fluid jacket warmers.
- Be careful of inducing hyperthermia because these foals *cannot* regulate body temperature effectively. Foals should be warmed slowly during the initial resuscitation phase to avoid compounding reperfusion injury, particularly in those having experienced peripartum hypoxia.

Self-Trauma

- Reduce risk of decubitus sores by providing soft bedding (e.g., synthetic sheepskin, pressure point pads, plenty of cushion, blankets, and pillows) for recumbent foals.

Metabolic Disturbances

- Monitor serum/plasma electrolyte concentrations.
- ***Practice Tip:*** *Hyponatremia and hypochloremia are the most common disturbances associated with renal and endocrine immaturity or dysfunction. Hyperkalemia and hypokalemia may also be present; hypocalcemia is common. Metabolic (organic and inorganic) and respiratory acidosis are also common in affected foals.*
- Guidelines for correction include the following:
  - Hypernatremia
    - Correct sodium slowly (0.5 mEq/h)
    - Rapid correction can result in brain edema
  - Hyponatremia
    - Correct sodium slowly (0.5 mEq/h)
    - Rapid correction can result in pontine dysmyelinolysis
  - Hyperkalemia
    - Calcium, dextrose, insulin, sodium bicarbonate, peritoneal dialysis, potassium-binding resins used as enemas
  - Hypokalemia
    - Supplement fluids with 20 to 40 mEq/L of KCl or KPO_4, and give supplemental potassium orally if needed
    - Do *not* exceed 0.5 mEq/kg/h of potassium in intravenous fluids.
  - Inorganic acidosis
    - Inorganic acidosis is caused by hyponatremia or hyperchloremia (strong ion acidosis with normal anion gap)
    - Treat with sodium bicarbonate slowly intravenously or orally
    - Amount to administer: 0.4 × base deficit × body mass (kilograms). Give half slowly, and then reassess. Monitor $PaCO_2$.
  - Organic acidosis
    - Organic acidosis is most commonly caused by lactic acidosis (high anion gap)
    - Treat with fluid volume, inotropes, and vasopressors

Nutrition

- Healthy foals ingest approximately 20% to 25% or more of their body weight in milk each day.
- In sick foals, begin enteral feedings cautiously at a rate of 5% or 10% of body weight in milk divided into 10 to 12 feedings per day. Volumes should be gradually advanced as they are tolerated; gastric residuals should be monitored before each subsequent feeding.
- If the foal cannot tolerate sufficient enteral nutritional support, supply additional calories using partial or complete PN.

Incomplete Cuboidal Bone Ossification

- See Chapter 21, p. 309.
- Most premature and some dysmature foals have varying degrees of incomplete cuboidal bone ossification.
- Obtain a radiograph of at least one carpus (dorsopalmar view) and tarsus (lateral and dorsoplantar view) to evaluate the degree of ossification.
- If the foal is active but has minimal cuboidal bone ossification, attempt to keep the foal non–weight bearing as much as possible and allow only short periods of controlled standing (~5 min/h), ideally with assistance. Foals should be kept in small foal stalls to discourage activity. When recumbent, they should be turned often (every 2 hours) and passive range of motion/physical therapy is used on all limbs.
- Physical therapy is an important component of managing these foals to prevent limb contracture and laxity.
- In general, sleeve casts should be used judiciously because they exacerbate lateral-medial instability by inducing additional joint laxity.

NEO

NEO

- If only mild incomplete ossification exists, restrict exercise and use corrective shoeing (heel extension for laxity and toe extension for contracture/flexure deformity) and balanced foot trimming as needed to maintain a proper weight-bearing axis. More severe cases, especially those with concurrent angular limb deformities, may require bandaging and splints or tube casts above the fetlock if standing unassisted. Keep foal off slippery surfaces, and provide assistance in rising.
- Use glue-on shoes with appropriate medial or lateral extension to help straighten limbs if valgus or varus is present.

Evaluate Serum Immunoglobulin G Concentration
- Check within 8 to 12 hours of birth. If IgG is <800 mg/dL, administer colostrum supplementation, plasma transfusion, or both.

Secondary Bacterial Infection
- Premature and dysmature foals are at increased risk of infection. Administer broad-spectrum, bactericidal antibiotic therapy (3 to 5 days) until the foal is up and nursing normally.

Botulism: Shaker Foal Syndrome
- Botulism manifests as generalized weakness, dysphagia, muscle fasciculations, and hypoventilation in the neonatal foal. Most affected foals are approximately 1 month of age, although foals with shaker foal syndrome can range from a few days of age to several months.
- The gait of affected foals is often stilted, and pupillary dilation with ptosis may be present. Foals may be found dead because of respiratory paralysis.
- Most often botulism in the newborn is caused by *C. botulinum*, type B, which is endemic in areas of the eastern United States. Shaker foal syndrome occurs when foals ingest spores that subsequently vegetate and colonize the GI tract, producing toxin. In addition to type B, types A and C are common on the West Coast.

⊙> WHAT TO DO

Botulism
- Foals may require mechanical ventilation because of hypoventilation associated with intercostal and diaphragm muscle fatigue. Either pressure support (PS) or synchronous intermittent mechanical ventilation (SIMV) with pressure support is usually adequate.
- Diagnosis is often presumptive and based on clinical findings. *Practice Tip: Positive fecal cultures are strongly supportive in foals.*
- Repetitive nerve stimulation of the common peroneal nerve is described as an aid in the diagnosis of botulism in foals. Botulism caused a decrease in the baseline M amplitudes with incremental responses at high rates.
- Treatment usually includes beta-lactam antimicrobials (*not* procaine penicillin or aminoglycosides because they may affect neuromuscular function) and botulism plasma containing antitoxin. Nutritional support is provided through a feeding (nasogastric) tube, unless ileus is present. Urinary catheters may be required if foals are unable to urinate voluntarily.
- *Important:* Prevention of type B botulism in foals is through vaccination of the mares. Mares in endemic and high-risk areas should be vaccinated.

⊙> WHAT NOT TO DO

Botulism
- Do *not* administer aminoglycosides because they inhibit neuromuscular function.
- Do *not* administer procaine penicillin G or tetracyclines.
- Do *not* allow the foal to nurse if dysphagia is apparent.

Uroperitoneum
- Rupture of the urinary structures can involve the bladder, urachus, urethra, ureters, or kidneys. Most commonly, the bladder or urachus is involved.
- Clinical findings include:
  - Lethargy
  - Abdominal distention
  - Lack of suckling
  - Stranguria
  - There is little to no observed urination, although the presence of a urine stream does *not* rule out the presence of uroperitoneum.
- Foals with urachal rents in particular often produce urine streams.
- Tachypnea is common because of restricted tidal volume from the abdominal distention.
- Urachal, urethral, and occasionally ureteral tears result in periumbilical, subcutaneous, and perineal edema, respectively.
- Diagnosis of uroperitoneum is through abdominal ultrasonography and abdominocentesis.
- Definitive diagnosis is the finding of an abdominal fluid creatinine that is twice or more the concentration of serum creatinine.
- Other means of diagnosis are through retrograde contrast radiography using sterile, water-soluble radiopaque material deposited in the bladder. Sterile methylene blue can also be instilled within the bladder with subsequent abdominocentesis to look for blue dye in the abdominal fluid. *Practice Tip: The contrast radiography and methylene blue techniques miss ureteral tears and some urachal ruptures; these techniques are seldom needed to diagnose uroperitoneum.*
- Cytologic examination of the abdominal fluid may be warranted to rule out other causes of abdominal effusion.
- Serum chemistries usually reveal azotemia, hyponatremia, hypochloremia, and hyperkalemia. Foals already hospitalized and treated with sodium-rich crystalloids before rupture can have normal serum sodium and chloride concentrations, and the serum azotemia may be slower to develop.
- Electrocardiography is an important preoperative evaluation for dysrhythmias or alterations in the electrocardiogram caused by hyperkalemia, including:
  - Tented T waves
  - Blunted or absent P waves
  - Prolonged QRS complex duration and PR interval
  - Shortened QT interval

- Thoracic radiography or ultrasonography should also be preformed preoperatively because some foals with uroperitoneum can have significant pleural effusion.
- Blood cultures and measurement of serum IgG concentrations are important adjunctive diagnostics.
- Urachal ruptures often develop secondary to urachitis. Culture of the resected urachus is particularly important in these cases.

⊙⟩ WHAT TO DO

Uroperitoneum

- Preoperative treatment consists of hemodynamic and metabolic stabilization.
- Treat with potassium-free fluids, such as 0.9% saline or isotonic (1.3%) sodium bicarbonate depending on plasma pH. These fluids may increase uroperitoneum volume unless an abdominal drain is placed.
- Means of lowering potassium in addition to dilution include provision of glucose (4 to 8 mg/kg per minute), sodium bicarbonate, and insulin therapy in more refractory cases.
- Calcium is rapidly cardioprotective from the effects of hyperkalemia and should be provided, diluted along with dextrose in the initial fluids administered.
- *Clinical Example:* Administer 20 mL/kg of 0.9% saline containing 5% dextrose and 0.5 to 1 mL/kg of 23% calcium borogluconate (diluted in saline at no more than 50 mL calcium gluconate per liter) at a rate of 4 to 6 mL/kg/h. If bolus fluid administration is required due to hypovolemia, then 20 mL/kg of 0.9% saline with 1% to 2.5% dextrose and 10 to 15 mL of 23% calcium borogluconate (or more, depending on plasma ionized calcium concentrations) can be administered over 20 to 30 minutes. After 1 L of fluids, if hyperkalemia is still present, additional saline containing dextrose and sodium bicarbonate (1 to 2 mEq/kg) can be administered. Calcium and sodium bicarbonate should *not* be diluted in the same bag of fluids because microprecipitation can occur.
- Urine removal from the abdomen is an important feature in relieving hyperkalemia and improving ventilation. Peritoneal drainage can be performed using teat cannulas or abdominal drains. These are best placed using ultrasound guidance because plugging with omentum is common. Surgery immediately following completion of abdominal drainage is recommended (once potassium has decreased to <5.5 meq/L). Removal of the teat cannula or drain may result in prolapse of omentum and/or subcutaneous accumulation of urine at the drain site.
- If significant pleural effusion is present and causing respiratory compromise, drain the pleural fluid.
- Broad-spectrum antimicrobials should be given because a high percentage of foals with uroperitoneum are septic.
- Colts with ruptured bladders should have indwelling urinary catheters left in place for 1 to 3 days in the postoperative period, or longer if bladder atony is believed to be present, until normal bladder function returns; otherwise, rerupture may occur.

Other Differential Diagnoses of Generalized Weakness

- Neonatal isoerythrolysis: foals present with icterus, hemolysis, anemia, and hemoglobinuria.
- Meconium impaction: foals present with colic, straining to defecate, tail flagging, and abdominal distention.
- Syndrome of inappropriate antidiuretic hormone secretion (SIADH): This is a condition of excessive antidiuretic release. SIADH is proposed to affect foals 12 to 48 hours of age with signs of decreased urine volume, concentrated urine, hyponatremia, and hypochloremia. Serum creatinine concentrations are variable. The foals gain excessive weight consuming a milk diet because of retention of free water within the vascular space. SIADH occurs secondary to brain injury in humans.
  - These foals are *not* in renal failure, and the treatment of choice is fluid and milk restriction with monitoring of urine output, urine specific gravity, and serum electrolyte values. Clinical signs are associated with electrolyte disturbances (hyponatremia), which can be severe. The key to diagnosis is concentrated urine and weight gain.
- Tyzzer's disease is an acute, fulminating hepatitis caused by *Clostridium piliforme*. Pertinent features are the following:
  - The disease affects foals 6 to 42 days of age.
  - Clinical findings include icterus, obtundation, greatly increased concentration of hepatocellular enzymes, severe hypoglycemia, and significant lactic acidosis.
  - Foals may be found comatose because of significant hypoglycemia and hypovolemic/septic shock.
  - This disease is often fatal, although there is one report of a surviving foal and another involving a suspected case, indicating survival is possible with early and aggressive support.
  - Early institution of antimicrobial therapy (aminoglycoside/beta-lactam combination or other) and parenteral nutrition along with supportive measures for liver failure appear to be the key treatments for a rare successful outcome.
- Neonatal EHV-1 infection: If the fetus survives an in utero infection with EHV-1, it may be born viremic at birth. Neonatal herpes infection has a very high mortality rate.
  - Clinical signs include respiratory distress, neurologic signs, icterus, and generalized weakness. Fundic examination may reveal retinal hemorrhages.
  - *Practice Tip: Bone marrow necrosis may result in pancytopenia and affected foals generally have severe lymphopenia and neutropenia with total WBC counts below 1200 cells/μL.*
  - Liver enzymes may be elevated but in some cases are normal.
  - Survival in neonatal foals in outbreaks has been rarely reported and associated with acyclovir administration. Current treatment is recommended with valacyclovir, recommended dose for adult horses, 30 mg/kg PO, q8h for 48 hours, then 20 to 30 mg/kg PO, q8 to 12 h; or acyclovir, 10 mg/kg IV q12h.
  - Diagnosis can be made with PCR testing of whole blood and nasopharyngeal swabs, or virus isolation from buffy coat.

- Affected foals should be managed with strict biosecurity; 20% or more of the infections may be due to the "neurovirulent" strain of EHV-1.
- Fescue toxicosis: Foals born to mares with fescue toxicosis are often dysmature or postmature as a result of prolonged gestational periods and abnormal placentation.
  - They are often large, thin, and have long hair coats, with behavior consistent with peripartum asphyxia.
  - Affected foals are treated with supportive care as described for foals with hypoxic-ischemic injury.
  - Because agalactia usually develops in the dam, foals must be fed alternative sources of colostrum and milk replacer.
  - Treatment of mares exposed to endophyte fungus–infested (*Neotyphodium coenophialum*) fescue antepartum consists of domperidone, 1 mg/kg PO q24h. Vitamin E supplementation of mares in the last 30 days of gestation may result in higher serum concentrations of IgG in foals nursing affected mares.

●》 WHAT TO DO

General Therapy for Septicemia
Cardiovascular Support

- Replacement Fluid Therapy
- *Fluid challenge* method of fluid replacement: To correct hypovolemia, administer crystalloids, 10 to 20 mL/kg over 10 to 30 minutes, depending on degree of shock, to manage hypovolemia and hypotension. Balanced electrolyte solutions, such as Plasma-Lyte A or 148, Normosol R, or LRS are optimal for rapid volume expansion. Sick foals usually require between 1 and 4 of these fluid boluses depending on the degree of hypovolemia. After each bolus, the foal's perfusion parameters (both clinical and laboratory) should be reassessed for additional volume administration.
- The clinical perfusion parameters include:
  - Mentation status
  - Jugular fill
  - Mucous membrane color
  - CRT
  - Extremity temperature
  - Heart rate (not as reliable in foals as in adults)
  - Pulse quality
- The laboratory indicators of perfusion status include:
  - Serial measurements of lactate
  - Acid-base status
  - Venous oxygen saturation and oxygen extraction ratio
  - PCV
  - Total protein concentration
- Monitoring tools that can indirectly indicate the perfusion status include:
  - Serial measurements of arterial blood pressure, indirect or direct
  - Measurement of urine output
- The crystalloid dose is repeated as needed until CVP is maximized (10 to 12 cm H_2O). **Practice Tip:** *CVP is* not *generally an accurate predictor of volume status, but it is a good guide to limiting fluid therapy. A normal CVP does* not *necessarily equate to normal blood volume status; however, a maximal CVP does provide an indicator that fluid bolus administration should be discontinued.*
- If the CVP limit is reached, and hypoperfusion is still evident based on clinical and laboratory parameters, then alternate means of

managing the hypoperfusion, including the use of inopressors, need to be considered.
- **Note:** Dextrose-containing fluids alone are *not* indicated or appropriate for rapid volume expansion unless hypoglycemia is present. Five percent dextrose in water is *not* a replacement fluid and should *not* be used as a fluid bolus treatment.
- The foal should be reevaluated after each bolus and before administration of the next. The goal is volume resuscitation but *not* overhydration or overloading with sodium.
- Maintenance Fluid Therapy: There are a minimum of two ways of providing maintenance fluid therapy:
  - *One:* Based on the fluid intake of normal neonatal foals and studies of fluid physiology, the maintenance fluid requirement in the neonatal foal is 4 to 6 mL/kg/h.
  - *Two:* An alternative means of maintenance fluid therapy is using the Holliday-Segar formula, regarded as a "dry" or more conservative means of fluid therapy. The minimum "dry" maintenance fluid rate is calculated as follows:
    - 100 mL/kg per day for the first 10 kg of body mass plus
    - 50 mL/kg per day for the second 10 kg of body mass plus
    - 20 to 25 mL/kg per day for the remainder of the body mass
- The Holliday-Segar formula provides the volume needed for a recumbent foal *not* consuming a milk diet for water maintenance and is approximately 94 mL/h for a 50-kg foal. This rate needs to be adjusted upward accordingly to meet losses incurred by the foal because of increased insensible (increased respiration, fever, physical activity) or sensible (increased urine output, gastric reflux, diarrhea) losses. Most foals actually begin at 1.5 to 2 times the calculated "dry" rate.
- If the foal is *not* receiving milk or total parenteral nutrition (PN) as an energy source, then dextrose can be added and the concentration or rate adjusted to provide 4 to 8 mg/kg per minute until dextrose needs are met.
- Normal sodium need for a growing neonatal foal is approximately 1.5 to 3 mEq/kg per day based on milk intake of normal foals and is generally met by the administration of a single liter of plasma or crystalloid containing 140 mEq/L.
- Monitor blood pressure, CVP (goal, 2 to 10 cm H_2O), urine output, heart rate, peripheral pulses, and respiratory function. There is no "magic" number for mean blood pressure in foals, but a mean pressure between 45 and 50 mm Hg is usually adequate if the pulse pressure difference is >30 to 40 mm Hg and clinical signs of perfusion are adequate, especially adequate urination. Other recommendations are to maintain mean arterial pressure at 60 mm Hg or greater.
- The physical examination and clinical condition are the most critical indicators of adequate perfusion:
  - Is the foal warm in its periphery?
  - Are peripheral pulses easily found?
  - Is the foal making urine, and what is the mental status of the foal?
  - If the answers to these questions are yes or adequate, then perfusion is acceptable regardless of the blood pressure readings.
  - A foal that is ambulatory and rises on its own likely has adequate perfusion.
- Adjunctives to Fluid Therapy: Plasma may be needed to maintain oncotic pressure and intravascular fluid volume.
  - Minimum volume to administer is 20 mL/kg (1 L for an average-sized foal) over 60 minutes, but foals with adequate fluid volume should be administered plasma at a slower rate.

- One liter of plasma provides the equivalent sodium load of a normal milk diet in a normal foal in a single day.
- Hetastarch or VetStarch may also be used by clinicians at an initial dose of 3 to 10 mL/kg body mass. *Note:* It is recommended *not* to use hetastarch at the higher doses until further safety studies are performed because of concerns in the human literature with the use of hetastarch products. Larger doses (more than 10 mL/kg) may cause or exacerbate coagulation abnormalities because they induce a von Willebrand's–like condition.
- Volume expansion alone usually is sufficient to correct mild to moderate metabolic acidosis. Severe metabolic acidosis, especially when caused by a strong ion acidosis (i.e., hyperchloremia or hyponatremia) may necessitate sodium bicarbonate supplementation. This is very common in diarrhea cases with ongoing bicarbonate losses, but be aware that for each milliequivalent of bicarbonate administered, a milliequivalent of sodium also is administered and the subsequent increases in pH decrease plasma potassium. The recommendation based on clinical experience is to administer sodium bicarbonate through an isotonic 1.3% solution, 150 mEq $NaHCO_3$ per liter.
- **Practice Tip:** *Sodium bicarbonate should* not *be administered to patients in cardiac arrest or that need considerable resuscitation efforts, until late in cardiopulmonary resuscitation (CPR) (after 5 to 10 minutes of unsuccessful CPR attempts). Ensure adequate ventilation before administering sodium bicarbonate because it increases $Paco_2$ in foals that are hypoventilating. Avoid rapid infusion of sodium bicarbonate: it is unnecessary and may lead to respiratory or paradoxical CNS acidosis.*
- **Vasopressive Therapy:** Sepsis-induced hypotension is difficult to manage if the foal is fluid refractory (septic shock) because some foals may be less responsive to adrenergic drugs. This may be simply a function of how they manifest sepsis with vasomotor dysfunction or adrenal insufficiency, or alternatively, it may be associated with developmental age.
- Treatment recommendations for hypotension with hypoperfusion in neonatal foals include the following:
  - **Step 1**: Isotonic fluids as indicated earlier
  - **Step 2**: Dobutamine: 2 to 15 µg/kg per minute as a continuous infusion
    - Dobutamine is used to treat patients with adequate volume expansion as a beta-adrenergic, inotropic agent to improve cardiac output and oxygen delivery.
    - Titrate dose to effect.
    - Discontinue administration if severe tachycardia develops (>50% increase).
  - **Step 3**: Pressor therapy: Norepinephrine, 0.01 to 3.0 µg/kg per minute
    - Norepinephrine is an alpha-agonist pressor agent.
    - Norepinephrine should always be used with dobutamine to minimize splanchnic hypoperfusion and to ensure maximum cardiac function.
    - Norepinephrine is one of the least offensive pressor agents in terms of GI hypoperfusion in other species.
  - **Step 4**: Vasopressin, 0.25 to 0.4 U/kg per minute
    - At this low dose, vasopressin provides support for adrenergic pressors without inducing renal effects, particularly in septic patients.
    - A potential concern with vasopressin in foals and other species is GI and splanchnic hypoperfusion.
    - Vasopressin should therefore *not* be used in primary GI cases until studied further, and is reserved for use after norepinephrine has been tried first.

- For unresponsive moderate-to-severe hypotension:
  - Epinephrine: 0.1 to 2.0 µg/kg per minute. **Practice Tip:** *Expect measured lactate concentration to increase substantially when this drug is used.*
  - Phenylephrine: 1 to 20 µg/kg per minute. Although this pressor almost always increases measured pressure, the generalized vasoconstriction produced is probably counterproductive in the treatment of the patient because of severely diminished peripheral perfusion due to excessive increases in systemic vascular resistance.
- **Practice Tip:** *Combinations of the aforementioned treatments are commonly used, and a good first-choice combination includes dobutamine-norepinephrine and dobutamine-vasopressin.*
- **Addressing Endocrine Dysregulation:** Relative or absolute adrenal insufficiency with hypothalamic-pituitary-adrenal axis dysfunction may also exist in some septic foals. It has been reported that hospitalized foals may have inappropriately low basal cortisol and an inadequate response to administration of cosyntropin.
- Cosyntropin is a synthetic derivative of adrenocorticotropic hormone (ACTH); it is used in the ACTH stimulation test for diagnosis of adrenocortical insufficiency. A failure for serum cortisol concentrations to increase after cosyntropin administration is consistent with adrenocortical insufficiency.
- Some foals have inappropriately high ACTH concentrations, and high ACTH : cortisol ratios. If the septic foal is unresponsive (i.e., remains hypotensive) to administration of IV fluids and routine pressor drugs, hydrocortisone sodium succinate can be tried: 1.3 mg/kg/day for 48 hours, then 0.65 mg/kg/day for 24 hours, and then 0.33 mg/kg/day for 12 hours. The total daily dose is divided into 6 doses and administered as an IV bolus every 4 hours. This dosage is based on an experimental study, which showed that this low dose of hydrocortisone ameliorates endotoxin-induced proinflammatory cytokine expression in neonatal foals without impairing their innate immune responses (Hart KA et al, 2011).

Respiratory Support

- The aim of therapy is to minimize ventilation-perfusion mismatching.
- Use cautious fluid therapy to maintain adequate left ventricular and atrial pressure and thus promote more uniform lung perfusion.
- Frequent repositioning of the foal reduces dependent lung atelectasis; encourage sternal recumbency.
- Use intranasal (IN) humidified oxygen therapy to manage hypoxemia (Pao_2 <70 mm Hg, oxygen saturation (SaO_2) <90%) if ventilation is adequate. Use oxygen flow of 2 to 10 L/min (40 to 200 mL/kg/min). The provided fraction of inspired oxygen (Fio_2) is unpredictable and depends greatly on the minute volume. Administer oxygen through a cannula positioned in the nasal passage with the end of the cannula at the level of the medial canthus of the foal's eye. Tape or suture nasal cannula in place. Oxygen tubes in both nostrils can be used to increase Fio_2. Be careful *not* to pass the nasal cannula into the esophagus; the resultant abdominal and GI distention is dangerous and develops rapidly.
- Mechanical positive pressure ventilation (PPV) is used to prevent alveolar collapse, reduce respiratory muscle fatigue, and address increased oxygen consumption associated with sepsis. Positive end expiratory pressure (PEEP; 4 to 8 cm H_2O) and pressure support (8 to 16 mm Hg) may be needed. PPV is indicated if IN oxygen therapy alone fails to correct hypoxemia and/or if $Paco_2$ >65 mm Hg with a pH <7.25 is unresponsive to respiratory stimulants (i.e., neurogenic hypoventilation occurring in foals with hypoxic-ischemic encephalopathy), and is *not* associated with metabolic alkalosis (i.e.,

not compensated or not compensatory). Peak airway pressure should be kept at a minimum level, preferably less than 30 cm H_2O to prevent barotrauma. Increased $Paco_2$ can be tolerated (permissive hypercapnia) as long as pH is acceptable and there are *no* signs of carbon dioxide narcosis or deleterious cardiovascular effects. Fio_2 should be kept as low as is practical to minimize oxygen toxicity of the lungs, eyes, and other organs. Prolonged Fio_2 at >50% to 60% may result in oxygen toxicity.

- Mild to moderate hypoventilation is treated with doxapram in foals with neurogenic-origin hypoventilation. This includes foals with peripartum asphyxia. A constant rate infusion of doxapram is used (0.01 to 0.05 mg/kg/min). Foals receiving doxapram should be monitored for hyperexcitation, agitation, and even seizures. Two studies have reported increased efficacy of doxapram in treating neonatal foal hypoventilation as compared with caffeine. Recent studies have shown doxapram to be a safer treatment for perinatal asphyxia and postanesthetic hypoventilation than once believed. It can have side effects such as increased pulmonary pressure and respiratory alkalosis, which should be avoided in foals with lung immaturity and cerebral injury, respectively.

- Caffeine administration has also been used to manage abnormally slow respiratory rate, hypoventilation, and respiratory acidosis resulting from central respiratory center depression. Administer 10 mg/kg PO or per rectum as a loading dose, followed by 2.5 to 3 mg/kg PO once daily as a maintenance dose. Therapeutic trough serum concentration is 5 to 25 μg/mL. Toxicity (CNS signs) is associated with concentrations greater than 40 to 50 μg/mL, but these concentrations are rarely achieved in foals.

- **Practice Tip:** *Caffeine is* not *as effective as doxapram for the treatment of hypoventilation.*

Nutritional Support

- Hypoglycemia is managed initially with a glucose infusion best administered as a constant infusion at a rate of 4 to 8 mg/kg per minute. This is accomplished by administration of dextrose in fluids as a 5% to 10% solution in maintenance fluids or as a 50% dextrose solution administered through a separate syringe piggy-backed into the maintenance fluid line. The 50% solution should *not* be administered without diluting in fluids because it is hypertonic and potentially injurious to the endothelium.

- **Clinical Example:** At this rate, a 50-kg foal would receive 120 to 240 mL of 10% dextrose per hour diluted in crystalloids. Do *not* give foals bolus infusions of 50% dextrose.

- Caloric requirements: A healthy foal consumes 15% to 25% (or higher) of its body weight daily in milk, which equals 81 to 135 kcal/kg per day. Sepsis and fever are believed to increase caloric requirements to 150 kcal/kg per day in ambulatory or active foals; however, this may not be true in all cases, and foals that are recumbent and weak likely have reduced caloric requirements even when septic. Many ill foals gain weight on 10% body weight equivalent feeding (~50 to 54 kcal/kg per day) likely because of decreased energy requirements associated with recumbency and lack of normal activity. Studies have suggested the energy requirement of recumbent, sick foals is as low as 43 to 55 kcal/kg/day.

- Enteral feeding: Use mare's milk, foal milk replacer, goat's milk, or a combination. **Practice Tip:** *Milk replacer may cause diarrhea and goat's milk may cause constipation. A diet consisting entirely of goat's milk can lead to metabolic acidosis; therefore, goat's milk should be mixed in equal volumes with milk replacer.*

- **Clinical Goal:** *The goal is 10% to 20% of body weight per day in milk administered in small volumes every 2 to 3 hours.* **Note:** *For sick foals (sepsis or peripartum asphyxia) the initial feeding goal is 10% of body weight per day.*

- If GI function is a concern, begin enteral feeding cautiously at 5% to 10% of the foal's body weight per day or less with gradual advancement of volume as it is tolerated. Supplement with PN if <10% of body weight in milk is fed daily for 2 consecutive days. Do *not* allow stuporous foals to nurse or drink from a bottle. Always feed foals standing or in sternal recumbency and maintain them in that position for at least 10 minutes after feeding is completed to prevent aspiration.

- **Important:** Never feed a cold, severely hypotensive foal. Make sure initial fluid replacement, glucose supplementation, and warming occur before the first feeding.

- **Parenteral nutrition (PN):** These solutions are hypertonic and must be administered continuously through large peripheral veins (e.g., jugular or cranial vena cava) and long catheters (>5 inches [12.5 cm] long) at precise flow rates. Central venous lines (20 cm) with 2 to 3 ports and lumens are ideal for administration of PN. One of the lines can be dedicated to PN administration. Use an infusion pump, dial-a-flow regulator, or a Buretrol[3] solution set to administer PN.

- Monitoring PN:
  - Target blood glucose concentrations should remain between 80 and 180 mg/dL.
  - Test blood for hyperglycemia and hypoglycemia frequently, and check urine for glucosuria to regulate the amount of glucose delivered.
  - The presence of persistent hyperglycemia suggests loss of glucose regulation and does *not* necessarily indicate that too much glucose is being administered. In these cases, insulin can be administered as a continuous infusion at 0.005 to 0.2 U/kg per hour. Use regular insulin, and pretreat all lines because insulin adsorbs to plastic. Changes in insulin and glucose rates should be made slowly and over many hours (~4 hours).
  - $Paco_2$ should be monitored because PN can increase tissue production of CO_2, which can compound respiratory acidemia in foals with hypoventilation.
  - Monitor serum for lipemia and triglyceride concentrations; lipids should *not* be administered if triglyceride concentrations are >200 mg/dL. The plasma is evaluated grossly for lipemia (white), although this rarely occurs except in severe sepsis. Foals with a serum triglyceride concentration >200 mg/dL should receive a lipid-free formulation.
  - Monitor PCV and total protein for signs of dehydration.
  - Nitrogen balance can be monitored with periodic assessment of BUN and blood ammonia concentrations.
  - Foals receiving PN should also be monitored for hypokalemia, hypercapnia, metabolic acidemia, nitrogen intolerance (high BUN or ammonia), and septic/catheter-related problems.

- Components of PN:
  - 50% dextrose
  - 8.5% or 10% amino acids
  - 10% or 20% lipids: use for long-term PN, >3 days
  - Companies that supply TPN components include: Baxter International, Fresenius Kabi, and Braun.

  Practice Tip: *Daily caloric requirements should be met primarily by dextrose and lipids.*

  - Lipid-free formulas are often used for short-term (<3 days) PN administration. Recent work in human critical care suggests lipids may be proinflammatory in sepsis.
  - For long-term (≥3 days) PN administration, lipids should be included to prevent fatty acid deficiency.

---

[3]Baxter International, Deerfield, Illinois.

- Lipids should contribute approximately 50% nonprotein calories.
- To ensure the amino acids are used for structural protein and *not* catabolized for energy, the ratio of nonprotein calories to grams of nitrogen should be maintained between 100 and 200.

Caloric density:
- Lipids, 9.0 kcal/g
- Carbohydrate (glucose), 3.4 to 4.0 kcal/g
- Protein (amino acids), 4.0 kcal/g

- Starting formula of PN for short-term use <3 days:
  - A lipid-free formula: Use a 1:1 solution of 50% dextrose and 8.5% amino acids can be used in foals, with a caloric content of 1.02 kcal/mL.
  - Target a caloric rate of 50 kcal/kg/day for recumbent, sick foals.
  - Begin with 25% of target rate, and increase every 4 to 6 hours until target is reached in 24 hours. During this 24-hour period, dextrose is supplemented at 4 mg/kg/min initially; a decrease by 25% of the rate occurs every 4 to 6 hours as the PN formula is increased.
  - Supply B and C vitamins separately; dilute in crystalloids.
- Starting formula of PN for longer-term use (≥3 days):
  - Potassium chloride is added to the parenteral formula if needed.
  - When first starting PN with lipids, begin at one fourth the desired flow rate. Check blood for lipemia and check blood and urine for hyperglycemia (blood glucose concentration, >180 mg/dL) at 3- to 4-hour intervals, and increase flow rate by one fourth until the final rate is achieved.
- **Clinical Example 1:** Sample calculation for 50-kg foal:
  - Dextrose: 10 g/kg per day = 500 g = 1 L of 50% dextrose
  - Amino acids: 2 g/kg per day = 100 g = 1 L of 10% amino acids or 1.2 L of 8.5%
  - Lipids: 1 g/kg per day = 50 g = 0.5 L of 10% lipids
  - Total volume: 2.5 L of PN. Caloric content is approximately 1.14 kcal/mL.
- **Clinical Example 2:** Another formula commonly used for ≥3 days in 50-kg foal:
  - 1 L of 50% dextrose
  - 1.5 L of 8.5% amino acids
  - 0.5 L of 20% lipids
  - Total volume: 3.0 L of PN. Caloric content is approximately 1.13 kcal/mL.
- To provide 50 kcal/kg to a 50-kg foal, approximately 2200 mL of this latter formula is required per day, equating to 91 mL/h. As tolerated, the PN can be increased to provide approximately 75 kcal/kg per day, or 140 mL/h.
  - Begin PN at 35 mL/h. Slowly increase the rate every 3 to 4 hours by 35 mL, frequently checking glucose concentrations of plasma/serum, until 90 to 140 mL/h is reached for an average-sized foal.
- **Note:** Human critical care studies suggest lipids may be proinflammatory in sepsis.

Antimicrobial Therapy for Sepsis
- Broad-spectrum, bactericidal antimicrobials are indicated. Treatment should be based on culture and sensitivity results whenever possible.
- Administer antimicrobial therapy for a minimum of 10 to 14 days in foals with documented bacteremia, provided that *no* localized areas of infection develop requiring more prolonged treatment.
- Specific sites of infection (e.g., pneumonia, meningitis, arthritis, and osteomyelitis) require prolonged antimicrobial therapy for 30 days or longer. Penicillin and aminoglycoside antimicrobials constitute a

popular combination that provides coverage against gram-positive and gram-negative aerobes and anaerobes.
- Antimicrobial dosages (see Appendix 9 for expanded drug dosage lists) are as follows:
  - Penicillin: 22,000 to 44,000 U/kg IV q6h or 22,000 U/kg IM q12h; use in combination with an aminoglycoside if renal function is adequate.
  - Ampicillin: 22 mg/kg IV q6-8h; use in combination with an aminoglycoside if renal function is adequate.
  - Amikacin: 21 to 30 mg/kg IV q24h in foals <7 days of age combined with therapeutic drug monitoring; ideally peak should be ≥10 times the minimum inhibitory concentration (MIC) of the cultured or suspected microbe. Peak concentrations should be ≥60 μg/mL at 30 minutes, or ≥40 μg/mL at 1 hour after administration. ***Practice Tip:*** *To minimize nephrotoxicity, the trough concentrations should be ≤1 μg/mL at 20 to 23 hours after administration. Serial measurement of plasma creatinine concentrations should be performed in foals receiving aminoglycosides.*
  - Gentamicin: 6.6 mg/kg IV q24h, and up to 10 mg/kg IV q24h in foals <7 days of age. Peak and trough concentrations should be monitored; ideally peak should be ≥10 times the MIC and trough <1 μg/mL at 20 to 23 hours after administration. If MIC data are not available, the 1-hour postadministration peak should be ≥20 μg/mL. **Note:** Gentamicin is believed to be potentially more nephrotoxic than amikacin in very young foals; use with caution and only in well-hydrated foals. Serial monitoring of plasma creatinine should be performed while foals are treated with gentamicin. **Note:** Many gram-negative organisms may be resistant to gentamicin.
  - Ceftiofur sodium: 2 to 10 mg/kg IV q12h; 5 mg/kg IV q 12 h for most uses; may also be administered SQ (Hall et al, 2011). In foals with renal insufficiency, longer treatment intervals are recommended because of reduced clearance. One can use ceftiofur in combination with aminoglycoside (i.e., amikacin) coverage for increased gram-negative and *Staphylococcus* spectrum.
  - Recently the continuous rate infusion (CRI) of ceftiofur has been described (Wearn et al, 2013). CRI administration is an alternative administrative method for ceftiofur in foals. Because it is a time-dependent antimicrobial, maintenance of plasma concentrations above the MIC of the microbe for the entire dosing interval is optimal. The recommended dose to achieve plasma steady-state concentrations of 2 μg/mL, based on experimental data (Wearn et al, 2013) is:
    ○ Bolus loading dose of 1.26 mg/kg
    ○ Follow immediately by a CRI of 2.86 μg/kg/min to maintain plasma concentrations of desfuroylceftiofur (DCA) ≥2 μg/mL (total daily dose, approximately 5.4 mg/kg/day). For more resistant bacteria (MIC >2 μg/mL), higher dose rates are required.
  - Ceftiofur crystalline-free acid[4] can also be used in foals. The labeled dose of 6.6 mg/kg, administered subcutaneously (SQ) q72h is effective against only 79% of bacterial isolates obtained from foals (it is expected to be effective against bacteria with a MIC ≤ 0.5 μg/mL (Hall et al, 2011). To increase the spectrum of activity, the dose needs to be increased and the administration interval may need to be decreased; requires additional pharmacokinetic studies. Swellings at the injection site are common.
  - Ticarcillin/clavulanic acid: 50 to 100 mg/kg IV q6h; indicated for *Pseudomonas aeruginosa* infections susceptible to the drug.

---

[4]Excede (Pfizer Animal Health, New York, New York).

NEO

- Trimethoprim-sulfonamide: 25 to 30 mg/kg PO or IV q12h. Do *not* administer if uncertain of GI function. Many gram-negative organisms may be resistant; therefore, it is not an optimal drug combination for treating a septic foal.
- Use third-generation cephalosporins if meningitis is suspected: cefotaxime, 40 to 50 mg/kg IV q6 to 8h. Many other cephalosporin choices include:
  - Ceftazidime: 50 mg/kg IV q6h
  - Ceftriaxone: 25 mg/kg IV q6h
  - Ceftizoxime: 50 mg/kg IV q6h
  - Cefotaxime: 40 mg/kg IV q6h (or CRI with loading dose of 40 mg/kg IV followed by CRI of a total daily dose of 160 mg/kg per 24 h)
  - Cefepime, a fourth-generation cephalosporin, 11 mg/kg IV q8h
- Imipenem-cilastatin sodium and meropenem: Broadest-spectrum beta-lactam bactericidal antimicrobials at 10 to 15 mg/kg slowly IV q6h. These carbapenem antimicrobials are reserved for foals with nonresponsive or highly drug-resistant sepsis.
- ***Practice Tip:*** *Imipenem-cilastatin sodium and meropenem are expensive, and rarely seizures are reported as an adverse effect. The carbapenem group of antimicrobials is excreted in the urine; therefore, an effort should be made to prevent the foal's mare from ingesting urine-contaminated hay.*
- Fluconazole for fungal infections:
  - 8.8 mg/kg PO q24h (loading dose)
  - 4.4 to 5 mg/kg PO q24h (maintenance dose)

Immune System Support: Colostrum Administration
- Feed only foals with normal cardiovascular status and body temperature.
- ***Practice Tip:*** *Foals should receive approximately 1 L of colostrum with a specific gravity >1.060 divided into 3 to 4 feedings during the first 8 to 10 hours of life. This dosage is equivalent to 1g of IgG per kilogram body mass.*
- Foals intolerant of feeding that do *not* receive colostrum during the initial 12-hour period postpartum require plasma transfusions, 20 to 40 mL/kg IV.

Coagulopathies in Sepsis
- Foals with sepsis commonly develop coagulopathies.
- It has been reported that the prothrombin time/partial thromboplastin time, whole blood decalcification, fibrinogen, fibrinogen degradation products, percent plasminogen, percent alpha$_2$-antiplasmin, and platelet activator inhibitor are increased in foals with septicemia.
- Protein C and antithrombin concentrations are decreased, consistent with reduced endogenous anticoagulants and subsequent hypercoagulation.
- There are a number of reports of digital, brachial, and aortoiliac arterial thromboses representing clinical evidence of coagulopathies such as DIC.
- Treatment of coagulopathies includes therapy aimed at sepsis, i.e., broad-spectrum antimicrobials, heparin, and plasma.
- Low-molecular-weight heparin is currently used in human patients and adult horses, and was recently studied in foals. Recommended doses for adult horses are:
  - Dalteparin: 50 IU/kg SQ q24h
  - Enoxaparin: 40 IU/kg SQ q24h
  - A report in foals suggests the dose of dalteparin be increased; additional research is needed to determine the optimal dose.

Plasma Transfusion
- Use plasma to manage failure of passive transfer (FPT) and to:
  - Provide opsonins
  - Improve immune response
  - Support oncotic pressure
  - Defend intravascular fluid volume
- Plasma also provides antithrombin and clotting factors for foals with coagulopathies.
- Fresh plasma contains platelets (platelet-rich plasma), which is an advantage for foals with neonatal alloimmune thrombocytopenia.
- Administer hyperimmune plasma from donors negative for red-cell antibodies and blood-borne diseases. This plasma is commercially available from several sources.
- If orally administered, serum-derived commercial IgG products can be used. One example is Seramune.[5] They should be mixed with colostrum to improve absorption. The same dose of 1 g/kg of IgG is recommended. *Absorption of these products can be erratic,* and foals should be reevaluated after administration of these products for IgG serum concentration.
  - Foals >18 hours old or foals with GI dysfunction may be unable to absorb sufficient colostral antibodies and may need a plasma transfusion.
- Minimum plasma volume to administer is 20 mL/kg. The volume of plasma required to manage FPT depends on the IgG in the recipient's blood and donor's plasma.
- Because of sepsis-induced protein catabolism, septic foals need a larger volume of plasma than healthy foals to increase serum IgG to the same concentration.
- Administer sufficient plasma to increase serum IgG >800 mg/dL for septicemia.
- Recheck serum and blood IgG every few days during treatment to ensure that concentrations remain adequate.
- Sources of commercial plasma with IgG concentration ≥2500 mg/dL:

HiGamm Equi	Polymune Plus	Immuno-Glo	Hypermune
Lake Immunogenics	PlasvacUSA, Inc	Mg Biologics	Veterinary Immunogenics Ldt.
348 Berg Road	1535 Templeton Rd	1721 Y Ave.	United Kingdom
Ontario NY 91451	Templeton, CA 93465	Ames, IA 50014	+44 (0) 1768 863881
800-648-9990	805-434-0321	515-769-2340	

General Nursing Care
- Provide warmth, using heating pads, warm fluids, radiant warmers, forced hot air blankets, and fluid jacket warmers (Thermal Angel Blood and IV Fluid Infusion Warmer[6]), a warm intravenous fluid pouch, and Safe and Warm[7] reusable instant heat measuring 7 to 9 inches (17.5 to 22.5 cm).
- Maintain sternal recumbency as much as possible. Frequent repositioning helps prevent decubitus sores and dependent lung atelectasis.

[5]Sera, Inc., Shawnee Mission, Kansas.
[6]Estill Medical Technologies, Inc., Dallas, Texas.
[7]Safe and Warm, Inc., Boulder City, Nevada.

- Apply sterile ocular lubricant to the eyes of foals that spend most of their time in lateral recumbency to prevent exposure keratitis and ulceration. Carefully evaluate both eyes daily for corneal ulcers.
- Gastroprotectants can be administered if warranted. Gastroduodenal ulcers in these patients may be associated with GI hypoperfusion rather than gastric pH. Critically ill foals may have an alkaline gastric environment and a blunted response to inhibitors of acid production; thus the use of histamine-2 (H_2)-antagonists may be of little use in the care of these patients. Milk in the stomach is alkalinizing to the gastric contents, and frequent feeding is protective if the foal is tolerant of enteral nutrition.
- A report (Furr M et al, 2012) described the use of antiulcer medications in hospitalized neonatal foals and an associated increased risk of diarrhea. Omeprazole, ranitidine, cimetidine, and sucralfate were all associated with an increased odds ratio of diarrhea.
  - Gastroprotectant options include:
  - Ranitidine, 6.6 mg/kg PO q8h, 1.5 mg/kg IV q8h, also a mild prokinetic, and/or
  - Famotidine, 2.8 mg/kg PO q12h or 0.3 mg/kg IV q12h or
  - Omeprazole, 2 to 4 mg/kg PO q24h +/−
  - Sucralfate, 20 mg/kg PO q6h

Dysphagia

- Dysphagia in foals is common and can manifest as:
  - Nasal regurgitation of milk
  - An inability to prehend (suckle)
  - Aspiration pneumonia
- Differential diagnoses for inability to prehend include:
  - Peripartum hypoxia
  - Significant hyponatremia
  - Botulism
  - White muscle disease
  - Craniofacial malformations
  - Cranial nerve deficits
- Differential diagnoses for nasal regurgitation of milk include:
  - Transient pharyngeal paresis associated with peripartum asphyxia
  - Selenium deficiency (white muscle disease) associated with dorsal displacement of the soft palate
  - Cleft palate
  - Epiglottic entrapment or persistent frenulum
  - Subepiglottic cyst
  - Botulism
  - Esophageal obstruction (choke)
  - Megaesophagus
  - Branchial arch defect
  - Homozygous state of HYPP
  - Idiopathic: Some foals cannot nurse without aspirating and none of the above possibilities defines the problem. Most of these affected foals drink successfully from a pan/bucket placed on the ground. There may be a breed predisposition for this problem.

- Pharyngeal paresis associated with peripartum asphyxia or selenium deficiency is usually a transient disorder and resolves with time and selenium supplementation if deficient.

●〉 WHAT TO DO

Dysphagia

- Treat the underlying cause, if known.
- Affected foals need to be fed through a nasogastric tube if too weak to voluntarily drink, or muzzled and allowed to drink milk from a bucket held in a dependent position to minimize the potential for aspiration. Most have a good prognosis with time, unless there is an irreparable congenital defect.
- Treat aspiration pneumonia.
- Foals homozygous for the HYPP gene are usually dysphagic and dysphonic as neonates.
  - Nasal regurgitation of milk, ptyalism, and stridor are common.
  - A DNA test for HYPP is available.
  - Many foals improve as they grow.
  - Severe cases need to be managed with acetazolamide (2 mg/kg PO q12h) and/or phenytoin (2.8 to 10 mg/kg PO q12h). Therapeutic drug monitoring should be performed for phenytoin (goal: 5 to 10 µg/mL). **Important:** Phenytoin minimizes clinical signs but does *not* prevent hyperkalemia, while acetazolamide modulates plasma potassium levels and aids in preventing hyperkalemia.

Colic

Signs of Colic in Newborn Foals

- Poor nursing behavior: "milk face" from milk streaming down the foal's face
- Rolling, treading
- Abnormal posture while recumbent
- Abdominal distention
- Teeth grinding
- Tachycardia, tachypnea
- Tenesmus

Common Causes

- *Meconium impaction:* This is generally confirmed with abdominal palpation and digital examination. Abdominal radiography or ultrasonography is used to visualize more orad impactions. Overzealous treatment for meconium impaction with repeated enemas can result in colic or straining because of proctitis or perineal irritation.
- *Ileus:* Associated with GI hypoxia from peripartum asphyxia or septic shock
- *Intussusception:* This is seen with ultrasonography ("target" lesion of intussusceptum invaginating into the intussuscipiens) and associated with intestinal hypoxia and resultant dysmotility.
- *Enteritis/peritonitis:* Frequently caused by clostridial microorganisms or viruses and accompanying bacteremia. Foals are often colicky before development of diarrhea.
- *Gastroduodenal ulceration:* This is uncommon as a primary cause of colic in the neonate but may be a primary problem

in the older foal. Many gastric ulcers are clinically "silent" in neonatal foals.

- *Intestinal volvulus:* **Important:** A true surgical emergency. Diagnosis is suspected based on clinical signs of severe pain, reflux, and abdominal distention. Ultrasonographic evaluation of the abdomen can confirm the presence of multiple loops of turgid, distended small intestine with minimal to *no* motility. Abdominal distention is often rapid and severe.
- *Chlyoabdomen:* Often transient and *no* cause identified.

Meconium Impaction

- *Practice Tip:* Meconium impaction is more common in colts than in fillies. It is not unusual for the foals to also have FPT of immunity; perhaps colostrum ingestion aids in meconium expulsion, or failure to absorb ingested IgG indicates intestinal malfunction.
- In addition to colic, abdominal distention, and poor nursing behavior, affected foals may have tenesmus, tail flagging, and an arched-back posture. If obstruction is complete, abdominal distention can develop rapidly.

Diagnosis

- Palpation of firm meconium in the rectum and pelvic canal on gentle digital examination
- A history of unsuccessful straining to defecate
- Firm fecal material in the pelvic inlet detected with abdominal palpation, plain radiography, or contrast radiography after a barium enema examination
- Sonographic detection of echogenic material in the distal colon and rectum

●》 WHAT TO DO

Meconium Impaction
Warm, Soapy (Ivory Soap) Water, Gravity Enemas
- Use a soft urinary catheter or small rubber feeding tube and enema bucket with 75 to 180 mL of the solution. If repeated enemas are needed, alternate soapy water with warm water or water mixed with J-lube or rectal lubricant to minimize excessive mucosal irritation. **Practice Tip:** *Dioctyl sodium sulfosuccinate (DSS) enemas should not be used because of irritation and secondary proctitis.* If repeated enemas are needed, the solution can be diluted to half-strength sodium chloride (a 1:1 ratio of 0.9% saline and water) made into a soapy water enema. This avoids excessive free water enemas and subsequent hyponatremia.
- Sodium phosphate[8] enemas made for humans can also be used in foals. However, *no* more than one "adult" sized or two "pediatric" sized enemas are used per day because of the potential for hyperphosphatemia.
- **Note:** Repeated enemas may lead to pathologic tenesmus and rectal edema!

Retention Acetylcysteine Enemas
- High, retention enemas are indicated in foals with high (orad) meconium impactions and in those with impactions that do *not* resolve with soapy water or sodium phosphate enemas.

- The foal is usually sedated for the procedure (e.g., diazepam ± butorphanol).
- Use Mucomyst or powdered N-acetyl-L-cysteine. If Mucomyst is used, add 40 mL of 20% solution to 160 mL water to make a 4% solution. If using the powder, add 8 g of powder and 1½ tbsp (~22.5 g) of sodium bicarbonate (baking soda) to 200 mL of water. Gently insert a lubricated Foley urinary catheter (30F with 30-mL balloon in most average-sized foals) with a balloon tip approximately 2 to 4 inches (5 to 10 cm) into the rectum (as long as it passes without resistance) and gently inflate the balloon. Slowly infuse 4 to 7 oz (120 to 200 mL) of acetylcysteine solution by gravity flow into the rectum. Occlude the catheter end for a minimum of 15 minutes (ideally 45 minutes). Deflate the balloon and remove the catheter. The retention enema can be repeated.
- Administer N-butylscopolammonium bromide[9] (0.3 mg/kg body weight slowly IV or SQ once)

Oral Laxatives
- Proximal (high) impactions require oral laxatives in addition to enemas. The safest, least irritating laxative is mineral oil (120 to 160 mL) administered through a nasogastric tube if the foal is >12 to 18 hours of age. Mineral oil lubricates around the impaction and reduces the risk of complete obstruction, which can rapidly result in severe and painful gas accumulation and abdominal distention. **Practice Tip:** *Milk of magnesia (60 to 120 mL) is an oral laxative that must be used conservatively.*
- **Do Not Use:** Castor oil or DSS administered orally is *not* recommended because of excessive mucosal irritation and increased risk of severe diarrhea and colic.

Intravenous Fluid Therapy
- Intravenous fluid therapy is useful in cases of refractory impaction. Dextrose supplementation is recommended if nursing is curtailed because of increasing abdominal distention and colic.
- In general, foals should *not* be allowed to nurse until the meconium begins to pass. Dextrose supplementation should be provided (4 mg/kg/min) and PN should be instituted if the colic and distention lasts longer than 24 hours.

Percutaneous Bowel Trocarization
- Bowel trocarization should only be used in rare cases. If severe abdominal distention develops before the impaction resolves, enough to cause severe, life-threatening respiratory compromise, consider the technique described for cecal trocarization if cecal dilation is present (see Chapter 18, p. 160, and p. 548). Trocarization often provides immediate pain relief without excessive medication and allows time for medical therapy and potential presurgical stabilization. Be aware of the risk of causing potentially fatal septic peritonitis. Broad-spectrum antimicrobials should be administered.

Surgical Management
- Surgical exploration and relief of the impaction may be indicated in foals with severe abdominal distention resulting in respiratory and cardiovascular compromise (intraabdominal hypertension with abdominal compartment syndrome).

Analgesics and Sedatives
- Analgesics and sedatives may be needed to prevent self-trauma in foals that are recumbent and rolling.
- Flunixin meglumine: 0.5 to 1.0 mg/kg IV q24 to 36h provided that renal function is normal; avoid repetitive doses because of its

[8]Fleet (C.B. Fleet Company, Inc., Lynchburg, Pennsylvania).

[9]Buscopan (Boerhinger Ingelheim Vetmedica, Inc., St. Joseph, Missouri).

potential for adverse effects on the GI tract and kidney. Alternatively, ketoprofen is used because it is believed to be safer (1 to 2 mg/kg IV q24h).

- Butorphanol: 0.01 to 0.04 mg/kg IV. This is an excellent first choice and usually highly effective. Administration can be repeated as needed at 1- to 4-hour intervals provided the foal is *not* excessively sedated.
- Xylazine: 0.1 to 0.5 mg/kg IV; use sparingly because of adverse effects on GI motility and hemodynamics. Some debilitated neonatal foals experience significant ileus or respiratory/hemodynamic compromise after use of xylazine. Administering butorphanol and xylazine together reduces the dosage of xylazine needed.

Ileus

- Decreased GI motility is associated with ischemic and hypoxic bowel damage resulting from sepsis/SIRS/septic shock or peripartum hypoxia and adverse events.
- Ileus may also be present with hypovolemia, hypoperfusion, and hypothermia.
- *Practice Tip: Small-intestinal intussusception can theoretically develop as a result of ileus or prokinetic drugs used to promote motility.*
- Premature foals may have ileus and intolerance of enteral feeding.

Clinical Signs

- Decreased or absent borborygmi
- Tympanic abdominal distention
- Colic
- Gastric reflux: Bloody, dark brown to black reflux suggests mucosal damage; consider administration of sucralfate in these cases
- Diarrhea or constipation

Diagnosis

- Based on results of physical examination and supported by several diagnostic techniques:
  - Transabdominal ultrasound examination shows distended or hypomotile bowel and lack of propulsive motility. If necrotizing enterocolitis is present, ultrasound examination may show gas echoes within the bowel walls.
  - Abdominal radiographs show generalized small- and large-bowel distention. Pneumatosis intestinalis (gas formation within the bowel wall) is observed with severe necrotizing enterocolitis.

◉〉 WHAT TO DO

Ileus

- Depends on the underlying cause

Severe Hypoxic/Ischemic Gut Damage with Gastric Reflux or Bloody Diarrhea

- Provide intestinal rest. Discontinue all enteral feeding until reflux, distention, and diarrhea resolve and borborygmi return. Severe cases may need up to 7 days of complete intestinal rest. Small amounts of easily digested enteral food (milk or commercial isotonic products) support enterocytes and enzyme production.
- Parenteral alimentation (see p. 556)

- Broad-spectrum, bactericidal antibiotics are recommended (see pp. 549 and 557).
- Sucralfate: 20 mg/kg PO q6h
- If a foal shows signs of endotoxemia, consider administering 20 to 40 mL/kg of hyperimmune plasma to provide opsonins and immunoglobulins to support the immune system.
- Slowly reintroduce enteral feeding, beginning with small volumes of colostrum or fresh mare's milk.
- Complications associated with necrotizing enterocolitis include:
  - Septicemia
  - Intussusceptions
  - Peritonitis
  - Anemia
  - Stricture formation
- Rule out *C. perfringens* and *C. difficile* infection.

Mild to Moderate Ileus, Mild Colic Associated with Feeding, Varying Amounts of Reflux, and Inconsistent Manure Production

- Decrease volume of enteral feedings temporarily (may require short-term discontinuation) and support with partial PN.
- Allow controlled exercise, short periods of turnout with dam in a small paddock.
- If constipation develops, treat with enemas, oral laxatives (mineral oil and psyllium in small amounts), and maintain hydration with orally or intravenously administered fluids.
- Give oral probiotic agents: commercial products or 2 to 3 oz (60 to 90 mL) of active culture yogurt PO q12 to 24h.
- Neostigmine 0.5 to 1 mg/50-kg foal can be administered SQ if there is gaseous distention of the large intestine and obstruction has been ruled out. Sedation may be needed if abdominal pain develops following the neostigmine. Metaclopramide IV, PO, or rectal suppository (see p. 548) can be used for generalized ileus.

Intussusception

- Colic caused by intussusception may be mild to severe, depending on the location and duration of obstruction and the level of mentation of the foal.
- Abdominal distention and reflux usually develop.
- The diagnosis often is made with transabdominal ultrasonography. Sonography shows "bulls-eye" target lesions that represent a cross-sectional view of intussuscepted bowel. The intussusceptum invaginates into the intussuscipiens. Contrast radiography may help identify the location of obstruction.

◉〉 WHAT TO DO

Intussusception

- Treatment is surgical.
- Prognosis for survival is guarded to grave if multiple intussusceptions are found, if there are large sections of compromised bowel, or if peritonitis is severe.
- Postoperative complications include:
  - Recurrent intussusceptions
  - Stricture formation
  - Intraabdominal adhesions

Enteritis: With or Without Peritonitis

- Enteritis may be caused by a primary GI disorder (e.g., rotaviral infection) or secondary to other systemic conditions, such as septicemia or peripartum hypoxia (see Chapter 18, p. 220, and pp. 542 and 547, respectively).

Clinical Signs

- Colic
- Abdominal distention, reduced or absent borborygmi, tympany
- Diarrhea ± blood, mucus
- Variable rectal temperature
- Injected sclera and hyperemic mucous membranes if enteritis is associated with endotoxemia
- Prolonged CRT, hypovolemia, and dehydration
- Tachycardia
- Leukopenia with neutropenia with or without immature (band) neutrophilia is common in foals with enteritis

Infectious Causes of Enteritis in Neonatal Foals

Bacterial

- *Salmonella* can cause acute to peracute diarrhea accompanied by peritonitis and endotoxemia in severe cases. Affected foals often are bacteremic and are at increased risk of developing septic osteomyelitis or arthritis.
- *E. coli* septicemia: *E. coli* isolates recovered from the blood of foals with diarrhea have *not* been shown definitively to be enterotoxigenic pathogens; many foals with *E. coli* bacteremia also have concurrent enteritis. Enterohemorrhagic (attaching and effacing) strains of *E. coli* have been associated with sporadic enteritis in foals.
- Clostridial enteritis *(C. perfringens, C. difficile)* can produce fetid diarrhea that is often bloody, particularly with *C. perfringens* infection. Affected foals often have concurrent septicemia. Lactase deficiency has been documented in foals with clostridiosis. Other clostridial species, such as *C. sordelli* or *C. welchii* may cause diarrhea; however further evidence is required.

Viral

- Rotavirus, coronavirus, adenovirus, and parvovirus have been isolated from foals with diarrhea.
- ***Practice Tip:*** *Rotavirus is the most common cause of viral diarrhea in neonatal foals.*
  - Rotavirus produces nonfetid, watery diarrhea that may be accompanied by fever and anorexia.
  - Anecdotally there is an increased incidence of gastroduodenal ulcer disease during some rotavirus endemics.
  - Rotaviral infections have been associated with lactase deficiency.
- Coronavirus appears to be an emerging pathogen in adult horses; it can commonly be found in feces of healthy foals.
  - In 2011-2012 there are a number of published and non-published outbreaks of febrile and enteric disease in adult horses in Japan and the United States.
  - The most common clinical signs include:
    - Fever
    - Lethargy
    - Diarrhea ranging from mild to severe

- The vast majority of these cases are adult horses; however, the increased incidence of coronavirus outbreaks raises awareness of its possible presence in foals and as a co-infection cause of diarrhea.

Parasitic

- *Strongyloides westeri* nematode larvae have been associated with mild neonatal foal enteritis in high numbers.
- *Cryptosporidium parvum* is another infectious cause of enteritis in foals. It can occur as both sporadic cases and outbreaks of diarrhea in foals. It may be a monoinfection or co-infection.
- *Giardia* is a potential protozoal cause of diarrhea in foals; its exact role in enteritis of horses and foals remains to be explained.

Nutritional

- Overfeeding can produce gastric distention, ileus, and diarrhea, particularly with milk replacer.
- If the gastric, digestive, and absorptive capacities are overwhelmed, a large, rapidly fermentable carbohydrate load reaches the colon, resulting in osmotic diarrhea.
- Sudden diet changes (e.g., changes from mare's milk to artificial replacer) can result in diarrhea.
- Lactase deficiency is associated with bacterial and viral enteritides. Primary lactase deficiency is believed to affect foals; however, this remains to be confirmed.

Other

- Enterocolitis is associated with hypoxic or ischemic intestinal damage. It is also associated with prematurity and intolerance to enteral feeding with bacterial overgrowth (e.g., necrotizing enterocolitis).
- Sand or dirt ingestion can induce a mechanical enterocolitis.
- "Foal heat diarrhea" is caused by physiologic and maturational changes occurring in the GI tract and usually results in self-limiting diarrhea that occurs between 5 and 14 days of age and lasts less than 5 to 7 days. Affected foals are *not* systemically ill and have normal clinical laboratory studies.

Diagnosis: General Guidelines

- Obtain a blood culture in foals with acute diarrhea if septicemia is suspected (e.g., *Salmonella, E. coli, Clostridium,* and other enteric organisms). ***Practice Tip:*** *Up to 50% of foals with enteritis are blood-culture positive.*
- Obtain a fecal culture for *Salmonella* sp. and clostridial organisms. Polymerase chain reaction can be used for *Salmonella* organisms, and toxin assays should be performed for clostridial infections (toxins A and B for *C. difficile;* alpha, beta, and epsilon toxins for *C. perfringens*). (See Chapter 18, p. 220).
- Perform fecal flotation and direct smear.
- Obtain a rotavirus test: Rotazyme[10] enzyme-linked immunosorbent assay, Rota Test[11] (latex agglutination), or fecal PCR.

---

[10]Abbott Laboratories, North Chicago, Illinois.
[11]Wampole Laboratories, Carter Wallace, Inc., Cranbury, New Jersey.

- Electron microscopy is useful for identifying viral infections, including rotavirus.
- Fecal PCR for *Salmonella*, rotavirus, coronavirus, *Cryptosporidium*, and *C. perfringens* toxins.
- Immunofluorescent antibody testing for *Cryptosporidium* and *Giardia*
- Abdominal radiography:
  - Enteritis, especially during the early stages, often is associated with varying degrees of ileus and generalized gas or fluid accumulation within the bowel lumen.
  - Intramural gas accumulation (pneumatosis intestinalis) occurs with severe necrotizing enterocolitis. Pneumoperitoneum occurs with bowel rupture.
  - Radiographs are useful to rule out sand- or dirt-induced enteropathy.
- Transabdominal ultrasonography:
  - An increased volume of intraluminal fluid and bowel wall edema may be present with enteritis.
  - Peritonitis is associated with an increased volume of echogenic peritoneal fluid with or without fibrin tags.
  - Intramural gas accumulation (pneumatosis intestinalis) casts bright white echoes and is associated with severe hypoxic intestinal damage.
- Hematology, chemistry:
  - Leukopenia and neutropenia are associated with endotoxemia.
  - Immature neutrophilia (bands) may be present.
  - Toxicity of cells may be evident on cytologic examination.
  - Secretory diarrhea usually results in hypochloremia, hyponatremia, varying degrees of metabolic acidosis, hemoconcentration, and variable potassium concentrations.
  - Protein-losing enteropathy can result in hypoproteinemia.
- Perform abdominocentesis if septic peritonitis is suspected.
  - Peritoneal fluid contains increased protein concentration and nucleated cell count, although often it is *not* specific in the information provided.
  - ***Practice Tip:*** *Be very cautious performing abdominocentesis in foals with enteritis because enterocentesis can have fatal consequences.*

●▶ WHAT TO DO

Neonatal Diarrhea (see Chapter 18, p. 220)
- Restore and maintain hydration using balanced, polyionic fluids such as Plasma-Lyte A or 148, Normosol R, or LRS.
- Monitor serum concentrations of electrolytes, glucose, and creatinine, acid-base balance (blood gases), lactate, PCV, and total protein.
- If the foal is anorectic, administer dextrose for the first 12 to 24 hours, and if the period of anorexia extends beyond this period, parenteral nutrition is instituted in the neonatal foal.
- Broad-spectrum, bactericidal, parenteral antimicrobial therapy is recommended for foals with severe diarrhea because of the increased risk of septicemia.

- ***Practice Tip:*** *Enterococcus sp. is the most common bacteria isolated in blood cultures from foals with diarrhea. Therefore, penicillin or ampicillin and amikacin should be part of the antimicrobial coverage when enteritis and sepsis are part of the clinical picture. If amikacin is administered, renal function must be monitored! Metronidazole is indicated for* C. difficile.
- Administer intestinal protectants: Biosponge or bismuth subsalicylate[12] 0.5 to 1 mL/kg PO q4 to 6h; kaolin and pectin, 4 to 8 mL/kg PO q12h.
- A Lactaid tablet mixed with 2 to 6 oz of yogurt can be administered orally q4h for possible lactase deficiencies.
- Nonsteroidal anti-inflammatory drug therapy is used by some clinicians if the foal shows signs of endotoxemia. A "low-dose" of flunixin meglumine, 0.25 mg/kg IV q8 to 12h, is preferred for short periods, because of the adverse risks to the kidneys and GI tract.
  - The conservative use of NSAIDs is advised because of their ulcerogenic potential and the possibility of disrupting normal renal function, reducing mucosal perfusion, and slowing healing of the gastrointestinal tract.
- Plasma administration benefits foals with FPT, hypoproteinemia, and potentially those with endotoxemia.
- Consider antiulcer medication: sucralfate, 20 to 40 mg/kg PO q6h; omeprazole, 4 mg/kg PO q24h. Foals with diarrhea are at increased risk for gastric ulceration.
- Metronidazole (see Equine Emergency Drugs; Appendix 9, p. 850) is recommended for foals with clostridial enteritis.
- For noninfectious causes: Administer loperamide, 4 to 16 mg PO q6h, beginning with the low-dose and increasing the dose in 2-mg increments every 2 to 3 doses. ***Practice Tip:*** *Loperamide (antidiarrheal) increases segmentation rate, slows transit time, and may enhance toxin absorption in cases of acute, infectious enteritis. Therefore, the use of loperamide is reserved for foals that do* not *have signs of severe endotoxemia or infectious enteritis.*
- Lidocaine may be beneficial for ileus and abdominal pain (see p. 549).

Congenital Malformations of the Neonatal Foal

- Hernias: umbilical, scrotal, diaphragmatic
- Hamartomas: congenital tumors and vascular proliferations
- Cleft palate
- Prognathia
- Brachygnathia
- Subepiglottic cysts
- Pharyngeal cysts
- Arthrogryposis
- Clubfeet
- Choanal atresia
- Congenital cataracts and other ocular defects
- Cardiac defects: ventricular septal defect; tetralogy of Fallot; others
- Kyphosis
- Scoliosis
- Mesodiverticular band

---

[12]Corrective Suspension (Phoenix Pharmaceuticals, Inc, St. Joseph, Missouri).

- GI malformations
- Renal dysplasia
- Biliary atresia
- Portosystemic shunt
- Congenital immunodeficiencies (selective IgM or IgG deficiency)
- Megaesophagus
- Ectopic ureter
- Ureteral dilation
- Bladder malformations
- Atresia ani/atresia coli

Genetic Disorders of the Neonatal Foal

- See Chapter 13, pp. 70-72.
- Polysaccharide storage myopathy of Quarter Horses and related breeds
- Equine polysaccharide storage myopathy of Draft horses (*not* clinically apparent in neonatal period)
- Recurrent exertional rhabdomyolysis of Quarter Horses and related breeds (*not* clinically apparent in neonatal period)
- Glycogen storage disease IV (glycogen branching enzyme deficiency) in Quarter Horses and related breeds
- HYPP (may *not* be apparent in neonatal period) in Quarter Horses and related breeds
- Atlanto-occipital-axial malformations of Arabians and other breeds
- Cerebellar abiotrophy of Arabians and Gotland ponies
- Anterior segment dysgenesis of Rocky Mountain Horses
- Equine night blindness (Appaloosas)

- Epitheliogenesis imperfecta (Saddlebreds and other breeds)
- Hereditary junctional mechanobullous disease of Belgian Draft horses
- Equine glucose-6-phosphate dehydrogenase deficiency (Saddlebreds)
- Cataracts (Thoroughbreds, Morgans, Quarter Horses, Belgians, possibly Arabians)
- Ileocecocolic aganglionosis; overo lethal white syndrome in Paint Horses and Pintos
- Hereditary equine regional dermal asthenia in Quarter Horses and related breeds—*not* clinically apparent in neonatal period
- Severe combined immunodeficiency syndrome of Arabians
- Fell Pony immunodeficiency syndrome
- Norwegian Fjord arthrogryposis
- Megaesophagus (Friesian horses?); *not* necessarily apparent at birth
- Juvenile epilepsy of Egyptian Arabians
- Lavender foal syndrome of Arabians
- Narcolepsy/catalepsy (American miniatures, others?)
- Dwarfism (American miniatures)
- Inhibitory glycine receptor deficiency in the spinal cord (myoclonus) of Peruvian Pasos
- Persistent hyperammonemia in Morgan horses

References

References can be found on the companion website at www.equine-emergencies.com.

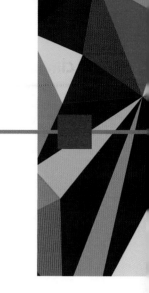

CHAPTER 32

Shock and Systemic Inflammatory Response Syndrome

Thomas J. Divers and Joan Norton

Shock and SIRS Terminology

Important definitions:

Shock: Inadequate tissue oxygenation, most often caused by decreased perfusion

Septic shock: Most commonly a result of bacteremia, endotoxemia associated with gram-negative sepsis or other pathogen-associated molecular patterns of gram-positive or gram-negative sepsis, which trigger a cascade of vasoactive and inflammatory mediators resulting in cardiopulmonary and vascular changes of shock; most commonly caused by enterocolitis, metritis, pleuropneumonia, clostridia or staphylococcal infection, and neonatal septicemia

Systemic inflammatory response syndrome (SIRS): The systemic response associated with release of vasoactive and inflammatory mediators that cause shock; initiated by the following:

- Bacteremia
- Endotoxemia (mostly gram-negative bacteria)
- Pathogen-associated molecular patterns (PAMPs) of gram-positive bacteria:
  - Flagellin
  - Lipoteichoic acid
- Traumatic shock
- Hemolysis
- Anaphylactoid-like reactions
- Localized infections
- Hyperthermia
- Hypothermia
- Dehydration
- Hypotension
- Any organ injury that causes hypoxia and release of vasoactive or inflammatory mediators. All of the above may activate chemokines, cytokines, prostanoids, neutrophils, myeloperoxidase and platelets.

Multiple organ dysfunction syndrome (MODS): Septic shock or SIRS causing dysfunction of one or more organs such that sequelae and signs from this organ dysfunction become clinically apparent. The most commonly involved organs in the horse are the following:

- Heart and cardiovascular system: weak pulses, tachycardia, initially bright red congested membranes that turn a purplish color, with progression of sepsis because of the deoxygenation of hemoglobin in "low flow" capillaries
- Renal system: depression from azotemia and electrolyte abnormalities; decreased urine production
- Intestinal tract: ileus, diarrhea, colic, trembling, tachycardia, fever, and depression caused by absorption of toxins and bacteria across compromised gut wall
  - When horses are given endotoxin, colic and cardiovascular abnormalities precede fever by 30 to 60 minutes.
- Lung: pulmonary edema or acute respiratory distress syndrome (ARDS) (these occur infrequently in adult horses)
- Coagulation system: most commonly hypercoagulation and thrombosis; however, with severe thrombocytopenia, bleeding may occur
- ***Important:*** *Feet: laminitis—the foot should be considered a shock organ in the horse!*
- Endocrine system: inappropriate cortisol production in some septic foals potentiating signs of hypotension. Glucose dysregulation often causes hypoglycemia in septic foals and hyperglycemia in septic adults. The hypoglycemia in foals is not related to excessive insulin production because their insulin levels are low.
  - Adiponectin, an anti-inflammatory and insulin-sensitizing adipokine, is diminished in sepsis, while resistin, a protein with proinflammatory properties and other proinflammatory cytokines are elevated (tumor necrosis factor–alpha [TNF-α]). These responses are likely exaggerated in horses with metabolic syndrome.
  - Many cytokines that mediate insulin resistance are elevated in sepsis.

Clinical Signs of Shock and SIRS

- In septic shock and SIRS, inadequate tissue perfusion and oxygenation are mostly a result of the following:
  - Intravascular fluid volume loss
  - Hypotension—poor vascular tone
  - Heart failure and/or insufficient cardiac output
  - Maldistribution of blood flow
  - "Leaky" capillary membranes and edema formation
  - Diminished oxygenation of hemoglobin
- Early in the course of septic shock and SIRS, the predominant cause of inadequate tissue perfusion-oxygenation is maldistribution of blood flow, frequently followed by systemic hypotension.
- Early maldistribution of blood flow results from the following:
  - Decrease in arteriovenous tone caused by endogenous release of beta-catecholamines and release of mediators such as nitric oxide, cytokines, and autocoids.
- Leaky vessels result from the following:
  - Arachidonic acid metabolism (cyclooxygenase-2 [COX-2]): prostanoids and leukotrienes
  - Macrophage procoagulant production and complement activation
  - Neutrophil and platelet adherence to vessels causing the release of inflammatory mediators, oxidative enzyme activity, and activation of proteases, oxidants, and other damaging enzymes such as matrix metalloproteinases
  - Release of autocoids (e.g., histamine and endorphins)
  - Microthrombosis: platelet aggregation; exposure of subendothelial collagen; and release of tissue factor, anaphylatoxins, and other procoagulants
- *Treatment is most successful during the early stage of shock and SIRS.* The early phase of shock is frequently called the "hyperdynamic" phase of shock and is associated with left ventricular dilation, increased heart rate, and increased cardiac output (mostly caused by increased heart rate and decreased vascular resistance). The mucous membranes are generally hyperemic during this phase.
  - ***Practice Tip:*** *This is the best time for fluid therapy!*
- Later stages of shock are associated with the following:
  - Decreased cardiac index, including myocardial depression
  - Diminished beta$_1$ and alpha response (inappropriate vasodilation)
  - Systemic hypotension: often refractory to most drugs
- Further maldistribution of blood flow occurs from the following:
  - Shunts
  - Sludging in capillaries
  - Further increase in vascular permeability: capillary leak syndrome
  - Vascular obstruction
- Diminished cellular oxygenation and increased cellular acid production occur, including increased tissue CO_2 and increased $Pv_{CO_2}:Pa_{CO_2}$ ratio.

- Free radical formation, increased intracellular Ca^{2+}, decreased adenosine triphosphate, and cellular death also result. Increased caspases cause apoptosis and cellular death resulting from either apoptosis or necrosis can further stimulate inflammation.
- Progression of the foregoing leads to MODS.
- At this stage the following occur:
  - Extremities are cold
  - Peripheral pulse is weak
  - Mucous membranes are dark
  - Capillary refill is slow (>3 seconds)
  - Mental alertness is altered
  - Petechiation may be present
  - Urine production is diminished or absent
- As a result of severe hypoperfusion/hypoxemia, the intestinal barrier is damaged, allowing systemic absorption of normal enteric endotoxin, flagellar proteins, or bacterial translocation (from the intestine to blood and other organs). Diminished hepatic phagocytosis of endotoxin and bacteria further exacerbates the systemic demise.
- ***Practice Tip:*** *In the horse, damage to the circulation of the intestines, lungs, kidneys, and feet (rare in foals) is the most life-threatening injury associated with septic shock and SIRS.*

Diagnosis of SIRS and MODS

- Historical evidence may include depression, anorexia, fever, and tachypnea.
- Physical examination reveals tachycardia, tachypnea, hypothermia or hyperthermia with weak pulse quality, and cool or cold extremities.
- Mucous membranes may be hyperemic or injected with a prolonged capillary refill time. Foals may present with ecchymosis or petechiae in the aural pinnae, nasal septum, or sclera, and hyperemic coronary bands.
- Laboratory data include:
  - Leukopenia (<4000/μL)
  - Leukocytosis (>12,000/μL) with immature band cells
- Hyperlactatemia occurs: >2.0 mmol/L
- Serum biochemistry alterations may occur, related to the underlying cause of SIRS or to the development of MODS
- Foals suffering from sepsis or SIRS may have failure of passive transfer and inadequate concentrations of circulating IgG.
- Hypotension is often seen with mean arterial pressure <65 mm Hg; low central venous pressure can indicate inadequate circulatory volume.
- Arterial blood gas abnormalities may include low Pa_{O_2} (<60 mm Hg) or saturation <92%.
- Urine production should be monitored as absence of or decline in urine production often indicates poor systemic perfusion and in some cases renal failure.
- Aerobic and anaerobic cultures should be obtained to identify an etiologic agent.

Management of Septic Shock and SIRS

Septic Shock and SIRS

- Goal: Reestablish tissue blood flow and oxygen delivery to normal or above-normal values without causing tissue edema or further oxidative injury. Hemodynamic targets should include some measure of the adequacy of cardiac preload, such as central venous pressure, and perfusion pressure, such as mean arterial pressure.
- ***Practice Tip:*** *These can be estimated in the field by speed of jugular fill when the vein is manually compressed in the caudal neck and palpation of the facial artery to estimate pulse pressure.*

Volume Support: The Best General Treatment

- Administer crystalloids: hypertonic saline solution, balanced electrolyte fluid, or both. Hypertonic saline solution (4 to 5 mL/kg IV followed by isotonic fluid therapy) has the advantage of causing a rapid increase in cardiac output and systemic arterial pressure with a decrease in pulmonary arterial pressure and only a brief reduction in vascular tone. Hypertonic saline may decrease polymorphonuclear adhesion molecules, lessening the damage from marginating neutrophils. Additional effects from hypertonic saline may include enhanced phagocytic activity via enhanced Toll-like receptor expression, decreased free radical formation, and diminished short-term tissue edema formation.
  - ***Important:*** Hypertonic saline should be used more cautiously in foals because of their inherent inability to regulate sodium as well as adults.
- The preferred polyionic, isotonic cystalloid: there is minimal or no evidence that lactated Ringer's solution is better than Plasma-Lyte or other crystalloids. Neonatologists generally prefer a fluid with some magnesium and calcium and lower sodium, such as half-strength lactated Ringer's solution (Na^+ = 65.5 mEq/L) or Plasma-Lyte 56 to prevent hypernatremia.
- Administer these fluids rapidly and ideally while measuring systemic arterial pressure, central venous pressure (CVP, see Chapter 10, p. 35), and colloidal pressure (most easily performed by measuring total solids although colloid osmometry is more accurate).
- ***Practice Tip:*** *The field response to fluid therapy is best assessed by monitoring pulse pressure, mucous membrane color, capillary refill time (CRT), heart rate, and urine production.*
- If pulmonary or cerebral edema is a concern (most often a concern in recumbent neonatal foals or foals with sodium abnormalities), then small boluses (2 to 3 mL/kg) should be administered at a time, with reassessment between each fluid bolus. For other age horses experiencing septic shock, rapid administration of 10 to 20 mL/kg can be given initially, followed by assessments previously described.
- Although more expensive, fluid therapy might include a combination of crystalloids and colloids. Colloids are theoretically important in treating septic shock and SIRS because of the vessel leakage that occurs and the inability of crystalloids to remain in the intravascular bed longer than 1 hour. Colloids help maintain colloidal intravascular pressure, which keeps fluids in the intravascular space. Colloids may plug some leaky capillary sites although small molecules may pass into the interstitial space and negatively influence intravascular homeostasis. It is difficult to confirm the potential benefits in spite of their positive effects on mortality in human medicine beyond what occurs with crystalloid therapy, and recent reviews suggest increased mortality with their use!

- Plasma and a synthetic colloid are ideally administered simultaneously because each has separate and potentially beneficial effects in treating sepsis beyond the colloid effects.

Plasma

- Albumin is comparable (slightly lower) with synthetic colloids in maintaining oncotic pressure. Although synthetic colloids have a higher molecular weight, plasma has the advantage of being negatively charged, which helps maintain cations and fluids secondarily in the intravascular space. Albumin may also have some anti-inflammatory and antioxidant properties not found in synthetic colloids.
- Antithrombin III is an important inhibitor of the coagulation cascade.
- Fibronectin enhances opsonization of endotoxin and prevents bacterial translocation.
- Proteins C and S serve to inactivate clotting factors and enhance fibrinolysis; protein C may have anti-inflammatory properties because there is significant "cross-talk" between inflammatory and coagulation events.
- Alpha$_2$-macroglobulin inhibits proteases.
- Antibodies against lipopolysaccharide or cytokines are of some benefit but less important than the other plasma factors in managing septic shock and SIRS.
- ***Practice Tip:*** *Mixing heparin in the plasma bag to activate antithrombin III is no longer recommended because of the potential for heparin to reduce the anti-inflammatory effects of protein C.*
- Dosage of plasma is 1 L or more for 450-kg adult.

Synthetic Colloids

- Hetastarch (6% hydroxyethyl starch 450/0.7),[1] 2 to 10 mL/kg, can be used immediately while plasma is thawing. Hetastarch may be effective in reducing the "vascular leak" syndrome. At high doses, >10 mg/kg, it may adversely affect coagulation and cause kidney disease.
- Hydroxyethyl starch (HES)[1] refers to a class of synthetic colloid solutions that are similar to glycogen.
  - For all HES products, the average molecular weight (kDa) and the proportion of glucose units on the starch molecule are replaced by hydroxyethyl units (typically 0.35 to 0.5) and listed numerically.
  - ***Example:*** Hetastarch average molecular weight is 450 kDa with 0.7 glucose units on the starch molecule being replaced by hydroxyethyl.
  - The greater the substitution on the starch molecule and the higher molecular weight equals a longer half-life.
  - There is a range of different-sized molecules in any given solution (e.g., 450 kDa weight of hetastarch is the average).
  - The substitution pattern is often listed on the products; the C2/C6 ratio is based on the location of hydroxylation. The higher the ratio of C2/C6, the slower the breakdown of starch.
- Pentastarch, although more expensive, in the United States, has a higher number of molecular weight particles in the 200,000 or 200 kDa-MW range, which are believed an ideal size for decreasing vessel leaking and more effective in "drawing" fluid from the interstitial fluid space. This has *not* been confirmed.
- VetStarch[1] (hydroxyethyl starch 130/0.4) is a lower molecular weight (average, 130,000) with higher oncotic properties than the previously mentioned and possibly has a decreased negative effect on coagulation. The product has a higher C2/C6 than hetastarch.

---

[1]VetStarch is a trademark of the Abbott Laboratories; hetastarch and pentastarch are available.

- All three products "leak" into the interstitial fluid space, then molecules less than 65 kDa are excreted in the urine, and the larger molecules are metabolized by amylase.
- Human albumin[2] (25%) provides the *greatest* osmotic pressure of all the colloids. Human albumin has been safely given to horses and temporarily reduces noninflammatory edema. Generally, human albumin is administered at 1 to 3 mL/kg per hour. ***Important:*** As with any foreign protein, anaphylaxis can occur. Duration of oncotic effect is generally only a few days. There are reports of 25% albumin causing immunosuppression in some species. Repeated dosing should *not* be administered after 5 days because antibodies may develop against the foreign protein.
- Dextrans have fallen out of favor because of their association with anaphylaxis-type reactions more so than other synthetic colloids in which reactions are rare. Dextrans might have an advantage over other colloids in horses at risk of platelet aggregation because of their potential to inhibit platelet aggregation. Whether dextran treatment is beneficial in septic disorders with a high risk of thrombosis (i.e., colitis; pleuritis; equine herpesvirus-1, vasculitis; the prodromal stages of laminitis) is unknown. Dose of dextran 70 is 5 to 10 mL/kg. Pretreatment with nonsteroidal anti-inflammatory drugs (NSAIDs) decreases adverse effects.
- Oxyglobin, 1 to 10 mL/kg, was an excellent colloid that may also improve oxygen delivery to end capillaries. *Currently it is not available.*

Pump Support

- If fluid therapy alone is unsuccessful in normalizing blood pressure, cardiac output, and perfusion but CVP is normal (6 to 12 cm H_2O) indicating sufficient preload, the use of beta$_1$-agonist therapy to improve pump function is indicated. ***Important:*** Use these drugs *only* if there is adequate preload. Administer dobutamine, 2 to 15 μg/kg per minute diluted in saline solution, for beta$_1$ activity; begin with 5 μg/kg per minute, which is shown to improve microcirculatory perfusion independent of changes in cardiac output or blood pressure.
- If volume and pump support (e.g., dobutamine) are *not* successful in maintaining adequate blood pressure and improving urine output, dopamine (2 to 15 μg/kg per minute diluted in saline solution) can be administered. A low-dose stimulates renal dopaminergic receptors and increases renal blood flow. A middle-dose also stimulates beta$_1$ receptors, and a high-dose causes beta$_1$- and alpha-receptor stimulation, which decreases renal perfusion.
- ***Practice Tip:*** *One of the best general indicators of successful perfusion of most organs is the production of a large volume of urine.*

Pressor Support

- Pressure support should only be used when the previous treatments used are unsuccessful in satisfactorily providing adequate blood pressure and urine production! If fluid therapy and beta$_1$-agonist therapy are unsuccessful in improving blood pressure for "forward flow" of blood and urine production, administer norepinephrine (beta- and alpha-agonist), 0.1 to 1.5 μg/kg/min. Administering norepinephrine at the highest recommended dose with *no* improvement in blood pressure and urine production in a volume replete/filled horse (normal CVP or near maximal intravascular volume expansion) means the alpha receptors are *no* longer responsive. Vasopressin, 0.05 to 0.8 U/kg per adult horse (acting via the V$_1$ receptors), should instead be administered, 0.5 to 1.0 mU/kg/min.
- Short-term use of vasopressin (i.e., hours) helps reach the goal of improving catecholamine-refractory hypotension and increasing

urine production (dose, 0.05 to 0.8 U/kg in a 450-kg horse). Minimal effect on intestinal perfusion or heart rate occurs at this dose in other species. Vasopressin at higher dosages can decrease heart rate and intestinal perfusion.
- ***Practice Tip:*** *Septic foals with "refractory hypotension" can be given hydrocortisone (0.5 to 2 mg/kg q8 to 12h IV) as a treatment for relative adrenal insufficiency.* Treatment with hydrocortisone may improve efficacy of vasopressors.
- Dobutamine therapy can be continued along with norepinephrine or vasopressin therapy and may even help maintain intestinal perfusion during the pressor (norepinephrine or vasopressin) therapy.

Oxygen Therapy

- Administer adequate oxygen to maintain normal or above normal Pao$_2$.
- ***Practice Tip:*** *Check the hemoglobin (Hgb) concentration as adjunct for effective O$_2$ therapy: maintain Hgb within normal range:*
  - *Too low (<3 to 7 g/dL) indicates need for transfusion.*
  - *Too high (variable) indicates need for additional fluids.*
- For most patients, insert an intranasal tube in one or both nostrils (depending on the degree of hypoxia) to administer humidified oxygen.
- Most adults and even some foals tolerate flow rates of 15 L/min as long as there is *not* a noticeable noise from the flow (see Chapter 25, p. 453, on procedures).
- If the patient is comatose, the oxygen is best administered via endotracheal tube with or without positive pressure.
- For a septic foal with respiratory distress that requires mechanical ventilation, administer positive pressure ventilation with 50% oxygen concentration.
- For persistent hypoxemia and probable pulmonary arterial hypertension, nitric oxide may be mixed in the oxygen line at a ratio of 1:5 to 1:9. ***Important:*** A special valve is needed to administer the nitric oxide at the proper ratio.
- ***Practice Tip:*** *Pao$_2$ should be maintained at >70 mm Hg (partial pressure of venous oxygen [PvO$_2$], >35 mm Hg; venous oxygen saturation [SvO$_2$], >60%; lactate, <2 mmol/L) and Pvco$_2$:Paco$_2$ ratio of close to 1.*

Antimicrobial Support

- Broad-spectrum coverage for gram-positive and gram-negative aerobes and sometimes anaerobes (e.g., intravenous penicillin and amikacin in foals; penicillin and gentamicin in adults; or enrofloxacin and penicillin or a third-generation cephalosporin [e.g., 5 mg/kg ceftiofur] with or without amikacin is recommended; see Appendix 9).
- If anaerobic coverage is important (i.e., intestinal, oral adult horse pneumonia, or reproductive tract "seeding"), metronidazole may need to be added to the treatment regimen.
- In adult horses, monotherapy (enrofloxacin or ceftiofur) is commonly used as an initial therapy, especially if there is concern about renal function, whereas combination therapy (beta-lactam and an aminoglycoside) is initial routine treatment in foals unless renal function is a concern.
- Imipenem, meropenem , or human group IV cephalosporin therapy is reserved mostly for use in foals with highly resistant organisms.
- The initial choice of antimicrobials should depend upon an understanding of which organisms are more likely present based on clinical signs, history, which organ systems are involved, sensitivity patterns in the practice area or farm, and potential toxicity.
- ***Practice Tip:*** *The earlier the antimicrobial therapy is started in septic or even severe hypotensive/hypoxemic shock, especially in foals, the better the prognosis.*

Surgical Treatment: Sepsis-Source Control

- Establish drainage, and resect and debride necrotic tissue.
- Bind toxin in intestinal tract with activated charcoal or Biosponge.
- ***Practice Tip:*** *If global perfusion pressure (determined by pulse pressure, CRT, urine production, and when available, Doppler monitoring of blood pressure), and global oxygenation (as determined by PvO_2 and SvO_2) have improved but lactate does not improve in 2 hours, strongly consider the possibility of a local perfusion/oxygen debt such as strangulated bowel.*

Prostanoid Inhibitors

- Administer flunixin meglumine, 0.3 mg/kg IV q8h, if there is no primary gastrointestinal disease and urination has occurred. Flunixin meglumine, 1 mg/kg IV, can be given as an initial treatment particularly if colitis/enteritis is *not* the cause of the sepsis.
- Meloxicam (0.6 mg/kg IV), which is very expensive as a parenteral preparation in the United States, and firocoxib are the best available COX-2 specific inhibitors for the horse, and they might be indicated for endotoxemia associated with severe gastrointestinal disease. The rather specific COX-2 inhibitory effect of these drugs (firocoxib is more specific than meloxicam) might allow the benefits of inhibition of inducible prostanoids on the cardiopulmonary system while allowing normal gut repair, though this is currently unproven.
- Carprofen (0.7 to 1.4 mg/kg IV) is a potent NSAID and a more selective COX-2 inhibitor than phenylbutazone, flunixin meglumine, or ketoprofen.
- Conversely, highly selective COX-2 inhibitors (i.e., firocoxib) may not block thromboxane and prostaglandin F2-alpha (PGF-2 alpha), which are believed detrimental in sepsis.
- ***Practice Tip:*** *Flunixin meglumine, 0.3 mg/kg IV q8h is still the preferred NSAID for equine sepsis unless there is severe intestinal disease. It can be administered simultaneously with firocoxib (0.09 mg/kg IV q24h).*

Endotoxin Inhibitors

- Administer hyperimmune plasma, 2 to 4 mL/kg IV. The antibodies against the core lipopolysaccharide may be of some benefit, along with other components of plasma previously discussed.
- Administer polymyxin B, 6000 units/kg IV q8h (6000 units = 1 mg/kg), over a minimum of 15 minutes and preferably after urination is noted; the dose can be repeated 3 to 5 times over 36 hours.
  - Polymyxin B may neutralize some circulating endotoxin; unfortunately, the cytokine cascade is established before treatment is begun in most patients, and the greatest benefit of treatment is known to occur if it is initiated before endotoxin challenge.
  - Polymyxin B treatment is frequently used in horses, and adverse effects (renal toxicity and neuromuscular weakness) are uncommon.

Additional Therapy

- Steroids: dexamethasone, 0.25 mg/kg IV. Most studies show little value in outcome, but corticosteroids inhibit arachidonic acid metabolism (prostanoids and leukotrienes) and are frequently used as a single dose early in severe septic shock that is judged to be imminently life-threatening.
- ***Practice Tip:*** *In foals, hydrocortisone, 0.50 to 2 mg/kg IV, should be administered in hypotensive shock that is* not *responsive to appropriate fluid and pressor treatment.*
- Pentoxifylline, 8.4 to 10 mg/kg PO or IV q12h, is commonly used to inhibit cytokines; it also improves deformability of red blood cells and protects several body organs from cytokine injury. Only an oral preparation is commercially available, but a powdered form can be purchased from Professional Compounding Centers of America (PCCA) (800-331-2498) and can be compounded for intravenous use (dose, 7.5 mg/kg).
  - Pentoxifylline has been used intravenously without adverse effects, but problems have been reported. It is unclear if the source or preparation of the pentoxifylline is responsible for these reported problems. Most pentoxifylline studies suggest the drug needs to be administered before endotoxin challenge to be effective.
- Platelet antagonism: Inhibition of platelet aggregation may diminish microvascular thrombosis and the inflammatory response associated with platelet aggregation.
  - ***Important:*** NSAIDs are not effective in inhibiting platelets.
  - Clopidogrel (Plavix), 4 mg/kg PO loading dose (first dose), then 2 mg/kg PO, q24h, can inhibit platelets exposed to endotoxin. This drug is now off-patent and is not prohibitively expensive.
- Dalteparin (low-molecular-weight heparin), 50 (adult) to 100 (foal) units/kg SQ q24h, does *not* have the red blood cell aggregation/low packed cell volume side-effect of regular (unfractionated) heparin.
  - At the higher dose in the horse, dalteparin has good activity against thrombin and, interestingly in other species, has been shown to have an anti-inflammatory effect via increased COX-1 activation and increased prostacyclin levels with a decrease in tumor necrosis factor and interleukin-12.
    - ***Note:*** Dalteparin is expensive in the United States.
- Lidocaine (1.3 mg/kg slowly IV followed by 0.05 mg/kg/min continuous rate infusion [CRI]) administration after correction of life-threatening fluid deficits) may have some advantages in treating septic shock (see Appendix 2, p. 804):
  - It *may* diminish leukocyte activation associated with endotoxemia, which *may* be helpful in preventing intestinal or other organ reperfusion injury.
  - It may also provide analgesic effects allowing less NSAID therapy in horses with damaged intestinal mucosa and help maintain intestinal motility.
  - It has a possible downside in that it might diminish neutrophil phagocytosis.
- ***Practice Tip:*** *Glycemic control: Glucose should ideally be maintained between 90 and 145 mg/dL in the adult or between 90 and 160 mg/dL in the foal.*
  - If the equine patient is hyperglycemic after correcting fluid deficits, controlling pain and/or anxiety, and ideally after rapidly restoring blood pressure and urine output, regular insulin can be started at 0.05 to 0.1 units/kg per hour while monitoring blood glucose potassium, and maintaining potassium therapy (unless hyperkalemia is present).
  - Insulin may have direct anti-inflammatory/anti-apoptotic effects independent of glycemic control. *The control of hyperglycemia in adult horses with insulin therapy is* not *proven and could have adverse effects.*
  - Foals that have a blood glucose <50 mg/dL can be given 1 mL/kg 10% to 50% dextrose.
- Ulcer prophylaxis is common in foals although there is some evidence this therapy may predispose the foal to infectious diarrhea. Therefore, only use sucralfate unless diarrhea is already present, in which case use either ranitidine, 1.5 mg/kg IV q8h, because it may have some motility-enhancing effects not found with other ulcer-prevention treatments, or if NSAIDs are expected to be used for several days, then proton pump inhibitors (omeprazole) are preferred.
- Cryotherapy (see Chapter 43, p. 712).

Additional Less Commonly Used or Unproven Treatments

- Ethyl pyruvate, 150 mg/kg IV, has been shown to decrease endotoxin-stimulated cytokine production in vitro, but clinical relevance of this is unclear.
- Oxygen free radical inhibitors:
  - Dimethyl sulfoxide, although commonly used, has *no* evidence for its use and therefore it is *not* recommended!
- There is evidence that hyperbaric oxygen treatment *is not indicated* in horses with endotoxemia.
- Vitamin E as an antioxidant to decrease production of reactive oxygen species; 10-20 IU/kg PO q24h (only PO; IM preparation is irritating)
- Allopurinol has little indication for use in the horse.
- N-acetylcysteine can be administered at 50 to 150 mg/kg IV slowly if liver enzymes are markedly elevated. The sterile nebulization product can be given intravenously but is expensive and efficacy is unproven.
- Furosemide is used to decrease pulmonary arterial wedge pressure (pulmonary edema), *but* it can cause systemic vasodilation and decreased cardiac output.
- Oral glutamine: Oral fluids with essential amino acids, including glutamine, are provided (when the gastrointestinal tract is functional) to support enterocyte function and to decrease endotoxin absorption and bacterial translocation.
- ***Practice Tip:*** *Sodium bicarbonate can be used when blood pH <7.1. Also consider Biosponge. Treatment is controversial. Do not use with respiratory acidosis (increased $Paco_2$), hypocalcemia, or hypokalemia.*
- Magnesium sulfate, 0.1 to 0.2 g/kg IV over 24 hours; it may have some cellular protective effects but at higher dosages may cause hypotension. Use in horses at increased risk of laminitis.
- Granulocyte colony-stimulating factor, 10 μg/kg IV q24h, has been given to some foals with severe neutropenia, septic shock, and SIRS. There is generally a response (increased granulocyte count) except in herpes infection, although the benefit on survival is doubtful.

Monitoring Treatment of Septic Shock and SIRS

Perfusion

- Heart rate
- Mucous membrane color, CRT, palpable pulse pressures
- Urine production: should be normal or increased after administration of intravenous fluids. Urine specific gravity can be used to help determine appropriate administration volume.
- Cardiac contractility: M mode may be used to *estimate* this value. Contractility should be 35% to 50%, and chamber size should appear normal in addition to clinical evidence of euvolemia and/or normal CVP. In some hospitals, cardiac output can be measured by lithium dilution or sonographic method.
- Arterial pressure: tail cuff or subjective digital pulse pressure. An arterial line can be established for recumbent foals (mean arterial pressure should be >65 mm Hg, ideally 120 to 130 mm Hg systolic pressure). The accuracy of the indirect monitoring of blood pressure using oscillometric measurements can vary depending on the following:
  - The ratio of bladder cuff width to tail circumference. No ideal ratio is known; however, a bladder width of 20% to 25% and length of 50% to 80% of the circumference of the tail is recommended. For foals, a 5.2-cm bladder width is recommended. The cuff can alternatively be placed over the metatarsus (great metatarsal artery) or the forearm (median artery) in foals.
  - The positional location of the cuff in relation to the level of the base of the heart. ***Practice Tip:*** *This affects blood pressure measurements, as does the standing patient's head position; if possible keep the head in the same neutral position each time blood pressure measurements are performed.*
- *At best,* the indirect measurement gives an acceptable mean pressure and an indication of trends when performed intermittently in the identical manner and on the same patient. An accurate heart rate on the monitor should be displayed when blood pressure measurements are computed.
- ***Practice Tips:***
  - *Mean arterial pressure <60 mm Hg without urine production is an indication for enhanced treatment and further monitoring.*
  - *Fluid therapy is the number 1 way of improving cardiac output and perfusion.*
- CVP should be 5 to 15 cm H_2O for adults and 2 to 12 cm H_2O for foals. Lower values are an indication for increased fluid rate, whereas high values are often, but not always, an indication for decreased fluid rate, pump therapy, and/or the possibility of renal failure. See Chapter 10, p. 35, for measurement of CVP.
- Administer plasma protein, to a goal of ≥4.2 g/dL, to maintain oncotic pressure and prevent edema formation.
- ***Practice Tip:*** *Oncotic (osmotic) pressure should remain greater than 18 mm Hg in adults and 15 mm Hg in foals in order for crystalloid therapy to be most effective and to prevent edema formation.*
- Packed cell volume should be 30% to 45%.

Oxygenation and Blood Gases

- Pao_2: keep close to 100 mm Hg. This can be accomplished with intranasal oxygen in most cases.
- In recumbent foals, pulse oximetry can be used on the tongue or rectum for frequent measurement of oxygen saturation.
- ***Practice Tip:*** *Saturation of >97% is assurance that Pao_2 is >70 mm Hg and can be used to reduce the number of arterial blood gas measurements needed.*
- It is more difficult to perform pulse oximetry in the awake horse, although some "shocky" horses allow measurements using the tongue or other mucous membranes. If the heart rate reported on the pulse oximetry is incorrect, then *do not* believe the saturation value.
- Pvo_2: goal is >35 mm Hg. Lower values indicate abnormal oxygen delivery or increased oxygen extraction.

- Svo_2: goal is saturation >60%. Monitor response to intranasal oxygen administration and for signs of improved perfusion.
- $Pvco_2 - Paco_2$ = <5 mm Hg as the goal of therapy
- Mucous membrane color indicates perfusion quality and tissue oxygenation at the site of recording.
- Blood pH: Determine metabolic or respiratory component of any abnormality, and treat accordingly.
- Anion gap or lactate reduction is used to detect increased unmeasured anions (if plasma protein level has decreased, lactate may be high with a normal anion gap).
- Most commonly, increased numbers of unmeasured anions are associated with lactic acidosis and/or renal failure. Blood lactate value can be measured with an I-Stat or, for minimal cost, with a Lactate-Pro (and should be <2 mmol/L). In the horse, levels can return to normal quickly (<2 hours) with correction of perfusion/oxygenation deficits to all organs.
- *Practice Tip: If the lactate remains high after resuscitation, then either more aggressive treatments are needed to combat systemic hypoperfusion/hypoxia, or there may be regional abnormalities, such as a section of diseased bowel (compare blood and peritoneal fluid lactate), in which case surgery should be considered. Clearance delays may also exist.*
- *Practice Tip: Measurement of lactate is so easy and accurate that this should replace trying to monitor venous oxygen or venous oxygen saturation as indicators of response to treatments.*
- For primary cardiopulmonary disease requiring ventilation therapy, a capnograph can be used to help determine shunt fraction. Normal = $P_{(et)}CO_2$ of 35 to 45 or 2 to 4 mm below plasma arterial or venous Pco_2. As shunt fraction increases, $P_{(et)}CO_2$ goes down and $Pvco_2$ and $Paco_2$ go up. $P_{(et)}CO_2$ also can be used to estimate the presence of cardiac output when trying to resuscitate after cardiac arrest.

Sepsis Control
- Monitoring the extent of infection and/or diseased tissue or organs
- Palpate and/or ultrasound diseased tissue to determine whether the infection/inflammation is being controlled
- Evaluate peritoneal and other fluids
- Other laboratory testing: complete blood cell count, chemistry panel

Miscellaneous Monitoring
- Obtain an electrocardiogram: Control arrhythmias.
- Monitor cardiac troponin: cTnI should be <0.1 ng/mL; if higher, this indicates myocardial disease and may be associated with ST depression on electrocardiogram.
- *Practice Tip: Similar to lactate, the elevation in cTnI on admission is not as important as the level following resuscitation!*
- Perform ultrasonographic examination of abdomen for bowel motility and fluid and of thorax for abnormal fluid or evidence of pneumonia. Cardiac function can also be estimated by ultrasound examination.

- If the horse is hydrated, has normal or high-normal CVP, and ventricular contractility is >35%, then one can "safely" *assume or estimate* cardiac output is normal. Lithium dilution can be used in foals for more precise measurement of cardiac output.
- Monitor digital pulses, lameness, and feet temperature.
- *Practice Tip: Cases at very high risk for laminitis, such as septic metritis, **should be maintained in ice boots** to a level above the fetlock until heart rate and mucous membranes are normal and neutrophilic bands and toxic changes are no longer present on bloodwork.*
- Monitor body temperature, mental attitude, manure production, and gastric size via ultrasound or presence of reflux and abdominal size.
- With intestinal disease, intraabdominal pressure can be monitored with a balloon catheter in the bladder where it is normally negative pressure (hence a vacuum sound upon entering the bladder). Greater than 7 cm H_2O indicates excessive abdominal pressure and the possible need for treatment to decrease pressure (i.e., motility-regulating drugs, lidocaine, or trocarization).
- Intravenous fluid lines and environmental conditions should be closely monitored.
- Monitor overall clinical appearance, attitude, and appetite.
- Carefully monitor the catheterized vein.
- Monitor the pregnant mare/fetus (discussed in Chapter 27, p. 497).
- Monitor the arrested/resuscitated horse/foal (discussed in Chapter 29, p. 514).
- Platelet count, neutrophil count, neutrophil morphology, plasma glucose, electrolytes, triglycerides (especially for ponies, donkeys, and miniature horses, but useful in all anorectic horses), and creatinine should be monitored as needed. These are prognostic and therapeutic markers.
- Therapeutic drug monitoring can be used to help determine whether appropriate dosages of a drug are being administered, e.g., for aminoglycosides.
- *Important: Although aminoglycoside nephrotoxicity is a common problem in critical care management of horses and foals, subtherapeutic administration is likely more of a problem and this may result in less than adequate sepsis control.*

Key Goal-Oriented Parameters for Treatment of Shock
- Heart rate decreasing toward normal range (not always a positive finding in septic neonatal foals)
- Mean arterial pressure at least 70 mm Hg adult; 65 mm Hg in neonatal foals
- Urine production normal or increased
- Mucous membrane color light pink to red with CRT <3 seconds
- CVP in normal range (equivalent to quick jugular distention when vein held off)
- Osmotic pressure >18 mm Hg adult; 15 mm Hg for foals
- Pao_2 near 100 mm Hg, and/or SaO_2 >95%; PvO_2 35 to 40 mm Hg or greater, and/or SvO_2 >60%

SIRS

- Blood lactate <2 mmol/L or with hyperlactatemia, a reduction of 20% to 50% every 1 to 2 hours
- Blood glucose in normal range; septic foals are often hypoglycemic, whereas septic adults are frequently hyperglycemic.
- No toxic changes in neutrophils or band neutrophils; platelet count and electrolytes within normal range
- No clinical evidence of laminitis
- Ideal patient comfort and no complications
- Patient looks and feels better

●❯ WHAT TO DO

Sepsis and Shock Summary
- Administer crystalloids: hypertonic saline solution, balanced electrolyte fluid, or both!!
- Administer plasma or sometimes a synthetic colloid if possible.
- Provide drainage for septic fluids, removal of necrotic tissue, and appropriate antimicrobial therapy (see pp. 568-569).
- Flunixin meglumine, 0.3 to 1 mg/kg IV
- For gram-negative sepsis, begin **cryotherapy** of the feet with ice boots, covering the foot to the mid-metacarpus/tarsus!

- Pentoxifylline (8.4 mg/kg PO or IV) and polymyxin B (6000 units/kg IV q8h) are commonly used and appear to have some benefit.
- Dalteparin (low-molecular-weight heparin), 50 (adult) to 100 (foal) units/kg SQ q24h if affordable
- Intranasal oxygen if possible
- Monitor pulse pressure, jugular vein refill, membrane color, CRT, heart rate, urine production, and clinical signs.
- ***Practice Tip:*** *Lactate concentrations are the single best laboratory indicator of treatment success. Glucose should be carefully monitored in foals.*
- If there is not an adequate response to the previously mentioned treatments (Be sure there is adequate fluid therapy to correct intravascular volume deficits!), then additional pump support (pressors, e.g., dobutamine, norepinephrine, vasopressin (see p. 568) should be used.

References

References can be found on the companion website at www.equine-emergencies.com.

CHAPTER 33

Temperature-Related Problems: Hypothermia and Hyperthermia

Thomas J. Divers

Heat Stroke

- Usually occurs in poorly conditioned horses that are overworked in hot and humid climates and/or in horses with anhidrosis, dehydration, or exhaustion syndrome.
- Can occur in individuals confined to poorly ventilated areas during hot and humid weather; this especially is a problem during shipping.
- It may also occur in otherwise healthy horses when the sum of temperature (in degrees Fahrenheit) and humidity have a value of 180 or more or in horses moved from cool to hot climates for competition without a sufficient acclimation time (several days).
- Older horses may be more prone to heat stroke due to decreased plasma volume with age.
- Also infrequently occurs among foals treated for *Rhodococcus equi* using a macrolide antibiotic such as erythromycin.
- Other causes include sick foals exposed to high environmental heat and humidity, horses having seizures and/or that have injury to the hypothalamic area of the brain, and horses with compartmental/compressive myopathy.
- Horses grazing endophyte-infected fescue may have decreased heat tolerance.
- *Note:* high fever, even up to 106°F, in horses with viral infections (e.g., influenza) rarely if ever causes heat stroke!

Diagnosis

- Early diagnosis is important for effective treatment.
- Diagnosis is based on the history and clinical signs.
- Heat stroke can trigger a systemic inflammatory response, disseminated intravascular coagulation, renal failure, neurologic dysfunction, and other forms of organ dysfunction.

Clinical Signs

- Poor sweating response
- Hot, dry skin signals the early onset of heat stroke
- Tachycardia with or without arrhythmia
- Tachypnea
- Elevated rectal temperature (41° to 43°C [106° to 110°F])
- Prolonged capillary refill time, muddy mucous membranes
- Depression
- Weakness
- May progress to collapse or ataxia
- Decreased appetite, refusal to work, ileus
- May progress to coma and death

●▸ WHAT TO DO

Heat Stroke

- Decrease the body temperature:
  - The more rapid the cooling and the earlier treatment is provided, the better the prognosis.
  - Move the affected horse to a shaded, well-ventilated area (use fans if available).
  - Apply cold or ice-water hydrotherapy (approximately 6°C [42.8°F]) to the entire body and repeat as needed. Use alcohol baths over the neck, thorax, and abdomen if cold water is not available. Evaporation of water may not be effective under humid environmental conditions so use of a fan or continually scraping off the cold water and reapplying may be needed.
  - Offer all three of the following: cold, lukewarm, and electrolyte-supplemented water in hopes of encouraging drinking.
  - Ice packs can be placed over the carotid area of the neck, but do *not* cover the entire neck.
  - Administer an antipyretic: dipyrone or flunixin meglumine (Banamine), which also is useful for its anti-endotoxin effect. *Many exhausted or heat stroke horses are endotoxic.*
    - This treatment should not be repeated without an evaluation of renal function.
- Restore blood volume:
  - Use any crystalloid fluid, but 0.9% saline solution *with potassium chloride, 20 to 40 mEq/L,* is recommended. Fluids should be no warmer than 16° to 21°C (60° to 70°F) and may be refrigerated to enhance the internal cooling effect. If the clinical signs of heat stroke are severe, 5 L/500 kg of a colder (45°F) intravenous fluid should be given while closely monitoring clinical signs and temperature.
  - Use hypertonic saline solution if the heart rate is rapid and the capillary refill time is prolonged; >5 seconds. Continuous administration of 3% saline for 24 to 48 hours is recommended if neurologic signs are present and are believed to be due to cerebral edema (see Chapter 22, p. 369). If neurologic signs develop, the horse can also be treated using hypothermia by administering chilled crystalloids; at 45°F; sedation with valium may be needed.
  - When the rectal temperature reaches 102°F, a comprehensive clinical examination is performed. If physical findings are

normal, hydration and urine color normal, and laboratory values for renal function, cTnI, and lactate are trending toward normal, additional intensive therapy can likely be stopped. Administer 2 L of hyperimmune plasma (antibodies against endotoxin) for more severe cases.
- Cool rectal fluids may be administered if proper precautions are provided (i.e., soft tubing, gravity flow).

◉〉 WHAT NOT TO DO

Heat Stroke
- Do *not* use wet towels or any fabric cover because these prevent heat convection!
- Do *not* force the horse to walk although voluntary movement in the shade is fine.
- Do *not* withhold water.
- Do *not* let the horse become hypothermic or develop severe shivering, *unless* there are associated neurologic signs and hypothermia is used as treatment for the neurologic signs!
- Do *not* administer alpha-agonist tranquilizers because they may cause respiratory distress.

Malignant Hyperthermia

- A potentially fatal disease in heavily muscled halter Quarter Horses with a mutation in the ryanodine receptor 1 gene.
- Hyperthermia is mostly stimulated by anesthesia or stress.

Clinical Findings
- Hyperthermia
- Tachycardia with ventricular arrhythmias
- Sweating
- Muscle rigidity and colic signs
- Protrusion of the third eyelid
- Electrolyte and acid-base imbalances including hyperkalemia and severe mixed acidemia
- Plasma creatine kinase is increased, but the peracute nature of the disease and rapid death may not allow time for marked increases.

Diagnosis
- History, signalment, anesthesia, clinical signs, hyperthermia with myopathy, and genetic testing.
- In addition to anesthesia, recurrent episodes of tying-up, exercise, and stress may "trigger" the malignant attacks.

◉〉 WHAT TO DO

Malignant Hyperthermia
Treatments
- Dantrolene, 2 mg/kg IV, followed immediately by oral treatment with 10 mg/kg and 1 hour later continue with oral dantrolene at 2 to 4 mg/kg every 2 to 6 hours until signs resolve.
- Acepromazine to sedate and relax the horse; preferred over alpha-agonist tranquilizers
- Fluid therapy (cold hypertonic saline) to correct electrolyte abnormalities and improve tissue perfusion

Anhidrosis

- Usually affects the exercising athlete and a few sedentary adult horses.
- Also occurs among stabled horses subjected to hot and humid environments for long periods.
- The condition represents an *inability to sweat* in response to normal stimuli.
- Exact cause is unknown but may be a result of decreased expression of aquaporin-5 (impairment of both β-adrenoceptor and purinoceptor pathways) in sweat gland cells.
- Can develop acutely but generally develops gradually.
- A form of anhidrosis also occurs among young, healthy foals especially Draft foals, with persistent tachypnea.

Clinical Signs
- Onset may be gradual or abrupt
- Failure to sweat with appropriate stimuli (heat, exercise)
  - *Note:* Some affected horses have patches of sweating under the mane, under the jaw, base of the ears, or in the pectoral or perineal regions.
- Tachypnea (some pant), decreased exercise tolerance, rectal temperature higher than normal after exercise (>40° C [104° F])
- Respiratory rate higher than heart rate
- The signs are progressive if affected horses are left in a hot environment.

Less Common Clinical Signs
- Depression, anorexia, weight loss, alopecia

Diagnostic Tests
Epinephrine or Terbutaline Challenge
- Administer 1:1000 and 1:10,000 epinephrine, 0.1 mL intradermally, using both concentrations. Affected individuals have little or no response (local sweating) within 1 hour.
- A quantitative test using adsorbent pads after intradermal terbutaline administration has been published (see MacKay, 2008).
  - *Practice Tip: Intravenous epinephrine administration exacerbates the problem and should be avoided.*
- Terbutaline, 0.5 mg intradermal injection, also can be used.
- There are different degrees of severity, but in the most severe cases, the disorder may be permanent.

◉〉 WHAT TO DO

Anhidrosis
- Administer an antipyretic agent, such as flunixin meglumine; initiate cold-water hydrotherapy; and provide shade, with a fan, if possible.
- The only proven prevention is to move the affected horse to a more temperate climate or place in an air-conditioned stall for an

extended time, although electrolyte supplementation (ONE AC[1] and lite salt) may have some preventative (not therapeutic) efficacy.
- Provide electrolyte supplementation to all horses exercising in hot weather.
- Clip body hair: This is sometimes useful in the care of otherwise healthy foals, especially draft foals, with persistent tachypnea.
- In milder cases, single or occasional administration of clenbuterol (5 mL PO/500 kg BW) may be effective.
- In cases that are nonresponsive to the above regimen, a large dose of methylprednisolone, 30 mg/kg IV, can be administered in addition to clenbuterol with the goal of making the sweat glands more responsive to sympathetic stimulation.
- House affected individual in an air-conditioned stall.

Exhaustive Disease Syndrome

- Multisystemic changes occur in horses subjected to brief maximal-intensity or longer submaximal-intensity exercise, especially during hot and humid weather.
- Problems develop in association with fluid and electrolyte losses, acid-base changes associated with exercise, and depletion of the energy stores of the body.
- A familial predisposition to the disease may occur in some cases.

Diagnosis

- Tachypnea[2] (>40 breaths/min after a 30-minute rest)
- Tachycardia[2] (>60 beats/min after a 30-minute rest)
- Elevated rectal temperature (40° to 41°C [104° to 106°F])
- Dehydration (may have fluid deficits of 20 to 40 L) and a lack of interest in water or food (despite the severe dehydration) are common findings. Fluid losses of 6% to 10% of body weight in endurance athletes can lead to heat exhaustion.
- Severe depression, decreased pulse pressure, decreased jugular distention, prolonged capillary refill time
- *Continued sweating* at reduced rate
- Cardiac irregularities (e.g., supraventricular or ventricular tachycardia)
- Muscle cramps or spasms and/or myopathy
- Colic with decreased or absent intestinal sounds, unless spasmodic colic develops; there is also increased incidence of small intestinal volvulus in these horses
- Lack of anal tone
- Synchronous diaphragmatic flutter, often associated with ileus
- Central nervous system signs
- Loss of >7% body weight

Laboratory Findings

- Hypochloremia, hypokalemia, hyponatremia, abnormally low ionized calcium value, azotemia, high packed cell volume and total protein, increased muscle and liver enzyme values, increased lactate and cTnI are variably

present. Hypochloremia and laboratory evidence of dehydration are the most consistent findings.
- With severe myopathy and renal failure, potassium may be increased.
- Variable bicarbonate concentration is found: normal or high with milder cases, low with severe cases.
- Glucose is usually normal or high and can be low with extreme exhaustion.

WHAT TO DO

Exhausted Horse
- Decrease body temperature.
  - Move the patient to a shaded, well-ventilated area.
  - Apply cold-water hydrotherapy frequently to entire body. Intermittent application may be preferred to continuous application because continuous application may cause such severe vasoconstriction of the skin that it interferes with the conduction and convection loss of heat.
- *Fluid therapy* goal for exhausted patients is to replace volume, correct electrolyte abnormalities, and provide a source of calories. To expedite rapid rehydration, use two IV catheters.
  - Lactated Ringer's solution and KCl, 20 mEq/L at 10 to 20 L/h, in more severe cases with suspected acidemia
  - 0.9% saline solution or Ringer's solution with KCl, 20 mEq/L and 20 mL of calcium borogluconate/L given at the rate of 10 to 20 L/h/500-kg horse, in less severe cases without acidemia
    - *With or without* 5 g dextrose/100 mL at 2 L/h: Glucose and calcium concentrations can be variable in exhausted or hyperthermic horses
- If urination does not occur after several liters of fluids have been administered, discontinue KCl. If urination is normal, KCl administration can be increased to 40 mEq/L.
- Hypertonic saline solution should not be used to treat exhausted endurance horses because these individuals may have significant deficits of intracellular fluids. If cerebral signs such as central blindness, head pressing, and coma develop, then a hyperosmotic, chilled fluid such as 3% saline and/or mannitol should be administered as treatment for suspected cerebral edema.
- If synchronous diaphragmatic flutter or intestinal atony is found on physical examination, administer 100 to 300 mL of 20% calcium borogluconate IV *slowly* over 30 minutes. Discontinue administration if cardiac irregularities develop or worsen (see Chapter 17, p. 145).
- If evidence of organ failure or severe metabolic acidosis (pH <7.1) is seen, administer bicarbonate solution if above crystalloid therapy does not improve pH.
- ***Practice Tip:*** *Sodium bicarbonate is contraindicated if synchronous diaphragmatic flutter is present and is not routinely used in the care of exhausted horses!*
- Oral fluids can be given as long as there is no intestinal dysfunction: 5 to 8 L of electrolyte solution q30min as needed.
- Prepare an electrolyte solution as follows:
  - 1½ tbsp (27 g) sodium chloride
  - 1 tbsp (18 g) KCl (Morton's Lite salt)
  - 0 to 40 g dextrose, depending on blood glucose value
  - 4 L water, osmolality of approximately 350 mosmoles (without dextrose)
  - Amino acids such as glutamine can be added
- The oral fluids listed earlier can be offered to the horse to drink before stomach tubing. If the horse refuses the electrolyte fluid then

offer cool water. Discontinue all oral fluids if abdominal discomfort or gastric reflux develops.
- Flunixin meglumine, 1 mg/kg IV initially and then 0.3 mg/kg q8h; this treatment may not be effective if the hyperthermia is not mediated by the hypothalamus.
- Hyperimmune plasma with antibodies against endotoxin: administer 2 L. **Note:** Exhausted athletes are at increased risk of endotoxemia.
- Administer antioxidants: vitamin E, 7000 U PO per adult.

SIRS

▶ WHAT NOT TO DO

Exhausted Horse
- *Do not* use phenothiazine tranquilizers. These patients are at high risk of cardiovascular collapse and death.
- *Do not* administer nonsteroidal anti-inflammatory drugs without appropriate fluid replacement.

Prognosis

Prognosis is generally good if appropriate therapy is instituted early. However, multisystemic complications develop in some patients 2 to 4 days after an exhaustion episode. These manifestations include the following:
- Myopathy
- Rapidly progressive laminitis
- Renal dysfunction
- Gastrointestinal ulceration
- Elevation in values of liver-derived enzymes and bilirubin
- Impaction colic

Hypothermia and Frostbite
- Common in cold climates, donkeys, and under certain clinical situations (i.e., postanesthesia, *septic and hypotensive foals,* hemorrhagic/traumatic shock, or debilitated and aged horses).
- Rare among adult horses but can occur in debilitated patients and is common in donkeys and weak foals exposed to extreme cold.

Diagnosis
- Mild hypothermia occurs between 93° and 97°F; body temperatures below 93°F indicate severe hypothermia.
- With severe hypothermia, shivering response may be lost and peripheral vasodilation may even occur, both of which may worsen the hypothermia. A cascade of systemic acidosis and coagulopathy may occur with severe hypothermia.
- Cold extremities with color change are present: white to deep purple skin may be warm and red if recirculation has started.
- Mild hypothermia may cause an increase in heart rate, whereas severe hypothermia may cause a bradycardia and diminished respiratory rate and effort. With severe hypothermia, depression is expected.

▶ WHAT TO DO

Hypothermia
- Initiate *core rewarming* to provide heat centrally; for extreme hypothermia, surface rewarming without core rewarming may in some cases cause a lowering of the core temperature.
- *Practice Tip: The speed of rewarming depends on the clinical condition of the patient, the primary illness, and specific laboratory findings. Trauma patients with bleeding are generally rewarmed rapidly. Septic patients or those with evidence of early organ failure, including the brain, are generally managed by warming more slowly because the hypothermia may have some benefit in organ preservation.*
- Use warm fluid therapy:
  - Warm crystalloids and colloids, especially plasma, provide antithrombin III and other anticoagulants. In addition to their rewarming effect, intravenously administered fluids may be needed to treat hypovolemia.
  - Initiate gastric or rectal administration of a warm, balanced isotonic electrolyte solution.
  - Administer thyroxine 0.1 mg/kg PO q24h to hypothermic donkeys and weak foals with clinical or laboratory evidence of hypothyroidism.
  - Rewarm extremities (surface rewarming). *Practice Tip: With peripheral rewarming alone, hypovolemic shock may occur as the result of peripheral vasodilation.*
  - Move affected individual to a heated area or at least out of the wind, and apply blankets to prevent convection (atmosphere) or conduction (ground) loss of heat while trying to institute a heating process that may include the following:
    - Circulating warm water heating pads or warm water bottles (100°F) and heating pads or heat lamps may be used, being careful *not* to burn the skin. Be careful with hair dryers!!
    - Forced-air warming blankets such as the Bair Hugger[3] can be set at different temperatures and are effective at warming hypothermic foals.
- Restore dermal microcirculation:
  - Antiprostaglandins: flunixin meglumine dose recommended IV
  - Pentoxifylline, 10 mg/kg PO q12h
  - Vasodilator: Use acepromazine, but only if hydration and pulse pressure are normal!
  - Platelet aggregation inhibitor: aspirin or clopidogrel[4]
  - Low-molecular-weight heparin, 50 to 80 U/kg subcutaneously (SQ) q24h
- Provide local treatment to frostbite areas:
  - Apply topical aloe vera gel three or four times per day.
  - Nitroglycerin ointment (2%) can be applied to small areas that are most severely affected, although absorption through the skin in the horse is not proven.
  - *Note:* Wear gloves when handling nitroglycerin ointment.
- Administer antimicrobial agents if necrosis is expected or to help protect against sepsis associated with hypothermia-induced immunosuppression.
- Provide analgesics.
- Administer broad-spectrum antibiotics to severely hypothermic foals because of the increased risk of bacterial translocation.

[3]Augustine Medical, Eden Prairie, Minnesota.
[4]Plavix (Bristol-Myers Squibb).

●〉 WHAT NOT TO DO

Hypothermia

- *Do not* attempt to rewarm septic, hypovolemic, and/or organ failure (including brain dysfunction) patients too fast or to above 101°F! The warming system(s) (see Neonatology, Chapter 31, p. 530) should not be higher than 105°F, and the rewarming process should be over 30 minutes. *Do not* place foals in a hot water bath tub.
- *Do not* burn patient with heat lamps or hair dryers; they may not have normal sensation and may not react to the high temperatures.
- Avoid rubbing, which damages frozen cells.
- *Do not* feed milk to a severely hypothermic foal.
- *Do not* allow horses and foals to become progressively hypothermic while recovering from general anesthesia.
- With severe hypothermia accompanied by hypotension, *do not* warm the skin and distal extremities without providing intravenous fluids (preferably of body temperature).

Prognosis

- Influencing factors are the following:
  - Duration of exposure
  - Temperature
  - Wind chill
  - Moisture on skin
- Circulatory status of patient
- Effectiveness of treatment
- Some patients slough skin or hooves in the affected limbs, whereas others have no additional signs once the limb is rewarmed.
- Edema and failure to rewarm usually are poor prognostic indicators for the limb.
- ***Practice Tip:*** *In cases of septicemia, especially in foals, a similar syndrome is caused by arterial thrombosis in one or more distal extremities. There may be no association with cold weather! If the thrombosis is known to be acute (hours), tissue plasminogen activator (tPA)[5] (2 to 5 mg) can be administered into the arterial thrombus or just proximal to the thrombus. It is unlikely to be effective, and the prognosis is grave.*
- Some foals may have seizures following the rewarming, requiring treatment to control seizures and the presumed cerebral injury (see Chapter 22, p. 372, and Chapter 31, p. 538).

References

References can be found on the companion website at www.equine-emergencies.com.

---

[5]Activase.

SIRS

PART III

Toxicology

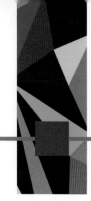

CHAPTER 34

Toxicology

Robert H. Poppenga and Birgit Puschner

Problem

A poisoning should be suspected if the following has occurred:

- Many horses are sick with no known exposure to infectious disease.
- Affected individuals have been exposed recently to a new environment.
- Affected individuals have recently been given medication.
- There has been a recent change in feed.
- There has been a recent change in water.
- There has been recent pesticide application in the horse's environment.
- There has been recent construction activity in the horse's environment.
- There are unusual weather conditions.
- The horse has inadequate feed or pasture.
- An uncommon clinical condition exists.
- There has been a potential threat for a malicious poisoning.
- An unexplained death has occurred.

Presentation

- Poisonings often affect many animals in a short time and thus attract substantial public attention and interest.
- Many indications for toxicology testing exist.
- Obvious cases involve sudden onset of disease in a number of horses.
- Finding of common feed or environmental conditions further supports a suspicion of poisoning.
- A toxicosis is also suggested in the animal that is found "suddenly dead."
- Other situations suggesting testing from a toxicology laboratory include drug testing in the racehorse industry, testing for nutritional adequacy (especially selenium and vitamin E status of horses), or providing testing in suspect cases of malicious poisoning.

●〉 WHAT TO DO

Poisoning

- Establishing an accurate diagnosis depends heavily on a systematic investigation because, unfortunately, there is no single comprehensive test for all possible toxicants. However, newer analytic methodologies allow broad-based screening of appropriate samples in cases in which exposure to a specific toxicant has not been identified.
- Even if a poisoning is suspected, the clinician has to be an objective observer, considering toxic and nontoxic causes of disease.
- Obtain a complete history, including data on breed, age, sex, body weight, reproductive status, vaccine history, current medications, medical history, housing facility and environment, and presence of other animals and any abnormalities in them.
- Perform a detective-like inspection of the premises. The horse's entire environment has to be evaluated for toxic sources and hazardous conditions, including the following:
  - Feed, including recent feed changes
  - Water source
  - Pest control measures in the environment of the horse
  - Recent application of pesticides or herbicides
  - Recent renovations of old buildings
  - Paint or solvent applications
  - Recent horse movements to a new environment
  - Location of farm chemicals
  - Recent animal management decisions

- Perform a complete physical examination.
- Perform an exposure assessment if possible. An exposure assessment is critical to the proper diagnosis and management of a toxicology case. In those instances in which the information is available at least to approximate an exposure and the veterinarian fail to do so, the case may be mismanaged, giving unnecessary treatment to a horse, and increasing the costs of treatment to an owner. In many instances, it is not possible to do a proper exposure assessment because of a lack of necessary information. A veterinary toxicologist can be consulted to perform an assessment accurately and interpret the data.
- If unexplained deaths occur, a complete postmortem examination in all suspect cases should be performed, including thorough gross inspection of the entire body and all gastrointestinal (GI) contents. Samples of all major organ systems and any gross abnormalities should be preserved in 10% neutral buffered formalin for histopathologic examination by board-certified pathologists whenever a field necropsy is conducted.
- Collect specimens suitable for toxicology testing (Table 34-1), including samples from affected, live horses; samples collected during necropsy; and samples collected in the environment of the affected horses.
- Consultation with a veterinary toxicologist aids in the workup of a poisoning case and can help provide a thorough background to help prevent recurrence.

Table 34-1	Samples That Are Needed for Analytic Toxicologic Analysis		
Sample Type	**Preferred Amount**	**Condition**	**Potential Analyses**
Environmental			
Hay, grain, concentrate feeds, mineral supplements	500 g plus; adequate, representative sample	In paper or plastic bags, glass jars; avoid spoilage during shipping	Insecticides, herbicides, heavy metals, salts, feed additives, antibiotics, ionophores, mycotoxins, nitrates, sulfate, chlorate, cyanide, plant toxins, botulinum, vitamins, rodenticides
Plants	Entire plant	Press and dry or freeze	Identification, alkaloids, tannins, grayanotoxins (rhododendron), cardiac glycosides (oleander, foxglove, adonis)
Mushroom	Whole	Keep cool and dry in paper bag	Identification; chemical test for amanitins
Water	1 L	Preserving jar	Pesticides, salts, heavy metals, blue-green algae identification, microcystins, anatoxin-a, sulfate, nitrate, pH
Environment	Source/bait	Freeze in bag	Try to obtain package label and send also, variety of toxicants
Live Animal			
Whole blood	5-10 mL	EDTA Anticoagulant	Cholinesterase activity, lead, selenium, arsenic, mercury, cyanide, some organic chemicals, anticoagulant rodenticides
Serum	5-10 mL	Spin and remove clot; use additioanl special tube for zinc	Copper, zinc (no rubber contact if testing for zinc), iron, magnesium, calcium, sodium, potassium, drugs, alkaloids, oleandrin, vitamins, anticoagulant rodenticides, monensin
Urine	50 mL	Send in plastic, screw-cap vial	Drugs, some metals, alkaloids, cantharidin (blister beetle), fluoride, paraquat, oleandrin
Ingesta/feces (collect at different time points)	100 g plus	Freeze	Plant identification (if not too macerated), seed identification, cardiac glycosides (oleander, foxglove, adonis), grayanotoxins (rhododendron), alkaloids (taxus), tannins, insecticides, drugs, cyanide, ammonia, cantharidin (blister beetle), 4-aminopyridine, petroleum hydrocarbons, antifreeze, heavy metals, ionophores, algal toxins
Biopsy specimens	For example, liver	Freeze	Pyrrolizidine alkaloids, metals, organochlorine insecticides
Hair	10 g	Tie mane/tail hair; note origin	Selenium (chronic exposure)
Postmortem			
Ingesta (collect contents of stomach, small intestine, and large intestine; keep separate)	500 g for each sample	Freeze	Plant identification (if not too macerated), seed identification, cardiac glycosides (oleander, foxglove, adonis), grayanotoxins (rhododendron), alkaloids (taxus), tannins, insecticides, drugs, cyanide, ammonia, cantharidin (blister beetle), 4-aminopyridine, petroleum hydrocarbons, antifreeze, heavy metals, ionophores, algal toxins
Liver	100 g	Freeze	Heavy metals, insecticides, anticoagulant rodenticides, some plant toxins, some drugs, vitamins
Kidney (cortex)	100 g	Freeze	Heavy metals, calcium, some plant toxins, antifreeze
Brain	Half of brain	Sagittal section, leave midline in formalin for pathologist	Cholinesterase activity, sodium, organochlorine insecticides
Fat	100 g	Smaller sample okay for biopsy samples in formalin	Organochlorine insecticides, polychlorinated biphenyls
Ocular fluid	1 eye	Freeze	Potassium, ammonia, magnesium
Injection site	100 g	Freeze	Some drugs, other injectables
Miscellaneous	100 g	Special tests, usually freeze	Special tests, such as spleen (barbiturates) and lung (paraquat)

EDTA, Ethylenediaminetetraacetic acid.

- It is important to keep in mind the possibility of future litigation in any suspected poisoning case; pictures and thorough documentation can help veterinarians recall case details long after an incident.
- Veterinary toxicology laboratories: Veterinary toxicology laboratories are accredited by the American Association of Veterinary Laboratory Diagnosticians (AAVLD). Accredited laboratories can be found on the AAVLD website (www.aavld.org). Not all accredited laboratories provide comprehensive toxicologic testing. Laboratories *routinely* performing toxicologic testing include the following:
- Analytical Sciences Laboratory, University of Idaho; 208-885-7900
- Animal Disease Diagnostic Laboratory, Oklahoma State University; 405-744-6623
- Animal Health Laboratory, University of Guelph; 519-824-4120
- Arkansas Livestock and Poultry Diagnostic Laboratory; 501-907-2430
- California Animal Health and Food Safety Laboratory System, University of California; 530-752-6322
- Clemson Veterinary Diagnostic Center, Clemson University; 803-788-2260
- Diagnostic Center for Population and Animal Health, Michigan State University; 517-353-0635
- Indiana Animal Disease Diagnostic Laboratory, Purdue University; 765-494-7440
- Livestock Animal Diagnostic Center, Lexington, KY; 859-257-8283
- Pennsylvania Animal Diagnostic Laboratory System, University of Pennsylvania; 610-444-5800
- Texas Veterinary Medical Diagnostic Laboratory, Texas A&M University; 979-845-3414
- Utah Veterinary Diagnostic Laboratory, Utah State University; 435-797-1895
- Veterinary Diagnostic and Research Center, Murray State University; 270-886-3959
- Veterinary Diagnostic Laboratory, Cornell University; 607-253-3900
- Veterinary Diagnostic Laboratory, Iowa State University; 515-294-1950
- Veterinary Diagnostic Laboratory, North Dakota State University; 701-231-8307
- Veterinary Medical Diagnostic Laboratory, University of Missouri; 573-882-6811
- Wyoming State Veterinary Laboratory, University of Wyoming; 307-742-6638

General Decontamination Procedures

- Relatively few antidotes exist for the toxicants most likely to poison horses. However, early and appropriate decontamination and vigorous symptomatic and supportive care often result in recovery.
- Decontamination after ingestion of a toxicant consists of the following steps:
  - Removal of material from the stomach: In horses, removal of material from the stomach is difficult because of the inability to administer an emetic and the time and effort required to perform gastric lavage.
  - Administration of activated charcoal (AC) to adsorb toxicant present in the GI tract: In most suspected intoxications, the best approach to decontamination is administration of an adsorbent such as AC with or without a cathartic as soon as possible after the ingestion. AC is administered as an aqueous slurry through a stomach tube at a dosage range of 1 to 2 g/kg body mass (~1 g of AC per 5 mL of water).
  - Administration of a cathartic to hasten elimination of contents from the GI tract: Commonly used cathartics include:
    - Sodium or magnesium sulfate (Glauber's salt and Epsom salt, respectively) can be administered at 250 to 500 mg/kg body mass mixed in the AC slurry.
    - Sorbitol (70%), also mixed in the AC slurry, can be administered at 3 mL/kg body mass.
    - There is little need to administer a cathartic if significant diarrhea is already present.
    - The efficacy of giving AC with a cathartic compared with giving AC alone has not been established; therefore, giving AC alone is acceptable.
    - Under no circumstances should a cathartic be given alone.
  - Bathing: Dermal or ocular exposure to a toxicant necessitates thorough bathing with soap (a dish soap such as Dawn is recommended) or copious irrigation with tap water (for dermal) or normal saline solution (for ocular).
- Self-protection precautions: Always observe appropriate precautions during decontamination procedures to avoid self-exposure or exposure of others to the toxicant.

WHAT NOT TO DO

Poisoning

- *Do not* rely on toxicologic testing of a single type of fluid or tissue sample to provide conclusive results; multiple samples may be required. Call a toxicology diagnostic laboratory for advice on appropriate sample collection if unsure.
- *Do not* delay decontamination procedures.
- Mineral oil often is given after suspected exposure to a toxicant. This practice should be *discouraged* because there is no evidence that mineral oil is an effective adsorbent for most toxicants. Mineral oil has a laxative, *not* a cathartic, effect. Mineral oil should not be administered with AC because of a possible diminution of the adsorptive capacity of the administered AC.
- *Do not* discard material that is suspected to contain a toxicant.

Toxicants Predominantly Affecting the Gastrointestinal Tract

Amitraz

- Amitraz is a formamide insecticide available in the United States as an acaricide dip or spray for cattle and hogs and is used in the management of canine demodectic mange.
- Horses are sensitive to this drug; it should *not* be used on horses.

Mechanism of Toxic Action

- Alpha$_1$- and alpha$_2$-adrenergic agonist activity

Clinical Signs

- Ingestion can cause impaction, colic, depression, tranquilization, and incoordination.
- All occur within 24 hours of exposure.

●〉 WHAT TO DO

Amitraz Toxicosis

- If dermal exposure, give a soap and water bath.
- If oral exposure, administer AC, 1 to 2 g/kg PO.
- Yohimbine and atipamezole are alpha₂-adrenergic antagonists. Appropriate dosages for reversal have *not* been determined; however, 0.15 mg/kg slowly IV is recommended for yohimbine, and 0.1 mg/kg slowly IV is recommended for atipamezole.
- Administer intravenous fluids.
- Give flunixin meglumine, 1 mg/kg IV q24h.

Atropine Toxicosis

- Atropine toxicosis most commonly occurs when atropine has been administered (often incorrectly) for suspected organophosphorus (OP) or carbamate insecticide poisoning.
- Plants such as Jimson weed (*Datura stramonium;* Fig. 34-1), nightshades (*Solanum nigrum, S. dulcamara, S. elaeagnifolium),* and belladonna (*Atropa belladonna*) contain related tropane alkaloids.
- Foliage of potatoes and tomatoes contains tropane and steroidal glycoalkaloids and can be toxic.

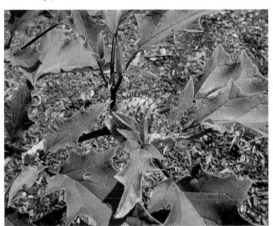

Figure 34-1 *Datura stramonium* seed capsule.

Mechanism of Toxic Action

- Competitive inhibition of muscarinic acetylcholine receptors at postganglionic parasympathetic neuroeffector sites
- High dosages can block nicotinic receptors at autonomic ganglia and neuromuscular junctions.

Clinical Signs

- Ingestion can cause bloat, colic, dry membranes, and dilated pupils (anticholinergic toxidrome).
- Steroidal glycoalkaloids cause gastroenteritis.

●〉 WHAT TO DO

Atropine Toxicosis

- After plant ingestion, AC, 1 to 2 g/kg PO
- Flunixin meglumine, 1.0 mg/kg IV
- Neostigmine, 0.01 mg/kg subcutaneously (SQ), repeated as needed. ***Practice Tip:*** *Use should be reserved for horses exhibiting extreme agitation or abdominal bloat.*

Black Locust *(Robinia pseudoacacia)*

- Ingestion of young sprouts, bark, or pruned or fresh leaves can cause illness. Potential toxicity of other *Robinia* species is not clear (Figs. 34-2 and 34-3).

Mechanism of Toxic Action

- One hypothesized toxic principle, *robin,* is a toxalbumin that inhibits protein synthesis. However, a number of bioactive constituents have been isolated; their role in disease pathogenesis is not known with certainty.

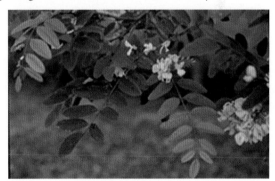

Figure 34-3 *Robinia pseudoacacia.*

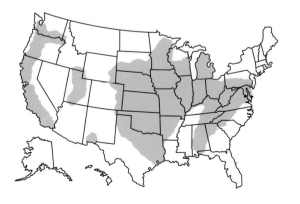

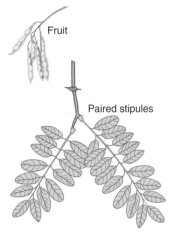

Fruit

Paired stipules

Figure 34-2 Distribution and drawing of *Robinia pseudoacacia* (black locust).

TOX

Clinical Signs

- Ingestion can cause anorexia, diarrhea (may be bloody), colic, depression, weakness, tachycardia, and irregular pulse.
- Rarely fatal, but laminitis can be a severe sequela.

●〉 WHAT TO DO

Black Locust Toxicosis

- Administer AC, 1 to 2 g/kg PO.
- Administer intravenous fluids.
- Provide nutritional support.

Blister Beetle

- Toxicosis is caused by ingestion of the blister beetle (*Epicauta* spp. and *Tegrodera latecincta*), which can be found in alfalfa that has been simultaneously cut and crimped (see Chapter 18, p. 237).
- Blister beetles usually are found in the Great Plains states, the Midwest, and occasionally in other parts of the country.
- Intoxication is more likely middle to late summer when the beetles are feeding on alfalfa.
- The toxic principle is *cantharidin.*

Mechanism of Toxic Action

- Cantharidin, a vesicant and irritant, initially affects the GI tract following ingestion. Once absorbed, it is eliminated via the kidneys. Elimination results in damage to the kidneys and urinary tract mucosa.
- Toxin directly damages the myocardium.
- Inhibition of phosphatase 2A occurs.
- Cause of hypocalcemia is unknown.

Clinical Signs

- Mucous membrane irritation, including oral cavity, GI tract, and urinary tract; mucosal ulcerations can develop
- Colic

- Hypocalcemia with synchronous diaphragmatic flutter
- Frequent urination
- Hematuria and/or hemoglobinuria
- Cardiac damage possible
- Shock
- Neurologic signs only in a few cases
- Sudden death

Diagnosis

- Compatible clinical signs, postmortem lesions (erythema and occasionally erosions of GI mucosa)
- Identification of blister beetles in hay or GI contents
- Measure cTnI to help determine severity of myocardial necrosis.
- Submit GI contents and urine for analysis for cantharidin.

●〉 WHAT TO DO

Blister Beetle Toxicosis

- Remove suspect feed; administer AC, 1 to 2 g/kg PO.
- Administer intravenous fluid therapy.
- Monitor serum calcium concentration, and supplement only if needed.
- Provide supportive care: analgesics, corticosteroids, and antibiotics.
- Administer proton pump inhibitors or H$_2$-receptor antagonists for mucosal ulcerations.
- There is no known antidote.

Prognosis

- Prognosis is guarded.
- With neurologic signs, the prognosis is poor.

Buckeye (*Aesculus glabra*)

- Buckeye is the most common species of *Aesculus* (Fig. 34-4).
- Buckeye is found in moist, well-drained soils of woods and thickets in the midwestern United States, southeast and California (Figure 34-4).

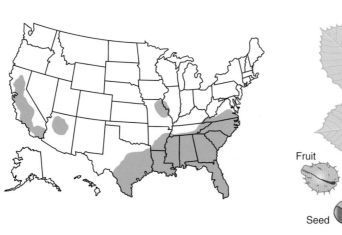
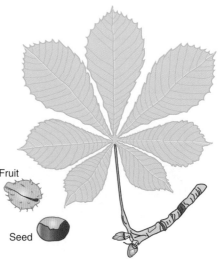

Figure 34-4 Distribution of *Aesculus glabra* (buckeye) and drawing of *A. hippocastanum* (horse chestnut).

- Toxic effects are believed to be caused by a number of saponins. See Horse Chestnut below.

Buttercups (*Ranunculus* spp.)

- The *Ranunculus* genus comprises several hundred species and is widely distributed. Buttercups are plentiful in many pastures.
- Horses almost *never* eat the plant in a pasture setting, and drying renders the plant nontoxic.
- The toxic principle is *ranunculin,* which releases protoanemonin when damaged.
- Cyanogenic glycosides are present in some species.

Mechanism of Toxic Action

- Protoanemonin is a potent vesicant.

Clinical Signs

- Ingestion can cause irritated oral mucous membranes, colic, anorexia, diarrhea, and muscle tremors that may proceed to excitement and convulsions.
- Contact with crushed plant can cause skin irritation.

●▶ WHAT TO DO

Buttercup Toxicosis

- Administer AC, 1 to 2 g/kg PO.
- Provide symptomatic and supportive care.

Castor Bean *(Ricinus communis)*

- Numerous cultivars are planted as ornamentals (Fig. 34-5). Typically, castor bean overwinters only in the middle and southernmost regions of the United States.
- Plants are grown commercially in California and Florida for castor oil.
- Seeds and foliage are poisonous.
- Ingested seeds that remain intact in the GI tract are not toxic. The seed contains the alkaloid *ricinine* and the glycoprotein *ricin.*

Mechanism of Toxic Action

- Ricinine can cause seizures through gamma-aminobutyric acid receptor type A antagonism; there is a possible neuromuscular effect.
- Ricin inhibits protein synthesis and secondarily, DNA and RNA synthesis; impairs sugar absorption; and is an irritant.

Clinical Signs

- Ingestion can cause colic, profuse and watery diarrhea, fever, incoordination, depression, sweating, terminal convulsions, and death.
- Signs may be delayed 12 hours or more after ingestion.

Diagnosis

- Identification of seeds in GI contents, evidence of consumption, and compatible clinical signs
- Detection of ricinine or ricin in GI contents, serum, or urine

●▶ WHAT TO DO

Castor Bean Toxicosis

- Administer AC, 1 to 2 g/kg PO.
- Provide sedation if needed (xylazine, 0.4 mg/kg); IV fluids (hypertonic saline solution), followed by polyionic isotonic fluids.
- Administer flunixin meglumine, 1.0 mg/kg IV.

Horse Chestnut *(Aesculus hippocastanum)*

- The horse chestnut is a garden and park tree in North America (see Fig. 34-4).

Mechanism of Toxic Action

- The mechanism of action is uncertain. Experimentally studied saponins, especially aesculin, are neurotoxic at low dosages and hemolytic at higher dosages. Saponins also have a hypoglycemic effect. Alkaloids may also contribute.

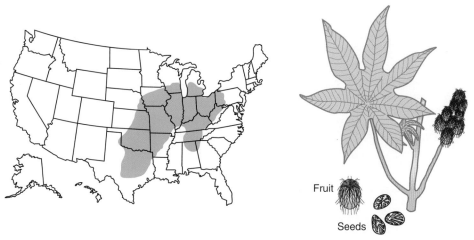

Figure 34-5 Distribution and drawing of *Ricinus communis* (castor bean).

Clinical Signs

- Ingestion can cause colic, inflamed mucous membranes, hyperesthesia, and ataxia followed by muscle tremors, paresis, dyspnea, convulsions, and death.
- Mortality is uncommon.

●> WHAT TO DO

Horse Chestnut Toxicosis
- Administer AC, 1 to 2 g/kg PO.
- Administer analgesics (parenteral), supportive fluids (intravenous), and symptomatic treatment.

Oak (*Quercus* spp.)

- Oaks compose a variety of native and introduced species that are widely distributed in the United States.
- Species range in size from shrubs 2 to 3 feet (60 to 90 cm) in height to large trees (Fig. 34-6).
- *Practice Tip: ALL species should be considered toxic.*
- Toxic principles are polyphenolic complexes called tannins, which are categorized as condensed or hydrolyzable. Hydrolyzable *tannins* such as gallotannins are responsible for clinical effects.
- Oak rarely causes poisoning in horses as opposed to cattle, although poorly fed horses may eat leaves, acorns, or oak buds.
- Relatively large amounts of the plant have to be ingested before clinical signs occur.

Mechanism of Toxic Action

- Tannins interact with and denature protein.
- Phenolic metabolites are likely responsible for GI; renal; and less commonly, liver damage.

Clinical Signs

- Anorexia, colic, sometimes bloody diarrhea, tenesmus, and depression are followed by frequent urination and constipation.
- Dependent edema may develop associated with protein-losing enteropathy.

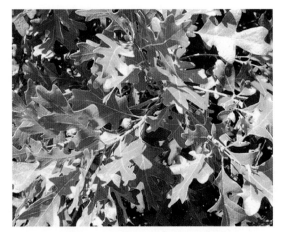

Figure 34-6 *Quercus gambelii* or scrub oak.

Diagnosis

- Evidence of plant consumption
- Detection of gallotannins in GI contents or urine

●> WHAT TO DO

Oak Toxicosis
- Administer fluids and nutritional and other supportive care.
- Evaluate for possible kidney damage.

Organophosphorus and Carbamate Insecticides

- Poisoning with OP and carbamate insecticides usually causes clinical signs of nervous and GI dysfunction.
- The most likely source of the poisoning is inappropriate or accidental oral or topical administration of an insecticide or anthelmintic containing OPs or carbamates. Clinical signs for both insecticides are similar.

Mechanism of Toxic Action

- Inhibition of acetylcholinesterase enzyme results in excessive cholinergic stimulation.

Clinical Signs

- Ingestion can cause colic, hypersalivation, sweating, diarrhea, muscle tremors, miosis, weakness, dyspnea, and convulsions.
- Typical mnemonics are SLUDGE or DUMBELS.
- OPs and carbamates increase the peristaltic activity of the intestines and cause bradycardia.
- Behavioral changes may occur and have recently been documented in horses fed tetrachlorvinphos (Equitrol[1]).

Diagnosis

- Horse has history of exposure and compatible clinical signs.
- Exposure is confirmed by measurement of whole blood, brain, or retinal cholinesterase activity. If significant OP or carbamate exposure has occurred, the cholinesterase or butyrylcholinesterase activity is much lower (50% of normal or below) than the normal range for the referring laboratory.
- *Note:* Blood should be collected in ethylenediaminetetraacetic acid (EDTA) and placed on ice and tested as soon as possible. Normal whole blood cholinesterase activity is approximately 2 to 2.5 µM/g/min but may vary between laboratories and handling of sample.
- *Practice Tip: If submitting samples to a laboratory for human beings, submit a control (unexposed) equine sample.*
- If submission of samples to the laboratory is delayed, samples collected in a case of carbamate insecticide exposure can exhibit a "regeneration" of active cholinesterase, resulting in a normal value.
- Submit GI contents and liver for detection of a specific OP or carbamate insecticide. Representative feed samples should be obtained and tested if the suspected source is

---

[1]Equitrol (Farnam Co., Phoenix, Arizona 85013).

feed. Concentrations of OPs and carbamates can be very high in feed and GI content samples. **Note:** These insecticides can penetrate plastic. Therefore, make sure that sample cross-contamination does not occur.

●〉 WHAT TO DO

Organophosphorus and Carbamate Insecticides

- Administer atropine, up to 1 mg/kg given to effect IV (repeat as required subcutaneously), to control clinical signs of OP and carbamate poisoning.
- There should be obvious improvement in the muscarinic effects (salivation, miosis, bronchosecretion, and sweating) soon after atropine treatment begins.
- Glycopyrrolate use may be associated with fewer adverse effects than atropine. **Note:** Glycopyrrolate is not approved for use in horses. Titrate dosage to effect (0.01 mg/kg IV).
- Pralidoxime hydrochloride (2-PAM) is specific for OPs and does not help in carbamate poisoning. Administer 20 mg/kg IV q4 to 6h, if needed.
- **Important:** If exposure is believed to be due to a cholinesterase inhibitor but it is unknown whether OPs or carbamates are involved, administer 2-PAM if available.
- Pass a stomach tube to remove any gastric reflux fluid.
- Administer AC, 1 to 2 g/kg PO, along with supportive care such as replacement fluids.
- Accurate diagnosis of OP or carbamate poisoning in horses is imperative because of the possible adverse effects of atropine administration. *High-dosage atropine used in OP or carbamate poisoning therapy should never be administered without clear historical, clinical, and preferably laboratory evidence that OP or carbamate poisoning is responsible for the clinical signs.*
- Transient abdominal pain following oral administration of OP anthelmintics is not uncommon; however, it is unusual that atropine treatment is required.

Red Clover (*Trifolium pratense*)

- Under certain environmental conditions a fungus, *Rhizoctonia leguminicola,* can grow on the clover and produce a mycotoxin, slaframine, which increases saliva production and causes slobbering.
- The fungus is seen as blackish brown spots on the clover.
- More commonly, the fungus affects horses grazing pastures containing some red clover or, less commonly, when red clover is in the hay.
- The same fungus may produce clinical signs in horses when present on other legumes, for example, white clover (*Trifolium repens*), alsike clover (*Trifolium hybridum*), or alfalfa (*Medicago sativa*).
- Fungus persists in vegetative tissue and seeds; therefore, once a pasture is infested, slobbers can be a recurring problem, especially when weather is cool and moist.

Mechanism of Toxic Action

- Cholinergic agonism

Clinical Signs

- Excess salivation occurs. This may occur within 1 hour of grazing infected clover and may persist for up to 24 hours

after removing the horse from the clover. Duration can be several hours for mild cases or continuous.
- In severe cases, diarrhea, frequent urination, and anorexia occur.

●〉 WHAT TO DO

Red Clover Toxicosis

- Remove affected individual from the pasture, or remove hay.
- Detoxification of contaminated hay is not possible.

Tobacco (*Nicotiana* spp.)

- Tobacco plants (commercial, wild, and ornamental) are extremely unpalatable; therefore, poisoning is uncommon.
- Poisoning may occur if horses are housed where tobacco is stored or where wild tobacco plants grow and there is little else to eat.
- Alkaloids are teratogenic.
- Toxic principles are nicotine and other alkaloids, such as anabasine.

Mechanism of Toxic Action

- Nicotine causes initial stimulation with subsequent depolarizing blockade of nicotinic receptors in sympathetic and parasympathetic ganglia, neuromuscular end plates, and the central nervous system.

Clinical Signs

- Ingestion can cause initial excitement, colic, diarrhea, incoordination, muscle tremors, and excess salivation followed by muscle weakness, recumbency, and stupor.
- Death may occur from respiratory paralysis.
- Survival beyond 12 hours is a good prognostic sign.

●〉 WHAT TO DO

Tobacco Toxicosis

- Administer AC, 1 to 2 g/kg PO.
- Provide fluid therapy and symptomatic treatment.

Other Gastrointestinal Poisonings

Salt Poisoning

- Salt ingestion can cause diarrhea, colic, and neurologic signs when salt-deprived horses are fed salt and do not have adequate water available.

Diagnosis

- Elevated serum or cerebrospinal fluid concentration of sodium

●〉 WHAT TO DO

Salt Poisoning

- Provide fluid therapy: 2.5% dextrose/0.45% saline solution or polyionic crystalloid; and dimethyl sulfoxide, 1 g/kg IV.
- *Do not* use 5% dextrose.
- For chronic poisoning (1 day or more), use 0.9% saline to slowly lower serum sodium.

Arsenic and Mercury

- Can produce sudden death with severe GI erosions

Clinical Signs

- Salivation
- Diarrhea
- Depression

Diagnosis

- Diagnosis is based on history plus testing of whole blood, GI contents, liver, and kidney for arsenic or mercury concentration.
- Any detectable concentration of arsenic or mercury is unexpected and is compatible with exposure to a source of the metal.
- Clinical signs plus hepatic and kidney arsenic concentrations >10 ppm are compatible with arsenic intoxication.

●〉 WHAT TO DO

Arsenic and Mercury Poisoning

- Administer dimercaprol, 3 to 5 mg/kg IM q8h on day 1 and 1 mg/kg IM q6h on days 2 and 3.
- Succimer is a newer, orally administered chelator that is effective for chelation of lead, arsenic, and mercury. Little information is available on its use in horses, but it has been demonstrated to be safe in other species for management of lead intoxication. Recommended dosage is 10 mg/kg PO q8h for 5 to 10 days.
- Measurement of blood concentration should be repeated several days after cessation of chelation therapy to assess the need for additional therapy.

Toxicants Predominantly Affecting the Nervous System

Ammonia Intoxication

- Ammonia intoxication most often occurs due to liver disease or inadequate glomerular filtration. Another potential cause is primary hyperammonemia from intestinal motility disturbances, inflammation, or increased intestinal ammonia production.
- If functional liver mass is inadequate, ammonia derived from the GI tract, catabolism, or skeletal muscle exertion cannot be converted to urea, resulting in plasma ammonia concentrations increasing.
- The cause of the primary intestinal hyperammonemia is unproven but may be related to intestinal overgrowth of ammonia-producing bacteria. This has occurred in both stalled and pastured adult horses.

Clinical Signs

- ***Practice Tip:*** *Primary ammonia intoxication should be strongly considered when horses have signs of acute encephalopathy, severe acidosis, normal liver enzyme values, and hyperglycemia.*
- Supportive treatment, fluids, oral neomycin, and sedation when needed can result in complete recovery within 72 hours in many cases.
- Colic and diarrhea also may be present.

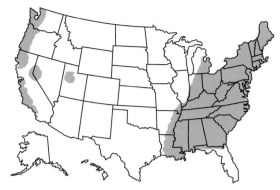

Figure 34-7   Distribution of *Hypochoeris radicata* (Australian dandelion).

Diagnosis

- Confirmation of the disorder is by measuring ammonia in blood or cerebrospinal fluid (CSF). If ammonia levels cannot be immediately measured, samples (serum/plasma/CSF/aqueous) should be quickly frozen or else the ammonia results are difficult to interpret.

Australian Dandelion *(Hypochoeris radicata)*

- The Australian dandelion causes outbreaks of stringhalt and roaring in horses in Australia.
- Similar outbreaks of unknown cause are reported in the western, southeastern, and mid-Atlantic United States (Fig. 34-7).
- Stringhalt also is associated with acute injury to the rear legs and hypocalcemia.
- The toxins have not been identified.

Mechanism of Toxic Action

- Unknown

●〉 WHAT TO DO

Australian Dandelion Toxicosis

- For severely affected individuals, phenytoin, 7.5 mg/kg PO q12h, may eliminate clinical signs.
- Fifty percent of horses recover within 8 months.
- Consider acupuncture (see Chapter 8, p. 28).

Avocado *(Persea americana)*

- Avocado is found mainly in Florida and California.
- Poisoning most commonly occurs when affected horses have access to pruned branches, which remain toxic when dried.
- Only the Guatemalan type and its hybrids are known to be toxic; toxic principle is believed to be persin and all parts of the tree are believed to be toxic, especially the leaves.

Mechanism of Toxic Action

- The mechanism of action is unknown, although administration of persin experimentally has caused mammary gland and myocardial necrosis.

Clinical Signs

- Ingestion can cause noninfectious mastitis, depression, mild tremors, and colic.

- Higher, repeated dosages are associated with cardiac arrhythmias and respiratory distress.
- Edema of the head, neck, and submandibular edema occurs.
- Death is uncommon.

Avocado Toxicosis
- Provide symptomatic and supportive care.
- Mastitis subsides within 1 week; however, no additional milk is produced during the lactation.

Botulism
- Botulism is caused by *Clostridium botulinum* and is mainly a clinical problem among foals 2 to 8 weeks of age; however, it can affect adults (see Chapter 22, p. 354, and Chapter 31, p. 552).
- Eight toxin types exist with variable regional distribution.
- In Kentucky, Pennsylvania, Maryland, New Jersey, Eastern New York, and Virginia, botulism is endemic and almost always caused by *C. botulinum* toxin type B. Forage contaminated with the toxin is the most likely cause.
- Type A botulism sporadically occurs west of the Mississippi River in Oregon, Idaho, Montana, Wyoming, Washington, California, and Nebraska.
- Type C occurs sporadically in horses that have ingested carcasses mixed in feed (i.e., carrion botulism).
- In adults, botulism is most often a result of ingestion of preformed toxin in vegetative matter. Rounds bale hay feeding is responsible for some cases. In foals, it is a toxic-infectious process caused by ingestion of *C. botulinum* type B spores.
- Wound botulism occurs among horses but is uncommon.

Mechanism of Toxic Action
- Inhibition of the release of acetylcholine causing presynaptic blockade of nerve impulses

Clinical Signs
- Generalized weakness
- Decreased tail, eyelid, and tongue tone

- Mydriasis and ptosis
- Trembling
- Lying down and recumbency
- Dysphagia (soft palate is usually displaced on endoscopic examination)—not always present with Type A
- Weakness that can progress to severe paresis with an inability to stand
- Respiratory difficulty

Diagnosis
- Although it is difficult to isolate the toxin, submit samples of serum, gastric, and intestinal contents; feces; and suspect feed for PCR analysis. A laboratory for testing is at the University of Pennsylvania, New Bolton Center (610-444-5800, ext. 6383 or 6245).
- In foals, culture of *C. botulinum* type B from the feces is strongly supportive of the diagnosis in the presence of dysphagia and weakness.

Botulism
- Administer antiserum (see Chapter 22, p. 355, and Chapter 31, p. 552).
- Avoid stress.
- Provide supportive care.

Bracken Fern (*Pteridium aquilinum*)
- Although frequently listed in textbooks, bracken fern poisoning is uncommon among horses because a large quantity of the unpalatable plant must be consumed (Figs. 34-8 and 34-9).
- Toxic principle is a type I thiaminase.

Mechanism of Toxic Action
- Competitive-type inhibition of thiamine cofactor activity

Clinical Signs
- Ingestion can cause unthriftiness, lethargy, ataxia, blindness, recumbency, and convulsions.
- Polioencephalomalacia can be found on postmortem examination.

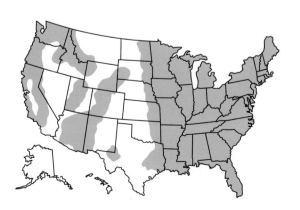
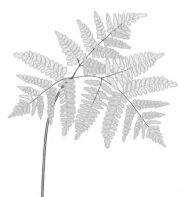

Figure 34-8 Distribution and drawing of *Pteridium aquilinum* (bracken fern).

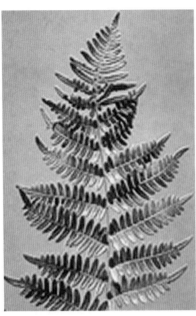

Figure 34-9 *Pteridium aquilinum.*

WHAT TO DO

Bracken Fern Toxicosis
- Administer thiamine hydrochloride, 5 mg/kg slowly IV or IM q6h for 5 days.
- Response to early treatment is dramatic.

Fumonisin Mycotoxins
- Fumonisins are mycotoxins produced by *Fusarium* spp. of fungus, are mainly found on corn, and can be present in high concentration in corn screenings; toxic concentrations of fumonisins occur sporadically.
- Fumonisins cause equine leukoencephalomalacia (or moldy corn poisoning).
- Several fumonisins have been isolated; fumonisin B1 is the most toxic, and fumonisins are primarily neurotoxic, but liver damage can occur as well.

Mechanism of Toxic Action
- Fumonisins inhibit sphingosine and sphinganine N-acetyltransferases, which are important for sphingolipid synthesis. Sphingolipids are important for normal cell structure, cell-cell communication, cell–extracellular matrix interactions, modulation of receptor kinases, and signal transduction.
- Sphinganine accumulation is cytotoxic, inhibits protein kinase C and other signal transduction pathways, and increases intracellular calcium concentration.

Clinical Signs
- Signs occur after the affected individuals eat the feed for several days.
- Ingestion can cause anorexia, ataxia, blindness, head pressing, decreased tongue tone and movement, depression, seizures, occasionally icterus, and death.
- Horse is afebrile.
- Bradycardia often is present.

Diagnosis
- See Chapter 22, p. 362, for more information.
- Nonspecific findings include high protein, albumin, immunoglobulin G concentrations, and increased albumin quotients in cerebrospinal fluid.
- Fumonisins may be detected in suspect feed.
- The maximum recommended concentration of fumonisins in horse feed is 5 ppm. Toxic dose is approximately 30 ppm.
- Malacia of the white matter of the cerebral cortex and in some cases hepatosis with elevation of serum hepatic enzymes may occur. The heart may also be affected.
- The contaminated corn usually appears normal on inspection.
- Many diagnostic laboratories test for fumonisins.

WHAT TO DO

Fumonisin Mycotoxins
- Provide supportive care. Affected individuals infrequently completely recover.
- *Do not* feed corn screenings to horses.

Horsetail (*Equisetum hyemale* and *E. arvense*)
- Horsetail ingestion is rarely reported as a toxicosis in horses *but* can occur if little else is available to eat.
- Toxic principle is a thiaminase, similar to bracken fern.

WHAT TO DO

Horsetail
Mechanism of Toxic Action, and Clinical Signs
- See Bracken Fern, p. 589.

Insulin
Hypoglycemic shock has been reported in horses inappropriately treated with insulin.

Diagnosis
- High-pressure liquid chromatography is used to identify the source of insulin in the serum; the test is performed by drug-testing centers.

WHAT TO DO

Insulin Overdose
- Provide continuous administration of 5% to 10% dextrose; polyionic crystalloids with 40 mEq/L potassium chloride; and dexamethasone, 0.2 mg/kg IV, initially followed by a decreasing dose for 2 to 3 additional days.

Prognosis
- Prognosis is poor.

Ivermectin/Moxidectin
- Ivermectin and moxidectin are macrolide endectocides that are commonly used in horses; intoxications are rare in adult horses because of large therapeutic indices (tenfold

safety margins are reported for adult horses) but can occur (mostly Quarter Horses).
- **Practice Tip:** *Solanum spp. plants may decrease toxic threshold of ivermectin in adult horses.*
- Moxidectin, unlike ivermectin, is toxic to foals <4 months of age and should not be used in this age group. On rare occasion, ivermectin given to a very young foal causes adverse effects similar to, but not as severe as, moxidectin.

Mechanism of Toxic Action
- All macrolide endectocides are gamma-aminobutyric acid (GABA)-agonists and intoxication occurs when a sufficient concentration of drug reaches the brain causing GABAergic receptor stimulation.
- Drugs bind to postsynaptic GABA-gated chloride channels resulting in inhibition of neuronal impulse transmission.
- Macrolide endectocides do not readily penetrate the mammalian blood-brain barrier because of a transmembrane, multidrug efflux pump (MDR1).

Acute Signs
- Signs have been well described in horses and include depression, ataxia, central blindness, mydriasis, and tremors of the lips.
- Signs may progress for 36 hours often followed by complete recovery.
- Foals <4 months of age that have received moxidectin are often comatose.

Diagnosis
- History of recent drug administration along with compatible clinical signs.
- Measurement of drug concentrations in plasma/serum (antemortem) or brain (postmortem)

● WHAT TO DO

Ivermectin Toxicosis
- No specific reversal agents are available although sarmazenil, 0.04 mg/kg IV q24h or 1.5 mL/kg of 20% Intralipid IV bolus, could be used to help reverse the effects. Evidence for the efficacy of using Intralipid for treating ivermectin or moxidectin intoxications is limited, and optimal dosing recommendations have not been established.
- Administer AC, 1 to 2 g/kg PO, as soon as possible after an oral exposure.
- Recumbent horses might require extensive nursing care in an intensive care setting.

Prognosis
- The prognosis is good for horses and mules that have clinical signs after receiving ivermectin at normal or near the normal dose.
- The prognosis for moxidectin toxicosis in foals is guarded.

Lead
- Lead poisoning is rare but can be caused by ingestion of lead paint, old batteries, or lead weights.

Mechanism of Toxic Action
- Lead interferes with a variety of enzymes, especially those with a sulfhydryl group.
- Lead replaces zinc as an enzyme cofactor.
- Lead inhibits several enzymes necessary for heme synthesis: delta-aminolevulinic acid synthetase, coproporphyrinogenase, and heme synthetase.

Acute Signs
- Ingestion can cause weakness, ataxia, depression, and convulsions.
- Laryngeal paresis, especially with exercise or excitement, may be present with chronic lead poisoning.

Diagnosis
- Whole-blood lead concentration is greater than 0.6 ppm (or greater than 0.3 ppm with compatible clinical signs).
- Liver or kidney contains 5 to 10 ppm (wet weight) or greater. **Practice Tip:** *To calculate and approximate a liver or kidney dry weight value from a wet weight value, multiply the wet weight value by 3.3. Alternatively, if a wet weight value is desired from a dry weight determination, divide the dry weight value by 3.3. This assumes tissue moisture content of approximately 70%.*

● WHAT TO DO

Lead Toxicosis
- Administer calcium EDTA, 75 mg/kg per day slowly IV, divided q12h. Treat for 2 or 3 days and then stop for 2 or 3 days and repeat if needed.
- Succimer is a newer, orally administered chelator that is effective for chelation of lead, arsenic, and mercury. Little information is available on its use in horses, but it has been shown to be safe in other species for management of lead intoxication. Recommended dosage is 10 mg/kg PO q8h for 5 to 10 days. Measurement of blood concentrations should be repeated several days after cessation of chelation therapy.
- Give thiamine, 5 mg/kg IV or IM.
- Magnesium or sodium sulfate, 1 g/kg PO via nasogastric intubation, helps remove lead from GI tract.
- Maintain adequate hydration of affected patient during treatment period.

Locoweeds (Certain *Astragalus* spp. and *Oxytropis* spp.)
- Locoweeds grow in central and western range lands of North America (Figs. 34-10 to 34-12).
- **Practice Tip:** *A large amount of the plant must be ingested (30% of body weight over 6 to 7 weeks).*
- Toxic principle is *swainsonine*. Horses eat the plant even when other forage is available and can become habituated to the plant.

Mechanism of Toxic Action
- Inhibits lysosomal alpha-mannosidase with subsequent intracellular accumulation of oligosaccharides, loss of cellular function, and cell death. Inhibition of Golgi mannosidase II results in the alteration of glycoprotein

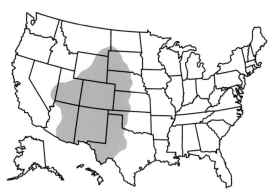

Figure 34-10   Distribution of *Astragalus mollissimus* (locoweed).

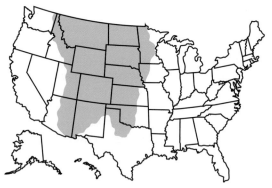

Figure 34-11   Distribution of *Oxytropis lambertii* (locoweed).

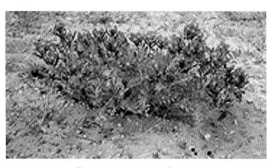

Figure 34-12   *Astragalus* spp.

synthesis, processing, and transport, which leads to dysfunctional membrane receptors, cellular adhesion molecules, and circulating hormones.
* Central nervous system, lymphoid tissue, endocrine tissues, and liver contain lysosomal vacuoles.

Clinical Signs
* Depression, tremors, ataxia, dysphagia, hyperexcitability, apparent blindness, emaciation, impaired reproduction, stringhalt-like gaits, paraplegia, and death

Diagnosis
* Swainsonine can be measured in serum samples. Contact the U.S. Department of Agriculture Poisonous Plant Research Laboratory in Logan, Utah (435-752-2941).
* Histologic changes in affected tissues are highly suggestive.

●› WHAT TO DO

Locoweeds Toxicosis
* No antidotes have been demonstrated to be effective; reserpine, 3.0 mg/450 kg q24h IM or 1.25 mg/450 kg PO for 6 days, has been reported to eliminate the clinical signs and allows safe handling.
* Horses should *not* be kept in areas where locoweeds grow.
* Recovery may occur in mild cases, but affected individuals should never be used for riding or work.

Marijuana, Hemp *(Cannabis sativa)*
* Marijuana is a tall annual herb of the hemp family.
* Occasionally, marijuana is fed to horses. Active ingredients are *d-tetrahydrocannabinol* and related *resinoids*.

Clinical Signs
* Ingestion can cause depression and drowsiness, with possible periods of excitement, hyperactivity, tremors, and hyperresponsiveness to touch and sound.
* Recovery usually occurs in a few to 24 hours.

●› WHAT TO DO

Marijuana/Hemp Toxicosis
* Administer AC, 1 to 2 g/kg PO, if ingestion was within previous 2 hours.
* Provide symptomatic and supportive care.

Phosphide Salts (Zinc or Aluminium Phosphide)
* Aluminum and zinc phosphide are used as insecticides and rodenticides.
* They are also used for grain fumigation due to the release of phosphine gas after contact with moisture.
* The released phosphine gas is colorless and has an odor of decaying fish.
* Acute poisoning can be caused by ingestion of phosphide containing salts that release phosphine upon contact with the acidic environment in the stomach, or by direct inhalation of phosphine.

Mechanism of Toxic Action
* Phosphine gas is responsible for the clinical signs. Phosphine inhibits cytochrome C oxidase, which is considered partially responsible for the toxicity. Mechanisms resulting in free radical formation and cholinesterase inhibition also play a role in the pathogenesis.
* Phosphide salts are corrosive.

Clinical Signs
* Profuse sweating, tachycardia, tachypnea, muscle tremors, pyrexia, ataxia, seizures
* Hypoglycemia and elevated liver enzymes.

Diagnosis
* Detection of phosphine gas in gastrointestinal contents is provided by certain toxicology laboratories.
* Phosphine detection tubes can be used to detect phosphine in the air.

- Postmortem findings include widespread hemorrhages in multiple organs, pulmonary edema, congestion of multiple organs, neuronal necrosis in the brain, and hepatic lipidosis.

●› WHAT TO DO

Phosphide Salts Toxicosis
- Caution veterinary staff about the risks of exposure to phosphine gas. Provide sufficient ventilation.
- There is limited evidence on the usefulness of decontamination. Sodium bicarbonate 0.1 g/kg PO may decrease hydrochloric acid and delay the conversion of phosphide salts to phosphine.
- Activated charcoal and di-tri-octahedral smectite have been given but there are no data on their efficacy.
- Provide supportive and symptomatic care.
- Prognosis is poor and most affected individuals will likely die within 24 hours.

Rye Grass *(Lolium perenne)*
- Rye grass is a common pasture grass of the southeastern United States and West Coast that can be parasitized by an endophytic fungus called *Neotyphodium lolii*.
- Rye grass staggers is caused by toxic alkaloids, especially lolitrem B, produced by the fungus.
- Rye grass staggers is a sporadic disease that occurs during years that are apparently conducive to fungal growth.
- The condition may rarely be seen with other grasses (e.g., Bermuda grass and Dallis grass).

Mechanism of Toxic Action
- The fungal toxin is believed to inhibit large conductance calcium-activated potassium channels and increase release of neurotransmitters.

Clinical Signs
- If at rest and left undisturbed, affected individuals can appear normal.
- If disturbed or forced to move: stiffness, tremors, weakness, and incoordination are apparent.
- Death usually is accidental (e.g., falling into water and drowning).

●› WHAT TO DO

Rye Grass Toxicosis
- Remove horse from pasture; recovery generally occurs rapidly.

Selenium Toxicosis
- Acute form of toxicosis results from inappropriate selenium injections (see Table 34-1) or feeding toxic amounts.
- Errors in feed formulation can occur but rarely cause problems.
- Toxicity is reported in horses administered 3.3 mg/kg PO (smaller amounts can be toxic).

Mechanism of Toxic Action
- Oxidative stress
- Displacement of sulfur in sulfur-containing amino acids

Clinical Signs
- Signs of acute selenosis include excess salivation, tremors, ataxia, apparent blindness, respiratory distress, diarrhea, inability to stand, and death.
- Signs of chronic selenosis include hair or hoof abnormalities, coronary band separation, and joint stiffness.
- If poisoning is suspected, measure selenium concentrations in the blood and liver samples.

●› WHAT TO DO

Selenium Toxicosis
- Provide symptomatic and supportive care.
- Acetylcysteine, beginning at 140 mg/kg IV and then 70 mg/kg IV q6h, is suggested for acute poisoning.

Sudan Grass *(Sorghum bicolor)*
- In addition to the risk of acute cyanide poisoning, grazing on Sudan grass for several weeks can cause equine cystitis and ataxia syndrome (Fig. 34-13).
- Toxicosis has occurred in the central and southern Great Plains of North America in pastures almost exclusively composed of sorghum species. Problems do not occur from eating dry, well-cured hay.
- Cyanide and nitriles are hypothesized to cause the cystitis and ataxia, although neither has been shown to reproduce the disease.

Mechanism of Toxic Action
- Unknown

Clinical Signs
- Ingestion can cause ataxia of the rear limbs, a hopping gait, and dribbling of urine (the bladder is enlarged).

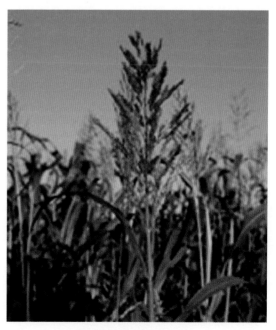

Figure 34-13 *Sorghum* spp.

TOX

- Abortion can occur at any time during gestation, dystocia may result from a deformed fetus, or the newborn foal may be deformed or weak.
- Acute poisoning (cyanide) frequently causes death.

Diagnosis

- Clinical signs, exposure, cyanide levels in gastric contents or forage

●〉 WHAT TO DO

Sudan Grass Toxicosis
- Remove horse from pasture and manage any bladder infection with antibiotics.
- Full recovery is unusual.
- See cyanide for appropriate treatment (p. 601).

White Snakeroot (*Eupatorium rugosum*)

- Toxic principle is unknown (older texts list *tremetol*), is cumulative, and can be passed in the milk (Figs. 34-14 and 34-15).
- ***Practice Tip:*** *White snakeroot grows in shady areas and is a problem in late summer and fall; it remains toxic after frost or when dried.*

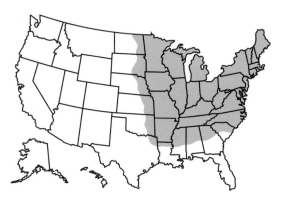

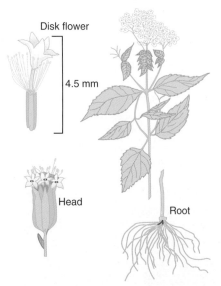

Figure 34-14 Distribution and drawing of *Eupatorium rugosum* (white snakeroot).

Mechanism of Toxic Action
- Not certain; metabolic alterations resulting from tricarboxylic acid cycle impairment and decreased use of glucose

Clinical Signs
- Ingestion can cause weakness, depression, trembling, sweating, salivation, and recumbency.
- Arrhythmias, jugular vein distention and pulsation, cardiac damage, and dependent edema are possible.
- Increases in serum values of lactate dehydrogenase and creatine kinase occur.

●〉 WHAT TO DO

White Snakeroot Toxicosis
- Provide symptomatic and supportive care.
- Remove horse from source.
- Horse may have long-term cardiac compromise.

Yellow Star Thistle (*Centaurea solstitialis*)

- Yellow star thistle grows predominantly in the western United States (Figs. 34-16 and 34-17).
- Russian knapweed (*Centaurea repens*) causes identical signs and is considered more toxic.

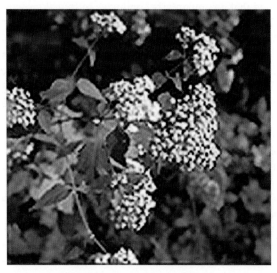

Figure 34-15   *Eupatorium rugosum.*

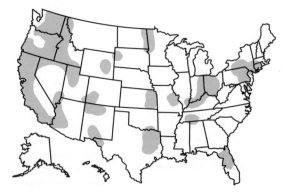

Figure 34-16   Distribution of *Centaurea solstitialis* (yellow star thistle).

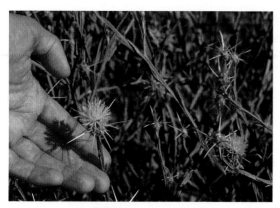

Figure 34-17 *Centaurea solstitialis.*

- Numerous sesquiterpene lactones and biologically active amines are present and are potentially involved in disease pathogenesis.

Mechanism of Toxic Action
- Lesions are restricted to the globus pallidus and substantia nigra.
- Several of the lactones have been found to be cytotoxic to neurons in vitro.

Clinical Signs
- Signs begin suddenly after chronic ingestion of the plant.
- Affected individuals can prehend food with their incisors but cannot move the food back into the mouth. They have difficulty in drinking water and may immerse the head deep into the water to swallow. The lips may be retracted from hypertonic facial muscles, and the tongue may protrude.
- Depression, ataxia, circling, and starvation may occur.
- Horse may have secondary aspiration pneumonia.
- Oxidative stress may play a role in neuronal degeneration causing neurologic signs.

Diagnosis
- Magnetic resonance imaging (MRI) can provide accurate and sensitive visualization of typical lesions seen in the brain.
- Nigropallidal encephalomalacia is found at necropsy.

●〉 WHAT TO DO

Yellow Star Thistle Toxicosis
- No specific treatment is available.
- Vitamin E should be administered.
- Affected individuals *do not* recover, but if not severely diseased, they may learn to accommodate.

Toxicants Predominantly Affecting the Liver
Aflatoxins
- *Aflatoxins B_1, B_2, G_1, and G_2 are produced by Aspergillus flavus and A. parasiticus,* which grow on corn, peanuts, cottonseed, and other small grains in warm, wet conditions.

- Aflatoxins have been reported to cause acute hepatic failure (neurologic signs and icterus) in horses.

Mechanism of Toxic Action
- Aflatoxins and their liver metabolites react with enzymes, RNA, and DNA within the hepatocytes, and the result is acute or chronic liver dysfunction.

Diagnosis
- Evidence of exposure (have feed tested for mycotoxins), clinical signs, laboratory findings of liver disease and failure

●〉 WHAT TO DO

Aflatoxicosis
- Remove horse from suspect feed.
- General therapy for hepatic failure (see Chapter 20, p. 277)
- Administer L-methionine, 25 mg/kg PO
- Administer vitamin E, 6000 to 10,000 units q24h PO, in the adult

Alsike Clover *(Trifolium hybridum)*
- Alsike clover is a pasture legume found mostly in Canada and the northeastern United States.
- *Practice Tip: A cluster of cases may occur among horses grazing alsike clover grown on clay soil during certain years, probably owing to wet weather conditions.*
- Alsike must be predominant feed for several days to several weeks to cause subacute intoxication.
- Longer-term ingestion is reported to be associated with liver damage and hepatogenous photosensitization (see Chapter 20, p. 274).
- The toxic principle has *not* been identified; it may be a plant toxin or more likely a mycotoxin growing on the clover.

Mechanism of Toxic Action
- Subacute intoxication: uncertain, but toxin may be a primary photosensitizer
- Chronic intoxication: uncertain, but toxin may be a hepatotoxin causing hepatogenous photosensitization

Clinical Signs
- Photosensitivity (erythema, swelling, edema, and sloughing of skin in lightly or nonpigmented areas)
- Icterus
- Neurologic signs indicative of hepatic encephalopathy

●〉 WHAT TO DO

Alsike Clover Toxicosis
- Remove alsike from diet.
- Protect patient from direct sunlight.
- Administer general therapy for photosensitization and liver failure (see p. 275).

Prognosis
- Good if identified early in the syndrome before significant liver damage has occurred

TOX

Iron Toxicosis

- Iron toxicosis may occur in horses given one large dose (overuse of a hematinic, oral or injectable) or may be caused by long-term accumulation (hemochromatosis).
- ***Practice Tip:*** *Foals receiving even small-dosage iron supplements before nursing may experience fatal hepatopathy. Foals receiving blood transfusions for neonatal isoerythrolysis may occasionally have hepatic iron overload and progressive liver disease.*

Mechanism of Toxic Action

- Oxidative cell damage

Clinical Signs

- Early signs associated with oral ingestion include colic, diarrhea, and melena.
- Intoxicated horses often present with anorexia, lethargy, and icterus.
- Signs of hepatoencephalopathy can be seen (see Chapter 20, p. 273).
- ***Important:*** Clinical signs of liver failure generally do not occur unless more than 60% to 75% of hepatic function is lost.

Diagnosis

- Laboratory findings of liver disease: increased serum gamma-glutamyl transpeptidase (GGT), alkaline phosphatase (ALP), total and conjugated bilirubin, bile acids, fibrinogen, fibrin degradation products (FDPs), and ammonia
- Thrombocytopenia, lymphopenia, and prolonged prothrombin time (PT) and activated partial thromboplastin time (aPTT)
- Liver iron concentration is >300 ppm; most horses with iron toxicosis have values threefold or more above the upper normal range.
- The concentration of iron in the liver can be abnormally high without liver disease (hemosiderosis), as in vitamin E deficiency
- Serum value of iron is frequently normal in chronic hemochromatosis and may be increased with acute toxicosis
- Elevation of serum and liver concentrations of iron is not specific for iron toxicosis and is found in a variety of liver disorders. Correlation with laboratory and histopathologic lesions is necessary.

●❯ WHAT TO DO

Iron Toxicosis

- Provide supportive therapy for hepatic failure.
- After oral exposure, administer magnesium hydroxide (milk of magnesia) to precipitate iron in the GI tract.
- Administer vitamin C, 0.5 g/kg PO, and deferoxamine, 10 mg/kg IM or slowly IV twice, 2 hours apart.
- If urine is reddish gold, additional treatment may be needed to hasten excretion in acute cases.

Klein Grass and Fall Panicum (*Panicum* spp.)

- Klein grass poisoning is primarily a problem in Texas and the southwestern United States, whereas fall panicum occasionally is a problem in the mid-Atlantic states.
- Liver damage is associated with the presence of saponins such as diosgenin; hepatogenous photosensitization results (see Chapter 20, p. 274).

Mechanism of Toxic Action

- Possible reaction of saponins with calcium results in precipitation of insoluble calcium salts in bile ducts.

Clinical Signs

- Chronic poor appetite and weight loss
- Depression; icterus; photosensitization; and more rarely, neurologic signs of hepatic encephalopathy

●❯ WHAT TO DO

Klein Grass and Fall Panicum Toxicosis

- General therapy for hepatic failure (see Chapter 20, p. 277)

Prognosis

- Prognosis is guarded if signs of hepatic failure are present, although some horses recover to normal appearance if the toxic hay is removed.

Pyrrolizidine Alkaloids

- Pyrrolizidine alkaloids are contained in the following plants: *Senecio* spp. (ragwort, groundsel; Figs. 34-18 and 34-19), *Crotalaria* spp. (rattlebox; Figs. 34-20 and 34-21), *Amsinckia* spp. (fiddleneck), *Echium vulgare* (viper's bugloss), *Heliotropium europaeum* (heliotrope), *Cynoglossum officinale* (hound's tongue; Figs. 34-22 and 34-23), and others.
- Intoxication from pyrrolizidine alkaloid–containing plants is a clinical problem mostly in the western United States, although some areas of eastern Canada and eastern United States have reported cases.

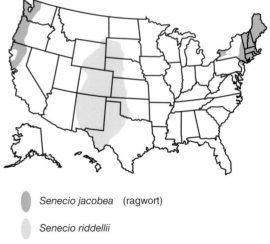

- Senecio jacobea   (ragwort)

- Senecio riddellii

Figure 34-18 Distribution of *Senecio jacobae* (ragwort; solid) and *S. riddellii* (stippled).

- Toxicity occurs from chronic ingestion of the plants, mostly in spring-cut alfalfa hay.
- Pyrrolizidine alkaloids produce a chronic hepatic disease, though the onset is often acute several weeks after ingestion.

Mechanism of Toxic Action

- Pyrrolizidine alkaloid liver metabolites interact with cellular constituents and cause a decrease of DNA-mediated RNA and protein synthesis.
- Cause hepatocyte degeneration, necrosis, and impairment of cell division, the latter resulting in megalocytosis.

Clinical Signs

- Signs consistent with hepatoencephalopathy: head pressing, circling, blindness, ataxia, icterus, photosensitization, and weight loss

Diagnosis

- Diagnosis may be difficult because exposure may have occurred long before the onset of clinical signs.
- Inspect the hay.
- Liver biopsy has characteristic findings of megalocytosis, centrilobular necrosis, portal fibrosis, and biliary hyperplasia.
- Suspect feed can be analyzed for alkaloids (Poisonous Plant Research Laboratory, Logan, Utah, or California Animal Health and Food Safety Laboratory, Davis).

⊙› WHAT TO DO

Pyrrolizidine Alkaloid Toxicosis

- Supportive care for hepatic failure (see Chapter 20, p. 273).
- Most affected individuals have signs of liver failure and die within days to several months after clinical signs develop.

Sensitive Fern *(Onoclea sensibilis)*

- The sensitive fern is found throughout eastern North America in open woods and meadows.
- Poisoning is rare because large quantities must be ingested over long periods.

Clinical Signs

- Ingestion can cause incoordination, anorexia, and hyperesthesia.
- Affected individuals have liver disease (fatty degeneration) and cerebral edema with neuronal degeneration.

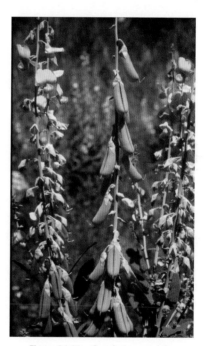

Figure 34-21   *Crotalaria spectabilis.*

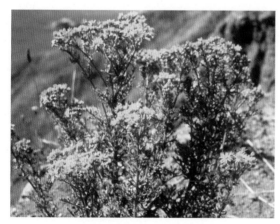

Figure 34-19   *Senecio jacobae.*

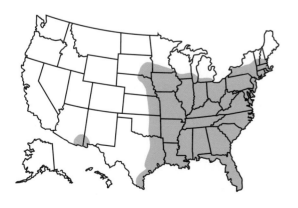
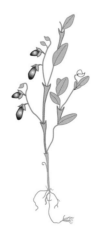

Figure 34-20   Distribution and drawing of *Crotalaria sagittalis* (rattlebox). Horses rarely eat the plant.

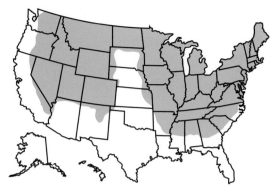

Figure 34-22   Distribution of *Cynoglossum officinale* (hound's tongue).

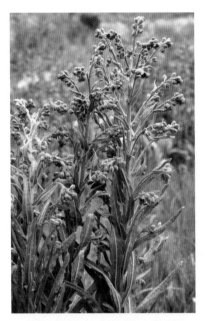

Figure 34-23   *Cynoglossum officinale.*

Blue-Green Algae (*Microcystis* spp., *Anabaena* spp., and Others)

- Intoxication of horses is rare, but algal toxins can cause sudden death.
- *Microcystis, Anabaena, Planktothrix, Nostoc, Oscillatoria,* and *Anabaenopsis* produce hepatotoxins (microcystins); most problems are associated with *Microcystis* spp.
- The *neurotoxic anatoxins* (anatoxin-a and anatoxin-a$_s$) are mainly produced by cyanobacteria in the *Anabaena* genus, but also by other genera, such as *Planktothrix, Oscillatoria, Microcystis, Aphanizomenon, Cylindrospermum,* and *Phormidium.*
- Algal blooms occur in water bodies when environmental conditions are conducive to rapid algal growth followed by toxin production.
- Algal blooms can be concentrated along the leeward side of the body of water, thus increasing the risk of ingestion.

Clinical Signs
- Microcystin-affected individuals can have a sudden onset of gastroenteritis, hemorrhagic diarrhea, and hypovolemic shock; acute liver failure and seizures precede death.

- Anatoxin-a is a nicotinic receptor agonist that causes muscle fasciculations followed by neuromuscular blockade, collapse, dyspnea, cyanosis, seizures, and death.
- Anatoxin-a$_s$ inhibits cholinesterase enzymes (see Organophosphorus and Carbamate Insecticides, see p. 586).

Diagnosis
- Detection of algal toxins in water samples and GI contents (via analytic detection)
- Identification of toxigenic algae in water (preserve algal bloom material in 10% formalin for microscopic examination)
- Identification of toxigenic algae in GI contents
- Characteristic liver lesions following microcystin exposure

●》 WHAT TO DO

Blue-Green Algae Toxicosis
- Administer AC, 1 to 2 g/kg PO, as early as possible.
- Provide symptomatic and supportive care.

Toxicants Predominantly Affecting the Skin
Snow-on-the-Mountain (*Euphorbia marginata*)
- *Euphorbia marginata* and other *Euphorbia* spp. are in the spurge family.
- Spurges contain an irritant milky sap that causes contact irritation of the skin, mouth, and GI tract.

●》 WHAT TO DO

Snow-on-the-Mountain Toxicosis
- Wash skin with water; apply topical steroids or antihistamine emollients.
- For oral exposures, administer demulcents or mineral oil PO.
- If severe clinical signs are present, administer parenteral steroids, antihistamines, and analgesics.

Stinging Nettle (*Urtica Dioica* and Others)
- Plants have stinging hairs containing formic acid, histamine, serotonin, and other constituents that cause local irritation.
- Affected individuals have been reported to exhibit ataxia, distress, and muscle weakness for several hours after extensive contact with nettle; the mechanism is unknown.

●》 WHAT TO DO

Stinging Nettle Toxicosis
- Give steroids, antihistamines, and analgesics.
- Local cleansing of affected area
- Topical emollients as needed

St. John's Wort (*Hypericum perforatum*)
- St. John's wort is found throughout the United States along roadsides and in abandoned fields and open woods (Figs. 34-24 and 34-25).

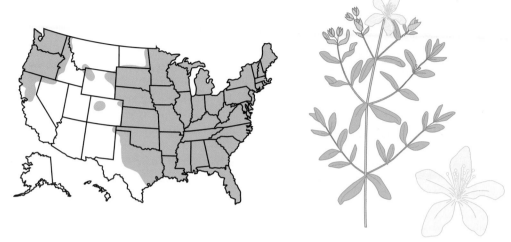

Figure 34-24   Distribution and drawing of *Hypericum perforatum* (St. John's wort).

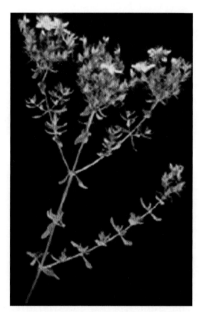

Figure 34-25   *Hypericum perforatum.*

- Toxic principle is *hypericin,* a pigment that directly reacts with light to cause primary photosensitization, often within 24 hours after ingestion.
- Buckwheat *(Fagopyrum esculentum)* also causes primary photosensitivity; however, exposure is unusual.
- Both plants remain toxic when dried.

Mechanism of Toxic Action
- Photodynamic agent (hypericin) activated by long ultraviolet light to a reactive compound; interaction of reactive compound with cellular constituents

Clinical Signs
- Clinical signs include dermatitis, pruritus, and ulceration, all of which are more severe in nonpigmented areas of the skin and areas of the body with more exposure to sunlight.

- Lacrimation, conjunctival erythema, corneal ulceration, and anorexia caused by irritation around the mouth also may occur.

●› WHAT TO DO

St. John's Wort and Buckwheat Toxicosis
- Remove the affected individual(s) from plant exposure and sunlight.
- Provide topical and systemic treatment of the dermatitis: antihistamines, glucocorticoids (prednisolone at 1.1 mg/kg q24h), flunixin meglumine at 1.0 mg/kg PO or IV q8 to 12h, and topical silver sulfadiazene.
- Administer ophthalmic antibiotics as needed.
- Administer systemic antibiotics in cases of severe dermatitis to manage secondary bacterial infections.
- Use surgical debridement to manage necrotic skin areas.

Photosensitization (Secondary)
- In primary photosensitization (e.g., St. John's wort), there is no biochemical evidence of liver disease.
- Secondary photosensitization involves failure of the liver to excrete a normal metabolite of chlorophyll, phylloerythrin, and subsequent accumulation of this substance.
- Phylloerythrin is a photodynamic agent that becomes reactive after activation by ultraviolet light.
- The differential diagnosis of secondary or hepatogenous photosensitivity includes hepatic failure (use biochemical tests, GGT, bilirubin) and ingestion of other plants such as alsike clover, panicum, and pyrrolizidine alkaloid–containing plants.
- Prognosis for horses with secondary photosensitization is worse than for primary photosensitization because of underlying liver disease.

Toxicants Predominantly Affecting the Musculoskeletal System
Black Walnut *(Juglans nigra)*
- Walnut and related hickories are important trees of eastern deciduous forests (Fig. 34-26).

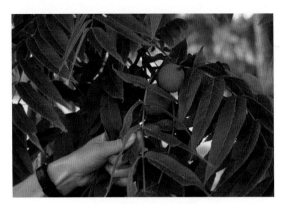

Figure 34-26 *Juglans nigra.*

- Problems arise after horses are bedded on wood shavings containing black walnut.
- The toxic principle of black walnut shavings is unknown.

Mechanism of Toxic Action

- Action is unknown, but toxin may enhance the vasoconstrictive actions of hormones such as epinephrine. Ingestion of the shaving is thought to be needed for the toxic effect, although some believe it can be absorbed through the skin; this is unproven.

Clinical Signs

- Laminitis often occurs within 12 to 24 hours of bedding on fresh black walnut shavings.
- As little as 5% black walnut shavings in the bedding can cause clinical disease.
- There may be considerable edema of all four limbs and mild pyrexia.
- Laminitis with edema of all four limbs affecting more than one horse on a farm should arouse suspicion of black walnut shaving toxicity.

Diagnosis

- Rule out other causes of laminitis.
- Black walnut can be identified in shavings by diagnostic laboratories or wood technologists.

◉ WHAT TO DO

Black Walnut Toxicosis
- Remove horse from the shavings.
- Wash legs with mild soap, and administer hydrotherapy.
- Administer magnesium sulfate, 0.5 mg/kg via nasogastric tube, as a cathartic.
- Treat for laminitis, for example, analgesics such as phenylbutazone, 4.0 mg/kg IV; flunixin meglumine, 1.0 mg/kg IV; or ketoprofen, 2.2 mg/kg IV (see Chapter 43, p. 709).
- Apply cryotherapy to the distal limbs (see Chapter 43, p. 706).
- Apply frog pads or place in sand bedding.
- Apply support wraps.
- Give pentoxifylline, 10 mg/kg PO q12h, and aspirin, 60 to 90 grains (10 to 20 mg/kg) PO every other day for a 450-kg adult (no evidence based benefit).
- Possibly administer acepromazine, 0.02 mg/kg IV or IM q6h, except in stallions (no evidence based benefit).

Prognosis
- Prognosis is generally better than for other causes of laminitis.

Day-Blooming Jessamine *(Cestrum diurnum)*
- Day-blooming jessamine is found in the southeastern United States, Texas, California, and Hawaii.
- Toxic principle is *cholecalciferol glycoside,* which causes hypervitaminosis D_3 (hypercalcemia).

Mechanism of Toxic Action
- Excessive vitamin D_3 causes increased absorption of calcium from the GI tract and renal tubules and increased osteoclastic activity, which results in hypercalcemia.
- Hypercalcemia can lead to metastatic tissue calcification.

Clinical Signs
- Signs are lameness, loss of weight, stiffness, and reluctance to move.
- Acute poisoning does not occur; however, chronic ingestion can cause calcification of tendons, ligaments, arteries, and kidneys.
- Serum calcium concentration is elevated.

◉ WHAT TO DO

Day-Blooming Jessamine Toxicosis
- Remove patient from source.
- Normal saline solution and furosemide diuresis with glucocorticoid administration may decrease calcium concentration.
- Provide symptomatic and supportive care.
- Evaluate kidney function.

Fescue Foot in Foals
- Arterial constriction in a limb is a rare occurrence in otherwise healthy foals grazing on fescue pasture.
- ***Practice Tip:*** *Most reported cases occurred during one summer; this finding suggests that unusual environmental conditions are needed.*
- Ergotism produced from the growth of *Claviceps purpurea* on grains has a similar presentation.

◉ WHAT TO DO

Fescue Foot in Foals
- Do nothing.
- Nitroglycerin cream can be applied over affected arteries (unproven efficacy).

Hoary Alyssum *(Berteroa incana)*
- A plant in the mustard family found throughout the Midwest and northeastern United States (Figs. 34-27 and 34-28).
- Hoary alyssum often grows in older alfalfa fields where considerable winterkill occurs; it remains toxic and palatable in dried hay.

Mechanism of Toxic Action
- Unknown

Clinical Signs
- Ingestion can cause acute onset of limb edema, along with lethargy, fever, and sometimes diarrhea.
- Joint stiffness, laminitis, and hematuria may develop.
- Clinical signs develop 18 to 36 hours after ingestion.
- Death is unusual.

●› WHAT TO DO

Hoary Alyssum Toxicosis
- Provide symptomatic and supportive care.
- When plant is removed from diet, remission of signs generally occurs within 2 to 4 days.

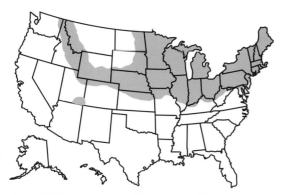

Figure 34-27 Distribution of *Berteroa incana* (hoary alyssum).

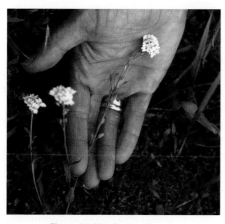

Figure 34-28 *Berteroa incana.*

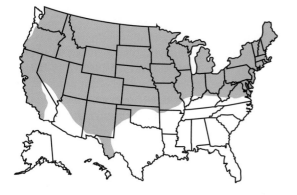

Toxicants Predominantly Affecting the Cardiovascular System
Foxglove *(Digitalis purpurea)*, Milkweed *(Asclepias* spp.), Yellow Oleander *(Thevetia peruviana)*, Dogbanes *(Apocynum* spp.), Lily-of-the-Valley *(Convallaria majalis)*, Summer Pheasant's Eye *(Adonis aestivalis)*
- These are potentially toxic plants that contain *cardiac glycosides.*
- Poisoning of horses by these plants is uncommon but can occur if the plants are mixed in hay and the affected individuals have little else to eat.

Mechanism of Toxic Action
- Action is inhibition of Na$^+$-K$^+$-ATPase with subsequent alteration of Na$^+$ and K$^+$ flux across membranes.
- Increase in intracellular Ca^{2+} levels result in alterations of cardiac conduction.

●› WHAT TO DO

Cardiac Glycoside Toxicosis
Clinical Signs and Treatment
- See Oleander, p. 603.

Cyanide
- Cyanide has been reported as a cause of sudden death among horses ingesting wild cherry (*Prunus* spp.) leaves, saplings, or bark (Figs. 34-29 to 34-31).
- Cyanide inhibits cytochrome C oxidase and disrupts the ability of cells to use oxygen in oxidative phosphorylation, resulting in tissue hypoxia.

Clinical Signs
- Hyperpnea
- Tachycardia
- Cardiac arrhythmias
- Seizures
- Apnea
- Coma
- Sudden death

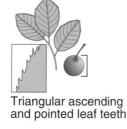

Triangular ascending and pointed leaf teeth

Figure 34-29 Distribution of *Prunus virginiana* (wild cherry).

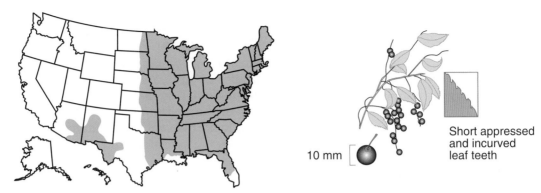

Figure 34-30   Distribution of *Prunus serotina* and drawings of *P. virginiana* and *P. serotina*.

Short appressed
and incurved
leaf teeth

10 mm

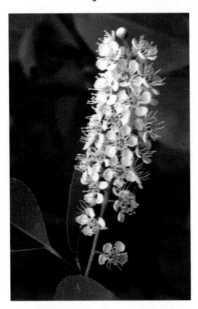

Figure 34-31   *Prunus serotina*.

Diagnosis

- Diagnosis is by detection of cyanide in appropriate samples such as GI contents, whole blood, and muscle tissue. ***Practice Tip:*** *Samples must be frozen immediately and stored in an airtight container.*
- Rapidity of onset of clinical signs and death combined with delay in obtaining test results precludes routine testing to assist in treatment.
- Blood can be bright red as a result of oxygen saturation.

●〉 WHAT TO DO

Cyanide Poisoning

- Rapid administration of sodium nitrate (20%) at 10 to 20 mg/kg IV followed by sodium thiosulfate at 30 to 40 mg/kg slow IV is antidotal.
- Rapidity of onset of clinical signs and death generally precludes use of cyanide antidotes.

Ionophore Antibiotic Poisoning

- Ionophore antibiotics are used in cattle and poultry feed to improve feed efficiency and as coccidiostats.
- These antibiotics are capable of carrying ions across biologic membranes.

- Common ionophores include monensin (Rumensin, Coban), lasalocid (Bovatec, Avatec), narasin (Monteban), laidlomycin (Cattlyst), and salinomycin (Sacox, Bio-Cox).
- Horses are extremely susceptible to ionophore antibiotics; the minimal lethal dosage of monensin may be as low as 1 mg/kg body weight.

Mechanism of Toxic Action

- Mediate an electrically neutral exchange of cations for protons across cell membranes
- Influx of cations, especially calcium, into cells
- Disruption of electrochemical gradients across mitochondrial membranes, leading to loss of cellular energy production

Clinical Signs

- Signs vary depending on the amount ingested and ionophore involved: anorexia, colic, diarrhea, depression, sweating, labored breathing, prostration, and death may precede any signs of heart failure.
- Cardiac arrhythmias may occur.
- Hyperventilation, jugular pulsation, tachycardia, and bright-red mucous membranes are found with cardiac failure (especially monensin).
- Sudden death has been reported, presumably from cardiac failure (especially with monensin).
- Weakness and recumbency occur in some cases without signs of heart failure (especially with salinomycin and lasalocid).
- Nervous system and muscle pathology may be present.
- Stranguria (straining) and excess urination (polyuria) are reported in some horses.

Diagnosis

- Echocardiography is an important adjunct to assess the presence and severity of myocardial damage; it is also useful for prognostic purposes (see Chapter 17, p. 153).
- Elevations in cardiac troponin I (cTnI) occur as rapidly as 18 hours and may peak 24 to 48 hours after ingestion.
- Send the suspect feed or GI (stomach and colon) contents to a laboratory. Most diagnostic laboratories can test for ionophores.
- Serum concentration of muscle enzymes generally is increased.
- Examine for histologic evidence of cardiac muscle lesions.

WHAT TO DO

Ionophore Antibiotic Poisoning
- Remove the suspect feed.
- Give AC, 1 to 2 g/kg PO, and magnesium sulfate.
- Administer intravenous polyionic fluids.
- Administer vitamin E and intramuscular selenium injection.
- Provide other supportive care.
- Minimize stress and physical activity.
- See Chapter 17, p. 154, for more details.

WHAT NOT TO DO

Ionophore Antibiotic Poisoning
- *Do not* administer digoxin.
- Mineral oil may increase absorption.

Yews (*Taxus* spp., including *T. cuspitata*, *T. baccata*, and *T. brevifolia*)
- Yews are common ornamental shrubs throughout the United States; the toxic principles are *taxine alkaloids,* especially taxines A and B (Fig. 34-32).
- *Practice Tip: Horses are most commonly exposed to yew plants when they are allowed to graze around show barns, offices, or homes or when clippings from the bushes are thrown into the pasture.*
- Ingestion of as little as 1.0 kg of Japanese yew leaves *(T. cuspitata)* can kill a 450-kg adult.

Mechanism of Toxic Action
- In vitro, taxines decrease cardiac contractility, maximal rate of depolarization, and coronary blood flow.
- In vivo, taxines slow atrial and ventricular rates with ventricles stopping in diastole.

Clinical Signs
- Ataxia, muscle trembling, and collapse occur.
- *Practice Tip: The heart rate is abnormally low.*
- Sudden death, within 1 to 5 hours of ingestion, can occur. If the individual survives, mild colic and diarrhea develop.

Diagnosis
- Compatible history and clinical signs
- Identification of leaf fragments in stomach contents and chemical analysis for plant constituents in GI contents and urine

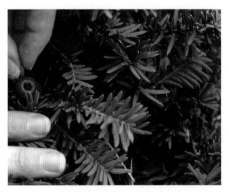

Figure 34-32 *Taxus cuspitata.*

WHAT TO DO

Yew Toxicosis
- If ingestion is suspected and no clinical signs are exhibited, administer AC, 1 to 2 g/kg PO, and place the patient in a quiet area.

WHAT NOT TO DO

Yew Toxicosis
- Administering any treatment after clinical signs are manifested can lead to excitement-induced death.

Oleander *(Nerium oleander)*
- Oleander was introduced into the United States and grows mostly in the southern states from California to Florida (Figs. 34-33 and 34-34).
- Oleander can be a potted houseplant in northern climates.
- Affected individuals become exposed from browsing on plants around buildings or eating dried leaves in the hay or discarded plant clippings.
- *Practice Tip: All parts of the plant are toxic, and as little as 1 oz (28 g or approximately 8 to 10 mid-sized leaves) of leaves can be lethal to a 450-kg adult.*
- Toxic principle is oleandrin, which remains toxic when the plant is dried.

Mechanism of Toxic Action
See Foxglove, p. 601.

Clinical Signs
- Signs include colic, muscle tremors, hemorrhagic diarrhea, recumbency, arrhythmias, weak pulse, and signs of cardiac failure.

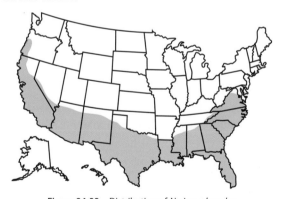

Figure 34-33 Distribution of *Nerium oleander.*

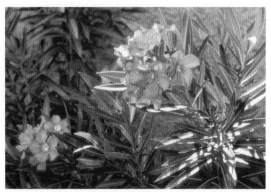

Figure 34-34 *Nerium oleander.*

- Renal failure may develop in horses that survive for several days.
- Onset of clinical signs may be delayed several hours after ingestion.
- Signs may persist for several days after last ingestion.

Diagnosis

- Evidence of consumption, compatible clinical signs
- Identification of leaf fragments in the stomach or GI contents: Some laboratories (California Animal Health and Food Safety Laboratory, Davis) test for oleandrin in the GI contents, urine, serum, liver, and heart.
- Histologic evidence of cardiac necrosis and possibly renal lesions

●〉 WHAT TO DO

Oleander Toxicosis
- Administer AC, 1 to 2 g/kg PO.
- Administer magnesium sulfate by mouth.
- Provide supportive care and confinement in a quiet area.
- Evaluate cardiac irregularities, and treat with appropriate antiarrhythmic drugs, if arrhythmia is life-threatening.

Toxicants Predominantly Causing Hemolysis or Bleeding

Moldy Yellow Sweet Clover (*Melilotus officinalis*), Moldy White Sweet Clover (*M. alba*)

- Sweet clovers are grown as forage crops, especially in northwestern United States and western Canada.
- Only when moldy are these plants toxic; the mold converts normal plant constituents to dicoumarol, an anticoagulant.
- Occurrence is rare among horses because horses are less likely than cattle to be chronically fed or ingest moldy sweet clover hay.

Mechanism of Toxic Action

- Interference with normal vitamin K_1 epoxide reductase function and resultant decline in vitamin K_1-dependent clotting factors (II, VII, IX, X)

Clinical Signs

- Bleeding abnormalities, as seen in anticoagulant rodenticide poisoning

Diagnosis

- History and clinical signs
- Prolonged PT or other abnormalities in coagulation profile
- Liver function otherwise normal

●〉 WHAT TO DO

Moldy Yellow Sweet Clover and White Sweet Clover
- Remove horse from suspect hay.
- See Anticoagulant Rodenticide Poisoning, p. 605.

Red Maple (*Acer rubrum*)

- Red maple is a common tree throughout eastern North America; also known as the swamp maple (Figs. 34-35 and 34-36).
- *Practice Tip: Red maple poisoning is the most common cause of hemolytic anemia among adult horses in the eastern United States.*
- The poisoning most commonly follows a storm that causes limbs to fall into the pasture or occurs when cut trees are left lying in a pasture.
- Wilted leaves are the most toxic; toxicity slowly decreases as the leaves dry. Fresh leaves are apparently *not* toxic.
- The putative toxic principle is *pyrrogallol,* which is derived from breakdown of gallotannins by esterases within the GI tract.
- Although not well documented, other *Acer* spp. should be considered potentially toxic.

Mechanism of Toxic Action

- Oxidative damage to red blood cells

Clinical Findings

- Ingestion can cause depression, red urine, jaundice, ataxia, and sometimes sudden death.
- Hemolysis, Heinz body formation, and methemoglobinemia occur, although one may predominate.

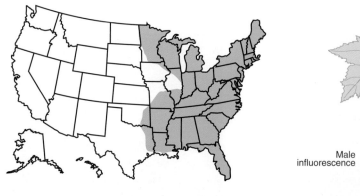 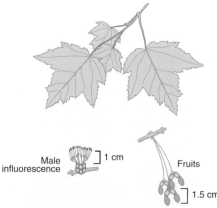

Figure 34-35 Distribution and drawing of *Acer rubrum* (red maple).

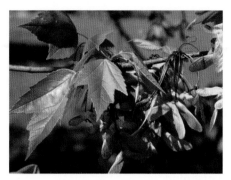

Figure 34-36 *Acer rubrum.*

- If hemolysis is the primary clinical finding of the disease, the course of the disease is 2 to 10 days.
- If methemoglobinemia predominates, then sudden death may occur.

Diagnosis
- Diagnosis is by history and clinical signs.
- Clinical pathologic examination reveals Coombs-negative hemolytic anemia with Heinz bodies and a variable degree of methemoglobinemia (8% to 50%).

● WHAT TO DO

Red Maple Toxicosis
- Perform a blood transfusion if packed cell volume is less than 11% over 2 days or more or if it is less than 18% in 1 day (see Chapter 20, p. 285)
- Large dosages of vitamin C (1 g/kg PO) may be of some benefit; however, the efficacy has *not* been demonstrated.
- Administer methylene blue, 8.8 mg/kg slowly IV, for individuals with methemoglobin over 20%; however, results may not be dramatic because of relatively low methemoglobin reductase activity in horses.
- Although clinical studies have not been performed, acetylcysteine, 50 to 140 mg/kg IV or PO may provide antioxidant treatment.
- Intravenous polyionic fluids are important to prevent hypovolemia, dilute red blood cell fragments that may trigger disseminated intravascular coagulation, and prevent renal tubular necrosis.
- Although the packed cell volume decreases with fluids, the number of red blood cells remains the same, and function may improve.

Anticoagulant Rodenticide Poisoning
- Anticoagulant rodenticide poisoning is caused by overzealous administration of warfarin in the management of navicular disease and by ingestion of anticoagulant rodenticides (e.g., warfarin, indanediones, and brodifacoum, among others).
- Newer anticoagulant rodenticides are 40 to 200 times as potent as warfarin and are much more commonly used.

Mechanism of Toxic Action
- Interference with normal vitamin K_1 epoxide reductase function and resultant decline in vitamin K_1-dependent clotting factors (II, VII, IX, X).

Clinical Signs
- Excessive bleeding from wounds and failure of blood to clot occurs.
- Often horse has pale mucous membranes from intraabdominal bleeding; hematomas may form or dyspnea may occur because of intrapleural bleeding.
- Clinical signs are delayed for 1 to 5 days after ingestion owing to persistence of functional clotting factors.

Diagnosis
- Diagnosis is by history and clinical signs.
- Patient may have prolonged PT or other abnormalities in coagulation profile (submit citrate sample with control).
- A specific anticoagulant rodenticide can be detected in serum, whole blood, or liver samples.
- Testing is widely available through diagnostic laboratories.
- Liver function is otherwise normal.

● WHAT TO DO

Anticoagulant Rodenticide Poisoning
- Administer vitamin K_1, 0.5 to 1 mg/kg SQ q4 to 6h for the first 24 hours.
- Follow with oral vitamin K_1, 5 mg/kg per day with food for an additional 7 days. With newer anticoagulants (indanediones, brodifacoum), vitamin K_1 is recommended for a minimum of 21 days.
- Administer fresh frozen plasma to affected individuals with clinical bleeding.

● WHAT NOT TO DO

Anticoagulant Rodenticide Poisoning
- *Do not* administer vitamin K_1 intravenously.
- *Do not* use vitamin K_3 in the treatment of horses.
- Avoid steroid use or other drugs that are highly protein bound because they can exacerbate the anticoagulant effects.

Wild Onions (*Allium* spp.), Domestic Onions (*A. cepa*)
- Wild onions are found in moist areas of most states, and the feeding of cull onions is associated with clinical problems.
- Onions cause Heinz body hemolytic anemia in horses ingesting large quantities of the plant or bulbs.
- The toxic principle is n-propyl disulfide.

Mechanism of Toxic Action
- Oxidative damage to red blood cells; hemoglobin denaturation

Clinical Signs
- Signs vary from a mild anemia to acute hemolytic anemia.
- Other signs occur as with red maple poisoning.
- Affected individuals often have a sulfur or onion odor to their breath.

TOX

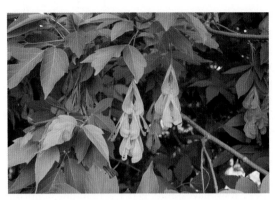

Figure 34-37 Ingestion of seeds from the *Acer negundo* (box elder) (U.S.) and *Acer pseudoplatanus* (Europe) is believed to cause atypical/pasture myopathy. The seeds (fruit) may linger on trees throughout the winter months. (Courtesy Dr. Mary Smith, Cornell University.)

●》 WHAT TO DO

Wild and Domestic Onion Toxicosis
- Remove onions from diet.
- Provide symptomatic and supportive treatment.
- Generally, toxicosis is not life threatening; significant anemia is unusual.

Toxicants Predominantly Affecting the Muscle

- Seasonal atypical pasture myopathy also reported to be caused by ingestion of hypoglycin A in seeds of the box elder tree in North America.
- Ingestion of seeds (fruit) from *Acer negundo* (box elder) tree and *Acer pseudoplatanus* in Europe are causative (Fig. 34-37). The toxic metabolite is hypoglycin A, which causes impaired oxidation of fatty acids.
- This disease is more common in Europe than in the United States and has been seen in horses in the Northeast and Mideast and possibly other areas.
- The disease is often fatal with horses having marked myoglobinuria. Riboflavin, carnitine, and CoQ10 can be used to treat cases, but prognosis is poor.
- Please see Chapter 40, p. 668, for more information on diagnosis and recommended treatments.

Toxicants Predominantly Affecting the Urinary System

Aminoglycosides
- ***Practice Tip:*** *Toxicity of aminoglycosides is especially common when used in dehydrated or hypotensive patients.*

Mercury
- Inorganic mercury may be ingested in toxic amounts when horses lick mercury poultices or blisters (mercuric iodide, mercuric oxide) applied to the legs.
- If mercury is ingested, severe tubular nephrosis and GI ulceration occur.

Mechanism of Toxic Action
- Direct reaction of mercury with cellular constituents

Clinical Signs
- Anorexia, weight loss, colic, stomatitis, and diarrhea
- Progressive signs of renal failure, laboratory findings of azotemia

●》 WHAT TO DO

Mercury Poisoning
- Administer intravenous fluids (see treatment of renal failure, Chapter 26, p. 486).
- Acute cases are managed with oral sodium thiosulfate, 0.5 to 1.0 g/kg slowly IV, and dimercaprol (BAL), 2.5 mg/kg IM q6h for 2 days and continued q12h for an additional 8 days.
- Succimer is a newer, orally administered chelator effective for chelation of lead, arsenic, and mercury. Little information is available on its use in horses; however, it has been shown to be safe in other species for management of lead intoxication. Recommended dosage is 10 mg/kg PO q8h for 5 to 10 days.
- Measurement of blood concentration should be repeated several days after cessation of chelation therapy to determine need for additional therapy.
- Provide supportive care with a GI protectant: sucralfate, 4 g PO q6h.

Nonsteroidal Anti-inflammatory Drugs

- All nonsteroidal anti-inflammatory drugs are potentially toxic; toxicity generally is dosage and duration dependent, but can be idiosyncratic.
- Mechanism of toxic action is probably related to inhibition of prostaglandin synthesis.
- Clinical signs include depression, bruxism, oral ulceration, polyuria, and less frequently, diarrhea.
- Therapy for intoxication is symptomatic and supportive.
- See Chapter 18, p. 232, for additional details.

Vitamin K$_3$ (Menadione)
- Signs of depression and renal failure may occur in affected individuals 3 to 4 days after parenteral administration of vitamin K$_3$ (no longer commercially available).

●》 WHAT TO DO

Vitamin K$_3$ Toxicosis
- Intravenous fluids (See treatment of renal failure, Chapter 26, p. 487.)

Toxicants Predominantly Affecting the Reproductive System

Please see Chapter 24, p. 447, for fescue toxicity in mares.

References

References can be found on the companion website at www.equine-emergencies.com.

Special Problem Emergencies

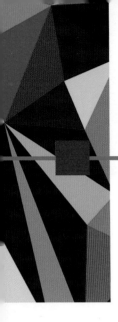

CHAPTER 35

Burns, Acute Soft Tissue Swellings, Pigeon Fever, and Fasciotomy

R. Reid Hanson, Earl M. Gaughan, Nora S. Grenager, and Janik C. Gasiorowski

Thermal Injury Burns

- Thermal injuries are uncommon in horses, with most resulting from barn fires; however, burns from wild fires seem to be increasing.
- Thermal injuries may also result from lightning, electricity, caustic chemicals, or friction.
- Most burns are superficial, easily managed, inexpensive to treat, and heal in a short time.
- Serious burns, however, can cause rapid, severe burn shock or hypovolemia with associated cardiovascular collapse. The large surface area of the burn injury dramatically increases the potential for loss of fluids, electrolytes, and calories.
- *Practice Tip: Burns covering up to 50% or more of the body are usually fatal, although the depth of the burn also influences mortality.*
  - Wound infection is almost impossible to prevent because of the difficulty of maintaining a sterile wound environment.
  - Long-term care is required to prevent continued trauma because burn wounds are often pruritic and self-mutilation is common.
- Burned horses frequently are disfigured, preventing them from returning to full function.
- Management of severe and extensive burns is difficult, expensive, and time consuming.
- Before treatment, it is recommended that the patient be carefully examined with respect to cardiovascular status, pulmonary function (smoke inhalation), ocular damage (corneal ulceration), and extent and severity of the burns; the prognosis should be discussed with the owner.

History and Physical Examination

- A complete history helps determine the cause and severity of burns.
- *Practice Tip: The extent of the burn depends on the size of the area exposed, while the severity relates to the highest temperature the tissue reaches and the duration of overheating.*

- This explains why skin injury often extends beyond the original burn. Skin typically takes a long time to absorb heat and a long time to dissipate the absorbed heat. ***Important:*** The longer the horse is exposed to the high temperature, the poorer the prognosis.
- Physical criteria used to evaluate burns include:
  - Erythema
  - Edema
  - Pain
  - Blister formation
  - Eschar formation
  - Presence of infection
  - Body temperature
  - Cardiovascular status
- In general, erythema, edema, and pain are favorable signs because they indicate that some tissue is viable, although pain is *not* a very reliable indicator for determining wound depth. Often, time must elapse to allow further tissue changes in order for an accurate evaluation of burn severity to be made (Figs. 35-1 and 35-2).
- It is important that the entire patient be examined, *not* just the burns.
- Burn patients frequently become severely hypovolemic and "shocky" and have respiratory difficulty; thermal injuries may cause serious suppression of the immune system.

Clinical Signs

- Skin burns—most common on the back and face
- Erythema, pain, vesicles, and singed hair (Figs. 35-3 and 35-4)
- Tachycardia and tachypnea
- Abnormal discoloration of mucous membranes
- Blepharospasm, epiphora, or both, which signify corneal damage
- Coughing, which may indicate smoke inhalation
- Fever, which signals or confirms a systemic response
- Special attention should be taken to identify injury to major vessels of the lower limbs and presence of ocular perineal, tendon sheath, and joint involvement

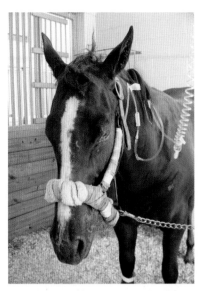

Figure 35-1 Burn injury to the muzzle, eyelids and burn edema along the ventral neck region in a horse 24 hours after burn injury due to a barn fire.

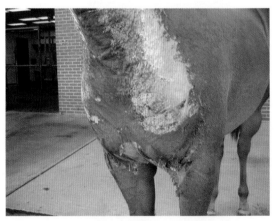

Figure 35-2 Same horse as in Fig. 35-1. The extent of the burn is more evident after the skin has sloughed as a result of the latent thermal injury to the skin.

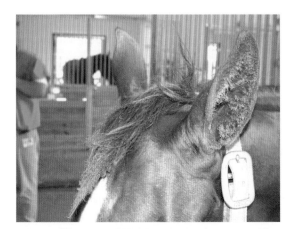

Figure 35-3 Singed forelock and ear hair due to heat generated from a barn fire.

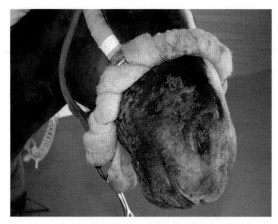

Figure 35-4 Severe erythema with loss of epithelium of the muzzle and nasal hair of the nostril of a horse due to a barn fire.

- ***Practice Tip:*** *Euthanasia is recommended for horses with deep partial-thickness to full-thickness burns involving 30% to 50% of the total body surface area.*

Laboratory Findings

- Shock supported by laboratory tests indicating a decrease in cardiac output, low total solids, increase in PCV (reduced blood volume) and decrease in plasma osmolality (increase in vascular permeability)
- Anemia may be severe and steadily progressive
- Hemoglobinuria
- Hyperkalemia initially, often followed by hypokalemia (associated with fluid therapy)

Classification of Burns

- Burns are classified by the depth of the injury.

First-Degree (Superficial) Burns

- First-degree burns involve only the most superficial layers of the epidermis.
- These burns are painful and characterized by erythema, edema, and desquamation of the superficial layers of the skin.
- Because the germinal layer of the epidermis is spared the burns heal without complication (Fig. 35-5).
- Prognosis is excellent unless there is ocular or respiratory involvement.

Second-Degree (Partial-Thickness) Burns

- Second-degree burns involve the epidermis and can be superficial or deep

Superficial Second-Degree Burns

- Superficial second-degree burns involve the stratum corneum, stratum granulosum, and a few cells of the basal layer.
- Typically, these burns are painful because the tactile and pain receptors remain intact.
- Because the basal layers remain relatively uninjured, superficial second-degree burns heal rapidly with minimal scarring, within 14 to 17 days (Fig. 35-6). Prognosis is good.

EMG

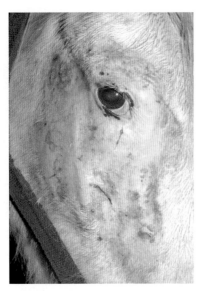

Figure 35-5   First-degree burn of the right facial and periocular area.

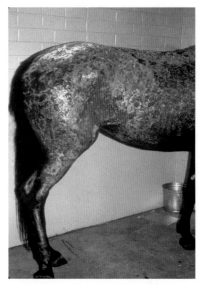

Figure 35-7   Deep second-degree burn of the right dorsum and right hind limb.

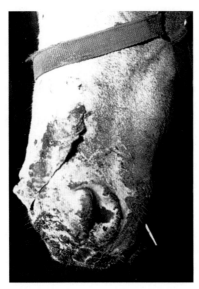

Figure 35-6   Superficial second-degree burn of the nose.

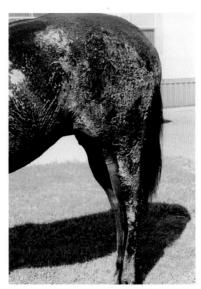

Figure 35-8   Deep second-degree burn of the left hind limb. The central burn area is surrounded by less severe skin burns illustrating the dissipating radiating effects of the heat and damage to the skin.

Deep Second-Degree Burns

- Deep second-degree burns involve all layers of the epidermis including the basal layers.
- These burns are characterized by erythema and edema at the epidermal-dermal junction, necrosis of the epidermis, accumulation of white blood cells at the basal layer of the burn, eschar (slough produced by a thermal burn) formation, and minimal pain (Figs. 35-7 and 35-8).
- The only germinal cells spared are those within the ducts of sweat glands and hair follicles.
- Deep second-degree wounds may heal in 3 to 4 weeks if care is taken to prevent further dermal ischemia that may lead to full-thickness necrosis.
- Prognosis: In general, deep second-degree burns, unless grafted, heal with extensive scarring.

Third-Degree (Full-Thickness) Burns

- Third-degree burns are characterized by loss of the epidermal and dermal components, including the adnexa and damage to underlying tissue structures.
- No cutaneous sensation occurs.
- The wounds range in color from white to black (Fig. 35-9).
- There is fluid loss; a significant cellular response at the margins of the wound and deeper tissue; eschar formation; lack of pain and shock; wound infection; and possible bacteremia and septicemia.
- Healing is by contraction and epithelialization from the wound margins or acceptance of an autograft.
- ***Practice Tip:*** *These burns are frequently complicated by infection.*
- Prognosis can be poor, depending on extent of tissue injury.

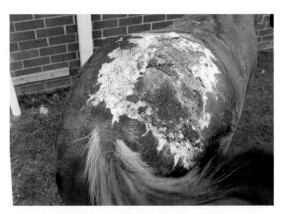

Figure 35-9 Third-degree burn of the dorsal gluteal region incurred during a barn fire resulting in hot asphalt roof shingles falling on the horse. The central burn area is surrounded by deep and superficial second-degree burns.

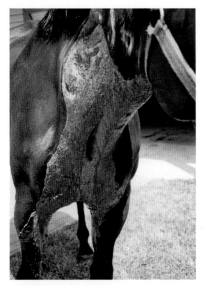

Figure 35-10 Fourth-degree burn of the right cervical neck region and pectoral area. Demonstrates involvement of the skin and underlying muscle, ligaments, fat, and fascia.

Fourth-Degree Burns

- Fourth-degree burns involve all of the skin layers and underlying muscle, bone, ligaments, fat, and fascia (Fig. 35-10).
- Prognosis is usually grave.

●❯ WHAT TO DO

First-Degree Burns

- Typically, first-degree burns are not life-threatening unless there is severe ocular and/or respiratory involvement.
- Immediately cool the affected acute burn area with cold water or cold packs to "draw" heat out of tissues and decrease continued dermal necrosis.
- Cold water application should continue for at least 30 minutes; if more prolonged, then body temperature must be monitored.
- If the burn is more than 3 hours old, cooling may not have any benefit.

- If there is minimal ocular and respiratory involvement, application of topical water-soluble antibacterial creams: aloe vera or silver sulfadiazine cream may be the only treatment required.
- Silver sulfadiazine:
  - A broad-spectrum antibacterial agent able to penetrate the eschar
  - Active against gram-negative bacteria, especially *Pseudomonas,* with additional effectiveness against *Staphylococcus aureus, Escherichia coli, Proteus,* Enterobacteriaceae, and *Candida albicans*
  - Relieves pain and decreases inflammation
  - Causes minimal pain on application but must be used twice a day because it is inactivated by tissue secretions
  - Decreases thromboxane activity
- Aloe vera:
  - Gel derived from a yucca-like plant
  - Has antithromboxane and antiprostaglandin properties
  - Relieves pain, decreases inflammation, stimulates cell growth, and kills bacteria and fungi
  - May actually delay healing once the initial inflammatory response has resolved
- Pain control is managed with flunixin meglumine (Banamine), phenylbutazone (Butazolidin), or ketoprofen (Ketofen). Continuous rate infusion (CRI) of lidocaine may be needed in addition to non-steroidal anti-inflammatory drugs (NSAIDs) for horses in severe pain.

●❯ WHAT TO DO

Second-Degree Burns

- Typically, second-degree burns are *not* life-threatening.
- Manage the initial burn the same as for superficial burns (cold water application, topical creams, and pain management, see above).
- Burn is associated with vesicles and blisters.
  - Vesicles should be left intact for the first 24 to 36 hours following formation because blister fluid provides protection from infection, and the presence of a blister is less painful than the denuded exposed surface.
  - After this interval, partially excise the blister and apply antibacterial dressing to the wound or allow an eschar to form (Figs. 35-11, 35-12, and 35-13).

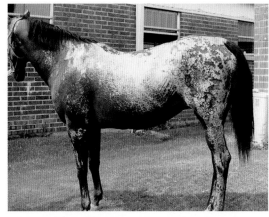

Figure 35-11 Deep second-degree and third-degree burns of the dorsum and left hind limb 8 days after injury. Marked erythema and early eschar formation is present.

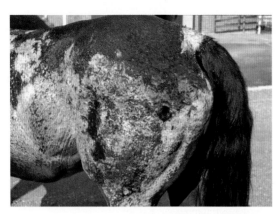

Figure 35-12   Same horse as in Fig. 35-11, 5 weeks after injury. The eschar is still present centrally. The wounds are cared for with twice-daily application of silver sulfadiazine and removal of the loose eschar. Notice the peripheral epithelialization of skin.

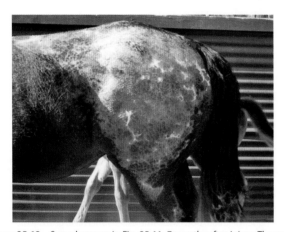

Figure 35-13   Same horse as in Fig. 35-11, 7 months after injury. The entire wound has epithelialized. The skin is thin and brittle because of a lack of sufficient subcutaneous tissue.

⦿ WHAT TO DO

Third-Degree Burns

- Because third-degree burns are potentially life-threatening, treatment of shock and/or respiratory distress should be the first priority (see "What To Do: Burn Shock").
- Destruction of the dermis leaves a primary collagenous structure called an *eschar.*
- Eschar excision and open treatment are not practical for extensive burns in horses because of the likelihood of environmental contamination and massive loss of fluid and heat.
- ***Practice Tip:*** *The most effective and practical therapy for large burns in horses is to leave the eschar intact, with continuous application of antibacterial agents.*
- Initially, the surrounding hair should be clipped and the wound debrided of all devitalized tissue. Attempt to cool the affected skin using an ice or cold-water bath. Copious lavage with a sterile 0.05% chlorhexidine solution is recommended.
- A water-based antibiotic ointment (e.g., silver sulfadiazene or Silvadene[1]) is applied liberally to the affected areas to prevent

[1]Silvadene (Dr. Reddy's Laboratories, Inc., Bridgewater, New York 08802).

heat and moisture loss, protect the eschar, prevent bacterial invasion, and loosen necrotic tissue and debris. This slow method of debridement allows removal of necrotic tissue as it is identified, thereby preventing possible loss of healthy germinal layers by mistake.
- The eschar is allowed to remain intact with gradual removal, permitting it to act as a "biological" bandage until it is ready to slough. Devitalized areas that appear necrotic or fetid should be debrided.
- Because bacterial colonization of large burns in horses is not preventable, the wound should be cleaned 2 or 3 times daily, and a topical antibiotic reapplied to reduce the bacterial load to the wound.
- Occlusive dressings should be avoided because of their tendency to produce a closed wound environment that encourages bacterial proliferation and delays healing.
- A shroud sheet soaked in antiseptic solution (0.05% chlorhexidine) and draped over the topline of the horse works well to protect burn areas in this region. Dry flakes of sterile starch copolymer can be mixed with silver sulfadiazine and applied as a bandage anywhere on the body.
- Systemic antibiotics do *not* favorably influence wound healing, fever, or mortality, and can encourage the emergence of resistant microorganisms in humans and in horses, antimicrobial resistance is becoming an important clinical concern. Additionally, circulation to the burned areas is often compromised, affecting therapeutic tissue levels of the antimicrobials at the wound site.

Burn Shock: Life-Threatening

- A profound hemodynamic and metabolic disturbance caused by a failure of the cardiovascular system to maintain adequate perfusion of vital organs and especially the skin.
- These burns usually exceed 15% of body surface area and require aggressive fluid therapy.
- This is associated with injury caused by contact with dry heat (fire), moist heat (steam or hot liquid), chemicals (corrosive substances), electricity (current or lightening), friction, or radiant and electromagnetic energy.
- ***Practice Tip:*** *Burns greater than 15% of body surface area are likely to require fluid therapy.*
- ***Important:*** Burn shock often occurs in the first 6 hours after the burn insult.
- Large volumes of lactated Ringer's solution may be needed.
- An alternative is to use hypertonic saline solution, 4 mL/kg, with plasma, hetastarch, or both, followed by additional isotonic fluids.
- If there is inhalation (smoke or heat) injury then crystalloids should be limited to the amount that normalizes circulatory volume and blood pressure.

⦿ WHAT TO DO

Burn Shock

- Attain venous access; this is especially important if the neck has been burned and progressive tissue edema/swelling in the jugular vein area is expected.
- Use lactated Ringer's solution unless electrolyte values dictate otherwise.

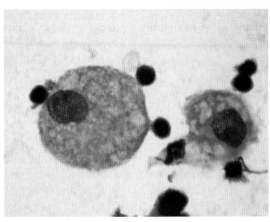

Figure 35-14 Carbon particles associated with alveolar macrophages in the bronchoalveolar wash as a result of inhalation smoke injury. Chemical injury continues as long as chemical-covered carbon particles remain attached to the airway mucosa, with the size of the particles determining where damage occurs within the respiratory tree.

- Administer flunixin meglumine, 0.25 to 1 mg/kg IV q12 to 24h.
- Administer pentoxifylline, 10 mg/kg PO q12h or IV in 500 mL saline q12h.
- Carefully monitor hydration status, lung sounds, and cardiovascular status.
- Administer plasma, 2 to 10 L IV per adult.
- **Practice Tip:** *As a general rule, for a 450-kg adult, 1 L of plasma increases the total solids 0.2 g/L.*
- Dimethyl sulfoxide (DMSO), 1 g/kg diluted to 10% solution IV for the first 24 hours, may decrease the inflammatory response and pulmonary edema.
- If pulmonary edema is present and is unresponsive to DMSO and furosemide (see Equine Emergency Drugs for dosage recommendations; Appendix 9, p. 835) treatment, administer dexamethasone, 0.5 mg/kg IV once only. If there is a rapid loss of plasma protein and pulmonary edema, 25% human albumin (1 mL/kg) can be administered (pretreat with flunixin) along with furosemide.
- If there are respiratory signs or smoke inhalation is suspected (most burns to the face have smoke or heat inhalation injury), begin systemic antimicrobial therapy.
  - With smoke or heat inhalation injury, large amounts of high protein exudate may exude into the nostrils and airways causing a gel-like obstruction.
    - These "pseudomembranous casts" may need to be removed by aspiration; nebulization with saline, acetylcysteine and heparin; and by manually stimulating a cough.
  - Administer penicillin intramuscularly for prophylaxis against oral contaminants colonizing the airway. Broad-spectrum antimicrobial therapy may encourage fungal superinfection.
  - If respiratory signs deteriorate, transtracheal aspiration should be performed, and additional broad-spectrum antimicrobial therapy administered according to the results of Gram stain, culture, and sensitivity (Fig. 35-14).

Chemical Burns
- Corrosive substances that come in contact with the skin can cause severe skin injury.
- Inhalation injury from toxic gases contained in smoke and carbon particles coated with irritating substances, can result in injury to the upper and lower airways.

● WHAT TO DO

Chemical Burns
- Read package label to identify the chemical[2] to guide the decision on specifically *what to do*!
- Brush powdered chemicals off the wound and hose with water for a minimum of 30 minutes.
- Irrigate burned eyes using a gentle stream of saline.
- Follow with appropriate treatment based on type and severity of burn, as previously described.

● WHAT NOT TO DO

Chemical Burns
- *Do not* let chemical spray contact you or other parts of the horse (i.e., eyes).
- *Do not* try to neutralize an acid with a base or vice versa.

● WHAT NOT TO DO

Skin Care for Burns
- Do *not* apply ice directly to the burn area because further tissue damage may occur; protected cold packs or cold water is preferred.
- Do *not* continually apply cold water without monitoring rectal temperature.
- Do *not* apply greasy ointments to the wounds.

Smoke Inhalation
- The onset of respiratory distress following thermal/smoke injury is often 12 to 24 hours; however, carbon monoxide poisoning has immediate effects and may cause acute death.
- For severe upper airway injury, a temporary tracheostomy may be required. Perform the procedure only if an obstruction is anticipated (also see Chapter 25, p. 456).

● WHAT TO DO

Smoke Inhalation
- Endoscopy of the trachea should be performed for prognostic purposes.
  - If there is obvious sloughing of the mucosa, aspiration should be performed.
  - Aspiration should last *no* longer than 15-second intervals because prolonged aspiration leads to hypoxemia.
- Supplemental humidified oxygen should be provided through an intranasal catheter.
- Nebulization with albuterol, amikacin (1 mL), and acetylcysteine should be performed every 6 hours. If large amounts of pseudomembranous casts are being formed, heparin can be added to the nebulization fluid.
- Systemic antioxidant therapy should include orally administered vitamins E and C.
- Flush mouth q4h with 0.05% chlorhexidine solution.
- The use of systemic antibiotics is controversial. One choice is penicillin alone as for burn shock. Another choice is ceftiofur (Naxcel[3]),

[2]The Animal Poison Center, 888-426-4435 or www.aspca.org/Home/Pet-care/poison-control.
[3]Zoetis/Pfizer/Pharmacia and Upjohn Co., New York, New York 10017.

EMG

2 to 4 mg/kg IV q12h, and metronidazole 15 to 25 mg/kg PO q6 to 8h.
- Flunixin meglumine, 0.25 to 1 mg/kg IV q12h, should be administered for its anti-inflammatory effect and with the goal of decreasing pulmonary hypertension.

Corneal Ulceration and Eyelid Burns

◑〉 WHAT TO DO

Corneal Ulceration and Eyelid Burns
- If the lids are swollen, apply ophthalmic antibiotic ointment to the cornea every 6 hours.
- Examine the cornea for ulceration initially and then twice daily.
- If damaged, debride necrotic cornea after tranquilization and application of a topical anesthetic.
  - Apply antibiotics and cycloplegics (atropine) topically. Do *not* use corticosteroids.
  - A third eyelid flap may be needed to protect the cornea from a necrotic eyelid.
- Silver sulfadiazine can be used topically on burns around the eyes.

◑〉 WHAT NOT TO DO

Corneal Ulceration and Eyelid Burns
- Do *not* use chlorhexidine around or in the eye!

Nutrition

- Assessment of adequate nutritional intake is performed with a reliable weight record.
- *Practice Tip:* Weight loss of 10% to 15% during the course of illness supports inadequate nutritional intake (see Chapter 51, p. 768).
- Early enteral feeding:
  - Decreases weight loss
  - Maintains intestinal barrier function by minimizing mucosal atrophy
  - Reduces bacterial and toxin translocation and subsequent sepsis

◑〉 WHAT TO DO

Nutrition
- Gradually increase grain; add fat in the form of 4 to 8 oz of vegetable oil and offer free-choice alfalfa hay to increase caloric intake (see Chapter 51, p. 769).
- Additional nutritional support includes parenteral and forced enteral routes; the latter being superior (see Chapter 51, p. 773).
- An anabolic steroid may be used to help restore a positive nitrogen balance.
- If smoke inhalation is a concern or there is evidence of burns around the face, the hay should be water-soaked and fed on the ground with good ventilation.

Complications

Wound Infection
- Severe burns become infected. Most infections are caused by normal skin flora.

- *Pseudomonas aeruginosa, S. aureus, E. coli,* beta-hemolytic streptococci, other *Streptococcus* spp., *Klebsiella pneumoniae, Proteus, Clostridium,* and *Candida* organisms are commonly isolated.
- It is appropriate to change topical antibacterial creams as needed to control infection.
- Silver sulfadiazine is effective against gram-negative organisms such as *Pseudomonas* and has some antifungal activity.
- Aloe vera is reported to have antiprostaglandin and antithromboxane properties (e.g., to relieve pain, decrease inflammation, and stimulate cell growth) in addition to antibacterial and antifungal activity.

Pruritic Wounds
- Healing burn wounds are pruritic.
- Significant self-mutilation through rubbing, biting, and pawing can occur if the horse is not adequately restrained or medicated.
- Usually the most intense pruritic episodes occur in the first weeks during the inflammatory phase of repair and during eschar sloughing.

◑〉 WHAT TO DO

Pruritic Wounds
- To prevent extreme self-mutilation, the horse must be cross-tied and/or sedated (e.g., acepromazine except in breeding stallions) during this time.
- Antihistamines, such as Benadryl, may be effective in some cases.
- Reserpine can be effective in decreasing the urge to scratch by successfully breaking the itch-scratch cycle.

Other Short-Term Complications
- Habronemiasis, keloidlike fibroblastic proliferations, sarcoids, and other burn-induced neoplasia can develop secondary to thermal injuries.
  - Chronic nonhealing areas should be excised and autografted to prevent neoplastic transformation.
- Hypertrophic scars, which commonly develop following deep second-degree burns, may form but generally remodel in a cosmetic manner without surgery within 1 to 2 years.
- Because scarred skin is hairless and often depigmented, solar exposure should be limited.
- Delayed healing, poor epithelialization, and complications of second intention healing may limit return of the horse to previous activities.

Acute Swelling: Edema

Earl M. Gaughan and Thomas J. Divers

- Acute edematous conditions in the horse most commonly result from:
  - Increased hydrostatic pressure
  - Septic inflammation
  - Local or general immune response (vasculitis)

- Acutely occurring hypoproteinemia is a less common cause.
- Inflammatory conditions, both septic and immunologic, usually are painful to the touch.
- Edema resulting from increased hydrostatic pressure is less painful and, in many cases, nonpainful.

Acute Onset of Edema in All Four Limbs of More Than One Horse

- This common occurrence can affect more than one individual on a farm, especially weanlings and yearlings.
- Fever often is present.
- Edema and fever affecting several horses often is caused by equine herpesvirus 1 or 4; influenza; equine rhinitis viruses; unidentified viruses; or less commonly, EVA.
- EVA can manifest as ventral edema and focal areas of painful edema elsewhere on the body. Vasculitis caused by EVA may result in sloughing of the skin. Other viral infections usually do not cause severe vasculitis.
- Babesiosis and equine infectious anemia (EIA) should be considered but would more commonly cause clinical signs in a single horse at a time.

Diagnosis

- Diagnosis is made with history, clinical signs, virus isolation, and serologic findings.
- Hoary alyssum (see Chapter 34, p. 600) poisoning is a toxic cause of limb edema, fever, and occasionally mild diarrhea affecting groups of horses in the north eastern and north central United States. A member of the mustard family, the plant is evidently palatable to horses. Clinical signs usually occur 18 to 36 hours after the horse consumes hay or pasture with large amounts of hoary alyssum and resolve within 2 to 4 days of removal of contaminated hay.

WHAT TO DO

Acute Vasculitis in Multiple Limbs/Multiple Horses

- Administer NSAIDs: dipyrone, 22 mg/kg IV or IM, or phenylbutazone, 4.4 mg/kg PO q24h, or flunixin meglumine, 1.1 mg/kg IV or PO q12 to 24 h, as supportive therapy for viral infection.
- Consider corticosteroids: dexamethasone, 0.04 mg/kg PO, IV, or IM q24h, if the edema is progressive or persists more than 7 days and there is no clinical or laboratory evidence of sepsis.
- Possibly administer antibiotics: ceftiofur, 2.2 mg/kg IV q12h or 4.4 mg/kg IM q24h.
- Provide cold hydrotherapy and leg wraps to reduce the swelling.

Acute Edema of Multiple Limbs Affecting Only One Horse

- Acute edema of all four limbs or the ventral abdomen, generally accompanied by fever, may affect a single individual.
- The differential diagnosis includes the following:
  - Equine infectious anemia
  - Anaplasmosis/ehrlichiosis
  - Babesiosis
  - Borreliosis (Lyme disease, which is probably a rare cause of leg edema)
  - *Onchocerca,* especially after anthelmintic treatments
  - Prefoaling or postfoaling ventral edema
  - Purpura hemorrhagica
  - Immune-mediated hemolytic anemia (see Chapter 20, p. 278)
  - Autoimmune thrombocytopenia
  - Right-sided heart failure (see Chapter 17, p. 149)
  - Ventral abdominal hernia
  - Acute septic cellulitis
  - Idiopathic or toxic conditions (see Chapter 34, p. 598)
- Further information on the some of these differential diagnoses follows.

Purpura Hemorrhagica

- *Practice Tip: Consider purpura hemorrhagica with any unexplained vasculitis and edema.*
- Edema is most common in the limbs and ventral abdomen and is often moderately painful to the touch. Edema can form elsewhere in the body, causing respiratory distress (laryngeal swelling and pulmonary edema), colic, heart failure (distress and trembling), or myositis (stiffness).
- Fever and petechiae of mucous membranes occur in approximately 50% of cases.
- Often the horse has a history of respiratory infection or exposure to *Streptococcus equi* (most frequent) or *S. zooepidemicus* in the preceding 2 to 4 weeks. In other cases, no incriminating infectious agent can be found.

Diagnosis

- Diagnosis is based on a complete blood cell count (CBC), measurement of creatine kinase (CK) and aspartate aminotransferase (AST), platelet count, measurement of serum immunoglobulin A, and serologic testing for serum streptococcal M protein antibody and immune complexes (performed at Gluck Equine Research Center, University of Kentucky).
- A skin specimen from an edematous area obtained with a 6-mm Baker biopsy punch[4] can be submitted in formalin to confirm vasculitis. Detection of immunoglobulin deposition is rare, and submission in special medium (Michel's) or snap freezing is recommended if a biopsy is to be performed. The biopsy specimen should *not* be harvested from an area over an important structure (e.g., tendon). In most cases, the biopsy does *not* help in the diagnosis or management of the case.
- Mature neutrophilia generally occurs, and CK and AST levels frequently are elevated with or without signs of myositis.
- A normal platelet count >90,000 cells/mL is expected. This can be helpful in separating purpura hemorrhagica (with fever and leg edema) from anaplasmosis where fever, thrombocytopenia, and sometimes leg edema are present.

EMG

[4]Baker Cummins Pharmaceuticals, Inc., Miami, Florida.

- An elevation in plasma protein measurement is common, as are an elevated immunoglobulin A level and a high antibody response to streptococcal M protein in some horses. However, a high antibody response to streptococcal M protein can occur in some healthy individuals.
- Severe proteinuria and even hematuria occur in some patients.
- Severe myopathy, mostly involving the pelvic limbs, may also occur in some horses (see Chapter 22, p. 358).

Differential Diagnosis

- Equine viral arteritis (EVA), equine herpesvirus 1 or 4, equine infectious anemia, leptospirosis, babesiosis, *Anaplasma phagocytophilum* infection, and other acute immune-mediated skin diseases are differentials for purpura hemorrhagica.
- Lyme disease may be considered a differential but rarely causes marked fever or limb edema. ***Practice Tip:*** *Be careful interpreting positive Lyme titers. Many normal horses in endemic areas have a titer to* Borrelia. *Additional testing with kinetic enzyme-linked immunosorbent assay), multiplex serology, immunoblots, and polymerase chain reaction (PCR; performed at Cornell University Diagnostic Laboratory) may be indicated.*
- Most Standardbreds are serologically positive for EVA. (For more information, see Chapter 52, p. 777.)

⬤❯ WHAT TO DO

Purpura Hemorrhagica

- Corticosteroids: Administer dexamethasone, 0.04 to 0.16 mg/kg IV or IM q24h.
  - Begin dexamethasone treatment at 0.08 mg/kg. If there is no response in 24 to 48 hours, the dosage should be increased or another diagnosis considered.
  - Continue at the clinical response dose for 2 to 3 days after signs abate and decrease the dosage over 7 to 14 days. Clinical signs may recur as the steroid dosage is decreased or withdrawn. If corticosteroids are contraindicated, *plasma exchange* can be tried.
  - Plasma Exchange Procedure: Remove 8 mL/kg of the patient's blood and replace it with 8 mL/kg compatible plasma.
- In mild cases, corticosteroids may *not* be needed.
- Antibiotics: Administer aqueous penicillin, 22,000 IU/kg IV q6h, or penicillin procaine, 22,000 IU/kg IM q12h, during steroid therapy.
- Administer furosemide, 0.5 to 1 mg/kg IV or IM q12 to 24h, for 1 to 2 days for severe edema.
  - Naquasone is an alternative to furosemide.
- Apply leg wraps and hydrotherapy for limb edema.
- Measure cardiac troponin I if there is pronounced tachycardia or arrhythmia.
- Perform a temporary tracheostomy for life-threatening laryngeal edema (see Chapter 25, p. 456).
- ***Practice Tip:*** *Purpura hemorrhagica is a serious disease with life-threatening complications in some cases. This can be a difficult diagnosis to make unless there is a good history of recent strangles exposure.*
- There is no single diagnostic test; purpura hemorrhagica is a clinical diagnosis.

- Owners should be informed of the risks of corticosteroid-associated laminitis, which is generally low except in horses with metabolic syndrome, and that laminitis can result from purpura-induced vasculitis.

Equine Infectious Anemia

- The acute clinical syndrome caused by equine infectious anemia is rare but can cause fever, edema, hemoglobinuria, jaundice, depression, and petechial or ecchymotic hemorrhage.
- Thrombocytopenia is usually clinically evident with the acute form of the disease.
- A PCR test for rapid results or serology (Coggins or ELISA) test can be performed, although seroconversion may *not* be present at the onset of the disease, necessitating retesting 10 to 14 days later.

⬤❯ WHAT TO DO

Equine Infectious Anemia

- EIA horses should be kept in a screened stall at least 200 yards (180 m) from other horses.
- EIA is a reportable disease.

Equine Anaplasmosis/Granulocytic Ehrlichiosis

- *Anaplasma phagocytophilum* infection is a common cause of edema and fever among horses in certain areas of the western United States (e.g., northern California), as well as the East Coast, Minnesota, and Wisconsin. The organism is spread by ticks (incubation period may be 1 to 9 days), which can frequently be found on the horse.
- Clinical signs are depression, anorexia, ataxia, limb edema in some horses, fever, and petechial hemorrhages.
- Laboratory findings include thrombocytopenia, leukopenia, and mild anemia. The organism (morula) is often seen on a blood smear during the febrile stage in the neutrophils with a Giemsa stain (Fig. 35-15).
- PCR testing (send sample to University of California-Davis, Cornell University, or other laboratory offering the test) is useful in early confirmation. PCR should be

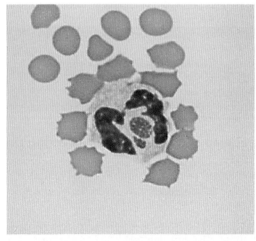

Figure 35-15   Wright-Giemsa stain of a blood smear of an adult horse from northern Virginia with fever and leg edema. The *light blue bodies* in the neutrophil are *Anaplasma phagocytophilum* morulae.

positive during the febrile stage of the disease; morula within granulocytes may not be observed during the early and late stages of the febrile period.

- If the disease has been present for several days, serologic testing can be performed, but *not* all horses have good seroconversion. Some horses do not undergo seroconversion for several weeks.
- The SNAP test seems to be positive during the febrile stage in approximately 50% of horses.

●》 WHAT TO DO

Equine Anaplasmosis

- Administer oxytetracycline, 6.6 mg/kg IV q12 to 24h for 5 to 7 days.
- Alternatively, minocycline, 4 mg/kg PO q12h or doxycycline, 10mg/kg PO q12h are often used but are not believed to be as effective as intravenous oxytetracycline.

Onchocerca

- Reaction to *Onchocerca cervicalis* larvae after anthelmintic therapy does not require treatment unless the ventral edema is very painful or the horse has a fever.
- In these cases, use dexamethasone, 0.05 mg/kg q24h, and an antibiotic such as ceftiofur, penicillin, or trimethoprim-sulfamethoxazole.

Prefoaling or Postfoaling Ventral Edema

- Rule out hernia, ruptured prepubic tendon (see Chapter 24, p. 437), mastitis (see Chapter 24, p. 448), hematoma, and cellulitis.
- If the mare is in good health and the edema is progressive, administer two dexamethasone (5-mg)/trichlormethiazide (200-mg) boluses PO q24h (ground up, mixed in molasses) or 1 to 3 doses of furosemide (1 mg/kg IV). The dose of dexamethasone is highly unlikely to cause abortion in late-term pregnant mares, but it is possible, and risk:benefit should be discussed with the owner!
  - This treatment should be used only when infectious causes have been ruled out and the edema is progressive.
- If there is a suggestion of a body wall defect before foaling, abdominal support using a "belly bandage" is recommended.
- Supportive care—cold water therapy, leg wraps, handwalking are recommended. Mild edema in late-term pregnant mares is not uncommon.

Idiopathic Condition

- Most individual cases are responsive to corticosteroids.
- If septic cellulitis or abnormal lung sounds are *not* present, but there is progressive edema with severe pain, treat with steroids.

Anaphylactoid Reactions Causing Edema

- *Practice Tip: Previous sensitization to an antigen is not always required for an anaphylactoid reaction. The most common drugs that can cause a reaction are plasma vaccines, injectible vitamin E and selenium, anthelmintics,*

penicillin, trimethoprim-sulfamethoxazole, anesthetics, and NSAIDs.

- Many of the reactions to parenterally administered penicillin, trimethoprim-sulfamethoxazole, and anesthetics that cause collapse are not immunologic in origin and are covered under Adverse Drug Reactions (see Appendix 4, p. 812). Anaphylactic reactions generally occur within minutes to 12 hours after exposure to an agent and may persist for several days.
- The clinical signs are urticaria, dyspnea, sweating, collapse, and occasionally laminitis.
- The diagnosis is based on a history of exposure.

●》 WHAT TO DO

Anaphylactoid Reactions

Urticaria Only

- Antihistamine: Administer diphenhydramine, 0.25 to 1 mg/kg *slowly* IV if signs are severe or rapidly progressive or IM, or doxylamine succinate, 0.5 mg/kg slowly IV or IM if cardiovascular status is stable.
- Urticaria persists in many cases and may have to be managed with oral prednisolone, 0.4 to 1.6 mg/kg PO q24h or every other day for several days.
- Dexamethasone, 0.1 to 0.25 mg/kg IV, may be used in addition to the treatments previously listed if the edema is rapidly progressive.

Respiratory Distress

- Administer epinephrine 1:1000 (as packaged), 3 to 6 mL/450 kg given slowly IV or 3 to 10 mL/450 kg IM in less severe cases. Epinephrine may also be given intratracheally (20 mL) or as a last resort by intracardiac route if the horse has collapsed and is nonresponsive.
- Perform a temporary tracheostomy (see Tracheostomy Procedure, Chapter 25, p. 456) if laryngeal edema is present.
- Administer furosemide, 1 mg/kg IV.

Cardiovascular Collapse and Hypotension (Weak Pulse, Pale Mucous Membranes)

- Administer epinephrine (as above), 2 L hypertonic saline solution or dobutamine, 50 mg/500 mL in dextrose solution administered over 10 to 20 minutes to a 450-kg adult (5 to 10 µg/kg per minute).
- Lastly, vasopressin can be administered 0.3 U/kg IV as a single dose if there is no response to the epinephrine/saline or dobutamine.

Idiopathic Urticaria

- Idiopathic urticaria occurs in a generalized or a local form.
- The generalized form frequently is a persistent problem, although the immediate response to corticosteroids or antihistamines is often good.
- Local edema (ocular, nasal, laryngeal) may occur without a known cause.
- Conjunctival edema of one or both eyes is the most common symptom.

●》 WHAT TO DO

Idiopathic Urticaria

Ocular: Palpebral Edema

- Ophthalmic corticosteroid administration after a careful and complete examination of the eye and fluorescein stain reveals no corneal erosion.

EMG

Skin Urticaria

- Administer antihistamines or corticosteroids: diphenhydramine 0.25 to 1 mg/kg slowly IV or IM; hydroxyzine hydrochloride, 1 to 1.5 mg/kg IM q8 to 12h; or either dexamethasone, 0.05 to 0.1 mg/kg IV, or prednisolone, 0.5 mg/kg PO q24h.
- This form of urticaria may recur for weeks or months.

Malignant Edema: Clostridial Myositis

- Malignant edema most commonly occurs:
  - On the chest from a wound
  - At the site of a non-antibiotic intramuscular injection
  - From perivascular injections
- The most common intramuscularly administered drug associated with malignant edema is flunixin meglumine, probably because it is the most frequently administered non-antibiotic drug with limited tissue irritation given intramuscularly.

Clinical Signs

- Acute painful swelling that is warm and soft then becomes cool and firm
- Subcutaneous crepitus in some cases
  - ***Practice Tip:*** *subcutaneous crepitus is absent in many cases of clostridial myositis.*
- Stiff neck after a cervical injection with inability to lower the head
- Rarely, ataxia

Diagnosis

- Diagnosis is made with needle aspiration and Gram stain in search of large, gram-positive bacilli.
- Place the fluid sample in anaerobic culture media (Port-a-Cul), and send a slide for fluorescent antibody examination.

WHAT TO DO

Malignant Edema: Clostridial Myositis

- Antibiotics
  - Administer penicillin, 22,000 IU/kg IV q4 to 6h. ***Note:*** A higher dose may be used, but it increases the risk of antibiotic-induced colitis.
  - Combine with metronidazole, 15 to 25 mg/kg PO q6h or 30 mg/kg per rectum q6h. An initial intravenous treatment with metronidazole, although expensive, may be helpful in slowing *C. perfringens* growth and toxin elaboration.
  - Oxytetracycline administered intravenously with metronidazole per os is an acceptable *second* choice. There is some evidence that oxytetracycline is more effective at inhibiting toxin production than penicillin, but there are no studies to confirm superior efficacy of either treatment protocol.
- Surgical incision and drainage or radical incision may be needed if the disease appears rapidly progressive or no improvement is seen after 24 hours of antimicrobial treatment.
  - ***Practice Tip:*** *It is better to incise too early than to wait until it is too late.*
- Hyperbaric oxygen may be useful, but is *not* a substitute for early surgical drainage! Hyperbaric oxygen does *not* prevent toxin proliferation. Oxygen can simply be diffused into the surgical wound but efficacy is unproven.

- Anti-inflammatory therapy: Administer phenylbutazone, 4.4 mg/kg PO q12 to 24h
- 1 to 2 L of equine plasma with antibodies against *C. perfringens* should be administered.
- Perform hydrotherapy.
- Administer tetanus prophylaxis.

Acute Swelling in a Single Limb

Trauma

- The presence of acute swelling in a single limb, associated with substantial or severe lameness must be considered and evaluated as an emergency. The affected limb must be carefully examined for possible decompensation of bone, joint, and/or tendon/ligament tissues.
- One should also explore carefully for wounds. This may require clipping hair and examination of the sole of the foot.
- Be careful using local anesthesia before a thorough evaluation of supporting structures is complete. Premature local anesthesia can result in catastrophic decompensation/failure of the musculoskeletal support system.
- The swelling should be characterized as edema or synovial effusion. Remember that edema presents as pitting skin surface upon palpation and synovial effusion has a "water balloon" appearance and texture, resuming its original appearance after digital palpation.

Diagnosis

- Pain with lameness
- Palpation characteristics: pitting edema versus effusion
- Ultrasonography can help determine edema from effusion, as well as characteristics of bone, tendon, ligament, and joint anatomic architecture.
- Radiography is indicated any time fracture or luxation is considered a rule-out!
- Contrast radiography and ultrasonography indicated any time a puncture wound or small laceration occurs in the region of a joint, tendon sheath, or bursa.

WHAT TO DO

Acute Swelling: Single-Limb Simple, Nonsynovial Wound

- Clean the wound.
- Administer NSAIDs: phenylbutazone, 2.2 to 4.4 mg/kg PO or IV.
- Administer antibiotics as indicated based on physical findings.
- Bandage the wound with a sterile primary layer and additional support as needed.

Synovial Wound

- Sample synovial fluid for culture and sensitivity testing. (See Chapter 21, p. 332).
- Avoid arthrocentesis through a large swelling to minimize the chance of introducing bacteria into the joint.
- Perform high-volume articular lavage. The preference is for arthroscopic-guided lavage. Alternatives include large-gauge through-and-through needle lavage, teat cannulas, and catheters. Lavage fluid should be saline or balanced polyionic fluids. Additives to lavage fluids include DMSO (0.5% to 10% solution) and antibiotics (0.5 to 1 g amikacin; others).

- Administer antibiotics: systemic, regional, and/or local.
- Administer NSAIDs: phenylbutazone, 2.2 to 4.4 mg/kg PO or IV.
- Provide physical support: Bandage with or without splint support typically is indicated.

Fracture/Luxation
(See Chapter 21, p. 314.)

- First-aid is essential. Appropriate assessment, support, and immobilization for transportation often determine prognosis for successful repair. Distal limb trauma (distal to midradius or distal tibia) should be supported with strong, firm bandaging and external coaptation splints or casts. Care must be exercised with fracture/luxation trauma of the proximal limbs. Poorly placed bandages, splints, or casts can add weight to the affected limb without adequate immobilizing of the fracture/luxation site. As close as possible, attempts should be made to immobilize the joints proximal and distal to the site of injury. If in doubt, do not bandage the distal limb.
- As a rule, transport the horse with the two sound limbs facing forward in the trailer or van (see Chapter 21, p. 314).
- Great care should be exercised when considering sedation and/or tranquilization of a horse with a limb fracture or luxation. An induced ataxia can create life-threatening complications with these injuries. Xylazine and detomidine can result in profound sedation and remove a horse's innate protective mechanism. Acepromazine likely does not provide the desired chemical restraint and analgesia for a horse with fracture/luxation trauma and may create hypotensive complications in these situations. *Important: Acepromazine should be considered as contraindicated for horses with fracture/luxation trauma.*
- Administer NSAIDs: Use an appropriate, but not excessive, dosage schedule (e.g., phenylbutazone, 2.2 to 4.4 mg/kg PO or IV).
- Administer antibiotics: Consult with potential referral center for preferences before referral. Broad-spectrum systemic antibiotics are indicated before surgery is started.

Cellulitis

Cellulitis of a Limb

- *Practice Tip: Septic cellulitis, the most common cause of painful inflammatory edema in horses, usually is associated with a wound, scratches, or a local reaction to an injection. However sometimes no inciting cause is identified when it affects a leg.*
- Scratches, or pastern dermatitis, can be very mild in horses, and it often respond well to conservative hydrotherapy, bandaging, and sometimes diclofenac, although some cases can be more aggressive, requiring systemic antibiotics and anti-inflammatory drugs.
- Pain and progressive swelling are the characteristic findings. Cases can range from mild swelling and pain to severe, rapid onset of lameness, swelling, and high fevers.
- Diagnosis is based on results of Gram stain and culture of a sample of fluid. Anaerobic culture tubes[5] are recommended.
- Explore the wound to establish drainage and to search for a foreign body.

---

[5]Port-a-Cul (Becton-Dickinson Microbiology Systems, Cockeysville, Maryland).

- Perform an ultrasound examination with a 7.5-MHz probe to localize and evaluate the fluid and to check for hyperechoic foreign bodies.
- *S. aureus* or *Clostridium* organisms are common causative agents of severe and often rapidly spreading cellulitis in horses.
- Staphylococcal infection may result from blunt trauma, such as that caused by a starting gate or a bruise to the hock, without a noticeable break in the skin.
- *Important:* Staphylococcal and clostridial infections are considered the most pathogenic causes of cellulitis in horses.

●〉 WHAT TO DO

Cellulitis
Antibiotics

- Administer penicillin, 22,000 IU/kg IV q6h, and gentamicin, 6.6 mg/kg IV q24h, if cellulitis is severe and rapidly progressive and if there is the probability of a mixed bacterial infection. *Practice Tip: If using gentamicin, check serum creatinine every 2 to 3 days and be sure the patient is well hydrated and producing urine.*
- If an anaerobic infection is suspected, because of the foul smell of the exudate or the presence of subcutaneous gas, add metronidazole, 15 to 25 mg/kg PO q6 to 8h, to the treatment regimen.
- In less severe cases or when only gram-positive cocci (staphylococci) are seen on Gram stain, ceftiofur, trimethoprim-sulfamethoxazole, or both may be used.
- Enrofloxacin, 7.5 mg/kg PO once a day or 5 mg/kg IV q24h, is an excellent choice for staphylococcal and gram-negative cellulitis but a poor choice for anaerobic or streptococcal infection.
- Hydrotherapy: For septic and aseptic (injection site) cellulitis, administer cold water therapy for the first 24 hours or until the pain subsides, followed by warm water therapy.
- DMSO may be useful for its antiedema and anti-inflammatory indications.
- Support: Wrap legs if an extremity is affected.
- NSAID: Administer phenylbutazone, 4.4 mg/kg PO q12h, for 2 to 3 days.
- Other anti-inflammatories and analgesic considerations are found in Chapter 49, p. 757.
- *Reminder:* When should tetanus toxoid or antitoxin or both be given to horses with a wound?
  - Tetanus toxoid is administered to most horses, especially young horses, with recent wounds. If vaccination prophylaxis is current, antitoxin is not given.
  - If the wound has occurred in an individual less than 2 years of age with questionable tetanus vaccination, use antitoxin (preferably a product with low incidence of serum hepatitis associated with it).
  - In areas of the world with Theiler's disease, antitoxin should be administered to adults only if there is no history of previous tetanus toxoid vaccination.
- Surgical drainage: Perform incision and drainage (I&D) when and where appropriate.
- If a limb is involved, lameness may be non–weight-bearing and every attempt (especially in larger horses) should be made to prevent support limb laminitis (SLL). Treatments that may prevent this include high-dose systemic analgesia, epidural (morphine), and intermittently slinging the horse (quick lift sling). (See Chapter 37, p. 636, and Chapter 43, p. 712.)

Lymphangitis

- Lymphangitis is an emergency!
- There is often an acute progressive swelling of one hind limb, with serum oozing through the skin.
- Fungal infections usually are nodular and slower to develop than are bacterial causes.
- Acutely affected patients have a fever and frequently are non–weight bearing.
- The longer the affected leg remains swollen, the more severe is the anatomic disruption of the lymphatic vessels.
- A wound may or may not be present on the leg.
- Diagnosis is based on clinical signs and results of ultrasound examination using a 7.5-MHz probe that reveals numerous dilated vessels (lymphatic vessels). The gross and ultrasonographic appearance of the limb is more uniform compared with that of cellulitis.
- Culture of the fluid should be attempted with a 22-gauge needle to minimize damage to the limb and avoid vessels; the etiologic agent generally is not identified.
- The best chance of obtaining a positive bacterial culture is in the untreated acute case.

●》 WHAT TO DO

Lymphangitis

- Administer antibiotics: Enrofloxacin, 7.5 mg/kg IV q24h, is the preferred antibiotic. Other options include trimethoprim-sulfamethoxazole, 20 to 30 mg/kg PO q12h; amikacin, 15-20 mg/kg IV q24h; oxytetracycline, 6.6 mg/kg IV q12h; or other antimicrobials effective against *S. aureus*. *Practice Tip: For an acute lymphangitis, antimicrobial coverage against* S. aureus *should be provided.*
- Administer anti-inflammatory drugs: phenylbutazone, 4.4 mg/kg IV or PO q12h.
- Provide aggressive hydrotherapy with cold water. Use a whirlpool bath or hydrotherapy tub or a cold boot[6,7] if available. If the patient can get its leg in the boot, the constant pressure of the water reduces the limb size. Prompt reduction in the soft tissue swelling may prevent long-term damage to the leg.
- Administer pentoxifylline, 10 mg/kg PO q12h, to improve circulation in the severely swollen leg.
- Support wrap the opposite leg and institute preventatives for contralimb laminitis (see Chapter 43, p. 712).
- Encourage moderate walking as comfort permits.
- Administer furosemide, 1 mg/kg IV or IM q12 to 24h, for two treatments or trichlormethiazide/dexamethasone (Naquasone) for recurrent cases without fever. If the leg swelling is rapidly progressive, a single dose of a steroid may be required.
- A support wrap with a nitrofurazone (Furacin) sweat can be applied to the affected leg in more chronic conditions.
- The owners should be advised that lymphangitis is a serious disease, the causative agent is rarely identified, the prognosis is guarded unless there is a rapid response to therapy, and recurrence is common.

Corynebacterium Pseudotuberculosis Infection

- *Corynebacterium pseudotuberculosis* is a bacterial infection characterized by external abscesses in the western

United States or ulcerative lymphangitis/cellulitis nationwide, and it can cause internal abscesses (see p. 622).
- There is typically progressive swelling in the pectoral area, mammary gland, ventral abdomen, inguinal area (causing swelling of one limb), or sporadically elsewhere on the body.
- Ultrasound examination reveals abscesses deep to the external swelling.

●》 WHAT TO DO

Corynebacterium Pseudotuberculosis **Lymphangitis**

- Incise and drain abscesses identified and localized on ultrasound examination.
- Systemic procaine penicillin, 20,000 to 44,000 IU/kg IM q12h
- Treat as per Lymphangitis.

Miscellaneous Causes of Edema

Hematoma

- Hematoma is an acute swelling caused by vessel rupture with a collection of blood. A common cause is a traumatic event (i.e., a kick).
- If the swelling is not progressive, the hematoma organizes, and surgical drainage is delayed.
- If the skin is injured, administer an antimicrobial agent such as penicillin.
- ***Practice Tip:*** *Rule out thrombocytopenia as the cause of hematoma before administering intramuscular injections by examining the mucous membranes for petechial hemorrhage.*
- If the hematoma is rapidly progressive, an artery or, in rare instances, a large vein may have been injured. Most rapidly progressive hematomas of the limbs are associated with a fracture, such as fracture of the pelvis (i.e., laceration of the iliac artery).
- Severe lameness also suggests a fracture. If *no* cause for hematoma is identified and the hematoma is progressive despite medical treatment, consider surgery to isolate and ligate the offending vessel.

●》 WHAT TO DO

Hematoma

- Administer phenylbutazone, 4.4 mg/kg PO q12 to 24h, because it has little or *no* effect on platelet function.
- Administer butorphanol, 0.01 to 0.02 mg/kg IV, 2 to 5 minutes after a low dose of xylazine, 0.2 to 0.4 mg/kg IV, if sedation is needed.
- Administer polyionic fluids if indicated: *no* hypertonic saline solution should be used when first examined.
- Apply a pressure wrap at the affected site, if possible.
- Whole-blood transfusion is used if bleeding is progressive, the patient's condition is deteriorating, or PCV decreases to <18% within 12 hours after the start of bleeding.
- ***Important:*** Caution is warranted in using PCV as a guide for transfusion because it can vary during the first 12 to 18 hours during or after hemorrhage. If thrombocytopenia is present, the blood should be freshly collected in a plastic container for transfusion (see Chapter 20, p. 285).

---

[6]P.I. Medical, Athens, Tennessee.
[7]Cool Systems, Equine Game Ready, www.gameready.com.

- Aminocaproic acid, IV administration, 20 mg/kg, mixed in 1 to 3 L of saline solution may be used to manage prolonged uncontrolled bleeding.
- Consider antibiotics:
  - Systemic antibiotic therapy may not be essential as a component of emergency treatment for hematomas.
  - Some reasonable argument is also made concerning the ability of systemically administered antibiotics to reach appropriate minimal inhibitory concentration (MIC) levels in the depths of a hematoma.
  - There is *no* better in vivo environment for bacteria to multiply than in blood, and therefore the potential for a hematoma becoming an abscess is considerable, *especially if an aspirate has been performed to confirm the diagnosis.*
  - Antibiotics are indicated for the treatment of a hematoma if skin abrasions, lacerations, or bacterial systemic illness is also present.
  - Appropriate systemic dosages should be administered, and drugs with a known ability to penetrate poorly vascularized tissue should be considered (e.g., chloramphenicol).

Nutritional Myopathy

- Acute muscle swelling caused by selenium deficiency is rare but can occur.
- Swelling of the masseter and pterygoid muscles (masseter myopathy) results in a severe swelling of the facial muscles and protrusion of the conjunctiva.
- Affected individuals appear stiff and reluctant to chew, but they can eat.
- The urine is frequently dark and strongly positive for occult blood (myoglobin) on urine dipstick examination.
- This form of myopathy usually is a disease of poorly fed horses.
- Blood (whole blood, plasma, or serum) is collected for measurement of selenium (normal, 15 to 25 mg/dL) and serum level of creatine kinase. Plasma selenium is usually <5 mg/dL and CK is very high in most cases.
- White muscle disease may occur in adults, newborn foals, or weanlings.
- Atypical myopathy (see Chapter 40, p. 668) should be considered in pastured horses with acute myoglobinuria.

●> WHAT TO DO

Nutritional Myopathy
- Administer selenium, 0.05 mg/kg IM; repeat in 3 days if the diagnosis is confirmed.
- Administer DMSO, 1 g/kg diluted IV, once as ancillary therapy.
- Apply warm compresses on the affected area.
- Provide nursing care for any tissue compromised by the swelling, such as the conjunctiva.
- Administer phenylbutazone, 4.4 mg/kg PO q12h.
- If indicated, administer intravenous fluids to correct hypotension, electrolyte abnormalities, and azotemia.

Snake Bite, Spider Bite, Bee Sting, and Other Causes of Acute Severe Dermatitis/Urticaria

- Bites and sting injuries occasionally result in severe swellings in horses.

- Snake bite is common on the noses of horses, causing airway obstruction and hemolysis (see snake bite, Chapter 45, p. 726).
- Bites of black widow spiders can cause hot, painful swelling.
  - The diagnosis is supported by finding the spider in the stall.
- Bites of fire ants can cause acute swelling, particularly of the distal limbs.
  - Fire ants are common in the southeastern United States, where they build large mounds (nests).
- Bee stings cause acute, painful swelling and can be fatal if they occur in large numbers. Bee stings may also affect several horses at once!
  - Bee stings are identified by circular areas of edema with a stinger in the center of the swelling.

●> WHAT TO DO

Bites and Stings
- Administer an antihistamine: diphenhydramine, 0.25 to 1 mg/kg slowly IV, IM, or SQ; or doxylamine succinate, 0.5 mg/kg slowly IV or IM; hydroxyzine hydrochloride, 1 to 1.5 mg/kg IM or PO.
- Administer corticosteroids: dexamethasone, 0.04 mg/kg IV/IM, if the injury and swelling are severe.
- Administer epinephrine, 3 to 7 mL (1:1000 solution) per 450-kg adult slowly IV or SQ, *only* in cases of systemic (anaphylactic) involvement and respiratory distress.
- Hyperbaric oxygen therapy (see Chapter 7, p. 25).
- Provide airway support:
  - Place a short endotracheal tube in the proximal nasal passages before the swelling becomes so severe a temporary tracheostomy is required. ***Practice Tip:*** *This is especially important in the treatment of individuals bitten on the nose by a snake.* One disadvantage is that severe nasal mucosal necrosis may occur; the alternative is to perform a temporary tracheostomy (see Chapter 25, p. 456).
- Administer broad-spectrum antibiotics for snakebite, such as penicillin, 44,000 IU/kg IV q6h, gentamicin, 6.6 mg/kg IV or IM q24h, and metronidazole, 15 to 25 mg/kg PO q6 to 8h or 25 to 30 mg/kg per rectum q8h. ***Note:*** Monitor serum creatinine, hydration status, and urine production when treating with an aminoglycoside antibiotic.
- Antivenin can be given for snake bites if the bite has occurred within 24 hours. Because of the size of the patient, the frequent time delay of >24 hours between the bite and clinical recognition of the problem, and the possibility of an adverse reaction, antivenin is rarely used. Recent evidence suggests that the usefulness of antivenin may extend beyond the initial 24-hour period.
- Administer tetanus toxoid.
- Administer NSAIDs for snake bite: flunixin meglumine, 1 mg/kg IV q12h for 3 days.
- Perform a fasciotomy if indicated (see p. 622).
- If gross swelling causes respiratory distress localized to the nares or muzzle and swelling prevents prehension of food/water and swallowing, fasciotomy should be considered.
  - This procedure is most often needed for a snake bite wound on the face.
- Similarly, acute bilateral jugular thrombosis may cause dramatic swelling of the head, obstructing nasal airflow.
- For head swelling associated with acute bilateral jugular vein thrombosis, if acute bilateral obstruction occurs, the head should

be raised, and the pressure points under the mandible caused by the halter should be padded. If the swelling is progressive, a fasciotomy can be performed, or after surgical scrub of the skin, several rows of needle sticks over both masseter muscles can be performed to allow fluid drainage.

Fly Bites

- Fly bites rarely require emergency treatment.
- Severe reactions to horse flies (core of necrotic tissue in the center of the swellings), stable flies, horn flies, or black flies (characteristic hemorrhagic center in the urticarial swelling) can occur.
- In very rare instances, large numbers of black fly bites lead to death.

Other Causes of Acute Dermatitis

- Contact dermatitis, photosensitivity, and drug eruptions can require emergency treatment.
- Photosensitivity is caused by ingestion of photosensitizing plants or liver disease, most commonly from toxic plants or less commonly from mycotoxins on the plants.
- Stinging nettle grows in moist fields, particularly on disturbed soil in many parts of the world and is extremely irritating to horses, people, and other animals when there is skin contact with the plant.
- Acute urticaria and extreme pruritus and pain may occur and last for 24 to 48 hours.
- Tranquilization may be required to control the horse during the intense pruritus and pain.
- Corticosteroids and antihistamines provide only limited relief.
- Drug eruptions in the form of multifocal dermatitis that are unusual in appearance or distribution can occur at any time during treatment or within several days of discontinuation of treatment.

●〉 WHAT TO DO

Contact Dermatitis

- Administer corticosteroids, topical or systemic (in severe cases only), for contact dermatitis or photosensitivity.
- Remove the causative agent.

Acute and Severe Pruritus

- Acute and severe pruritus is most common in the summer months owing to acute *Culicoides* hypersensitivity.
- Drug eruptions, reaction to stinging nettle, and bites by fire ants and other insects can cause intense pruritus.
- Consider neurologic disorders such as rabies or self-mutilation syndrome in stallions.

●〉 WHAT TO DO

Acute Severe Pruritus

- Corticosteroids: Dexamethasone, 0.05 to 0.1 mg/kg IV, or prednisolone, 2 mg/kg PO, to control itching in severe cases
- Diphenhydramine, 0.25 to 1 mg/kg slowly IV or IM

Fasciotomy

- Fasciotomy is a surgical procedure in which the skin, subcutaneous tissue, and fascia are incised for the purposes of drainage and/or decompression of deeper tissues.
- Fasciotomy minimizes the sequelae associated with "compartmental syndrome" and the compromise of vital neurovascular structures.
- The procedure has been described for treatment of:
  - Clostridial myositis
  - Severe thrombophlebitis (especially when the airway is compromised)
  - Acute swelling associated with envenomation, injection, or vaccination
  - Nerve compression associated with compartmental syndrome
- Incisions vary in size based on their intended function. Injection site abscesses or snake bites require simple 1-cm stab incisions, whereas diffuse myonecrosis associated with acute clostridial infection necessitates long, deep cuts.
  - In these cases sonographic guidance is a useful adjunctive tool to better define the affected area and large blood vessels before fasciotomy.
  - To treat compartmental syndrome, fasciotomy can be performed through a small incision but extended to the deeper fascial planes using Metzenbaum scissors without enlarging the skin incision.

Equipment

- Clippers
- Material for sterile scrub
- 2% local anesthetic, 5- to 50-mL syringe, and 22-gauge, 1½-inch needle
- Sterile gloves
- #10 scalpel blade and handle

Procedure

- Clip hair and prepare skin with aseptic technique as the situation warrants.
- Inject local anesthetic into the subcutaneous tissues.
- Incise the skin over the area to be drained or decompressed. Incisions should be at least 1 cm in length. If the affected area is extensive, lengthen the incision(s) parallel to the lines of maximal resting skin tension (if possible) to afford the necessary drainage or decompression.
- If treating infection, copiously lavage the incised tissues.
- Cover fasciotomy sites with bandage material to absorb drainage and minimize gross contamination.
- Allow the incision(s) to heal by second intention.
- Fasciotomy for nerve decompression has been described for the suprascapular, medial, and lateral palmar/plantar metatarsal and deep branch of the lateral plantar nerves. These specific procedures are beyond the scope of an emergency text.

EMG

Complications

- Some degree of bleeding is expected.
- Severe bleeding may occur with inadvertent incision or transection of large vessels.

Pigeon Fever

- Pigeon fever is a *Corynebacterium pseudotuberculosis* infection typically characterized by deep subcutaneous or external abscesses that are common to the western United States and occasionally ulcerative lymphangitis/cellulitis nationwide.
- *C. pseudotuberculosis* can also cause internal abscesses.
- The name, pigeon fever, is derived from the external abscesses caused by *C. pseudotuberculosis* that classically occur in the pectoral region, giving the horse a pigeonlike appearance.

Etiopathogenesis

- Pigeon fever is caused by the gram-positive, intracellular, pleomorphic, rod-shaped, facultative anaerobic bacteria *Corynebacterium pseudotuberculosis,* which is thought to enter the skin through fly bites, abrasions, or wounds.
- It is contagious, with an incubation period of 1 to 4 weeks.
- Incidence of disease varies annually and is seasonal and sporadic, with most cases of external abscesses occurring during dry summer to fall months in the southwestern–western United States.
- Approximately 8% of horses develop an internal infection, usually 1 to 2 months after peak numbers of external infection are seen.

Clinical Signs

For Deep Subcutaneous or External Abscesses

- Single or multiple maturing swellings in classic locations such as the pectoral region, along the ventral midline, prepuce, mammary gland, and axilla, though abscesses can occur in any location. The abscesses contain copious tan, odorless, purulent exudate.
- Sometimes horses present with fever, edema, lameness, weight loss, and depression.

For Internal Infection

- Anorexia, fever, lethargy, weight loss, and signs referable to the location of the infection (i.e., respiratory signs, colic signs, or hematuria).

For Ulcerative Lymphangitis

- See Cellulitis, p. 619.

Diagnosis

External Abscesses

- History and clinical signs in a horse in the appropriate geographic location and time of year are suggestive.
- If the clinician is not sure pigeon fever is the cause of the swelling, it can be aseptically aspirated for gross and cytologic evaluation and culture of the sample.

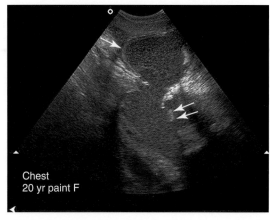

Figure 35-16   Transdermal ultrasound of external abscess; note the thick hyperechoic capsule *(one arrow)* and deeper abscess pocket *(two arrows).* (Photo courtesy of Matthew Durham.)

- Culture: The bacteria grow rapidly and easily on blood agar within 1 to 2 days.
- Ultrasound: Ultrasound of mature abscesses typically reveals a thick-walled capsule surrounding exudate of mixed echogenicity (Fig. 35-16).
  - Ultrasound is most useful for evaluating undetermined swelling, determining maturity of an abscess, and finding the best location to establish drainage.
- Serology: The synergistic hemolysis inhibition (SHI) test measures immunoglobulin G to exotoxin of *C. pseudotuberculosis.* The accuracy of serum titers with external abscess(es) is controversial. In general, titers ≥1:160 are indicative of active infection; however, some horses have no appreciable titer with external abscesses.
  - The SHI test is available at the California Animal Health and Food Safety Laboratory System in Davis, California (see Chapter 34, p. 582).
- Other laboratory abnormalities: Classic changes that occur in approximately 40% of horses include anemia of chronic disease, neutrophilic leukocytosis, hyperfibrinogenemia, and hyperproteinemia.

Internal Infection

- History and clinical signs in a horse in the appropriate geographic location are suggestive.
- Serology: Titers ≥1:512 are highly specific for internal infection in the absence of external disease. With concurrent external disease, titers ≥1:1280 are more specific for internal infection.
- Ultrasound is useful for identifying affected organs (most commonly liver, kidneys), to determine the extent of pulmonary disease or peritonitis, or to help obtain aspirates or body fluid samples.
- Other laboratory abnormalities: Classic changes that occur in approximately 40% to 76% of horses include anemia of chronic disease, neutrophilic leukocytosis, hyperfibrinogenemia, and hyperproteinemia. Results of abdominocentesis or transtracheal wash may be consistent with bacterial infection.

EMG

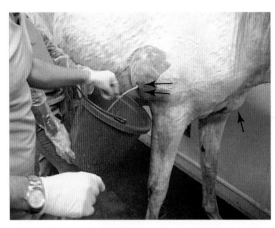

Figure 35-17 Appropriate drainage of an external abscess in the triceps muscle area *(two arrows)* with second maturing abscess in pectoral region *(one arrow).* (Photo courtesy of Matthew Durham.)

Ulcerative Lymphangitis
- See Cellulitis, p. 619.

Treatment
External Abscesses
- Once the abscess is "mature," indicated by a soft area of overlying skin, clean the skin and incise and drain (lance) the abscess with a #15 scalpel blade (Fig. 35-17).
  - Wear gloves, collect the abscess contents and lavage solutions, and dispose of all materials associated with the procedure to prevent further environmental contamination and transmission of the disease to other horses.
  - Many abscesses open and drain on their own.
  - If the abscess is immature, use serial ultrasound examinations to determine when to drain the abscess. The owner can be instructed to apply warm compresses daily or a topical poultice, such as ichthammol or furacin with DMSO, to hasten abscess maturation.
- Flush the abscess pocket with dilute povidone-iodine (Betadine), 0.1% solution (1 mL of povidone-iodine per 100 mL of clean water), the color of "weak tea," or dilute chlorhexidine, 0.05% solution (2.5 mL of 2% chlorhexidine solution per 100 mL of clean water), using a 60-mL catheter-tip syringe or teat cannula until the drainage fluid is clear. It may be necessary to manually break down fibrous tissues inside the abscess cavity.
  - It is generally unnecessary to anesthetize the skin unless the abscess is deep within the muscle. Fractious or very sensitive horses require sedation for safety of the equine patient and treating personnel during the procedure.
- After drainage and lavage of the abscess, the tissues ventral or distal to the abscess should be cleaned to minimize risk of subsequent infections on the exposed skin.
- The owner should be instructed on how to flush the abscess once or twice daily in the same manner until the abscess heals from within. For biosecurity, the owner should wear gloves and be careful in disposing of the lavage fluid and associated materials.

- Hydrotherapy helps decrease associated edema.
- Topical therapy: The application of a topical antimicrobial around the incision is recommended, and appropriate fly control measures for all horses are critical.
- Anti-inflammatories: Some horses benefit from NSAIDs.
- Antimicrobial therapy is generally not necessary for external abscesses and is believed to potentially prolong resolution of the abscesses. Exceptions include horses with signs of systemic illness, abscesses deep within muscular tissue, or abscesses in other hard-to-access locations. See therapy for internal infection (following section).
- Tetanus prophylaxis: Administration of appropriate tetanus prophylaxis is important because the wound is open.

Internal Infection
- Administer antimicrobials: Either procaine penicillin (20,000 U/kg IM, q12h), sodium ceftiofur (2.2 mg/kg IV q12h or 4.4 mg/kg IM q24h), or trimethoprim-sulfa (30 mg/kg PO, q12h), with rifampin (2.5 to 5 mg/kg PO, q12h) are the most efficacious in vivo, although many antibiotics are efficacious in vitro.
  - Most often horses are started on a parenteral antimicrobial in combination with rifampin to improve penetration of the abscess capsule and because of the intracellular location of the bacteria, and then are switched to all oral medications after 2 to 3 weeks.
  - Duration of antimicrobial therapy is variable from one to several months.
- Administer additional treatments appropriate to the body system/organ affected. For example, this may include percutaneous drainage of the abscess or peritoneal lavage.

Ulcerative Lymphangitis
- See Cellulitis, p. 619.

Prevention
External Abscesses and Internal Infection
- An equine vaccine is currently in development.
- Good sanitation and fly control: Complete quarantine of affected horses is not generally necessary because the bacteria resides in the soil and is transmitted by flies, but strict attention to good biosecurity and fly control may reduce the incidence of new cases.
- There is no known way to adequately decontaminate the environment.
- Typically, natural immunity follows after infection.

Ulcerative Lymphangitis
- See Cellulitis, p. 619.

Prognosis
External Abscesses
- Drainage and wound healing generally occur in 2 to 4 weeks, although horses can develop recurrent or persistent infections for more than 1 year.
- Mortality rate is <1%.

Internal Infection
- Mortality rate is 30% to 40% in treated horses and 100% in untreated horses.

Ulcerative Lymphangitis
- See Cellulitis, p. 619.

▶ WHAT TO DO

Pigeon Fever
- Incise and drain the abscess if clinically ready and debride and lavage the abscess cavity after drainage; collect and properly dispose of all infected material to minimize environmental contamination.
- Facilitate abscess "maturation" if it is not ready to be opened and drained; use warm compresses and topical poultices. Ultrasonography is helpful to determine abscess status/maturity and timing of surgical drainage.

- Administer NSAIDs if the horse is clinically depressed or in pain.
- Use appropriate fly control.
- Administer tetanus prophylaxis if not current or vaccination status is questionable.

▶ WHAT NOT TO DO

Pigeon Fever
- Do *not* attempt to open and drain the abscess prematurely.
- Do *not* put a horse with immature external abscess on antimicrobials unless there are signs of systemic illness or the abscess is too deep to safely and effectively drain.

References
References can be found on the companion website at www.equine-emergencies.com.

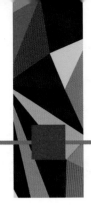

CHAPTER 36

Caring for the Down Horse

Rachel Gardner

- Initial evaluation of the recumbent horse involves assessment of the entire situation, including the location of the horse and safety of the horse and all involved personnel.
- A complete history should be taken that includes signalment, history of recent health or performance problems, recent treatments and onset (acute vs. chronic) of the recumbency.
- Knowledge of diet and management practices, recent travel, and vaccination history are also important.

Clinical Examination

- A physical examination, as complete as possible, and assessment of hydration should be performed if safe.
  - The limbs, head, and neck should be carefully palpated for evidence of pain or fracture.
  - A systematic neurologic exam should be performed, and if abnormalities are detected a neuroanatomic diagnosis should be formulated.
  - The general mentation of recumbent horses can be difficult to discern because of the stress of recumbency, inability to react normally, and potential exhaustion following prolonged struggling.
  - The neurologic exam should also include evaluation of the cranial nerves, skin sensation, cutaneous trunci reflex, patellar reflexes, and withdrawal reflexes. Tail and anal tone should be assessed, although anal tone may be altered in the down horse. Bladder tone and size may be evaluated via rectal examination (see Chapter 22, p. 339).
  - Muscle tone, including that of the eyelid and tongue, should be evaluated carefully, as weakness is a characteristic finding with botulism.
  - *Practice Tips:*
    - *If the horse is able to rise into a dog-sitting position, then injury to the spinal cord caudal to T2, myopathy, or injury to the peripheral nerves of the hind limbs should be considered.*
    - *If the horse is unable to raise the head and respiratory pattern is abnormal, either a lesion in the proximal cervical spinal cord or diffuse neuromuscular disease is likely.*
    - *If the horse only lies on one side, then vestibular disease should be considered.*
  - The eyes, or at a minimum the accessible eye, should be evaluated completely.

- When the recumbent physical and neurologic exams fail to elucidate a cause for the recumbency, attempts should be made to assist the horse to stand, which may make musculoskeletal injury or ataxia more apparent.

Diagnostic Testing

- Initial diagnostic evaluation should include a complete blood count, serum biochemistry panel, and urinalysis.
- Alterations in the leukogram may be suggestive of an inflammatory or infectious process, although it is important to distinguish these changes from those secondary to recumbency.
- Evaluation of a blood smear may provide further evidence of toxemia, alterations in red blood cell morphology, evidence of neoplastic cells, or *Anaplasma phagocytophilum*.
- Alterations in the serum biochemistry panel may provide evidence of a primary disease or changes secondary to recumbency.
- *Practice Tip: Significantly elevated creatine phosphokinase (CK), aspartate aminotransferase (AST), and lactate dehydrogenase (LDH) concentrations occur with rhabdomyolysis, and generally to a lesser degree with recumbency alone (see Chapter 22, p. 358).*
- Electrolyte concentrations should be evaluated for the purposes of diagnosis of the primary cause of recumbency and for guiding therapy. Lactate concentrations can be used as a marker for tissue hypoxia, disease severity, and tissue perfusion.
- *Practice Tip: Measurement of blood ammonia may be indicated to evaluate for hepatic encephalopathy or primary hyperammonemia. Ammonia samples must be evaluated immediately or within 1 hour if kept on ice.*
- If central nervous system (CNS) signs are observed on examination or a neurologic cause of the recumbency cannot be ruled out based on exam findings, evaluation of cerebrospinal fluid (CSF) may be indicated.
- *Practice Tip: CSF is most easily and reliably obtained via atlanto-occipital (AO) puncture in the recumbent horse (see Chapter 22, p. 340).*
- Because general anesthesia is often required for AO sampling, this should only be performed on a stable patient in which a vertebral fracture is not suspected.
- *Practice Tip: Short-term general anesthesia using xylazine, diazepam, and ketamine provides 20 to 25 minutes of*

anesthesia time, which is adequate for the procedure (see Chapter 47, p. 744). If a short-acting anesthetic is used to remove the horse from the transporting van/trailer, then movement of the horse and CSF collection can be performed with a single anesthetic procedure.

- If the patient is unstable or if general anesthesia is not desired, lumbosacral (LS) puncture may be performed. This procedure is more challenging but may be assisted via the use of ultrasound to identify the LS space. Placing an object between the hind feet so that the limbs are positioned a normal distance apart may help ensure a successful centesis.
- Cytologic evaluation should be performed on fresh CSF samples. Samples may also be cultured or tested for specific antibodies/organisms.
- Radiography using handheld machines is useful to identify the presence and extent of fractures in the limbs, head, and neck. More robust fixed machines may be used to evaluate the caudal neck, ribs, thoracolumbar vertebrae, or pelvis.
- Computed tomography and magnetic resonance imaging require general anesthesia but may provide further diagnostic information regarding the head, cranial neck, and distal limbs (see Chapter 14, p. 107).
- Ultrasonography can be used to evaluate soft tissue structures, superficial bone integrity, and for the presence of body cavity effusions or hemorrhage (see Chapter 14, p. 81).
- Endoscopy can be used for evaluation of the upper airway, guttural pouches, and stylohyoid bones.
- An electrocardiogram is indicated in horses whose recumbency may be related to arrhythmias or in whom an arrhythmia is auscultated (see Chapter 17, p. 124).
- Myelography is indicated to evaluate for cervical spinal cord compression, although focal lateral sites of compression can be inapparent on routine myelography due to difficulty in obtaining diagnostic ventral-dorsal views in adult horses (see Chapter 22, p. 345).
- Muscle biopsy may be indicated if a myopathy is suspected (see Chapter 6, p. 24).
- Transcranial magnetic stimulation is used to measure abnormal nerve conduction along the descending motor tracts to determine the presence of spinal cord or peripheral nerve injury. Electromyography may help classify neuropathies, myopathies, or neuromuscular disorders. Electroencephalography can be used to complement the clinical examination in identifying functional disturbance in brain activity.

Differential Diagnoses for Recumbency

- Accurate diagnosis is critical in forming a therapeutic plan and reasonable prognosis.
- *Practice Tip: A poor prognosis should not be assumed based on recumbency alone.*
- Differential diagnoses for recumbency are summarized subsequently although more complete descriptions of each problem are found in other parts of this book.

Musculoskeletal Disorders

- Musculoskeletal disorders are one of the most common causes for recumbency.
- Long bone, pelvic, or axial skeletal fractures may cause recumbency. Depending on the site, fracture stabilization may be adequate to assist the horse to rise. The prognosis is variable and depends on the site and severity of the fracture.
- Laminitis commonly results in a disproportionate time in recumbency, and in severe cases can result in complete recumbency. Abaxial nerve blocks may help facilitate standing and further diagnostic evaluation. When severe enough to cause complete recumbency, the prognosis for laminitis is generally poor.
- Generalized weakness, due to old age, chronic disease, severe degenerative joint disease, or cachexia, commonly results in recumbency. Treatment with anti-inflammatories; analgesics; and in the case of hind-limb degenerative joint disease, epidural administration of medications, may be sufficient to assist a patient to stand. The long-term prognosis tends to be poor unless the underlying problem is addressed with proper analgesics or appropriate nutrition.
- Myopathies are a relatively common causes of recumbency in the horse. Exertional myopathies may be severe enough to cause recumbency in exhausted horses or horses that are cast for prolonged periods.
- Horses with polysaccharide storage myopathy (PSSM) may also become recumbent following a severe episode (see Chapter 22, p. 360). Muscle sensitivity, firmness on palpation, and trembling may be observed; pigmenturia may be present.
- Atypical myopathy results in peracute onset of clinical signs and has a poor prognosis.
- Monensin intoxication results in skeletal and cardiac myopathy. Additional clinical findings include tachyarrhythmias, heart failure, and acute death.
- Salinomycin toxicity may produce recumbency without cardiac failure.
- White snakeroot ingestion may lead to recumbency due to severe myonecrosis.

WHAT TO DO

Musculoskeletal

- Treatment should include intravenous fluids to correct dehydration and provide diuresis as prophylaxis against pigment nephropathy.
- If hypochloremia and alkalosis are present, 0.9% NaCl with supplemental potassium is recommended.
- Analgesics (phenylbutazone or flunixin meglumine), intravenous dimethyl sulfoxide (DMSO), acepromazine, and methocarbamol may be used.
- Recumbent PSSM horses should be treated with corn oil (6 oz/450 kg) via nasogastric tube or an intravenous lipid product.
- If recumbency follows general anesthesia and malignant hyperthermia is a concern, treatment should include dantrolene or phenytoin.

EMG

- Myopathy due to selenium deficiency may involve the masseter and/or pterygoid muscle groups. Diagnosis is by whole blood selenium concentrations or glutathione peroxidase activity. If selenium deficiency is suspected, an intramuscular injection of vitamin E/selenium should be given while awaiting laboratory confirmation and is unlikely to cause harm if selenium levels are later determined to be adequate. If the diagnosis is correct, a second treatment 3 days later is recommended.
- Immune-mediated myositis can occur following infection with Streptococcus equi or viral infection. Diagnosis is by historical findings and consistent histopathologic changes in muscle biopsies. Additional treatments include corticosteroids (prednisolone or dexamethasone) and penicillin. If the immune-mediated myopathy is severe and rapidly progressive, large doses (0.2 mg/kg) of dexamethasone may be required.
- *Anaplasma* myopathy is best treated with tetracycline intravenously and has a good prognosis.
- Subcutaneous fluid or gas crepitation is suggestive of *clostridial myonecrosis*. Specific treatments include anti-endotoxic medications, properly dosed penicillin, metronidazole, and surgical fenestration (see Chapter 35, p. 618).

Central Nervous System (CNS)

- CNS disorders are common causes for a down horse. CNS trauma may involve the brain, brainstem, or spinal cord.
  - Young horses are susceptible to CNS trauma following basisphenoid fracture from rearing and flipping over, resulting in head tilt, balance loss, blindness, recumbency, epistaxis, and/or hemorrhage from the ear.
  - Horses are prone to vertebral fracture and spinal cord injury after a fall.
  - A favorable prognosis is given if neurologic signs are secondary to edema/hemorrhage rather than direct neuronal damage.
- *Cervical compressive myelopathy (CCM)* may cause recumbency from cervical stenosis exacerbated by acute trauma or severe flexion of the neck such as following a myelogram.
  - The history may include clumsiness or tripping, or neck stiffness in older patients.
  - If attempts are made to stand, symmetric ataxia may be apparent.
  - Intravertebral and intervertebral sagittal diameter ratios should be calculated on survey radiographs and may suggest vertebral canal stenosis (see Chapter 22, p. 346).
  - Osteoarthritis of the articular processes, most commonly C5-6 and C6-7 in older horses is suggestive, but not necessarily diagnostic, of the disease. CSF is typically normal.
  - Compression can also occur from other causes, including neoplasia, hematoma, abscess, granuloma, and cysts. CSF analysis varies.
  - Definitive diagnosis for cervical compressive myelopathy is by myelography.

EMG

● WHAT TO DO

Cervical Compressive Myelopathy

- Treatment depends on the cause of the compression and commonly includes high doses of dexamethasone in cases of acute onset or exacerbation of signs.
- Surgical arthrodesis or decompression may be indicated.
- The prognosis is guarded if significant improvement does not rapidly occur with treatment.

- *Encephalomyelitis* due to infection with the viral encephalitides can cause recumbency.
  - Eastern equine encephalitis (EEE) and Venezuelan equine encephalitis (VEE) are clinically indistinguishable and patients commonly show cerebral signs and remain afebrile. CSF analysis reveals mononuclear to mononuclear and neutrophilic pleocytosis, elevated protein, and xanthochromia. Antemortem diagnosis is by demonstrating rising serum titers. Treatment is supportive (see Chapter 22, p. 363), although dexamethasone may be helpful in early or progressive cases.
- *Equine herpesvirus-1 (EHV-1)* causes respiratory disease, abortion, and neurologic disease.
  - Recumbency may occur because of severe CNS vasculitis.
  - Older adult horses in situations of high "stocking" density or increased movement are more commonly affected and outbreaks are common.
  - Affected horses are usually febrile and demonstrate a rapid onset of symmetric ataxia that may progress to recumbency.
  - Hind limbs are typically more affected and may result in "dog sitting."
  - Urinary bladder paralysis and urine dribbling are common, and fecal retention may occur in recumbent patients.
  - CSF is commonly xanthochromic with an elevated protein level.
  - Treatment is largely supportive (see Chapter 22, p. 348). Moderate to high dose dexamethasone is recommended in rapidly progressive or severe cases.
  - Strict quarantine measures should be taken when EHV-1 is suspected, and all horses at risk should have temperature monitored at least twice daily.
  - *Practice Tip: Any horse in which rabies or EHV-1 remains a differential diagnosis should be treated with strict biosecurity measures (see Chapter 53, p. 791). Human exposure should be limited and a list should be kept of all individuals who have had contact with the horse. Gloves should be worn and all specimens from the patient labeled with "Rabies Suspect." Commercial vaccines are effective for prevention of rabies, but not EHV-1.*
  - *Practice Tip: Diagnosis may be confused with anaplasmosis because of paresis and recumbency with xanthochromic CSF. Botulism, moldy corn poisoning, atypical myopathy, and ionophore toxicity may also be causes of multiple horses developing recumbency but without fever.*

- Horses occasionally become recumbent because of *equine protozoal myeloencephalitis (EPM)* (see Chapter 22, p. 343).
  - Recumbency with EPM is more commonly associated with peracute or acute onset of signs and may be accompanied by vestibular signs, cranial nerve signs, or signs of lower motor neuron disease of the limbs.
  - Ataxia before recumbency is commonly asymmetric and horses remain afebrile. CSF analysis is typically normal.

▶ WHAT TO DO

Equine Protozoal Myeloencephalitis
- Treatment is with antiprotozoal medications such as ponazuril, diclazuril, or a sulfadiazine-pyrimethamine combination in addition to supportive care.
- Double doses of ponazuril are commonly used for the first week of therapy; treatment is recommended while awaiting laboratory confirmation of infection.
- Corticosteroids and DMSO may be useful in the rapidly progressing case.
- The prognosis is poor once recumbency occurs and in survivors, relapse following cessation of treatment may occur.

- Severe *vestibular disease* results in recumbency due to balance loss (see Chapter 22, p. 350).
  - Temporohyoid osteoarthropathy (THO) commonly results in vestibular signs.
  - Affected horses may have a history of unusual chewing behavior or an incident causing sudden head elevation.
  - Horses with acute onset of peripheral vestibular signs demonstrate nystagmus (fast phase away from the lesion) and a head tilt, and preferentially lie on the side of the lesion.
  - Circling and leaning toward the side of the lesion are observed if the horse is assisted to stand.
  - Strength is maintained and contralateral hypertonia may occur. Mentation remains normal and ipsilateral facial nerve paralysis commonly occurs.
  - Endoscopy of the guttural pouches, which can be difficult in the recumbent horse, or dorsoventral radiographs reveal enlargement and possible fracture of the proximal stylohyoid bone on the affected side.

▶ WHAT TO DO

Vestibular Disease
- Treatment consists of supportive care and anti-inflammatory therapy (see Chapter 22, p. 351).
- Otitis media and interna can cause similar signs or may occur concurrently with THO; therefore, antibiotic treatment with trimethoprim-sulfa, enrofloxacin, or chloramphenicol is often recommended.
- If facial paralysis is present, frequent ophthalmic lubrication or tarsorrhaphy is recommended.

- Denervation muscle atrophy, especially of type 1 (postural) muscle fibers due to *equine motor neuron disease (EMND)* (see Chapter 22, p. 355), results in excessive recumbency.
  - In subacute stages, horses may show signs of weakness, trembling, base-narrow stance, weight loss, and sweating before recumbency.
  - Ophthalmic evaluation reveals fundic lesions from lipofuscin accumulation in approximately 30% of cases.
  - Diagnosis is made by history and clinical findings, as well as demonstration of denervation muscle atrophy in a biopsy of the sacrocaudalis dorsalis muscle.

▶ WHAT TO DO

Equine Motor Neuron Disease
- Affected horses should be administered 5000 to 7000 IU vitamin E daily, although the prognosis is poor for the uncommon down horse.

- *Equine anaplasmosis,* caused by infection with *Anaplasma phagocytophilum,* occasionally causes ataxia, which can progress to recumbency.
  - Horses are febrile and may exhibit depression, anorexia, edema, icterus, petechiae, and orchitis.
  - Diagnosis is by observation of inclusions in neutrophils, polymerase chain reaction (PCR) testing on whole blood, or rising serum titers.

▶ WHAT TO DO

Equine Anaplasmosis
- Treatment consists of tetracycline and supportive care.
- Response to treatment tends to be rapid, and the prognosis is good.

- *Tetanus* may result in skeletal muscle spasticity causing stiffness, trembling, spasm, and recumbency.
  - Masseter muscle stiffness, eyelid retraction, and flared nostrils are commonly present, and clinical signs are exacerbated by excitement.
  - Diagnosis is based on clinical signs in an unvaccinated horse with a history of soft tissue injury 1 to 3 weeks before.

▶ WHAT TO DO

Tetanus
- Treatment is with antitoxin administration, which binds residual circulating endotoxin.
- Intrathecal administration of antitoxin may be performed in early cases that remain ambulatory.
- Supportive care in a quiet environment should be provided, and sedation should be used before performing procedures.
- If a wound is present, it should be debrided to improve perfusion and oxygenation.
- Concurrent vaccination is indicated, but the prognosis for recumbent horses is grave.

- Recumbency may occasionally occur secondary to *hepatic encephalopathy* or *primary hyperammonemia.*

EMG

- Acute cerebral signs, including behavior change, blindness, circling, seizures, and recumbency may be present.
- Horses with hepatic encephalopathy have elevated liver enzyme concentrations, abnormal hepatic function tests, and icterus.
- Horses with primary hyperammonemia commonly have a history of gastrointestinal disease, most commonly colic or diarrhea.
- Definitive diagnosis is by measurement of elevated blood ammonia >150 μmol/L.
- Concurrent metabolic acidosis and hyperglycemia are supportive findings.

>> WHAT TO DO

Hepatic Encephalopathy/Primary Hyperammonemia
- Treat liver disease, if present (see Chapter 20, p. 268).
- Sedate with phenobarbital or small doses of xylazine, if needed.
- Oral neomycin or oral magnesium sulfate may be administered.
- IV fluid therapy will likely be indicated.
- The prognosis for hepatic encephalopathy is poor; however, primary hyperammonemia has a more favorable prognosis.

- Bracken fern ingestion, moldy corn toxicity (ingestion of fumonisin B1), and adverse reactions to fluphenazine decanoate may also cause recumbency because of their toxic effects on the CNS. Inadvertent intracarotid injection of medications may result in hyperexcitability, collapse, seizure, or coma.

>> WHAT TO DO

Central Nervous System—General Guidelines
- General supportive and nursing care
- Intravenous fluids
- Anti-inflammatory treatment:
  - Corticosteroids
  - Nonsteroidal anti-inflammatory drugs (NSAIDs)
- Mannitol or hypertonic saline
- Intravenous DMSO
- Vitamin E supplementation for antioxidant purposes

Peripheral Nervous and Neuromuscular Systems
- Peripheral nerve disorders may cause recumbency secondary to:
  - Mechanical injury
  - Trauma
  - EPM
  - Neoplasia
  - Abscess
  - Caudal aortic thrombosis
  - Iatrogenic causes
- Abnormalities of major *peripheral nerves* results in muscle weakness (paresis or paralysis), hyporeflexia or areflexia, hypotonia or atonia, and neurogenic atrophy. Examples include:
  - Femoral nerve paralysis secondary to EPM
  - Dystocia and obturator nerve paralysis following severe hind limb abduction.

- In horses with caudal aortic thrombosis, the pelvic limbs are cold, associated muscles are firm on palpation, and no femoral pulse is present.
- The prognosis is guarded for horses recumbent because of a peripheral nerve disorder or thrombosis, although recovery may occur if early and aggressive treatment is pursued in cases of EPM.
- Recumbency due to *botulism* (see Chapter 22, p. 354) may be acute or chronic in onset.
  - Trembling occurs during standing as a result of weakness, and resolves during recumbency.
  - Dysphagia is a common presenting complaint and persists once down.
  - The history commonly includes feeding of poorly stored forages, especially round bales.
  - Diagnosis is based on history and clinical signs.
  - Diagnosis can be confirmed by the presence of botulism toxin in feed, serum, gastrointestinal (GI) contents, or wound contents, or the presence of spores in intestinal contents.

>> WHAT TO DO

Botulism
- Treatment consists of administration of specific or multivalent antiserum *early* in the course of the disease and supportive care.
- Type B botulism can be prevented by vaccination with a type B toxoid.
- The prognosis is poor in adult horses once recumbency has occurred, although recovery is possible with good nursing care and time.

Metabolic Disorders
- Disorders that lead to *electrolyte abnormalities*—hyponatremia, hypocalcemia, hyperkalemia—and may result in recumbency.
  - Hyperkalemia is most commonly observed during episodes of hyperkalemic periodic paralysis (HYPP) in Quarter Horses or Quarter Horse crosses, or it may occur secondary to uroperitoneum or renal failure.
  - Additional clinical signs include muscle stiffness, fasciculations, weakness, respiratory stridor, and death.
  - Cardiac arrhythmias may be present.
  - Preliminary diagnosis is based on clinical signs and serum potassium concentrations >6 mEq/L. Genetic testing is available to confirm diagnosis.

>> WHAT TO DO

Hyperkalemic Periodic Paralysis
- Slow IV administration of calcium borogluconate, $NaHCO_3$, or dextrose solution (see Chapter 22, p. 357)
- Long-term management includes:
  - Dietary management
  - Potassium-wasting diuretics such as acetazolamide

- *Exhaustion* from overwork, especially in hot, humid conditions, can cause recumbency.

- Clinical signs include:
  - Severe sweating
  - Tachycardia
  - Tachypnea
  - Severe dehydration
  - Cardiac arrhythmias
  - Synchronous diaphragmatic flutter
  - CNS signs
- Electrolyte abnormalities and serum biochemical abnormalities are frequently present.

●〉 WHAT TO DO

Exhaustion
- Decrease body temperature.
- IV or oral fluid resuscitation
- Electrolyte replacement
- NSAIDs following fluid replacement
- Anti-endotoxic therapy (see Chapter 32, p. 567)
- Prognosis is good if the initial response to treatments is productive; however, delayed onset of myopathy, laminitis, and organ failure is possible.

- *Hypoglycemia* rarely causes recumbency in the adult horse. ***Practice Tip:*** *When present, it is most commonly secondary to neoplastic disease/tumors.*

Respiratory and Cardiovascular Disorders
- *Cardiovascular collapse,* especially when acute, may result in recumbency.
- *Hemorrhage,* whether external or internal, may result in cardiovascular collapse.
  - Internal bleeding occurs most commonly in the abdomen, although bleeding into the thorax and uterus may occur.
  - Initial diagnosis is based on history, mucous membrane pallor, tachypnea, tachycardia, abdominal discomfort or respiratory compromise, and low blood pressure.
  - Further diagnosis is achieved by ultrasound examination and/or abdominocentesis or thoracocentesis.

●〉 WHAT TO DO

Cardiovascular Collapse
- Judicious administration of intravenous fluids
- Blood transfusion
- Intravenous aminocaproic acid
- NSAIDs
- Intranasal oxygen insufflation
- Quiet environment

- *Severe shock* (see Chapter 32, p. 565) may also cause recumbency, whether due to decreased perfusion or secondary to sepsis. Diagnosis is based on history and clinical signs of dark mucous membranes with prolonged capillary refill time, poor peripheral pulses, and cool extremities.

Gastrointestinal Diseases
- Horses with abdominal pain may present down, but clinical examination and response to analgesics usually indicates that abdominal pain is the cause of the recumbency—*an unwillingness to stand rather than inability to stand.*
- Horses with severe parasitism and starvation may be examined because of recumbency. Treatment is discussed in Chapter 50, p. 764, but the prognosis is poor for the down horse with these disorders.
- Similarly, horses with neoplasia and/or organ failure may be examined because of recumbency.
  - Clinical examination, ultrasound exam, serum chemistries, complete blood count (CBC), and cytology of body fluids or tissue often reveal a cause.

●〉 WHAT TO DO

Down Horse
Transport
- Transport of the down horse is challenging and potentially dangerous.
- In a quiet or depressed horse, transport may be carried out without the use of sedation/anesthesia; however, some degree of sedation is typically necessary.
- The horse should be protected with padded leg wraps and a helmet, if available.
- Horses can be moved on a flat surface with a coordinated effort by several people simultaneously pushing/pulling the horse in the same direction. Ropes can be tied to the down limbs to allow more distance between the limbs and people for safety.
- More effectively, a horse can be moved using a Large Animal Rescue Glide[1] (see Chapter 37, p. 638). The glide is a large sheet of durable, conformable plastic with handles and areas to hook ropes along the edges. The plastic slides easily over a variety of surfaces, and the edges can be folded to accommodate stall and trailer doorways.
- An effective method for moving a recumbent horse is to place the UC Davis Large Animal Lift[2] on the horse and use it to pull the horse onto the Large Animal Rescue Glide. The glide can then be pulled into the trailer and left under the horse to facilitate moving the horse off the trailer and into a hospital stall.

Basic Supportive Care
- Management of the down horse includes treatment of the primary disease (when known or working cause) and intensive supportive care.
- Bedding should be compressible, comfortable, and absorbent. It should be cleaned and aerated each time the horse is moved or turned. Wood shavings as a base-layer, with a thick covering of straw works well. Sheets or blankets may be placed on top to prevent abrasions, and the head should be slightly elevated. When the horse stands or is assisted with a sling, ensure that bedding is not slippery or excessively deep.
- Positioning is critical in the down horse. Ideally, the horse should remain in sternal recumbency, propping with straw bales as necessary. The horse should be turned every 2 to 6 hours, even if it is able to remain in sternal recumbency. Turning helps prevent decubital ulcers, compressive myelopathy and neuropathy, and supports ventilation.

---

[1]Large Animal Rescue Glide (L.A.R.G.E., Greenville, South Carolina).
[2]Large Animal Lift (Large Animal Lift Enterprises, Chico, California).

EMG

- ***Practice Tip:*** *Turning is ideally achieved by placing in sternal recumbency and pushing the body over the limbs; however, this is difficult in a full-sized horse. The advantage of this technique is that it allows the atelectic "down-side" lung to become inflated before being placed in lateral recumbency with the opposite lung down.*
- Alternatively, with the horse in lateral recumbency, ropes may be tied to the down limbs and pulled by individuals on the opposite side of the horse while one person assists the head. *Caution* should be used because horses typically struggle when the procedure is first performed.
- Many recumbent horses can bear some weight and spend considerable time upright with the assistance of a sling. Decreasing recumbent time minimizes the effects of prolonged recumbency and some muscle mass can be maintained.
- The sling also provides the clinician with the opportunity to better evaluate the patient.
- Horses with abnormal mentation are poor candidates to sling, and fractious or nervous horses may require light sedation or tranquilization. The sling must be properly adjusted to prevent pressure sores and the horse should be monitored closely while in the sling.
- The amount of time the horse stands in the sling should be gradually increased, if well tolerated. Horses with botulism should *not* be assisted to stand with a sling unless necessary because of complications of recumbency.
- ***Practice Tip:*** *Excessive movement of horses with botulism depletes acetylcholine stores.*
- Use of a sling:
- To use a sling safely in a stall environment, a cross-beam and hoist capable of supporting at least 2000 to 4000 lb (900 to 1800 kg) should be available, depending on the size of the horse, sling, and hoist. The UC Davis Anderson sling provides the most support in the most stable and balanced manner (see Chapter 37, p. 638). The sling consists of a rectangular overhead support, which provides level support, abdominal support, and additional leg supports alleviating excessive pressure on the abdomen and thorax/sternum. Disadvantages of this sling are that it is expensive and can be difficult to place on the horse, especially in a down patient without sedation or anesthesia.
- The Liftex sling[3] is simpler to use, containing an abdominal support, as well as tail and chest supports. It is less expensive and easier to place on the recumbent patient.
- The UC Davis Large Animal Lift is the most affordable and lightweight of the slings. It is intended to be used for lifting and moving horses, rather than providing ongoing support for a horse unable to stand unassisted, although it can be used in this manner. The device is relatively simple to place on a recumbent horse and can be used with a tractor or winch for lifting.
- ***Practice Tip:*** *There should be even "tension" on the bar or it may bend as the horse is being lifted.* If a horse needs continued support for standing, the Anderson sling may be placed over the UC Davis Large Animal Lift once the horse has been lifted to a standing position, then the Large Animal Lift can be removed.
  - On an especially quiet horse, the individual may be lifted using the sling and positioned in a bovine float tank.[4] The horse must be monitored closely, and there is a risk of injury when confined to the tank.

- The Enduro NEST,[5] recently developed by Enduro Medical Technology, supports the horse with a sling containing an abdominal support and leg supports. The sling is supported by a self-contained metal frame providing customized support or for lifting the horse. A horse can be placed under, and recover from, general anesthesia safely while being continuously supported in a standing position. The device can be used in a fixed position to provide variable limb support or is mobile to assist a weak, injured, or neurologic horse to walk.
- *Self-trauma and decubital ulcers* can be minimized with attention to good nursing care—bedding and skin care.
  - Leg wraps are recommended to protect the distal limbs and shoes should be wrapped to alleviate sharp edges.
  - Well-fitting head bumpers help prevent head trauma, which commonly occurs during failed attempts to get into sternal recumbency.
  - Horses should be groomed frequently and damp areas from sweat or urine should be dried thoroughly because wet skin is more prone to pressure sores and ulceration.
  - Wounds should be kept clean and dry, and antibiotics or topical medications used if necessary.
- *Ophthalmic care* of the recumbent horse includes:
  - Lubrication with an artificial tear ointment should be performed bilaterally at least q3-4h.
  - Corneas should be stained at least q24h to monitor for corneal ulceration.
  - Corneal ulcers should be treated aggressively and a temporary tarsorrhaphy considered if necessary.
- *Nutritional support* is an integral and challenging aspect of supportive care (see Chapter 51, p. 768).
  - Horses that are not dysphagic should be positioned in sternal recumbency and offered water, long-stem forage, and grain.
  - Horses are more likely to eat when standing, so feed and water should always be offered at a comfortable height when horses are assisted to stand.
  - Horses that are dysphagic or inappetent for several days require enteral or parenteral nutritional support.
  - Enteral feeding may be provided by nasogastric tube, and the tube can be left indwelling or passed several times daily.
  - Enteral diets may be formulated using complete feeds or alfalfa meal, or a commercial equine enteral diet may be used.
  - Feedings should be divided into 4 to 6 small meals per day while the horse is sternal or standing.
  - In horses with adequate gastrointestinal function, maintenance fluids may be administered by nasogastric tube.
  - In horses with gastrointestinal dysfunction in which enteral feeding is not possible, parenteral nutrition with dextrose, amino acids, and lipid solutions should be considered.
  - Maintenance fluid requirements must also be met using intravenous fluids in horses on parenteral nutrition.
- *Intravenous catheter care* is challenging because of an unavoidably contaminated environment and frequent movement at the catheter site (see Chapter 3, p. 9).
  - Polyurethane, over-the-wire jugular catheters are recommended because they are less likely to cause thrombosis than over-the-needle catheters.
  - Routine catheter care—i.e., flushing the catheter with heparinized saline q6h is recommended.

---

[3]Liftex Large Animal/Equine Sling (Liftex Corporation, Philadelphia, Pennsylvania).
[4]Aqua Cow Rise System (Aqua Cow/North America, Saint Johnsbury, Vermont).

[5]Enduro N.E.S.T. (Enduro Medical Technology, South Windsor, Connecticut).

- A neck wrap of elastic tape with dry gauze placed over the base of the catheter is recommended to prevent friction and gross contamination, and should be replaced daily or more often if soiled.
- The vein and the catheter insertion sites should be inspected at least two times a day for evidence of skin swelling, heat, or thickening of the vein. If any abnormalities are detected, the catheter should be removed and the tip cultured.
- In the event of a compromised jugular vein, hot-packing the catheter site and vein several times a day, followed by topical application of DMSO/furacin sweat, ichthammol or Surpass[6] are recommended to minimize thrombophlebitis. Antibiotic therapy is typically indicated.
- *Urinary catheterization* is necessary in horses with neurologic disorders that cause an atonic bladder, such as EHV-1, and in horses not urinating appropriately.
  - Some down horses, especially mules, may choose not to urinate even with normal bladder and spinal cord function.
  - Catheterization may be performed several times a day or the catheter may remain indwelling.
  - Indwelling catheters are useful for keeping the bedding and patient dry and helping to prevent decubital ulceration.
  - An indwelling Foley catheter should be placed under aseptic conditions and urine collected using a closed system. IV tubing and empty sterile IV fluid bags placed deep in the bedding below the level of the bladder can be easily and inexpensively used to collect urine.
  - Securing the catheter and/or tubing to the skin on the ventral body wall (males) or tail (mares) using elastic tape or suture, respectively, alleviates pressure on the catheter when the horse struggles or is turned.
  - The urinary collection system should be monitored for obstructions and urine collection bags emptied at least several times a day.
  - ***Practice Tip:*** *The most common complication of urinary catheterization is cystitis due to ascending bacterial infection.*
  - Cytologic and dipstick evaluation of urine is easy and inexpensive, and should be performed every few days. If cystitis is suspected, a urine culture and colony count should be performed and antibiotic therapy instituted.
- *Large colon impactions* are common in down horses because of poor gastrointestinal motility.
  - It is essential to monitor fecal production closely in these horses.
  - Easily digestible feeds should be offered and mineral oil administered by nasogastric tube.
  - Manual evacuation of the rectum may be necessary, especially in horses with EHV-1.

[6]Surpass (Boehringer Ingelheim Metmedica, Inc., St. Joseph, Missouri).

References

References can be found on the companion website at www.equine-emergencies.com.

EMG

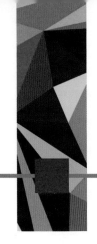

CHAPTER 37

Disaster Medicine and Technical Emergency Rescue

Rebecca M. Gimenez

Individual Situations

- Clinicians frequently equate everyday emergencies with "disasters," or at a minimum, some complex emergencies (e.g., six horses injured in an overturned trailer) are referred to as "disasters."
- Emergencies, such as a trailer wreck on a highway, are defined as incidents that require immediate response, are usually resolved within several hours, and seldom exhaust the local resources.
  - The owner's involvement may be minimized on scene to maintain safety protocols.
- In a typical clinical emergency (colic, laceration, choke), the clinician and staff work with the owner to help the patient.
  - Traditionally, contact between the emergency services and provider is made via the clinic's phone number or e-mail.
- In an emergency involving other emergency services personnel (fire/rescue, law enforcement, paramedics, and animal control), the clinician and staff work as part of a team under the Incident Command System to extricate, treat, and assist the patient.
  - In this case, communication is initiated and sustained thru 911 dispatch or emergency communication coordination offices.
- Any situation that entails clinical involvement longer than a few hours, spanning days or weeks after the initial incident, is identified as a disaster.
- There are two categories of disasters:
  - Human-caused/technologic (e.g., electrical grid failure, nuclear release)
  - Natural (e.g., hurricanes, floods)
- From an analytic perspective, the biggest difference between "emergencies" and "disasters" is the number of resources (especially personnel) involved.
- In a disaster, the veterinarian works with emergency services at local, state, and federal levels and other specified rescue personnel as a member of a team under the Incident Command System to assist the patient.
  - The owner is rarely present.
- Based on the nature and scope of the incident, the coordination occurs through local, county, state, and/or federal response teams using a variety of communications services.

- Technical emergencies include:
  - Hallmarks involving confined space (overturned trailers, earthquake, or hurricane destruction)
  - Structural collapse (snow collapse, earthquake, and tornado destruction)
  - Hazardous materials (HAZMAT) and/or chemical, biologic, radiologic, nuclear (CBRNE) (diesel leaks, septic tanks, nuclear release)
  - Unstable ground (septic tanks, mud entrapment, surface ice, flood waters)
  - Fire (barn and wildfire)
- These are specialty forms of rescue within the emergency services that should *not* be attempted without all of the following:
  - Training
  - Correct personnel protective equipment (PPE)
  - Teamwork

Knowing How to Proceed, Perform, and Interact with Other Responders in an Emergency/Disaster

- Whether it is a single incident (e.g., trailer overturn on the road) or a large-scale disaster (e.g., wildfire), the practitioner is one member of a group of emergency responders.
- In the case of a single, smaller incident, local responders include firefighters, law enforcement, and possibly animal control and paramedics.
- In the case of both small- and large-scale events, it is essential for the professional practitioner to know how to interact with other emergency response individuals from county, state, federal, and private emergency response organizations. Examples of these organizations include:
- County Agricultural/Animal Response Team (CART)
- County Emergency Response Team (CERT)
- State Animal Response Team (SART)
- Office of the State/Commonwealth Veterinarian
- State Department of Agriculture
- Federal Emergency Management Agency (FEMA)
- National Disaster Medical System (NDMS)
  - National and State Veterinary Response Teams (NVRT)
- American Veterinary Medical Association (AVMA)
  - Veterinary Medical Assistance Teams (VMAT)

- Non-Governmental Organizations (AHA, HSUS, ASPCA, CODE-3, NARSC, etc.)
- U.S. Armed Forces (Army, Navy, Marines, Air Force) and U.S. Coast Guard
- Law enforcement personnel (local and from different states)
- Fire department personnel (local and from different states)
- Animal Control; Agricultural/Cooperative Extension
- Regardless of the type of emergency or disaster, all individuals and organizations involved respond under a common protocol known as the Incident Command System (ICS), and National Incident Management System (NIMS), under the National Response Plan (NRP). The ICS was developed more than 25 years ago by the U.S. Forestry Service to respond to wildfires in a safer and better coordinated manner in order to avoid losing lives on the fire ground. In 2014 the National Fire Protection Association (NFPA) promulgates the first ever standards for Technical Animal Rescue (large and small animals) in their Standard 1670 "Standard on Operations and Training for Technical Search and Rescue Incidents" for emergency responders, and includes ICS as the basic framework for a TLAER scene. The basic principles of the ICS are fully applicable to animal incidents and include the following:
  - Planning: An incident action plan must be developed for every incident (simple and verbal, or complicated and written) depending on the size and length of response.
  - Team Approach: Every responder acts as part of a team and knows their job.
  - One Coordinator: The Incident Commander (IC) coordinates the incident response; he/she is the leader and shoulders the responsibility for the entire scene.
  - Span of Control: One person can only coordinate the activities of five to seven responders.
  - Safety: Safety, for the victim and the rescuers, is the primary reason for the team approach.
  - No Freelancing: Individuals responding/acting on their own constitute a risk and a liability to others on the scene. The IC has the authority to forcibly remove them from the scene.
- In today's world, the equine practitioner *is* an emergency responder. Therefore, it is imperative for the practitioner and staff to understand and communicate using the emergency response "language" of ICS.
  - The best online training source for the ICS is the Emergency Management Institute, under FEMA.
- There are different levels of ICS training.
- The basic level, ICS 100 and NIMS 700, give the equine practitioner the basic qualifications to help respond in an emergency/disaster of any size, locally or nationally.
  - The basic ICS 100 and NIMS 700 courses (IS-100 Introduction to the Incident Command System and IS-700 National Incident Management System [NIMS], An

---

Box 37-1   **Additional Animal-Related Disaster Courses**

- Federal Emergency Management Agency: *FEMA Independent Study Program: IS-10 Animals in Disaster, module A&B; and Livestock in Disasters,* Emmitsburg, MD, 2008, Emergency Management Institute. The following course descriptions and objectives were retrieved January 26, 2012, from http://training.fema.gov/IS.
- **IS-11.A: Animals in Disasters: Community Planning at http://training.fema.gov/EMIWeb/IS/IS11a.asp**

Course Description

This course provides information for groups to meet and develop meaningful and effective plans that improve the care of animals, their owners, and the animal-care industries in disasters.

Course Objectives

The objectives of this course are to learn how to develop a community plan for managing animals in an emergency, identify hazards and threats most likely to affect your community and ways to minimize their impact on animals, indicate how communities use the Incident Command System (ICS) to respond effectively to an incident involving animals, describe resources available to help communities recover from a disaster, and develop community support for a disaster preparedness plan involving animals.

- **IS-111.A: Livestock in Disasters at http://training.fema.gov/EMIWeb/IS/is111a.asp**

Course Description

This course combines the knowledge of livestock producers and emergency managers to present a unified approach to mitigate the impact of disasters on animal agriculture.

Course Objectives

The objectives of this course are to learn and understand issues that arise when disasters affect livestock, determine a farm's susceptibility to hazards, and identify actions to reduce economic losses and human and animal suffering in disasters.

Introduction) can be completed online in about 4 hours.
- In disaster situations, failure to possess this certification could result in dismissal from the response scene. In localized emergencies, it may result in your failure to coordinate with the team.
- After taking a simple online test, one can receive a certificate of completion.
- Other animal-related disaster content courses are available (Box 37-1).

Types of Emergencies/Disasters

- *Road emergency* (trailer and towing vehicle accidents, loose horses, rider and/or horse hit by a vehicle)
- *Off-road emergency* (falls, entrapment, entanglement or entrapment in mud)
- *Competition emergency* (3-day event, rodeo, show jumping, endurance, etc.)
- *Barn fires* (accidental or arson)
- *Natural and technologic disasters* (hurricane, flood, tornado, blizzard, wildfire, earthquake, nuclear, electrical) that require evacuation or shelter in place
- *Hazardous spills* (evacuation or shelter in place)

- Veterinarians are creative and independent. This creativity allows clinicians to help horses in difficult situations by being able to process many "helpful" suggestions.
- However, the independence frequently results in humane destruction of patients that could have been helped by a well-organized team.
- Technical emergency rescue performed in a way that is safe for the rescuers and the equine patient requires training in technical aspects of rescue procedures for all emergency responders, including the veterinarian.
- This training has been offered for over 17 years in the United States (see Additional Animal-Related Disaster Courses, p. 645) and is now being offered on four other continents.

Planning

- Planning for emergency or disaster response requires detailed protocols and training at several levels. The basis of disaster medicine is sharpening standard emergency skills rehearsed in routine clinical emergencies.
- Emergencies where other responders share the scene are more difficult to plan for, necessitating training and preparation in coordination with a team of rescuers.
- Written emergency protocols are mandatory, and "emergency kits" must be prepared for sometimes unimaginable scenarios. For example, a horse:
- Is stuck in mud at the bottom of a steep ravine, has been there for 12 hours
- Has fallen into a tire feeder and only his hind feet are sticking out
- Has survived a horrific trailer roll on the interstate and is tied with a trailer tie, now lying under the divider of a two-horse trailer
- Is hanging from a railroad trestle by one leg
- The emergency kit should contain everything needed for a specific type of emergency. The kit should be portable, clearly marked, and readily accessible. These kits can serve several functions in routine practice:
- Crash kit: For chemical restraint, resuscitation, or euthanasia, with dosages of each drug listed. This kit is most valuable at the side of an anesthetized patient and in the management of adverse drug reactions (see Chapter 47, p. 738).
- Catheter kit: Contains all the materials for placing an intravenous catheter and for fluid administration (several boxes of fluids readily available). The catheter kit saves valuable time in an emergency and facilitates routine catheter placement in nonemergency situations (see Chapter 47, p. 735).
- Respiratory kit: Contains tracheostomy equipment and instruments and includes tubing for oxygen delivery, a humidifier, and a small oxygen tank (see Chapter 47, p. 736).
- Splint kit: Contains pre-cut polyvinyl chloride pieces, tape, bandage material, hack saw, and cast material, all of which can be tailored to the specific type of limb problem (see Chapter 21, pp. 319-324).
- Emergency kits can be kept in the ambulatory clinician's vehicle and stored as part of the hospital's inventory. Plastic inventory tags and reflective stickers with your name on each bag or kit facilitate rescue operations and ensure that the equipment is returned.

Preparation and Training

- The universal principle to follow in any incident is to determine, then use, the simplest approach that results in an efficient and safe extrication.
- Training in the use of specialized technical large animal rescue equipment is beyond the scope of this chapter, but always encourages that the horse be allowed or assisted to "self-rescue" when possible.
- Veterinarians and other emergency responders should attend one of the equine technical disaster and emergency rescue courses at the Awareness or Operations level available through training organizations (e.g., Disaster Animal Response Team and Sheltering, www.hsus.org; Technical Large Animal Emergency Rescue, Inc., www.tlaer.org; and Large Animal Rescue Company, www.largeanimalrescue.com).

Disaster Equipment

- Equipment used for equine emergencies and disasters can be classified into the categories in Box 37-2.
- Some specialized large-animal rescue equipment (Large Animal Lift,[1] Nicopolous Needle,[2] Becker Web Sling,[3] Mud Lances,[4] A-Frame,[5] etc.) is commercially available. Research on the use of these best practices and resource typing of equipment is ongoing at www.tlaer.org and veterinary schools (Louisiana State University, Mississippi State University, University of California at Davis, North Carolina State University). Many of the most useful items are simple to make or to convert from conventional or human rescue systems. It has been suggested that an investment of less than $7000 USD could completely outfit a team with basic and many advanced technical rescue items for a local supply.
- Larger and more expensive equipment needs for a community should be proposed and purchased by the community and used under the direction of a veterinarian skilled in large-animal rescue techniques, and perhaps maintained on the local fire/rescue equipment; alternatively it can be funded privately and coordinated by a team under a nonprofit designation.

The Large Animal Lift[6]

- The Large Animal Lift (LAL)[7] is a device used for lifting downed horses and relies on the skeletal system and lightweight equipment that is more easily applied to a recumbent horse.

---

[1]Large Animal Lift Enterprises, Chico, California.
[2]TLAER, Inc., Pendleton, South Carolina.
[3]Hast, Inc., Floyd, Virginia.
[4]TLAER, Inc., Pendleton, South Carolina.
[5]TLAER, Inc., Pendleton, South Carolina.
[6]The editors acknowledge and thank Dr. John Madigan from the University of California for supplying the figures and description of the LAL.
[7]Large Animal Lift Enterprises, Chico, California.

- Use of the LAL without specific training can be dangerous to the operator and rescued horse.
- The LAL uses include the following:
- Lifting recumbent horses in the field using a back hoe, mechanical system, or other overhead device
- Anesthesia recovery assist; body recovery

- Lifting the weak geriatric horse that is unable to stand unassisted or supporting starve/neglect horses for several days after authorities take control of them
- Preventing horses with pelvic injuries or other orthopedic injuries from lying down

---

Box 37-2   Equipment for Equine Emergency and Disaster Response

Protective Equipment
- Gloves
- Boots
- Protective headwear (helmet or hard hat)
- Goggles
- Ear protection
- Protective clothing (durable, long sleeves and pants)
- Rappelling gear (harness, helmet, gloves)
- Water rescue gear (personal flotation device, dry suit, boots, and specialized helmet)
- Surface ice rescue gear (ice rescue suit, specialized helmet, harness)
  Note: Do *not* attempt to perform a rescue operation in surface ice, mud, swift or floodwater without training.
- Biosecurity suit (i.e., Tyvek suit) in preparation for a chemical disaster.

Critical Equipment
- Halters of different sizes (nylon, sturdy hardware)
- Lead ropes (10 foot [3-m] cotton, sturdy hardware and chain shank)
- Two 35-foot (10.7-m) sections of ½-inch (1.3-cm) kernmantle static rescue rope
- Two 20 foot (6 m) of 3-inch (7.6-cm) nylon web with a loop on each end (forward assist sling) (Fig. 37-1)
- Two 4 to 6 feet (1.2 to 1.8 m) of 5-inch-wide (12.7-cm) web with loops sewn on each end
- Spread bar with 2 lift points (with snap shackles for release)
- Fleece-lined breast collar (sturdy hardware)
- Two sets of fleece-lined hobbles
- 1 gallon (3.8 L) of lubricant
- Six 6-foot (1.8-m) loops of ½-inch (1.3-cm) rescue rope with mariner's knots
- Protective gear for the horse's head
- 12 large steel carabiners
- One leg-handling cane, heavy duty aluminum

- Cotton horse earplugs
- Canvas or plastic tarps (minimum 8 × 8 feet [2.4 × 2.4 m])
- Camera/Video capability (batteries, extra storage cards)

Important Equipment
- One containment portable fence (e.g., 5 foot × 110-foot [1.5 × 33.5-m] Polygrid fence)
- One 4:1.5 rope anchor system (with 2 double pulleys and Prusik loops [Fig. 37-2])
- One 3:1 Z-rig rope anchor system (with two single pulleys and Prusik loops)
- 300 feet (91.4 m) of ½-inch (1.3-cm) rescue rope
- One human class III full body harness
- Two canvas or plastic tarps (at least 12 × 12 feet [3.7 × 3.7 m])
- Blankets (horse type and reflective surface heat saving type)
- Hand tools (Cutting saws, axes, shovels)
- Boat hook (extendable)
- Documentation, forms, identification
- Portable screen (for competition or public rescues)
- Emergency lights, reflective and signage
- Large rubber mat, or Rescue Glide set (Fig. 37-3) with ratchet straps and hobbles

Mechanized Equipment
- Four-wheel drive truck with fixed winch (minimum 8000 lb [3629 kg]), CB or two-way radio and public-address system; capable of towing trailer or ambulance
- Portable winch (minimum 3000 lb [1361 kg])
- Wrecker, crane, or rough-terrain forklift (minimum 10-foot [3-m] boom clearance above ground)
- Equine "ambulance," such as a converted horse trailer (with intravenous fluid capability)
- When helicopter rescue is the only option: Anderson sling with cable, web connector, frame (Fig. 37-4)
  Note: Helicopter rescue of horses is considered to be a last resort; it is dangerous and should *not* be attempted without proper training in ground procedures for helicopter rescue.

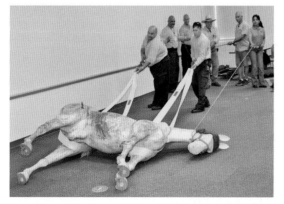

Figure 37-1   The backwards drag is practiced in a classroom so that safety and the manipulation learning experienced are maximized for students. A 20-foot (6-meter) strap is useful for many of these types of manipulations and minimizes injury to the horse. (Courtesy Miami-Dade Fire Rescue.)

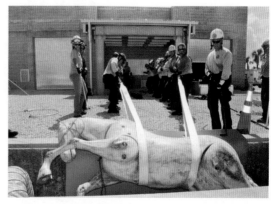

Figure 37-2   The sideways drag out of a trench with edge protection is practiced by students representing veterinarians, animal control, fire department, and police personnel with Randy the Rescue Horse Mannequin. (Courtesy University of Florida VETS Team.)

Continued

Box 37-2   Equipment for Equine Emergency and Disaster Response—cont'd

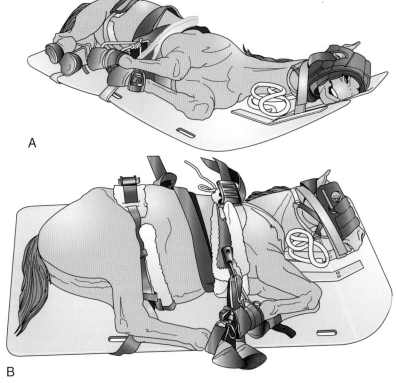

Figure 37-3   Rescue glide set. **A** Side glide. **B,** Top glide. (Courtesy Dr. Rebecca Gimenez, TLAER.org.)

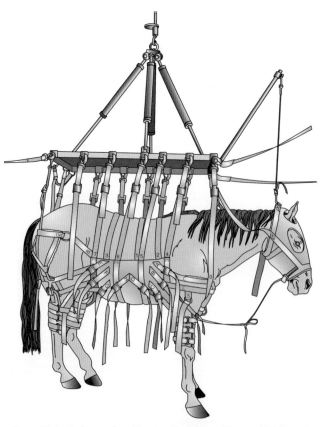

Figure 37-4   Anderson sling. (Courtesy Dr. Rebecca Gimenez, TLAER.org.)

- Please refer to Fig. 37-5, which offers a step-by-step demonstration of the application of the LAL on an equine mannequin.

Personnel

- Disaster planning is a positive and nonthreatening way to bring together many different relevant organizations and persons working as a team (preferably *before* a disaster occurs.)
- Area veterinarians can share ideas on how to respond to various problems, and possible solutions with governmental agencies, law enforcement, animal control, and emergency management personnel.
- Volunteer groups, such as Red Cross, volunteer fire personnel, colic or foal treatment teams in academic institutions, can be organized and given a chance to hone and practice relevant skills. Any volunteer group is a means to involve persons of various skills, including local and emergency professionals.
- Practice drills for all types of imaginable emergency and disaster situations ensure a trained team that is interested in and up to date on disaster medicine skills.

Chronologic Walk-Through of a Disaster

Step at Which Decisions Must Be Made	Specific Considerations at Step
Assessment of the situation during initial contact	If humans are injured, need for emergency medical services (EMS); whether EMS has been called to the scene Physical access to patient; need for police escort, need for Fire/Rescue Additional equipment needs Additional personnel needs
Development of a mental protocol on the way to the scene	**Restraint:** Calming techniques (massage, voice) Physical (earplugs, blindfold, twitch) Chemical (drugs and dosages) **Physical Examination:** Procedures for special circumstances, stay out of the operational area **Scene Security:** "Onlooker" recruitment or dispersal Jobs to fill: traffic control, animal handler, owner control person, operational personnel, safety, Incident Commander (IC)
Arrival on the scene	Meeting with Incident Commander (chief emergency worker on scene) Assessment of overall situation: Whether the horse's rescue is a primary or a secondary concern (people are rescued first) Prioritize and triage scene
Assessment of the patient's situation	Whether the horse is dead or alive, whether it is being treated or euthanized Attitude: quiet, sulking, or depressed Struggling: coordinated or uncoordinated Concept of self-preservation Obvious medical problems (e.g., wounds and shock) Less obvious problems (e.g., temperature, pulse, respiration; neurologic and musculoskeletal status) Legal: whether owner or authorized agent wants documentation (photographs, video, written account); notification of insurance company (for humane destruction cases)
Finalization of team plan	Specific equipment and personnel needed Coordination with IC about rescue options and avenues of approach to extrication Additional specialized equipment needed (e.g., Jaws of Life) Specific treatment and restraint (none, sedation, anesthesia, humane destruction); when in doubt, be conservative Whether rescue workers understand their jobs (everyone should) and communication Safety first: check and recheck; use a checklist
Rescue/Extrication	Technical steps of rescue performed as prescribed by Emergency Rescue personnel
Aftermath of rescue	Examination, assessment Treatment of patient
Debriefing, review after rescue	Transport of patient Sharing of written information Thanking all participants Review of entire protocol, mental and written procedures Scheduling follow-up examinations

EMG

EMG

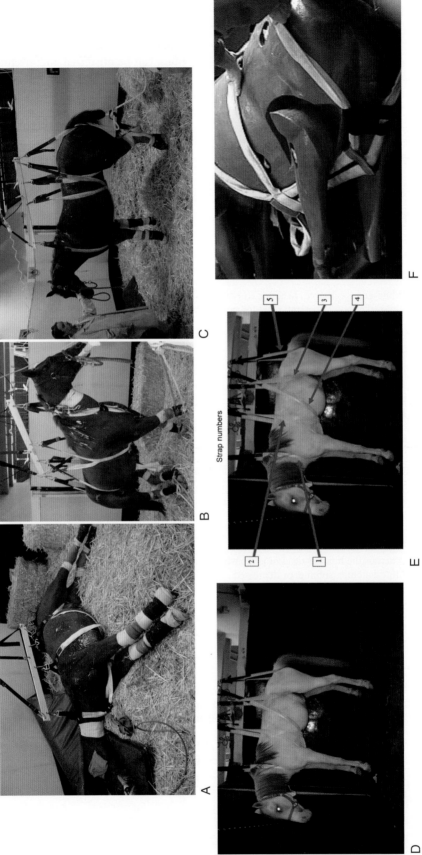

Figure 37-5 Application of the Large Animal Lift (LAL). **A** to **C,** Views of LAL ready for lifting. **D,** LAL on a lifted horse. **E,** Strap numbers 1 to 5 are indicated. **F,** Front section placed.

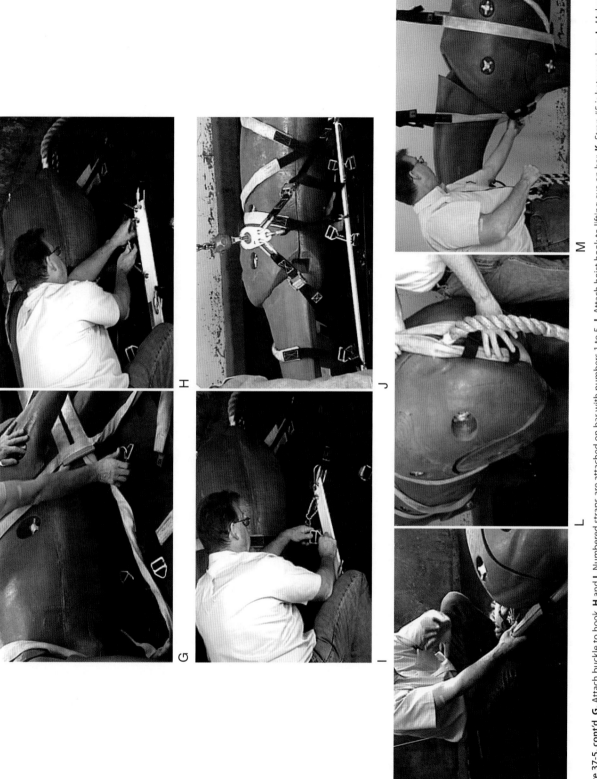

Figure 37-5, cont'd G, Attach buckle to hook. **H** and **I,** Numbered straps are attached on bar with numbers 1 to 5. **J,** Attach hoist hook to lifting eye on bar. **K,** Strap #5 is between legs. **L,** Make sure rear straps (holding #5) stay between rear legs during attach and lift. **M,** Make sure pad and strap are not cutting off airway. (Courtesy Dr. John Madigan, University of California.)

EMG

Practice and Community Involvement

- Dealing with the effects of large-scale natural and human-created disasters involves more personnel and equipment than a clinical or technical emergency.
- Responding to a disaster requires knowledge of how the state's emergency preparedness and response divisions are organized and how individual veterinarians and volunteers should work within that system from call out to response to retiring.
- Within the scope of a disaster are numerous emergencies. Training in technical aspects of large animal rescue, organizing emergency kits (see Box 37-2), relevant experience and education, and planning all ready the clinician for specific situations within each disaster.
- Counterproductive thinking (e.g., "These things happen in other places, not here!") is to be avoided. Everyone is stressed and excitable, irritable, and tired. Work to provide leadership, a calm and positive work environment for those working around you, and realize that no one can do it all. Delegate tasks to qualified individuals.
- The goal of practitioners should be to facilitate the preparedness of horse owners ahead of time. There is no substitute for owners taking responsibility for their horses and facilities. Many owners have never thought about how difficult it is simply to help their horses survive in the absence of electricity, communication, city water, and appropriate food.
- A clinician involved in disaster planning should understand four specific points:
- Assess the present level of interest and organizational skills of the local equine community.
- Learn the office of emergency management and planning's role in community response and its relationship to other emergency response groups (e.g., fire/rescue, police, emergency medical services, and hospitals (human and animal).
- Learn the veterinary skills and personal contacts for those personnel available at the local, state, and national levels that can be leveraged in a disaster.
- Learn the national, state, and local emergency preparedness and response systems that are in place and how to work with and within those systems to get tasks completed.
- To accomplish disaster preparedness and response successfully, all four areas must be carefully considered, and the most probable types of disasters that can occur in your community must be prioritized. Use the disaster curve (Fig. 37-6) to determine the time needed for specific catastrophes.

Involvement of the Horse Community

- Veterinarians are ideal leaders in the animal disaster planning of a community (Fig. 37-7). Clinicians interested in disaster preparedness and response will organize their practices around, or be involved in, routine clinical emergencies expandable to all levels of disaster preparedness.
- An ALL-HAZARDS approach to disaster planning involves evacuation and shelter-in-place strategies for any

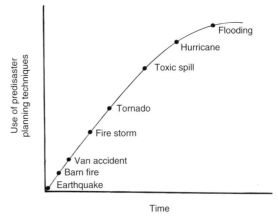

Figure 37-6   Disaster curve. (Courtesy Dr. Richard Mansmann.)

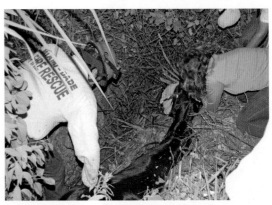

Figure 37-7   Horse trapped in a ditch is attended to by a team of firefighters and a veterinarian. Here they are coming up with a plan to provide medical stabilization and possible sedation before attaching simple manipulation methods (webbing and edge protection). (Courtesy Miami-Dade Fire Rescue.)

disaster type that might be expected to hit a specific community.
- Groups need 6 to 12 owners with basic skills and interest to form an organization with other local owners.
- Close coordination with trained emergency rescue personnel (e.g., police, fire, emergency medical services [EMS], and animal control) in the early stages of development of an organization greatly facilitates rescue-related training and practice opportunities. Ask them to share their experiences with rescuing large animals. What worked? What did not? Once the emergency community knows that you are interested, trained, equipped, and available, prepare to be used regularly (Figs. 37-8, 37-9, and 37-10).
- Disaster response can be a unifying experience for different horse groups.

Involvement of the Local Office of Emergency Services

- For success, a strong working relationship and trust must be developed between local volunteer groups of animal owners and the office of emergency planning for the community; this is the most critical component for any animal group doing community emergency work.

EMG

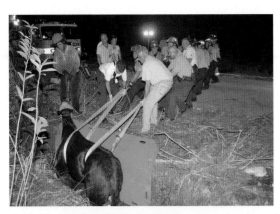

Figure 37-8   The horse is sedated, blindfolded to protect the eyes and calm it, a Rescue Glide is used for edge protection, and webbing is placed in a sideways drag configuration for a manual simple vertical lift with webbing. Notice the owner is clear of the rescue effort. (Courtesy Miami-Dade Fire Rescue.)

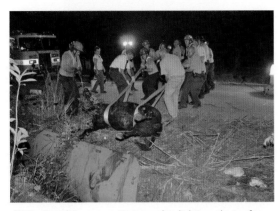

Figure 37-9   Complete success. Having a plan, lighting, plenty of manpower, and a teamwork attitude results in a professional technical rescue. (Courtesy Miami-Dade Fire Rescue.)

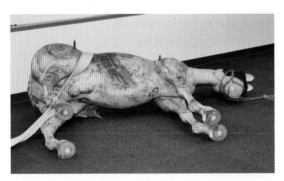

Figure 37-10   The Hampshire Slip configuration of the sideways drag features the use of webbing around the downside limbs of the horse, preventing it from rolling over while being manually extricated. (Courtesy John Haven, University of Florida VETS Team.)

- The issue of incorporating animals in disaster planning can be organized into local efforts by representatives attending emergency services and town hall and county planning meetings.
- Owners and veterinarians must learn the local protocols and laws that govern local emergency preparedness and response for both people and animals.
- Organizations such as humane societies, extension offices, and the American Red Cross are excellent resources for training and help.

- Large facilities such as racetracks, fairgrounds, and show facilities should develop shared needs planning for an emergency to include large animal sheltering.
- Insurance for volunteers who work in a disaster environment may be available through county emergency services.
- A complete definition of funding, responsibilities, and roles of all animal-related organizations in various types of disasters is still undetermined. Every veterinarian, horse owner, and community is responsible to work within the framework of existing emergency planning to help reduce losses in disasters and identify the necessary funding, equipment, and roles played in emergency management.

The American Association of Equine Practitioners and Disaster Medicine

- An important role of the American Association of Equine Practitioners (AAEP) service to members and horse owners is to provide the equine practitioner with information that helps them in emergencies and/or disasters affecting the practitioner and their clientele.
- Through its standing Disaster Committee, the AAEP provides emergency/disaster information on an ongoing basis through their website: www.aaep.org/emergency_prep.htm (see Inside Back Cover for additional emergency resources).

Available Emergency Services

- The American Veterinary Medical Association (AVMA) created the Veterinary Medical Assistance Team (VMAT) program after Hurricane Andrew in 1992. In 1993, the AVMA and the U.S. Department of Health and Human Services signed a Memorandum of Understanding (MOU) with the AVMA establishing the VMAT program as a public-private partnership to assist in providing veterinary emergency preparedness and response.
- AVMA and federal government worked together in a public-private partnership for disaster response needs from 1993-2007, with teams housed by AVMA responding as federal employees.
- In 2008, changes in federal government policy led to the creation of two separate and complementary Veterinary Disaster Response Team programs: the federal government's National Veterinary Response Team (www.phe.gov/Preparedness/responders/ndms/teams/Pages/nvrt.aspx; see Inside Back Cover for additional emergency resources) and AVMA's Veterinary Medical Assistance Team (VMAT) program.
- The AVMA Executive Board approved a new state-focused program, and the AVMF Board of Directors authorized a grant to fund it. The new VMAT program allows for more flexibility, seeks and maintains MOUs for response efforts with individual states, and provides emergency and disaster response training on issues relative to animals in disasters.
- VMAT (www.avma.org/VMAT) members serve as first responders to ensure high-quality care of animals during disasters and emergencies by augmenting existing

EMG

veterinary resources in the impacted area. The VMAT program serves three primary functions when its help is requested by state authorities: Early Assessment Volunteer Teams, Basic Treatment Volunteer Teams, and Training Programs.

- Numerous state veterinary medical associations are involved in their states' emergency and disaster planning. Contact your state veterinary association for specifics.
- State Animal Response Teams (SART; www.ncsart.org) are interagency state organizations dedicated to preparing, planning, responding, and recovering during animal emergencies in the United States. SART is a public–private partnership, joining government agencies with private concerns around the common goal of animal issues during disasters. SART programs train participants to facilitate a safe, environmentally sound and efficient response to animal emergencies on the local, county, state, and federal levels. The teams are organized under the auspices of state and local emergency management utilizing the principles of the Incident Command System (ICS). Over 20 states now have this program in place, and others are in development.
- The American Humane Association (www.american humane.org) is a national nonprofit providing emergency services and disaster response capabilities on a nationwide basis and provides training in large animal sheltering and disaster response.
- HSUS (www.humanesociety.org/issues/animal_rescue/ ndart/ndart.html) provides National Disaster Animal Response Team (NDART) and Emergency Animal Sheltering (EAS) training for volunteers through Humane Society University.
- The National Animal Rescue and Sheltering Coalition, or NARSC (www.narsc.net/resource-library) is a U.S. 501(c) 6 organization comprised of 13 national nonprofit organizations. NARSC works to improve the welfare of animals throughout the United States by identifying, prioritizing, and finding collaborative solutions to major human-animal emergency issues. Several NARSC agencies provide animal disaster response and emergency training opportunities.
- FEMA (http://training.fema.gov/emicourses) has a physical campus and online educational training:
    Emergency Management Institute (EMI)
    16825 South Seton Ave.
    Emmitsburg, MD 21727
- There are several communities that have equine-specific ambulance services available for organized events, local animal controls, and emergency and disaster work:
    - Moore County, NC (www.mceeru.com)
    - MSPCA at Nevins Farm, MA (www.mspca.org/ adoption/methuen-nevins/equine-safety–ambulance -program)
    - SPCA in Aiken, SC (http://aikenspca.org/equine -ambulance)
    - CODE 3 (http://code3associates.org/disastersvcs.php)
- Several states have animal, large animal, or equine-specific emergency rescue volunteer organizations. Contact your

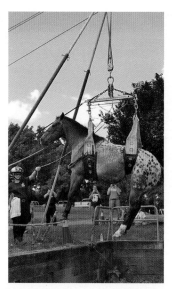

Figure 37-11   Trained horse in a simple vertical lift configuration using a Becker sling, demonstrating the good support provided the horse with the wide webbing directly behind the front legs and supported by a chest piece to keep it in place, and directly in front of the back legs. Two lift points balance the load, minimizing struggling, and allows the horse to more easily be placed into and taken out of the sling. (Courtesy Dr. Rebecca Gimenez.)

state emergency operations/preparedness division. Fire departments, USAR/Special Operations teams (www .fema.gov/emergency/usr) and fire academies in several states are conducting training of their personnel in this specialty aspect of heavy rescue, and may have a team in your area. A contact list of links is available at http:// firelink.monster.com/education/articles/2621.

Product Manufacturers of Emergency Equipment

Simple Vertical Lift (Becker) Sling (Fig. 37-11)
Dr. Kathleen Becker, DVM
becker@hast.net
(518) 302-0784; Fax: (540) 745-4036
http://rescue.hast.net

Equine Sked Stretcher (Rescue Glide)
Ben McCracken
(864) 270-1344
benmccracken@rescueglides.com
www.rescueglides.com

MSPCA—Nevins Farm
Roger Lauze
978-687-7453 ext. 6124
rlauze@mspca.org
http://www.mspca.org

Dealers for All Brands and Types of Rescue Equipment
Technical Rescue
(800) 771-5342
www.technicalrescue.com

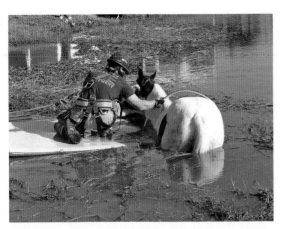

Figure 37-12 Trained horse in the mud is being accessed above the rescue environment using an inflatable rescue path. Mud lances inject air into the mud around the horse's legs, "freeing" the legs before removal using the sideways drag manipulation method. (Courtesy Dr. Rebecca Gimenez.)

CMC Rescue Equipment
(800) 235-5741; Fax: (800) 235-8951 US
(805) 562-9120; Fax: (805) 562-9870 International
www.cmcrescue.com

Karst Sports
(800) 734-2851
www.karstsports.com

Rock-n-Rescue
(800) 346-7673
www.rocknrescue.com

TLAER Nicopolous Needle, A-Frame, Quick Release Spread
    Bar, Mud Lances
(Fig. 37-12)
Dr. Tomas Gimenez
tlaer@bellsouth.net
(864) 940-1717
www.tlaer.org

Protective Clothing
Cascade Fire Equipment
(800) 654-7049
www.cascadefire.com

Forestry Suppliers, Inc.
(800) 647-5368
www.forestry-suppliers.com

Galls
(800) 477-7766
www.galls.com

The Rescue Source
(800) 45-RESCUE
www.rescuesource.com

Portable Fence
Polygrid Ranch Fence
(800) 845-9005
www.jerrybleach.com

Helicopter Sling (Anderson Sling) and Large Animal Lift
Large Animal Lift Enterprises
Chico, CA 95926
530-320-2627
www.andersonsling.com

Aluminum Leg Splint
Kimzey Veterinary Products
www.kimzeymetalproducts.com

Safety Personal Protective Equipment
Tychem SL
(800) 645-9291
www.lakeland.com

Vertical Lift Spread Bars, Pulleys
www.boatliftdistributors.com

Horse First Aid Storage System
(877) 487-4677
www.madewithhorsesense.com

Load Release, Snap Shackles
www.seacatch.com
www.catsailor.com

Technical Rescue Training Resources

Technical Large Animal Emergency Rescue, Inc. (TLAER)
    Training
Dr. Rebecca Gimenez
delphiacres@hotmail.com
www.tlaer.org
(214) 679-3629

Large Animal Rescue Company, Inc. Training
Cpt. John and F.F. Debra Fox
tlar@got.net
www.largeanimalrescue.com
(831) 635-9021

Sierra Rescue / Rescue 3 West—Rope and Water Training
Julie Munger
www.sierrarescue.com
(800) 208-2723

RESCUE 3—Rope and Water Training
Jenny@rescue3.com
(916) 687-6556
www.rescue3international.com

Surface Ice Training
Team Lifeguard Services, Inc.
http://teamlgs.com
(845) 657-5544

Equine and Bovine Rescue Training Mannequins
www.resquip.com

References

References can be found on the companion website at www.equine-emergencies.com.

EMG

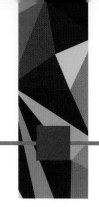

CHAPTER 38

Emergency Treatment of Mules and Donkeys

Alexandra J. Burton, Linda D. Mittel, and Jay Merriam

Introduction: Important Facts

- Donkeys and mules are often medically treated as horses; however, there are significant differences that are important in emergency and critical care of the donkey and mule.
- Donkeys and mules are very stoic and may *not* exhibit severe signs of pain with gastrointestinal disease or laminitis.
- *Practice Tip: Anorexia in a donkey can rapidly lead to hyperlipemia, a life-threatening complication with any disease.*
- *Practice Tip: Donkeys, both foals and adults, are prone to hypothermia in cold weather!*
- *Important:* Donkeys bond strongly with each other and with other animals and therefore critically ill donkeys should *not* be separated from their companions during treatment if at all possible.
  - Simply removing a donkey from its usual surroundings and herd mates can lead to pining and anorexia.
  - Two options:
    - Continue treatment in the field.
    - Bring a companion to the hospital if intensive therapy is needed.
- Donkeys are often longer-lived than horses, often reaching their 30s and 40s.
- Many of the common medical problems in developed countries are related to old age and domestication, most importantly overfeeding; donkeys have lower energy requirements than horses.
- Normal vital signs—temperature, pulse, and respiration—for donkeys are in Table 38-1.
- Gestation length is variable (11 to 13 months) but average is 365 days; twins may be seen more frequently than in horses.

Clinical Pathology

- *Practice Tip: Donkeys and mules often have muscle covering the middle third of the jugular vein; samples are best collected from the proximal one third of the vein. This is especially true when they resist handling; broken and bent needles may occur.*
- Donkeys have some differences in their hematologic and biochemical data:

- They have a higher mean corpuscular volume and mean corpuscular hemoglobin, and a variable red blood cell count.
- Packed cell volume may be somewhat higher in younger donkeys.
- Donkeys *do not* usually show an increase in packed cell volume until they are significantly (12% to 15%) dehydrated.
- Creatinine and total bilirubin are lower, and alkaline phosphatase is higher than in horses.
- Triglycerides can also be higher and more variable in normal donkeys; triglyceride values correlate with body condition score (i.e., thin donkeys have the lowest level and obese donkeys the highest). The same is true for very-low-density lipoproteins.
- Insulin levels are lower (2.1 ± 2.05 μU/mL), and adrenocorticotropic hormone (ACTH) levels are higher (66.7 ± 20.7 pg/mL) in donkeys.
- Normal values for thyroid hormone (T_3 and T_4); vary depending upon the laboratory method and are *not* greatly different from normal horse values.
- The serum is paler in color in donkeys and mules than in horses.

Commonly Encountered Conditions
Colic

- *Practice Tip: Large-colon impactions are the most common cause for colic in donkeys. The most common sites in decreasing order are:*
  - Pelvic flexure
  - Cecum
  - Small colon/rectum
- Donkeys with impactions are often depressed or dull with reduced appetite and frequently *do not* exhibit the typical signs of colic.
- The mortality rate from large-colon impaction in donkeys is reported to be high at approximately 50%.
- Risk factors identified for large-colon impaction in donkeys include:
  - Dental pathology
  - Recent weight loss
  - Concentrate feeding
  - Reduced access to pasture and an increased tendency to ingest gravel, sand, etc.

Table 38-1	Normal Temperature, Pulse, and Respiratory Rate	
	Young Donkey <2 Years	**Mature Donkey**
Pulse (beats/min)	44-80	44-68
Respiration (breaths/min)	28-48	13-31
Temperature °F/°C	99.6-102.1/37.6-38.9	98.8-100/37.1-37.8

- Donkeys should be fed high-fiber and high-concentrate feeds, *not* lush pasture or hay.
- The typical "colic" signs shown with more severe gastrointestinal pain are the following:
  - Rolling from sternal to lateral
  - Kicking at the abdomen
- Donkeys develop diarrhea readily with stress and small changes in feed.
- Liver pain from hyperlipemia may also present as colic.
- Colic in donkeys and mules may be similar to that in horses although mules are more stoic.
- With severe parasitism, donkeys frequently develop rectal prolapse (see Chapter 18, p. 215).
- Colic is also associated with severe parasitism (may be large and small strongyles) and is seen in both developed and underdeveloped countries.

●〉 WHAT TO DO

Colic in Donkeys
- Treatment for colic in donkeys is the same as for horses (see Chapter 18, p. 190).
- ***Practice Tip:*** *Use caution when holding "fat" donkeys off feed because of the tendency to develop hyperlipemia. Unlike horses, keeping a small amount of hay available to colicky donkeys allows one to monitor status and limit the hyperlipemia.*
- Withholding feed from donkeys, especially those that are overweight and for more than 24 hours, requires that intravenous supplementation (glucose or partial parenteral nutrition) be given.
- Use a smaller-diameter nasogastric tube because the ventral meatus is smaller than in a pony of similar stature.
- Donkeys have a very thick body wall; therefore, a 3½-inch (8.75-cm) spinal needle or metal teat cannula or bitch catheter may be needed for abdominocentesis.

Laminitis
- The foot of a donkey is normally more upright than that of a horse, with thicker soles and hoof walls.
- Donkeys rarely require shoes even in work because the horn is tough and hard.
- ***Practice Tip:*** *Hoof testers are* not *a reliable diagnostic tool in donkeys; a mule's foot is similar to a horse.*
- Donkeys are at risk for laminitis, especially if overweight.
- Clinical signs include reluctance to move, slow "stiff" movement, and weight shifting. ***Note:*** Many nonlaminitic, normal donkeys are also reluctant to move in unfamiliar situations or surroundings!

- Older donkeys may have chronic laminitis in all four feet because of previous disease, which goes unnoticed because of the donkey's stoic nature.
- Unilateral founder after a severe lameness (e.g., foot abscess) in the contralateral limb is also common.
- Insulin resistance (IR) may be an important factor associated with laminitis; insulin levels are useful in identifying donkeys at risk for laminitis.
- Laminitis is rarely seen in developing countries, and hoof problems there are usually due to neglect, lack of trimming, and lack of trained farriers.
- The radiographic anatomy of the donkey foot and the changes with laminitis *do not* follow those seen in the horse.
  - Comprehensive measurements are available in a manuscript by Collins et al, 2011 (see Bibliography).
  - The main differences are:
    - Dorsal hoof wall slope (steeper)
    - Alignment of the phalanges
    - Position of the third phalanx (P3) relative to the hoof wall
  - The third phalanx is *not* in line with the coronary band in the laminitic donkey foot because it is positioned more distally in the hoof capsule than in the normal horse.
- ***Practice Tip:*** *The laminitic donkey's foot has increases in angular deviation between the dorsal aspect of P3 and dorsum of the hoof wall, phalangeal rotation, and increased distal displacement of P3.*

●〉 WHAT TO DO

Laminitis
- If sole padding is used, support the sole and *do not* elevate the heel.
- Provide deep bedding, sand, or a soft paddock.
- Nonsteroidal anti-inflammatory drugs (NSAIDs) are well tolerated in adult donkeys. A dosage of 4.4 mg/kg phenylbutazone q12h for long treatment periods generally has few clinical side effects. However, mild anorexia and diarrhea was reported in a small number of miniature donkeys receiving phenylbutazone at 4.4 mg/kg IV q12h for 12 days in an experimental model. Firocoxib (Equioxx[1]), 0.1 mg/kg PO q24h is an alternative especially in older donkeys because of its excellent safety profile.
- In acute laminitis, on a short-term basis, NSAIDs may need to be dosed more frequently (q8h) because NSAIDs are excreted more rapidly in donkeys than in horses. The pharmacokinetics of NSAIDs in mules is similar to horses.
- Lidocaine constant rate infusion (CRI) at one half the dose for horses (i.e., 0.025 mg/kg/min) may be used as adjunctive analgesia in severe cases.

●〉 WHAT NOT TO DO

Laminitis
- Foot radiographs should *not* be interpreted with reference baselines for horses.

[1]Equioxx (Merial LLC, Duluth, GA 30096-4540).

- Elevating the heel in a laminitic donkey may make the patient more uncomfortable. If in doubt, leave barefoot on deep bedding.
- Scapulohumeral (shoulder) joint arthritis often complicates treating laminitis in older donkeys.

Hyperlipemia

- *Practice Tip: Hyperlipemia in donkeys, triglycerides >500 mg/dL (5.6 mmol/L), is probably the most common critical illness in donkeys in developed countries because of overfeeding and obesity.*
- Mortality rates are reported from 60% to 80% and increase with increasing peak serum triglyceride concentration. Serum triglyceride levels in donkeys are variable and generally run higher than in horses.
- *Practice Tip: Triglycerides normally are <200 mg/dL (2.26 mmol/L), and in healthy donkeys the highest triglyceride values are reported to be 144 mg/dL (1.6 mmol/L).*
  - Hyperlipemia is accelerated by:
    - Reduced appetite or anorexia (commonly due to dental disease or laminitis)
    - Stress
    - Pregnancy
    - Lactation
    - Pituitary pars intermedia syndrome (PPID; Cushing's syndrome)
  - In a case-control study of 449 donkeys with clinical hyperlipemia, concurrent disease (present in 72% of cases) was the greatest risk factor for development of hyperlipemia.
  - In some studies, older, obese females are reported to be most at risk, but no sex or body condition score predilection was identified.
- Hyperlipemia is considered relatively common in sick miniature donkey foals.
  - Donkeys that had suffered a weight loss of ≥10 kg (22 lb) in the preceding 6 months had more than six times an increased the risk of developing hyperlipemia.
  - *All donkeys are most likely to develop hyperlipemia after moving to a new environment and population of animals, which is a stressful situation.*
- Risk factors for hyperlipemia include:
  - Sporadic feeding of concentrate meals
  - *Practice Tip: Donkeys are "trickle eaters," eating 14 or more hours per day, and thus feeding concentrate may interrupt this pattern.*
  - Bedding on cardboard or paper, which may provide bulk when ingested but no energy
  - A donkey brought into a strange hospital environment with a concurrent illness
- The clinical signs are the same as in ponies but more subtle. **Important:** In developing countries these clinical signs may signal other illnesses because hyperlipemia is rarely seen due to the low weight and poor condition of donkeys:
  - Reduced appetite or anorexia
  - Depression/lethargy

- Intermittent abdominal pain
- Elevated temperature
- Weakness and incoordination
- Signs of liver failure: icterus, ventral edema, hepatic encephalopathy (circling, head pressing, seizures) (see Chapter 20, p. 268)

●› WHAT TO DO

Hyperlipemia

- Treatment is the same as for horses and consists of enteral feeding and intravenous administration of glucose with or without insulin (see p. 272).
- Mild to moderate cases of hyperlipemia are better managed in the field because the donkey is less stressed and more likely to begin eating again.
- Enteral nutrition: commercially prepared critical equine care meals or homemade gruels consisting of alfalfa meal, KCl, baking soda, and glucose solutions are easily prepared in the emergency situation (see Enteral Treatment to follow).
- *Practice Tip: If using a commercial diet, feed only 50% of the calculated requirements initially, working toward 100% of the intended requirements by day 4; this decreases the risk of gastrointestinal upset.*
- Anabolic steroids (stanozolol, 0.5 mg/kg IM once a week) are used in donkeys that are persistently anorectic to stimulate appetite and counteract catabolism.
- *Important:* A complicating factor in donkeys with hyperlipemia is the development of pancreatitis in the more severe cases, as in dogs and humans. The pancreas becomes inflamed and edematous with adhesions to the surrounding organs. Peritonitis with red/brown cloudy fluid is found on abdominocentesis. Plasma amylase and lipase concentrations may also be elevated. **Note:** *Pancreatitis carries a grave prognosis.*
- *Note:* For severe cases, regular insulin given PRN or CRI is preferred (see p. 273)

Enteral Treatment Guidelines

- If plasma triglycerides (TG) are 200 to 500 mg/dL (2.26 to 5.65 mmol/L), use the following:
  - 100 g glucose, 5 g sodium bicarbonate powder plus an oral multivitamin preparation PO q12h
  - 30 IU protamine zinc insulin SQ once or twice daily
- If plasma TG are 500 to 800 mg/dL (5.65 to 9.0 mmol/L) and the plasma is cloudy, use the following:
  - 100 g glucose, 5 g sodium bicarbonate powder plus an oral multivitamin preparation in 2 to 3 L water by nasogastric tube q12h
  - 30 IU protamine zinc insulin SQ q12h
- If plasma TG are 800 to 1500 mg/dL (9.0 to 17.0 mmol/L) and the plasma is off-white, use the following:
  - 2 L balanced electrolyte solution and 200 mL 50% dextrose IV q24h
  - Drench or stomach tube q12 to 24h with enteral nutrition or homemade gruels as recommended previously.
  - 30 IU protamine zinc insulin q12h SQ
  - Flunixin meglumine, 1.1 mg/kg
  - Broad-spectrum antibiotics

- If TGs are more than 1500 mg/dL (17.0 mmol/L) (often cloudy orange color due to hyperlipemia and icterus), then treatment is more aggressive, using both enteral support and insulin treatments (see p. 272 and supportive care fluids, etc.).

Respiratory Disease

- Donkeys normally have a higher respiratory rate than horses, and their pulmonary dynamics are more similar to cattle, with increased total pulmonary resistance and a reduced dynamic compliance.
- Donkeys can be infected with equine influenza virus and develop more severe illness than horses.
- Risk of secondary bacterial pneumonia is high with viral respiratory diseases and therefore early prophylactic antimicrobial treatment is recommended.
- Chronic interstitial fibrosing pneumonia (pulmonary fibrosis) is relatively common in donkeys; because of their nonathletic nature, loss of lung function can be significant before clinical signs are evident.
- Donkeys may suffer from recurrent airway obstruction (RAO).

●〉 WHAT TO DO

Lower Respiratory Disease
- Aggressive supportive therapy (see Chapter 25, p. 474):
  - Oxygen
  - Anti-inflammatories
  - Bronchodilators
  - Antibiotics for secondary bacterial pneumonia
  - Ensure that the donkey continues to eat and *if not,* enteral or parenteral nutrition should be given.

Tracheal Collapse
- ***Practice Tip:*** *As in Miniature Horses, tracheal collapse can occur in donkeys and is more common in older donkeys.*
- The condition is more likely in the presence of pulmonary fibrosis or other diseases causing increased respiratory effort and negative pressure (e.g., RAO).
- The site of collapse is most commonly in the distal cervical trachea at the thoracic inlet because the tracheal rings are more dorsoventrally flattened in this location.
- Tracheal endoscopy is difficult in donkeys because they swallow quickly when the larynx is touched/stimulated.
- Donkeys have more pharyngeal collapse than horses on inspiration and become distressed with soft palate displacement.
- Acute clinical signs:
  - Anxiety/distress
  - Difficulty breathing, attempted oral/mouth breathing
  - Respiratory stertor and honking, increased noise on tracheal auscultation
  - Palpable tracheal vibrations
- Chronic clinical signs:
  - Increased inspiratory and expiratory effort
  - Chronic cough

- Tracheal narrowing can be identified on radiographs. In mild and/or chronic cases, endoscopy may be useful in the diagnosis.

●〉 WHAT TO DO

Tracheal Collapse
- Oxygen
- Corticosteroids (IV and/or inhaled)
- Bronchodilators (see Chapter 25, p. 475)
- IV atropine and furosemide are given for rapid bronchodilation and reduction of airway edema in an acute crisis.
- ***Note:*** Because tracheal collapse is more likely to occur in conjunction with lower respiratory disease, it is recommended to identify, treat, and manage any underlying conditions such as RAO, pulmonary fibrosis, or bacterial pneumonia.

Neonatal Isoerythrolysis
- Clinical neonatal isoerythrolysis (NI) occurs in approximately 10% of mule foals, and it is likely that all mare-donkey matings produce sensitization with subclinical NI.
- Nearly all recognized cases are mule foals born from mares that have delivered previous mule foals.
- Mule foals may also suffer immune-mediated thrombocytopenia with or without NI.
- ***Important:*** All multiparturient mares (or mares with unknown history) bred to jacks should have their blood tested for antidonkey red blood cell antibodies at 2 to 3 weeks before foaling. Send mare serum to the University of California, Davis for testing (530-752-1303). Gestation is 365 days, and twins may be seen more frequently than in horses.

●〉 WHAT TO DO

Neonatal Isoerythrolysis
- Treatment is the same as horse foals with NI (see Chapter 20, p. 280).
- ***Practice Tip:*** *Donkeys, mules, and even zebras can be administered horse whole blood or plasma but a cross match is recommended.*

Castration and Wound Problems
- There are many references suggesting donkeys and mules have a greater tendency to bleed after castration than do horses because of the relatively large testicles, thicker scrotum, and larger blood vessels, all of which increase the chance of hemorrhaging.
- It is generally *not* recommended to do standing castrations. Many veterinarians prefer to use an emasculator with a crushing action separate from the cutting surface. Cutting off the bottom of the scrotum may cause increased bleeding. The use of the Henderson castration device has almost totally eliminated postoperative bleeding when done as a closed procedure. Use of a modified scrotal ablation is also helpful as there are many more scrotal vessels in the skin than in horses or mules. Stripping of the cord is also more difficult. The use of lidocaine locally is very helpful in relaxing the cord and prolongs anesthesia.

- Donkeys should be vaccinated for tetanus; this disease is seen commonly in developing countries.
- Donkeys commonly receive bite wounds or other skin injuries such as dermatophilosis and ulcerative lymphangitis. Treat these problems as in horses (see Chapter 19, p. 241).
- Saddle sores and deep wounds tend to fibrose more than in horses and mules.

Reproduction/Foaling

- Donkeys are similar to horses in breeding and foaling with several notable differences:
  - The gestation length is about 370 days with a range from 360 to 380 days.
  - Miniature donkey gestation length varies from 342 days to 13 months (390 days).
  - Twins may be seen more frequently.
  - Donkey mares foal in either day or night.
- Characteristics of premature donkey foals are:
  - Weakness
  - Low birth weight
  - Delays in standing
  - Ears flopped downward and backward; this occurs with most donkey illnesses.
- Donkey foals are *not* very hardy and require shelter for the first 2 to 4 weeks of life.
- A rain-soaked donkey foal that develops hypothermia can rapidly progress to death.
- *Practice Tip: Donkeys (all ages) are prone to hypothermia! These donkeys may have hypothyroid dysfunction predisposing them to hypothermia.*
- *Note:* Dystocia is increased in Miniature donkeys because of their larger domed heads.

⏺❯ WHAT TO DO

Foaling
- Make sure the donkey foal is dry, has warm shelter, and nurses within 2 to 2.5 hours postpartum. Provide additional heat if needed.
- Check IgG 12 to 18 hours after birth to determine adequate IgG absorption (>800 mg/dL).
- If the donkey foal has difficulty maintaining body temperature, check thyroid function.

Pharmacology

- Pharmacokinetics of drugs is often different compared with horses, although many compounds have *not* been studied specifically in donkeys.
- *Practice Tip: Elimination of flunixin meglumine after a single dose, 1.1 mg/kg IV, is significantly faster in donkeys than in horses and mules.*
  - Controlled studies have *not* been done, but recommendations are a shorter dosing interval for flunixin meglumine when used in donkeys.
- Similarly, phenylbutazone clearance after a single dose, 4.4 mg/kg IV, is fivefold greater in donkeys compared with

horses (mules not studied), and the dosing interval is usually shortened. Mules are believed to have clearance values more like horses.
- In donkeys requiring more analgesia, phenylbutazone is dosed at 4.4 mg/kg IV q8h in the short term.
- Clearance of a single dose of sulfamethoxazole, 12.5 mg/kg, and trimethoprim, 2.5 mg/kg, is twice as fast in donkeys as in mules or horses, thus the need for shorter dosing intervals in donkeys.
- *Practice Tip: When administering a lidocaine constant rate infusion for analgesia, start with half the dose for horses (i.e., only 0.025 mg/kg per minute) to avoid ataxia; some donkeys will need a slightly higher dose. A possible explanation for this phenomenon is delayed hepatic clearance in cases of hepatic lipidosis although* no *evidence-based studies have been done.*

Differences in Pharmacology
Anesthesia of Donkeys and Mules

- A 50% increase in sedative dose is frequently needed to provide acceptable sedation in a mule or feral/unhandled donkey: xylazine, 1.6 mg/kg IV, or detomidine, 0.03 mg/kg IV.
- Domesticated donkeys appear to require a similar dosage to horses.
- Butorphanol, 0.4 mg/kg IV, or diazepam, 0.3 mg/kg, should be combined with alpha$_2$-drugs for increased sedation.
- *Practice Tip: Ketamine, 2 to 3 mg/kg IV, is the most commonly used injectable anesthetic. The half-life of ketamine is shorter in donkeys and mules; therefore, repeated dosing or continuous administration of a triple drip (see Chapter 47, pp. 738 and 744) may be required for procedures lasting more than 10 to 15 minutes.*
- Donkeys require *less* guaifenesin than horses; the guaifenesin concentration in the triple drip should be reduced by 40%.
- Miniature donkeys are reported to be more difficult to anesthetize than other donkeys, and therefore after sedation with xylazine and butorphanol, Telazol[2] (tiletamine and zolazepam), 1.1 to 1.5 mg/kg IV, or propofol, 2 mg/kg IV, may be used in place of ketamine. When donkeys receive alpha-agonists for tranquilization, sneezing may occur; this is likely a unique feature in donkeys and not other equines although nasal besnoitiosis should be ruled out as a cause.
- *Note:* Intubation is more difficult than in the horse because the larynx is tilted more caudally with a shorter epiglottis.
- Donkeys have a very narrow trachea for their size; the average 180-kg (396-lb) donkey requires approximately a 16-mm internal diameter endotracheal tube (range, 14 to 18 mm).

---

[2]Telazol (Fort Dodge Animal Health Division of Wyeth, a subsidiary of Pfizer, Inc., 235 E. 42nd St., New York, New York, 10017).

- The weight of donkeys and mules can be estimated by heart girth measurement using tapes intended for horses.

Vaccinations

- Donkeys and mules should be vaccinated similarly to horses. Rabies, tetanus, and other infectious diseases are seen as real threats in developing countries.

Humane Destruction

- Donkeys and mules are humanely destroyed the same as with horses, but additional euthanasia solution may be needed.
- If a donkey must be euthanized and has been stabled with an inseparable companion, it is recommended to let the healthy donkey spend 30 minutes or so with the euthanized companion to prevent excessive pining and searching for his companion, which may lead to hyperlipemia.
- *Note:* Donkeys and mules are the backbone of developing countries and are the sole providers for many families. Many of the diseases and conditions seen in developed countries are not recognized in these developing countries and vice versa.

References

References can be found on the companion website at www.equine-emergencies.com.

EMG

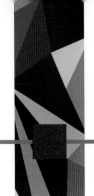

CHAPTER 39

Emergency Problems Unique to Draft Horses

Samuel D. A. Hurcombe

Important Clinical Points—Draft Horses

- Draft horses are large, heavy breeds of horses characterized by tall stature (>16 hands), heavy muscular build, and large body size (>1400 lb). Common breeds include Percheron, Belgian, Shire, and Clydesdale, and they are often used in pulling, plowing, and farm labor.
- Breed differences exist regarding specific conditions, challenges in diagnostics, and treatment of the critically ill Draft horse, when compared with lighter breeds. These differences are often attributable to the Draft horse's large size, heavy body weight, and often stoic nature.
- Draft horses may express pain in subtle, less violent ways compared with other breeds, and veterinarians should interpret changes in behavior or physiologic parameters (i.e., elevated heart rate, respiratory rate) with greater scrutiny.
- When dosing medications and fluids to large breed horses, the veterinarian should consider using a low end of a dosing range and be somewhat conservative with dosing on a per-kilogram or per-pound basis.
- If not conservative in "routine" dosing practices, overdosing of medications/fluids may result, compared with a more accurate, but less practical dosing based on body surface area. Conservative dosing is especially recommended for the following: cardiovascular medications, tranquilizers, sedatives, and anesthetic agents.

Colic

- Gastrointestinal emergencies occur in Draft breeds as with any other type of horse.
- Intact males have a predisposition for inguinal/scrotal hernia causing intestinal obstruction and pain and as such, palpation of the inguinal rings and scrotum is important when evaluating male horses for colic.
- The clinical signs of abdominal pain can be subtle in Draft breeds, and any suspected signs of colic should not go without further investigation.
- Draft horses undergoing colic surgery have a higher mortality rate than light breed horses. One study found that horses weighing >680 kg had longer duration of anesthesia, more postoperative morbidity, and an overall short-term survival rate of 60% compared with horses weighing <680 kg.
- The most common surgical lesions are related to the ascending colon (right displacement and large-colon volvulus). It is theorized that colonic displacements/volvulus

may occur more commonly in Draft breeds because of their large body size and an increased potential for colon movement, although this is not evidence based.
- Nonsurvival in Draft horses undergoing colic surgery was associated with the horse having a small intestinal lesion or developing postoperative complications including myositis, peripheral neuropathy, ileus, diarrhea, and endotoxemia.
- One of the most significant determinants of survival from surgical colic is early referral and thus intervention, which is true for all horses and particularly with Draft breeds.

Clinical Signs and Diagnosis of Colic

- As for any other horse with colic
- Abnormalities on rectal examination may be difficult to palpate; palpate inguinal rings
- Complete a thorough evaluation including nasogastric intubation, even if signs are subtle or intermittent

●〉 WHAT TO DO

Colic

- Refer horse with any of the following to a surgical facility: moderate to severe and/or persistent pain; small-intestinal distention, and/or enterogastric reflux; tight colonic taenial bands on rectal examination; scrotal enlargement; serosanguineous and/or turbid abdominocentesis; any horse with pain refractory to analgesics.
- Transport the horse with a long, indwelling nasogastric tube left in place with the end facing away from the eyes. If capped, have owners stop to decompress or cover end of the tube with an exam glove from which the fingers have been cut off (to act as a Heimlich valve).
- Assess degree of dehydration and/or shock and begin intravenous fluid therapy if >5% dehydrated and continue en route to a referral facility if possible (see Chapter 18, p. 190).
- Early referral is of paramount importance to help maximize the patient's prognosis for survival.

◇〉 WHAT NOT TO DO

Colic

- Do not misinterpret outward subtle clinical signs of low-grade pain. Some horses have severe life-threatening lesions and display minimal signs.
- Do not administer acepromazine as an analgesic agent to a horse with colic.

Castration and Postcastration Emergencies

- Male Draft horses, along with Tennessee Walking horses and Standardbreds, are at higher risk of congenital and acquired inguinal herniation of bowel compared with many light breeds because of the large size of the inguinal canal and rings.
- Because of the large inguinal rings and canal, routine open castration poses a risk of intestinal evisceration. In one study of 568 juvenile Draft colts (4 to 5 months of age), small-intestinal evisceration occurred in 4.8% and omental herniation was observed in 2.8% (7.6% of all colts either eviscerated or herniated). Therefore, many clinicians prefer to castrate at a young age before sexual maturity and adopt a semiclosed or closed castration technique ensuring that the common vaginal tunic is closed.
- A study of 131 Draft colts undergoing routine field castration in which the common vaginal tunic was ligated in addition to routine Serra emasculation reduced the incidence of omental herniation/intestinal evisceration (1/131; 0.76%).
- Strict adherence to sterile technique is required, particularly if the vaginal tunic is closed with absorbable suture, to minimize infection and development of scirrhous cord.
- If referral is an option, external ring closure may also assist in reducing the risk of bowel herniation through a castration site and is best performed under general anesthesia.

Postcastration Herniation/Evisceration

For what to do and what not to do, see Chapter 24, p. 432, Stallion Reproductive Emergencies.

Conditions Related to Recumbency Including General Anesthesia

- Because of their large size, specific problems can occur in Draft horses as a consequence of prolonged recumbency. As such, every effort should be made to minimize anesthesia times (i.e., during field procedures such as castration) as well as quickly addressing any reason why the equine patient might not be standing (e.g., musculoskeletal/neurologic disorders, colic, etc.).
- The clinician should always consider if a procedure can be performed safely and effectively in the standing patient; however, if general anesthesia is required, every effort should be made to minimize surgery times and optimize oxygen delivery and perfusion.
- Anesthesia-related complications of particular importance include:
  - Ventilation-perfusion mismatch contributing to hypercapnia and hypoxemia
  - Myositis due to pressure and poor perfusion
  - Myelitis/neuropathy related to compression and/or poor perfusion
- Since perfusion is critical to the delivery of oxygen and nutrients to the tissues, every effort should be made to optimize cardiac output and perfusion pressures when Draft breeds are anesthetized:

- Intravenous fluids (balanced isotonic electrolyte solution)
- Inotropic support using dobutamine
- As low as possible flow/administration rates of depressant anesthetic agents (particularly inhalant drugs)
- Time is likely the most significant factor in reducing anesthetic-related complications and should be kept as short as possible.
- Decubital ulcers, pleuritis/pneumonia, and traumatic keratitis may occur in the recumbent patient, and preventative measures such as soft bedding, fluorescein eye staining, and the judicious use of antimicrobials may be indicated.

The Recumbent Patient

For what to do and what not to do for the recumbent Draft horse, see Chapter 36, p. 626.

- Anesthetic recovery can be challenging for Draft horses especially with a musculoskeletal injury, neurologic disease, prolonged anesthesia, and weak/underweight patients.
- In many instances, assistance may be required for certain patients using a hoist and sling to assist the patient to stand. This requires a team approach and should be implemented *before* the patient fatigues too quickly from repeated ineffective attempts to stand.
- Provision of intravenous glucose and calcium is advocated by some to "recharge" the muscle with energy and myocontractile nutrients, particularly in weak or exhausted horses. If polysaccharide storage myopathy (PSSM) is suspected, intravenous lipids (0.1 g/kg) are administered over 30 minutes with the goal of supplying a "useable" energy source.

◉› WHAT TO DO

The Recumbent Draft Horse Having Difficulty Rising

- Use low-dose sedative/tranquilization to minimize struggling and overexertion.
- If indicated, use a sling if the horse has made several failed attempts to stand. Do not remove sling support too quickly; allow sufficient time (30 minutes to several hours) for reperfusion of compressed tissues and for potential neurapraxia from nerve compression to resolve. Time may also be dictated somewhat by the temperament of the patient and acceptance of sling application.
- If the horse is weak/exhausted, provide intravenous volume support to maintain perfusion, notably to compressed muscles/nerves. The addition of dextrose (2% to 4% solutions) and calcium (calcium gluconate—4 g/1000 mL isotonic fluids = 20 cc of 23% solution/1 L crystalloid solution).
- Provide analgesia for compression myositis/exertion in the form of NSAIDs; flunixin meglumine at 0.5 to 1.0 mg/kg IV.
- Wrap distal limbs with support bandages to minimize self-trauma during attempts to stand.
- When sling assistance is unavailable and the horse is fatigued, some experienced clinicians have advocated the use of doxapram hydrochloride as a general central nervous stimulant following adequate

IV fluid and analgesia administration. Although this treatment may cause adverse cardiac and neurologic effects, one or two doses of doxapram, 0.1 to 0.2 mg/kg IV, may stimulate the horse to make a more deliberate attempt to stand and has been used with variable success by the author and colleagues. Multiple repeat dosing is not recommended (personal communication).

◉❯ WHAT NOT TO DO

The Recumbent Draft Horse Having Difficulty Rising

- *Do not* use excessive force/coercion if the horse is clearly unable to make effective attempts to stand. Muscle fatigue, sweating, myositis, hyperthermia, and exhaustion can occur quickly. These horses are best managed by rest and supportive measures until assistance by way of a sling can be implemented.

Myopathies in Draft Horses

- Several myopathies can affect Draft horse breeds resulting in significant pain, lameness, recumbency, and other associated sequelae.
- Polysaccharide storage myopathy (PSSM), atypical myopathy, exertional myopathy, and other suspected myopathies including the "shivers" can be problematic. PSSM is more common in European–origin Draft breeds (i.e., Percheron, Trekpaard, Comtois, Breton, and Belgium breeds) and uncommon in United Kingdom–origin Draft breeds (i.e., Shire and Clydesdale).

Clinical Signs

- Stiffness or soreness on palpation of large muscle groups (e.g., gluteals)
- Reluctance to ambulate or stiff gait with short strides
- Sweating, tachycardia, tachypnea, hyperthermia
- Pigmenturia
- Horses with shivers may show weakness, exaggerated hind limb flexion during ambulation that may worsen if asked to move sideways (laterally), tail elevation, difficulty backing up, difficulty keeping the hind feet held up during foot examination/farriery work

◉❯ WHAT TO DO

Myopathies in Draft Horses

- Establish intravenous access.
- Improve tissue perfusion: intravenous fluids such as isotonic, polyionic balanced electrolyte solutions are best at 1 to 2 times maintenance (i.e., 40 to 80 mL/kg/day) provided that the individual is able to produce urine. Hypertonic saline at 2 mL/kg IV helps recruit volume quickly but should be followed by isotonic fluids (see Chapter 32, p. 567).
- Administer analgesics: Nonsteroidal anti-inflammatory medications; flunixin meglumine, 0.5 to 1.0 mg/kg IV q12 to 24h or phenylbutazone, 2.2 to 4.4 mg/kg IV q12 to 24h.
- If hyperthermic, start external cooling strategies using fans, alcohol baths, cool water sponge baths, and ice packs over regions of high-volume blood flow (e.g., jugular veins and carotid artery). Cool intravenous fluids can lower core body temperatures.

- If PSSM is suspected, oral fats (vegetable oil) should be administered mixed in alfalfa pellets or via nasogastric tube ($\frac{1}{2}$ to 1 cup of oil for an adult Draft horse).
- See treatment as for exertional rhabdomyolysis (see Chapter 22, p. 359).

◉❯ WHAT NOT TO DO

Myopathies in Draft Horses

- Do not administer acepromazine for anxiolysis (to reduce anxiety). Resultant hypotension may decrease perfusion pressures.

Specific Reproductive Emergencies

- Draft horses are at risk of certain reproductive-/parturition-related emergencies compared with light breed horses.
  - Twinning in mares has been reported in Draft mares, notably Belgian mares. Draft mares may already be at risk of developing prepubic tendon rupture and body wall hernias, and twin pregnancy may be additive to the risk.

Dystocia

- Dystocia caused by malpresentation of the fetus to the birth canal can occur in Draft mares.
- In one study, transverse presentation was more commonly observed in Draft horses than other breeds. Transverse presentation can be particularly challenging to correct and may require fetotomy or cesarean section if assisted or controlled vaginal delivery fails (see p. 504).
- For any dystocia, controlled vaginal delivery may be the preferred method of dystocia correction despite the requirement of general anesthesia. This helps uterine relaxation and provides the manipulator a means of control and the ability to more easily manipulate the foal in the most expedient time frame.
- Quick resolution of the dystocia may negate the potential risks of general anesthesia and recovery.
- The mare should receive blood volume +/− blood pressure support throughout the procedure.
- For "simple" dystocia (i.e., dorsosacral anterior presentation with slight fetlock/carpal flexion), assisted vaginal delivery with the use of epidural anesthesia may be most appropriate and removes the concerns of general anesthesia and recovery in large mares.

Hypocalcemia

- Lactational hypocalcemia may occur in heavily lactating mares toward the end of the lactation period.
- Weakness, tachycardia, synchronous diaphragmatic flutter (thumps), and muscle fasciculations may be observed as a prolonged extracellular calcium drain occurs through lactation.
- If clinical signs of hypocalcemia/hypomagnesemia are present (see Chapter 17, pp. 144 and 145), serum ionized fractions of both calcium and magnesium should be determined to confirm the diagnosis.

EMG

- Supplemental calcium as calcium gluconate and weaning the foal is usually sufficient to correct the electrolyte derangement.
- Most cases are observed toward the end of the lactation period and therefore, weaning is usually not problematic for the foal.

Specific Neonatal Conditions

- Draft neonatal foals are at risk of common conditions such as septicemia, failure of transfer of passive immunity, neonatal maladjustment syndrome, and isoerythrolysis similar to other breeds.

Idiopathic Hyperthermia

- Disorders of temperature regulation can occur secondary to inflammatory conditions affecting the hypothalamus and thermoregulatory center.
- A peculiar condition, seen in some Draft breed foals in which hyperthermia of unknown origin occurs, has been recognized. Draft foals may be overrepresented in these cases as anecdotal reports have indicated.
- The term "idiopathic hyperthermia" has been suggested and is essentially characterized by a persistent rectal temperature >39°C (102°F), often exceeding 40° to 40.5°C (104° to 105°F) with no other apparent cause.
- Affected foals are often tachypneic without evidence of pulmonary pathology but otherwise are bright, alert, and still maintaining vigor during nursing and other interactions with the mare.
- The diagnosis is by exclusion; that is, ruling out another source of inflammation/infection such as septicemia, is important.
- Treatment is largely symptomatic; external cooling strategies may be employed to help reduce core temperatures. Although technically less effective than internal cooling methods, external cooling can be helpful. Evaporative cooling by using fans and water or isopropyl alcohol baths is the most practical.
- Room temperature to slightly cooled intravenous crystalloid fluids may offer an easy method of internal cooling to help reduce body temperature in these cases.
- Affected foals respond well to supportive treatment, and the condition usually resolves in 7 to 14 days.

Hereditary Diseases

- Junctional epidermolysis bullosa is a mechanobullous disease documented in neonatal Belgian foals characterized by basal epithelial cell layer cleft formation between the lamina densa of the basement membrane zone along the lamina lucida of the skin.
- Hemidesmosome and basement membrane protein disruption leads to cleft formation; erosion; and detachment of the skin, especially at pressure points.
- Clinical features in affected foals may include coronary band separation, sloughing of hooves, and erosions at mucocutaneous junctions and oral cavity.
- A homozygous mutation occurs in the LAMC2 gene that encodes for the production of a truncated laminin-γ2 protein, resulting in defective laminin-5, a protein distributed in the basement membrane of epithelial tissues.
- The mode of inheritance is believed to be autosomal recessive because both males and females can be affected.
- Genetic testing is available (see Chapter 13, p. 70).
- Affected foals are humanely destroyed because of skin and hoof loss in the neonatal period; the disease carries a grave prognosis for survival.

Specific Dermatological Conditions

- Pastern dermatitis, thickened skin, and edema of the distal hind limbs in Shires, Clydesdales, Belgian Draft horses, and less commonly in Gipsy Vanners, is usually due to chronic progressive edema.
- Chronic progressive edema may begin at an early age, is progressive, and almost certainly a genetic disease although no genetic test is currently available. Treatment is comprised of clipping the leg feathers, gently cleaning the area, treating bacterial dermatitis with antibiotics, oral administration of ivermectin, and application of fipronil[1] spray (every 1 to 2 weeks) if chorioptic mange mites are present.

References

References can be found on the companion website at www.equine-emergencies.com.

[1]Frontline (Merial Limited, Duluth, Georgia).

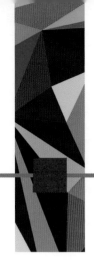

CHAPTER 40

Emergency Diseases Outside the Continental United States

Alexandre Secorun Borges, Tim Mair, Israel Pasval, Montague N. Saulez, Brett S. Tennent-Brown, and Andrew W. van Eps

AUSTRALIA AND NEW ZEALAND

Brett S. Tennent-Brown and Andrew W. van Eps

Actinobacillus equuli Peritonitis

- *Actinobacillus equuli* is a commonly recognized cause of acute sepsis and enteritis in neonatal foals.
- The organism is generally regarded as an opportunist in adult horses. However, in Australia, *A. equuli* is a relatively common cause of peritonitis; it is also common in the United States.

Epidemiology

- *A. equuli* is a normal inhabitant of the equine gastrointestinal and respiratory tracts; however, the source of infection in cases of peritonitis is unclear.
- No age, breed, or gender predilection is apparent.

Clinical Signs and Diagnosis

- There appear to be two forms of the disease:
  - Acute form—more common and may recur months or years later in the same horse
  - Chronic infection
- In the acute form, horses typically have signs of lethargy and mild to moderate abdominal pain.
- Horses with chronic infection have weight loss.
- Other reported signs include:
  - Depression
  - Reduced fecal output
  - Diarrhea
  - Straining to urinate or defecate
- Heart and respiratory rates are mildly to moderately increased, and the majority of affected horses have an increased rectal temperature.
- Gastrointestinal sounds are reduced or absent in most cases; rectal examination may reveal inspissated feces within the rectum or large intestine but is often unremarkable.
- Most horses have a normal peripheral white cell count but some have a leukocytosis or occasionally a leukopenia.

- Mild hemoconcentration is common, and plasma fibrinogen concentration is often increased; hypoproteinemia appears to occur only occasionally.
- Abdominal fluid from affected horses is grossly turbid with a greatly increased nucleated cell count and protein concentration.
- ***Practice Tip:*** *Abdominal fluid often has a characteristic orange, red, or brown color; the white cell count is commonly greater than 100,000 cells/mL, and nondegenerate neutrophils may predominate.* In one report, bacteria were seen in approximately half the cases in which fluid was examined cytologically.
- Diagnosis is based on clinical findings and results of the abdominocentesis. Definitive diagnosis requires a positive culture from the abdominal fluid; a pure growth of *A. equuli* was obtained in more than 70% of cases in one series.

●› WHAT TO DO

Actinobacillus equuli

- Treatment should initially consist of broad-spectrum antibiotics such as a beta-lactam/aminoglycoside combination, although the organism is often sensitive to penicillin and trimethoprim-sulfas.
- Culture and sensitivity results may be used to tailor antimicrobial therapy when they become available. Horses typically respond rapidly to antimicrobial therapy; however, recurrence has been reported in a few instances, and longer therapy—2 to 4 weeks—may be indicated.
- Anti-inflammatory drugs, such as flunixin meglumine, may be beneficial, although additional supportive care is often unnecessary.
- ***Note:*** Duration of treatment should be guided by:
  - Sequential peritoneal fluid white cell counts
  - Plasma fibrinogen concentration
  - Improved color of peritoneal fluid
- Most horses have an excellent prognosis if treated appropriately.

Balclutha Syndrome

- In 1998, 11 of 26 horses at a single training stable in New Zealand's southern South Island developed ulcers on the lingual and gingival mucosal surfaces.

- Two additional epidemics on 10 properties were subsequently identified.
- An infectious cause was strongly suspected, and transmission by direct contact seemed most likely.
- No age, gender, or breed predilection was identified.
- Although vesicles were occasionally observed, lesions progressed directly to ulcers in most horses.
- No lesions were observed outside the oral cavity, and affected horses remained afebrile, bright, and alert.
- Toxins, contact irritants, and other food- and water-related causes of the clinical signs were ruled out.
- Multiple diagnostic specimens were collected and submitted, but no causative agent was identified.
- Similar outbreaks of ulcerative stomatitis were also reported in New Zealand in the late 1980s and early 1990s. These also occurred in the autumn (fall), and a definitive diagnosis was not made in either case.
- *Practice Tip: The importance of this type of ulcerative condition is its resemblance to vesicular stomatitis (VS).*
- VS is a viral disease of horses and other livestock characterized by vesicular lesions on the tongue and oral mucous membranes. Lesions may also occur on the mammary glands, external genitalia, and coronary bands. The initial vesicular lesions of VS are often missed, and affected horses are usually first examined when they have ulcerative or erosive lesions.
- VS is classified by the Office International des Epizootics as a list A disease primarily because of its resemblance to foot-and-mouth disease. **Important:** Foot-and-mouth disease does not occur in equids.
- The implications of an outbreak of an ulcerative disease that could affect multiple species for countries that rely heavily on export of agricultural produce are obvious.
- It is essential that the appropriate regulatory authorities are contacted and quarantine procedures instituted should one encounter any type of ulcerative or vesicular condition in livestock.

Crofton Weed Poisoning (Numinbah Horse Sickness, Tallebudgera Horse Disease)

- Ingestion of the plant *Eupatorium adenophorum (Ageratina adenophora)* causes a pulmonary toxicosis characterized by increased respiratory effort.
- The plant is native to Mexico but now occurs as an intractable weed in many parts of the world, including Australia and New Zealand.
- In the 1940s, outbreaks of chronic respiratory disease in horses in New South Wales and Southern Queensland were linked to consumption of large quantities of *E. adenophora.*

Epidemiology

- In Australia, there are a large number of farms infested with *E. adenophora* with a history of pneumotoxicosis in horses.

- Respiratory disease caused by *E. adenophora* has also been reported in New Zealand.
- In initial reports, horses of both sexes aged between 18 months and 12 years were affected.
- The putative toxins appear to be absorbed from the gastrointestinal tract, and inhalation of plant material (e.g., pollen) is not required for disease.
- Ingestion of large amounts of plant material is required for intoxication, and *E. adenophora* are readily ingested by horses.
- *Practice Tip: Feeding studies have shown that flowering stages of the plant are more toxic than nonflowering stages.*
- Most cases appear in the summer after ingestion of plants in the spring and a minimum of 2 months after first exposure.
- *E. riparium* is a perennial weed in Queensland and New South Wales. Although feeding samples of *E. riparium* produce lesions similar to *E. adenophora*, field cases have not been reported.

Clinical Signs

- The first and most prominent clinical sign is coughing, exacerbated by exercise.
- Decreased exercise tolerance is seen.
- Rapid, heaving respiration with a double expiratory effort may occur.
- Adventitial sounds, often increased after exercise, are heard on auscultation of the lungs.
- In severely affected chronic cases, there may be weight loss and cyanosis.
- Cardiac arrhythmias develop in some horses and can result in sudden death.

Pathology

- The pneumotoxin of *E. adenophora* is unknown.
- Pyrrolizidine alkaloids (PAs) are suspected because of the similarities of lesions to *Crotalaria*-associated lung disease ("jaagsiekte") of horses in South Africa and Northern Australia.
- Pulmonary fibrosis is seen at necropsy, and there may be cavities within the pulmonary parenchyma containing necrotic material.
- In some cases the lung septa are distended with edema.
- In historic descriptions, the lungs of chronically affected horses were firm and did not collapse upon opening of the thoracic cavity.
- The visceral pleura is white and thickened, and there are focal adhesions to the parietal pleura.
- In cases of sudden death, there may be hydrothorax, pulmonary edema and emphysema, hydropericardium, and dilation of the heart.
- Histopathologic examination is confirmatory and reveals sheets of epithelial-like cells lining the alveoli. In most chronic cases, clumps of inspissated protein are present in the alveoli. Many bronchioles and surrounding alveoli are filled with eosinophils and neutrophils.

EMG

●> WHAT TO DO

Crofton Weed Poisoning
- The condition is irreversible, and no effective therapy is recognized.
- Antibiotics and corticosteroids have improved some cases.

Hendra Virus

- In September 1994, infection with Hendra virus (HeV; formally equine morbillivirus) caused acute respiratory disease and death in 14 horses and one human in Brisbane, Australia.
- Including this original outbreak, there were 14 subsequent separate incidents of HeV until 2011.
- In 2011, there were an additional 18 separate HeV incidents (10 in Queensland and 8 in New South Wales), which represented a marked increase in incidence and a wider distribution than previously reported into Western Queensland and further south into New South Wales.
- In total, confirmed natural infections have been documented in 56 horses, 1 dog (seroconversion with no clinical signs), and 7 humans (4 human deaths).
- The original outbreak manifested clinically as acute respiratory disease, whereas the overwhelming clinical presentation in all cases since the 2008 Redlands outbreak has been acute neurologic disease.

Epidemiology

- HeV is closely related to Nipah virus, and together they form the genus *Henipavirus* in the family Paramyxoviridae.
- *Practice Tip: Epidemiologic evidence indicates that fruit bats (flying foxes or Pteropodidae) are the natural reservoir for HeV, with sporadic "spill-over" of HeV to horses being the cause of natural horse infections.*
- HeV has been found in the urine, uterine fluids, placental material, and aborted pups of infected fruit bats, and it has been suggested that ingestion of feed or water contaminated with these materials may be the primary means by which horses become naturally infected.
- The majority of horse cases have occurred from June to December, showing some correlation with the mid-late pregnancy/birthing period of the major flying fox species.
- The index case on most occasions has been a horse kept outside in an area attractive to flying foxes.
- Horse-to-horse spread has occurred most efficiently when horses have been stabled together but can less commonly occur in a paddock situation.
- *Practice Tip: Spread from horse-to-horse, and horse-to-human, appears to require close contact with body fluids, particularly respiratory secretions. HeV may also survive on fomites for a period of hours.*
- HeV utilizes cell surface protein receptors (ephrin-B2 and ephrim-B3) that are widespread in vascular endothelium.
- Vasculitis, particularly in the respiratory and central nervous systems, leads to respiratory and/or neurologic signs.

- A minor genetic change in the virus structure may have led to the predominance of neurologic signs in cases after 2008.
- *Important:* The serious zoonotic risk that HeV presents to veterinarians in the eastern states of Australia necessitates vigilant attention to biosecurity when working with diseased horses in these areas.
- It should also be noted that while transmission risk increases with disease progression in horses (being maximal at terminal/postmortem stages), experimental evidence suggests that horses may excrete HeV in nasopharyngeal secretions even before the development of clinical signs of disease.
- *Practice Tip: Adoption of personal protective equipment (PPE) for procedures involving contact with (particularly) airway secretions and careful exclusion of HeV through testing is advised.*
- Up-to-date information can be found through the Queensland Government website at www.dpi.qld.gov.au/4790_13371.htm.

Clinical Signs

- Experimentally, the incubation period ranges from 5 to 16 days; in fatal cases, the disease course is typically short, lasting only about 2 days.
- Initial clinical signs include:
  - Pyrexia and restlessness (weight shifting between limbs)
  - Progression to depression
  - Ultimately signs of acute respiratory and/or neurologic disease
- Approximately 25% of horses may survive acute infection.
- *Practice Tip: There are no pathognomonic signs for HeV infection; however, sudden death in one or more horses in an affected region should be treated with high suspicion.*
- Affected horses present with acute disease onset with rapid deterioration. Commonly reported clinical signs in natural cases have included:
  - Pyrexia
  - Tachycardia
  - Weight shifting/restlessness
  - Tachypnea and respiratory distress
  - Weakness and collapse/inability to rise
  - Ataxia
  - Altered mentation and central blindness
  - Head tilt and circling
  - Muscle twitching
  - Facial swelling/edema
  - Urinary incontinence
  - Frothy nasal discharge

Pathology

- The most significant gross lesions in affected horses are:
  - Edematous lymph nodes (submandibular and bronchial)
  - Dilated pulmonary lymphatic vessels

- Subpleural hemorrhages
- Pulmonary consolidation
- Edema
- Edema of other tissues has also been observed. The airways in field cases are often filled with thick, occasionally blood-tinged, foam.
- *Note:* The characteristic histologic lesion confirming HeV infections is the presence of systemic vasculitis, particularly evident in tissues of the respiratory tract, brain, and meninges.
- Edema, syncytial cells, viral inclusion bodies, and alveolitis are observed in pulmonary tissues.
- Nonsuppurative encephalitis characterized by perivascular lymphocyte cuffing, neuronal necrosis, and focal gliosis has been observed.

Diagnosis

- *Practice Tip: HeV infection should be considered in horses exhibiting a high fever and signs of acute lower respiratory tract or neurologic disease in a region where the virus is known to occur or may have been introduced.*
- Differential diagnoses include:
  - Plant poisonings (e.g., Crofton weed, avocado)
  - Ionophore toxicity
  - Intestinal lesions (colitis and other causes of colic)
  - Bacterial pneumonia
  - Viral encephalitis/meningoencephalitis (including equine herpesvirus-1 (EHV-1), flavivirus infection, exotic encephalitides)
  - Purpura hemorrhagica
  - Snake bite envenomation
  - Tick paralysis *(Ixodes holocyclus)*
- Laboratory testing is *essential* for confirmation and includes:
  - Virus isolation
  - Detection of viral nucleic acid in body fluids or tissues
  - Demonstration of specific serum antibodies
- Detailed guidelines are available from local government sources for sample collection when testing for Hendra virus.
- *Important:* Stringent precautions including adequate personal protective equipment (protective eyewear, particulate mask, impervious gloves, and gown) should be taken when sampling horses if there is a suspicion of HeV infection.
- In live or dead horses, blood, nasal swabs, oral swabs, or rectal mucosal swabs are appropriate samples for submission for polymerase chain reaction (PCR) testing.
- Serology and virus neutralization tests may also be used to detect antibodies.
- Necropsy should be avoided until receipt of (negative) preliminary results in suspect cases.

●▶ WHAT TO DO

Hendra Virus

- It is critical to exclude HeV as a potential cause of acute disease/death in horses from an affected area.

- It is essential for veterinarians working in affected areas to be familiar with appropriate biosecurity measures, including appropriate PPE.
- *Important:* Veterinarians faced with highly suspicious HeV cases (including cases of sudden death) should contact local government authorities immediately for advice.
- A subunit vaccine against Hendra virus is approved for use in horses. In experimental trials, as part of the safety testing, the vaccine was extremely effective in preventing infection and appears to be very safe.

Indigofera Linnaei Poisoning (Birdsville Horse Disease)

- *Indigofera* spp. plants are widespread in tropical and temperate parts of the world including Australia.
- *Corynocarpus* spp. (Karaka) plants containing the same family of toxins occur in New Zealand.

Epidemiology

- *Indigofera linnaei* (Birdsville indigo) occurs extensively in northern Australia, dominating vegetation in some regions.
- Poisonings occur mostly in western Queensland, northern South Australia, and the Northern Territory when *I. linnaei* composes the major portion of the diet.
- *Practice Tip: Cases occur most commonly between November and March when rainfall is sufficient to stimulate growth of I. linnaei but insufficient to allow growth of other forage plants.*
- Experimentally, horses must consume 4.5 kg of plant material per day for at least 2 weeks before clinical signs appear.
- *Note:* A similar condition has been described in horses in Florida ("grove disease") grazing *I. hendecaphylla*.
- The closely related species *I. spicata* (creeping indigo) recently caused an outbreak of neurologic disease in southeast Queensland.

Pathophysiology

- The toxic principle appears to be a nitrotoxin, which is hydrolyzed to 3-nitropropanoic acid (NPA).
- NPA inhibits succinate dehydrogenase and other mitochondrial enzymes, impairing cellular energy production within the nervous system.
- The hepatotoxin indospicine does *not* contribute to the neurologic signs in horses.

●▶ WHAT TO DO

Indigofera Linnaei Poisoning

- Treatment is supportive.
- Most horses recover if removed from the causative plant.
- Some recovered horses "roar" as a result of laryngeal paralysis.
- A chronic condition may develop, characterized by ataxia, particularly of the hind limbs.

EMG

Clinical Signs

- Clinical signs include the following:
  - Inappetence
  - Weight loss
  - Somnolence
  - Affected horses tend to segregate themselves from herd mates
  - Neurologic signs include the following:
    ○ Hypermetric forelimb gait
    ○ Apparent hindquarter weakness: the haunches are carried low, the hocks are extended, and the individual tends to drag the hind feet.
    ○ The head is carried abnormally high and the tail is stiff and extended.
    ○ Difficulty when turned in tight circles, tending to pivot on the forelimbs.
- As the condition progresses, horses may suddenly lose control of their hindquarters.
- In some cases, there is a bilateral ocular discharge, corneal opacity or edema, stomatitis, and dyspnea.
- If not removed from the source of toxin, affected horses may become recumbent with intermittent tetanic convulsions shortly before death.

Flavivirus Infection

- Members of the genus *Flavivirus*, including Kunjin virus (a subtype of West Nile virus), Murray Valley encephalitis virus (MVEv), and Japanese encephalitis virus (JEv) are mosquito-borne viruses that have caused disease in horses and human beings in Australia.
- Although many infections are subclinical, severe disease may occur in immunologically naive horses.

Epidemiology

- Kunjin virus is a strain of West Nile virus that is indigenous to Australia.
- It causes disease in human beings and has occasionally been reported to cause neurologic disease in horses.
- Kunjin virus is endemic in the tropical north of Australia, and serologic evidence of its presence has been detected in western New South Wales.
- In 2011, an unprecedented outbreak of neurologic disease in horses attributed primarily to Kunjin virus occurred in New South Wales, Victoria, and Queensland, with more than 1000 horses affected.
- Clinical signs during the outbreak were similar to those reported with West Nile Virus infection in North America and there was a mortality rate of 10% to 15%.
- MVEv is also endemic in Northern Australia; an increase in cases of MVEv infection in horses was documented in 2011, in association with unusually heavy rainfall, and there have been other outbreaks noted in association with similar climatic conditions in the past.
- The insect-borne alphavirus, Ross River virus, has also been implicated in outbreaks of muscle soreness and arthropathy in horses with a similar geographic distribution to Kunjin virus and MVEv.

- In 1995, three cases of human Japanese encephalitis were reported on an island in the Torres Strait north of the Australian mainland.
- Serologic evidence of recent JEv infection was subsequently found in human beings, dogs, pigs, and horses on islands in the region.
- No disease was reported in any of the horses that had antibodies against JEv. In 1998, a case of human Japanese encephalitis was reported on the Australian mainland, and serologic evidence of infection in pigs was detected in the same area. Papua New Guinea is thought to be the most likely source of virus.

Clinical Signs

- Clinical signs of Kunjin virus and MVEv infection in horses are similar to those reported for West Nile virus infection in North America:
  - Initial clinical signs include profound depression and mild colic.
  - Increased responsiveness to touch and sound
  - Muscle fasciculations
  - Facial paralysis, twitching, and difficulty masticating
  - Ataxia, including proprioceptive deficits and dysmetria
  - Weakness, recumbency
- Most horses recover slowly over 1 to 3 weeks, but a mortality rate of 10% to 15% is reported.
- Japanese encephalitis cases in horses are usually sporadic or occur in small clusters.
  - Although subclinical infections are most common, case-fatality rates of 5% to 15% are reported in endemic areas.
  - Mortality rates up to 30% to 40% have been observed in seasonal epidemics in Japan, and high mortality rates should be anticipated in immunologically naive horses.
  - Three clinical syndromes have been described:
    ○ *Transient type:* Clinical signs include:
      - Fever (up to 104°F [40°C] for 2 to 3 days)
      - Anorexia
      - Sluggish movement
      - Congested or jaundiced mucous membranes
    ○ *Lethargic type:* Clinical signs include:
      - Fluctuating fever (101.8° to 105.8°F [38.8° to 41°C])
      - Lethargy
      - Anorexia
      - Nasal discharge
      - Dysphagia
      - Jaundice
      - Ataxia
      - Petechial hemorrhages may be observed.
    ○ *Hyperexcitable type:* This is the *least* common manifestation and occurs in less than 5% of cases. Clinical signs include:
      - Demented behavior, may be uncontrollable
      - High fever (>105.8°F [>41°C])
      - Aimless wandering
      - Shying at imaginary objects

- Blindness
- Profuse sweating
- Bruxism
- Muscle twitching
- Collapse and death are common in severe cases
- Horses may demonstrate ataxia that progresses to recumbency and death over 5 days to 6 weeks

Pathology
- There are no characteristic gross lesions in the brain.
- Histopathology lesions include:
  - Diffuse nonsuppurative encephalomyelitis with phagocytic destruction of nerve cells and focal gliosis
  - Perivascular cuffing
  - Engorged blood vessels containing many mononuclear cells

Diagnosis
- *Practice Tip: Flavivirus encephalitis should be considered if there is a geographic and temporal clustering of a disease characterized by neurologic signs, particularly in association with climatic conditions conducive to amplification of mosquito vectors (high rainfall).*
- Laboratory confirmation is essential for a definitive diagnosis.
- Acute and convalescent (7 days and 3 weeks post) blood samples should be submitted for serologic analysis.
- Hendra virus infection should be considered an important differential diagnosis and therefore should be ruled out in all cases.
- *Note:* The epidemiology, clinical signs, and recovery rate are similar to West Nile encephalitis in North America.

⏩ WHAT TO DO

Flavivirus Infection
- No specific treatment exists for viral encephalitis in horses.
- Hendra virus infection should be ruled out in all cases.
- Therapy is primarily supportive.

Lolitrem Toxicity (Perennial Ryegrass Staggers)
- Ryegrass staggers occurs chiefly in New Zealand and to a more limited extent in southeastern Australia.
- The condition is caused by tremorgenic (quivering) mycotoxins produced by the endophytic (proliferating) fungus *Neotyphodium (Acremonium) lolii*, which infects perennial ryegrass *(Lolium perenne).*

Epidemiology and Pathophysiology
- The mode of action of the lolitrems has *not* been defined; because of the transient nature of the disease, the nervous signs are assumed to be caused by a reversible biochemical toxicosis. Spontaneous and complete recovery is generally rapid once horses are allowed to graze uncontaminated pasture.

- The endophyte *N. lolii* produces peramine, which is repellent to insects and reportedly improves persistence of infected cultivars.
- Of the tremorgens produced, lolitrem B is the most abundant, with others present in only small quantities.
- Lolitrem B is concentrated in the leaf sheaths near the base of the plant so that disease is most likely to occur at the end of summer or early fall when pasture is short and horses are forced to graze close to the ground.
- Horses may also be poisoned when fed seed cleanings of *L. perenne,* and toxicity persists in hay.
- Ryegrass staggers may affect a variable number of horses within a herd, and individuals appear to vary in their susceptibility.
- Ryegrass staggers is primarily a disease of inconvenience because affected individuals are difficult to move.
- Death, if it occurs, is due to misadventure.
- The disease has been seen in the southeastern United States.

Clinical Signs and Diagnosis
- Clinical signs appear within 1 to 2 weeks of exposure to a toxic sward.
- Signs may not be apparent during quiet grazing but are obvious when the horse is disturbed or moves.
- Early clinical signs in horses include the following:
  - Fine muscle tremors
  - Head weaving
  - Ataxia
  - Hypersensitivity to stimuli
  - Inability to move quickly because of limb and trunk stiffness in mildly affected horses
  - Collapse with brief tetanic spasms and limb paddling in more severely affected horses
  - Tenesmus may be seen in severely affected horses.
- Clinical signs usually resolve rapidly if horses are left alone. Pasture may be tested for the presence of endophyte (Poppi stain) or lolitrem B (high-performance liquid chromatography assay).

⏩ WHAT TO DO

Lolitrem Toxicity
- There is no specific treatment.
- Affected individuals should be gently removed from the affected pasture as soon as possible.
- Rye grasses make up the majority of pasture in many areas, and because of the high prevalence of endophyte infection, finding safe pasture can be difficult under some circumstances.

Pyrrolizidine Alkaloid Poisoning
- Numerous plants within a large number of botanical families produce pyrrolizidine alkaloids (PAs), and disease caused by them occurs in grazing horses in most countries.
- Several hundred PAs have been identified and characterized.

EMG

- Not all PAs are toxic, but of those that are, most are hepatotoxic with a few being pneumotoxic or nephrotoxic (see Chapter 34, p. 596).

Epidemiology

- Pyrrolizidine alkaloidosis is now less common in horses; however, it continues to remain a risk because of the prevalence of PA-containing plants within or adjoining grazed areas.
- *Practice Tip: Plants most commonly associated with PA toxicity in New Zealand and Australia include* Senecio *spp. (e.g., ragwort [tansy ragwort], groundsels, and fireweeds),* Heliotropium *spp. (e.g., common and blue heliotropes),* Echium *spp. (e.g., Paterson's curse), and* Crotalaria *spp. (e.g., Kimberley horse poison and the various rattlepods).*
- These plants are not very palatable and are usually only eaten in sufficient quantity to cause disease when feed availability is short or when they have been accidentally included in preserved feeds. PA toxicity is not significantly reduced by conversion to hay, ensilage, or pellets.

Pathophysiology

- PAs are *not* toxic in themselves, but their metabolites are highly reactive alkylating agents that bind to DNA and other cellular components.
- In most affected species, the liver is primarily affected, but in some circumstances toxins may escape into the circulation and damage the lungs and kidneys.
- PAs are cumulative toxins resulting in chronic disease, and clinical signs may *not* appear until weeks or months after ingestion ceases.

▶▶ WHAT TO DO

Pyrrolizidine Alkaloid Poisoning

- Once clinical signs become apparent, treatment is unlikely to be successful.
- The antimitotic effect of cross-linking of DNA and the bridging fibrosis make regeneration of the liver difficult.
- Treatment is largely supportive, with emphasis on dietary management to reduce hepatic workload.
- Patients that recover clinically may never regain their former physical fitness, and any exertion is likely to lead to rapid exhaustion.

Clinical Signs

- Clinical signs of PA toxicosis in horses are those of liver failure and include the following:
  - Weight loss and behavioral changes
  - Icterus may or may *not* be present.
  - Signs of hepatic encephalopathy are common and include the following:
    - Depression
    - Ataxia
    - Yawning
    - Head pressing
    - Compulsive walking
    - Stertorous breathing (laryngeal dysfunction)
  - A photosensitive dermatitis may be present.

- Although clearly a chronic condition, many horses present acutely in fulminate liver failure.

Diagnosis

- Diagnosis is based on clinical signs of liver disease and a history of exposure to PA-containing plants.
- Access to plants by affected individuals can be difficult to establish because of the lag between ingestion and onset of clinical signs.
- Contributory evidence for exposure to PAs includes increases in hepatic enzyme activity, although these enzymes may have returned to normal by the time clinical signs become apparent.
- A liver biopsy should be performed in cases of liver disease to assist in diagnosis and assess prognosis.
- Characteristic histopathologic changes in PA toxicosis include:
  - Hepatocyte megalocytosis (as a result of inhibition of mitosis)
  - Biliary duct hyperplasia
  - Fibrosis of the portal triads
- *Note:* Hepatocyte megalocytosis may also be seen in cases of aflatoxicosis and may be absent in some cases of PA toxicosis.
- Horses with evidence of bridging fibrosis usually do *not* survive longer than 6 months.

Snake Bite

- Venomous snakes most commonly implicated in snake bites in Australia are *Notechis scutatus* (tiger snake) and *Demansia textilis* (common brown snake).
- Although mortality is rare, bites from these snakes may cause significant morbidity in adults and foals (see Chapter 45, p. 724).

Epidemiology

- Most bites occur during the summer on the muzzle.

Pathophysiology

- Snake venom contains a number of neurotoxins and myotoxins, the exact composition of which depends on the species of snake involved.
- Secondary bacterial infection may occur at the bite site and contribute to pathologic effects.

Clinical Signs

- Clinical presentation depends on the species of snake, size of affected horse, and location of the bite.
- Although horses appear to be more susceptible than other large animal species, there is generally insufficient venom to cause rapid death in adults.
- It is uncommon to detect a bite mark; however, local swelling may be considerable.
- Clinical signs may include the following:
  - Pupillary dilation that is unresponsive to light
  - Muscle tremors and weakness
  - Agitation

- With brown snake bites, adult horses may be dysphagic with accumulation of feed material in the mouth.
- Foals may appear drowsy with partial paralysis of the lips, tongue, and eyelids.
- Respiratory distress, sweating, dysphagia, recumbency, and death may occur in foals.
- *Important:* The venom of some snakes may affect coagulation.

Diagnosis and Treatment

- Diagnosis is usually based on clinical signs.
- Diagnostic kits are available for the identification of specific venoms in blood, urine, or tissue.

●》 WHAT TO DO

Snake Bite

- Antivenin may be beneficial acutely, particularly in foals.
- Specific (i.e., Tiger or Brown) antivenins are available; in many cases, a combination Tiger-Brown antivenin is used because the offending snake is unknown.
- Antivenin should be administered intravenously. A single unit may be sufficient for foals and adult horses, but adults may require up to five units.
- *Practice Tip: Respiratory effort should be carefully monitored, and a tracheostomy or nasotracheal intubation should be performed if swelling within the upper airways causes obstruction* (see Chapter 25, p. 456, and Chapter 45, p. 726).
- Broad-spectrum antibiotic treatment should be initiated to prevent secondary bacterial infection. *Important:* The antibiotic regimen should include penicillin because clostridial infections are common.
- Tetanus prophylaxis (toxoid and/or antitoxin) should be administered.
- Supportive therapy includes intravenous administration of fluids and anti-inflammatory drugs.

Stringhalt

- Stringhalt is an involuntary, exaggerated flexion of one or both hocks.
- *Note:* In contrast to classic stringhalt, which is traumatic in origin, Australian stringhalt is likely the result of toxicity.
- The condition is usually bilateral, occurring in Australia and New Zealand, although it is also described in California and South America.

Epidemiology

- Outbreaks of Australian stringhalt are associated with grazing pasture heavily infested with *Hypochoeris radicata* (flatweed, catsear, false dandelion).
- However, a causal role of a plant toxin has *not* been proven, and feeding studies have *not* yet reproduced the disease.
- A number of other plants have been suggested to cause identical clinical signs, although strong evidence for their involvement is lacking.

- A similar flatweed-associated outbreak of stringhalt has been seen in Virginia, Georgia, and possibly other states in North America.
- Multiple (10% to 15%) individuals within a herd are often involved, although single cases are *not* uncommon.
- Disease usually occurs in the summer-autumn (January to March) period in the southern hemisphere.

Pathophysiology

- The pathologic lesion is a distal axonopathy affecting long, large-diameter myelinated axons of the peripheral nervous system.
- Neurogenic myofibril atrophy is present in the muscles innervated by affected nerves.
- There may be some changes in electromyography studies of affected muscles.
- There are no abnormal clinical pathologic findings.

Clinical Signs

- Adult horses, particularly larger individuals, are most commonly affected; however, the condition may occasionally occur in foals.
- Affected horses appear normal at rest but display characteristic hyperflexion of the hock when moving.
- *Note:* Both hind limbs are usually affected, and in severe cases, the horse may be unable to rise without assistance.
- In its mildest form, abnormalities are only observed when the horse begins to move, is backed, or turned.
- In some cases, hock flexion is so exaggerated that affected horses kick themselves in the abdomen; the limb is then held in flexion momentarily before being slapped down.
- Clinical signs may vary from day to day; they may be more severe when the horse is frightened or excited, after a period of rest, or during cold weather.
- The horses' general health is usually unaffected, although there is selective (neurogenic) wasting of the muscles of the digital extensor group (gaskin) and inner thigh.
- In some horses (usually Draft breeds), there are gait abnormalities and muscle atrophy of the forelimbs.
- Respiratory distress may occasionally be observed as a result of laryngeal dysfunction.
- Many patients show progressive deterioration over several weeks, followed by stabilization of clinical signs, and then gradual recovery.

●》 WHAT TO DO

Stringhalt

- Most horses recover spontaneously without treatment once they have been removed from infested pasture.
- Recovery is presumed to occur by axonal regeneration, a process that may take up to 18 months. Median recovery time is reported to be 6 to 12 months, although some horses may improve much more quickly.
- Treatment with phenytoin (15 mg/kg PO for 14 days) may reduce the severity of clinical signs and decrease the time until recovery in some horses.

- Sedation of affected horses may reduce the clinical signs and allow horses to move and be transported more easily.

Tick Paralysis

- The tick *Ixodes holocyclus* is a common cause of paralysis in companion animals in some regions of Australia.
- Infestations of five or more ticks may cause an ascending flaccid paralysis in foals and adult Miniature horses/ponies, as well as occasionally in full-size adult horses.
- Death from respiratory failure, such as occurs in dogs, can occur in horses.

●》 WHAT TO DO

Tick Paralysis
- Removal of the ticks and supportive care usually results in rapid and full recovery (often less than 3 days).
- There is some anecdotal evidence to suggest that commercial tick antiserum, administered intravenously at 0.5 to 2 mL/kg may be associated with reduced mortality.
- Chemical prophylaxis (topical synthetic pyrethroids or fipronil spray) may be required in endemic areas.

●》 WHAT NOT TO DO

Tick Paralysis
- Avoid preparations marketed for cattle that contain amitraz, which can cause fatal gastrointestinal ileus in horses.

EUROPE

Tim Mair

Equine Grass Sickness

- Equine Grass Sickness (EGS) is a dysautonomia/polyneuropathy of grazing Equidae (horses, ponies, donkeys, and exotic Equidae) with damage to neurons of the autonomic, enteric, and somatic nervous systems.
- The disease occurs throughout the United Kingdom and many northern European countries, including Norway, Sweden, Denmark, France, Belgium, Switzerland, Austria, Hungary, and Germany.
- It affects predominantly young horses with access to pasture in the springtime.
- Mal seco (dry sickness) is a similar condition that occurs in the Patagonia region of Argentina, Chile, and the Falkland Islands.
- The acute and subacute forms of the disease are fatal; however, a proportion of horses with the chronic form may survive.
- The cause of EGS remains uncertain, although a natural neurotoxin, either ingested or produced within the gastrointestinal tract, is probably involved.
- There is some evidence to suggest that EGS may be a toxico-infectious disease associated with exotoxins produced within the gastrointestinal tract by *Clostridium botulinum*.
- Low circulating antibody levels for both *Clostridium botulinum* type C and *Clostridium botulinum* type C toxoid are associated with an increased risk of devloping EGS.

Signalment and Epidemiology
- All ages can be affected, but the highest incidence occurs among 2- to 7-year-olds.
- Usually it affects only individuals in good body condition.
- Although the disease can occur at any time of year, the highest incidence in the northern hemisphere occurs in the spring and summer (April to July). In the southern hemisphere, the highest incidence occurs in October to February.
- EGS usually affects grazing horses.
- Disease often recurs on certain premises or pastures.
- Recent movement to a new pasture or new premises is a predisposing factor.
- Occurrence of the disease has also been related to other stresses such as foaling, castration, or breaking-in.
- Cool (7° to 10°C/46 to 50°F]), dry weather tends to occur in the 10 to 14 days preceding outbreaks.

Subdivisions of the Disease
- Acute
- Subacute
- Chronic

Clinical Signs
Acute
- Depression and somnolence
- Inappetence
- Colic
- Tachycardia (heart rate up to 100 beats/min)
- May be pyrexic (up to 40°C [104°F])
- May have bilateral ptosis
- Muscle fasciculations of the triceps and quadriceps muscle groups
- Generalized sweating, or localized to the flank, neck, and shoulder regions
- Dysphagia
- Dribbling of saliva
- Dehydration
- Small-intestinal distention
- Gastric reflux with nasal discharge of malodorous green or brown fluid
- Reduced or absent bowel sounds
- Abdominal distention
- Most patients die or require humane destruction within 2 days

Subacute
- The clinical signs are similar to, but less severe than, those of acute cases.

- Dysphagia
- Persistent tachycardia
- Patchy sweating on flanks, neck, shoulders
- Muscle tremors (triceps and quadriceps)
- Weight loss and development of marked "tucked-up" abdomen
- Ptosis
- Nasogastric reflux and episodes of colic are possible
- Most patients die or require humane destruction within 7 days

Chronic

- The clinical signs in the chronic form are insidious in onset. Survival of chronic grass sickness is possible in some appropriately selected and managed cases.
  - Severe weight loss with the development of a "tucked-up" abdomen
  - Base narrow stance and adoption of an "elephant on a tub" posture
  - Weakness and toe dragging
  - Ptosis
  - Persistent tachycardia (up to 60 beats/min)
  - Muscle tremors
  - Patchy sweating
  - Mild colic
  - Mild dysphagia and accumulation of food in the mouth
  - Rhinitis sicca with accumulation of dry mucoid discharge around the nares and the presence of a distinctive "snuffling" sound during breathing
- There are a few anecdotal, but unconfirmed, reports of recurrence in horses that have survived after the chronic form.
- It is postulated that subclinical disease may also occur, but this is not well documented.

Diagnosis

- Epidemiologic characteristics, signalment, clinical signs, and results of rectal examination allow a tentative diagnosis.
- *Practice Tip: Confirmation of grass sickness can be made only by demonstrating histopathologic lesions in the autonomic or enteric ganglia at postmortem examination or by ileal biopsy at laparotomy.*
- Exploratory laparotomy and ileal biopsy may be needed to differentiate acute grass sickness from surgical diseases causing small-intestinal obstruction (especially anterior enteritis, ileal impaction, and idiopathic focal eosinophilic enteritis).
- Phenylephrine eye drops (0.5%) cause a greater increase in the size of the palpebral fissure (as measured by the change in the angle of the eyelashes with the head observed from a frontal view) than occurs in normal horses. *Note:* This test should be performed in nonsedated horses.
- Endoscopic examination of the distal esophagus of patients with acute or subacute grass sickness may reveal longitudinal linear ulceration of the mucosa.

- Contrast esophagography (barium swallow) may show abnormal esophageal motility.
- Examination of enteric ganglia in rectal biopsies has proven to be unreliable for diagnosis.
- The value of histopathologic examination of nasal mucosal biopsies is currently being evaluated.

●〉 WHAT TO DO

Equine Grass Sickness
- The majority of cases of EGS do *not* survive.
- Acute and subacute grass sickness should be managed with humane destruction.
- Individuals with mild chronic disease may survive after prolonged treatment and nursing care.
- Treatment should *only* be considered in cases fulfilling the following:
  - Criteria for selection of chronic cases:
    - Some ability to swallow
    - Some appetite present
    - Some intestinal motility present
    - Heart rate less than 60 beats/min
  - Management of selected chronic cases:
    - General nursing care with frequent human contact, frequent grooming, and regular hand walking and grazing is important.
    - Hand walking may help stimulate appetite and intestinal motility.
    - Palatable high-energy, high-protein feeds are offered 4 to 5 times a day. Grass, apples, and fresh vegetables should be offered. A variety of different compounded feeds and forages should be available.
    - A deep, clean bed should be available to encourage the horse to lie down.
    - Cisapride, 0.5 to 0.8 mg/kg PO q8h for 7 days may help intestinal motility; its efficacy is uncertain.
    - Flunixin meglumine, 0.5 to 1.1 mg/kg IV, or phenylbutazone, 2.2 to 4.4 mg/kg IV, may be administered as necessary to control abdominal pain.
    - Diazepam, 0.05 mg/kg IV q2h, can be administered as an appetite stimulant.
    - Fecal output should be monitored, and enteral fluid therapy used if necessary to soften fecal consistency.
    - Mineral oil may also be helpful to aid fecal transit.
    - Probiotics may be helpful; their efficacy has *not* been evaluated.
- Cases likely to survive generally gain weight in the first 5 weeks after diagnosis, with return to normal body weight taking an average of 9 months.
- A proportion of surviving horses retain residual signs including:
  - Poor appetite
  - Degrees of dysphagia
  - Mild colic
  - Sweating
  - Coat abnormalities—textural or color changes

Prevention

- Studies are currently evaluating the immunogenicity and safety of a recombinant protein-based type *C. botulinum* toxin vaccine.

African Horse Sickness

- African horse sickness is a noncontagious arthropod-borne viral disease that can cause a mortality rate of 90% in naive horse populations.
- Although the disease is generally restricted to tropical and subtropical Africa south of the Sahara, it regularly spreads southward to South Africa and northward to other parts of the African continent.
- It has occasionally spread to Asia (as far as Pakistan and India) and to southern Europe (Portugal and Spain).
- It is believed that its geographic spread could increase as a result of changes to vector biology due to climate change.
- African horse sickness virus is transmitted by *Culicoides* spp., of which *C. imicola* and *C. bolitinos* have been shown to play an important role in Africa.
- The disease has a seasonal occurrence and its prevalence is influenced by climatic and other conditions which favor the breeding of *Culicoides* spp.

Signalment

- The horse is the most susceptible host.
- Mules and European donkeys are susceptible, but less so than horses.
- African donkeys and zebras are generally resistant (infection is subclinical).

Clinical Signs

- Four forms of the disease are recognized:
  - Pulmonary
  - Mixed
  - Cardiac
  - Horse sickness fever
- The *pulmonary* form ("Dunkop" form) is peracute or acute and is usually rapidly fatal following an incubation period of 3 to 4 days; this form usually occurs in naive, fully susceptible horses.
- The *cardiac* form ("Dikkop" form) usually is subacute and has an incubation period of up to 3 weeks.
- The *mixed* disease is a combination of pulmonary and cardiac forms.
- *Horse sickness fever* is a mild condition caused by less virulent strains of the virus and is characterized by pyrexia and edema of the supraorbital fossae.

Pulmonary Form

- May result in "sudden death"
- Depression and fever (39° to 41°C [102° to 106°F])
- Respiratory distress with flared nostrils and tachypnea (respiratory rate may exceed 50 breaths/min)
- Paroxysmal coughing
- Head and neck extended
- Profuse sweating
- Recumbency
- Frothy nasal discharge (terminally)
- Death usually occurs within a few hours of the onset of clinical signs.

- Only about 5% of horses affected by the pulmonary form survive.

Cardiac Form

- Fever (39° to 41°C [102° to 106°F]) that persists 3 to 4 days
- Edema of the head (starting with the supraorbital fossae), neck, and chest
- Conjunctival congestion
- Petechial hemorrhage on mucous membranes
- Colic
- Dyspnea
- Death (mortality rate, 50%) usually occurs within 4 to 8 days after the onset of fever.
- In cases that recover, swellings gradually subside over a period of 3 to 8 days.
- Paralysis of the esophagus may be a complication, resulting in dysphagia.
- Piroplasmosis may complicate recovery, resulting in icterus, anemia, and constipation.

Mixed Form

- Although the mixed form is the *most common form* of African horse sickness, it is rarely diagnosed clinically because of the peracute onset and rapid progression often resulting in death.
- Initial pulmonary signs of a mild nature that do not progress can be followed by edematous swellings and effusions; death results from cardiac failure.
- More commonly, the subclinical cardiac form is suddenly followed by marked dyspnea and other signs typical of the pulmonary form.
- Death usually occurs 3 to 6 days after the onset of the febrile reaction.

Horse Sickness Fever

- This is the *mildest* form of African horse sickness and is not frequently diagnosed in the clinical setting because of the none specific signs.
- The incubation period is between 5 and 9 days, after which the temperature gradually rises over a period of 4 to 5 days to 40°C (104°F), followed by a drop in temperature to normal, then recovery.
- Apart from the febrile reaction, other clinical signs are rare and inconspicuous.
- Some horses may be depressed with partial loss of appetite, congestion of the conjunctivae, slightly labored breathing, and increased heart rate, but these signs are transient.

Diagnosis

- Virus isolation from blood or tissues (spleen, lung, liver, heart, lymph nodes)
- Serology: Agar gel immunodiffusion (AGID), enzyme-linked immunosorbent assay (ELISA), complement fixation (CF) test, or virus neutralization tests

African Horse Sickness
- Treatment is symptomatic and supportive.
- Horses that survive should be rested for at least 4 weeks following recovery before being returned to light work.
- See p. 674.

Prognosis
- The mortality among susceptible horses is 80% to 90%.

Equine Encephalosis
- Equine encephalosis is an orbivirus infection of horses that usually presents with mild or subclinical signs.
- The virus is transmitted by species of *Culicoides,* which are endemic to the temperate regions of Africa.
- The epidemiology is very similar to African horse sickness, and there remains a threat of its introduction into Europe.

Clinical Signs
- Incubation period is 3 to 5 days.
- Ninety percent of infected horses show either no obvious signs of infection or develop only very mild clinical signs.
- Mild fever (39° to 41°C, or 102.2° to 105.8°F)
- Listlessness and inappetence
- Mild icterus
- Swelling of the eyelids and supraorbital fossae may be observed.
- Rarely, neurologic signs

Diagnosis
- Serologic conversion

Glanders (Farcy, Enzootic Lymphangitis)
- Glanders is a highly contagious disease of equidae caused by the gram-negative bacterium *Burkholderia mallei.*
- The disease is currently confined to some areas of Asia, the Middle East, Africa, and South America, but it has been occasionally introduced into Europe in imported horses.
- It is zoonotic.

Clinical Signs
- The incubation period is 3 to 14 days (latent infections and carrier states can also occur).
- Respiratory and cutaneous and acute and chronic forms are described, but there is considerable overlap.
- An acute and fatal bronchopneumonia is usually seen in donkeys and mules, whereas a chronic cutaneous form is more common in horses.
- Purulent ocular nasal discharge and nasal ulceration are seen.
- Subcutaneous and ulcerating nodules of the ventral abdomen, distal limbs, face, and neck occur.
- Weight loss is seen.
- The animal may be in respiratory distress.
- Death occurs in 1 to 4 weeks (more rapidly in donkeys).

Diagnosis
- The organism can be cultured from swabs from cutaneous lesions/postmortem material.
- Abscesses may not contain large numbers of organisms (and are often contaminated by other bacteria species, especially *Pseudomonas* spp. and *Pasteurella* spp.), so multiple cultures are recommended. Glanderous subcutaneous abscesses usually contain good numbers of pathogens, whereas ulcers are usually free of *B. mallei.*
- ***Important:*** Because glanders is *zoonotic,* all samples must be handled with great care in a laboratory that meets the requirements for "containment group 3" pathogens.
- Suspected material should be inoculated intraperitoneally into a male adult guinea pig to confirm diagnosis.
- PCR technique has recently been fully validated.
- Serology available includes complement fixation test, competitive ELISA.
- Malleinization detects the delayed hypersensitivity of infected horses to *B. mallei.* The mallein-purified protein derivate (PPD) is currently available in the Netherlands, Turkey, and Romania. Intradermo palpebral and intradermal methods are possible.

Borna Disease
- Borna disease is a sporadically occurring, usually fatal disorder caused by the highly neurotropic Borna disease virus.
- The disease occurs in endemic areas of Germany, Switzerland, Liechtenstein, and Austria.

Clinical Signs
- Disease may be subclinical, peracute, acute, or subacute.
- Incubation period ranges from 2 to several months.
- Alterations in behavior, lethargy, somnolence, hyperexcitability, aggressiveness
- Recurrent fever
- Head tilt and ataxia
- Torticollis, compulsive circling, head tremor, blindness, nystagmus, facial paralysis
- Convulsions

Diagnosis
- Detection of antibodies in serum and/or CSF via Western blot analysis or indirect immunofluorescence assay
- Cerebrospinal fluid (CSF) has lymphomonocytic pleocytosis

Dourine
- Equine trypanosomiases are acute or chronic infectious diseases caused by protozoan blood parasites.
- Depending on the parasite species involved, three diseases can be distinguished:
  - Nagana
  - Surra
  - Dourine

EMG

- Nagana is caused by infection with *Trypanosoma congolense, T. vivax,* and/or *T. brucei,* and occurs in sub-Saharan Africa.
- *Trypanosoma evansi* is the causal agent of Surra, which occurs mainly in North and Northeast Africa, Latin America (except Chile), the Middle East, and Asia.
- Dourine is the result of a venereal infection with *Trypanosoma equiperdum;* the parasite is cosmopolitan, and although Western Europe, Australia, and the United States are considered to be free from Dourine, sporadic introduction of the disease into Europe (recently Germany and Italy) occurs.

Clinical Signs
- Chronic infections occur that can persist for 1 to 2 years.
- Clinical signs usually appear within a few weeks of infection but, in some cases, may be prolonged.
- Appearance of clinical signs may be accelerated by stress.
- Clinical signs in mares include: vaginal discharge; edema of the vulva that then extends along the perineum to the udder and ventral abdomen; vulvitis and vaginitis; polyuria; abortion.
- Clinical signs in stallions include: edema of the prepuce and glans penis, spreading to the scrotum, perineum, and ventral abdomen and thorax; vesicles or ulcers on the genitalia.
- Conjunctivitis and keratitis are seen.
- Cutaneous "plaques" develop, especially over the ribs.
- Progressive anemia is seen.
- Neurologic signs include: restlessness, weakness, incoordination, paralysis (mainly of the hind legs), paraplegia, and death.

Diagnosis
- Serology—complement fixation test

●⟩ WHAT TO DO

Dourine
- International regulations of the World Organization for Animal Health (OIE) impose the slaughtering of complement fixation test (CFT)-positive horses.

Louping III
- Louping ill is an acute encephalitis caused by a tick-borne flavivirus.
- The disease is seen in certain areas of the United Kingdom and Ireland and affects mainly sheep, but it can rarely affect horses.
- The natural vector of the virus is the castor bean tick (sheep tick), *Ixodes ricinus.*

Clinical Signs
- Inappetence
- Pyrexia

- Ataxia and gait abnormalities
- Muscle tremors of the neck and facial areas
- Altered head carriage and opisthotonos
- Depression
- Avoidance of bright light
- Abnormal behavior, including constant exaggerated chewing
- The majority of affected horses recover following symptomatic and supportive therapy.

Diagnosis
- Serology—serum neutralization assay, complement fixation assay, and hemagglutination inhibition test

Atypical Myopathy (Atypical Myoglobinuria)
- Atypical myopathy has been reported in the United Kingdom, continental Europe, and Australia.
- It typically occurs in horses and ponies on pasture.
- Affected individuals usually are on a low plane of nutrition and are either *not* being exercised or are only minimally exercised.
- Adverse climatic conditions (heavy rain and gales) often occur before an outbreak.
- One or more individuals in a group may be affected.
- The cause of atypical myopathy is unknown, but an association with toxins of *Clostridium sordelli* has been suggested; in the United States, seeds of the box elder tree have been linked to the toxin.
- The disease is associated with the development of a multiple acyl-CoA dehydrogenase deficiency, which blocks several steps in mitochondrial lipid metabolism.
- Respiratory capacity of mitochondrial complexes of the electron transport system is significantly decreased.
- A severe rhabdomyolysis is seen, especially in muscles that contain a high proportion of oxidative type I fibers and the myocardium.

Signalment
- Any age, however most common among young horses (<6 years)

Clinical Signs
- May be found dead or recumbent
- Less severely affected individuals may have a sudden onset of stiffness, which may progress over several hours to recumbency.
- Usually no signs of pain or distress
- Appetite and thirst normal, even in recumbent individuals
- Temperature, heart rate, and respiratory rate are normal.
- Dark brown or red urine

Diagnosis
- Epidemiologic characteristics and clinical signs
- Marked elevations of creatine kinase (CK) and aspartate aminotransferase (AST) values

- Raised serum troponin I levels
- Myoglobinuria
- Some patients have elevations of sorbitol dehydrogenase and γ-glutamyl transferase.
- Some patients have hypocalcemia, especially in terminal stages.
- Muscle biopsy with immunohistochemistry to demonstrate excessive intramuscular lipid storage in type I myofibers
- Increased concentrations of acylcarnitines and organic acids in urine and/or blood

●》 WHAT TO DO

Atypical Myopathy
- If the patient can still stand, it should be transported to a well-bedded stable where intensive therapy can be administered.
- Provide symptomatic treatment of recumbent patients and management to limit further muscle damage.
- Prevent hypothermia if the patient is recumbent in a cold environment.
- Attempting to place recumbent patients in slings is rarely helpful.
- Correct fluid-electrolyte imbalances and acid-base abnormalities.
- Monitor urea and creatinine values to assess renal function.
- Digoxin (0.0022 mg/kg IV or 0.011 mg/kg PO) might be considered in cases that demonstrate reduced myocardial function. If severe arrhythmias occur, administration of antiarrhythmic drugs may be considered.
- The horse should be encouraged to eat a diet low in lipids and rich in carbohydrates (grass, good quality hay, alfalfa, grains, molasses, sugar water, carrots, and apples). Assisted enteral nutritional support (via nasogastric intubation) may be needed if the horse is anorectic or dysphagic (e.g., soaked alfalfa pellets or commercial liquid foods).
- Supplement with riboflavin in the form of a vitamin B complex.
- Treat hyperlipemia, if present.
- Prednisolone, 0.5 to 1 mg/kg PO q24h, may help in some cases.

Prognosis
- Mortality is high, up to 100% in some outbreaks.
- Improved prognosis is associated with ability to remain standing most of the time, normothermia, normal mucous membranes, and continued defecation.
- A poor prognosis for survival is associated with recumbency, sweating, anorexia, dyspnea, tachypnea, tachycardia, high packed cell volume (PCV), low chloride concentration, low arterial partial pressure of oxygen (Pa_{O_2}), and/or respiratory acidosis.
- Horses that are stiff but remain standing after 2 to 3 days have a good prognosis.
- Prognosis shows poor correlation with degree of elevation of CK and AST.
- Nonsurvivors usually die or are euthanized within 72 hours of the onset of clinical signs, but can remain alive for up to 10 days.

Foal Immunodeficiency Syndrome in the Fell and Dales Ponies
- The Fell and Dales are rare native U.K. pony breeds.
- Foal immunodeficiency syndrome (FIS) in these breeds is a lethal Mendelian recessive disease that manifests as a B-lymphocyte immunodeficiency.
- Approximately 10% of Fell ponies born each year die from this disease.
- A mutation of the sodium/myo-inositol cotransporter gene (SLC5A3) has been identified.

Clinical Signs
- Affected foals may appear normal at birth.
- At 2 to 3 weeks of age they commonly develop diarrhea (may be associated with cryptosporidiosis), cough (may be associated with adenovirus bronchopneumonia), and failure to suckle.
- Frequent chewing movements and halitosis associated with a pale pseudomembranous lingual covering
- Severe anemia
- Lymphopenia
- Dry, dull coat
- Deterioration usually results in death or euthanasia at 1 to 3 months

●》 WHAT TO DO

Foal Immunodeficiency Syndrome
- Symptomatic only
- No effective therapy

Prevention
- Genetic testing (mane or tail hair samples to be sent to Animal Health Trust, Newmarket, UK) and selective breeding

Plant Toxins
See Chapter 34, p. 580.

Deadly Nightshade *(Atropa belladonna)*
- Deadly nightshade contains atropine, which is a muscarinic antagonist of acetylcholine.

Clinical Signs
- Mydriasis and impaired vision
- Anorexia
- Hyperexcitability
- Shivering and muscle spasms
- Ataxia
- Polyuria, occasionally with hematuria
- Convulsions

Diagnosis
- History and clinical signs
- Identification of plant fragments in stomach and intestinal tract

EMG

●〉 **WHAT TO DO**

Deadly Nightshade
- Neostigmine, 0.005 to 0.01 mg/kg IM or SQ
- Activated charcoal by mouth
- Supportive care

Hemlock *(Conium maculatum)*
- Hemlock is widely distributed in the United Kingdom.
- It contains the alkaloid coniine.
- *Practice Tip: Only fresh plant material is toxic because drying inactivates the alkaloid.*

Clinical Signs
- Pupillary dilation
- Weakness
- Ataxia
- Bradycardia followed by tachycardia
- Bradypnea with increased respiratory effort
- Death due to respiratory arrest

Diagnosis
- Compatible history and clinical signs
- Identification of plant fragments in the stomach or intestinal contents

●〉 **WHAT TO DO**

Hemlock
- Activated charcoal by mouth
- Supportive care

Rhododendron *(Rhodendron ponticum)*
- Rhododendron is a widely distributed naturalized species in the United Kingdom and is poisonous because of its content of the polyol andromedotoxin.
- Poisoning usually occurs in winter when snow interferes with grazing or in summer when pastures are scorched by drought.

Clinical Signs
- Hypersalivation (ptyalism/sialorrhea)
- Retching
- Colic
- Diarrhea
- Excitement
- Depression
- Cardiovascular collapse
- Ataxia
- Death after several days due to respiratory depression and failure

Diagnosis
- Compatible history and clinical signs
- Identification of plant fragments in the stomach or intestinal contents

●〉 **WHAT TO DO**

Rhododendron
- Activated charcoal by mouth
- Supportive care

Water Dropwort (*Oenanthe* spp.), Water Hemlock (*Cicuta virosa*)
- These plants are toxic because of their content of resinous toxins oenanthetoxin and cicutoxin.
- The roots are particularly toxic and are usually eaten when they are dug up during ditching operations and left on the banks.

Clinical Signs
- Hypersalivation
- Abdominal pain
- Pupillary dilation
- Muscle spasms
- Seizures
- Death often occurs within a few minutes of the onset of clinical signs because of respiratory failure.

Diagnosis
- Compatible history and clinical signs
- Identification of plant fragments in the stomach or intestinal contents

●〉 **WHAT TO DO**

Water Dropwort/Water Hemlock
- Activated charcoal by mouth
- Supportive care
- In most cases, death occurs before treatment can be initiated.

THE MIDDLE EAST

Israel Pasval

- The equine diseases described in this section refer to the Middle East countries (ME) that are members of the Office of International Epizootics (OIE) and include Algeria, Bahrain, Egypt, Iran, Iraq, Israel, Jordan, Kuwait, Lebanon, Libya, Morocco, Oman, Palestine, Qatar, Saudi Arabia, Sudan, Syria, Tunisia, Turkey, United Arab Emirates, and Yemen.
- According to the OIE yearbooks, the most important equine emergencies are African horse sickness, equine piroplasmosis (EP; equine babesiosis), equine influenza (EI), surra, and horse mange (HM; Table 40-1).

African Horse Sickness
- African horse sickness (AHS) (see pp. 666 and 674) was the most important disease in the ME in the early 1960s. Because of successful implementation of eradication and vaccination measures, no cases of this disease have been reported since 1993. AHS is a highly fatal, viscerotropic,

EMG

Table 40-1 Horse Diseases in the Middle East According to OIE Data

Country	African Horse Sickness A110	Dourine B202	Epizootic Lymphangitis B203	Equine Infectious Anemia B205	Equine Influenza B206	Equine Piroplasmosis B207	Equine Rhinopneumonitis B208	Glanders B209	Equine Viral Arteritis B211	Horse Mange B213	Surra (Trypanosoma Evansi) B215
OIE Classification A–B*											
Yemen	–	–	–	–	–	–	–	–	–	–	–
United Arab Emirates	–	–	–	–	–	06+ 07+ 10+	–	–	–	–	–
Turkey	–	–	–	–	–	–	–	–	–	–	–
Tunisia	–	–	–	–	–	–	–	–	06	–	–
Syria	–	–	–	–	–	–	–	–	–	–	–
Sudan	–	–	–	–	–	–	–	–	–	–	09
Saudi Arabia	–	–	–	–	–	–	–	–	–	–	–
Qatar	–	–	–	–	–	06+? 07+? 08+?	–	–	–	–	09+
Palestine Auton Territory	–	–	–	–	–	–	–	–	–	–	–
Oman	–	–	–	–	–	–	–	–	–	–	–

Continued

EMG

Table 40-1 Horse Diseases in the Middle East According to OIE Data—cont'd

	African Horse Sickness	Dorine	Epizootic Lymphangitis	Equine Infectious Anemia	Equine Influenza	Equine Piroplasmosis	Equine Rhinopneumonitis	Glanders	Equine Viral Arteritis	Horse Mange	Surra (Trypanosoma Evansi)
Morocco	-	-	-	-	06	06+ 07+ 08+ 09+ 10+	06+ 07+ 08+ 09+ 10+	-	06+ 07+ 08+ 09+ 10?+	-	-
Libya	-	-	-	-	-	-	-	-	-	-	-
Lebanon	-	-	-	-	-	-	08?	11	-	-	-
Kuwait	-	-	-	-	08	-	-	09+ 10	-	-	-
Jordan	-	-	-	-	-	06+ 07+ 08+ 09+ 10+	-	-	-	-	09
Israel	-	-	-	-	06 07	06 07 08 09 10	06 08 11	-	-	-	-
Iraq	-	-	-	-	-	-	-	-	-	-	-
Iran	-	-	-	-	-	-	-	07+? 08? 09 10 11	-	-	-
Egypt	-	-	-	-	-	-	-	-	-	-	-
Bahrain	-	-	-	-	09? 10? 11?	-	-	10 11	-	-	-
Algeria	-	-	-	-	-	-	-	-	-	-	-

Data from the Office of International Epizootics (OIE).

*List A diseases are defined as transmissible diseases that have the potential for serious and rapid spread, irrespective of national borders, that are of serious socioeconomic or public health consequence, and that are of major importance in the international trade of animals and animal products. List A diseases must be reported to the OIE as soon as possible. List B diseases are defined as transmissible diseases that are considered to be of serious socioeconomic and/or public health importance and that are significant in the international trade of animals and animal products. List B diseases are also reportable, but these reports are of intervals.

Note: The numbers following the A and B listing designate the disease number in the OIE listings.

†The numbers mentioned in the table are the last two digits of the year.

? Suspected but not confirmed.

EMG

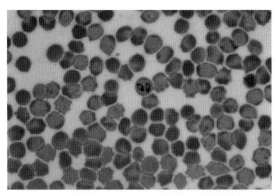

Figure 40-1 Intraerythrocytic *Babesia caballi* in blood smear stained with Giemsa (merozoites vary in size from 2 to 5 μm in length by 1 to 1.5 μm in width).

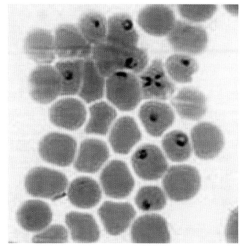

Figure 40-2 Intraerythrocytic *Theileria equi* merozoites in blood smear stained with Giemsa (1.5 to 3 μm) show the characteristic Maltese cross form.

insect-borne viral disease. The clinical signs are characterized by an impairment of the respiratory and circulatory systems causing fever, cardiac failure, edema, pulmonary edema, and respiratory distress.

●> WHAT TO DO

African Horse Sickness
- There is no treatment for AHS.
- The preventive measures include quarantine and precautions at frontiers and inside the country.
- When the disease is introduced into a region, the population should be surveyed for infection, and affected equidae should be humanely destroyed and the carcasses disposed of properly.
- Nonaffected equidae should be vaccinated. Vaccines have been developed for all nine serotypes.
- Control of vectors using insecticides, repellents, and the destruction of mosquito breeding areas is advised.
- See p. 669.

Equine Piroplasmosis
- During the last decade equine piroplasmosis (EP; also called equine babesiosis) cases have been reported repeatedly by Bahrain, Egypt, Israel, Jordan, Morocco, Tunisia, and United Arab Emirates.
- EP is caused by protozoa—*Babesia caballi* (Fig. 40-1) or *Theileria equi* (Fig. 40-2)—and is transmitted by ticks, particularly in countries with a hot climate.
- The signs of this disease range from acute fever, inappetence, and malaise to anemia and jaundice, sudden death, or chronic weight loss and poor exercise tolerance.
- See p. 683.

●> WHAT TO DO

Equine Piroplasmosis
- Confirmation of the diagnosis by microscopic examination (Giemsa stain) of blood smears is required.
- A number of serologic tests are available for the detection of carrier horses. There is *no* vaccine.
- Treatment using Imizol, imidocarb, or Berenil is usually effective (see p. 685).
- Tick control should be implemented.

- Quarantine for horses imported from countries where the disease is enzootic is recommended.
- See p. 683.

Equine Influenza
- Outbreaks of equine influenza (EI) have been reported repeatedly during the last decade by Israel, Morocco, and Tunisia.
- EI is an acute, contagious respiratory disease.
- EI is caused by two distinct subtypes of influenza A viruses.
- The clinical signs are fever, dry to moist cough, serous nasal discharge, lethargy, and anorexia; secondary infection of the upper respiratory tract can be fatal in foals.

●> WHAT TO DO

Equine Influenza
- Because influenza could be introduced by importation of infected horses, quarantine and other precautions at frontiers are necessary.
- No chronic carriers exist, and incubation is short, so it is likely that the disease would be recognized at quarantine inspection.
- Influenza vaccines are widely available and are routinely used in competition horses.
- In democratic countries, vaccination should remain prohibited except for sport horses participating in international events.

Surra
- Surra cases have been reported during the last decade by Egypt, Iraq, Jordan, Morocco, Oman, Saudi Arabia, Tunisia, and Yemen.
- The name "surra" comes from Sudan and is Arabic by origin.
- Surra is a disease of vertebrate animals, including horses and mules, is caused by the protozoa *Trypanosoma evansi*, and is transmitted by horseflies and vampire bats.
- The clinical signs are fever; weakness and lethargy; petechial hemorrhages (eyelids, nostrils, and anus); edematous swellings of the legs, briskets, and abdomen; urticarial

EMG

eruption of the skin; progressive loss of weight; anemia; and jaundice.

- In some animals, surra is fatal unless treated.

●〉 WHAT TO DO

Surra

- Identification of the protozoa is performed on a blood smear. Serologic tests are available.
- Use ELISA to declare disease-free status and card agglutination test to retest suspect samples.
- No vaccination is available.
- Treatment in horses includes diminazene aceturate (3.5 to 5.0 mg/kg IM, as a single dose and repeat in 5 weeks; see Appendix 9, p. 835).
- Importation from infected countries should be prohibited.

Horse Mange

- Horse mange (HM), or scabies, is an endemic disease in most of the ME.
- HM is caused by the infestation by microscopic arthropod parasites, generally called mites. Many different types of mites cause disease, but only sarcoptic mange due to *Sarcoptes scabiei* var. *equi* is considered an OIE disease.
- HM is a contagious zoonosis.
- Clinical signs include skin lesions that begin on the head, the neck, and the shoulders and constant pruritus.
- Lesions are small papules that develop into vesicles and then crusts. Progressively, there is alopecia and significant skin lignifications.
- If untreated, HM can lead to emaciation, weakness, and anorexia.

●〉 WHAT TO DO

Horse Mange

- Effective treatments include ivermectin and carbaryl (see Appendix 9, p. 835).
- No vaccine is available.
- Quarantine, movement control, and other precautions at frontiers and inside the country are recommended.

●〉 WHAT NOT TO DO

Horse Mange

- Do not use amitraz in horses.

Disease Management

- The activities of the Food and Agriculture Organization of the United Nations Regional Conferences for the Near East and the OIE Conferences of Regional Commission for the Middle East have significantly improved the equine health status in this region.
- Since 1990, increased attention to equine health in the ME has taken place with the foundation of the World Arab Horse Organization because of enhanced interest in the famous Arabian purebred horse.
- In the comprehensive report *Equine Health Status in the Middle East,* presented by G. Yehya to the OIE Regional

Commission (OIE Press Release, 1997), the author summarizes the animal disease control measures and import regulations. The reported control measures included the following:

- Setting up control programs inside the country
- Control of nonvertebrate vectors and wildlife reservoirs
- Quarantine measures at frontiers
- Epidemiologic surveillance campaigns with laboratory tests for the most important equine diseases
- The list of the reported import regulations consists of the following requirements:
  - An official health certificate complying with international standards is required by the majority of countries for the importation of horses.
  - Quarantine measures for horses imported from countries where diseases are enzootic are implemented in the majority of countries.
  - Some countries, such as United Arab Emirates, only allow horses to be imported directly by air.

SOUTH AFRICA

Montague N. Saulez

African Horse Sickness (AHS)
Etiology and Epidemiology

- African horse sickness is a noncontagious disease of equids caused by an orbivirus (nine serotypes exist) that is transmitted by *Culicoides* midges (especially *C. imicola* and *C. bolitinos*) (see pp. 666 and 670, Europe and Middle East).
- It is endemic in eastern and central Africa and occurs in South Africa. Initial reports refer to an outbreak of AHS in Yemen (1327), and horses imported to East Africa from India (1569). Also, there are reports of "perreziekte" following colonization of the Cape of Good Hope by settlers of the Dutch East India Company after introduction of horses (1652).
- AHS can also be found in North Africa, the Middle East, and Spain. This disease has not been identified in Mauritius and Madagascar. Outbreaks of AHS have been recorded in the following countries: Egypt, Palestine, Portugal, Lebanon, Jordan, Iran, Iraq, Cyprus, Syria, Libya, Afghanistan, Pakistan, India, Turkey, Tunisia, Algeria, Morocco, Saudi Arabia, and the Cape Verde Islands.
- Horses affected by AHS typically have pyrexia and inappetence with widespread edema affecting the subcutaneous, intermuscular, and pulmonary tissues. Mules, donkeys, and zebras may also be affected.
- ***Practice Tip:*** *Dogs may acquire AHS through ingestion of AHS-infected equine carcasses.*
- Depending on climatic conditions, AHS typically starts in northern regions of South Africa (December through January) before spreading southwards, especially when climatic conditions are favorable (early rain followed by

hot, dry periods are the most suitable conditions for the breeding of *Culicoides* midges).

- Following the first frost (April to May), which disrupts the *Culicoides* midge lifecycle, no new reports of AHS occur. In the Kruger National Park, AHS virus is continually transmitted between *Culicoides* midges and zebras. Zebras (and possibly donkeys) may act as a large reservoir for AHS virus in Africa.

Subdivisions of the Disease
- "Dunkop" or pulmonary form
- "Dikkop" or cardiac form
- "Mixed form"
- AHS fever

Clinical Signs
"Dunkop" or Pulmonary Form
- Fever
- Tachycardia, tachypnea, dyspnea, coughing
- Nasal discharge which is serofibrinous and frothy
- Sudden death
- Pulmonary form has the highest mortality rate in excess of 70%.

"Dikkop" or Cardiac Form
- Subcutaneous edema of the head and neck
- Edema of the supraorbital fossa
- Eyelids, cheek, tongue, neck may also be affected by edema
- Fever
- Petechiae of the conjunctiva and ventral tongue
- Inability to swallow due to esophageal paralysis
- Restlessness
- Mortality rate is 50%.

"Mixed Form"
- Most common form
- Dyspnea
- Widespread edema
- Mortality rate is 70%.

AHS fever
- Mild form
- Pyrexia
- Short episodes of tachycardia, dyspnea, and inappetence
- ***Practice Tip:*** *Due to presumed immunosuppression, infected horses may also acquire babesiosis with clinical signs of inappetence, icterus, and anemia.*

Pathology
"Dunkop" or Pulmonary Form
- Lung edema; trachea and bronchi filled with froth (Figs. 40-3, 40-4, and 40-5); hydrothorax
- Petechiae and ecchymoses on pleura and trachea
- Hemorrhage of the endocardium and epicardium
- Congestion of the glandular portion of the stomach; petechiation of the serosa and mucosa of the intestines

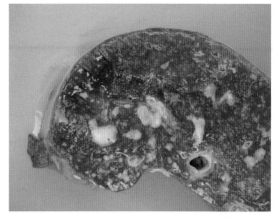

Figure 40-3 "Dunkop" form of AHS. Gelatinous edema and froth exuding from bronchi. (Courtesy of Prof. M. N. Saulez, Section of Equine Medicine, Department of Companion Animal Clinical Studies, Faculty of Veterinary Science, University of Pretoria, South Africa.)

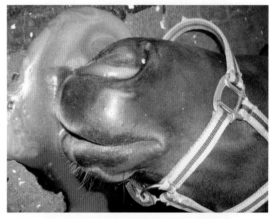

Figure 40-4 Pulmonary or "dunkop" form of AHS. Large quantity of frothy serofibrinous fluid from the nostrils of a horse that died acutely. (Courtesy of Prof. M. N. Saulez, Section of Equine Medicine, Department of Companion Animal Clinical Studies, Faculty of Veterinary Science, University of Pretoria, South Africa.)

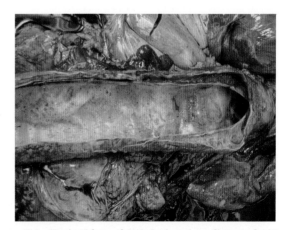

Figure 40-5 "Dunkop" form of AHS. Froth and serofibrinous fluid in the trachea of a horse that died. (Courtesy Prof. M. N. Saulez, Section of Equine Medicine, Department of Companion Animal Clinical Studies, Faculty of Veterinary Science, University of Pretoria, South Africa)

EMG

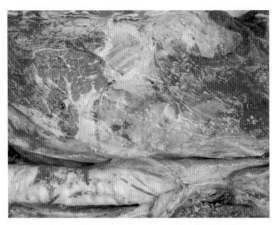

Figure 40-6   Edema of the intermuscular connective tissues in a horse with the "Dikkop" form of AHS. (Courtesy of Prof. M. N. Saulez, Section of Equine Medicine, Department of Companion Animal Clinical Studies, Faculty of Veterinary Science, University of Pretoria, South Africa.)

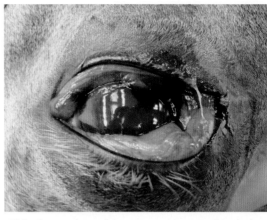

Figure 40-8   Severe edema of the upper and lower eyelids of a horse with AHS. (Courtesy of Prof. M. N. Saulez, Section of Equine Medicine, Department of Companion Animal Clinical Studies, Faculty of Veterinary Science, University of Pretoria, South Africa.)

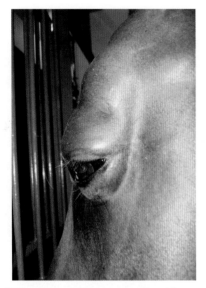

Figure 40-7   "Dikkop" form of AHS. Severe swelling of the supraorbital fossa. (Courtesy of Prof. M. N. Saulez, Section of Equine Medicine, Department of Companion Animal Clinical Studies, Faculty of Veterinary Science, University of Pretoria, South Africa.)

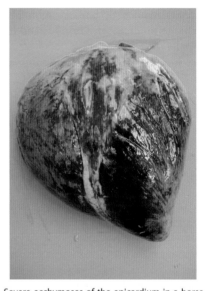

Figure 40-9   Severe ecchymoses of the epicardium in a horse affected with the "dikkop" or cardiac form of AHS. (Courtesy of Prof. M. N. Saulez, Section of Equine Medicine, Department of Companion Animal Clinical Studies, Faculty of Veterinary Science, University of Pretoria, South Africa.)

"Dikkop" or Cardiac Form
- Edema of the subcutaneous and intermuscular connective tissue, including the head and neck (Fig. 40-6). Supraorbital fossa (Fig. 40-7), eyelids (Fig. 40-8), cheeks, and tongue
- Hydropericardium and hemorrhage of the epicardium (Fig. 40-9)
- Congestion and petechiation of the cecum, colon, and rectum

"Mixed form"
- Similar to lesions observed in both "Dunkop" and "Dikkop" forms

Diagnosis
- Provisional diagnosis possible based on epidemiology, clinical signs, and macropathologic changes

- Virus isolation from blood, lungs, spleen, lymph node
- Serotyping of AHS isolates using virus neutralization tests
- Circulating antibody titers indicate recent infection.
- PCR-based assays to detect AHS virus and to differentiate between various AHS serotypes

Differential Diagnoses
- Equine encephalosis
- Babesiosis
- Purpura hemorrhagica
- Equine viral arteritis

●> WHAT TO DO

African Horse Sickness
- Provide symptomatic and supportive therapy in a stress-free environment.

- Antibiotics: benzyl penicillin (22,000 IU/kg IV q6h) and gentamicin (6.6 mg/kg IV q24h) for possible secondary infection
- NSAIDs: flunixin meglumine (1.1 mg/kg IV q12h or 0.25 mg/kg IV q6h)
- Dimethyl sulfoxide (DMSO) (10% solution IV q12 to 24h)
- Diuretics: furosemide (1 mg/kg IV as required)
- Tracheostomy and oxygen support (O_2, 10 L/h)
- Maintain blood pressure: 6% hydroxyethyl starch 130/0.4[1] (Voluven,[2] 0.5 to 1 mL/kg, IV q12 to 24h)
- Partial or total parenteral nutrition
- Vector control:
  - Stabling of equidae from dusk to dawn
  - Insect repellents
  - Application of insecticides

Prevention

- Immunize using attenuated strains prepared in a trivalent (serotypes 1, 3, and 4) and quadrivalent (serotypes 2, 6, 7, and 8) live polyvalent vaccine, 3 weeks apart.
- Prophylactic immunization in endemic regions in late winter or early summer
- Horses that recover may develop cross-immunity to other serotypes.
- Foals that have received adequate colostral transfer of antibodies from vaccinated dams should be vaccinated at 6 months of age

West Nile Virus (WNV)

- See Chapter 22, p. 349.

Etiology and Epidemiology

- WNV is a mosquito-borne flavivirus that may cause encephalomyelitis in horses and humans.
- It belongs within the Japanese encephalitis sero-complex of the family Flaviviridae that includes Japanese encephalitis, Kunjin, Murray Valley encephalitis, and St. Louis encephalitis viruses.
- Birds are the amplification hosts of WNV while mammals are mostly dead-end hosts.
- WNV isolates fall into five lineages, of which the most important are:
  - Lineage 1:
    - North America
    - North Africa
    - Europe
    - Australia
  - Lineage 2:
    - Southern Africa
    - Madagascar
    - Europe
- Although it was thought that the pathogenicity of lineage 1 strains was greater than lineage 2 strains, both

neuroinvasive and mild strains of WNV occur in both lineages.
- Up to 70% of horses are seropositive for WNV in South Africa. Although initially thought not to cause neuroinvasive disease in horses in South Africa, recent investigations indicated that 14% to 21% of cases of neurologic disease in horses may be due to WNV with a mortality rate of >40%.
- All reverse transcription polymerase chain reaction (RT-PCR) or virus isolation–positive cases were shown to be associated with lineage 2 WNV except for a single case detected in 2010 in a pregnant mare and her aborted fetus.

Clinical Signs

- Fever
- Ataxia, progressive weakness in forelimbs and hind limbs, recumbency
- Muscle fasciculations progressing to seizures

Diagnosis

- Virus isolation or RT-PCR from brain, spinal cord, CSF, or blood
- IgM antibody capture ELISA (MAC-ELISA) and plaque neutralizing titer (PRNT) in serum

Treatment

- Supportive therapy

Control

- Use of commercially licensed vaccines
- Vector control:
  - Horses should be kept in screened stables.
  - Use of mosquito repellents
  - Eliminate mosquito-breeding locations (drain stagnant water and discard used tires).
- ***Practice Tip:*** *Coinfection with African horse sickness and Sindbis virus can occur; differential diagnoses include Middleburg virus, Shuni virus, and Wesselsbron virus.*
- ***Practice Tip:*** *Public health consideration: The potential exists for zoonotic and laboratory infections.*
- Horses vaccinated for Eastern, Western, and Venezuelan equine encephalitis will *not* have protection from WNV.

Sindbis Virus
Etiology and Epidemiology

- This is an alphavirus that is transmitted by *Culex* mosquitoes.
- It has been identified in Kwazulu-Natal Province, Cape Town, and Gauteng Province.

Clinical Signs

- Fever
- Mild ataxia
- Neurologic symptoms may be present when there is coinfection with WNV.

---

[1]The colloid solution is identified by the molecular weight (130) and molar substitution (0.4). These are highly relevant to the pharmacokinetics of the different colloid products.
[2]Voluven (Fresenius Kabi, Halfway House, South Africa).

Diagnosis
- No serologic tests are yet available.
- Virus isolation or RT-PCR of brain, spinal cord, CSF, blood, or spleen

Treatment
- Supportive therapy

Wesselsbron Virus
Etiology and Epidemiology
- This is an acute, arthropod-borne flavivirus infection that historically affects sheep, cattle, and goats throughout sub-Saharan Africa.
- Isolates have been recovered from ostriches and a foal.
- Recent reports have identified Wesselsbron virus in the Western Cape and North West Province in two horses.

Clinical Signs
- Similar to WNV

Diagnosis
- Virus isolation and RT-PCR from brain, spinal cord, CSF, blood, liver, and spleen
- Serologic cross-reaction exists with WNV in IgG/IgM tests; confirm with neutralization assay if possible.

Treatment
- Supportive therapy

Control
- Vector control
- Avoid flood water regions where *Aedes* mosquitoes are found.
- ***Practice Tip:*** *The potential exists for zoonotic infections.*

Differential Diagnoses
- WNV
- Sindbis virus
- Middleburg virus
- Shuni virus

Middelburg Virus
Etiology and Epidemiology
- This is an alphavirus that is transmitted by *Aedes* mosquitoes.
- It has been identified in Kwazulu-Natal, Swaziland, North West, Gauteng, Karoo, and Northern and Western Cape in horses, livestock, and wildlife with neurologic symptoms.

Clinical Signs
- Fever
- Ataxia, progressive weakness in thoracic and pelvic limbs
- Recumbency
- Muscle fasciculation, seizures
- Affected horses have a lower mortality rate compared with horses with WNV.
- There can be coinfection with Wesselsbron virus.

Diagnosis
- RT-PCR from brain, spinal cord, blood, or CSF

Treatment
- Supportive therapy

Control
- Vector control as mentioned previously

Shuni Virus (SHUV)
Etiology and Epidemiology
- This is an orthobunyavirus transmitted by mosquitos and possibly *Culicoides.*
- In the 1960s, SHUV was isolated from cattle, sheep, and *Culicoides* midges; in 1977 it was found in the brain of two horses suffering meningoencephalitis (one each from South Africa and Zimbabwe). Thereafter, SHUV has been identified in *Culex theileri* mosquitoes caught in Johannesburg and from cattle and a goat in KwaZulu-Natal Province.
- In 2008-2010, two horses died from fatal encephalitis due to SHUV, as well as four others with neurologic symptoms.
- SHUV has been identified in Gauteng Province, Northern Cape, Karoo, and Limpopo Province.

Clinical Signs
- Fever, depression
- Ataxia, progressive weakness in forelimbs and hind limbs, recumbency
- Muscle fasciculation, seizures
- May be fatal

Diagnosis
- No serologic tests are available yet.
- RT-PCR of brain, spinal cord, CSF, or blood
- Cytologic analysis of CSF: lymphocytic pleocytosis may suggest infection.

Treatment
- Supportive therapy
- ***Practice Tip:*** *The potential exists for zoonotic infections and coinfection with Middleburg virus.*

Differential Diagnoses
- WNV
- Middleburg virus
- Wesselsbron virus

Equine Encephalosis Virus (EEV)
- See p. 667 for additional details.

Etiology and Epidemiology
- This orbivirus (seven serotypes exist) is transmitted by a variety of *Culicoides* spp. and is associated with African horse sickness.

- It is closely related to bluetongue and epizootic hemorrhagic disease viruses and infects equidae of southern Africa including Botswana, Kenya, and South Africa. Horses, donkeys, and zebra frequently have antibodies to EEV.

Clinical Signs
- Incubation period is 3 to 6 days.
- Most horses are asymptomatic.
- Pyrexia, inappetence, tachycardia, tachypnea
- Congestion and icterus of mucus membranes
- Infrequent swelling of eyelids and supraorbital fossa
- Progressive neurologic dysfunction leading to ataxia followed by recumbency
- Abortion
- Edema of the limbs

Macropathology
- Edema of lung, hydropericardium
- Petechiae of the serosa of the gastrointestinal tract, congestion of the glandular portion of the stomach
- Cerebral edema degeneration of cardiac myofibers

Diagnosis
- Most infections are subclinical.
- The virus can be isolated from blood, spleen, liver, lung, and brain.
- Circulating antibody titers are detected by serum neutralization assays and ELISA.

Differential Diagnoses
- African horse sickness
- Neurologic symptoms may be confused with:
  - WNV
  - Wesselsbron virus
  - Middleburg virus
  - Shuni virus

⊙› WHAT TO DO

Equine Encephalosis Virus
- Vector control (as in AHS)
- Symptomatic and supportive therapy

Toxic Plants of South Africa Affecting a Specific Organ or Body System
Liver
Seneciosis
- *S. latifolius* (Fig. 40-10) and *S. retrorsus* (Fig. 40-11) are the most important pyrrolizidine alkaloid-containing plants that are found in eastern regions of South Africa.
- Poisoning may result from eating fresh plant material or *Senecio*-contaminated hay.
- *Practice Tip: Flowering plants are the greatest risk.*

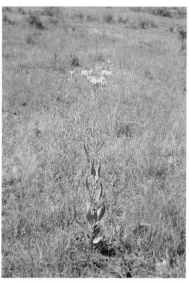

Figure 40-10   *Senecio latifolius.* (Courtesy of Professor C. J. Botha, Department of Paraclinical Studies, Faculty of Veterinary Science, University of Pretoria, South Africa.)

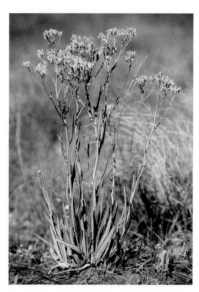

Figure 40-11   *Senecio retrorsus.* (Courtesy of Professor C. J. Botha, Department of Paraclinical Studies, Faculty of Veterinary Science, University of Pretoria, South Africa.)

Clinical Signs
- Acute:
  - Depression, inappetence, weight loss
  - Icterus
  - Petechiae, ecchymoses
  - Colic
- Chronic:
  - Also known as "*dunsiekte*"
  - Head pressing, yawning, aimless wandering ataxia

Diagnosis
- Liver biopsy: histopathology may reveal hepatic necrosis, inter- and intralobular fibrosis, hepatocellular megalocytosis and karyomegaly, central vein fibrosis, and bile duct proliferation.

EMG

●› WHAT TO DO

Seneciosis

- Supportive therapy: provide good-quality palatable feed and water.
- Although there is no proven efficacy the following may be used:
  - Colchicine (0.03 mg/kg PO q12 to 24h) to decrease liver fibrosis
  - S-Adenosylmethione (20 mg/kg PO q24h)
  - Pentoxifylline (10 mg/kg PO q12h)

Lupinosis

- Lupins are cultivated in the Western Cape as a green compost and fodder crop.
- They may be parasitized by a fungus, *Phomopsis leptostromiformis (Diaporthe toxica)* (Fig. 40-12).
- The principal toxin is phomopsin A, a cyclic hexapeptide.

Clinical Signs
- Colic, weakness, and icterus

Diagnosis
- Fungus may be visible on the lupine pods and seeds

Treatment
- Supportive therapy

Respiratory System

Crotolariosis

- *Crotalaria dura* and *C. globifera* are found in KwaZulu-Natal.
- They contain pyrrolizidine alkaloids and have been responsible for recent outbreaks.
- Associated with feeding of *Themeda* hay contaminated with *C. dura* or ingestion of fresh plants

Clinical Signs
- Dullness, restlessness, persistent walking and circling
- Chronic form (also called "Jaagsiekte") causes fever, polypnea, and dyspnea.

Diagnosis
- Liver biopsy and histopathology (see p. 679)

Treatment
- Supportive therapy

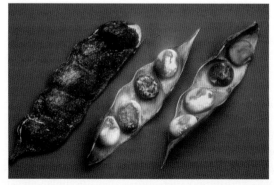

Figure 40-12 Lupinosis: *Phomopsis leptostromiformis* infection of lupine pods and seeds. (Courtesy of Professor C. J. Botha, Department of Paraclinical Studies, Faculty of Veterinary Science, University of Pretoria, South Africa.)

Differential Diagnosis
- African horse sickness
- Pneumonia

Ageratina Adenophora (Eupatorium Adenophorum)

- Also known as crofton weed, this plant was implicated in the death of horses in Zimbabwe.
- This plant is palatable and readily consumed by horses.
- *Chromolaena odorata (Eupatorium odoratum)* is closely related and may cause similar problems.

Clinical Signs
- Coughing, exercise intolerance, and dyspnea

Diagnosis
- Postmortem: macropathology of the lung may reveal interstitial and subpleural fibrosis

Treatment
- Supportive therapy

Nervous System

Leukoencephalomalacia (LEM)

- This is a fatal neuromycotoxicosis of horses that causes irreversible focal liquefactive necrosis of the cerebral white matter.
- LEM is caused by a saprophytic fungus, *Fusarium verticillioides (Fusarium moniliforme)* that grows on corn.
- Prevalence increases in wet months and can especially infect cobs when insect damage has occurred.
- The principal mycotoxin is fumonisin B_1, which alters sphingolipid synthesis.
- ***Practice Tip:*** *Fumonisin B_1 has been associated with anterior enteritis.*

Clinical Signs
- Latent period
- Restlessness, hypersensitivity, and icterus
- Ataxia, short-stepping, or goose-stepping gait
- Paralysis of lips and tongue, difficulty eating
- Convulsions

Diagnosis
- Postmortem: macropathology may reveal edema and yellow, swollen regions in the brain.
- Histopathology of the brain: liquefactive necrosis and hemorrhage of the subcortical region of the cerebral white matter
- Occasionally histopathology of the liver reveals hepatic necrosis.

Treatment
- No treatment exists.

Cynanchum

- *Cynanchum ellipticum* (Fig. 40-13), more commonly known as "monkey rope," occurs in coastal bush and wooded valleys.
- The principal toxins are glycosides ("cynanchoides").

Clinical Signs
- Ataxia, rocking forward and backward
- Recumbency

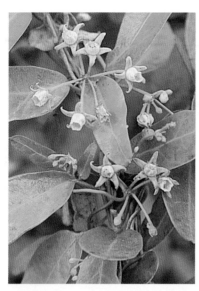

Figure 40-13 *Cynanchum* sp. (Courtesy of Professor C. J. Botha, Department of Paraclinical Studies, Faculty of Veterinary Science, University of Pretoria, South Africa.)

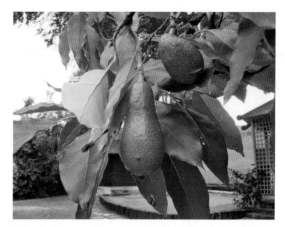

Figure 40-14 *Persea* sp. (Courtesy of Professor C. J. Botha, Department of Paraclinical Studies, Faculty of Veterinary Science, University of Pretoria, South Africa.)

Diagnosis
- Evidence of recent exposure

Treatment
- Supportive therapy
- Horses may recover once removed from contaminated pastures.

Cardiovascular System

Avocado
- *Persea americana*, especially of the Guatemalan race (Hass, Fuerte, and Nabal), has been implicated.
- The principle toxin is an unidentified cardiotoxin and persin.
- Horses can be exposed by eating fruit, seeds, and particularly leaves (Fig. 40-14).

Clinical Signs
- Severe edema of the head (masseter muscles, eyelids, and tongue), neck, and ventrum
- Tachycardia, polypnea, dyspnea, coughing, and arrhythmia
- Anorexia, weakness, and recumbency
- Lactating mares: noninfectious mastitis and agalactia

Diagnosis
- Access to avocado groves
- Postmortem: histopathology of the heart reveals myocardial degeneration and necrosis of the ventricle wall and septum

Treatment
- Supportive therapy
- Diuretics: furosemide
- NSAIDs

Cardiac Glycosides
- Plants such as *Nerium oleander* (oleander) and *Thevetia peruviana* are ornamental shrubs that often are planted close to stables and paddocks.

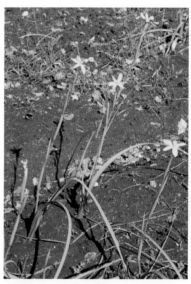

Figure 40-15 *Homeria* sp. (also referred to as the Transvaal yellow tulp). (Courtesy of Professor C. J. Botha, Department of Paraclinical Studies, Faculty of Veterinary Science, University of Pretoria, South Africa.)

- These plants are highly toxic and contain cardenolides.
- Bufadienolide cardiac glycosides are found in *Homeria* (Fig. 40-15) and *Moraea* species of "tulp."
- These plants are also contaminants of *Eragrostis* hay and lucerne (Fig. 40-16).

Clinical Signs
- Severe colic
- Weakness, depression, and icterus
- Inhibition of Na^+/K^+-ATPase, increased intracellular Ca^{2+} causing bradycardia, paroxysmal tachycardia, and arrhythmias (AV block, ectopic beats, and gallop rhythm with dropped beats)
- Yellow-green diarrhea

Diagnosis
- Analysis of gastrointestinal tract (GIT) content or urine
- Postmortem: histopathology of the heart may reveal myocardial necrosis and fibrosis.

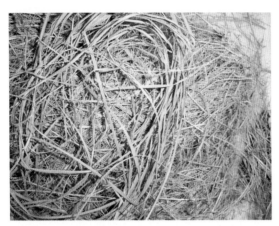

Figure 40-16 Contamination of hay with "tulp." (Courtesy of Professor C. J. Botha, Department of Paraclinical Studies, Faculty of Veterinary Science, University of Pretoria, South Africa.)

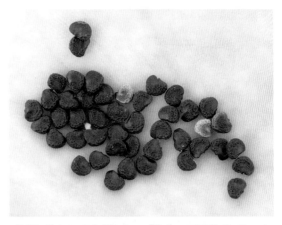

Figure 40-18 *Datura* seeds. (Courtesy of Professor C. J. Botha, Department of Paraclinical Studies, Faculty of Veterinary Science, University of Pretoria, South Africa.)

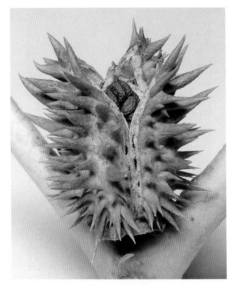

Figure 40-17 *Datura* seed pod; notice the prickly capsule. (Courtesy of Professor C. J. Botha, Department of Paraclinical Studies, Faculty of Veterinary Science, University of Pretoria, South Africa.)

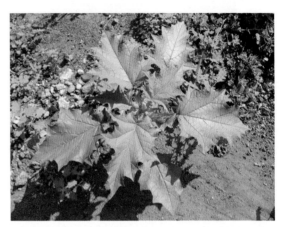

Figure 40-19 *Datura* sp. (Courtesy of Professor C. J. Botha, Department of Paraclinical Studies, Faculty of Veterinary Science, University of Pretoria, South Africa.)

Signs
- Ileus and intestinal impaction
- Colic

Diagnosis
- Tropane alkaloids in urine and stomach content

●》 WHAT TO DO

Datura
- Administration of polyionic fluids (PO/IV)
- NSAIDs: Flunixin meglumine (0.5 mg/kg IV q6h)
- Activated charcoal (1 g/kg PO q12h) alternating with mineral oil (4 L PO q12h)
- Cholinergic stimulants: physostigmine

Ornithogalum
- Chincherinchee *(Ornithogalum thyrsoides)* is found in the Western Cape Province close to water sources (Fig. 40-20).
- This popular cultivated flower is highly toxic and may be easily discarded and contaminate hay or fresh fodder.
- The principal toxin is cholestane glycosides.

Clinical Signs
- Anorexia, depression
- Watery diarrhea

●》 WHAT TO DO

Cardiac Glycosides
- Activated charcoal, 1 g/kg PO immediately
- Atropine and propranolol

Gastrointestinal System

Datura
- Found throughout South Africa, especially in cultivated lands with annual crops.
- These seeds are highly toxic to equidae.
- Horses are exposed through ingestion of concentrate contaminated with *Datura* seeds (Fig. 40-17 and 40-18) or hay contaminated by *Datura* plant material (Fig. 40-19).
- *Datura* contain parasympatholytic alkaloids, hyoscyamine (atropine), and hyoscine (scopolamine).

EMG

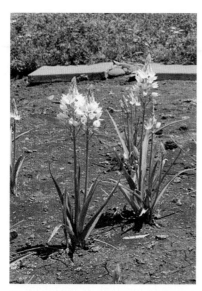

Figure 40-20 *Ornithogalum* sp. (Courtesy of Professor C. J. Botha, Department of Paraclinical Studies, Faculty of Veterinary Science, University of Pretoria, South Africa.)

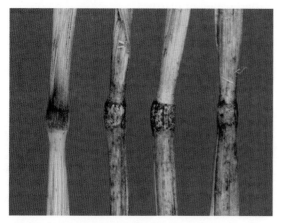

Figure 40-21 Bedding contaminated with *Stachybotrys atra.* (Courtesy of Professor C. J. Botha, Department of Paraclinical Studies, Faculty of Veterinary Science, University of Pretoria, South Africa.)

Diagnosis
• Exposure to contaminated feed
Treatment
• Supportive therapy

Skin/Integument

Stachybotryotoxicosis
• Outbreaks have occurred in Western Cape Province in stabled horses because of bedding contaminated by a fungus, *Stachybotrys atra* (Fig. 40-21).
Clinical Signs
• Necrosis of the nostrils and fetlocks
• Mucopurulent nasal discharge
• Eczema of the muzzle and edema of the head
Diagnosis
• Isolation of *Stachybotrys atra* from contaminated bedding
Treatment
• Supportive therapy

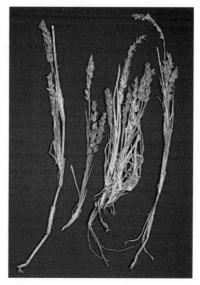

Figure 40-22 *Schmidtia* sp. (Courtesy of Professor C. J. Botha, Department of Paraclinical Studies, Faculty of Veterinary Science, University of Pretoria, South Africa.)

Sour Grasses
• Microscopic droplets of irritant acid can be secreted by *Schmidtia kalahariensis* (located in the Kalahari region of Botswana and Namibia) (Fig. 40-22) and *Enneapogon cenchroides* (widely spread) during active growth.
Clinical Signs
• Dermatitis, eczema, and alopecia of the muzzle and distal limbs
Diagnosis
• Exposure to contaminated pastures
Treatment
• Self-limiting
• Remove from contaminated pasture

SOUTH AMERICA

Alexandre Secorun Borges

Babesiosis

• Equine babesiosis, also known as equine piroplasmosis, is caused by tick-borne hemoprotozoan parasites: *Theileria equi, Babesia caballi,* or both. *Theileria equi* was previously known as *B. equi* and was reclassified in 1998 to the genus *Theileria* as a result of molecular analysis and confirmation of preerythrocytic stages inside lymphatic cells during its life cycle.
• *Theileria equi* and *B. caballi* are endemic in 90% of the world (South and Central America, the Caribbean, Africa, the Middle East, and Eastern and Southern Europe).
• These parasites are transmitted naturally by ticks of the genus *Amblyomma, Dermacentor, Rhipicephalus (Boophilus microplus* is now included in this genus), and *Hyalomma* (this latter genus is not present in Brazil).
• This disease can also affect donkeys, mules, and zebras.

- *B. caballi* is passed transovarially from one tick generation to the next, and therefore, the tick is important as a reservoir for this parasite.
- The same does *not* occur with *T. equi,* and the horse is the major reservoir for this agent.
- **Practice Tip:** T. equi *is more pathogenic than B. caballi.*

Epidemiology

- No sex or breed predilection is known.
- The disease is more common in horses older than 6 months of age.
- Neonatal foals can contract the disease by intrauterine transmission, especially with *T. equi;* vertical transmission with *B. caballi* is unlikely to occur.
- The disease is common in regions where the vector is present in higher numbers or when horses with no prior contact with the agent are introduced into an endemic area.
- Horses in pastures are at higher risk because of their permanent contact with ticks.
- Infected horses can remain carriers for long periods.
- Tick-borne transmission can be transstadial,[3] intrastadial,[4] or transovarial[5] for *B. caballi. T. equi* transmission can be either transstadial or intrastadial.
- **Practice Tip:** *Babesiosis can be iatrogenically transmitted by contaminated blood or surgical instruments; only a small volume of blood is needed for infection to occur.*

Clinical Signs

- Incubation for *T. equi* is 12 to 19 days, and 10 to 30 days for *B. caballi.*
- Severity depends on whether the horse was previously exposed to the agent and its immune status.
- Usually, *B. caballi* presents with lower parasitemia than does *T. equi.*
- Although the disease does *not* usually cause severe health problems in horses routinely exposed to *B. caballi* and *T. equi,* stressed horses or those without prior contact with the agent (i.e., naïve mature individuals) can contract a peracute form of the disease and are usually more severely affected, become very ill, or die.
- In the rare peracute case, the affected horse may be found dead.
- *Acute* infection is more common, and affected individuals usually have the following clinical signs:
  - Anorexia and fever are usually the first signs.
  - Anemia
  - Lethargy or depression
  - Weakness

- Icteric mucous membranes (jaundice); pale mucous membranes can be present in some horses during the initial phase of the disease.
- Tachycardia and tachypnea are usually present and depend on the severity of the anemia.
- Limb and abdominal edema in some cases
- Abnormal locomotion is typically secondary to weakness.
- Hemoglobinuria, which causes abnormally colored urine (dark red, black, or orange), secondary to hemolysis.
- *Subacute* cases can present with the following signs:
  - Intermittent fever
  - Inappetence
  - Weight loss
  - Mild abdominal pain
  - Mild edema of the distal limbs
  - Mucous membranes that are pink, light pink, or yellow and have petechial hemorrhages
- Other clinical signs/presentations to look for are the following:
  - Constipation or diarrhea
  - Horses with chronic infections are also anemic and usually perform poorer than horses without chronic infection.
  - Weight loss is observed in chronically affected horses.
  - Many cases in endemic areas can have a spontaneous recovery.
  - Severely affected mares can abort during the course of the clinical disease or soon thereafter.
  - Horses in areas with a high disease prevalence or prior exposure to the agents can have clinical babesiosis following another disease process that creates a secondary stress.
  - Strenuous exercise can convert a subclinical infection to an acute infection.
  - Permanent carriers can be asymptomatic.
  - Foals infected in utero are usually born weak, anemic, and jaundiced.

Diagnosis

- A suggestive history includes:
  - Tick infection
  - Travel to endemic areas
  - Blood transfusion
- History of contact with blood or with ticks from horses in endemic areas is important for individuals living in disease-free areas.
- Confirm hemolysis by checking the PCV and total plasma protein (TPP) levels.
- Low PCV and normal-to-high total protein values suggest hemolysis.
- Changes in plasma color (pink or icteric) with a low PCV are also suggestive of hemolysis.
- Air-dried and fixed methanol blood smears or whole blood collected with anticoagulants is used for

---

[3]Transstadial—pathogen remains with the vector from one developmental stage to the next.

[4]Intrastadial—agent can be transmitted by the same tick stage that acquired the parasite.

[5]Transovarial—disease-causing agent can be transmitted from parent arthropod to offspring arthropod or vectors may be able to pass the agent on to their own offspring transovarially.

identification of the agents using routine Romanowsky stains (Giemsa).

- *T. equi* have small erythrocytic stages reaching only 1.5 to 2.5 mm in length.
- *B. caballi* organisms in the erythrocytic stages are generally 3 to 6 mm.
- Maltese cross is a finding in *T. equi* infections (merozoites connected in a tetrad; see p. 673).
- ***Practice Tip:*** *Microscopic identification of parasites on routinely stained blood smears in subacute and chronic cases is uncommon because of the low number of parasites; however the smear is a useful and important test in acute cases. Even in acute cases, the absence of parasites on blood smears does* not *rule out the disease, and other specific tests must be performed.*
- Infected horses that remain carriers usually do *not* have parasites detected in Giemsa-stained blood smears because of the small numbers in the blood.
- Collecting blood from small vessels for direct examination has been suggested to increase the chances of identifying the agent (abnormal red blood cell morphology and higher adherence to capillary walls result in difficult passage through small vessels), especially for *B. caballi.*
- ***Practice Tip:*** *Collecting blood during a febrile episode from a small-diameter vessel (e.g., a facial vein) increases the chance of identifying the agent.*
- The indirect fluorescence antibody test, complement fixation (CF) test, and competitive enzyme-linked immunosorbent assay (cELISA) are performed to confirm the presence of antibodies to the organisms (2 weeks postexposure for CF and 7 to 10 days for cELISA).
- Endemic areas have a high prevalence of babesiosis; therefore, one must be careful when interpreting serum titers as a diagnostic test for active disease in horses.
- PCR (available in some laboratories) blood analysis confirms the presence of the parasite.
- Postmortem findings include the following:
  - Icterus
  - Enlarged spleen and liver
  - Petechial hemorrhages in the kidneys and heart
  - It is useful to perform a spleen imprint and look for the parasite inside red blood cells.
- ***Note:*** There are horses with mixed infections of *T. equi and B. caballi.*
- Foals younger than 3 months old from seropositive mares can have maternal antibodies to *T. equi* and *B. caballi* after colostrum ingestion.

▶▶ WHAT TO DO

Piroplasmosis

- Acute and subacute cases are treated promptly; otherwise, the disease can result in death.
- Blood transfusion is necessary in acute cases with a rapid decline in PCV (<18% within 24 hours) (see Chapter 20, p. 287). Horses with subacute babesiosis resulting in anemia usually receive a transfusion if the PCV level is <12%. Horses with poor hydration can have a higher measurable PCV despite their anemia.

- Check stained blood smears to evaluate for a large number of red blood cells with parasites, which usually indicates that the PCV is likely to drop further despite the initial treatment.
- Monitor hydration; fluids are important to prevent renal damage from hemolysis.
- *T. equi* is more refractory to treatment than *B. caballi,* although both respond to babesicidal drugs.
- Administer diminazene diaceturate: 4 mg/kg IM q12h over a 24-hour period, or
- Administer imidocarb dipropionate:
  - *Babesia caballi:* 2.2 mg/kg IM q24h for 2 days.
  - *Theileria equi:* 4 mg/kg IM q24h for 2 days. A third treatment is sometimes needed 72 hours after the first treatment.
  - Treated horses can have side effects of:
    - Restlessness
    - Abdominal pain
    - Sweating
- ***Note:*** Both drugs are hepatotoxic to horses. Imidocarb is more likely to cause nephrotoxic side effects; renal function monitoring is recommended during treatment.
- ***Practice Tips:***
  - *Use caution when treating donkeys with imidocarb because they are more likely to have side effects with these drugs.*
  - *The administration of N-butylscopolammonium bromide (Buscopan[6]) before treatment with imidocarb ameliorates the adverse cholinergic effects (e.g., colic).*

Differential Diagnoses

- Because equine infectious anemia is present in some South American countries, serum for Coggins test should be harvested for analysis, especially in endemic areas.
- Autoimmune hemolytic anemia is possible.
- Purpura hemorrhagica can be a differential diagnosis, particularly in subacute cases.
- Neonatal isoerythrolysis is a differential diagnosis in young foals with icterus. Other causes of icterus in foals are possible, but they usually present with a normal PCV level.

Prognosis

- Prognosis for survival is good in horses treated at the first signs of the disease.
- Prognosis is guarded when the disease is introduced in new areas and when there is no prior immunity in the affected horses

Prevention

- There is no cross-immunity between *B. caballi* and *T. equi* in horses.
- Control of equine babesiosis is important to keep the international market open to the horse industry. ***Important:*** Horses with antibodies to *T. equi* or *B. caballi* are restricted from entering areas that are disease-free.
  - ***Practice Tips:*** *Once a horse is infected, the carrier state may persist for long periods during which the horse may act as an "infection" reservoir.*

- *After recovery, horses may become carriers for long periods of time, 1 to 4 years for B. caballi and probably lifelong for T. equi.*
- ***Practice Tip:** High doses of imidocarb dipropionate are effective for treatment of Babesia caballi.*
- Disease-free areas should test horses before entry into their territory. Tests required may vary among countries for the identification of the organisms; usually, complement fixation and/or cELISA are used. ***Practice Tip:** The cELISA is more sensitive than CF in detecting chronically infected horses.*
- Equine babesiosis can be spread through contaminated needles, syringes, whole blood, or serum/blood plasma; iatrogenic transmission is important in specific situations.
- ***Practice Tip**: Check blood donors for B. caballi and T. equi before using their blood for a transfusion.*
- *T. equi* and *B. caballi* are endemic to South America, but outbreaks of clinical disease in adults are *not* common.
- *B. caballi* is transmitted transovarially and persists in its vectors for many generations. The tick is the major reservoir of this agent. The opposite is true for *T. equi,* which persists in vertebrate hosts over their lifetime, and intrauterine transmission is common. Therefore, the vertebrate host is the major reservoir.
- ***Practice Tip:** Tick control is the key point in keeping horses free of the parasite or reducing exposure to the disease.*
- ***Note:** Medications directed at the hemoprotozoan parasite are reported not to clear the chronic infection/carrier state in horses.*

●▸ WHAT TO DO

Prevention
- Horses living in endemic areas are at a higher risk of becoming carriers, and it is very difficult to maintain a disease-free population of horses in these areas. With the establishment of a comprehensive vector control program and the isolation of horses from cows, it is possible for horses to remain seronegative. This is important for horses that need to test negative to travel to parasite-free areas. This also avoids disease after stressful events, such as intensive competitive activities.
- Because *Rhipicephalus (Boophilus) microplus* is the most important vector for *B. equi* in Brazil, tick control on cattle, and avoiding contact between horses and cattle in areas where rigid control exists, help keep unexposed horses disease-free.
- Horses living in areas without good tick control are best managed with premonition—infection immunity; this practice protects them from the severe form of the disease. They have permanent titers for the infectious organisms, which are useful for protection in endemic areas.
- ***Important:*** Equine piroplasmosis is considered a foreign animal disease in the United States, but positive cases have recently been identified. For additional details on this disease in the United States and diagnostic test interpretation, refer to USDA, 2011. Equine Piroplasmosis Domestic Pathways Assessment 2011: Pathways Assessment for the Spread of the Causative Agents of Equine Piroplasmosis from Movement of a Horse from Quarantined Premises Within the Contiguous United States. USDA : APHIS:VS : CEAH: National Center for Risk Analysis. Fort Collins, CO. March, 2011, 62 pages; and Schwint ON, Ueti MW, Palmer GH, Kappmeyer LS, Hines MT, Cordes RT, Knowles DP, Scoles GA: *Antimicrobial Agents and Chemotherapy* 53(10):4327- 4332, 2009. Imidocarb dipropionate clears persistent *Babesia caballi* infection with elimination of transmission potential.

References

References can be found on the companion website at www.equine-emergencies.com.

CHAPTER 41

Flood Injury in Horses

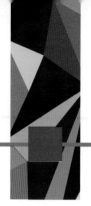

Rebecca S. McConnico

Introduction

- Floods are common weather-related disasters threatening the lives of people and horses.
- The yearly financial loss due to floods in the United States averages multiple billions of dollars causing damage to infrastructure and loss of economic activity.
- Flood-related livestock injuries and death make up a major part of these losses, impacting the economic and emotional welfare of livestock producers including horse owners.

Planning/Prevention

- Horse owners must take a fundamental and proactive role in protecting the livestock under their care.
- Advanced planning can help horse owners minimize the loss of life and the health problems associated with disasters such as floods.
- Horses that undergo evacuation relating to a disaster response associated with floods are stressed and likely to commingle with other horses and livestock.
- Herd biosecurity is breeched, which makes increasing herd immunity imperative.
- Pneumonia and abortions should be anticipated and can be minimized with proper herd nutrition and vaccination.
- *Practice Tip: Before storm seasons, horses should be vaccinated with current strains for equine herpesvirus 1 and 4 and appropriate equine influenza Clade(s) in addition to the encephalitides (eastern equine encephalomyelitis [EEE], western equine encephalomyelitis [WEE], West Nile virus [WNV]), rabies, and tetanus.*
- Individual identification is important, because it is important to be able to identify the herd of origin if horses are evacuated and commingled, or escape and are later captured. Many horses look alike, so brands, lip tattoos, or electronic identification unique to each individual horse or farm/ranch is vital.
- Single microchips should be implanted deep in the horse's nuchal ligament halfway between the poll and the withers on the left side. Pictures and/or videos of horses may also help identify them later.
- Horses should have two forms of identification:
  - Permanent microchip, lip tattoo, or brand
  - Visible tag or marking with owner name and current contact information

- Guidelines for predisaster identification marking of horses should include, as a minimum: a legible current contact telephone number or e-mail address with the owner's name that is plainly visible. Copies of herd records, proof of ownership, and registration papers should be stored in a safe and secure location.

Response

- In flood situations, horse owners are often frantic and demanding. It is important for communities to have a "livestock plan" that includes trained personnel and resources so that reasonable decisions can be made quickly to save lives and meet the urgent health-related needs of flood-affected horse victims.
- Horse owners should do their part to evacuate ahead of a flooding situation and be sure their horses are haltered and lead.
- Equine emergency response personnel should be current in medical triage; the response should be executed by an experienced team of individuals including veterinarians, first responders, and trained animal technician handlers.
- With equine rescue, responders are at risk for injury, and the horse may sustain additional injuries during the rescue activities.
- *Practice Tip: A basic guideline is to use the simplest, safest, and a "low tech" approach to minimize injury to horse and rescuers.*
- Stressed and injured horses are unpredictable and can significantly endanger people.
- Decisions regarding the appropriate type of response (rescue, field medical treatment, sheltering, or simply provision of feed and water) should be made with the primary objective being the safety of response personnel (see Chapter 37, p. 634).

Triage and Medical Treatment

- When horses are stranded in a flood, stress is an important contributor to flood-related medical problems. These conditions commonly include:
  - Colic
  - Diarrhea
  - Dehydration
  - Neurologic disease
  - Respiratory disease

- Laminitis
- Sole abscesses
- Skin abrasions
- Cellulitis
- Lacerations
- Fractures
- Corneal injuries
- The innate equine "fight or flight" response often accentuates even minor medical problems into life-threatening conditions. If possible, injured horses are examined by a field veterinarian and stabilized before transporting.
- Stabilization may include sedation to prevent further traumatic injury to the patient and handlers. Transporting fractious patients makes the situation worse, especially if the horse is improperly restrained.
- Horses that are severely dehydrated or exhibiting signs of cardiovascular shock may benefit from large-volume bolus of intravenous fluid therapy in the field before transporting (isotonic polyionic fluids, 50 mL/kg IV initially; 20 to 30 L/450-kg adult horse).
- During heightened stress, such as floods and rescue, it is important to move the patient to a quiet area for initial triage and assessment as soon as possible.
- Equine flood victims should be decontaminated by bathing with a detergent soap and thorough rinsing to remove toxins, debris, or microorganisms from the skin and to identify other sites of injury.
- Recommended bathing products include Dawn or Ivory dishwashing soap, or human or animal shampoos without additives.
- The hooves should be cleaned and examined for puncture wounds.

Handling and Restraint

- Chemical restraint is generally indicated to calm a horse, safely manage the rescue, or medically evaluate and treat the flood-stranded horse.
- Chemical restraint minimizes further injury to the patient and prevents human injury to allow rescue activities, including trailer extraction or helicopter sling rescue. Sedative agents used judiciously include:
  - Acepromazine (0.02 to 0.08 mg/kg IV)
  - Xylazine (0.5 to 1 mg/kg IV)
  - Detomidine (5 to 20 μg/kg IV)
  - Butorphanol (0.01 to 0.02 mg/kg IV)
- Adverse response to sedation and tranquilization produces:
  - Hypotension
  - Decreased gastrointestinal motility
  - Exacerbation of cardiovascular shock
- Experienced veterinarians recommend detomidine sedation (5 to 20 μg/kg) followed by butorphanol (0.01 to 0.02 mg/kg IV) for sedation if needed for air lift or trailer extraction.
- Yohimbine (0.1 to 0.15 mg/kg slowly IV) is indicated for alpha$_2$-agonist reversal in the event of significant bradycardia and hypotension.

- **Practice Tip:** *Horses rescued by flat or pontoon boats require general short-acting anesthesia using the "triple-drip" method—guaifenesin/ketamine/detomidine.* (See Chapter 47, p. 744.)
- Triple drip is commonly comprised of:
  - Guaifenesin 5%
  - Ketamine, 2 mg/mL
  - Detomidine, 5 μg/kg
- The horse or pony is premedicated with detomidine (10 to 20 μg/kg), induced with detomidine (10 μg/h and ketamine (2 mg/kg) IV bolus, and maintained on the triple drip (2 mL/kg/h) (see Chapter 47, p. 738).
- If a 15 drop per milliliter infusion set (typical primary IV set) is used, the rate is one to two drops per second of the triple drip solution to maintain the 500-kg horse under general anesthesia. This needs to be titrated in response to the individual patient's level of anesthesia.
- Recovery usually occurs 35 to 40 minutes after discontinuing the infusion. Providing a safe space for recovery is important and adds to the challenge of a disaster flood recovery.

Typical Injuries in Flood Victims
Integument and Musculoskeletal Injury

- Extremity, head, neck, and trunk lacerations and abrasions are commonly seen in equine flood victims.
- Limb lacerations are especially common and may be compicated by fractures and/or tendon lacerations.
- A horse exhibiting moderate to severe lameness requires a comprehensive examination to localize the lameness and prevent further exacerbation whether it is due to a fracture, soft tissue injury, nail penetrating the foot, or a combination of injuries.
- It is beneficial to have splinting devices, such as a Kimsey splint for lower limb splinting, readily available (see Chapter 21, p. 319).
- Flood-affected horses may develop dermatitis and cellulitis from breaks in the skin and standing in contaminated water for long periods.
  - Contaminants include:
    - Chemicals associated with an oil spill
    - Sewage
    - Minerals from mining or rock quarries
    - Elevated salinity—gulf, ocean, or brackish waters
- Flood waters with high saline content are more likely to cause diseases associated with ingestion and inhalation of water such as colitis, pneumonia, or neurologic disease.
- Mild to moderate cases of dermatitis and cellulitis can lead to more serious complications such as septic tenosynovitis or septic arthritis, and if *not* treated appropriately may result in severe lameness, loss of use, and even be life threatening.
- Early recognition and diagnosis of cellulitis enables rapid aggressive intervention for an improved outcome.

- Horses with cellulitis have swelling and heat in affected areas, show signs of pain and lameness, and often are febrile (102° to 104° F [39° to 40° C]).
- Horses with more severe infections become anorectic and painful.
- Cellulitic limbs are painful when touched and the horse may display moderate to severe lameness.
- Systemic antimicrobial therapy is indicated in cases of cellulitis and should provide broad-spectrum coverage with good tissue penetration.
- Beta-lactam antimicrobials are recommended because of the possibility of clostridial and other anaerobic bacterial infections.
- Dosing of ceftiofur sodium (2.2 to 4.4 mg/kg IV or IM q6 to 12h), procaine penicillin G (22,000 IU/kg IM q12h), or penicillin G potassium (22,000 IU/kg IV q6h) combined with an aminoglycoside *and* oral metronidazole (20 to 25 mg/kg PO or per rectum q8h) offers excellent coverage for the vast majority of bacterial organisms.
- Antimicrobial treatment for cellulitis should continue for 10 to 14 days, and possibly longer if necessary.
- Proper tetanus vaccination should be administered.
- Horses exposed to flood waters are also at increased risk for extremity dermatitis and cellulitis-associated fungal or fungal-like diseases such as equine pythium or basidiobolus.
  - In horses, fungal skin infections can be invasive, rapidly progressive, and result in proliferative pyogranulomatous disease.
  - Lesions can be ulcerative and oozing with a foul odor.
  - The growing "mass" may be especially pruritic, and affected horses are stressed and agitated, leading to self-mutilation in an attempt to relieve the discomfort.
  - The lesions grossly may be confused with exuberant granulation tissue. Fungal skin disease requires definitive diagnosis by biopsy and fungal culture[1] for determination of appropriate treatment.
  - If skin lacerations, dermatitis, or cellulitis fail to respond to standard care, including systemic antibacterial therapy, fungal infection needs to be ruled out by skin biopsy and fungal culture.
  - Treatments include a combination of surgery, antifungal treatments, and immunotherapy.

Hoof Problems
- Horses that have been standing in mud or water for long periods may suffer from thrush, soft soles, and loss of the frog compromising the integrity of the hooves' support structures and resulting in sole bruising and other hoof problems.
- When dried, the hooves may be more susceptible to separation of the laminae and subsequently white line disease, laminitis, or foot abscesses.

- The horse's feet should be cleaned using a hoof pick and brush as soon as possible to remove sharp objects capable of puncturing the hoof wall or sole.
- These horses may require "medical" farriery (podiatry) to treat thrush, hoof/sole defects, coronitis, or laminitis.
- Application of iodine-based hoof preparations can help to toughen soft soles and remove some of the moisture from soft hooves.
- Thrush-fighting products found in farm supply and tack stores can effectively treat minor cases of thrush if used as directed. See Chapter 42, p. 693, for more information on foot emergencies.
- Proper tetanus vaccination should be administered.

Ophthalmic Injuries
- Ophthalmic injuries, especially traumatic and foreign body corneal ulceration and uveitis, are common medical emergencies seen in equine flood victims due to flying storm debris and damaged stable and pasture environment.
- Animal handlers and first responders may *not* initially recognize ophthalmic injuries because they are concentrating on the more obvious injuries and rescue activities.
  - ***Practice Tip:*** *This is especially true for foals that may be hard to catch and examine; foals do not demonstrate eye pain to the same degree as adult horses.*
- A thorough ophthalmic exam with early recognition of injury and treatment are important for preventing more serious conditions. Please see Chapter 23, p. 396, for a comprehensive coverage of ophthalmic injuries such as:
  - Corneal defects
  - Corneal abrasions
  - Fungal keratitis
  - Corneal ulceration
  - Uveitis
- Ocular pain is also managed using the nonsteroidal anti-inflammatory drugs phenylbutazone, flunixen meglumine, and firocoxib (see Chapter 23, p. 414).
- Corticosteroid therapy should *not* be included in treating traumatic corneal ulceration in the horse.

Gastrointestinal Dysfunction
- Horses that are stressed from being stranded, injured, or unattended during a flood situation or have ingested contaminated water can develop colitis, colic, and systemic toxemia requiring medical care. Salmonella outbreaks have occurred in flood-stranded horses.
- Frequently, affected horses show signs of lethargy, inappetence, and colic, and some may develop mild to severe diarrhea. Death is possible from peracute colitis without the horse exhibiting diarrhea.
- Physical examination may reveal increased respiratory rate and heart rate due to abdominal discomfort and an increased body temperature due to toxin absorption.
- Signs of abdominal pain range from mild (such as recumbency or inappetence) to severe (rolling, thrashing); see

[1]Fungal culture (Pythium Lab, Louisiana State University).

Chapter 18, pp. 185 and 231, for a comprehensive coverage of colic and colitis in adult horses, respectively.

- Cases of colitis may be confused with other large-bowel disorders including large-colon torsion or volvulus.
- Systemic absorption of endotoxin can result in peripheral arteriovenous shunting and classic "brick red" mucous membranes.
- Hypovolemia and subsequent circulatory shock causes congested mucous membranes and weak peripheral pulses.
- Treatment for colitis is supportive and aimed at:
  - Plasma volume replacement (crystalloid fluid replacement)
  - Analgesic and anti-inflammatory therapy
  - Anti-endotoxin therapy
  - Antimicrobial therapy if indicated
  - Nutritional support
- Aggressive intravenous polyionic fluid therapy should be instituted immediately in horses showing signs of toxemia, colic, clinical dehydration, and/or colitis.
- *Practice Tip:* *Total fluid deficits should be calculated based on clinical assessment of dehydration (e.g., for 8% or moderate dehydration, 0.08 × 450 kg body weight = 36 L) and replacement fluids should be administered rapidly (up to 6 to 10 L/h per 450-kg adult horse).*
- Many horses with colic, dehydration, and electrolyte imbalances voluntarily drink electrolyte mixtures. Electrolyte mixtures in water should be offered in addition to a clean water source. Plain water must always be available!
  - Mixtures to consider providing include:
    - Water with baking soda (10 g/L)
    - Water with NaCl/KCl ("Lite" Salt) 6 to 10 g/L
    - Water with a commercial electrolyte solution
  - Horses with nasogastric reflux should *not* be offered water until normal transit of fluid and ingesta is reestablished.
- Horses unresponsive to symptomatic treatment should be referred to a surgical facility capable of intensive care and treatment.
- Horses with signs of toxemia (elevated heart rate, brick red mucous membranes, and clinical dehydration) absorb large amounts of endotoxin from the diseased intestinal mucosal barrier and therefore are at increased risk for:
  - Laminitis
  - Thrombophlebitis
  - Disseminated intravascular coagulation (DIC)
- Specific treatment for endotoxemia is important for patient survival (Table 41-1).
- The choice of treatment is based on:
  - Severity of disease
  - Renal function
  - Hydration status
- Goals of anti-endotoxin treatment include:
  - Neutralization of endotoxin before it interacts with inflammatory cells

Table 41-1	**Anti-Endotoxin Therapy**
Product	**Dosing Information**
Endoserum or	1.5 mL/kg body weight IV diluted 1:10 or 1:20 in sterile isotonic saline or lactated Ringer's solution
Hyperimmune (endotoxin) plasma	1-3 LIV
Polymyxin B	1000-6000 IU/kg body weight IV q8-12h for up to 3 days. Because of the possibility of causing nephrotoxic side effects, polymyxin B should be used judiciously and its use in azotemic patients is NOT recommended.
Flunixin meglumine	0.25 mg/kg IV q6-8h
Corticosteroid therapy	A single dose of a short-acting corticosteroid (prednisolone sodium succinate [1 mg/kg IV]) may be effective during acute endotoxemia without increasing the risk of laminitis
Dimethyl sulfoxide	0.1 g/kg IV q12-24h diluted to less than 10% solution (higher doses have been associated with exacerbating intestinal reperfusion injury in horses)
Allopurinol	5 mg or more/kg IV q4-6h for 1-2 days
Pentoxyphylline	8 mg/kg PO q8h

  - Prevention of the synthesis, release, or action of mediators
  - General supportive care
- The use of broad-spectrum intravenous antibiotics in colic and colitis cases is *not* always indicated.
- Mild and transient neutropenia or fever may *not* justify the use of broad-spectrum antimicrobials unless concurrent problems needing treatment are identified and a persistent neutropenia is present that increases the risk for:
  - Peritonitis
  - Pneumonia
  - Cellulitis
  - Thrombophlebitis
  - Disseminated intravascular coagulation
- Oral broad-spectrum antimicrobial medications are *not* recommended because they may disrupt the normal intestinal microbial population.
- Oral metronidazole (10 to 15 mg/kg q8h) is indicated when *Clostridium* spp. are suspected in the pathogenesis of the disease; metronidazole may also have local anti-inflammatory effects and may be effective in treating acute equine colitis of unknown etiology.
- Horses with diarrhea may benefit from treatment with oral adsorbents such as activated charcoal or smectite powder (see Chapter 18, p. 235).
- Flood-affected and injured horses often have a ravenous appetite and should be allowed to eat good-quality hay and fresh green grass, if available.
- Fresh water should be provided in small amounts initially then ad libitum.

- Reestablishment of normal feeding and watering should occur over 48 to 72 hours.

Neurologic Disease

- Equine flood victims are at increased risk of developing head and neck injuries and are more susceptible to infectious diseases such as viral encephalitides or clostridial infections (tetanus and botulism).
- Physical examination findings suggestive of central neurologic disease during patient triage requires immediate action, including:
  - Prevention of further progression of neurologic abnormalities
  - Emergency treatment aimed at treating inflammation (corticosteroid or nonsteroidal anti-inflammatory therapy)
  - Additional nursing and supportive care
- Vaccinating against encephalitides or viral and bacterial respiratory diseases may be contraindicated because the immune response in a stressed horse is minimal and vaccination may contribute in raising the stress level even further. Tetanus prophylaxis is the *only* vaccine indicated in rescued horses; it should be administered if the vaccination status of the patient is unknown or questionable.
- If ingested water contains elevated salt levels from a coastal storm surge, treating potentially salt-intoxicated horses must be done with caution to prevent exacerbation of the salt poisoning.
  - ***Practice Tip:*** *Ingestion of water containing over 7000 mg/L of total dissolved salt has the potential to cause acute salt poisoning.*
  - Salt poisoning may occur secondarily to water deprivation when horses are left unattended for several consecutive days.
  - ***Practice Tip:*** *The basic principles of treating salt intoxication include:*
    - *Replenishing plasma volume hydration more slowly than in standard cases of hypovolemia*
    - *Close monitoring of serum Na⁺ or osmolality* — Na^+
    - *Close monitoring of clinical neurologic signs*
  - Treatment with systemic anti-inflammatory medications including corticosteroid therapy (dexamethasone phosphate at 0.05 to 0.1 mg/kg q24h) may minimize signs of cerebral edema.
  - Hyponatremia may occur if the horse ingests a large volume of fresh water.

Respiratory Disease

- Aspiration in horses exposed to flood waters may cause acute pulmonary edema, acute lung injury, and pneumonia is usually life-threatening.
- Small amounts of aspirated water may cause inflammation, loss of surfactant, atelectasis, and lung consolidation. Seawater aspiration may pull fluid into the alveolus by osmosis, causing noncardiogenic pulmonary edema. If the water is grossly contaminated with bacteria or debris, a primary pulmonary infection can occur.

- Secondary severe septic pneumonia or pleuropneumonia is not uncommon.
- Horses stranded or "stuck" in ponds, deep mud, or flood waters and struggling and flailing for periods of time can develop upper respiratory tract (URT) inflammation (see Chapter 25, p. 461), such as:
  - Chondritis
  - Pharyngitis
  - Laryngitis or laryngospasms
- Emergency tracheostomy may be needed in horses that develop URT obstruction secondary to struggling (see Chapter 25, p. 456).
- Aspiration pneumonia may also occur secondary to laryngeal dysfunction.
- Treatment of these acute cases includes:
  - Aggressive anti-inflammatory therapy
  - Systemic broad-spectrum antibiotics
  - Furosemide, if *not* dehydrated
  - Systemic intravenous therapy with 10% DMSO (1 g/kg IV q24h) is believed to be effective in treating respiratory tract edema.
- Horses that are evacuated or rescued following a flood event may be commingled and become infected with respiratory infections such as:
  - Equine influenza virus
  - Equine herpes virus
  - *Streptococcus equi* subspecies *equi*
- ***Practice Tip:*** *Preventative health programs aimed at optimizing herd immunity before storm season help minimize herd outbreaks in the event of a disaster.*
- Complete submersion of a horse into a body of water causes asphyxia and severe cerebral hypoxia.
  - Cold-water submersion causes an immediate reflex shunting of blood to the heart and brain in addition to lowering the metabolic demand of these organs. Therefore the chances of survival may be increased in a horse quickly removed from a cold body of water.
  - Treatment for these cases includes:
    - Antimicrobials
    - Anti-inflammatories
    - Bronchodilators
    - Diuretics
    - Humidified oxygen
    - Surfactant transplant

Summary

- The majority of horses evacuated/rescued simply need good footing, water, hay, and to be dried off.
- There is no way to prepare for every situation that occurs in a flood situation.
- Veterinarians working closely with other producers and agricultural leaders can lessen the impact of a disaster on an equine operation.

- Preparation and detailed planning are the most important aspect of preventing flood-related injuries to horses.
- It is critical to encourage the horse-owning public and animal care professionals to have an evacuation plan for their families, including pets and other animals, and knowledge of local and regional disaster authorities (see Chapter 37, p. 634).

- Educational programs that empower communities to be responsible for caring for their own people and horses are needed for the future of a successful disaster response.

References

References can be found on the companion website at www.equine-emergencies.com.

EMG

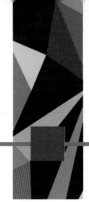

CHAPTER 42

Foot Injuries

Robert Agne

Infections of the Foot

- Infections of the foot can occur anytime the protective hoof capsule is compromised. Some common causes of foot infections include, but are not limited to:
  - Ascending infections from an imperfection in the white line (e.g., gravel)
  - Puncture wounds (e.g., foreign body, horseshoe nail)
  - Hoof cracks
  - Trauma to the hoof capsule such as hoof wall avulsions or laceration of the sole and/or frog
- Infections of the foot are classified as superficial or deep.
  - Superficial infections involve only the underlying dermis and are limited to the area just beneath the sole (subsolar) or just beneath the wall (submural).
  - Deep infections involve structures such as the distal phalanx, DIP (distal interphalangeal) joint, digital cushion, navicular bone/bursa, deep digital flexor tendon (DDFT) and sheath, and collateral cartilage (quittor).
- All foot infections can potentially become serious, even career ending or life threatening, if not treated appropriately.
- Clinical signs include acute, often non–weight-bearing lameness, increased digital pulse, and heat on palpation of the hoof.
  - Submural infections may be sore to palpation of the coronary band if the infection has migrated proximally.
  - Subsolar infections may eventually be sore to palpation of heel bulbs if the infection has migrated caudally along the sole.
  - However, infection should not be ruled out if palpation of coronary band or hoof tester examination is negative.

Ascending Infections from a White Line Defect (Gravel)

- The etiology is usually a defect in the white line, such as an old horseshoe nail tract, a stretched white line (secondary to a flare or dish in the hoof wall), or chronic laminitis.
- Infection, exudate, and sometimes gas can migrate under the hoof wall and/or the sole.

● WHAT TO DO

Foot Infections with Drainage

- Localize the area of infection with hoof testers.
- Remove the shoe by individually removing each nail with creased nail pullers.
- Scrub and clean the solar surface of the foot to remove the superficial exfoliating layer of sole and debris using a wire brush, hoof knife, and rasp.
- Defects in the white line, where bacteria may penetrate, are often characterized by a black or gray area. Once localized, drainage is established by following the tract using a sharp hoof knife or curette. Only a small hole is needed for drainage; if possible, limit the debridement to the white line so that the opened abscess tract can be protected/covered by a shoe once the infection resolves.
- Once drainage is established, the foot should be poulticed (e.g., Animalintex)[1] and bandaged.
- Maintain foot hydration using a moist poultice for at least 4 to 5 days or until drainage has stopped.
- The draining hole should then be protected until the defect has healed using a dry bandage, protective boot, or shoe covering the abscess tract.
- It may be necessary to use a leather or plastic pad with the shoe to protect a tract(s) in the sole or frog region.
- Before application of a dry bandage or shoe, with a hospital plate (made of 1/16- to 1/8-inch [0.16- to 0.32-cm] aluminum material anchored to the shoe) to protect the sole, pack the abscess tract with iodine-soaked cotton to reduce the risk of reinfection.
- Administer tetanus prophylaxis if it has been more than 3 months since tetanus vaccination.

● WHAT TO DO

Foot Infection Without Drainage

- If drainage is not easily established with routine debridement of the hoof wall/sole defect, radiographs should be taken to rule out other causes of acute foot lameness (e.g., fracture or laminitis) and to help locate submural or subsolar gas/fluid pockets using a light exposure radiographic technique with good soft tissue detail for best detection.
- Gentle exploration of the tract with a blunt probe frequently establishes drainage. Do not use sharp instruments or excessive force, which may seed the deeper tissues with infection.

---

[1]Animalintex (3M Animal Care Products, 3M Center, 275-5W-05, St. Paul, MN 55144).

- Often an overnight poultice, repeated for several days, helps "mature" the abscess and promote drainage.
  - A poultice can be made using an empty 5-L intravenous fluid bag and filling it with a generous handful of Epsom salt, bran mash, 10 mL of Betadine solution, and enough warm water to create a semisolid consistency. The foot is placed in the bag and incorporated into a lower limb bandage and left on for 24 hours.
- If the horse shows signs of tenderness over the coronary band or heel bulb, a similar poultice arrangement helps promote abscess drainage from those locations.
- Unless a deeper infection is suspected, the administration of systemic antibiotics is generally not recommended.
- As with any severe non–weight-bearing lameness, the opposite limb should be treated prophylactically to prevent contra lateral limb laminitis by mechanically supporting the sole and frog and the goal should be to improve the horse's comfort as soon as possible.
- Administer tetanus prophylaxis if it has been more than 3 months since tetanus vaccination.

◉❭ WHAT NOT TO DO

Foot Infections
- *Do not* open an abscess tract more than what is necessary for drainage. This creates a sole defect that may be difficult to protect once the abscess is resolved and *prolongs* healing time.
- *Do not* allow the hoof to dry excessively or intentionally desiccate horn tissue before resolution of the abscess because this may prematurely close the abscess tract and allow the abscess to reform.
- *Do not* allow the abscess tract to become contaminated with dirt or debris because this may prematurely close the abscess tract and reinfect the wound.
- *Do not* flush the abscess tract with a caustic agent because this may cause necrosis of submural or subsolar tissue.

Puncture Wounds to the Foot

- Any puncture wound of the foot is considered an emergency and should be evaluated immediately.
- Any delay in treatment of wounds that involve the susceptible synovial structures of the foot (e.g., DDFT sheath, navicular bursa, and DIP joint) increases the morbidity and mortality.
- Additionally, any delay in treating a puncture wound to the foot, even when a synovial structure is not involved, increases the recovery time and risks spread of infection to a synovial structure.
- These injuries are usually caused by a metal object, such as a roofing or fencing nail, wire, a tough wooden stem from a recently cleaned field, farm equipment, or a clip or nail from a lost shoe.

◉❭ WHAT TO DO

Puncture Wound to the Foot
- Scrub and clean the solar surface of the foot to remove the superficial exfoliating layer of sole and debris using a wire brush, hoof knife, and rasp.
- If the foreign object is still imbedded in the foot, radiographs should be taken while the foreign material is still in place to determine the depth and position within the foot.

- If the foreign body has been removed or is not present, the foot should be radiographed, starting with anteroposterior, lateral, and dorsoventral views. The foot should then be anesthetized with 2% Carbocaine using an abaxial sesamoid block or midpastern block (see Chapter 21, p. 290), scrubbed, and prepped for exploration and a contrast study/fistulogram. Five milliliters of contrast material is injected into the entry site using a teat cannula, an 18-gauge catheter, or a Tomcat[2] catheter threaded into the puncture site. Any contrast material that leaks onto the hoof wall or sole is removed with alcohol-soaked gauze, followed by a lateral and horizontal/dorsopalmar/plantar (DP) standing radiographic series. The puncture wound tract should be outlined with the fistulogram on the radiographs and an appropriate treatment plan initiated.
- If a puncture wound is suspected but the wound is not readily apparent, careful examination of the trimmed frog and sulci is recommended because the frog tissue easily closes over the puncture site, making the wound hard to find.
- Superficial puncture wounds are treated in a similar manner to a foot abscess, using "light" debridement of the wound tract (see p. 685); an antiseptic dressing; and protecting the wound with a bandage or hospital plate shoe, fabricated with an aluminum or plastic plate that can be easily removed to access the sole lesion. The wound should heal from the "inside-out" to prevent an abscess from forming.
- Deep puncture wounds to the central portion of the foot frequently involve the DIP joint, navicular bone/bursa, or DDFT/sheath and should be referred to a hospital facility immediately for debridement, lavage, regional perfusion (see Chapter 5, p. 16) and intravenous antibiotic therapy. If in doubt as to where the location and depth of the puncture wound, referral for further workup to assess the DIP joint, navicular bursa, and DDFT sheath should be recommended to the owner. If a referral center is not readily available, regional limb perfusion with amikacin/crystalloid solution (see Chapter 21, p. 303) is performed and the patient placed on systemic penicillin and gentamicin. The DIP joint and tendon sheath should be aseptically aspirated for fluid analysis and culture and treated with intrasynovial amikacin. If the navicular bursa is suspected to be involved, bursal fluid is obtained using ultrasonographic or radiographic guidance. After intrabursal needle placement is achieved, the bursa is lavaged with sterile crystalloid and treated with amikacin.
- Discuss with the referral center clinician whether systemic antibiotics should be administered before shipping the horse. This likely depends on duration of the injury and length of time before horse arrives at the facility.
- Additionally, the foot can be disinfected with a chlorine-based foot soak (Cleantrax)[3] and bandaged until shipping to a referral center is possible. The bandage should include a foot wrap with a moist poultice pad (e.g., Animalintex) to keep tissues hydrated, opened, and draining. Drying agents are contraindicated because dehydration of the tissue may prematurely close the draining tract.
- Case-specific therapeutic shoeing includes a treatment plate allowing wound access and mechanical support to raise the heel and reduce the strain on the injured tissues.
- The owner should be advised of the serious nature of this type of injury, the potential complications, and given a guarded prognosis.
- Frequently these cases are clinically comfortable for the first few days after injury until the infection becomes well established. For

---

[2]Tomcat is a generic name for a semirigid 18-gauge, 4.5-inch catheter.
[3]Cleantrax (Equine Technologies, 416 Boston Post Road, Sudbury, MA 01776).

the first 1 to 2 weeks after a puncture wound, it is important that these cases be treated aggressively with antimicrobials, wound and synovial lavages, and regional limb perfusion regardless of the clinical comfort.

- Administer tetanus prophylaxis if it has been more than 3 months since tetanus vaccination.

WHAT NOT TO DO

Puncture Wound of the Foot

- If the puncture wound is suspected to involve the coffin joint, navicular bursa, or tendon sheath, *do not* delay antibiotic administration. The prognosis for return to soundness diminishes rapidly when treatment of synovial structures is delayed.
- *Do not* allow horn tissue to become excessively dry or intentionally desiccate the hoof because this may seal the wound tract and cause abscess formation.
- If the foreign body remains in the foot, *do not* ship before removing the foreign body, marking its location or "protecting" it from loading, because direct weight-bearing and ambulation on the foreign body may cause further penetration of deeper structures.
- *Do not* aggressively explore the wound tract with a sharp or rigid "tool" because this may penetrate synovial structures.

Traumatic Injuries of the Foot

Contusions

- Nonpenetrating traumatic injuries to the foot can cause bone and/or soft tissue damage, and lesions are at times difficult to identify.
- Causes include working on hard and/or irregular surfaces, stone bruises, kicking hard objects, and hyperflexion or hyperextension of the coffin joint.
- Presenting clinical signs include acute lameness of a variable degree, heat and swelling, and an increase in the intensity of the digital pulse.
- Hoof tester examination is helpful to isolate the affected area, and a distal limb flexion test commonly exacerbates the lameness.
- In the case of bruising, bleeding may not be evident in the sole or wall for several weeks.

WHAT TO DO

Traumatic Injuries of the Foot

- Clean the foot and perform a comprehensive hoof tester examination to rule out infection or reduce the suspicion of an infection.
- Radiograph the foot to rule out fractures and laminitis. If radiographs are negative, they should be repeated in 1 week if the equine patient is still lame because some fractures do not show up on radiographs for 1 to 3 weeks until the fracture margins demineralize.
- Once a diagnosis of a contusion is confirmed, based on rule-outs, the horse should be stall rested and the following performed:
  - Start on anti-inflammatories (e.g., phenylbutazone, firocoxib, or flunixin meglumine).
  - Soak the foot in ice water for 15 to 20 minutes q12h for 72 hours; cryotherapy/cold therapy decreases inflammation.
  - Pack the sole with a paste made of epsom salts and DMSO, then cover with cotton. Be careful to not let the cotton packing

extend beyond the contact surface of the shoe to minimize sole pressure and possible subsequent lameness.
- If the individual does not show clinical improvement after 10 days and radiographs are negative, magnetic resonance imaging or nuclear scintigraphy are other diagnostic modalities that can be used to better assess the foot for inflammatory and soft tissue changes. Some cases have inflammation and edema in all three phalanges.
- Elimination of lameness secondary to traumatic injuries can take several weeks to resolve.
- When the horse is sound for turnout and/or return to work, a pad and soft packing is recommended for extra sole protection.

WHAT NOT TO DO

Traumatic Injuries of the Foot

- Do not move the equine patient from the stall if a fracture of the coffin bone is suspected and ruled out.
- Fracture displacement decreases the prognosis and the chances for return to athletic soundness.

Avulsions

- Avulsion of the hoof wall can occur in the following situations: an interference injury from another limb, from another horse in a close contact sport (racing, polo), driving, kicking a fence, getting a hoof stuck in a cattle guard, or from farm equipment in the field.
- Most avulsions occur in the heel region and vary from tearing the heel bulb to loss of a large portion of the hoof capsule.
- The depth of the injury also varies, from involving just hoof capsule separation from the dermis to injury of the underlying dermis (corium), coffin bone, collateral cartilage, or digital cushion.

WHAT TO DO

Avulsions of the Hoof Wall

- The equine patient should be sedated if agitated.
- Anesthetize the foot with an abaxial sesamoid block.
- Take radiographs to rule out a third phalanx lesion.
- Meticulously clean the affected area of debris.
- Trim the unattached wall using a hoof knife or hoof nippers.
- Lavage and soak the foot in a Betadine/water solution and wrap the foot in a well-padded bandage with a nonadherent dressing soaked in an antiseptic solution to cover the exposed corium.
- If the avulsion is clean and only involves the hoof capsule with no involvement of deeper structures, topical antiseptics may be all that are needed to prevent infection. Most avulsions epithelialize in 7 to 10 days.
- If there is sufficient hoof wall for a shoe, a bar shoe with frog support is recommended for protection and support of the affected area until healing occurs. More serious avulsions, where a shoe cannot be attached, require a foot cast (see Chapter 21, p. 333) to protect the underlying sensitive tissues until the foot cornifies.
- If the avulsion involves injury to the coronary band or pastern region, the patient should be referred to a hospital for surgical repair.
- Hoof wall instability is managed with hoof wall reconstruction once the affected hoof wall tissue is free of infection and healing.

EMG

⊙〉 WHAT NOT TO DO

Avulsions of the Hoof Wall

- When removing unattached hoof wall and debriding the wound, *do not* damage or remove healthy coronary band tissue. This may result in dystrophic hoof wall growth.

Lacerations

- Lacerations of the hoof capsule are not common but occur from kicking a wire fence or stepping on a sharp metal object.
- Lacerations can occur on the sole, frog, hoof, pastern, or heel bulb.

◐〉 WHAT TO DO

Lacerations of the Hoof Capsule and Wall

- Radiograph the foot to rule out a third phalanx injury or the presence of a foreign body.
- Promptly stabilize a full-thickness laceration of the wall to reduce swelling of the underlying corium, which can prolapse through the hoof defect and cause additional submural separation.
- Anesthetize the foot with 2% carbocaine using an abaxial sesamoid block or midpastern block (see Chapter 21, p. 290) and place a tourniquet at the level of the fetlock if there is excessive bleeding.
- Stabilize the injured wall using an aluminum plate ($\frac{1}{4}$ inch wide × $\frac{1}{8}$ inch thick × 3 inches long), conforming to the wall and bridging the laceration. These plates can be secured to the hoof wall with an adhesive or small wood screws that penetrate no deeper than the stratum medium. Adhesives should not contact the sensitive tissue or inhibit drainage of the wound.
- Stabilize the lacerated hoof wall in the non–weight-bearing position.
- Use a bar shoe or some type of therapeutic shoe for stability.
- Scrupulously scrub and pack the wound using an antiseptic and bandage.

- Systemic, broad-spectrum antimicrobials are recommended to reduce the chances of a submural infection.
- Administer anti-inflammatories/nonsteroidal anti-inflammatory drugs (NSAIDs), for analgesia and to reduce swelling of the corium.
- Stabilization of the hoof capsule is used until new hoof wall growth from the coronary band reaches at least one half the distance from the ground surface of the hoof wall.
- Administer tetanus prophylaxis if it has been more than 3 months since tetanus vaccination.

Lacerations of the Sole and Frog

- Radiograph the foot to rule out a third phalanx injury or presence of a foreign body.
- Scrupulously scrub and soak the foot in Epsom salts, Betadine, and water, or a commercially available chlorine-based foot soak (e.g., CleanTrax).
- Apply a shoe with a removable treatment plate to protect the injured area and treat the wound with an antiseptic dressing.
- Parenteral antimicrobial administration depends on the severity and depth of wound, chronicity, and potential for contamination.

Laceration of the Pastern or Coronary Band

- Moderate to severe lacerations of the pastern or coronary band should be referred to a surgical facility, especially if the wound is located in the palmar/plantar region of the pastern because involvement of the DDFT and/or tendon sheath is possible.
- Initial treatment should include copious wound flushing and cleaning the wound with a disinfectant scrub, then bandaging to protect the wound during shipping.
- If the DDFT or the extensor tendon has been completely severed, a fiberglass or Kimsey splint may be needed to facilitate ambulation and minimize additional injury to surrounding structures.

References

References can be found on the companion website at www.equine-emergencies.com.

CHAPTER 43

Laminitis

Amy Rucker and James A. Orsini

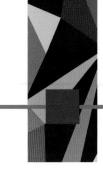

- Laminitis is defined as inflammation of the hoof lamellae/laminae.
- The distal phalanx (P3/coffin bone) is attached to the hoof capsule by the interdigitation of the dermal and epidermal lamellae, which extend through the bars, heels, quarters, and toe of the hoof capsule (Fig. 43-1).
- There are 550 to 600 primary epidermal lamellae (PEL), and 150 to 200 secondary epidermal lamellae (SEL) surrounding the perimeter of each primary epidermal lamellae.
- Epidermal basal cells are attached to a basement membrane (BM), and attach to P3 by collagenous connective tissue fibers running through the lamellar dermis.
- The dermis/corium, composed of arteries, veins, lymphatics, connective tissue, and nerves, is described by its location (i.e., coronary, lamellar, solar, and frog).
- Both the coronary and solar dermis have papillae projecting into the tubular horn. Each papilla has a central artery, vein, and capillaries. Terminal papillae, at the distal border of the dermal lamellae, are responsible for the epidermal cells that fill the space between the primary lamellae, forming the white line.
- Medial and lateral palmar digital arteries and veins anastomose within a terminal arch in the center of P3. Multiple osseous foramina allow smaller vessels to branch through the bone to the sublamellar vascular bed of the dermis.
- The solar surface of P3 has *no* perforating vascular canals. The circumflex artery is located distally and peripherally to the distal border of P3. Arterial branches and venous plexus course within the dermis between P3 and the sole of the hoof capsule.
- "Founder" is characterized by failure of the attachment of the epidermal lamellar cells to the underlying basement membrane of the dermal lamellae and is more appropriately termed "chronic laminitis."
- Laminitis from all causes has similar histopathology including:
  - Disruption of the basement membrane
  - Lengthening and narrowing of PEL and SEL
  - Alterations of the epidermal cells
  - Leukocyte infiltration in association with abnormalities of the secondary dermal lamellae and basement membrane, but the timing and degree varies according to the etiology
- *Practice Tip: Clinical treatment is aimed at preventing and minimizing displacement of P3 to allow healing before structural damage to the lamellae occurs. This prevents structural*

collapse and compression of the coronary and solar dermis, changes in hoof capsular growth, and bone remodeling.

Classification of Laminitis
Developmental Phase

- The developmental phase lasts from the time of exposure to causative agent through the onset of clinical signs, lasting 24 to 60 hours.
- Changes at a cellular level initiate lamellar separation.
- Current proposed pathways:
  - Sepsis/inflammatory pathway—a systemic injury or generalized inflammatory state results in lamellar failure
  - Carbohydrate overload—initiates a *"trigger factor"* mechanism resulting in BM separation and lysis
  - A histopathology scale grading the degree of *lamellar damage* explains why some cases easily recover while others have overwhelming damage refractory to treatment.
  - Endocrinopathic—hyperinsulinemia induces lamellar lesions, including SEL lengthening, primarily in the abaxial and middle regions of PEL and epidermal cell proliferation at the axial aspect. **Note:** There is less BM disintegration at the lamellar tips compared with the carbohydrate overload models.
  - Traumatic or weight-bearing—alterations of metabolic/vascular/lymphatic systems secondary to excessive mechanical load/avascular/trauma mechanism
- *Practice Tip: Prevention of clinical laminitis is possible in the developmental phase if the risk is recognized immediately. Continuous cryotherapy blocks lamellar inflammatory events, reducing the severity of clinical laminitis. At-risk horses should have their legs immersed in ice water (5° to 10°C) from the carpus/tarsus distally for 24 to 72 hours until resolution of clinical signs of disease and laboratory tests of systemic inflammation resolve.*
- Many clinical diseases result in laminitis. The "cause" is traced back to one of the four primary pathways listed previously:
  - Systemic inflammatory states such as colitis, metritis, sepsis with endotoxemia, and pneumonia can induce laminitis via pathologic signaling events.
  - Grain overload is similar to the carbohydrate overload model.
  - Endocrinopathic laminitis includes horses that are insulin resistant (IR) or suffering from equine Cushing's disease/pituitary pars intermedia dysfunction (PPID).

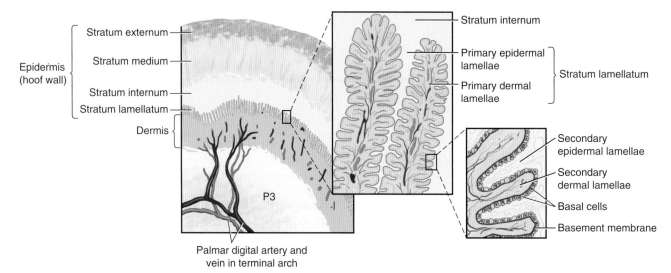

Figure 43-1   The hoof wall or epidermis consists of the stratum externum (thin layer, extending from the periople), stratum medium (majority of the wall, containing tubules and intertubular horn), stratum internum, and stratum lamellatum. The keratinized primary epidermal lamellae and primary dermal lamellae interdigitate in the region of the stratum lamellatum. Arteries and veins present in the sublamellar vascular bed of the dermis anastomose with vessels from the terminal arch of the palmar digital vessels, located in the center of the distal phalanx (P3). Microscopic examination reveals numerous secondary lamellae (dermal and epidermal) at the margins of primary lamellae. At the coronary band, proximal hoof wall, and terminal lamellae at the white line, proliferation of the epidermal basal cells form keratinized cells responsible for the growth of the hoof wall. Throughout the secondary epidermal lamellae, nucleated epidermal basal cells are attached to the basement membrane by hemidesmosomes. The basement membrane is attached to P3 by bands of connective tissue within the dermis.

- Support limb laminitis may develop secondary to any painful contralateral limb lameness.
- *Note:* Medical therapies (vaccinations or steroid injections) may inadvertently lead to laminitis. Attempts to induce laminitis in healthy horses with administration of steroids are *not* reproducible: for example, neither dexamethasone, 1 mg/kg/d for 9 days in ponies or a single injection of triamcinolone acetonide, 0.2 mg/kg, approximately 80 mg IM for an adult horse, caused laminitis in research settings. However triamcinolone injected at 0.2 mg/kg IM induced hyperglycemia and hyperinsulinemia for more than 6 days. It is believed that corticosteroids may influence cellular death, vascular function, the immune system, or the effects of other hormones, and be part of a multifactorial cause of laminitis in these cases, especially horses with equine metabolic syndrome (EMD).

Acute Phase

- The acute phase begins with the onset of clinical signs, lasting 72 hours.
- Clinical signs include varying degree of lameness, heat, bounding digital pulses, and +/− response to hoof testers.
- Response to treatment and control of inciting cause may determine if the horse becomes subacute (minimal lamellar damage) or chronic (collapse of suspensory apparatus of the third phalanx resulting in structural changes).

Subacute Phase

- Clinical signs resolve and mild lamellar changes result in a sound horse with *no* radiographic evidence of mechanical failure or injury to the third phalanx.

- The time line from the acute to subacute phase is generally 72 hours after onset of clinical signs.

Chronic Phase

- Failure of lamellae at the basement membrane results in structural changes of the foot due to loss of the attachment between P3 and the hoof capsule. Depending on the degree of collapse, alterations include:
  - Compression and distortion of the coronary dermis
  - Separation of the dermal and epidermal lamellae with lengthening of the dermal lamellae
  - Compression of the solar dermis
- Long-term sequelae for P3 include:
  - Widening of the osseous canals within P3
  - Remodeling of the distal border and apex

Chronic Phase: Compensated

- Clinical evidence of laminitis is apparent when examining the foot:
  - Widened white line
  - Growth rings that are *not* parallel
  - Changes in appearance of sole (loss of concavity)
- Radiographic changes include:
  - Remodeling of the apex and distal border of P3
  - Dorsal wall is altered ("rotational displacement"); the width of the proximal wall is less than the distal wall.
  - Sole depth (SD) >10 mm distal to the apex of P3 is the goal in the "stable" chronic compensated laminitis case.
- Venogram has contrast material evident around the remodeled apex of P3, distal to P3 in the circumflex and solar vessels, and at the coronary band. The pattern is mildly altered, often with a small volume of contrast material evident "feathering" into the dorsal lamellar scar.

- Horses require routine hoof care and are relatively sound, but should continue to be monitored.

Chronic Phase: Uncompensated

- Horses remain lame with periodic "flare-ups," which present as an acute exacerbation of laminitis.
- There is instability in the bond between the distal phalanx and the hoof capsule (lamellar wedge contributes to chronic lameness and irregular hoof growth; lamellar wedge describes the pathologic tissues that compose the lamellar region [stratum lamellatum] of the chronic laminitis foot; the pathologic horn is also described as "scar horn" or a second or ectopic white line).
- Bone disease/chronic osteitis or areas of damaged lamellae may cause recurrent foot abscesses.
- Venogram supports lamellar instability with contrast material "feathering" into the sublamellar vascular bed and replaced with lamellar wedge. During weight bearing, contrast material is reduced or absent distal to the apex of P3. ***Practice Tip:*** *There are important differences in the appearance of the weight-bearing and non–weight-bearing venogram because instability causes venous compression during the weight-bearing study.*
- Sole depth is usually inadequate to protect distal P3 (SD <10 mm). The sole dermis is compressed, resulting in poor sole growth. The sole may be soft with subsolar seromas.
- In cases of significant collapse, the sole may protrude distally and the apex of P3 or the solar dermis may penetrate the sole.
- The white line is wide and unorganized at the toe, often allowing debris to pack into the white line during breakover, which can result in abscessation. Heel growth exceeds growth at the toe pillars. The dorsal hoof wall grows outward instead of "downward" and may approach a horizontal position in orientation. In cases of neglect, the hoof capsule grows forward and upward, having the appearance of an "elf shoe."

Evaluation of the Laminitic Horse

History

- Duration of clinical signs and any previous episodes
- Known inciting cause and success of any treatments
- Orthopedic injuries/infections and resulting support-limb (contralimb) laminitis have delayed clinical signs and radiographic changes for 4 to 6 weeks
- Age: Recovery is easier for a 4-year-old than a 24-year-old patient
- Any recent medications administered, work load, and diet
- Assess surroundings/housing on farm, including:
  - Stall size and bedding: Ideally the stall is 20×20 feet and bedded with 2 feet of fluffy shavings. Closed-cell foam[1] padding, lining the stall floor, provides increased comfort for the acute and chronic laminitic horse.
  - Turnout lots: Assess size, footing, and available forage.

- Work area available for farrier and veterinarian should include a flat surface, good lighting, a power source, and be close to a stall.
- Location of stall in barn: A quiet location encourages the horse to lie down.

Physical Examination

- Evaluate the degree of lameness while standing, turning, and walking.
- A painful horse:
  - Has an elevated heart rate
  - Is constantly weight shifting
  - Stands with the back feet placed under the abdomen and resists movement
- ***Practice Tip:*** *A foot may have significant damage and not appear clinically painful. Conversely, the foot may be incredibly painful and show no gross clinical abnormalities.*
- Evaluate digital pulses: Normal vs. bounding; may increase in response to walking the horse.
- Evaluate the ease of lifting each foot: How comfortable is the horse, and can it stand with a foot raised?
- Perform laboratory studies: Complete blood count (CBC) and chemistry profile are performed at presentation to help determine the cause of laminitis.
- If IR or PPID is suspected, once the patient is more comfortable, measure ACTH, cortisol, insulin, leptin, and glucose hormones (triiodothyronine [T_3] and thyroxine [T_4]). (See medical management, p. 710.)

Evaluation of the Hoof

Hoof Capsule

- Growth rings: Uniform diameter vs. wider at the heel (suggests clubfoot or chronic laminitis)
- Previous rate of growth: Wide (7 to 10 mm) growth rings suggest rapid foot growth
- Wall thickness: A sound foot with lots of sole has a wall that is "heavy/wide" through the quarters
- Sole: Concave is good; flat indicates a weak foot or P3 is sinking/rotating; prolapsed indicates P3 is rotating/sinking or penetrating the sole
- White line: Uniform thickness is normal; wider at the toe indicates clubfoot or previous laminitis
- Clubfoot: The patient may already have compression of the solar dermis distal to the apex of P3 and tearing of the dorsal lamellae at the dorsal and distal aspect of P3 with bone damage/remodeling of the distal rim of P3 at the apex

Coronary Band

- Hair normally points distally in line with the face of the wall
- Record any areas of drainage or separation that indicate distal displacement of P3
- The coronary band should not have a palpable "rim/cleft" at the top of the hoof capsule that permits palpation of the inside surface of the coronet

Farrier

- The farrier routinely evaluates the patient's feet every 4 to 6 weeks; ask the farrier if any noticeable changes have occurred in the hoof in the last 6 months.

---

[1]American Foam Products, Painesville, Ohio. Distributed by Stoltzfus Equine and Supply, Gap, Pennsylvania; Phone: 717 442-8280.

Hoof Tester Evaluation

- The hoof tester evaluation is often misleading. The horse may be negative to hoof testers if it has a thick sole or if the hoof capsule is getting ready to slough.
- Be *gentle* when applying pressure and stop at the slightest pain response.

Heat

- Acute laminitis is associated with an increase in submural blood flow. Heat may be measured by digital palpation or thermography.

Radiographic Evaluation of the Foot

- A standardized radiographic technique is critical for comparison purposes. Radiographs are used to evaluate initial injury, devise a treatment plan with the farrier, measure response to treatment, and monitor the foot going forward.
- Meticulously clean the feet. A hoof pick or wire brush may be needed to remove dirt from deep within the frog sulci.
- Equipment: Two wooden foot blocks, with a radiopaque wire impeded in the top of the blocks as a point of reference, are needed. The blocks should be 0.75 inch (2.0 cm) shorter than the center of the collimator of the radiographic machine, resulting in the focal point of the x-ray beam centered at the distal border of P3. The low beam provides measurements of sole depth and P3 medial to lateral balance within the hoof capsule. Apply barium paste[2] (radiopaque marker) to conform to the dorsal hoof capsule from the hair on the coronary band to the toe for the lateromedial projection.
- Position the foot blocks according to the conformation of the horse (wide chest/toe in, narrow chest/toe out, etc.) with the metacarpi/metatarsi perpendicular to the ground and the head and neck facing forward. Careful positioning is needed for evaluation of digital alignment and joint loading.
- The x-ray cassette is placed parallel to the sagittal plane of the foot with the x-ray machine perpendicular to the cassette to avoid image distortion on the lateral-to-medial projection. The cassette touches the foot to eliminate image magnification. The technique allows evaluation of soft tissue detail including the hoof capsule, sole depth, and radiolucencies within the dermis (seromas), lamellar wedge, or epidermis (air or dirt seen with white line disease). On the zero-degree dorsopalmar projection, note the position of the distal phalanx (P3) within the capsule and the loading of joint surfaces. A 65-degree dorsopalmar projection may be taken in cases of chronic laminitis to evaluate the degree of bone disease at the distal rim of P3.
- Hind-feet radiographs are more challenging to obtain, but a baseline lateral view is mandatory. Hind-limb lamellae also show inflammatory changes after laminitis induction models, but laminitis is often less severe than in the forelimbs; this is thought to be due to factors such as weight bearing.

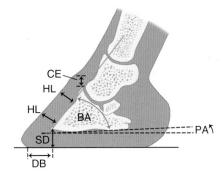

Figure 43-2 Radiographic measurements. Coronary-extensor distance (CE), horn-lamellae width (HL), sole depth (SD), digital breakover (DB), palmar angle (PA), and bone angle (BA). (Distances are measured in millimeters.)

Radiographic Measurements

See Fig. 43-2.

Coronary Extensor Distance (CE)

- Vertical distance, in millimeters, measured from a horizontal line drawn at the proximal dorsal coronary band to the extensor process.
- The range of normal varies, extending from 0 to 30 mm in sound horses, with an average of >12 to 15 mm.
- *Practice Tip: The CE is most useful as a comparison, increasing as disease progresses.*
- A rapid increase in CE occurs if P3 displaces distally—"sinker."
- A gradual increase occurs over weeks if the foot undergoes mechanical collapse.

Horn:Lamellar Distance (HL)

- A line perpendicular to the face of P3 is measured to the dorsal hoof capsule (as marked by the barium paste) for horn:lamellar distance. Measurements are made distal to the extensor process and at the distal tip of P3.
- The numbers should be the same proximally and distally. If the HL distance is asymmetric (greater distally), suspect displacement/rotation of P3 away from the epidermis.
- *Note:* A nonlaminitic clubfoot may have a disparity in the HL measurement (e.g., 15 mm proximally and 19 mm distally), especially if the farrier has been trying to stretch the toe to match the foot angle on the opposite foot.
- The HL varies with age and breed:
  - Weanlings: Proximal HL > distal HL as the first new foot grows out.
  - Yearlings: Proximal and distal HL are equal.
  - 2-to 4-year-old light breed horses in training (e.g., Quarter Horses, Arabians).
  - Thoroughbreds: HL is 17 mm:19 mm proximal and distal).
  - Occasionally a large-framed horse may have an HL measurement of 16 mm:16 mm. Two-year-old to 4-year-old Standardbreds in training have an HL of 20 mm:20 mm. Warmbloods may have an HL of up to 20 mm:20 mm, depending on their size.

---

[2]Intropaste (Mallinckrodt Inc., St. Louis, Missouri).

- Aged training or performance horses have a gradual increase in HL. The HL may become 17 mm:17 mm in light breed horses.
- Retired or bloodstock horses may have an even greater HL but never have developed laminitis.
- **Practice Tip:** *Suspect laminitis if the HL is greater than the range of normal for a particular age/breed. Example: A 5-year-old, 450-kg Quarter Horse has an HL distance of 18 mm:18 mm; consider the increase may be due to separation of the dermal and epidermal lamellae along the entire hoof capsule (distal displacement) if the horse has consistent clinical signs, perform a venogram to confirm the diagnosis.*
- **Practice Tip:** *Obtain baseline lateromedial radiographs to determine what is normal for the individual, and periodically update the information. In horses that are at high risk for laminitis, annual examinations are recommended.*

Sole Depth (SD)

- Sole depth refers to the distance measured perpendicularly from the apex of P3 to the ground.
- If the sole is concave, the air space appears black on the image. Record the sole in two ways: sole depth and concavity.
- Record the location or depth of radiolucencies in the sole (seromas or abscesses associated with P3).

Digital Breakover (DB)

- The horizontal distance measured from a line drawn from the apex of P3 to the most dorsal point of the toe is the "digital breakover."

Palmar Angle (PA)

- The angle measured between the palmar surface of P3 and the ground surface is the palmar angle.
- This angle may need to be measured twice if the medial and lateral wings are *not* symmetric.
- If the apex of P3 is remodeled, the measurement is made by drawing a straight line at the distal border of the wings and central P3.
- **Practice Tip:** *Structural collapse of the foundered foot must occur before any changes are evident on radiographs. This may take hours to days to occur, resulting in a delay in recognizing the severity of disease on radiographs.*
- The palmar angle (PA) and horn:lamellar distance (HL) have replaced measuring the degrees of P3 rotation.

Venographic Evaluation of the Foot

- The digital venogram uses radiopaque contrast injected into the palmar digital vein.
- The images of dermal vasculature detail changes within the foot before plain radiographic changes are evident.
- Dermal injury is manifested by changes in the appearance of the contrast pattern.
- Venous compression causes filling defects of contrast material; the defects on the venogram are treated by farriery and possibly surgery.

- **Practice Tip:** *Support-limb (contralimb) laminitis may have venographic and magnetic resonance imaging changes within 1 to 2 weeks; clinical lameness and radiographic changes are delayed for 4 to 6 weeks. These cases usually have a moderate to severe amount of lamellar damage.*

Venogram Procedure

- **Practice Tip:** *Plain radiographs of the study feet are taken before performing the venorgram for comparative purposes.*
- If the horse is shod, consider removing shoes before the venogram. If the shoes elevate the palmar angle more than 10 degrees, remove the shoe (including glue and any putty placed in the sole), clean the foot, and place it in a new plastic shoe with a heel wedge for the venogram. **Note:** *Do not* take a laminitic foot from an elevated palmar angle and stand it flat on the ground. This increases the tension of the deep flexor tendon and potentially damages the dermis.
- Perform local anesthesia of both front feet using an abaxial nerve block (see Chapter 21, p. 289). Inject 3 mL mepivacaine[3] hydrochloride subcutaneously over the medial and lateral palmar nerves at the base of the proximal sesamoids (abaxial sesamoid block).
- Organize all equipment needed to perform the study before bringing the horse to the radiographic area; when ready, clean the feet and stand the horse on the x-ray blocks.
- Sedate the patient with detomidine hydrochloride,[4] 1 to 3 mg IV.
- Clip the hair on the medial and lateral pastern so that both palmar digital veins are evident. If the leg has thick hair, then clip the palmar aspect of the fetlock (including over the palmar neurovascular bundle) at the point the tourniquet is applied.
- Fill two 12-mL Luer-Lok syringes with radiopaque contrast material[5] for an average 12.5-cm-wide foot. If you are working in a cold environment, keep the syringes warm to facilitate injection.
- Clip and aseptic prepare the venogram site is recommended.
- The veterinarian kneels in front of the foot to be studied, facing caudally. The radiographic machine is positioned for a lateral view. The assistant is behind the x-ray machine, lateral to the horse. All equipment should be within reach.
- Four-inch tape is wrapped around the fetlock to secure the tourniquet. *Do not* extend the tape onto the pastern.
- The recommended tourniquet is a 50-cm-length × 2.5-cm-wide strip of rubber inner tube. Fasten one end of the tourniquet to the 4-inch tape. The tourniquet is applied at the widest point of the fetlock, at the base of the sesamoids.

---

[3]Carbocaine (Pharmacia Upjohn Company, New York, New York).
[4]Dormosedan (Pfizer Animal Health, New York, New York).
[5]Diatrizoate meglumine and diatrizoate sodium (Bracco Diagnostics, Princeton, New Jersey).

Practice Tip: It is important that the palmar wraps of the tourniquet are applied as tightly as possible. Once the entire tourniquet has been stretched around the fetlock, it is secured with 2-inch tape wrapped several times around the fetlock. The end of the tape is left free on the outside of the fetlock (if the lateral vein is being used for injection).

- A 21-gauge × ¾-inch (0.8- × 19-mm) butterfly catheter with 30-mm tubing[6] is used. The palmar digital vein is relatively straight in the proximal pastern, but tortuous distally. A 2-cm straight section is identified mid-pastern, and the needle is inserted bevel-side out. Once blood flows freely (flashback), stop advancing the needle. The assistant should attach a Luer-Lok injection port on the catheter, using care *not* to dislodge the needle.

- Procedure for lateral palmar digital vein catheterization: The clinician's inside arm wraps around the limb in a medial-to-lateral direction, with the shoulder in direct contact with the dorsal carpus. The clinician's outside hand remains in contact with the butterfly catheter, applying light digital pressure to the vein and preventing the needle from backing-out as contrast is injected. The assistant inserts the needle of one syringe of contrast into the injection port and places the syringe in the veterinarian's inside hand. Using the thumb on the plunger, the veterinarian lightly aspirates for flashback followed by rapid injection of the contrast. Monitor for injection resistance and a subcutaneous injection, rechecking frequently to be sure the needle is still in the vein. The assistant removes the first syringe and attaches the second syringe. Flashback usually occurs when the needle is inserted into the injection port. During injection of the second syringe and using the inside hand and arm, the carpus is gently flexed. The goal is *not* to remove the foot from the block, but to flex the leg to relieve the tension of the deep digital flexor tendon and partially unload the foot. The assistant can help in keeping the foot on the block and turning the horse's head away from the foot being imaged to allow ease in flexion of the limb.

- When the injection is completed, the syringe and needle are removed, and the injection port and tubing are secured under the free end of tape.

- The contrast material is hyperosmolar, and it rapidly diffuses into the tissue. All radiographic images should be completed within 45 seconds after the injection to avoid "diffusion" artifacts. Lateromedial, dorsopalmar, and non–weight-bearing lateromedial views complete the study series. Additional views (65-degree dorsopalmar or oblique images) can be taken to highlight areas of interest. *Note:* If additional views are taken >45 seconds after injection, the contrast may create diffusion artifacts.

- After the images are obtained, the tourniquet is removed, and then the butterfly catheter is removed from the vein and a folded gauze compression bandage covering the medial and lateral veins is applied. *Do not* leave the compression bandage on for >15 minutes.

[6]Surflo Winged Infusion Sets (Terumo Corp, Somerset, New Jersey).

Trouble Shooting the Venogram

- *Do not* distort the skin on the pastern as the tape and tourniquet are applied.
- If the needle is placed in the vein and blood flows freely then stops, back the needle out 1 to 2 mm. If flashback doesn't resume, then redirect the needle.
- If "the vein blows" after the constrast injection is begun, and <3 mL of contrast has been injected, remove the tourniquet and the needle and place digital pressure on the vein. Wait 10 minutes and then use the opposite vein for the procedure. When performing the venogram, an assistant must maintain digital pressure on the first venipuncture site, only removing the hand during the radiographic imaging.
- If >3 mL of contrast is injected before a problem arises, stop the injection and take the radiographs. The images may still be diagnostic in spite of filling deficits due to inadequate contrast volume. Do not attempt to catheterize the other vein at this time. If the second vein is injured by the injection technique, the foot may be severely compromised. Delaying the procedure for 24 hours may be the best approach.
- From start-to-finish, bilateral venograms should be completed in 30 minutes. A longer procedure potentially compromises the laminitic patient by making the patient stand on a hard surface with both feet blocked.

Normal Venogram Findings

- See Fig. 43-3.
- The *terminal arch (TA)* of the palmar digital vessels courses through P3. It supplies many branches through osseous canals to the *sublamellar vascular bed (SLVB).* The SLVB is a distinct line located within 4 mm from dorsal P3.
- The *coronary plexus* is rounded in a crescent shape and located proximal and dorsal to the extensor process. Papillae of arteriovenous anastomosis of the horn tubules are parallel to dorsal P3.
- The *circumflex vessels* are peripheral and distal to P3. Many solar papillae are evident, and they are also in the same plane as the dorsal border of P3. On a normal foot with 20-mm sole depth, the circumflex vessels and solar papillae extend 10 mm distal to the palmar rim of P3.

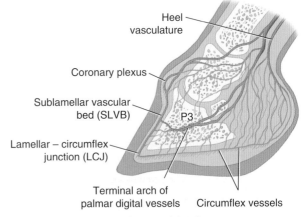

Figure 43-3 The normal digital venogram.

- The *lamellar-circumflex junction* mirrors the angle of the apex of P3 and gives rise to the terminal papillae of the white line.
- The *heel vasculature* arises from a branch proximal to the hoof capsule and is seldom changed by laminitis.
- On the dorsopalmar views of a normal foot, the SLVB remains within 4 mm of the dorsal, lateral, and medial borders of P3; the lamellar-circumflex junction is at the same angle as the distal rim of P3; the circumflex vessels are seen distal and peripheral to P3; the TA is visualized within P3; and the cunneate vessels of the frog are located distal to the terminal arch. The filling of the coronary plexus is *not* symmetric medial to lateral because of hoof asymmetry.

The Laminitic Venogram: Mild Compromise

- See Fig. 43-4.
- The lamellar-circumflex junction is folded.
- Terminal papillae are no longer oriented in same plane as dorsal face of P3.
- Solar papillae are *not* evident.
- Contrast may be reduced in the circumflex and solar vessels.
- Coronary papillae are usually *not* evident, but if present they are *not* oriented in the same plane as the dorsal face of P3.

The Laminitic Venogram: Moderate Compromise

- See Fig. 43-5.
- The coronary plexus is distorted and elongated. Contrast may be reduced or absent.
- SLVB may be widened as the dermal and epidermal lamellae detach. Alternatively, venous compression may result in areas void of contrast.
- Contrast is absent from portions of the circumflex and solar vessels.
- The lamellar-circumflex junction is folded and located proximal to the apex of P3.

The Laminitic Venogram: Severe Compromise

- See Fig. 43-6.
- Contrast is evident in the heel.

- If present, contrast in the terminal arch is reduced.
- Vessels are bluntly truncated at the coronary band.

The Laminitic Venogram: Distal Displacement (Sinker)

- See Fig. 43-7.
- The coronary plexus is mildly distorted.
- The SLVB is widened.
- Contrast is reduced or absent distal to P3 in the circumflex and solar vessels.

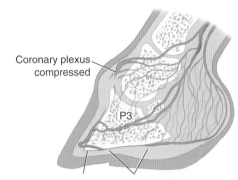

Figure 43-5   Laminitic venogram with moderate compromise. *LCJ,* Lamellar-circumflex junction.

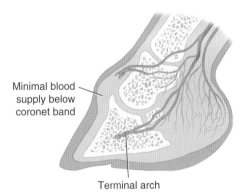

Figure 43-6   Laminitic venogram with severe compromise. Contrast is only evident proximal to the coronary band, with minimal contrast in the heel and terminal arch. This pattern is consistent with a severe sinker or with chronic progression of injury and resultant collapse.

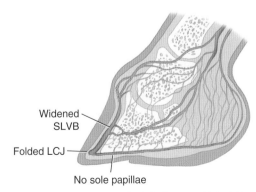

Figure 43-7   Laminitic venogram—distal displacement (sinker). Acute widening of the SLVB (sublamellar vascular bed) in the toe, quarters, and heels is evident with separation of the dermal/epidermal lamellae. The solar vessels are compressed and the LCJ (lamellar-circumflex junction) folded. This pattern may progressively worsen (see Fig. 43-6).

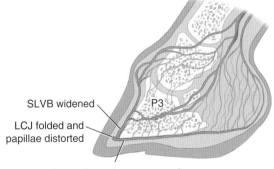

Figure 43-4   Laminitic venogram with mild compromise. *LCJ,* Lamellar-circumflex junction; *SLVB,* sublamellar vascular bed.

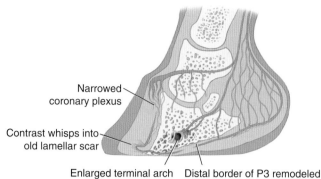

Figure 43-8   Laminitic venogram—chronic laminitis.

- The lamellar-circumflex junction may be mildly folded or may be proximal to the apex of P3.
- As damage progresses, the distal foot displacement has the appearance of the venogram shown in Fig. 43-6.

The Laminitic Venogram: Chronic Laminitis
- See Fig. 43-8.
- The coronary plexus is narrow and elongated. Papillae are *not* parallel to the dorsal face of P3, and the new wall growth is in the same plane as the papillae.
- The SLVB is widened; contrast "feathers" into the lamellar wedge. A fine line may be evident at the dorsal-most

border of the lamellar wedge at the interface with the epidermis.
- The apex of P3 is remodeled secondary to osteitis. Bone resorption may be due to avascularity or pressure/load on the solar dermis and epidermis. The lamellar-circumflex junction is remodeled around the apex. The terminal papillae are disoriented.
- Contrast is reduced in the circumflex and solar vessels. Solar papillae distal to the apex of P3 are only evident if the sole depth is >10 mm. Solar papillae may be present in the heel.

Technical Errors: Venogram
- Low volume of contrast material results in:
  - Vessels appear to taper and thin. Any "loaded" area is void of contrast.
  - *Practice Tip:* *Tourniquet failure may be secondary to vessel "padding" by hair on the palmar fetlock or by using too much tape.*
- Perivascular injection of contrast ("blown vein") may result in low volume of contrast material.
- A radiograph can be obtained at midcarpus to check for contrast above the tourniquet.
- It is important to place the tourniquet as described around the widest part of the fetlock, not at the metacarpus as would be done for a distal regional limb perfusion.

●❯ WHAT TO DO

Laminitis: Principles in Treating the Laminitic Foot
Internal Forces of the Foot (Fig. 43-9)
- *Gravity* forces P3 distally and is counteracted by *ground forces.* The larger the weight-bearing surface of the bottom of the foot, the better the weight distribution (pounds per square inch). The heels

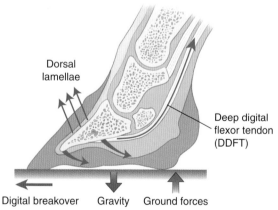

Figure 43-9   Internal forces of the foot. Failure of lamellar attachment may be treated by addressing other forces within the foot. Elevation of the palmar angle or tenotomy reduces the pull of the DDFT. Trimming the heel increases the weight-bearing surface area. Shoeing changes reduce digital breakover.

are trimmed to increase the surface area caudally. A pour-in pad[7] or composite putty[8] is placed on the sole to recruit the frog, heels, bars, and sole in the quarters for additional weight distribution.
- *Digital breakover* acts as a fulcrum over which the hoof capsule must move to relieve pressure of lamellar distraction within the foot. Dorsal, medial, and lateral breakover are all altered to reduce tearing of the diseased lamellae.
- With disruption of the *lamellae,* there is little to counteract the forces of gravity and the deep digital flexor tendon (DDFT) pulling P3 distally.
- The *heel* is often the healthiest portion of the foot. This may be due to the *digital cushion* and the ligaments of the collateral cartilages helping to support the wings. Use the heel in the treatment plan for the laminitic foot (see p. 705).
- Depending on the conformation of the horse (width of chest, rotational and angular limb deformity, clubfoot, or low heel), one or more parts of the foot may be stressed before the development of laminitis. *Important:* Consider this when formulating a treatment plan because the weak area may complicate treatment.
- For successful treatment, think of the forces within the hoof capsule. Questions to consider:
  - Where is the greatest area of load on the dermis?
  - Where has the dermal-epidermal junction failed?
  - Which plan has the greatest chance of "unloading" the compressed dermis and reducing strain on the diseased tissue?

---

[7]Equi-Pak (Vettec, Oxnard, California).
[8]Advance Cushion Support (Nanric, Lawrenceburg, Kentucky).

⬤〉 WHAT TO DO

Altering the Palmar Angle: Treating Acute Laminitis

- Elevating the palmar angle reduces the strain of the DDFT is one option for treatment of the acute laminitis case. Trim the heel to the widest part of the frog so that P3 is parallel to the ground surface.
- "Float" the quarters to reduce weight bearing and therefore wall strain.
- Bevel the toe at the white line to allow access to the lamellae if a seroma/abscess needs to be drained.
- Place the foot in a 20-degree elevated heel shoe[9] (Fig. 43-10).
- **Caution:** *Do not* trim the heels and then stand the horse without heel support; lowering the palmar angle increases the strain of the DDFT.
- Composite putty is mixed and placed in the inside of the shoe; the shoe is placed on the foot while the putty cures. When cured, remove putty from the solar surface directly opposite the anterior rim of P3, reducing sole pressure.
- Soft-ride boots, foot/hoof casts, stryrofoam, and silicone impression materials are other good treatment options commonly used for the acute laminitis case.

- The shoe may be secured to the foot with bandage material for routine treatment. Alternatively, the shoe may be fixed to the foot using glue[10,11] or 2-inch cast tape. **Note:** Shoes should *not* be nailed to the acutely painful foot.
- Computer modeling supports that increasing the PA places more strain on the dorsal lamellae. However, this seems inconsistent with clinical observations (see Figs. 43-11, *A*, and 43-11, *B*). Elevating the PA may increase forces on the quarters and increases weight bearing in the heels. However, "sacrificing" the heel and quarters may be necessary to treat the acute laminitis case. A horse with a low, crushed heel should have its heel monitored while in the shoe. Forces may be reduced if heel elevation is applied with a foot cast to decrease wall strain.
- The owner may begin with 2-inch-thick industrial Styrofoam bandaged to the foot as interim padding while the horse is waiting for emergency care. The Styrofoam may be "stacked" in the heel to reduce DDFT strain.

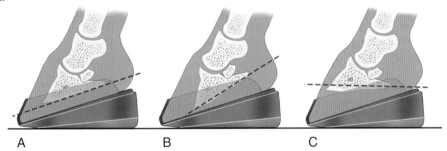

A   B   C

Figure 43-10   Elevated heel shoe for acute laminitis. **A,** Correct application: palmar surface of P3 is parallel to the top of shoe that includes a 20-degree heel wedge. The shoe is beveled at the perimeter, encouraging dorsal, medial, and lateral breakover. The point of breakover is directly distal, or slightly caudal, to the apex of P3. Putty is added to the sole after the shoe is placed to distribute weight bearing on the heel, bars, and frog. The putty is "cupped" in a convex pattern from the sole directly distal to the apex of P3. **B,** Incorrect application: wedging the foot with a positive palmar angle does not correctly load the foot. Potentially, putty could be used to elevate the wall at the toe pillars and establish a correct angle. The dorsal wall could be "dressed" to more appropriately fit the cuff of the shoe and reduce breakover. The bottom of the shoe could be "ground back" at the beveled toe to reduce breakover. **C,** Remove and reapply and monitor the foot with radiographs. Note: Most feet grow sole and in time lose the 20-degree palmar angle (PA); the pull of the deep digital flexor tendon (DDFT) is no longer reduced. Overloading of the heel can result in abscess or seroma formation.

⬤〉 WHAT TO DO

Developing a Hoof Treatment Plan

- Ideally, treatment is initiated well within 24 hours of clinical signs of laminitis. The longer the delay in treatment, the more cumulative tissue damage and associated change noted on the radiographs or venograms. If there is overwhelming damage and cumulative damage, the tissue repair may *not* allow recovery and a pain-free existence.
- Assess each foot independently and develop a treatment plan based on clinical signs, radiographs, venograms, owner capabilities, and underlying cause and duration of disease. Identify the area and degree of damage and select a shoe and technique to treat the specific problems.
- **Practice Tip:** *Use benchmarks for progress: Sole depth should increase 2 to 3 mm every 7 to 10 days. The venogram should improve such that the contrast pattern shows no areas of contrast voids.*
- **Practice Tip:** *Each case of laminitis and each hoof is different, so one type of hoof support and management does not work in every case. It is important to re-assess and amend the plan as frequently as needed.*

⬤〉 WHAT TO DO

Subacute Laminitis

- Classification criteria for subacute laminitis:
  - Mild to *no* lameness
  - *No* apparent radiographic or venogram changes
  - *No* palpable abnormalities of hoof capsule
- The horse should be on strict stall rest in deep bedding and closecell foam padding lining the stall floor for 2 weeks.
- After 2 weeks, the laminitis patient should be sound, with all antiinflammatory medications discontinued.
- If a shoe is used in the treatment, *do not* remove the shoe or lower the palmar angle until the radiographs are normal for 3 weeks.
- If all goals are reached, the lower wedge is removed from the shoe. After the palmar angle is reduced from 20 to 10 degrees, the horse should have normal digital pulses and remain sound in the stall.
- At 6 weeks, if the laminitis patient remains sound and there are *no* new radiographic changes, the horse may be regularly shod, turned out, and transitioned to a normal routine over 3 to 4 weeks.

---

[9]Ultimate (Nanric, Lawrenceburg, Kentucky).

[10]Super Fast Equi-Thane (Vettec, Oxnard, California).
[11]Equilox (Equilox International, Pine Island, Minnesota).

●〉 WHAT TO DO

Acute Laminitis

Mild Damage

(See Figs. 43-4, 43-11)

- Elevated heel shoe (see Fig. 43-10, p. 705) or alternative foot support (e.g., Soft-Ride boots or foot casts[12]) are applied.
- Mechanical support of the foot can be made on clinical experience of the veterinarian and farrier, foot radiographs and response to anti-inflammatory agents if venograms are not an option.
- Perform venogram at initial evaluation and repeat in 3 days to 3 weeks depending upon:
  - Clinical comfort
  - Control of cause of laminitis
  - Improvement in clinical signs (digital pulse, limb edema, heat, appearance of coronary band)
  - Measurable increase in sole depth on radiographs
- If the patient has *not* met the above goal metrics, repeat the venogram to screen for treatment failure with further collapse of the foot.
- Evaluate the horse at 4 weeks for:
  - Normal digital pulses
  - Soundness on *no* medications
  - Radiographic improvement in sole depth and the venogram
  - If the three above parameters are true, then the horse may be hand-walked a short distance every day or turned out to graze in a small round pen with good footing.
- If the venogram has contrast filling in all areas and sole papillae are evident after 6 weeks, then the horse may be shod.
- Digital breakover should be distal to the apex of P3, and the palmar angle should *not* be lowered to <10 degrees.
- Exercise is restricted to hand walking initially and then turnout in a small paddock with good footing.
- If clinical comfort is stable for 10 to 14 days, the laminitis patient should be sound at the walk and on no pain medications. During follow-up shoeing, short-term pain medication may be needed for several days; clinical comfort should remain stable on discontinuation of the medication.
- Increases in sole depth should be measurable on radiographs.
- Growth rings should be parallel, indicating normal hoof growth.
- The new dorsal wall growth should be parallel to the face of P3, and any abnormal toe should be incrementally trimmed at the solar surface as the shoe is reset.
- When the new wall growth reaches the level of the shoe, the horse may be returned to light work, approximately 6 to 9 months from disease beginning.
- After the foot has grown a second full cycle, the horse may return to regular use and competition.

Moderate Damage

- See Fig. 43-5 for an example of moderate damage.
- If the duration is less than 1 week, apply an elevated heel shoe, Soft-ride boots, foot casts, or other foot "appliance" for the best mechanical support for the injured hoof.
- Perform venogram at initial evaluation and repeat in 3 days to 1 week to make certain the foot is responding to treatment; if it is *not*, consider a DDF tenotomy.
- If patient presents with a history of several weeks' duration of disease, consider DDF tenotomy.
- If the venogram suggests mild to moderate damage (apex of P3 is even with the circumflex vessels with little contrast distal to P3) it

may be difficult to decide to treat with shoeing or shoeing in conjunction with the DDF tenotomy.

- If the horse presents on the first day of clinical signs, place the feet in elevated heel shoes (see Fig. 43-10) and repeat the venogram 5 days later. If on day 5 there is minor improvement or the condition is *no* worse, continue treatment and repeat the venogram on day 10. The case may be monitored with repeated venograms; a

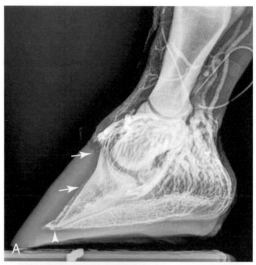
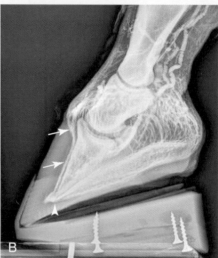

Figure 43-11 Laminitis of 2 weeks' duration with mild damage. **A,** Initial radiograph taken after contrast injection. Contrast is absent in the coronary plexus and proximal dorsal sublamellar vascular bed *(arrows)*. The lamellar-circumflex junction (LCJ) is distorted, and the terminal papillae are not parallel to dorsal P3 *(arrowhead)*. The apex of P3 is at the level of the circumflex vessels and contrast is reduced distally *(arrowhead)*. **B,** Second series of radiographs taken 10 seconds after contrast injection and placement of the foot in a 20-degree heel elevation shoe. Contrast has returned to the coronary plexus and proximal dorsal sublamellar vascular bed *(arrows)*. The lamellar-circumflex junction (LCJ) has a more normal orientation, and contrast has increased distal to the apex of P3 *(arrowhead)*. The terminal papillae remain incorrectly oriented. Note that the palmar rim of P3 is parallel to the top of the shoe confirming correct application of the elevated heel shoe. The shoe should be "fixed" to the foot and the venogram repeated in 1 week. Progress is marked by improvement of the appearance of the LCJ and orientation of the terminal papillae. Within 2 weeks, no compression of the circumflex vessels should be evident and within 3 weeks, solar papillae should be obvious. If the second venogram reveals worsening of the contrast pattern, shoeing and a deep digital flexor tenotomy would be considered. (Radiographs courtesy of Dr. Thomas Wagner)

[12]Soft-Ride Boots (Soft-Ride Corporation, Vermillion, Ohio).

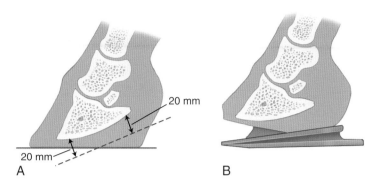

Figure 43-12   Shoeing in conjunction with a deep digital flexor tenotomy. **A,** A line is drawn on the radiograph 20 mm distal to the palmar surface of P3. The heel is trimmed so the palmar surface of P3 is parallel to the top of the 5-degree shoe. **B,** Putty is placed in the heel over the frog, bars, and sole for support. Glue secures the shoe to the foot and fills in the space at the toe pillars between the shoe and hoof wall. No putty or glue contacts the foot at the sole or toe.

decision is made for a DDF tenotomy *no* later than the end of week 3. If contrast still has *not* improved distal to the apex of P3 and sole depth is *not* increasing, then a DDF tenotomy is indicated. Closely monitoring the case assures that minimal bone damage occurs.

- If the patient presents with changes in the apex of P3 (osteitis), consider DDF tenotomy. Horses may return to intended use with a tendon scar but seldom are sound with significant bone damage. ***Note:*** Horses are *not* usually candidates for racing or jumping after tenotomy.

- ***Practice Tip:*** *Monitor the foot on the dorsopalmar radiographs and venograms. Many horse conformations stress one portion of the foot more than another. Generally, this is the medial wall in Thoroughbreds and the lateral wall on broad-chested Quarter Horses. A laminitis patient may have as much damage in the quarter as it does in the dorsal lamellae.*

Severe Damage

- See Figs. 43-6 and 43-7 for examples of severe damage.
- The foot is often painful and does *not* respond to regional anesthesia (nerve blocks).
- The severe (see Fig. 43-6) venogram pattern does *not* respond to shoeing alone. Shoeing in conjunction with a DDF tenotomy or humane destruction is recommended.
- If a severe (see Fig. 43-6) venogram pattern occurs after several days of clinical laminitis, the horse may respond to treatment including a DDF tenotomy and possibly wall resection in conjunction with a transfixation pin cast to temporarily decompress the lamellae. If the horse has a history of several weeks of laminitis, then the damage may be irreversible, and humane destruction should be considered.
- The severe (see Fig. 43-7) venogram pattern is that of a sinker. The foot may respond to treatment with an elevated heel shoe if treatment is initiated within hours to days of the development of laminitis. A venogram is repeated in 3 to 5 days to assess the response to shoeing. If the contrast pattern is improved on the venogram, conservative treatment (shoeing) is continued. The foot should initially be monitored with weekly venograms to make certain that dermal compression is resolving (sole depth should increase). If the response is *not* as expected, a DDF tenotomy is recommended.
- ***Practice Tip:*** *The DDF tenotomy is only successful if performed in conjunction with corrective trimming and shoeing.*
  - Shoe the horse with a 5-degree elevated heel aluminum shoe[13] (Fig. 43-12). Place breakover directly below the apex of P3. A heel extension prevents luxation of the distal interphalangeal joint. Trim the heel parallel to the distal border of P3. Often the only part of the foot touching the shoe is the heel.

- Secure putty elasomer under the foot and place the shoe on the heel positioned so the distal border of P3 is parallel to the shoe. The putty should have *no* contact with the sole below the apex of P3. Once the putty is cured, remove the edge of the putty in contact with the bars of the heel.

- Apply Equilox to the bar and place a "bed" from the heel to the toe pillar, making sure *not* to extend onto the sole; no glue is applied to the toe. Place the shoe on the foot, held at the correct angle by the cured putty. Impregnate strips of woven fiberglass cloth with glue and wrap the hoof from the wall distally over the medial and lateral edge of the shoe.

- Once the glue has cured, place an elevated heel shoe on the foot beneath the aluminum shoe (a 20-degree heel wedge is an alternative choice, with the glue-on aluminum shoe) to reduce strain on the DDF during surgery.

- Deep digital flexor tenotomy:
  - Perform a high four-point block of the palmar and palmar metacarpal nerves just below the carpus to anesthetize the leg (see Chapter 21, p. 288). A dorsal ring block may be performed subcutaneously to eliminate skin sensation.
  - After a sterile prep, maintain a sterile field and make a 2-inch vertical incision over the DDFT at midmetacarpal region. Use metzenbaum scissors to bluntly separate the DDFT from the suspensory ligament, and introduce a curved retractor. Withdraw the metzenbaum scissors and separate the DDFT from the superficial digital flexor tendon (SDFT). Insert a second curved retractor and withdraw the scissors. The curved ends of the dorsal and palmar retractors come in contact on the medial aspect of the DDFT and should overlap to protect adjacent neurovascular structures. Apply pressure on the retractors to elevate the DDFT slightly out of the incision, allowing complete exposure for transection with a scalpel blade.
  - Remove the elevated heel shoe to allow inspection of the transected proximal and distal ends of the DDFT (transected tendon ends should separate ≈2 cm). Close the skin incision and apply a sterile bandage to the leg. Change the bandage as needed and maintain the limb in a bandage for 3 months to minimize scar formation at the surgical site.
- Place gauze sponges soaked in Betadine solution between the lamellae at the toe and the shoe. The Betadine helps "toughen" the tissue and allow keratinization of any exposed dermis if P3 has penetrated the sole.
- Antibiotic prophylaxis is instituted based on risk of post operative infection. Tetanus prophylaxis should be current within the previous 6 months.
- Poultice any area along the white line that is draining edematous fluid.

---

[13]4-Point Tenotomy Railbar Shoe (Nanric, Lawrenceburg, Kentucky).

- Reevaluate the case 1 month after DDF tenotomy is performed. At the time of reexamination, the sole should cover any exposed bone if the sole was penetrated; there should be *no* drainage from the sole or lamellae. In cases without penetration, the sole depth should have doubled. The venogram should have contrast material distal to P3, including the apex of P3. The new wall growth at the coronary band should be uniform and adjacent to the face of P3.
- At 1 month post-tenotomy, contrast material should fill distal to P3 on the venogram, otherwise severe lamellar damage has probably occurred. Consider that this patient (severe lamellar damage) may survive but *not* live a pain-free existence or return to the previous routine.
- The entire care of the laminitis patient should be reviewed and short-term goals established or the horse should be humanely destroyed.

Chronic Laminitis with Acute Lameness

Abscess

- Fig. 43-8 represents a venogram that supports an increased risk for a foot abscess.
- ***Practice Tip:*** *Always think "abscess" first when a chronic laminitis case becomes acutely non–weight-bearing lame on one foot.* Clinical signs include:
  - Increased digital pulses
  - Increased heart rate
  - Severe pain that may last several days
- Plain radiographs are recommended to rule out other causes for the acute non-weight-bearing lameness.
- The abscess may be due to septic osteitis of P3. The diseased bone and associated septic discharge travels the path of least resistance and may travel along the solar plane to open at the heel bulbs and/or travel up the wall and open at the coronary band.
- Use a poultice to encourage drainage. Monitor the coronary band and heel bulbs for soft areas that open and drain. Make sure the coronary band does *not* prolapse over the top of the hoof wall,

compromising the blood supply of the coronet and causing further tissue injury.
- Occasionally the sole is soft with multiple seromas associated with compression of the solar dermis; the sinus tracts travel distally and anteriorly through the sole. ***Practice Tip:*** *Do* not *establish drainage by removing sole, which exposes important dermal tissue.*
- Some abscesses occur from retrograde contamination entering the "seedy" separations in the lamellae at the widened white line. A sharp hoof knife is used to follow the separation and debride the lamellar wedge until a fluid tract is opened or sensitive tissue is encountered; apply a poultice "plug" filling the tract q12h.
- The suspected area is poulticed q12h to encourage drainage, and then packed with Betadine solution when drainage stops. Consider adding systemic antibiotics (trimethoprim-sulfa +/− metronidazole) to the treatment regimen if drainage continues for several days or appears purulent.
- With advanced bone disease, surgical curettage is performed. An alternative is the use of sterile maggots to selectively debride the unhealthy tissue.[14]

Endocrinopathic Laminitis

- IR/PPID horses usually have an insidious onset with incremental tissue damage occurring over time. Lamellar attenuation and elongation associated with hyperinsulinemia helps explain why many horses have multiple mild episodes of laminitis with gradual widening of the white line. The damage is cumulative and eventually one episode seems to push the foot past the "tipping point" of mild disease and easy recovery.
- Survival is dependent on the diseased tissue recovery, but also the owner's ability to manage the underlying disease and the horse long-term. Successful treatment depends on nutritional and medical modifications with concurrent foot treatment.
- Recurrent bouts of laminitis eventually result in instability of the lamellar attachment. The foot becomes refractory to treatment.

●》 WHAT TO DO

Shoeing for Acute Lameness Associated with Chronic Laminitis

- Use the same principles of shoeing to relieve stress (Fig. 43-13):
  - Reduce breakover to decrease shear forces at the toe
  - Increase the weight-bearing surface of caudal portion of foot
  - Provide solar support or protection if needed
  - Achieve digital alignment
  - Relieve pulling of the DDFT and strain on the compromised lamellar tissue
- The shoe application corresponds to the degree of tissue instability in the foot: Increased instability requires enhanced breakover and adjustments to the palmar angle. Use the radiographs to devise a "blueprint" for treatment:
  - How is the foot trimmed?
  - Where is the point of breakover?
  - How should the palmar angle be adjusted?
- Chronic mild cases may *only* need a leather or plastic pad between the shoe and hoof for ground protection. A steel shoe with a beveled/rolled toe can be nailed on the foot if the horse is *not* painful. Elevating the flattened sole off the ground and giving it a

mechanical barrier offers some protection to P3. If the owner is reluctant to use shoes as part of the treatment protocol for the laminitic patient, turnout boots are an alternative to "cushion" the hoof sole.[15]
- If the foot continues to grow excessive heel and the horse is *not* sound, then wedge pads are incorporated. Measure the palmar angle on radiographs and trim the heel to increase the surface area of the weight-bearing heels. The total palmar angle cannot be lowered to avoid increasing the pull of the DDFT. Any "heel height" removed when trimming the foot is replaced using a wedge pad or elevated heel shoe (see Fig. 43-13). Reduce breakover by lightly dressing the toe and using a beveled toe shoe.
- The foot should have uniform foot growth. If the foot is growing more at the heel than toe, increasing the palmar angle between shoeing, then adjust the shoe to address internal forces of the foot. The palmar angle must be further elevated and digital breakover reduced. (see Fig. 43-13, *C*).
- Follow-up radiographs should support increases in sole depth. Ideally the sole should double in depth during the first 6- to 8-week shoeing cycle and eventually maintain a "heavy/thick" sole. Most

---

[14]Monarch Labs, 17875 Sky Park Circle, Suite K, Irvine, CA 92614. Phone: 949-679-3000; FAX: 949-679-3001; e-mail: info@MonarchLabs.com; www.monarchlabs.com.

[15]Soft-RideBoot (Soft-Ride Inc., Bacliff, Texas).

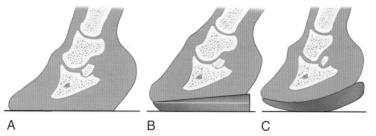

Figure 43-13   Shoe application for chronic laminitis. **A,** Generally, the heel "out-grows" the toe and the toe grows dorsally instead of distally, with minimal growth of wall at the toe pillars. The sole is compressed internally, so it does not grow sufficient mass to protect the distal rim of P3. Minimal treatment includes "dressing" the toe to reduce breakover. A protective boot with a soft sole insert is placed on the affected foot each day before turnout. At night, the horse is stall confined in dry shavings to encourage a "stronger" foot. Alternatively, the foot is shod with a beveled-toe shoe, a pour-in, or a leather pad. **B,** The toe is "dressed" to reduce breakover, and the heel trimmed to increase the weight-bearing surface area. A wedge pad is applied so that the overall palmar angle (PA) is not reduced (do *not* drop the PA; this increases the pull of the deep digital flexor tendon (DDFT), compressing the solar dermis and straining the dorsal lamellar attachment.) **C,** A rocker-rail shoe moves breakover behind the apex of P3. The heel is trimmed parallel to the palmar surface of P3, further increasing the surface area in the heel. The palmar angle is not decreased and the loading forces on the heel are increased. The center of the shoe "balance point" is located directly below the center of the distal interphalangeal joint. The phalanges are in alignment.

laminitic horses with a sole depth of 20 mm or greater are sound. The exception is a horse with poor lamellar attachment of P3 to the wall, or a horse with chronic osteitis.

- Aluminum shoes are often used because they are lightweight; a thicker shoe with beveled edges, to facilitate breakover, can be fabricated and is easy to apply with glue or cast tape. Aluminum shoes are manufactured with wedge or rail heels, cuffs for glue attachment, and adjustable rails. Plastic or polymer shoes are also available in a variety of sizes and styles.
- The Steward Clog[16] has beveled edges to reduce dorsal/medial/lateral breakover and a cupped sole at the toe. Composite putty is placed between the palmar sole and the clog. Screws are drilled through the hoof wall into the clog, allowing the horse to stand during the application. An alternative method is to use screws at the periphery of the wall and then use cast tape to secure the shoe.
- Rasping/sanding the dorsal wall until it is parallel to the dorsum of P3 has a nice "cosmetic" look, but does nothing to reduce internal

forces. Instead, reduce breakover of the shoe to decrease abnormal forces. Rasping/sanding the dorsal wall to the lamellar scar may actually weaken the hoof capsule.
- Bone disease with remodeling of the distal margin and apex of P3 may contribute to chronic pain. If bone remodeling reaches the osseous canal of the terminal arch of the palmar digital vessels, then the horse suffers recurrent abscesses and septic osteitis. Drainage is encouraged at the dorsal lamellar/sole interface with the goal of maintaining healthy sole and heel.
- ***Practice Tip:*** *Laminitis cases with mild bone disease and minimal lamellar wedge (the pathologic tissues that compose the lamellar region [stratum lamellatum] of the chronic laminitis foot; the pathologic horn is also described as "scar horn" or a second or ectopic white line) have the best prognosis.*
- A large lamellar wedge causes lameness because of instability of the bone-wall attachment and sole compression.
- If aggressive shoeing treatment does *not* return the foot to health and the horse to soundness, consider a DDF tenotomy.

●❯ WHAT TO DO

Medical Management of the Acutely Laminitic Horse
- Treatment is aimed at the underlying disease to prevent continued lamellar damage.
- Specific treatments may be indicated depending on the primary disease: Examples include intravenous DMSO (controversial) to decrease inflammation, +/- antioxidant (controversial efficacy); polymyxin B for endotoxemia; nasogastric administration of mineral oil for acute grain overload; antibiotics for sepsis, etc.
- Medical care also includes fluid therapy in the developmental and acute phases of laminitis to minimize hypovolemia, multiple organ dysfunction, or renal injury when administering potentially nephrotoxic doses of anti-inflammatory medications.
- ***Caution:*** Complete elimination of pain allows the horse to move freely or stand for prolonged periods, further contributing to the mechanical separation of the lamellar tissue. It is important to find a balance between the comfort of the horse and restriction of movement.

- ***Note:*** many medications and treatments used in laminitis have multi-modal mechanisms of action (e.g., phenylbutazone is anti-inflammatory and analgesic).

Anti-Inflammatory Medications
- Initial treatment goals with nonsteroidal-anti-inflammatory drugs (NSAIDs) are to control pain and reduce inflammation in the lamellar tissue. The NSAID selection may be based on the type of disease (e.g., COX-2 inhibitors/firocoxib for black walnut exposure and flunixin for colic/colitis cases). Once treatment has been started with a specific NSAID, a different drug may be used for long-term anti-inflammatory treatment. The higher initial dosages are reduced slowly over time in an attempt to minimize adverse side effects.
- Flunixin meglumine: 0.5 to 1.1 mg/kg IV or PO q12 to 24h; a nonselective COX inhibitor used to prevent systemic inflammatory response syndrome (SIRS) and for analgesia.
- Phenylbutazone: 2.2 to 4.4 mg/kg IV or PO q12h initially; a nonselective COX inhibitor used as an anti-inflammatory and analgesic. Reduce dose for long-term treatment to decrease adverse side effects.
- Firocoxib: 0.09 mg/kg IV q12h for 3 doses then 0.1 mg/kg PO q24h maintenance; a COX-2 inhibitor, it has empirically less initial pain

---

[16]Equine Digit Support System, Inc., Penrose, Colorado.

relief than phenylbutazone or flunixin. It may be indicated as an antihyperalgesic agent in central nociceptive sensitization due to COX-2 localization in the spinal cord dorsal horn. In chronic laminitis COX-2 is preferentially upregulated and therefore firocoxib is the preferred NSAID.

- Ketoprofen: 1.1 to 2.2 mg/kg IV q12 to 24h

Modification of Blood Flow/Vessels

- Pentoxifylline: 10 mg/kg IV or PO q12h; inhibits pro-inflammatory cytokine production, is anti-endotoxic and improves blood flow and red blood cell deformability.
- Acepromazine: 0.04 mg/kg IM q2 to 4h; decreases vascular resistance and may contribute to hypotension. *Caution:* A heavily tranquilized horse may *not* move or shift its weight, eliminating or reducing the important "pumping" mechanism of the foot.
- Low-molecular-weight heparin[17]: potentially decreases neutrophil-derived myeloperoxidase production in endothelial cells and may reduce the possibility of laminitis in postsurgical colic cases.
- Cryotherapy: prevents laminitis when started before the developmental phase of laminitis and is also used in the acute phase of the disease for additional anti-inflammatory and analgesic effects. It is continuously administered for 24 to 72 hours beyond resolution of clinical disease.
- Clopidogrel (Plavix), 4 mg/kg PO on day 1 then 2 mg/kg PO q24h thereafter for platelet inhibition.

Pain Medications

- See Chapter 49, p. 749 for comprehensive pain management.
- Sensory nerve terminals are located at the base of the dermal lamellae and may *not* be affected during developmental laminitis. Sensitization during the acute phase may develop secondary to locally released inflammatory mediators. Neurogenic inflammation may potentiate central hyperalgesia and in turn increase the excitability of dorsal horn neurons. Disruption of the lamellae may damage sensory neurons and produce spontaneous impulse discharges.
- Pain may become a pathologic problem by itself. Multimodal treatment aims include:
  - Reduce nociceptive signaling by sensory nerve terminals (NSAIDs and hoof treatment)
  - Suppress peripheral hyperalgesia (NSAIDs, local anesthesia, and analgesia)
  - Inhibit afferent nociceptive signaling to the central nervous system (CNS) (regional anesthesia)
  - Inhibit spinal nociceptive signal transmission (local anesthetics, opioids, alpha$_2$-agonists) and central hyperalgesia (opioids, alpha$_2$-agonists, ketamine, NSAIDs, gabapentin, pregabalin)
  - Prevent or inhibit neuropathic pain (systemic lidocaine, opioids, NSAIDs, gabapentin, pregabalin)
- The treatment objective is to achieve optimum pain control while incurring minimal side effects, recognizing that no single medication for neuropathic pain is 100% effective.
- Gabapentin and pregabalin cause a change in the release of neurotransmitters within the CNS. Gabapentin exerts analgesic properties primarily in the sensitized or hyperalgesic states. Oral bioavailability of gabapentin is poor, but pregabalin at a dosage of 2 to 3 mg/kg PO q8h is almost 100% bioavailable.
- Fentanyl/opiod agonist: 2 to 3 10-mg patches changed q3d, can be administered with sedatives
- Morphine: 0.2 to 2 mg/kg IV/IM q4 to 6h, administered with sedatives
- Butorphanol: 0.01 to 0.4 mg/kg IV/IM q2 to 4h, or IV continuous rate infusion (CRI) at 13 to 24 µg/kg/h (see Appendix 2, p. 805). May be

used in combination with an alpha$_2$-agonist, but adverse effects include reduced intestinal motility and reduced movement/stupor.

- Lidocaine: 1.3 to 1.5 mg/kg IV over 5 minutes as a loading dose, followed by 50 to 100 µg/kg/min CRI (see Appendix 2, p. 805). Lidocaine has analgesic, antihyperalgesic, and anti-inflammatory properties.
- Ketamine: Peripheral nerve stimulation leads to larger than normal postsynaptic potentials at the dorsal horn of the spinal cord, contributing to central hyperalgesia, synaptic plasticity, and chronic pain. Ketamine is antagonistic at the nerve receptors and is used to modulate central sensitization at a low-dose CRI as adjunctive therapy. Ketamine is administered using an initial bolus at 100 to 150 µg/kg and followed with a CRI of 60 to 120 µg/kg/h (see Appendix 2, p. 805).
- Pain may be modified using intermittent boluses or infusions of anesthetic agents including regional anesthesia using repeated injections of local anesthetics, topical local anesthetics (lidocaine patches), percutaneous catheterization adjacent to the palmar nerves for anesthetic administration, and caudal epidural catheterization for pelvic limb laminitis pain control. There is increased risk associated with these analgesic drugs when used in a horse that *does not* lie down; prolonged loading of the diseased feet may contribute to the collapse of the foot.

Regenerative Therapies

- Stem cells are injected into the laminitic foot via retrograde venous infusion, intraosseous delivery (see Chapter 5, p. 16), or injection directed into the coronary band. Although some practitioners report favorable responses in growth and comfort, the treatment recommendations are *not* evidence based.

Supportive Therapy

- Place the horse in a large box stall (i.e., 20 × 20 feet). The horse must have enough room for comfort, and bed the stall using a minimum of 2 feet of shavings, keeping the bedding "fluffed." Closed-cell foam padding, lining the stall floor, provides additional comfort for the horse with laminitis and may encourage the horse to lie down. The stall should be kept meticulously clean and be in a quiet location to encourage the horse to lie down.
- If the horse is recumbent for long periods, monitor for "bed-sores." Clean the wounds three times a day with Betadine scrub or witch hazel. When dry, apply silver sulfadiazine cream, A&D ointment with zinc oxide (petroleum base, allows to breathe), or diaper ointment[18] with lanolin.
- Feed the horse small meals several times a day. Place hay in several locations to encourage eating when recumbent. Offer water when in sternal recumbency.
- Provide supportive care for intestinal health to encourage normal gut microbes (prebiotics and probiotics) and prevent ulceration (omeprazole/GastroGard/UlcerGard[19]).
- Use periodic laboratory tests (blood urea nitrogen [BUN], creatinine, total protein, and albumin) to monitor kidney and intestinal health while on NSAIDs.

●▸ WHAT TO DO

Endocrinopathic Laminitis

- This category includes horses that develop laminitis secondary to IR, PPID, pasture turnout, or treatment with steroids.

---

[17]Lovenox (Sanofi Aventis-US, Bridgewater, New Jersey).
[18]Super-Duper Diaper Doo (Doctor's Best, Springfield, Missouri).
[19]Omeprazole (Merial, Duluth, Georgia).

- The term *equine metabolic syndrome* (EMS) is often used to describe the overweight, laminitic, IR horse that exhibits specific areas of regional adiposity. However, *not* all IR horses are overweight, *not* all overweight horses are IR, and some horses are both IR and PPID.

Endocrine Testing

- Testing for PPID: Measure endogenous ACTH. ACTH values increase in the late summer and fall; testing is representative of real ACTH values if using the correct reference range. ACTH concentrations may also increase because of acute disease, laminitis, and acute abdominal diseases (though ACTH should return to normal within several days of an isolated stressful event). (See Online Appendix 3 for reference values.)
- Blood is collected and placed in an EDTA tube; plasma separated and put in plastic tube within 8 hours for ACTH testing. Sample should be shipped chilled (ice packs) by overnight mail.
- ***Practice Tip:*** *Insulin sampling: Withhold grain the night before and allow only a flake of low carbohydrate hay for the late feeding. A fasting blood sample is obtained in the morning before feeding to minimize inaccurate insulin measurements.*
- Testing for Insulin Resistance: measure resting fasting insulin and glucose concentrations. The horse should be fasted for insulin testing. Feed one flake of low NSC hay no later than 10 PM the night before sampling. Collect blood in the morning before the barn is fed to reduce the stress of hearing the feed cart. A resting insulin level >20 μU/mL is considered diagnostic for IR. Dynamic testing, using glucose tolerance or a combined glucose-insulin test may be more accurate, but these tests require the horse to be hospitalized. The Oral Sugar Test is a dynamic test that can be easily and quickly performed in the field. Administer 0.15 ml/kg Karo light syrup PO, at 60 to 90 after administration, a blood glucose >125 mg/dl or insulin >45 μU/ml suggests insulin resistance (IR).
- ***Practice Tip:*** *Testing the acutely laminitic patient is difficult because stress and pain lower insulin sensitivity and could increase resting glucose and insulin concentrations. Endotoxemia and carbohydrate overload also reduce insulin sensitivity. Therefore, it is often necessary to institute management of suspected endocrinopathy before confirming via blood tests.*
- Endocrinopathic laminitis cases increase in the spring and fall because of seasonal variation of pasture forage and increased concentrations of nonstructural carbohydrates (NSC) (fructans, simple sugars, and starches). Glucose and insulin concentrations peak seasonally on pasture-grazing horses. Cool season grasses that live in climates with severe cold or frequent drought are more prone to NSC accumulation. The NSC varies over time, generally being lower in the morning and higher in the afternoon.
- Leptin results are interpreted in conjunction with insulin testing for EMS.[20] Normal reference range for leptin is 1 to 4 ng/mL; intermediate, 4 to 7 ng/mL; high >7 ng/mL. Leptin is unique because results are not adversely affected by feeding or stress, and therefore it is useful in ruling out other causes of hyperinsulinemia. The higher the leptin value, the more likely clinical EMS is a diagnosis. If the horse has an intermediate to high leptin value without hyperinsulinemia, consider obesity, increased risk for EMS, or treatment for EMS as likely differentials diagnosis.
- If endocrine test results are ambiguous, clinicians can use clinical findings to help determine if the patient needs treatment. IR may occur in horses as young as 4 years old (unusual) and should be considered if the horse is obese with abnormal fat deposits. PPID more often occurs in the horse that is >15 years of age with hirsutism, polyuria/polydipsia, and loss of muscle mass.

Endocrinopathic Medications

- Pergolide mesylate,[21] 0.001 to 0.003 mg/kg PO q24h, is a dopamine receptor agonist that is used to treat PPID. Horses of average size are usually started on 1 mg daily, with dose adjustment after at least 1 month guided by response to therapy and follow-up testing. ***Note:*** Some horses and ponies may require up to 0.01 mg/kg PO q24h.
- Cyproheptadine, 0.25 mg/kg PO q12 to 24h, may be used as an alternative or concurrently with pergolide in the PPID horse. Cyproheptadine may decrease corticotropin secretion, and is a serotonin, acetylcholine, and histamine antagonist.
- L-Thyroxine, 0.1 mg/kg PO q24h, hypothesized to increase insulin sensitivity; recommended dosage ranges from 48 mg/day per large pony or horse and 24 mg/day for small ponies and Miniature horses. This dosage is continued for several months in combination with dietary restrictions and exercise to encourage weight loss. L-thyroxine must be tapered before discontinuing, so 0.5 mg/kg PO q24h is administered for 14 days, then the dose is reduced to 0.25 mg/kg PO q24h for 2 more weeks before stopping treatment.
- Metformin, 15 to 30 mg/kg PO q12 to 24h, suppresses gluconeogenesis, increases glucose uptake in peripheral tissues, and reduces plasma triglyceride (insulin-sensitizing effect). It is usually used short-term (2 to 3 weeks) during a hyperinsulinemic crisis.
- Pioglitazone, 1 mg/kg PO q24h is a thiazolidinedione class of drugs with hypoglycemic action used to treat Type II diabetes. Plasma concentrations are lower and more variable compared to those considered therapeutic in humans.

Management

- Pay strict attention to dietary management and possibly increase drug doses as seasonal risk increases. If a horse is overweight, it should be in a dry lot and *only* turned out on pasture wearing a grazing muzzle, if at all.
- Grasses are highest in NSC: as they develop seed heads; under cool conditions, if stressed; and if growing in direct sunlight. To minimize sugar levels in a pasture, fertilize for rapid growth, avoid stressed grass, control high sugar weeds, and allow grazing *only* in the shade during the morning, if at all.
- Exercise in conjunction with appropriate dietary management can improve insulin sensitivity. ***Caution:*** *Do not* exercise laminitic patients if the foot is unstable. A program of 2 to 3 exercise sessions per week, 20 to 30 minutes per session, building in intensity and frequency is recommended.
- Hay cut before the development of seed heads and cut on overcast days may be lower in NSC. All hay should be tested before feeding. Hay is initially provided at 1% to 1.2% of current body weight/day to encourage weight loss. After 4 weeks, a 5% to 7% reduction in body weight is expected.
- Monitor body weight and regional adiposity. Body weight is calculated by measuring the length of the horse from the point of the shoulder to the point of the buttock and by measuring heart girth.

$$\text{Body weight (pounds)} = \frac{[\text{heart girth}^2 \text{ (inches)} \times \text{body length (inches)}]}{330}$$

The goal for weight loss is 1% of body weight per week. The circumference of the neck is measured in three places and monitored for reduction in fat deposits.

---

[20]Leptin test can be performed at Cornell University Animal Health Diagnostic Center, 240 Farrier Road, Cornell University, Ithaca, NY 14853. Phone: 607-253-3900; FAX: 607-253-3943; http://diagcenter.vet.cornell.edu.

[21]Prascend (Boehringer Ingelheim Vetmedica, Inc., St. Louis, Missouri).

- Some IR horses are underweight; ribs are evident with a cresty neck, and these horses will obviously have different dietary needs. ***Practice Tip:*** *To increase caloric intake while minimizing a glycemic response, feed multiple small meals of low NSC hay and commercial low-NSC feed. Soaked nonmolasses beet pulp (0.5 to 1.5 lb/1.1 to 3.3 kg q24h) or vegetable oil (½ to 1 cup q12 to 24h) may be added to the diet to increase non-NSC calories.*

Summary of What to Do and What Not to Do for Laminitis

●》 WHAT TO DO

Laminitis

- *Prevention!* Prevent laminitis from developing in the at-risk horse.
- If developmental phase of disease is suspected or the equine patient is at-risk for laminitis, consider the following preventive measures:
  - Take baseline radiographs
  - Support the foot:
    - Reduce breakover
    - Elevate the palmar angle to decrease pull of the DDFT and improve digital alignment
    - Support the sole with a putty elastomer
  - Administer **cryotherapy:** Place the feet in an ice-water *slurry* up to the carpus (knee) and tarsus (hocks). *Do not* remove until 48 to 72 hours after clinical and laboratory abnormalities stabilize.
- *Treat the primary disease.* Administer anti-inflammatories and medical supportive treatments as indicated.
- *Endocrinopathic disease.* Rule out or treat insulin resistance (IR) and/or pituitary pars intermedia dysfunction (PPID)/Cushing's disease; treat and manage the nutritional needs.
- *Be aware of historical foot and health issues* that may complicate treatment.
- *Standardize radiographic technique* for soft tissue measurements.
- *Use venograms* to assess the severity of the laminitis.
- *Bedding* in a stall should be deep.
- *Develop a treatment plan* based on history, physical examination, radiographs, and venogram; include medical, surgical, nutritional, pain, and foot management.
- Administer anti-inflammatories.
- *Manage pain* but *not* at the expense of decreasing long-term recumbency.
- Immediately provide hoof support as previously discussed.
- ***Practice Tip:*** *Unloading the foot reduces the mechanical collapse of the suspensory apparatus of the third phalanx.*
- Restrict exercise.
- *Setting goals:* Establish short- and long-term objectives including:
  - A time-line and metrics for anticipated goals of progress
  - Measure radiographic improvement (increase in sole depth, new growth parallel to the face of the distal phalanx (P3), and uniform foot growth)
  - Improvement in the venogram
  - Discuss progress or lack of progress with the support team
  - After the first month of treatment:
    - Foot should double in sole depth
    - Foot should grow a centimeter of uniform growth ring at the coronet (heel should *not* outgrow the toe)
    - There should be improvement in the appearance of the venogram contrast in the circumflex and solar vessels and the lamellar-circumflex anastomosis at the apex of P3

Note: It is important to frequently reevaluate the treatment protocol and prognosis for recovery.
- Owner's long-term expectations for the horse should be reviewed.

●》 WHAT NOT TO DO

Laminitis

- Do not exercise the horse: *restrict movement!*
- Do not overly sedate the horse so that it stands without shifting its weight.
- Do not take more than 1 hour for the initial evaluation and treatment. *Forcing a horse to stand for prolonged periods on hard footing affects treatment success. Make certain everything you need is close at hand before you begin.*
- Do not assume that because the radiographs appear "normal" there is *no* soft tissue damage. *Do a venogram!*
- Do not presume the horse is "stable" when its pain level is reduced. *The foot must have radiographic and venographic improvement if it is to recover.*
- Do not presume a laminitic horse that is only "maintaining" is going to survive. *Long-term survival depends upon progress.*
- Do not expect that a horse with advanced bone disease is going to be sound. *Even a mild degree of remodeling of the distal border of P3 may prevent the horse from returning to work. If osteitis and reabsorption has extended to the terminal arch, the horse will have chronic pain and recurrent foot abscesses/infections.*
- Do not shape the toe and lower the heels so the foot looks "normal" on radiographs. *Lowering the heel/palmar angle increases the pull of the deep digital flexor tendon.*
- Do not nail a shoe on a painful foot. *Use glue!*
- Do not place an acute laminitic horse in an environment where the bedding packs in the soles and is firm (wet sand, shavings, etc.). *Laminitic cases require strict attention to cleanliness and "fluffability" of their stall bedding.* ***Practice Tip:*** *Closed-cell foam padding is an excellent and inexpensive stall floor covering to manage the acute and chronic laminitic horse.*
- Do not cut a hole in the bottom of the sole searching for a foot abscess. *Alternatively, enter the foot through the separated lamellae at the white line of the toe, or apply a poultice to the hoof, including the coronary band and heel, to encourage drainage.*
- Do not neglect to ask the owner if the horse is insured. *Make certain the owner has contacted the insurance company immediately, and the agent contacts you for a report.* Detail your treatment plan and expected outcome barring any unforeseen setbacks.
- Do not presume that because you are happy with case progress that the owner is also happy. Written records of goals and expectations help clarify the course of therapy. *Owners become discouraged after a few weeks of treatment because they have* no *experience and lack long-term vision. Charting radiographically measurable progress helps the team stay focused and gives them hope.*
- Do not forget to reevaluate the status of endocrine disease as treatment progresses. *This may include confirming disease with more in-depth testing, or just evaluating the success of treatment.*
- Do not plan to return the horse to work before the foot has grown a minimum of one full cycle. *The foot should grow two cycles before returning to strenuous exercise.*
- Do not induce right dorsal colitis or renal disease with NSAIDs.

References

References can be found on the companion website at www.equine-emergencies.com.

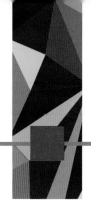

CHAPTER 44

Emergencies of the Racing Athlete

Patricia M. Hogan, Jennifer A. Wrigley, and James A. Orsini

Important Considerations for the Racing Athlete

- Racehorses generally experience the same types of emergencies as other horses and are treated similarly.
- There are several features that are unique to, or more of a concern in, racehorses and warrant special consideration.
- Types of racing athlete breeds include:
  - Thoroughbreds
  - Standardbreds
  - Quarter horses
  - Arabians
- Emergency conditions in racehorses occur at the racetrack either during a race or race training or immediately afterwards, which creates an unusual situation in administering emergency care.
- These circumstances add a component of physical and psychological stress that may *not* be present with, and are dissimilar to, other medical and surgical conditions in other horses.
- Injuries that occur during racing or training usually are more severe than in other disciplines because they occur at high speed and with greater energy. Interference by other horses in congested racing "traffic," "occult" injuries, and variability in racing surfaces are other recognized risk factors.
- Other components that are factored into the management of emergencies in racehorses include:
  - Presence of the public and media
  - Monetary value of the horse
  - Breeding value of the horse
  - Complex ownership of the horse (e.g., syndicate or corporation)
  - Inability to contact the principal owner at the time of emergency treatment
  - Mortality insurance

⦿ WHAT TO DO

Special Considerations
Postexercise Recovery
- Racing is an intense athletic pursuit that taxes almost every body system.
- *Practice Tip: In the absence of concurrent disease or ongoing stress, all clinically relevant changes in cardiopulmonary and metabolic indices, fluid and electrolyte balance, and body temperature typically* have returned to resting values by 60 to 90 minutes after the completion of intense exercise.
- The white blood cell differential may still reflect a stress leukogram at >90 min.
- Most of these changes return to resting values faster when the athlete is regularly walked after intense exercise, typically within 60 min in mild ambient conditions.
- If injury or other circumstances force the horse to remain quiet during this postexercise period, then the return to resting values is delayed.
- The transitional or postexercise recovery period is factored into the clinical assessment of the racehorse if the athlete is examined within an hour after a race or training session.

Sedation and General Anesthesia

- In an emergency situation, sedation or general anesthesia may be required immediately after a race or a training injury when the horse is still under the influence of exercise-induced catecholamine release and various exercise- and competition-associated physiologic and psychological disturbances.
- Sedation and general anesthesia can be safely performed within minutes after the conclusion of intense exercise; however, some precautions are needed.

Sedation
- The commonly used sedative drugs may safely be given to horses immediately after intense exercise, at the following dosages:
  - Xylazine: 0.2 to 1.1 mg/kg IV
  - Romifidine: 0.04 to 0.1 mg/kg IV
  - Detomidine: 0.01 to 0.02 mg/kg IV
  - Acepromazine: 0.02 to 0.03 mg/kg IV
  - Butorphanol: 0.02 to 0.04 mg/kg IV
- The cardiopulmonary depression routinely seen in resting horses is *no* greater than when these drugs are given immediately after intense exercise.
- *Practice Tip: The alpha$_2$-agonists, xylazine, romifidine, and detomidine, and acepromazine—an alpha-adrenergic antagonist—can delay the recovery from exercise-induced hyperthermia.*
- When hyperthermia is a clinical concern in a patient requiring sedation immediately postexercise, alternative methods for cooling the horse, such as hosing or sponging with cold water or alcohol or the use of electric fans, should be considered.

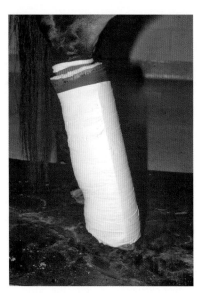

Figure 44-1   Dorsal splint incorporated in the bandage to stabilize the fetlock and pastern region after a racing injury.

- Opiates, such as butorphanol, should be administered with care because they may cause excitement or restlessness, often manifested as a persistent desire to walk, and ataxia when used alone or in higher doses (e.g., 0.1 mg/kg IV).
  - This effect is especially important to avoid in horses that have sustained musculoskeletal injuries.
  - High doses may also suppress gastrointestinal activity for up to 24 hours.

General Anesthesia
- When general anesthesia is induced immediately after strenuous exercise, such as to safely remove an injured horse from the track or extricate the horse from a horse trailer accident the following combination is recommended:
  - Sedation with xylazine, 1.1 to 2.2 mg/kg IV, with or without acepromazine, 0.02 to 0.04 mg/kg IV
  - Induction with ketamine, 2.2 mg/kg IV, and diazepam, 0.1 mg/kg IV
- The combination of tiletamine[1] hydrochloride and zolazepam hydrochloride, 1.1 to 2.2 mg/kg IV—also is an acceptable induction agent in this situation, although recovery can be more prolonged and rough in comparison to the previously mentioned combination (see Chapter 47, p. 744).
- *Practice Tip: Ketamine alone is* not *recommended, because it may* not *provide an acceptable quality of anesthetic induction, cardiopulmonary stability during anesthesia, and recovery.*
- Once any emergency measure has been undertaken (e.g., hemostasis for bleeding wounds, splinting of an injured limb [Fig. 44-1]), the anesthetized athlete must be moved to a safe location for recovery or its present setting made

safe by the removal of anything likely to cause injury during recovery.
- Support should be provided for the horse's head and tail to avoid further injury when the horse rises and until it is steady on its feet.
- These precautions are especially important if the horse has an injury to a limb or the spine.

Antimicrobial Drugs
- Generally, the same antimicrobial drugs recommended for use in other horses and conditions (see Chapter 21, p. 316), may be used in racehorses.
- *Practice Tip: There is some evidence that antimicrobial-induced colitis is more common in racehorses than in other horses, particularly with ceftiofur, and less commonly, enrofloxacin.*
- *Caution:* There is potential for increased nephrotoxicity when using the aminoglycosides gentamicin and amikacin in stressed, dehydrated patients that may also be given nonsteroidal anti-inflammatory drugs (NSAIDs) concurrently (Geor, 2007).
  - Correct fluid deficits as soon as possible to reduce the nephrotoxic potential of the aminoglycoside class of drugs.
  - Usage of the once-daily dosage regimen (see Chapter 21, p. 316) renders aminoglycosides safer in at-risk patients such as the racing athlete.

Nonsteroidal Anti-inflammatory Drugs (NSAIDs)
- Given the high incidence of gastrointestinal ulceration in racehorses (up to 90% in some studies), NSAIDs should be used with care in racehorses.
- *Note:* Stress or occupation-related gastric ulceration in horses primarily involves the squamous portion of the gastric mucosa especially along the margo plicatus, whereas NSAID-induced gastric ulceration seems to principally occur in the glandular mucosa.
- Because NSAIDs are an important basis of pain management in horses, avoiding them is *not* advised, unless the individual horse has demonstrated a particular sensitivity to them; instead, care with dosing and gastric ulcer prophylaxis is recommended.
- Except in individuals with idiosyncratic NSAID sensitivity, the risk for gastric ulceration is both dose and time dependent and also is dictated by the drug's relative selectivity for the COX-1 isoenzyme of cyclooxygenase (COX). Therefore, use the lowest effective dose for the shortest period necessary, and as soon as practical, switch to an NSAID that has demonstrated good selectivity for the COX-2 isoenzyme in horses (e.g., firocoxib).

Ocular Medications
- Corneal abrasions, contusions, and ulceration are relatively common in the racing athlete.
- Treatment as outlined in Chapter 23, p. 400, is suggested. *Important:* Use the lowest effective dose of atropine in

racehorses; gut motility may already be altered by stress and intense exercise. Butorphanol and other opiates should also be used with care for the management of eye pain.

Drug Rules

- In cases where the emergency condition may *not* prevent the horse from racing within the next week, or when long-acting drugs such as corticosteroids are considered, it is important to factor in drug withdrawal times and advise the owner and trainer accordingly.

Musculoskeletal Injuries

- Table 44-1 lists the more common causes of acute lameness in the racing athlete and Table 44-2 lists the most common musculoskeletal injuries by racing breed.
- Most musculoskeletal injuries in racehorses occur during racing or training.
- Because of the influence of exercise-induced catecholamine release, these patients typically are agitated beyond that caused by the pain of the injury. Therefore, the first step is to calm the patient sufficiently to prevent further

Table 44-1	Common Causes of Acute Lameness in the Racing Athlete Requiring Emergency Treatment by Anatomic Structure
Condition	**Comments**
Bone	
Fracture—complete	Potentially catastrophic
Fracture—incomplete/stress	Easily missed; may become catastrophic if allowed to propagate to a complete fracture
Fracture—articular	Chip, slab, other configurations of relatively small osteochondral fragments
Fracture—avulsion	May be intraarticular or extraarticular
Joint	
Synovitis/capsulitis	When severe, usually accompanied by capsular tear, hemarthrosis, fracture, or other intraarticular lesion
Hemarthrosis	May be spontaneous and the only finding on examination
Sepsis	Secondary to intraarticular injection or penetrating wound
Periarticular desmitis/desmopathy	Desmitis, rupture, or avulsion of periarticular ligaments such as collateral ligaments and patellar ligaments
Intraarticular desmitis/desmopathy	For example, intracarpal ligaments, cranial +/– caudal cruciate ligaments of the stifle
Luxation/subluxation	Usually secondary to periarticular desmopathy
Cartilage or meniscal injury	Cracks, flaps, or tears in these intraarticular soft tissues can cause acute joint pain
Tendon/Ligament	
Tendonitis of the superficial or deep digital flexor (SDFT and DDFT, respectively)	Degree of lameness is highly variable, but because it is a potentially career-ending injury, tendonitis still requires emergency care
Desmitis of the suspensory ligament	Lesions may occur at the origin, body, or branch(es), and may involve an avulsion fracture at the origin or insertion
Desmitis of an accessory ligament	For example, accessory ligament of the SDFT (proximal or superior check ligament), DDFT (distal or inferior check ligament), annular ligaments of the fetlock or digit, navicular suspensory ligaments, impar ligament
Desmitis of the distal sesamoidean ligaments	May be accompanied by avulsion fracture
Traumatic disruption of the suspensory apparatus	May involve bilateral sesamoid fracture, avulsion or rupture of the branches or body of the suspensory ligament or the distal sesamoidean ligaments, or rupture of the SDFT
Tenosynovitis	Effusion, hemorrhage, fibrosis, or sepsis within the common digital tendon sheath
Tendon rupture	Chronic tendonitis may result in sudden rupture of a flexor tendon, usually at the musculotendinous junction or at its insertion
Muscle	
Exertional rhabdomyolysis	"Tying up," when severe, may make the horse unwilling or unable to walk
Tear	Tearing of the muscle tissue, overlying fascia, or tendon of origin or insertion may occur from external trauma or from a slip or fall that causes overextension
Abscess	Injection-site abscesses can cause acute, severe lameness
Clostridial myonecrosis	Most often secondary to an IM injection, this septic condition is life-threatening
Nerve	
Spinal injury	Occasionally, spinal injury such as a cervical fracture presents as an acute lameness; paresis or paralysis may instead occur distal to the lesion

Continued

Table 44-1 **Common Causes of Acute Lameness in the Racing Athlete Requiring Emergency Treatment by Anatomic Structure—cont'd**

Condition	Comments
Peripheral nerve damage	Bruising, compression, laceration, or avulsion of a peripheral nerve, such as the suprascapular, radial, or peroneal nerve, can cause lameness or gait deficits; brachial plexus injury can cause complete loss of use of that forelimb
Integument/Subcutis	
Wounds	For example, rundown injuries to the flexor tendons or heel bulbs; lacerations over a tendon or joint require emergency care; deep puncture wounds to the solar surface of the foot need immediate care
Folliculitis	Bacterial (usually *Staphylococcus* spp.) infection of the skin can cause painful dermatitis
Cellulitis	When severe, the edema that may accompany acute injury can be sufficient to cause lameness; bacterial cellulitis typically causes severe edema and lameness
Foot abscess	Submural or subsolar abscess may cause acute, severe lameness that causes the horse to be "fracture lame"
Sole bruise, other foot bruising	Submural or subsolar bruising or hematoma may cause acute, severe lameness; deep bruising of the heel bulbs as a result of rundown injury can cause lameness
Laminitis	Acute laminitis can be a life-threatening condition and requires immediate care

Table 44-2   **Common Causes of Acute Lameness in the Racing Athlete Requiring Emergency Treatment by Racing Discipline**

	Thoroughbred	Standardbred	Quarter Horse	Arabian
Bone	Dorsal MCIII disease; condylar fx of MCIII and MTIII; proximal sesamoid fx; proximal phalanx fx; carpal slab fx; humeral or tibial stress fx	Condylar fx of MCIII and MTIII; proximal sesamoid fx; splint bone fx; tarsal slab fx; proximal phalanx fracture; carpal slab fracture, P3 fx	Dorsal MCIII disease/ stress-related bone injury (SRBI); tibial stress fx; osteochondral fragmentation of carpus	Dorsal MCIII disease (SRBI); osteochondral fragmentation of carpus (emergency treatment for carpal chips?); humeral or tibial stress fx
Joint	MCPJ associated with condylar fx; medial femorotibial joint; C-3 slab fx of carpus	Synovitis of carpal joint; T-3 slab fx of tarsus	Synovitis of carpal joint	Tarsocrural osteochondrosis (OCD)
Tendon	Tendonitis of SDFT	Tendonitis of SDFT	Tendonitis of SDFT	Tendonitis of SDFT
Ligament	Suspensory desmitis—branch or body of; traumatic disruption of the suspensory apparatus (TDSA)	Suspensory desmitis	Proximal suspensory desmitis	Proximal suspensory desmitis
Muscle	Recurrent exertional rhabdomyolysis (RER)	RER	RER	RER; back pain associated with hind end lameness
Foot	Abscess; bruising; P3 extensor process fx; underrun heels—risk factor for suspensory injury	Abscess; bruises	Abscess; bruising; underrun heels—risk factor for suspensory injury	Abscess; bruising

fx, Fracture; *MCIII,* third metacarpal; *MTIII,* third metatarsal; *MCPJ,* metacarpophalangeal joint; *OCD,* osteochondrosis; *SDFT,* superficial digital flexor tendon.

injury and to allow proper examination and treatment, which may require the patient be transported to an equine hospital for surgical treatment. The management of specific orthopedic emergencies is discussed in detail in Chapter 21, p. 314.

●》 WHAT TO DO

Musculoskeletal Injuries

Calm or Restrain the Patient

- Depending on the individual horse and the circumstances, the following methods of calming and restraining the patient may be used:

- Physical restraint by experienced personnel who know the horse
- Nose chain, lip chain, or stallion bit
- Nose twitch or skinfold grip (neck "twitch")
- Placing the horse in a quiet, dark stall *if the horse can be safely moved*
- IV sedation and analgesia (see p. 713)
- When selecting a sedation protocol, avoid dosages that are likely to cause ataxia or profound sedation.
- Although the patient is very excited, begin at the lower end of the dosage range and incrementally increase the dose as needed.
- Ataxia increases the risk of further injury and makes loading and transporting the horse to an equine hospital more difficult and hazardous, as can deep sedation.

- A safe and useful protocol is a combination of an alpha$_2$-agonist and butorphanol. The choice of alpha$_2$-agonist is made according to the duration of sedation required, with xylazine having the shortest effect (15 to 20 min) and detomidine the longest (50 to 60 min).
- Intravenous administration of a NSAID, such as phenylbutazone, is advisable at time of initial stabilization for pain relief.

Hemostasis If Needed

- If the injury involves an open wound that is bleeding, apply firm pressure over the wound or vessel until the bleeding stops.
- If a large vessel is lacerated, apply a tourniquet or direct pressure over the course of the vessel proximal to the wound and carefully explore the wound.
- If the lacerated vessel is identified, ligate it; if not possible, apply a firm pressure bandage over the wound before releasing the tourniquet.
- *Do not* leave the tourniquet on for longer than 30 minutes.

Perform a Physical Examination

- Although the injury may be obvious, perform a rapid and thorough physical examination to check for other injuries and for systemic problems, especially if the injury occurred during intense exercise.
- Cardiac or respiratory distress, dehydration, and hyperthermia may influence the choice or dose of drugs used in these patients; and in some cases treatment of the systemic disturbance may be indicated (e.g., IV fluid therapy; see Chapter 32, p. 565).
- If the horse is recumbent and unable to rise, consider a spinal cord injury and perform a limited neurologic examination (see Chapter 22, p. 341).
- If neurologic deficits are present and the horse is still on the track, then arrange to have the patient carefully moved from the track for further evaluation and limit movement of the spine in the process.
- The head should remain elevated if there is a suspicion of head trauma.
- If anesthesia is required to move the horse, ventilation should be carefully monitored, an endotracheal tube passed, and ventilatory support provided using an Ambu bag and oxygen.

Treatment or Humane Destruction?

- Depending on the severity of the injury, it may be necessary to make an immediate decision between treatment and euthanasia.
- In this high-pressure situation, where the owner or agent may *not* be present and the public and media may be observing, the guiding principle must be one of "animal welfare": is it humane to keep the horse alive?
- Because this is a life-or-death decision, it is especially important to perform a comprehensive examination of the patient and the injury. Euthanasia should be *considered* in the following circumstances:
  - If survival is unlikely—the injury is so severe that the horse probably *cannot* survive to treatment.
  - If permanent and severe debility is likely—the injury is so severe that recovery is likely to be long, painful, and incomplete, such that the horse will not even be pasture sound.
  - If complications are likely—the risk for complications is high and those complications would adversely impact survival or long-term comfort.

- If effective pain management is unlikely—the injury is so severe that it is difficult to effectively manage the horse's pain during treatment and recovery.
  - If severe spinal cord or brain damage has occurred.
- Euthanasia options and techniques are discussed in Chapter 48, p. 746.
- *Note:* The presence of the public may guide the best method as much as any other factor.

Stabilize the Injury

- Assuming that the decision is made for treatment, the injury must be stabilized to prevent further damage and pain caused by movement (see Fig. 44-1).
- Immediate stabilization also limits swelling and tissue injury that may compromise blood flow to the region and distal to the injury.
- This aspect of emergency care for racing injuries is particularly important with traumatic disruption of the suspensory apparatus, i.e., a "breakdown" injury, whether from suspensory damage, distal sesamoidean ligament avulsion, or bilateral sesamoid fractures.
- Unless the fetlock is stabilized in such a way as to align the dorsal cortices of the lower limb (i.e., walking on the toe or use of a Kimzey splint), the digital ischemia that may occur when the fetlock sinks can cause an otherwise successful surgical procedure to fail (see Fig. 44-1).
- Wrapping the lower limb with a Robert Jones type bandage with/without an underlying Gel-Cast[2] also helps by limiting swelling that may occlude blood flow through the palmar digital arteries and veins.
- Emergency care and splinting for specific orthopedic injuries is covered in Chapter 21, p. 319.
- *Practice Tip: If fetlock arthrodesis is planned, starting the equine patient on low-molecular-weight heparin,[3] 50 to 100 U/kg SQ q24h, and clopidogrel,[4] 2 mg/kg PO q24h, is recommended to inhibit platelet aggregation.*
- If the injury involves a break in the skin (an open fracture or a "rundown" injury to the flexor tendons), carefully clean gross contamination, minimizing further contamination of the wound. Cover the wound with a sterile, nonadherent dressing and postpone further exploration and treatment of the wound until the horse reaches a surgical facility.
  - Begin broad-spectrum antimicrobial therapy, such as a Beta-lactam (penicillin/cephalosporin) and aminoglycoside combination.
- Send a written record of all medications given—including dosage, route, and time of administration—with the horse to the surgical facility.

Less Severe Injuries

- Many musculoskeletal injuries sustained during racing or race training and causing sudden onset of lameness *do not* require immediate hospitalization for surgical treatment.

---

[2]Jorgensen Laboratorie, Loveland, CO 80538. www.jorvet.com.
[3]Dalteparin/Fragmin (Pfizer Inc., New York, New York).
[4]Plavix (Sanofi Aventis, Paris, France).

- The outcome for return to racing soundness may be improved by prompt and appropriate emergency treatment.
- Such conditions include:
  - Tendonitis of the superficial or deep digital flexor tendon
  - Desmitis of the suspensory origin, body, or branches
  - Synovitis of a high-motion joint (carpus, tarsus, fetlock)
  - Small, intraarticular (chip) fractures
- Emergency treatment should include the following:
  - Stall rest until the injury is fully assessed
  - NSAID therapy (phenylbutazone or firocoxib)
  - Cold therapy (cold pack, ice boot, GameReady[5] cryotherapy boot)
  - Firm, well-padded bandage as appropriate for injuries distal to the carpus/tarsus
  - Corticosteroids may be appropriate for some of these injuries; it is generally best to wait until the injury has been fully evaluated with radiographs, ultrasonography, or other diagnostic imaging tools.

Core Lesions

- Healing of anechoic lesions within the central matrix of the flexor tendons or suspensory branches may be facilitated by draining the blood or serum from these core lesions in the first 24 to 48 hours after injury. This procedure, "tendon splitting," involves making multiple small fenestrations through the tendon or ligament to the core lesion using a scalpel blade or needle and is aseptically performed in the standing horse under sedation and local anesthesia.
- Tendon "splitting" should be delayed until ultrasonographic examination confirms a core lesion; this surgical procedure requires ultrasonographic guidance for best results.
- This older procedure is being replaced by newer regenerative therapies:
  - Platelet-rich plasma (PRP)—growth factors
  - Autologous cells—mesenchymal stem cells

Stress Fractures

- The presentation for a stress fracture in a racing athlete can be variable. There may be an acute, severe lameness after exercise, with little or *no* other signs of injury, or the horse may present with a chronic low-grade lameness that becomes more pronounced with exercise and responds to rest.
- Examination may reveal pain on digital pressure directly over the fracture site.
- Some soft tissue and joint injuries may initially present with little or no swelling, heat, or other signs of inflammation.
- ***Practice Tip:*** *All acute lameness cases should be treated as a possible fracture, and a stress fracture in particular, until ruled out.*

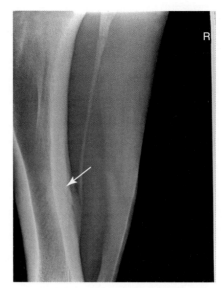

Figure 44-2   Digital radiograph of a healing tibial stress fracture *(arrow)* in a Thoroughbred racehorse. Increased radiopharmaceutical uptake was localized to the proximal tibia on nuclear scintigraphy.

- Initial treatment includes strict stall rest for suspected stress fractures below the carpus or tarsus and a firm support bandage.
- ***Practice Tip:*** *When a stress fracture proximal to the carpus/tarsus is suspected, such as in the tibia (Fig. 44-2), radius, humerus, or femur, it is recommended to cross-tie the patient to prevent the horse from lying down until further assessment is made, which may involve repeat radiography and/or nuclear scintigraphy.*
- NSAIDs are indicated for pain management in severe cases, but the importance of controlling the horse's activity *cannot* be overemphasized.
- There is the potential risk of these stress fractures becoming complete, comminuted fractures if the horse is permitted *unrestricted* activity.

◉› WHAT TO DO

Trauma to the Head and Neck

- In this emergency situation, a short-acting corticosteroid such as dexamethasone, 0.1 to 0.2 mg/kg IV, or Solu-Delta Cortef (prednisolone sodium succinate), 2 to 10 mg/kg q6h, is given and the horse is either allowed to remain quiet or is carefully moved to a safer location for further assessment.
- Emergency treatment for horses with early signs of neurologic dysfunction should include a short-acting corticosteroid such as dexamethasone, 0.1 to 0.2 mg/kg IV, or prednisolone sodium succinate,[6] 2 to 10 mg/kg IV. Additional treatments are dictated by the findings of diagnostic imaging (see Chapter 22, p. 367).
- Emergency treatment should include anti-inflammatory therapy, and application of an ice pack can help reduce periocular swelling.
- Intravenous NSAIDs, such as flunixin meglumine, are preferable to corticosteroids until a thorough ocular examination has been performed by an ophthalmologist.

---

[5]Game Ready Equine (Cool Systems, Concord, California).

[6]Solu-Delta Cortef (Pfizer, www.pfizer.com).

- *No* ointments or other ocular medications should be applied to the cornea until the eye has been thoroughly examined and stained for evidence of corneal epithelial damage.

Skull Fractures

- Skull fractures occasionally occur as a result of high-speed collisions, falls, or from flipping over when the horse rears or pulls back, loses its balance, and falls over backwards.
- Because of the shape of the horse's skull, the brain is located dorsally and is well protected; therefore brain injury is relatively uncommon in cases of head trauma.
- Most commonly, damage is to the paranasal sinuses, the bony orbit, the nasal bones, or the mandible. Examination and treatment are as described in Chapter 21, p. 324.
- More insidious than these facial fractures are those involving the base of the skull.
- Basilar skull fractures can cause serious neurologic and even vascular damage and are potentially fatal with few outward signs of injury.
- A thorough neurologic examination, focusing on the cranial nerves (see Chapter 22, p. 364), is indicated with all head injuries in the racing athlete.
- Loss of consciousness is a BAD sign, even if temporary, as is the inability to rise.

Spinal Injuries

- Because of the amount of force sustained during a high-speed fall or collision, the cervical spine may be injured along with, or instead of, the skull.
- The resulting degree of neurologic deficit depends on the severity of damage to the spinal cord or swelling within the spinal canal (e.g., hemorrhage).
- Death may result from respiratory paralysis with severe proximal cord damage, a complete vertebral luxation, or fracture.
- More often, the equine patient is conscious but down and unable to rise.
- In the first 30 minutes after such an injury it can be difficult to distinguish between "spinal shock," which is a temporary deficit in neural transmission, and permanent spinal cord damage.

●❯ WHAT TO DO

Sucking Chest Wounds

- Injury to the chest wall or thoracic inlet with penetration of the pleural cavity must immediately be closed to minimize the development of pneumothorax.

Wound Closure

- Suture the wound closed, including at least one layer of muscle and the skin, to create a temporary airtight seal.
- Exploration of the wound, lavage and drainage of the pleural cavity, and proper wound closure can be performed once the patient is stabilized and transported to an equine hospital.
- If suture material is *not* readily available, immediately cover the wound with a gloved hand, to prevent further aspiration of air into the pleural cavity.

- Filling the wound with an antiseptic cream is a helpful emergency measure to provide a seal and then cover the wound with a sterile or clean dressing.
- Use multiple rolls of Elastikon,[7] wrapped circumferentially around the horse's chest, or a surcingle to hold the dressing in place and maintain an airtight seal until the horse reaches the hospital.

Pneumothorax

- If signs of respiratory distress occur and lung sounds are difficult to hear or absent on auscultation, a pneumothorax is likely present. Seal the wound and aspirate as much air from the pleural space as possible to allow the lungs to reinflate using a 14-gauge needle attached to a 30- or 60-mL syringe (see Chapter 46, p. 730).
- ***Practice Tip:*** *To avoid puncturing the heart, great vessels, or lungs, insert the needle in the dorsolateral aspect of the eleventh or twelfth intercostal space.*
- A 3-way stopcock between the needle and syringe makes this procedure easier to perform.

Penetrating Abdominal Wounds

- Wounds of the abdominal wall that expose or allow eventration of omentum or gut should immediately be covered with a sterile dressing or closed with stay sutures until the horse can be safely transported to an equine hospital for complete evaluation and primary wound closure.
- If necessary, make a belly band using Elastikon or a surcingle to keep the dressing in place during transport.

Thoracic or Abdominal Injuries

- Penetrating injuries to the chest or abdomen are *uncommon* but can occur in racing athletes because they typically are caused by a fall or collision at high speed.
- The most common offending objects are broken guardrails, hurdles, or sulky shafts (i.e., metal or wood).
- Managing these injuries is similar to that discussed earlier for musculoskeletal injuries; however, some additional aspects are unique to the chest and abdomen. A comprehensive presentation of chest and abdominal wounds is in Chapter 46, p. 728.
- Because the mediastinum in most adult horses is incomplete, a large or unattended penetrating chest wound may result in pneumothorax and cause severe respiratory distress.

Ocular Emergencies

- Ocular and periocular injuries are relatively common in racehorses.
- Careful examination of the bony orbit and the globe itself is indicated with any trauma to the eye region.
- Examination and treatment of eye conditions are covered in Chapter 23, p. 387.
- Injuries in racing athletes are most often caused by:
  - Blunt-force trauma
  - Being struck in the eye by a whip
  - Flying debris

---

[7]Elastikon (Johnson and Johnson Medical, New Brunswick, NJ 08933. www.jnj.com).

Cardiopulmonary Distress

- Tachycardia and tachypnea are expected immediately and for several minutes after the conclusion of intense exercise.
- Neither should persist in a well-conditioned (i.e., fit) horse in the absence of disease, and neither should be accompanied by physical or behavioral signs of distress.

Cardiac Dysrhythmias and Murmurs

- Cardiac dysrhythmias are relatively *common* during intense exercise in racing athletes, generally transient, apparently asymptomatic (except atrial fibrillation), and disappear once exercise ceases (see Chapter 17, p. 124).
- *Practice Tip: Dysrhythmias that persist beyond the end of exercise and are accompanied by persistent tachycardia and signs of discomfort or distress are indications of a potentially serious electrical disturbance.*
- Heart murmurs are also relatively common and *not* always significant in racing athletes.
- Murmurs that persist after the end of exercise and are associated with persistent tachycardia and signs of discomfort or distress generally indicate a serious structural problem.
- *Practice Tip: Aortic chordae tendineae rupture may also be accompanied by acute respiratory distress, cough, moist rales, and frothy fluid at the nostrils (pulmonary edema). Rupture of the chordae tendineae often causes a "honking" sound on heart auscultation.*

●> WHAT TO DO

Cardiopulmonary Distress
Emergency Treatment
- In all cases of cardiac distress, carefully move the horse to a quiet stall and allow 5 to 10 minutes for the horse to relax before reassessing.
- Even if the dysrhythmia or murmur persists, as long as the patient is calm and signs of cardiac or respiratory distress have abated, then nothing more is needed at that time.
- Electrocardiography and/or echocardiography can be performed later to clarify the problem and direct treatment. See Chapter 17, p. 124, for additional information on emergency equine cardiology.
- If the patient remains agitated, then administer "light" sedation with an alpha$_2$-agonist (e.g., xylazine, 0.2 to 0.5 mg/kg IV, or diazepam, 0.05 to 0.1 mg/kg IV). The addition of butorphanol, 0.02 to 0.04 mg/kg IV, is worth adding if the horse remains uncomfortable.
- Signs of pulmonary edema are immediately treated with furosemide, 0.5 to 1 mg/kg IV. Avoid overhydration if administering fluids to correct dehydration.
- As soon as practical, transport the patient to an equine hospital for further workup, monitoring, and supplemental oxygen therapy.

Exercise-Induced Pulmonary Hemorrhage (EIPH)
- Although exercise-induced pulmonary hemorrhage (EIPH) is *common* in Thoroughbred racehorses, seldom does it present as a "true" emergency requiring further treatment other than quiet stall rest.

- Aspiration of blood into unaffected parts of the lung may cause temporary respiratory distress or agitation, but bleeding generally stops once the heart rate decreases and exercise-associated hypertension resolves.

●> WHAT TO DO

Exercise-Induced Pulmonary Hemorrhage
Emergency Treatment
- If the horse does *not* relax after a few minutes in the stall, administer "light" sedation, using xylazine or acepromazine at recommended dosages (see p. 713).
- In addition to calming the horse and lowering blood pressure, sedation encourages the horse to lower its head, facilitating blood removal from the lower airway.
- Once the horse has cooled down and recovered from sedation, provide food and water at ground level to encourage clearance of blood and secretions from the lower airways.
- After the race, administration of furosemide is likely to be helpful *only* if there is evidence of pulmonary edema, such as:
  - Persistent tachypnea with respiratory distress
  - Cough
  - Moist rales
  - Frothy fluid at the nostrils
- *Practice Tip: During an episode of epistaxis, the presence of bloody froth at the nostrils is not, on its own, evidence of pulmonary edema.*
- However, if furosemide is given before the race to prevent EIPH, it should *not* be repeated within 6 hours of the first dose. Flunixin meglumine, aminocaproic acid, clenbuterol, and various other drugs have been used after racing for severe EIPH, but evidence of their efficacy is limited.
- Antibiotic prophylaxis is recommended in moderate to severe cases of EIPH to safeguard against abscess formation at the site of bleeding.
- Sudden death from severe EIPH has been reported, although it is extremely *uncommon*.
- These deaths are impossible to predict because there may be relatively little blood at the nares. Move the horse in respiratory distress to a quiet stall, limit further activity in and around the stall, and lower the horse's blood pressure with xylazine or acepromazine; this may do more to prevent this *uncommon* occurrence than more involved means of investigation and treatment.

Upper Airway Obstruction
- Dynamic or intermittent upper airway obstruction is relatively *common* in racing athletes, because it has several possible causes including:
  - Laryngeal paresis/paralysis
  - Arytenoid chondritis (Fig. 44-3)
  - Epiglottic dysplasia or entrapment
  - Dorsal displacement of the soft palate
  - Axial deviation of the aryepiglottic folds
  - Pharyngeal collapse
  - Epiglottitis (Fig. 44-4)
- Typically, improved breathing is restored once exercise stops, so these conditions *do not* present as an emergency. The *exception* is a severe case of arytenoid chondritis in distress after exercise (see Fig. 44-3).
- Static or persistent upper airway obstruction, in comparison, is *uncommon* and when it does occur, it can present

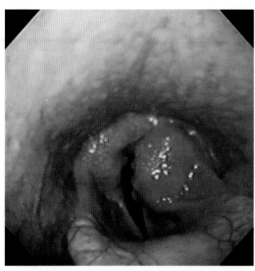

Figure 44-3 Severe left arytenoid chondritis causing exercise intolerance and respiratory distress.

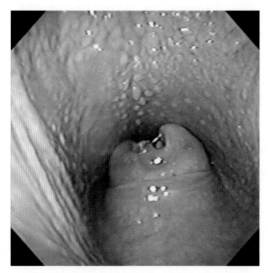

Figure 44-4 Acute epiglottitis. The chief complaint was making an upper airway noise and exercise intolerance. Endoscopic examination revealed a large soft tissue mass beneath the epiglottis.

as a true emergency requiring an emergency tracheostomy (see Chapter 25, p. 456).

- Causes of static or persistent upper airway obstruction include:
  - Arytenoid chondritis or chondropathy is the most common cause (see Fig. 44-3).
  - Subepiglottal abscessation (Fig. 44-5)
  - Trauma to the ventrum of the neck causing tracheal compression or collapse
  - Choke, or esophageal obstruction, is a less common cause (see Chapter 18, p. 177).

◉〉 WHAT TO DO

Emergency Tracheostomy
- If the horse is showing signs of respiratory distress at rest, accompanied by respiratory stridor, then tracheostomy should be considered (see Chapter 25, p. 456).

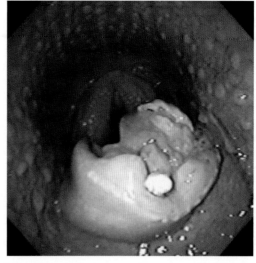

Figure 44-5 Subepiglottic abscess causing an upper respiratory tract noise and exercise intolerance.

- It is important to differentiate between upper and lower airway causes of respiratory distress.
- *Practice Tip: Performing a tracheostomy does* not *improve airflow if the cause of the respiratory distress is the lower airway.*
- Helpful information to make a decision on whether to perform a tracheostomy in a racing athlete may be obtained from the following:
  - History
  - Palpation and auscultation of the throat and neck
  - Thoracic auscultation
  - Endoscopy of the upper airway; endoscopy is definitive for an upper airway obstruction.
  - *Caution:* Use sedation judiciously and only if needed in cases for upper airway endoscopy, to avoid exacerbating the obstruction.

Metabolic Emergencies
Heat Stroke

Important: Heat stroke is a true medical emergency in any equine athlete.

◉〉 WHAT TO DO

Heat Stroke
- The hyperthermic horse must be cooled as quickly as possible:
  - Cold water hosing, sponging, or alcohol bath
  - Airflow: Electric fans and natural breeze over the body lower the core temperature faster than either electric fans or moving air alone, using the principle of radiant and evaporative cooling.
  - Air-conditioned stall: ***Practice Tip:*** *Air conditioning is not as effective at rapidly lowering body temperature in horses as it is in humans.*
  - Ice packs over the path of the carotid arteries (jugular groove) lower the temperature of the blood supplying the brain.
- ***Practice Tip:*** *Most important is to lower the horse's core temperature to <102° F (<39° C) as quickly as possible by cooling the entire body.*

Fluid Therapy

- Fluid therapy with chilled or room-temperature fluids is *not* an efficient way of lowering the core temperature in a hyperthermic horse after exercise.
- Intravenous or oral fluid therapy is recommended to correct any fluid and electrolyte deficits associated with sweating and to prevent the nephrotoxic effects of myoglobinuria secondary to hyperthermia.
- *Practice Tip: An IV fluid rate of 1.5 times maintenance (see Chapter 33, p. 573) is a good starting point.*
- Generally a balanced polyionic solution without potassium or bicarbonate is recommended as the initial fluid choice.
- Transient hyperkalemia normally occurs during maximal exercise as potassium ions "temporarily" shift from the intracellular to the extracellular fluid compartment.
- Metabolic acidosis is another hallmark of intense exercise in horses and resolves spontaneously at the end of exercise as accumulated lactate is metabolized.
- Anhidrosis confounds heat stroke (see Chapter 33, p. 574).
- For detailed information on heat stroke, see Chapter 33, p. 573.

Thumps

- Synchronous diaphragmatic flutter, or "thumps," is a condition in which the diaphragm and the flank contract or twitch synchronously with the heartbeat.
- Thumps is less common in racehorses than in endurance horses, where it is more often associated with dehydration, hyperthermia, hypocalcemia, and hypochloremic metabolic alkalosis.
- The frequent use of furosemide in racing athletes may result in fluid and electrolyte disturbances that predispose to thumps when other predisposing conditions are present, e.g., exercising in hot or humid conditions.

●〉 WHAT TO DO

Thumps
Fluid Therapy

- In most cases, thumps abates once the horse is rested and cooled and the fluid and electrolyte shifts associated with intense exercise normalize.
- If the patient is clinically dehydrated, then IV or oral fluid replacement is indicated (see Chapter 33, p. 575).
- Polyionic solutions usually are recommended because sodium, potassium, and chloride are the major ions lost in sweat.
- There is less need for the addition of calcium to rehydration fluids for racehorses with thumps compared with endurance horses.
- When administering calcium borogluconate IV in the absence of laboratory data on the horse's serum ionized calcium concentration, it is best to do the following:
  - Use a conservative dosage, 100 to 200 mL of a 23% calcium borogluconate solution.
  - Dilute the calcium borogluconate 1:4 in isotonic saline or dextrose solution. **Note:** Do *not* add calcium to fluids containing bicarbonate (i.e., lactated Ringer solution).
  - Administer the solution *slowly* IV while monitoring the horse's heart rate and rhythm.
- *Practice Tip: Stop the IV calcium once the diaphragmatic flutter ceases and if an unexpectedly high or low heart rate or dysrhythmia develops. If thumps persists, then resume calcium infusion at a slower rate.*

Exertional Rhabdomyolysis

- Exertional rhabdomyolysis, "tying up," is common in racehorses. When severe, it can present as an emergency because the horse may be unwilling or unable to move, and the associated myoglobinuria may cause acute renal failure.

●〉 WHAT TO DO

Exertional Rhabdomyolysis

- Emergency treatment includes the following:
  - Rest in a stall or small paddock.
  - Analgesics and anxiolytics: Administer an alpha$_2$-agonist (xylazine, romifidine, or detomidine) with or without acepromazine; butorphanol may also be added if needed (see p. 713 for dosages).
  - NSAIDs: Administer IV phenylbutazone or flunixin meglumine; phenylbutazone empirically appears more effective for musculoskeletal pain.
  - IV fluid therapy: Administer isotonic solution at 1.5 times maintenance (see Chapter 32, p. 567) until the urine is clear.
- Muscle relaxants such as diazepam, methocarbamol, phenytoin, and dantrolene are of limited benefit when effective analgesic and anxiolytic therapy is used.
- As soon as the horse is able, short periods of slow hand walking may facilitate faster recovery. Exertional rhabdomyolysis is discussed in Chapter 22, p. 359.

●〉 WHAT NOT TO DO

Exertional Rhabdomyolysis

- Diuretics are contraindicated because IV fluid therapy can safely and effectively induce diuresis without contributing to fluid loss by using a diuretic.
- Corticosteroid use is controversial, although a single dose of a short-acting drug such as dexamethasone, 0.05 to 0.1 mg/kg IV, may *not* be harmful.

Miscellaneous Emergencies
Colic

- Colic is relatively common in racing athletes and is caused by the same factors present in other performance horses with colic.
- Emergency examination and treatment are described in Chapter 18, p. 157.
- Other conditions that may mimic or present as colic in racing athletes include:
  - Pleuropneumonia ("shipping fever")
  - Thoracic or abdominal wall trauma
  - Spinal trauma
  - Myositis (including rhabdomyolysis)
  - Acute laminitis

Clostridial Myonecrosis

- Clostridial myonecrosis in racing athletes most often results from intramuscular injection of a substance/drug such as flunixin meglumine or a repository product such as an oil-based hormone and less often, secondary to a deep, penetrating wound.

- ***Practice Tip:*** *Subcutaneous emphysema, which is the presence of gas underneath the skin, is a cardinal sign of clostridial infection.*
- Sucking wounds (a penetrating wound through which air is drawn in and out) or upper airway lacerations may trap air in the subcutaneous tissues, but seldom do they cause the systemic signs of toxemia that are characteristic of clostridial myonecrosis.

⬤〉 WHAT TO DO

Clostridial Myonecrosis

- Clostridial myonecrosis can be life-threatening and should be treated aggressively because of the potent exotoxins produced by this obligate anaerobe.
- Systemic antimicrobial therapy: Choose a drug with an excellent spectrum of activity for *Clostridium* spp., such as crystalline Na$^+$ or K$^+$ penicillin IV (see Appendix 9, p. 835, for dosages).
- Debridement: Make a skin incision to expose the contaminated muscle tissue to air and debride any necrotic tissue; leave the wound open to drain with daily wound care (see Chapter 35, p. 618).
- IV fluid therapy: Administer balanced polyionic solution at a rate of administration to support cardiovascular requirements.
- Administer analgesics as needed: e.g., intravenous flunixin meglumine.

Bacterial Cellulitis

- Bacterial cellulitis occasionally occurs in racehorses and most often involves a hind limb.
- Affected limbs can be very painful and may present as an emergency.
- Bacterial thrombophlebitis may occur as a result of repeated use of the same jugular vein in racehorses.

⬤〉 WHAT TO DO

Bacterial Cellulitis

- Broad-spectrum antimicrobial therapy is directed against *Staphylococcus* spp. or by specific culture and sensitivity results. *Staphylococcus* spp. are commonly isolated from septic cellulitis around the jugular vein. Enrofloxacin is often used as first-line therapy pending culture and sensitivity results.
- Administer anti-inflammatory therapy: NSAIDs and sometimes corticosteroids.
- In severe cases of limb cellulitis, multiple superficial skin fenestrations of the affected limb can be made with a #15 scalpel blade for

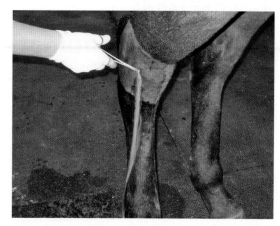

Figure 44-6 Severe hind limb cellulitis treated with multiple stab incisions and drainage of subcutaneous purulent material.

drainage of the exudates and edematous fluid (Fig. 44-6) (see Chapter 35, p. 622). Hot poultices are applied to the affected area several times a day to enhance drainage of septic fluid and/or purulent exudate.

- ***Practice Tip:*** *Laminitis of the contralateral/support limb is an important concern in cases of severe hind limb cellulitis in the Thoroughbred racehorse. If profound lameness is present, rapid resolution is needed and support of the contralateral/support limb is required for laminitis prophylaxis.*
- Mechanical stimulation of lymphatic resorption and outflow: Provide limited hand walking, especially if lameness is severe. Hot compresses and sweats alter the consistency of the exudate and assist in drainage along with bandaging and pneumatic wraps.
- Administer wound care for any primary lesion or secondary breaks in the skin.
- If the jugular vein is compromised because of the cellulitis (i.e., thrombophlebitis), anticoagulants such as aspirin, 0.25 grains/kg PO q48h, and clopidogrel,[8] 2 to 3 mg/kg PO q24h, may be indicated to inhibit platelet aggregation and prevent additional thrombus formation. If one jugular vein is severely compromised, it is imperative to maintain patency of the opposite vein.

References

References can be found on the companion website at www.equine-emergencies.com.

[8]Plavix (Sanofi Aventis, Paris, France).

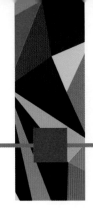

CHAPTER 45

Snake Envenomation

Benjamin R. Buchanan

Introduction

- Venomous snakes fall into two groups:
  - Coral snakes
  - Pit vipers
- Coral snake envenomation has *not* been reported in the horse and it is unlikely to occur.
- There are multiple species of pit vipers in North America including:
  - Several species of Rattlesnakes (*Crotalus* spp.)
  - Copperhead *(Agkistrodon contortrix)*
  - Cottonmouth/Water Moccasin *(Agkistrodon piscivorus)*
- The Cottonmouth, also called a Water Moccasin:
  - Is commonly found in the Eastern United States
  - Can attain a maximum length of 6 feet
  - Is colored a brown olive to grayish black
  - Prefers lowland swamps and areas near water
  - Is named the Cottonmouth from its characteristic white mouth, which it opens when disturbed
- Copperheads:
  - Are commonly found from Massachusetts to Nebraska and Florida to Texas
  - Can attain a maximum length of 4.5 feet
  - Are colored copper to orange-pink with brown/red bands on the back
  - Are found near water on wooded hillsides with rock outcrops and on the edge of swamps
- Rattlesnakes are common across North America in multiple habitats with different geographic areas having specific species.
  - Rattlesnakes vary in length from 15 inches to 8 feet.
  - All have a series of modified scales on the tail that emit a rattle sound when vibrated.
- *Practice Tip: Knowing the species in one's area is important because potency of the venom, clinical signs, and prognosis may vary.*
- Bites have been reported on most areas of the horse's body.
- *Practice Tip: The majority of cases presenting acutely occur on the face and head. Most bites are reported in the summer and many present >12 hours after envenomation.*
- Clinical signs and laboratory abnormalities are dependent on the snake involved and duration of time since envenomation.
- *Practice Tip: Rattlesnake bites are the most severe, with Cottonmouth and Copperhead being less serious (Table 45-1).*

Clinical Signs

Acute

- The initial clinical sign is significant pain and swelling at the bite site with petechiae and ecchymosis or discoloration of the skin, colic, and hemolysis noted in blood samples.
- Clipping the hair in the region of swelling may be helpful in identifying the bite wound.
- Single or multiple, painful, bleeding puncture wounds may be found indicative of a snake bite.
- Severity of clinical signs depends on the species of snake and the location of the bite.
- As local swelling increases, reduced blood flow slows venom uptake.
- Bites to the head can lead to a compromised airway requiring an emergency tracheostomy (Fig. 45-1, *A* and *B*).
- Bites to the body wall allow venom to be absorbed more rapidly. *Important:* Bites to the tongue are equivalent to intravascular dosing.
- *Practice Tip: Hypotension is an early complication of envenomation, along with tachycardia, arrhythmias, reduced borborygmi, dysphagia, epistaxis, and depression.*

Chronic

- The onset of chronic signs may be delayed for several hours.
- Long-term complications include cardiac disease, pneumonia, laminitis, and wound complications including significant tissue necrosis (Fig. 45-2).

Pathophysiology

- The mechanisms and effect of envenomation are dependent on the snake.
- As connective tissue is broken down by hyaluronidase, other components of the venom spread into the surrounding tissues.
- Myotoxins damage skeletal muscle and cardiac tissue.
- Hemorrhagic toxins affect coagulation and may cause hypercoagulation or hypocoagulation, depending on the specific venom.
- Some venoms also cause hyperfibrinogenolysis and "dissolve" clots as they form.
- Metalloproteases induce local pain and tissue necrosis.

Table 45-1	Approximate LD$_{50}$ and Venom Yields of Selected North American Pit Vipers	
Snake	**LD$_{50}$**	**Venom Yield (mg)**
Mojave Rattlesnake	0.23	113
Eastern Diamondback	1.68	590
Western Diamondback	2.18	500
Timber Rattlesnake	2.68	140
Cottonmouth	4.17	130
Copperhead	10.92	60

From Plumlee KE: *Clincal veterinary toxicology,* St Louis, 2003, Mosby, p 108.

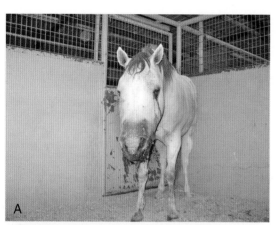

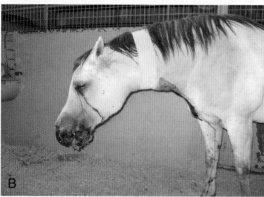

Figure 45-1 **A,** Facial swelling in a Quarter horse after a presumed Rattlesnake bite. **B,** Facial swelling and permanent tracheostomy in a gelding after a suspected Rattlesnake bite. (Photos courtesy of Dr. Will Evans.)

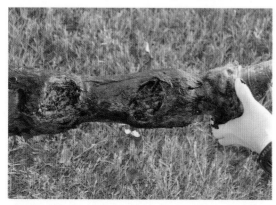

Figure 45-2 Severe necrosis of a distal limb approximately 2 weeks after a suspected snake bite.

- Additional nonenzymatic polypeptides that include potent neurotoxins are present in the venom of the Mojave Rattlesnake.

Diagnosis

- Diagnosis is presumptive and based on clinical signs and laboratory abnormalities.
- Common laboratory abnormalities can include:
  - Thrombocytopenia
  - Leukopenia
  - Neutropenia
  - Hemolytic anemia
  - Prolonged prothrombin time (PT) and partial thromboplastin time (PTT)
  - Hypoproteinemia
  - Hyperlactemia
  - Elevated cardiac troponin I (cTn I)
- Many of the clinicopathologic abnormalities are nonspecific and indicative of significant systemic inflammatory response syndrome (SIRS); coagulation and clotting abnormalities are common with both SIRS and severe envenomation.
- ***Practice Tip:*** *Echinocytes (spiculated RBCs) are reported in peripheral blood smears of nonequine species after pit viper envenomation but* not *in horses. Therefore, clinical signs and nonspecific laboratory changes are relied upon for evidence the horse was bitten by a pit viper.*

Treatment

- General management of envenomation should focus on supportive care and counteraction of the toxin.
- Initial treatment for snake bites to the head centers on maintaining an airway. In acute envenomation with facial swelling, a flexible tube is inserted into the nostrils to maintain the airway although severe nasal necrosis may occur as the swelling progresses. Placement of a temporary tracheostomy is needed in 75% of cases.
- Fluid therapy in the form of crystalloids is used to treat hypovolemia.
- Administration of inotropes and vasopressors is used in cases of refractory hypotension.
- Administration of plasma is useful for treatment of coagulopathies and colloid support.
- Nonsteroidal anti-inflammatories are indicated in almost all cases. Some cases may require additional analgesics.
- Monitoring for renal damage secondary to the envenomation and hypotension is recommended.
- Antibiotics in envenomation are controversial and have *not* shown any benefit in humans.
- Horses appear to be more susceptible to clostridial infections; antimicrobials to prevent clostridial infections and treat secondary tissue damage should be considered.
- Tetanus toxoid should be administered to horses without a recent history of vaccination.
- Antihistamines have *no* direct benefit against snake venom or its effects. Current studies in the horse neither support

EMG

Table 45-2	**Rattlesnake-bite Severity Scoring System for Horses**	
Variable	**Score**	**Signs**
Respiratory	0	Unremarkable
	1	Mild signs of respiratory distress
	2	Tachypnea present and increased work of breathing
	3	Severe respiratory distress with or without cyanosis
Cardiovascular	0	Unremarkable
	1	Mild tachycardia (50-60 beats/min)
	2	Moderate tachycardia (60-80 beats/min) or blood lactate concentration 2.5-4.0 mmol/L
	3	Severe tachycardia (>80 beats/min) or blood lactate concentration >4.0 mmol/L
Wound Appearance	0	No swelling
	1	Mild swelling involving only the nose or distal portion of the limb
	2	Moderate swelling involving the entire head or distal portion of the limb
	3	Severe swelling spreading to the neck or trunk
Hemostasis	0	No abnormalities
	1	PT and PTT higher than reference limits but a >25% increase or <120,000 but >100,000 platelets/µL of blood
	2	PT and PTT >25% but <50% higher than reference limits or <100,000 but >50,000 platelets/µL of blood
	3	PT and PTT >50% but <100% higher than reference limits or <50,000 but >20,000 platelets/µL of blood
	4	PT and PTT >100% higher than reference limits or <20,000 platelets/µL with signs of spontaneous bleeding

PT, Prothrombin time; *PTT,* partial thromboplastin time.
From Fielding CL, Pusterla N, Magdesian KG, Higgins JC, Meier CA: Rattlesnake envenomation in horses: 58 cases (1992-2009), *J Am Vet Med Assoc* 238: 631-635, 2011.

nor refute the use of antihistamines in the treatment of snake bites.

- **Practice Tip:** *Corticosteroids are known to increase mortality in people and should be avoided and reserved for treatment of an allergic reaction to antivenin.*
- The *only* proven treatment against pit viper envenomation is intravenous administration of antivenin.
- **Practice Tip:** *The earlier the antivenin is administered, the better the expected outcome; there is some evidence to support a benefit even when the administration is delayed.*
- A recent retrospective report suggests a reduced mortality with antivenin with *no* reactions in nine horses; however, there are *no* evidence-based studies evaluating the effect of antivenin in equine envenomation.
- A dose for the horse has *not* been established: 1 or 2 vials (10 to 20 mL) of Antivenin (Crotalidae[1]) Polyvalent is commonly administered.
- This dose is substantially lower than the human doses recommended, but studies in the dog have shown significant benefit with much lower dose than that used in humans.
- The high cost of the therapy may limit the use of Antivenin (Crotalidae) Polyvalent. CROFAB is an ovine polyvalent antivenin. Antivenin (Crotalidae) Polyvalent, Wyeth, is a refined and concentrated preparation of serum globulins

obtained by fractionating blood from healthy horses.[2] Crotalid Antivenin-Equine Origins,[3] Crotalus Atrox Toxoid[4] are additional antivenin preparations available for the horse.

●> WHAT TO DO

Snake Bite

- Emergency treatment of snake bites is basic supportive care.
- Obtaining and controlling the airway should be the *first* priority.
- A flexible tube in the nostrils may prevent suffocation from nasal and facial swelling.
- An emergency tracheostomy may be needed (see Chapter 25, p. 456).
- Treatment of hypotension is the *second* objective in emergency treatment of a snake bite.
- Intravenous therapy with crystalloids, colloids, inotropes, and vasopressors may be needed.
- Administration of broad-spectrum antibiotics and nonsteroidal anti-inflammatory drugs is indicated.
  - Antibiotics should include penicillin, metronidazole, and an additional antibiotic for gram-negative coverage.
- Tetanus toxoid should be administered.
- Proper wound care is important for healing (see Chapter 19, p. 241).

[1]Antivenin (Crotalidae) Polyvalent (E. Fougera & Co. and Savage Labs, both divisions of Nycomed US, Inc., Melville, NY 11747).

[2]CROFAB, (Wyeth, part of Pfizer).
[3]Crotalid Antivenin-Equine Origins (Lake Immunogenics, 348 Berg Rd., Ontario, NY 14519; 800-648-9990).
[4]Crotalus Atrox Toxoid (Red Rock Biologic, Woodland, CA; 866-897-7625).

EMG

- Routine laboratory evaluation is recommended to monitor systemic response to the snake bite.
- If the envenomation is believed due to a pit viper, intravenous administration of antivenin is given; the earlier the antivenin is administered the better.
- Horses should be monitored closely for 6 to 24 hours for a delayed reaction after an acute snake bite.
- Circumferential measurements over and adjacent to the area of the swelling allow for monitoring the progression of local swelling.
- Progression of swelling can be used as an indicator of local progression of the envenomation.

WHAT NOT TO DO

Snake Bite

- Many first-aid techniques have been advocated for acute snake bite treatment; however, many have *not* been proven and may be detrimental.
- The use of cold packs, ice, tourniquets, incision and suction, electroshock, and alcohol should be avoided.
- Corticosteroids are known to increase mortality in human studies and should *not* be used in the initial management of an envenomation.

Prognosis

- The prognosis depends on the degree of envenomation, the snake involved, and the duration of time before treatment.
- Mortality from envenomation is 10% to 25% although chronic complications such as laminitis may ultimately lead to humane destruction.
- A Rattlesnake-bite severity score (RBSS) has been proposed for horses (Table 45-2). The RBSS is significantly associated with outcome; a score >8 had a 50% mortality in one published study.

References

References can be found on the companion website at www.equine-emergencies.com.

EMG

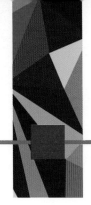

CHAPTER 46

Thoracic Trauma

Rolfe M. Radcliffe

- Thoracic injury in horses is uncommon, but not rare, and may follow blunt or penetrating trauma.
- When it does occur, management of thoracic injury frequently requires rapid treatment decisions to save horses from life-threatening sequelae.
- Such complications include:
  - Pneumothorax
  - Pneumomediastinum
  - Hemothorax
  - Hemorrhagic shock
  - Diaphragmatic hernia
  - Pleuritis
  - Damage to the lungs, heart, blood vessels, or other structures including the abdomen
- *Practice Tip: The primary objective is patient stabilization through triage of cardiovascular and pulmonary compromise and pain management before either medical or surgical treatment.*
- Management decisions should be based on several factors, including location, type, and extent of thoracic injury, anesthetic concerns, and treatment response.

Clinical Signs

- Clinical signs result from damage to internal and/or external thoracic structures.
- Internal damage may include pneumothorax or hemothorax, as well as injury to the lungs, heart, or blood vessels with resultant respiratory distress.
- External injury often involves the chest wall (rib fracture, muscle damage, damage to nerves and blood vessels) with associated pain.
- Shock may be a problem in either case with significant blood loss or respiratory compromise.
- Nostril flaring, dyspnea, tachypnea, marked respiratory effort, and cyanotic mucous membranes are common clinical signs in these patients.
- In horses with pneumothorax, the effort in breathing is increased because of elevated intrathoracic pressure and decreased lung compliance. A characteristic shallow, rapid breathing pattern results in an effort to minimize the work of breathing.
- *Practice Tip: Because the mediastinum is often incomplete in the horse (except when blocked by another inflammatory condition such as pleuropneumonia), pneumothorax can be bilateral and therefore associated with significant respiratory compromise.*

- Damage to intercostal blood vessels; thoracic wall muscles; and the lungs, heart, or other vessels often leads to hemothorax and associated signs of hypovolemic shock and pain.
- Blunt thoracic trauma often results in:
  - Closed pneumothorax
  - Pulmonary contusions
  - Flail chest
  - Other internal organ damage
- Open pneumothorax following penetrating thoracic injury results in:
  - Cardiac tamponade
  - Subcutaneous emphysema
- Besides respiratory and cardiovascular structures, trauma involving the gastrointestinal, neurologic, and musculoskeletal systems may also occur.
- *Practice Tip: Clinicians should have a high index of suspicion for concurrent abdominal injury with deep wounds and those located caudal to the sixth rib.*
  - These horses may present with signs of colic associated with damage or rupture of internal viscera, diaphragmatic hernias, or other organ injury.

●》 WHAT TO DO

Emergency Management of Thoracic Trauma

- Patient stabilization is foremost in effective emergency triage and be the focus during initial evaluation before other management steps.
- Oxygen supplementation is indicated in most cases of respiratory distress for the treatment of hypoxemia ($PaO_2 < 80$ mm Hg). Provide nasal O_2 insufflation at a flow rate of 15 L/min in adult horses. Intratracheal oxygen administration increases the fraction of inspired oxygen and may also help speed the absorption of air from the pleural cavity in cases of pneumothorax.
- *Practice Tip: Five conditions to immediately address in horses:*
  - Pneumothorax
  - Flail chest
  - Hemothorax
  - Hemorrhagic shock
  - Abdominal injury
- Follow emergency triage treatment **ABC** protocol:
  - **A**irway
  - **B**reathing } To restore alveolar ventilation, oxygenation and treat shock
  - **C**irculation
- Control wound hemorrhage if possible, and begin oxygen supplementation, fluid therapy (including blood transfusion if necessary), antibiotics and anti-inflammatory medications.

- Once the patient is stabilized, collect arterial blood from the facial (preferred) or carotid artery to assess ventilation and gas exchange. Normal blood gas parameters in the awake adult horse breathing room air are the following:
  - Arterial pH: 7.4 +/− 0.2
  - $PaCO_2$ (mm Hg): 40 +/− 3
  - PaO_2 (mm Hg): 94 +/− 3
  - Base excess (mEq/L): 0 +/− 1
  - SpO_2 (%): 98 to 99
- *Practice Tip:* Perform pulse oximetry to evaluate the oxygen saturation of hemoglobin and for continued monitoring of oxygenation and ventilation. Based on the oxyhemoglobin saturation curve, an oxygen saturation of <91% corresponds to inadequate arterial oxygen content.
- Administer broad-spectrum antibiotics for horses with open or penetrating thoracic trauma: penicillin potassium, 22,000 to 44,000 IU/kg IV q6h, in combination with gentamicin, 6.6 mg/kg IV q24h, or ceftiofur, 3 to 5 mg/kg IV q12h.
  - If the horse is in severe respiratory distress, enrofloxacin should replace gentamicin since gentamicin has the potential to cause weakness of skeletal muscle (e.g., intercostal muscles).
- Tetanus prophylaxis

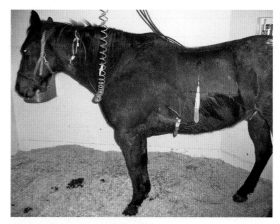

Figure 46-1 An 18-year-old Appaloosa gelding with a history of impaling itself on a fence post in the axillary region of the right forelimb. The horse presented in severe respiratory distress with multiple rib fractures, flail chest, bilateral pneumothorax, and hemothorax. Emergency management included intranasal oxygen administration (15 L/min), removing the pleural air and fluid, and analgesic and fluid therapy. Note placement of the two chest tubes: one for removal of pleural air (caudodorsal), the other for removal of fluid and blood (cranioventral).

Pneumothorax

- Pneumothorax results when a communication occurs between the atmosphere and the pleural space.
- A pressure gradient between the negative pressure of the pleural space and the alveolar or atmospheric pressure forces air into the pleural cavity, collapsing the lung and compromising pulmonary gas exchange.
- In horses, pneumothorax is a reported complication following open or closed thoracic trauma, pleuropneumonia, and surgery of the respiratory tract.
- Three types of pneumothorax are reported:
  - Open
  - Closed
  - Tension pneumothorax
- *Open* pneumothorax occurs when a thoracic wound allows air to pass both into and back out of the chest cavity.
- *Closed* pneumothorax develops when air enters the thorax from within the chest cavity, such as following ruptured bullae in cases of pleuropneumonia or penetrating injury to the lung parenchyma secondary to displaced rib fractures.
- *Tension* pneumothorax, which is an exaggerated form of closed pneumothorax, occurs when air enters but does not leave the chest, such as with a pleurocutaneous fistula acting as a one-way valve.
- Any condition (i.e., damage to the chest wall, airway, or lung) causing a pneumothorax can create a tension pneumothorax; air enters and gets trapped within the pleural space. Pressure builds up in the chest cavity leading to lung collapse, decreased blood return to the heart, and shock.
- Because of steadily increasing intrathoracic pressure that exceeds atmospheric pressure, *rapid* cardiopulmonary

collapse with severe hypoxia and sudden death has been reported with this problem.
- Emergency treatment of pneumothorax is directed at patient stabilization by closure of thoracic wounds and immediate removal of pleural air (Fig. 46-1).
- Lung laceration may occur following displaced rib fractures in horses, leading to closed pneumothorax.
- Bronchial ligation and closure of the damaged lung parenchyma may be performed by suture or staple techniques.
- Horses with axillary wounds require special consideration, even though most of these injuries do *not* initially involve the thoracic cavity.
  - Because these wounds allow for the one-way entrance of air, marked subcutaneous emphysema often develops, with potential migration of air into the mediastinum and eventually the thorax, with a few cases developing pneumothorax.
  - To prevent life-threatening pneumothorax, these horses should be managed by packing the axillary wound, strict stall confinement, and respiratory tract monitoring.
- *Practice Tip:* Auscultation and percussion of the chest wall helps distinguish pneumothorax from hemothorax. In patients with pneumothorax, lung sounds are absent with increased resonance percussed dorsally, whereas reduced lungs sounds ventrally and percussion of a fluid line are typical of hemothorax.
- Palpation of the chest wall and wounds aids in identification of rib fractures and thoracic penetration.
- Thoracic radiography and ultrasonography are useful to confirm chest involvement, including rib fractures, pneumothorax, pneumomediastinum, hemothorax, diaphragmatic hernias, and foreign bodies (Fig. 46-2).

EMG

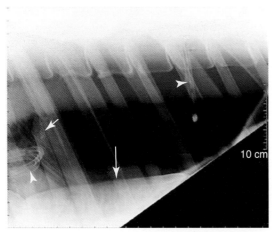

Figure 46-2   Lateral thoracic radiograph of the horse shown in Fig. 46-1 demonstrating bilateral pneumothorax. This is an example of open pneumothorax secondary to a large wound in the right cranioventral thorax. Note the dorsal margin of the left and right collapsed lungs *(large arrow),* the fractured rib *(small arrow),* the placement of a dorsal chest tube *(right arrowhead)* for removal of pleural air and fluid, and an anesthetic soaker catheter *(left arrowhead)* over the fractured ribs of the right hemithorax for pain management.

◉❯ WHAT TO DO

Pneumothorax

- Close and/or bandage chest wounds immediately to reduce the severity of pneumothorax. Seal the chest with temporary wound closure or packing, application of petrolatum dressings, or cover the wound with plastic wrap (Fig. 46-3).
- Immediately after "sealing" the chest cavity, remove pleural air to improve ventilation and oxygenation. Insert a sterile teat cannula, 14-gauge catheter or thoracostomy tube into the dorsal thorax at the eleventh to fifteenth intercostal space. To remove the air, use an extension set, three-way stopcock and 60-mL syringe, or alternatively connect the chest tube to an active suction pump. Place a thoracostomy tube (24F to 36F) ventrally at the seventh to eighth intercostal space for removal of large volumes of pleural fluid or blood (see Fig. 46-1).
- Remove air from the chest cavity slowly, applying a pressure of −20 mm Hg or less to avoid re-expansion pulmonary edema. This

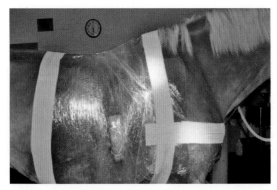

Figure 46-3   A 7-year-old Belgian Draft horse mare following treatment for a severe pleuropneumonia. The horse had an exploratory thoracotomy by rib resection for treatment of localized abcess and adhesion formation. Following surgery, the incisions were left open for drainage, covered with stent bandages, air removed by suction, and the thorax wrapped with cellophane to seal the chest wall. A similar technique to seal the thorax is indicated following penetrating thoracic trauma. (Photo courtesy of Dr. Sally Ness, Cornell University.)

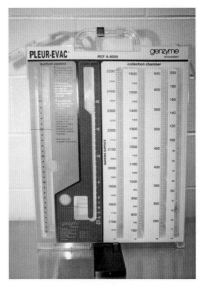

Figure 46-4   Pleur-Evac (Genzyme Biosurgery, Fall River, Mass), a pressure-regulated chest drainage unit designed for the evacuation of air and fluid from the thoracic cavity in humans. Note the three chambers: suction control, water seal, and the collection chamber. The suction control chamber *(blue)* is connected to suction, and the collection chamber *(white)* to the patient. The water seal chamber *(red)* allows air to exit the pleural cavity, and acts as a manometer, reflecting the amount of negative pressure in the patient's chest. (Photo courtesy of Dr. Jan Hawkins, Purdue University.)

complication leads to secondary hypoxemia, hypotension, and reduced cardiac output, and is more likely following pneumothorax of an extended duration and with application of extreme negative pressure.
- If tension pneumothorax is present, immediately convert to an open pneumothorax by opening the wound that is acting as a one-way valve, or placing a teat cannula to allow intrathoracic pressure to return to atmospheric pressure.
- ***Practice Tip:*** *An open pneumothorax is less detrimental than a tension pneumothorax.*
- After removal of pleural air and fluid, attach a Heimlich or other one-way valve to allow continuous exiting flow. Alternatively, continuous-flow chest evacuation may be used via connection to the J-Vac[1] or Pleur-evac[2] vacuum drain systems (Fig. 46-4). Advantages of the Pleur-evac device include a large collection chamber (2500 mL capacity) for evacuation of fluid from the chest cavity, a water seal chamber for the one-way exit of air from the thorax, and the ability to control and monitor the level of suction pressure.
- Pack axillary wounds with saline-soaked roll gauze, recommend strict stall confinement, and monitor closely for respiratory distress. Because such wounds often act as a one-way valve when horses move, marked subcutaneous emphysema frequently develops, possibly leading to pneumomediastinum and pneumothorax.
- Emergency or delayed thoracotomy may be indicated for severe thoracic injury, displaced rib fractures, flail chest, hemothorax, and lung laceration.
- Place overlapping horizontal mattress and simple continuous suture patterns to seal lacerations of the lung margin and central lung parenchyma, respectively, using monofilament, absorbable suture material with swaged-on, atraumatic needles.

[1]Ethicon, Somerville, New Jersey.
[2]Teleflex, Research Triangle Park, North Carolina.

Flail Chest

- Flail chest develops when two or more adjacent ribs are fractured in multiple planes, often secondary to blunt thoracic trauma. ***Practice Tip:*** *This is most common in foals with fractured ribs.*
- An unstable section of chest wall results from the contiguous rib fractures, causing paradoxical respiratory movement.
- Such abnormal movement prevents full expansion of the lungs, quickly leading to severe ventilator compromise and decreased oxygenation.
- Because severe pain limits chest wall excursion following thoracic injury, particularly in patients with rib fracture, analgesia is an important goal of therapy.
  - A combination strategy is best, incorporating systemic and local analgesic techniques.
- Rib fractures may also damage the underlying pulmonary tissue, further impairing ventilation and gas exchange.
- ***Practice Tip:*** *Rib fractures may also lacerate major arteries in the chest.*
- Importantly, the pulmonary contusion and parenchymal injury following blunt chest trauma may be the primary cause of respiratory dysfunction; treatment in human medicine has been redirected toward:
  - Pulmonary physiotherapy
  - Analgesics
  - Selective endotracheal intubation
  - Ventilation
  - Close observation for respiratory decompensation.
- In humans, flail chest is stabilized when there is:
  - The presence of a fixed thoracic impaction: displaced rib fractures directly compressing airway bronchi and/or lung parenchyma
  - Massive chest wall instability
  - During thoracotomy for management of other problems
- Because of the severe injury required to create a flail chest in adult horses, underlying pulmonary and other thoracic damage is likely, and similar to human management, initial patient stabilization is the priority.
- With severe thoracic injury in horses, an emergency or delayed exploratory thoracotomy may be indicated to restore normal ventilatory function associated with a large flail segment and for the treatment of other injuries.
- Conservative and surgical methods of flail chest stabilization are reported in horses depending on the extent of chest wall damage.
- An external splint may be fabricated in cases of closed thoracic injury with intact soft tissues. The splint may be comprised of a metal or plastic base with vertical aluminum rods for wiring of the unstable rib bones to the plate (Fig. 46-5). Open reduction and internal fixation of the fractured ribs is another viable option.
- Septic pleuritis may be a complication of this technique if the orthopedic wires enter the pleural cavity.
- In cases of extensive thoracic injury, surgical treatment is indicated for control of severe bleeding, repair of lung or

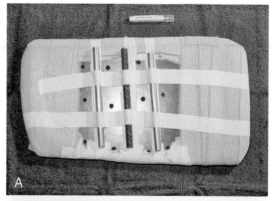
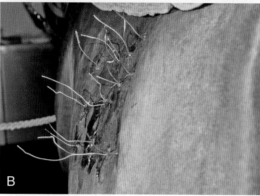

Figure 46-5 An external splint applied to the chest wall of a horse with thoracic trauma for stabilization of flail chest. **A,** The splint (made of a metal or plastic base with vertical rods), extending over adjacent nonfractured ribs, bridges the flail segment and allows anchoring of fractured ribs to the plate. **B,** Wires are placed around or preferably through the ribs. (Photo courtesy of Dr. Norm Ducharme, Cornell University.)

other intrathoracic organ damage, and to accomplish tissue debridement, rib fracture stabilization, and reconstruction of the chest wall.
- When penetrating thoracic injury also involves the abdomen, surgical exploration of the peritoneal cavity may also be indicated.

● WHAT TO DO

Flail Chest

- Stabilize patients with flail chest using analgesics, oxygen supplementation, fluid therapy, blood transfusion if necessary, and wound management.
- Provide analgesia for horses with thoracic wounds, especially with rib fractures, because pain limits chest wall excursion and impairs normal ventilation. Systemic analgesics must be used carefully to avoid compounding respiratory depression.
  - Block the intercostal nerves (caudal to rib) with 0.5% bupivacaine dorsally and for two intercostal spaces cranial and caudal to the thoracic wound.
    - Alternatively a "soaker catheter" may be placed subcutaneously above the injury to allow for regional perfusion of local anesthetics (Fig. 46-6). Any flexible indwelling catheter that is imbedded near the wound or in surgical sites can be used to deliver continuous infusions of local anesthetics.
- In horses with severe thoracic trauma, stabilize large flail chest segments to help restore normal ventilation. Surgical treatment is

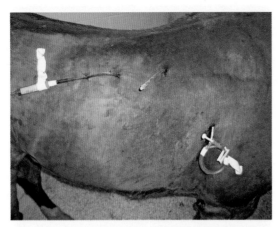

Figure 46-6   Right thorax of the horse shown in Fig. 46-1 demonstrating the use of a "soaker catheter" *(center)* for control of severe pain associated with multiple rib fractures and secondary flail chest. Note also the dorsal thoracic tube for removal of pleural air *(left)*, and an oxygen line *(right)* to help prevent anaerobic infection in the deeper aspect of the wound.

indicated in cases of severe fracture or soft-tissue injury to debride the wound, stabilize rib fractures with orthopedic wire or plates, and reconstruct the chest wall. Place an external splint if necessary for minor damage where the chest wall is intact.

- General anesthesia with positive pressure ventilation is essential in complicated cases because it maintains normal respiratory function with an open chest cavity, allowing for surgical exploration and management.
- ***Practice Tip:*** *Objective guidelines of respiratory failure help determine the need for endotracheal intubation and mechanical ventilation:*
  - Respiratory distress or progressive respiratory fatigue, tachypnea, or bradypnea
  - PaO_2 <60 mm Hg at FiO_2 >0.5 (intranasal oxygen even at 15L/min generally provides an FiO_2 <0.35
  - $PaCO_2$ >55 mm Hg at FiO_2 >0.5
  - PaO_2 to FiO_2 ratio <200
  - Severe head or other injury needing ventilator support

⬤❱ WHAT NOT TO DO

Flail Chest
- *Do not* apply a bandage to patients exhibiting flail chest respiratory movement.
- Bandaging of the thorax causes inward stabilization of the flail segment, secondary pulmonary injury, and additional ventilatory compromise.

⬤❱ WHAT TO DO

Fractured Ribs—Neonatal Foal
- Diagnosis soon after birth based on clinical signs of increased respiratory rate and thoracic cage asymmetry, palpation, and ultrasound examination (see Chapter 14, p. 84).
- Primary treatment—conservative management if no evidence of flail chest, hemothorax, lung contusions, and no fractures displaced toward and overlying the heart.
- Surgical stabilization of the fractures are recommended if any of the above are evident on evaluation.

⬤❱ WHAT NOT TO DO

Fractured Ribs—Neonatal Foal
- Do not overly restrain the newborn foal until fractured ribs are ruled out.
- Remember—fractured ribs are more common in the primiparous mare and with dystocias.
- Don't forget—75% of rib fractures occur on the left side of the thorax just dorsal to the costochondral junction of ribs 3 to 8.

Hemothorax and Hemorrhagic Shock

- Hemorrhagic shock develops with significant blood loss in thoracic trauma patients and may be associated with damage to the heart, and large thoracic, pulmonary, or intercostal vessels.
- Hemothorax usually is the end result and the clinical signs—tachycardia, tachypnea, weak arterial pulses, pale mucous membranes, cold extremities, respiratory distress, trembling, weakness and sweating—are referable to hypovolemic shock.
- Emergency treatment is directed toward restoring intravascular fluid volume, cardiac output, and tissue perfusion. Several different fluids may be used for volume replacement, including polyionic crystalloids, hypertonic saline, whole blood, and colloids such as plasma or hetastarch.
- ***Caution:*** Hypertonic saline should be used cautiously when treating patients with uncontrolled bleeding, and large volumes of hetastarch (20 mL/kg) are contraindicated because of potential coagulopathies.
- The administration of fresh-frozen plasma may be beneficial in replacing lost clotting factors, and aminocaproic acid may help stabilize clot formation by decreasing fibrinolysis.
- Yunnan Baiyao (15 mg/kg PO q12h) may enhance coagulation.
- Whole-blood transfusion is indicated with severe or ongoing hemorrhage and should be based on clinical signs of hypovolemia (i.e., high heart rate, poor pulse quality, pale or white mucous membrane color, cool extremity temperature, depression, and general weakness).
- ***Practice Tip:*** *Packed cell volume is not a useful test in judging the need for whole-blood transfusion in peracute bleeding because significant decreases usually do not occur for 8 to 12 hours after blood loss. Blood lactate, arterial or venous oxygen saturation, and blood pressure are useful in assessing hypovolemia.*
- Approximately 6 to 8 L of blood (30% to 40% of the estimated or calculated blood loss) should be transfused in an adult horse.
- Autotransfusion may also be performed after the sterile collection of blood from a body cavity, providing the bleeding was not associated with neoplasia, sepsis, or other bacterial contamination.
- If the affected horse has labored breathing or other signs of respiratory distress, draining of large volumes of blood and fluid from the pleural cavity may be indicated to

EMG

improve ventilation and perfusion matching and decrease intrapulmonary shunting of blood.

- Do not remove blood from the chest unless it is needed for autotransfusion or the volume of blood is believed to inhibit lung expansion. Leaving the blood in the chest may inhibit bleeding if the bleeding site is below the "blood line." In addition, some of the red blood cells in the thoracic cavity will autotransfuse.
- Thoracic surgery is usually reserved for the control of severe or continued bleeding despite medical therapy.
- Emergency thoracotomy in people is reserved for serious problems:
  - Evacuation of pericardial tamponade
  - Control of massive intrathoracic hemorrhage
  - Air embolism
  - Open cardiac massage
  - Perforation of the main aerodigestive tracts

⏺ WHAT TO DO

Hemothorax and Hemorrhagic Shock

- Immediately begin aggressive intravenous fluid therapy using polyionic crystalloids (20 to 80 mL/kg) over several hours. The goal of treatment should be to maintain slightly low systemic blood pressure to ensure organ perfusion without disrupting blood clots (permissive hypotension). Hypertonic saline (4 mL/kg IV) and equine plasma (2 to 4 L/450 kg) or hetastarch (10 mL/kg) may also be considered for rapid intravascular volume expansion and treatment of low colloid oncotic pressure, respectively (see Chapter 20, p. 284).
- Stop or slow bleeding if possible. With a history of trauma, surgery is indicated if bleeding is severe or continues despite medical therapy. Emergency thoracotomy is supported in horses for management of:
  - Severe hemorrhage
  - Flail chest
  - Repair of significant lung damage
- Perform a whole-blood transfusion when indicated. In peracute cases of bleeding, the goal of treatment is to replace 30% to 40% of the estimated blood lost. *Practice Tip: Heart rate, blood pressure, and mucous membrane color may not change until 30% or more of blood volume is lost. Blood lactate increases with a 20% loss. Blood volume (L) = body weight (BW) (kg) × 0.08.*
- Place a thoracostomy chest tube (based on auscultation, radiography, or ultrasound examination) to remove large accumulations of blood and fluid from the chest to improve ventilation/perfusion matching and when deemed appropriate for autotransfusion. With open thoracic wounds, removing free blood may also help prevent the development of septic pleuritis and adhesions.
- Administer aminocaproic acid (25 to 40 mg/kg mixed in 0.9% saline and given slowly IV every 6 hours) to help stabilize blood clots through its binding and inhibition of plasminogen activation.

Abdominal Injury

- In penetrating thoracic wounds in horses, abdominal or spinal injury occurs concomitant with thoracic trauma in ≈20% of cases.
- Severe injury of the colon (perforation), renal trauma, and spinal luxation can result in humane destruction.

- Abdominal involvement with less severe injury can also occur and these horses have a better prognosis after treatment, particularly when abdominal organs are not injured.
- Injury to the abdominal cavity is more likely following penetrating wounds of the caudal chest in horses, but even cranial thoracic trauma may involve the abdomen because the cupula of the diaphragm extends to the sixth rib during expiration.
- *Practice Tip: Abdominal involvement is possible with any thoracic wound caudal to the sixth rib and other deep penetrating wounds of the thorax, and a comprehensive evaluation of the abdomen is required.*
- Abdominocentesis, ultrasonography, local wound exploration, and laparoscopy or exploratory celiotomy are standard techniques in the diagnosis of abdominal cavity involvement.
- Emergency abdominal surgery may be indicated after patient stabilization for cases where abdominal organ damage is suspected or confirmed.

Diaphgragmatic Hernias

- Diaphragmatic hernias may develop in horses following injury to the thorax or abdomen.
- Trauma, dystocia, and strenuous activity are the most common causes of acquired diaphragmatic hernias in adult horses.
- Clinical signs depend on the size of the defect and abdominal structures displaced.
- Strangulation of the small intestine usually occurs through small defects of the diaphragm resulting in acute severe colic; colonic displacement occurs through large defects leading to pulmonary compression and respiratory dyspnea.
- Successful repair of diaphragmatic hernias have been reported with direct suturing and mesh herniorrhaphy.
- Preoperative diagnosis of herniation through the diaphragm may be difficult; however, thoracic ultrasonography and radiography may be useful, and may reveal:
  - Abdominal organs (such as gas-filled intestine) in the chest cavity
  - An inability to see the diaphragmatic outline
  - Cranial displacement of the diaphragm
- Ultrasound evaluation may provide valuable information on the location and size of the defect, and the type and size of abdominal organs displaced into the thoracic cavity.

⏺ WHAT TO DO

Abdominal Injury

- Evaluate the abdomen of horses having deep penetrating thoracic injury and when wounds are located caudal to the sixth rib.
- Diaphragmatic hernias may occur with either thoracic or abdominal injury. Preoperative diagnosis may be obtained via thoracic ultrasonography or radiography. Image the diaphragm with a 5 +/-MHz transducer; evaluate each intercostal space, beginning ventrally and following adjacent and parallel with the body wall until the diaphragm diverges dorsally and medially behind the lung. Look for

evidence of disruptions of the diaphragm or abdominal visceral within the thoracic cavity.

- Emergency celiotomy is indicated for abdominal organ injury, and for diaphragmatic hernias with strangulating intestinal obstruction, colon, or other organ displacement.

- Although the prognosis for survival is guarded with large diaphragmatic hernias and varies depending on the location of the defect, closure of the defect may be performed with large-gauge suture (#2 polyglactin 910, Vicryl, Ethicon) or mesh repair via a celiotomy, thoracotomy, laparoscopy, and/or thoracoscopy.

Conservative Treatment, Surgery, and Anesthesia for Thoracic Trauma

- Most cases of thoracic injury may be managed successfully with conservative treatment following the primary patient stabilization steps outlined previously.

- Knowing when to refer a patient or when to intervene with emergency thoracotomy or thoracoscopy are important considerations in patient management.

- Generally, conservative management should pertain to horses with:
  - Simple rib fractures
  - Small chest wounds
  - Controlled pneumothorax
  - Hemothorax
  - Patients *without* severe contamination:
    - Rib fractures
    - Lung lacerations
    - Deep penetration

- Surgical intervention is reserved for:
  - More severe injury
  - Improved exploration
  - Lavage of the thoracic and abdominal cavities
  - Control of bleeding
  - Repair of lung laceration or damage
  - Stabilization of multiple or complicated rib fractures and flail chest
  - Appropriate wound closure

- For most horses with severe thoracic injury, simply enlarging the existing traumatic wound provides the best exposure of the ribs, muscles, heart, lungs, diaphragm, and pleura.

- Reported surgical approaches to the equine thorax include lateral thoracotomy either via an intercostal or rib resection technique, and thoracoscopy.

- Anesthetic considerations depend not only on the choice of conservative versus surgical management, but also on other factors including:
  - Patient stability
  - Location

- Type and extent of trauma
- Anesthetic concerns
- Clinician experience
- Response to initial treatment

- General anesthesia should be avoided until after the trauma patient has been stabilized, and standing wound management techniques are preferred over recumbency to avoid further respiratory and cardiovascular compromise.

- Intercostal perineural anesthesia or other local nerve blocks are often sufficient to provide effective analgesia for standing thoracic procedures.

- Care must be taken to avoid tension or bilateral pneumothorax during standing thoracic treatment because these problems are difficult to manage without mechanical ventilation.

- General anesthesia has the advantage in the following circumstances:
  - Controlled positive-pressure ventilation in horses with open pneumothorax
  - Deep penetrating wounds
  - Severe chest wall damage
  - Complicated rib fractures
  - Extensive lung lacerations
  - Foreign bodies
  - Severe contamination requiring aggressive thoracic lavage
  - Hemorrhage
  - Pneumothorax
  - Hypoxemia that persists despite conservative medical treatment

- ***Practice Tip:*** *The basis of emergency management of horses with thoracic trauma is primary patient stabilization through the assessment and support of respiratory and cardiovascular functions.*

Prognosis

- The prognosis for horses suffering from thoracic injury depends on many factors including:
  - Type and severity of thoracic damage
  - Occurrence of secondary complications and sequelae
  - Response to conservative or surgical treatments

- Without extrathoracic injury, or severe complications, horses are reported to have a favorable prognosis for survival.

References

References can be found on the companion website at www.equine-emergencies.com.

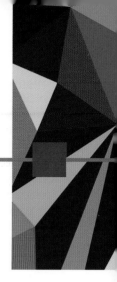

SECTION II Anesthesia

CHAPTER 47

Anesthesia for Out of Hospital Emergencies

Stuart C. Clark-Price

- Emergencies requiring anesthesia away from a hospital setting occur often and require a clinician to be familiar with techniques for rendering a patient unconscious.
- The focus of this chapter is on methods to provide short-term (<45 minutes) general anesthesia when analgesia, unconsciousness, and complete immobility are needed, and inhalant anesthesia is not practical. Standing sedation using constant rate infusion (CRI) is described; however, emergencies requiring only local anesthesia, sedation, and tranquilization are not discussed (see Chapter 49).
- The goal of emergency anesthesia is usually one or more of the following:
  - To enable immediate, definitive treatment to be administered on site (e.g., suture laceration and control of bleeding)
  - To allow life-threatening conditions to be stabilized before and during transportation to a surgical facility (e.g., long-bone fractures)
  - To prevent further injury to the patient and personnel while the patient is evaluated and plans are formulated for treatment
  - To immobilize a patient for safer removal from a hazardous environment (e.g., trailer accident)
- Normal risks associated with general anesthesia are amplified when anesthesia is administered in an emergency away from the hospital. Increased risk may be caused by the following:
  - The compromised condition of the patient
  - Unsatisfactory environment for administering anesthesia, including increased risk of injury to personnel
  - Minimal time for planning
  - Minimal ability to monitor physiologic parameters
- *Practice Tip: Risk and unfavorable outcomes can be reduced by preparing standard emergency anesthetic protocols that are understood by everyone involved and by having necessary materials assembled for easy transportation. "Up front" investment in time and resources results in higher quality emergency care.*

We recognize and appreciate the original contributions in previous editions to this chapter of Ann Townsend and Dr. Robin Gleed.

Basic Emergency Anesthesia Kit

- An emergency anesthesia kit can be preassembled and stored in a clinic or ambulatory vehicle for quick access. The kit should be examined monthly for expired drugs and completeness.
- A large plastic storage box can be used to hold all equipment with a smaller fishing tackle box to hold needles, syringes, and small medication vials placed inside. Equipment for the kit can be divided into required equipment and suggested additional equipment.

Required Equipment

- Three halters (foal, adult, and extra-large sizes)
- Lead ropes
- Two 30-foot ropes (nylon climbing ropes are suggested as these are less likely to break if used to move anesthetized horses, and can also be used as head and tail rope)
- Four endotracheal tubes with functional cuffs (26-, 20-, 14-, and 8-mm internal diameter)
- Sterile surgical lubricant
- Two-inch-long (5-cm) polyvinyl chloride pipe mouth gag (wrapped with porous white tape and inserted between incisor teeth to prevent damage to endotracheal tubes)
- 60-mL syringe to inflate endotracheal tube cuffs
- Tackle box (containing needles, syringes, injection caps, extension sets, IV catheters [10-, 14-, 18-, and 20-gauge], 2-0 nylon suture on a straight needle, white medical tape, 4- × 4-inch gauze, heparinized saline solution, and drugs). Advance labeling of essential syringes minimizes confusion during emergency anesthesia.
- Cordless clippers
- Surgical scrub and isopropyl alcohol
- General surgical pack
- Sterile ophthalmic eye lubricant
- Paper towels
- Large cotton towels
- Blankets (aluminum space blankets take up less space than horse blankets but provide minimal padding)
- IV crystalloid fluids and administration sets

Suggested Additional Equipment

- This equipment should be included in practices that offer emergency ambulance services to specialty or referral hospitals or for clinicians wanting to offer advanced life support.
- Protective padded hoods
- Body slings
- Tracheostomy tubes, 8- to 26-mm inner diameter (ID) with functional cuffs (regular endotracheal tubes can be used for tracheostomies also)
- Equipment necessary to provide ventilatory assistance (Figs. 47-1 and 47-2):
  - Oxygen, medical grade, size E tanks. **Note:** A single E tank holds 660 L of oxygen at 1900 psi.
  - Oxygen regulator—two-stage, downstream pressure set at 60 psi for use with the demand valve
  - Oxygen flow meter
  - Oxygen demand valve
  - Oxygen hose, 20 to 40 feet (6.1 to 12.2 m)
- Multiparameter monitors (i.e., electrocardiogram [ECG], pulse oximeter, and indirect blood pressure capabilities)

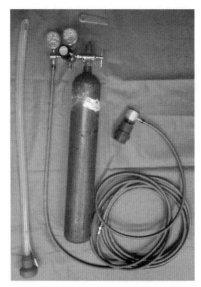

Figure 47-1   Example of equipment needed to provide ventilatory support to horses in the field. Included is an E size cylinder of oxygen, a cylinder key, a two-stage regulator, oxygen hose, a demand valve with an adaptor, and an endotracheal tube.

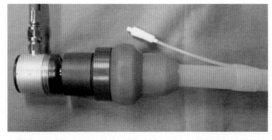

Figure 47-2   Close-up view of a demand valve attached to a large animal endotracheal tube with an adaptor.

- Cable hoist puller, come-along
- Hobbles
- Pole syringe injection system
- Fluid bag pressure infuser
- Extension cord, 100 feet (30.5 m)
- Equine rescue glide for transport of anesthetized or down horses (Large Animal Rescue Glide Equipment, *www.rescueglides.com;* see Chapter 37, p. 638)

Analgesic, Anesthetic, and Restraint Drugs

- Acepromazine, 0.02 to 0.03 mg/kg IV (*do not* exceed 20 mg), is a centrally acting tranquilizer that exerts its effect through dopamine receptor blockade. Use of acepromazine has been associated with improved recoveries from general anesthesia because of its anxiolytic effects. Acepromazine has a long duration of action (>3 hours) and provides no analgesia. Side effects, previously reported, include dose-dependent penile paralysis and a reduction of seizure threshold. Use of acepromazine has been largely replaced by the alpha$_2$-agonists, xylazine, romifidine, and detomidine. Acepromazine can cause profound hypotension because of alpha-receptor blockade in the peripheral vasculature. Use of epinephrine in horses that have received acepromazine can result in "epinephrine reversal" and result in worsening of hypotension from epinephrine action on vascular beta-receptors. **Practice Tip:** *The use of acepromazine in horses with conditions that may be associated with shock, hypotension, or seizure is* not *recommended.*
- Butorphanol, 0.01 to 0.04 mg/kg IV, is an opioid that produces unreliable sedation when used alone. Butorphanol has opioid-agonist and -antagonist properties. Butorphanol can produce excitement or dysphoria when it is the only agent used in some individuals. Butorphanol potentiates the analgesic effects of alpha$_2$-agonist drugs and can be used in conjunction with alpha$_2$-agonist to produce analgesia and chemical restraint (e.g., butorphanol, 0.01 to 0.02 mg/kg, plus xylazine, 0.6 mg/kg IV).
- Detomidine, 5 to 20 µg/kg IV or 20 to 40 µg/kg IM, is an alpha$_2$-agonist that produces reliable sedation and analgesia. Detomidine has a long duration of action (up to 2 hours). Because of the profound cardiovascular depressant effects of detomidine, use it carefully in the care of patients with cardiovascular compromise. **Practice Tip:** *Detomidine and other alpha-agonists may cause aggression after sedation in a small number of horses. Be careful! They may also cause marked, but transient, tachypnea when given to febrile horses.* **Important:** Draft breeds are more dose sensitive to the effects of detomidine than are other horses. Conversely, mules may need larger doses. Donkeys may assume sternal recumbency. Detomidine can be administered as a CRI for prolonged sedation and analgesia for standing procedures (see p. 738).
- Diazepam, 0.1 to 0.2 mg/kg IV, is a sedative frequently administered to promote muscle relaxation with drugs such as ketamine. Diazepam can produce excitement in adults when used on its own. In foals up to 4 weeks of age,

diazepam has sedative effects and can be used as a pre-anesthetic. ***Practice Tip:*** *A primary use of diazepam is to manage seizures.*

- Euthanasia solution. Approved for humane destruction *only*. Because this solution often produces transient motor activity and gasping, it may be advisable to sedate the horse before administering (e.g., with xylazine).
- Guaifenesin, 40 to 100 mg/kg IV to effect, is a centrally acting muscle relaxant used in conjunction with the anesthetic drugs ketamine, thiopental, and propofol to induce and maintain anesthesia. Guaifenesin has no analgesic or anesthetic properties. Overdosage causes ataxia, apnea, and profound muscle relaxation. Guaifenesin usually is administered as a 5% solution. Solutions greater than 10% may result in hemolysis. One-liter vials or IV bags of pre-mixed 5% solutions are available from pharmaceutical companies and compounding pharmacies. Peak effect is reached 10 minutes after administration. Guaifenesin should be administered through an IV catheter. Extravasated guaifenesin is exceptionally irritating to tissues and causes necrosis and sloughing.
- ***Important:*** Mules and donkeys may be more dose sensitive to guaifenesin than are horses.
- Ketamine, 2.2 mg/kg IV, is a dissociative anesthetic and is the most commonly used induction agent in equine anesthesia. Ketamine increases heart rate and overrides the bradycardia caused by xylazine and detomidine tranquilization. Ketamine causes increased cerebral and ocular pressure and may be contraindicated when cerebral and intraocular pressures are a primary concern. Its use in people anesthetized following head trauma has not resulted in an increased mortality compared to other anesthetics. Ketamine may cause excitement and even seizure-like activity if administered without preexisting central nervous system (CNS) depression; therefore, precede administration with a sedative (e.g., xylazine).
- Dexmedetomidine, 5 to 10 µg/kg IV, is an alpha$_2$-agonist that induces more profound sedative and analgesic effects with smaller doses than xylazine, romifidine, or detomidine. As with other alpha$_2$-agonist drugs, use care when using dexmedetomidine in patients with cardiovascular compromise. Used alone as a sedative, dexmedetomidine administration can result in severe ataxia. Dexmedetomidine can be useful when combined with other drugs for total intravenous anesthesia through a CRI (see the following protocol, p. 738). The increased cost associated with the use of dexmedetomidine may preclude its use in some cases.
- Methadone, 0.1 mg/kg IV or IM, is a pure mu-agonist opioid that can be used similarly to butorphanol for analgesia. Methadone is unique in that it also has *N*-methyl-D-aspartate (NMDA) antagonist properties that extend its analgesic properties and thus it may be more appropriate for severe pain such as bone fractures. Similar to other opioid use in horses, methadone may cause excitability and should be administered in conjunction with sedatives such as xylazine or acepromazine.

- Midazolam, 0.1 to 0.2 mg/kg IV, is a benzodiazepine that is similar to diazepam regarding uses and side effects. Unlike diazepam, which is delivered in a propylene glycol base, midazolam is water soluble. Propylene glycol can cause tissue irritation and cardiac dysrhythmias, thus potentially making midazolam the preferred drug in septic, neonatal, or compromised patients. However, the duration of action of midazolam may be shorter.
- Morphine, 0.05 to 0.1 mg/kg IV or IM, is another pure mu-agonist opioid that can be used for pain management. Morphine is known to cause excitatory behavior in horses, particularly in doses >0.1 mg/kg. However, adverse behavior can be limited with the concurrent use of a sedative such as xylazine or acepromazine.
- Propofol, 2 to 4 mg/kg IV, is a nonbarbiturate short-acting anesthesic agent that has been used in horses for induction and maintenance of anesthesia through CRI (see p. 744). Propofol administration can result in depressed ventilation and profound hypotension. Additionally, often large volumes are needed for induction of anesthesia that cannot be delivered at a rate sufficient to prevent excitement and ataxia that are often seen in the adult horse when propofol is used for induction. However, horses that receive guaifenesin (90 mg/kg IV) before induction do not tend to experience excitement and have smooth inductions. ***Important:*** The combined effects of guaifenesin and propofol can profoundly reduce ventilation, and horses induced with this combination should be intubated and have assisted ventilation! The smaller dose volume used to induce anesthesia in foals and weanlings decreases this adverse effect and makes it a satisfactory agent in these patients. ***Practice Tip:*** *Propofol reduces cerebral metabolic oxygen consumption, and had previously believed by some to be the preferred drug for patients with brain injury, seizures, or increased intracranial pressure. It may also decrease cerebral blood flow, which may have an unwanted effect (good or bad) on the patient. The higher cost of propofol and its potentially adverse effect on ventilation may prohibit its use in some cases.*
- Romifidine, 40 to 120 µg/kg IV, is an alpha$_2$-agonist that has preanesthetic and tranquilizing effects similar to those of other alpha$_2$-agonists. Romifidine can be combined with diazepam and ketamine for short-duration intravenous anesthesia. The sedation and analgesia achieved with romifidine are not as good as those achieved with detomidine. However, individuals sedated with romifidine may not drop their head or become as ataxic compared with horses sedated with xylazine or detomidine. This clinical effect could be beneficial when tranquilizing a horse with head or cerebral edema!
- Telazol, 1 to 2 mg/kg IV, is a proprietary 1:1 combination of the dissociative anesthetic, tiletamine and the benzodiazepine, zolazepam. Tiletamine and zolazepam have a longer duration of action than the similar drugs ketamine and diazepam, respectively. Cardiovascular profile and side effects are similar to anesthesia with ketamine and diazepam/midazolam. Recovery is often prolonged

and can be rough. For short-term anesthesia and a smoother recovery, telazol is often not recommended. Combination of low-dose telazol with ketamine and detomidine provides a superior induction and recovery of anesthesia than with telazol alone.

- Thiopental sodium, 4 to 10 mg/kg IV alone, or 3 to 4 mg/ kg IV with 5% guaifenesin, is an ultrashort-acting barbiturate used for rapid induction of anesthesia after bolus administration. Transient apnea often occurs. *Note:* Thiopental is currently not available in many countries.
- *Practice Tip: Use with caution in emergency situations because thiopental sodium depresses ventilation, cardiac output, and systemic blood pressure. Thiopental also can be used at 3 to 4 mg/kg, mixed with guaifenesin or as a bolus after pretreatment with guaifenesin or a benzodiazepine (diazepam or midazolam). As with propofol, thiopental reduces cerebral blood flow and metabolic consumption of oxygen and can be used in neurologic cases in a similar manner to propofol.*
- Xylazine, 0.2 to 1.1 mg/kg IV, is an alpha$_2$-agonist that produces reliable sedation and analgesia. Xylazine also causes bradycardia and reduces cardiac output. Use xylazine with caution in the treatment of patients with cardiovascular compromise. To some extent, the adverse effects of xylazine on the cardiovascular system are ameliorated by ketamine. ***Important:*** Draft breeds are more sensitive to xylazine than are other horses. Mules may need higher dosages than do donkeys or horses.

- Analgesic, anesthetic, sedative, and urgent drugs for an equine emergency kit are categorized in Table 47-1.

Constant Rate Infusion (CRI) Drugs for Anesthesia and Sedation/Analgesia

CRI General Anesthesia

- "Triple Drip": ketamine, alpha$_2$-agonist, and guaifenesin. Dilute 2 g ketamine plus one of the alpha$_2$-agonists in 1 L 5% guaifenesin; administer at a rate of 1 to 3 mL/kg per hour after induction.
- "Double Drip": thiopental (where thiopental is available) and 5% guaifenesin. Dilute 2 g thiopental into 1-L vial of 5% guaifenesin; administer at a rate of 1 to 2 mL/kg per hour after induction.
- **"Alternative Triple Drip":** in 1 L of crystalloid fluids (i.e., lactated Ringer's solution), dilute 2 g ketamine, 100 mg of midazolam, plus one of the alpha$_2$-agonists. Administer at 1 to 3 mL/kg per hour to effect. It is recommended to recover horses that have been anesthetized with this combination in a padded recovery stall or an open area with no obstacles because a small number of these horses are more ataxic when standing than when receiving the formula with guaifenesin.
  - Xylazine, 500 mg
  - Detomidine, 20 mg
  - Romifidine, 50 mg
  - Dexmedetomidine, 1.75 mg
  - *Note:* Guaifenesin may be difficult to obtain in some areas and can be substituted with midazolam in the formula.
- Propofol, 0.2 to 0.4 mg/kg per minute (can be used in combination with ketamine or dexmedetomidine) is another general anesthesia protocol for out of hospital emergencies. There must be the ability to ventilate the patient if propofol is used.

Standing Sedation/Analgesia Protocols

- Detomidine, 8.4 µg/kg IV loading dose, followed by 0.5 µg/kg per minute. This can be accomplished by adding 5 mL of 10 mg/mL detomidine to a 500-mL bag of 0.9% sodium chloride. Using a microdrip fluid set (60 drops/ mL) start with an administration rate of 0.005 drops/kg per second. The rate can then be adjusted as needed to maintain effective sedation.
- Romifidine, 80 µg/kg IV loading dose, followed by 15 to 30 µg/kg per hour.
- Xylazine, 1 mg/kg IV loading dose, followed by 0.65 mg/ kg/hour.
- Dexmedetomidine, 5 µg/kg IV loading dose, followed by 2.0 µg/kg per hour.
- The addition of butorphanol may reduce the amount of the alpha$_2$-agonist necessary and reduce head drooping

Table 47-1	Suggested Analgesic, Anesthetic, Sedative, and Emergency Drugs for an Equine Emergency Kit
Drug Category	**Drug***
Sedative	Xylazine Detomidine Romifidine Acepromazine
Analgesic	Butorphanol (controlled substance)
Muscle Relaxant	Midazolam or diazepam (controlled substance) Guaifenesin (5%)
Induction Agent	Ketamine (controlled substance) Propofol
Intravenous Fluids	Crystalloid (lactated Ringer or other balanced electrolyte solution) Colloid fluid (hetastarch, Vetstarch) Hypertonic saline solution
CPCR Drug	Epinephrine Atropine Lidocaine Vasopressin
Miscellaneous	Euthanasia solution (controlled substance) Flunixin meglumine Dobutamine Atipamezole or yohimbine Prednisolone sodium succinate

*Some of these drugs are controlled substances in many countries and have specific storage requirements.

and ataxia. Butorphanol, 17.8 µg/kg loading dose, followed by 0.38 µg/kg per minute.

Cardio-Pulmonary-Cerebral Resuscitation (CPCR) Drugs and Support Drugs

- Atipamezole, 0.05 to 0.2 mg/kg IV, is a synthetic alpha$_2$-adrenergic antagonist. ***Practice Tip:*** *For all alpha$_2$-antagonists, administer slowly and monitor the effect carefully.* This drug can produce adverse cardiac effects and excitement and reverse analgesic effects and sedation. It is advisable to start by administering one half the calculated dosage.
- Atropine, 0.01 to 0.02 mg/kg IV, is used to manage sinus bradycardia. ***Caution:*** Ileus can result from use and horses should be monitored closely for signs of colic.
- Dobutamine, 0.001 to 0.008 mg/kg per minute (1 to 8 µg/kg per minute) IV, is a beta$_1$-agonist that increases mean cardiac output and arterial blood pressure. Dobutamine has a short half-life and is best used in an infusion (50 mg in 500 mL of 0.9% saline solution equals 0.01% solution or 0.1 mg/mL or 100 µg/mL). *Do not* mix with lidocaine, aminophylline, furosemide, calcium, or sodium bicarbonate. Overdosage produces tachycardia, tachydysrhythmia, and hypertension. ***Note:*** In hypovolemic patients, *do not* use dobutamine as a substitute for intravascular volume replacement. Dobutamine produces severe sinus tachycardia when used with atropine.
- Doxapram, 0.2 mg/kg IV, is a respiratory stimulant that works by having an effect on central respiratory centers and on carotid and aortic chemoreceptors. Doxapram is considered by some to be *contraindicated* if severe hypoxia has already occurred because use of the drug could result in neurologic and cardiac complications. In an emergency, resuscitation by positive pressure ventilation with 100% oxygen is the preferred management of apnea. If doxapram is used, intubation and oxygen supplementation should be provided. Doxapram or aminophylline (1 to 2 mg/kg) have been used to combat anesthetic-induced respiratory depression when mechanical ventilation was unavailable.
- Ephedrine, 5 to 10 µg/kg IV, has indirect and direct effects on blood pressure. Direct effects are through weak adrenergic stimulation of alpha$_1$-receptors. Indirect effects are through systemic release of epinephrine.
- ***Practice Tip:*** *Exhausted horses may have depleted levels of catecholamines and have a reduced response to ephedrine administration. In these cases, vasopressin 0.4 U/kg IV may be more appropriate to increase vascular tone.*
- Epinephrine *(Adrenalin),* 0.02 mg/kg IV or 0.2 mg/kg by intratracheal route and repeated as necessary, *is a drug of choice for cardiopulmonary resuscitation.* Epinephrine is a mixed alpha- and beta-sympathomimetic agent that produces peripheral vasoconstriction and cardiac stimulation. Through the jugular vein, inject this agent in conjunction with fluid therapy to ensure that the drug reaches the central compartment.

- ***Important:*** Intracardiac injection of any drug is *not* recommended. Myocardial damage and/or laceration of a cardiac vessel can occur.
- Flunixin meglumine, 0.25 to 1 mg/kg IV, is a nonsteroidal anti-inflammatory drug that also possesses anti-endotoxin properties.
- Hetastarch or Vetstarch, 2 to 10 mL/kg per hour, are a synthetic colloid solutions that has a high and low molecular weight respectively. High doses of hetastarch may cause platelet dysfunction and acute kidney injury.
- Hypertonic saline solution (7%), 4 mL/kg over 5 minutes (3 L maximum dose to a 450-kg adult), is used principally as a short-term (<30 minutes) blood volume expander to manage shock; it causes hypernatremia because of the high sodium concentration in the solution.
- ***Important:*** *Hypertonic saline solution is contraindicated in cardiogenic shock.* The mechanism of action is to shift intracellular and interstitial water into the intravascular space. Therefore, hypertonic saline solution is viewed as *emergency treatment only;* administer in conjunction with conventional replacement fluids.
- Balanced electrolyte solution (lactated Ringer solution, Normosol-R, Plasma-Lyte), 10 to 40 mL/kg per hour, is an isotonic crystalloid solution used to correct hypovolemia, dehydration, shock, and acidosis. Lactated Ringer solution can be used with colloidal or hypertonic saline solutions (see Chapter 32, p. 567).
- Lidocaine, 0.5 to 1 mg/kg IV, is used to manage ventricular tachydysrhythmias. These are relatively uncommon in horses, but prompt treatment may be critical when they are present in anesthetized horses.
- Prednisolone sodium succinate, 2 to 5 mg/kg IV, is used to stabilize cell membranes during shock and after resuscitation.
- Vasopressin, 0.05 to 0.9 U/kg IV, CRI 0.0001 to 0.05 U/kg/min, is used to increase peripheral vascular resistance and blood pressure. Its use in CPCR in humans and small animal patients may result in more favorable outcomes and it may be important in restoring blood pressure in hypovolemic shock. Its use in horses is under investigation.
- ***Note:*** As the pH of blood decreases, catecholamine receptors become less functional. During CPCR, particularly in foals, vasopressin use may increase vascular tone better than epinephrine. The use of both vasopressin and epinephrine together during CPCR is gaining traction in veterinary medicine.
- Yohimbine, 0.1 mg/kg IV, is used to reverse the effects of alpha$_2$-agonists, xylazine, and detomidine.
- ***Practice Tip:*** *Yohimbine can cause excitement and cardiac arrhythmias; so minimize this effect by administering one half of the calculated dosage slowly. Administer the second half of the dosage only if necessary. Use when early termination of an alpha$_2$-agonist is desirable or to manage inadvertent alpha$_2$-agonist overdosage. Repeated dosage may be needed.*

General Anesthetic Considerations

Induction of Anesthesia

- The method and techniques used for induction of anesthesia greatly depend on the condition of the horse.
- Down horses can be induced where they are situated and then moved under anesthesia (see Chapter 36, p. 631, and Chapter 37, p. 634). Extreme caution should be used with down horses, particularly those with neurologic disease because unpredictable movement, including paddling, can be dangerous to personnel. These patients may need to have sedation administered intramuscularly via pole syringe before administration of any intravenous medications.
- Standing horses should be induced in a manner that best controls their movement to recumbency. When possible, induction next to a strong, smooth wall with attendants standing on the side of the horse away from the wall can be used (Fig. 47-3). Induction can also be performed against a wall inside of a large trailer; this eliminates the need to load an anesthetized horse if transporting to a hospital.
- If no surface is available to anesthetize a horse, a large paddock or pasture can be used. The horse should be directed to gently move in a circular motion by leading with a halter and lead rope after the induction agents are given. This minimizes the chances of a horse moving forward or backward into obstacles during induction and allows the clinician to have some control of the horse's descent and prevent the horse's head from striking the ground.

Depth of Anesthesia

- Distressed horses in emergency situations are likely to have different sensitivity to anesthetics compared with nondistressed horses. Therefore, depth of anesthesia should be monitored closely by trained personnel. Excessive depth may lead to decreased blood pressure, decreased cardiac output, and hypoventilation or apnea.
- Fever, sepsis, low blood pH, or endotoxemia may have local effects on drug receptors, increasing or decreasing their affinity for a particular drug.
- Drug dosages should be adjusted according to patient condition.
- Pain and distress increase sympathetic tone and circulating catecholamine levels. These increases can cause a hyperdynamic cardiovascular state characterized by increased cardiac output. Drug requirements may greatly increase under these circumstances, but use caution to prevent an overdosage when catecholamine levels decline.
- In hypovolemic horses, the reduced volume of distribution of injected drugs can increase susceptibility.

- Exhaustion also can complicate an emergency because it is often associated with muscle damage, dehydration, electrolyte imbalance, and decreased circulating levels of catecholamines.
- ***Practice Tip:*** *Of particular importance is the careful use of alpha$_2$-agonist drugs in patients with compromised cardiovascular systems. In many cases, the sedative effects may be more pronounced and the reduction in cardiac output that accompanies the use of this class of drugs may overwhelm a horse's natural compensatory mechanisms.*

Monitoring

- A pulse oximeter provides continuous evidence of a pulse and is used to measure oxygen saturation. Portable units are available with various probe clip sizes that accommodate horses of different sizes. Areas of placement include the tongue, vulva, prepuce, light colored ears, and flank folds. Patients with an SpO_2 measurement less than 92% are candidates for supplemental oxygen.
- Multiparameter monitors are available in many sizes and shapes. Portable, battery-powered units can be especially useful. Electrocardiograms can be used for the detection of dysrhythmias and to monitor response to treatment. Indirect blood pressure measurement should be undertaken in any horse receiving pressor agents. Mean blood pressure measurement is a useful indirect measurement of perfusion pressure. Adult and juvenile horses (particularly recumbent horses) should have a mean blood pressure of at least 70 mm Hg and foals should have a mean blood pressure of 55 to 60 mm Hg.
- ***Practice Tip:*** *Blood pressure cuffs should be placed on the base of the tail for the most accurate readings. The width of the cuff should measure at least 40% of the circumference of the tail to give the most accurate readings (Fig. 47-4). The average of three successive readings, 1 minute apart, should be used because indirect blood pressure measurement can vary widely and generally tends to read slightly lower than actual blood pressure. If the heart rate is reported along with the blood pressure, check by auscultation to make sure the heart rate is correct: if the heart rate is not correct then the blood pressure measurement is likely incorrect also.*
- Point of care units (e.g., VetScan i-STAT 1 Portable Clinical Analyzer, Abaxis, Inc.; see Chapters 10 and 15) can be used to measure various blood values, including acid-base status, electrolytes, lactate, and blood gas values.
- ***Note:*** *Baseline and serial lactate measurements can be useful in determining initial and ongoing treatments. Elevated lactate levels should be observed to decline during appropriate fluid and resuscitation therapies and can be monitored during anesthesia.*

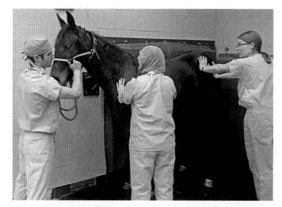

Figure 47-3 Example of placement of a horse for induction of anesthesia. After sedation, the horse is induced next to a wall to allow for a controlled movement to recumbency.

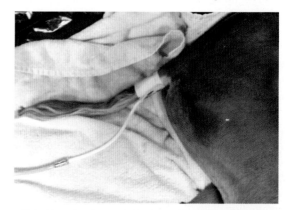

Figure 47-4 Example of proper placement of a tail cuff for indirect blood pressure measurement of a foal. Placement in adult horses would be similar and can be applied while the horse is standing or recumbent.

- An accurate anesthetic record is the best defense against claims of negligence. The best way to ensure safe anesthesia and an accurate record is to designate someone to be personally responsible for anesthesia and supportive care. Drugs administered, time administered, dose, and route of administration should be included in any anesthesia record.

Respiratory Support

- Orotracheal intubation is the best method to ensure airway patency and is mandatory if ventilation is controlled.
- A demand valve attached to a two-stage regulator valve and type E oxygen cylinder is suitable for controlling ventilation with oxygen. Demand valves allow spontaneous ventilation to be supplemented with oxygen. For larger horses, the regulator may have to be adjusted to 60 psi to maintain sufficiently high inspiratory flow.
- E cylinders contain approximately 660 gaseous liters; therefore, 3 or 4 cylinders may be needed to ventilate a 450-kg adult for 30 minutes.
- A 30-foot (9.1-m) length of hose allows isolation of the compressed gas cylinder from the patient. A dolly also helps secure the cylinder.

Cardiovascular Support

- A 14-gauge (or larger), 5½-inch (14-cm) over-the-needle catheter should be secured (with cyanoacrylate glue [superglue or tissue glue] or suture [2-0 nylon]) in a peripheral vein; the jugular vein is preferred. Other veins that can be used include the cephalic vein, lateral thoracic vein, and the saphenous vein.
- If the patient is hypovolemic, administer balanced electrolyte solution at a rate of 10 to 20 mL/kg IV. Use 7% hypertonic saline solution at a rate of 4 to 6 mL/kg if hypovolemia is severe.
- **Practice Tip:** *A 450-kg adult should receive no more than 3 L of 7% hypertonic saline solution. Hetastarch (2 to 10 mL/kg) or Vetstarch can be used with other crystalloids to manage hypovolemia. Doses of hetastarch higher than 10 mL/kg may interfere with platelet numbers or function and prolong prothrombin and partial thromboplastin times and should be used with caution in patients with coagulopathies.*
- Dobutamine, vasopressin, or ephedrine in conjunction with fluid therapy should be used only with adequate preload and monitoring of the heart rate, rhythm, and systemic blood pressure. Increasing the heart rate in a ventricle that is not full increases the cardiac oxygen requirements and may be detrimental to the patient.

Positioning and Padding

- Pad pressure points (shoulder, hips) and large muscle groups during anesthesia.
- Protect the eyes, especially when moving the patient. Application of sterile ophthalmic eye lubricant can be used to decrease corneal abrasions and desiccation associated with reduced tear production.

Ileus

- Horses that require emergency anesthesia may have a full gastrointestinal (GI) tract. The reduction in GI motility caused by anesthetic drugs can predispose these patients to ileus and colic. A full GI tract can complicate ventilation and result in hypoxemia during anesthesia.
- Many anesthetic and tranquilizing drugs decrease intestinal motility; therefore, consider the risk of postanesthesia colic.
- Minimizing positional changes while the patient is recumbent may decrease the risk of intestinal torsion.

Hyperkalemic Periodic Paralysis

- Hyperkalemic periodic paralysis (HYPP) is a genetic disorder among Quarter horses. Stress is a primary factor in the disease.

- In the emergency setting and with anesthesia, it is important to recognize and manage HYPP immediately (see HYPP/nervous system Chapter 21, p. 311, and Chapter 22, p. 357).
- Treatment with intravenously administered calcium, dextrose-containing solutions, and sodium bicarbonate can be performed while the patient is anesthetized.

Hypothermia

- Hypothermia usually is a problem only in foals. However, monitor body temperature in all emergencies when shock and environmental temperature extremes are possible.
- Keeping patients wrapped in blankets not only reduces the loss of body heat but may also provide padding.
- In some situations application of external heat sources such as warmed fluid bags and forced warm air blankets may be useful.
- **Practice Tip:** *Avoid use of heat lamps because they provide limited usefulness and can result in severe thermal burns.*

Recovery from Anesthesia

- Upon completion of an anesthetic procedure, horses must be recovered in as safe a manner as possible.
- In general, horses tend to recover with better-coordinated muscle activity after injectable anesthesia than after inhalational anesthesia.
- Other factors that impact recovery include:
  - Disease process
  - Duration of anesthesia
  - Cardiovascular status
  - Acid-base and electrolyte status (particularly ionized calcium levels)
  - Anesthetic/analgesic drugs administered
- Exhausted, neurologic, geriatric, neonatal, or horses with orthopedic injury may require assistance during recovery. Assistance can be given with the use of tail and head ropes (Fig. 47-5).
- Recoveries should be performed in an area free of obstacles to prevent further injury. An open field or a well-padded, solid wall stall can be used. Extra shavings or straw can be added to a stall to provide padding (shavings should be used with caution because small particles can be inhaled or irritate the cornea). Corals and stalls with pipe panels or wire should be avoided.

Euthanasia

- Humane or economic considerations may necessitate destruction of the equine patient. Anesthesia (Adult Protocol 1 or 2) makes euthanasia easier to accomplish and more humane.

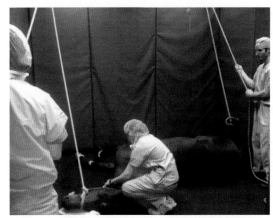

Figure 47-5 Example of head and tail ropes being used to assist the recovery of a horse from anesthesia. Ropes can be slung over beams or rafters in a barn or stout tree limbs in a field setting. Acepromazine is being administered to reduce anxiety and facilitate a smoother recovery.

ANESTH

Specific Clinical Situations

- In some cases requiring emergency anesthesia, sedation or tranquilization and local anesthesia may be all that is necessary initially to stabilize a patient.
- General anesthesia should be considered for patients that need complete immobilization. Minimizing general anesthesia time decreases the incidence of complications.

Severe Lacerations

- Determining the volume of blood lost after a laceration is often difficult. Horses with tachycardia (heart rate >50 beats/min in the adult horse) should be presumed to be hypovolemic until proven otherwise, and should be treated with crystalloid and/or colloidal solutions for volume replacement. Consider placement of an IV catheter and stabilization therapy before administration of any sedatives or anesthetic agents.
- **Practice Tip:** *Heart rate increases and blood pressure drops when 25% or more of the blood volume is lost and indicates the need for volume replacement therapy.*
- When possible, control bleeding with bandages or compression wraps before induction of anesthesia.
- The cardiodepressant effects of alpha$_2$-agonists and barbiturates can be dangerous in hypovolemic patients. Adult Protocol 1 or 2 (see p. 744) is often preferred for induction because either one causes minimal depression of the cardiovascular system. Standing sedation and local anesthetic protocols may be useful in surgical closure of laceration of the thorax or abdomen.

Fractures

- It is often necessary to stabilize fractures before transporting the patient to a surgical facility.
- Considerations are the same as those for severe lacerations and Adult Protocol 1 or 2 (see p. 744) can be used. Internal hemorrhage and volume depletion may occur with fractures, particularly with long bone fractures. Intravenous volume replacement therapy should be considered.
- Ameliorate pain with opioid administration. Low doses of acepromazine may help reduce anxiety.
- When hypovolemia is not evident or volume replacement therapy has been administered, alpha$_2$-agonists can be used for additional analgesia and sedation.
- Higher-than-normal dosages may be required in excitable horses because of elevated catecholamine levels.
- Induction of anesthesia and immobilization on a rescue glide may facilitate easier transport to a surgical facility. A controlled induction with the horse placed against a solid surface, such as a smooth wall, may help prevent further damage to a fractured bone. Long bone fractures can be splinted with the horse standing and then the horse anesthetized for transport to minimize weight bearing on the fractured bone (see Chapter 21, p. 319).

Seizures and Neurologic Diseases

- Horses with neurologic disease may present in various states including depressed mentation or exhibiting focal or widespread seizure activity, or they may be recumbent and quiet or recumbent and frantic (i.e., paddling and thrashing).
- Down horses may require general anesthesia to facilitate movement from dangerous situations and transport to a treatment facility (see Chapters 36 and 37).
- Treat a patient with seizures by administering diazepam/midazolam, 0.1 to 0.4 mg/kg IV. Anxious, recumbent, or frantic horses may require administration of an alpha$_2$-agonist to prevent injury to themselves and personnel. **Practice Tip:** *Midazolam has a shorter half-life than diazepam.*
- If anesthesia is needed for transport and/or diagnostic testing, a protocol based around thiopental (where available) or propofol is recommended by some. Either induction agent should be preceded with the use of 5% guaifenesin (Adult Protocol 3 or 4, p. 744).
- In foals and small horses, propofol may be the induction agent of choice if ventilation is available and blood pressure is normal.
- The use of dissociative anesthetics like ketamine has in the past been considered contraindicated because of their ability to induce seizurelike activity and increase intracranial pressure. Although use of ketamine may increase intracranial blood flow, its use in humans with head trauma has not resulted in increased mortality when compared to other anesthetics.

Dystocia

- General anesthesia can be used to produce sufficient vaginal and uterine relaxation to facilitate manipulation of malpositioned foals.
- Elevating the caudal end of the anesthetized mare briefly (<20 min) allows abdominal viscera to move cranially and improves the ease of fetal manipulation. The increased pressure of the viscera on the diaphragm reduces the size of the thoracic cavity and the ability of the lungs to expand. Controlling ventilation with a demand valve can be used to minimize ventilatory compromise.
- Adult Protocol 1 or 2 is usually satisfactory for these situations, followed by maintenance with a "triple drip."
- General anesthesia for field cesarean section rarely results in a live foal and places the mare at increased risk; extensive manipulation per vagina increases the risk of complications during cesarean section. Rapid stabilization and transport to a surgical facility usually results in the best chance for a favorable outcome.

Uterine Torsion

- Anesthesia for nonsurgical correction of uterine torsion can be performed safely in many field situations. The "plank in the flank" procedure can be performed after induction of anesthesia with Adult Protocol 1 or 2 (see p. 744). Maintenance of anesthesia with "triple drip" can be performed (see p. 738) if multiple attempts are performed. However, it is not recommended to make more than two attempts.
- As with other obstetric emergencies, if distress is observed in the mare or fetus, rapid medical stabilization and transport to a surgical facility may be best.

Colic

- Horses with severe colic are frequently unresponsive to analgesics and are unmanageable to the point at which they can injure themselves and are dangerous to transport. Injectable anesthesia may be needed before definitive treatment or transportation to a surgical facility.
- Intravenous fluids and other supportive treatment usually are needed in these situations.
- A benzodiazepine with ketamine combination is a suitable induction technique.
- Abdominal distention may necessitate controlled ventilation. Trocarization may be helpful in relieving gas distention if it can be localized to the cecum or possibly the large colon (see pp. 18, 160, and 161).
- Correcting nephrosplenic entrapment of the large colon can be attempted in the field by administration of phenylephrine and walking or jogging up and down a slope, or less commonly, by "rolling" the patient from right to left lateral recumbency under general anesthesia. Adult Protocol 1 or 2 (see p. 744) is generally used for this purpose. Appropriate medical therapy is important in conjunction with "rolling," if previous attempts using phenylephrine and controlled exercise are unsuccessful.

Extrication/Entrapment

- Horses may need to be anesthetized for safe removal from dangerous situations.
- It is difficult to assess accurately the physiologic status of these patients.

- In difficult or unsafe situations where getting close to the patient is not possible, the use of a pole syringe may allow intramuscular administration of sedative drugs.
- The use of Telazol-ketamine-detomidine (TKD) (see Protocol 2, p. 744) may be preferred over other protocols because the small volume of drug may be easier to give in these situations. Intramuscular administration of TKD (5 to 6 mL/450 kg) via a pole syringe can be performed to provide profound sedation in horses and minimize risk to personnel.
- Skills and equipment needed for safe removal of horses are important in disasters such as hurricanes, floods, and trailer accidents (see Chapter 37, p. 634).

Cardio-Pulmonary-Cerebral Resuscitation (CPCR)

- Emergency field anesthesia can result in respiratory and cardiac arrest, for example, from:
  - Hypovolemia
  - Upper airway obstruction
  - Pneumothorax
  - Hypokalemia
- Careful, continuous monitoring and early intervention are the keys to success in CPCR. Fig. 47-6 is a guide for patient evaluation.
- Box 47-1 is a guide for CPR.

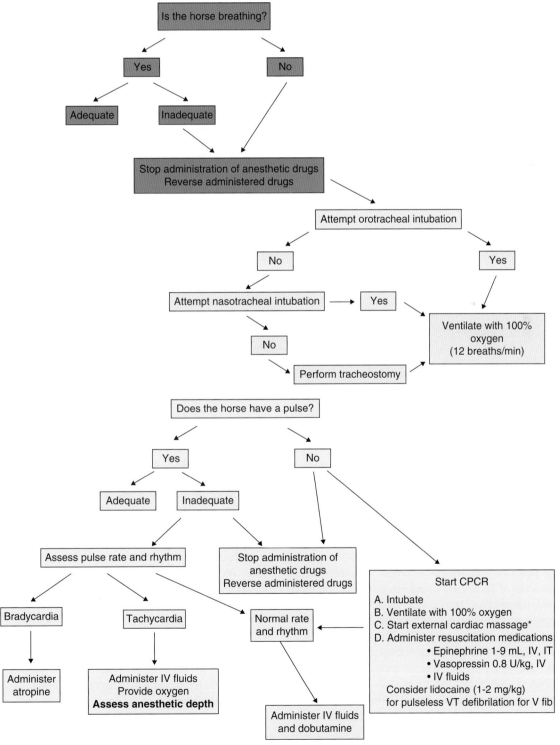

Figure 47-6 Guide for patient evaluation for cardiopulmonary resuscitation following anesthetic induction.
*May be initial treatment for foals.
IT, Intratracheal; *IV,* intravenous; *V fib,* ventricular fibrillation.

Box 47-1	**Cardio-Pulmonary-Cerebral Resuscitation (CPCR)**

- Verify arrest, discontinue anesthetics, and note time of arrest.
  A: Airway: Place an orotracheal or nasotracheal tube.
  B: Breathing: Start positive pressure ventilation with 100% oxygen.
  C: Circulation: Establish external cardiac massage at 30 pumps/min by "knee drops" on chest.
- Administer epinephrine: 0.02 mg/kg intravenously or intratracheally.
- Administer fluids (lactated Ringer's solution, physiologic saline solution) at shock dosage to improve cardiac output (40 mL/kg). A capnograph and pulse oximeter can be used to monitor results of resuscitative efforts.

◉❯ WHAT NOT TO DO

Dystocia

- In dystocia cases, *do not* maintain the Trendelenburg (head-down) position for long periods because it is associated with reduced ventilation and cardiac output.

Selected Protocols for Emergency Anesthesia

Protocols for Adult Horses

Protocol 1

- Premedication:
  - Xylazine, 0.3 to 1.1 mg/kg IV
  - One opioid of choice:
    - Butorphanol, 0.01 to 0.04 mg/kg IV
    - Morphine, 0.1 mg/kg IV or IM
    - Methadone, 0.1 mg/kg IV or IM
  - Wait 3 to 5 minutes for peak effect
- Induction (given in rapid succession):
  - Diazepam or midazolam, 0.05 to 0.1 mg/kg IV
  - Ketamine, 2.2 mg/kg IV
- Maintenance: "Triple drip" or "alternative triple drip" CRI (see p. 738). Titrate carefully to produce the desired level of anesthesia (1 to 3 mL/kg/h).
- *Practice Tip:* With a standard 15-drops/mL administration set, this equates to 1 to 2 drops per second for a 450-kg adult.

Protocol 2

- Premedication:
  - Xylazine, 0.3 to 1.1 mg/kg IV
  - One opioid of choice (see Protocol 1)
- Induction:
  - 3 mL/450 kg of TKD (Telazol, ketamine, and detomidine) solution
- *Practice Tip:* TKD solution can be prepared by reconstituting a 5-mL vial of Telazol with 4 mL ketamine (100 mg/mL) and 1 mL detomidine (10 mg/mL). Induction is as rapid and smooth as ketamine/benzodiazepine and results in a smooth recovery with minimal cardiorespiratory depression. This method results in profound muscle relaxation for induction but does not provide surgical anesthesia. Following recumbency, additional administration of anesthetic/analgesic drugs (ketamine, thiopental, "triple drip") may be needed before surgical procedures. An additional benefit is the small volume of drug needed for induction compared with other protocols.

- Maintenance:
  - "Triple drip" or "alternative triple drip" as described on p. 738

Protocol 3 (Not Available in the United States)

- *Caution:* This protocol is not recommended in cases of hypovolemia and shock. An IV catheter must be placed.
- Premedication:
  - Xylazine, 0.3 to 1.1 mg/kg IV
  - Wait 3 to 5 minutes for peak sedation
- Induction:
  - 5% guaifenesin administered to effect—the patient becomes ataxic after approximately 0.6 to 1 mL/kg IV (60 to 90 mg/kg) (A single dose of diazepam or midazolam, 0.1 to 0.2 mg/kg, can be substituted for the guaifenesin)
  - Then administer a bolus of thiopental, 3 to 4 mg/kg IV
- Maintenance:
  - 2 g thiopental in 1 L of 5% guaifenesin titrated to approximately 1 to 2 mL/kg/h

Protocol 4

- *Important:* The use of propofol as an induction agent may result in excitement during induction. This protocol is suggested for patients exhibiting neurologic signs of seizures or increased intracranial pressure. Propofol may be cost prohibitive in large horses but should be considered in neurologic patients, especially in areas where thiopental is unavailable.
- Premedication:
  - Xylazine, 0.3 to 1.1 mg/kg IV
  - 5% guaifenesin administered to effect—the patient becomes ataxic after approximately 0.6 to 1 mL/kg IV (90 mg/kg)
- Induction:
  - Propofol, 2 to 4 mg/kg IV
- *Important:* The use of guaifenesin is necessary to prevent excitement during induction with propofol and provides additional muscle relaxation.
- Maintenance:
  - Propofol, 0.2 to 0.3 mg/kg per minute, administered via a syringe pump or IV bolus at 5- to 15-minute intervals as needed based on depth of anesthesia.
- *Caution:* Propofol induction may cause profound apnea and should be used only when intubation and ventilator support are available. It may also reduce cerebral blood flow.

Protocol 5 (for Severely Depressed or Debilitated Patients)

- *Caution:* In healthy individuals, this induction can cause excitement. This protocol is indicated only in cases of severe hypovolemia, endotoxic shock, or CNS depression.
- Premedication: none
- Induction:
  - Diazepam or midazolam, 0.1 to 0.2 mg/kg IV
  - Ketamine, 2.2 mg/kg IV
- Maintenance:
  - "Triple drip" or "alternative triple drip" as described on p. 738
- *Important:* These patients should be administered high volumes of crystalloid fluids before and during anesthesia.

Protocols for Foals Less Than 4 Weeks of Age

Protocol 1

- Premedication:
  - Midazolam or diazepam, 0.1 mg/kg IV. Wait for peak sedation to take effect. The foal may lie down.
- Induction:
  - Ketamine, 2.2 mg/kg IV
- Maintenance:
  - A modified "triple drip"—1 L of 5% guaifenesin with 125 to 250 mg xylazine and 1g ketamine titrated to approximately 0.5 to 1 mL/kg per hour

Protocol 2

- The use of propofol in foals provides for an excellent induction and smooth recovery. Vigilant cardiorespiratory monitoring is essential because propofol can cause apnea and hypotension. These side effects are dose and rate responsive and can be minimized by administering propofol slowly "to effect."
- Premedication:
  - Midazolam or diazepam, 0.1 mg/kg IV. Wait for peak sedation to take effect. The foal may lie down.
- Induction:
  - Propofol, 2 to 4 mg/kg IV
- Maintenance:
  - Propofol, 0.2 to 0.3 mg/kg per minute, administered via a syringe pump or IV bolus at 5- to 15-minute intervals as needed based on depth of anesthesia.
- *Practice Tip:* Nasal insufflation with oxygen or intubation and assisted ventilation are highly recommended with this protocol.

References

References can be found on the companion website at www.equine-emergencies.com.

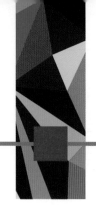

CHAPTER 48

Euthanasia/Humane Destruction*

Thomas J. Divers

- Properly performed euthanasia is important to ensure humane destruction of terminally ill or distressed horses and is particularly important when viewed by the client.
- Before administering any euthanasia solution:
  - Properly identify the patient being humanely destroyed, and recheck that this is the correct horse and owner/insurance company consent is verified.
- Things to consider:
  - Location
  - Distracting noise
  - Surface
  - Surrounding objects!
  - Adequate restraint
  - Condition of the jugular veins
  - Placement of the needle or catheter
    - Needle stick injuries to humans can occur during a rushed euthanasia!
  - Safe handling and disposition of the carcass
    - Location of burial
    - Possibility of consumption of the destroyed horse after barbiturate euthanasia. This must be avoided.
  - Physical condition of the halter, shank, and holder, and clear safety instructions for the handler
  - Possible emotional reactions of people viewing the humane destruction
  - Always *think* "what could go wrong?"

Performing Humane Destruction Without Tranquilization

- This can readily be performed in a calm horse.
- Prepare two 60-mL syringes of approved euthanasia solution; one syringe may contain 40 mg of succinylcholine (expensive) if one wants to prevent agonal gasping or paddling.
- *Practice Tip: Dose may vary depending on the size of the horse; generally 120 mL of a 390 to 392 mg/mL pentobarbital solution is adequate for a 450-kg horse.*

*Note: Veterinarians' right to legally transport controlled substances to farms and barns is coming under scrutiny. Veterinary Medicine Mobility Act of 2013 (H.R. 1528) is the legislature under consideration to amend the controlled substance act (CSA) that currently prohibits veterinarians from transporting controlled substances to treat animal patients outside of their registered location.

- Insert a 12- or 14-gauge, 2-inch (5-cm) nondisposable needle or 14-gauge, 5.25-inch (13.3-cm) intravenous catheter in the jugular vein (catheter preferred) with an extension set.
- After blood aspiration, to ensure that the needle or catheter is properly positioned in the vein, *rapidly* inject the syringe with 50 to 55 mL of the euthanasia solution first into the jugular vein.
- Immediately attach the second syringe (60 mL) making sure the needle is still in the lumen of the vein and inject quickly.
- If the jugular veins are easy to access and the horse has minimal reaction to the first needle insertion, it is sometimes easier to make rapid back-to-back needle insertions and injections. This is the advantage of the catheter and extension set system and especially in cases when less experienced assistants or owners are present.
- The horse usually falls within 30 seconds after injection of the two doses.
- Death should be confirmed by auscultation for an absence of a heartbeat and determining that the corneal reflex is lacking and pupils are dilated and fixed.
- *Important:* When using commercial euthanasia solutions at the proper dose, the most common reason for a delayed or ineffective response is that some of the drug was not administered intravenously or earlier tranquilization reduced cardiac output.

Performing Euthanasia with Tranquilization

- Tranquilization should be used in excited, apprehensive horses or when surroundings/situations are not considered ideal for humane destruction.
- To ensure a tranquil state during administration of the euthanasia solution:
  - Heavily sedate the patient with detomidine, 0.01 to 0.02 mg/kg IV, or xylazine, 0.5 to 1.0 mg/kg IV.
  - Once sedation is established, administer the concentrated pentobarbital solution, as described in the preceding section, through a 12-gauge needle or a 14-gauge, 5.25-inch (13.3-cm) catheter properly placed in the jugular vein and an extension set attached and secured.
  - Tranquilized horses are slower to collapse than nontranquilized individuals and may require an additional volume of euthanasia solution for more immediate effect.

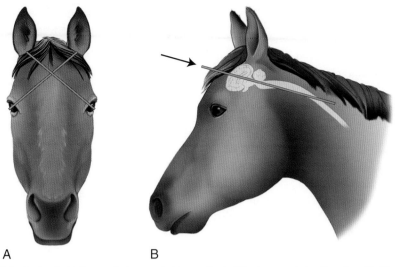

Figure 48-1   Anatomic site for gunshot or penetrating captive bolt for humane destruction of equids. The point of entry is the center of two intersecting lines drawn from the lateral canthus of the eye and the base of the opposite ear. The ballistic is directed so that it penetrates the brain and brainstem. **A,** Frontal view. **B,** Lateral view. (Adapted from Jan Shearer, Iowa State University.)

Nervous or Needle-Shy Patient

- Heavily sedate the individual with detomidine, 0.02 mg/kg (10 mg/500 kg) IV, or 10 to 30 mg IM. (Use an injection pole if necessary, or detomidine can be "squirted" in the mouth using 10 to 20 mg or more.)
- If the horse allows you to open its mouth, detomidine gel (0.4 mg/kg) can be placed under the tongue. *Caution:* Avoid human eye or skin contact with detomidine gel.
- Place a 14-gauge, 3.5- or 5.25-inch (8.9- or 13.3-cm) catheter in the jugular vein with an extension set and administer euthanasia solution, rapidly.

Euthanasia Under Anesthesia

- This procedure can be performed with the administration of an approved euthanasia solution or the alternative is to administer concentrated potassium chloride IV—approximately 10 mEq/kg bolus—30 g/500-kg horse.

Euthanasia of Patients with Thrombosed Jugular Veins

- Place a 14- or 16-gauge, 3.5-inch (8.9-cm) catheter in the lateral thoracic vein. An extension set makes the injection procedure easier.
- Tranquilize the patient and administer the euthanasia solution.
- If the lateral thoracic vein cannot be catheterized, use detomidine, 20 mg IV, injected into the cephalic vein, or 40 mg IM.
- Once the patient is sedated, intracardiac administration of euthanasia solution and +/-succinylcholine can be performed with a 16-gauge, 3.5- to 6-inch (8.9- to 15.2-cm) needle and 60-mL syringe.

Humane Destruction of Horses at Public Events or When Unpredictable Movement of the Horse May Cause Human Injury or Unexpected Events

- In these cases, succinylcholine is mixed in the first syringe of concentrated barbiturate and administered to the horse, followed immediately with the second 60 mL of euthanasia solution.

Bullet Euthanasia

- On rare occasion it may be necessary to use "bullet" euthanasia by either a veterinarian or police officer who is trained and licensed in the proper use of the technique. Ideally, the horse is heavily sedated first; though this may not be an option.
- A 0.22 or a 0.32 caliber lead bullet is directed into the center of the forehead (just above the intersection of two lines drawn from the eyes to the opposite ears) and aimed toward the foramen magnum and down the neck. See Fig. 48-1.
- The firearm should be placed very near or against the forehead before discharge/firing.
- The possibility of bullet ricochet, public scrutiny, and a terrifying noise should be considered in choosing the venue before the procedure.

For More Information

- For further reading, please refer to www.avma.org/KB/Policies/Documents/euthanasia.pdf for the American Veterinary Medical Association (AVMA) Guidelines for the Euthanasia of Animals 2013. Also useful are the American Association of Equine Practitioners (AAEP) Guidelines for Euthanasia 2011, supplied here.

ANESTH

- The AAEP recommends that the following guidelines be considered in evaluating the need for humane destruction of a horse.
- The attending veterinarian is often able to assist in making this determination, especially regarding the degree to which the horse is suffering. It should be pointed out that each case should be addressed on its individual merits and that the following are guidelines only. It is not necessary for all criteria to be met.
- Horses may be euthanized at an owner's request for other reasons, as the owner has sole responsibility for the horse's care.
- Before humane destruction, clear determination of the insurance status of the horse should be made as this policy constitutes a contract between the owner and insurance carrier.
- In accordance with AVMA's position on euthanasia of animals, the AAEP accepts that humane destruction of unwanted horses or those deemed unfit for adoption is an acceptable procedure once all available alternatives have been exhausted with the client. A horse should not have to endure conditions of lack of feed or care eroding the horse's quality of life. This is in accord with the role of the veterinarian as animal advocate. See Box 48-1.

Box 48-1	**Guidelines to Assist in Making Humane Decisions Regarding Horse Euthanasia**

- A horse should *not* have to endure continuous or unmanageable pain from a condition that is chronic and incurable.
- A horse should *not* have to endure a medical or surgical condition that has minimal chance of survival.
- A horse should *not* have to remain alive if it has an unmanageable medical condition that renders it a hazard to itself or its handlers.
- A horse should *not* have to receive continuous analgesic medication for the relief of pain for the rest of its life.
- A horse should *not* have to endure a lifetime of continuous individual box stall confinement for prevention or relief of unmanageable pain or suffering.

From AAEP Guidelines for Euthanasia (2011) © American Association of Equine Practitioners. Assessed August 2013 at www.aaep.org/health_articles-view.php?id=364.

References

References can be found on the companion website at www.equine-emergencies.com.

CHAPTER 49

Pain Management

Bernd Driessen

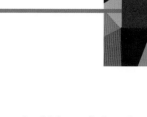

- Pain has been defined by the International Association for the Study of Pain (IASP) as an "unpleasant sensory and emotional experience" in a conscious subject. More appropriately for horses, pain may be described as "an aversive sensory and emotional experience representing awareness by the animal of damage or threat to the integrity of its tissues."
- It is generated after neuronal signal processing within the brain (especially cerebral cortex) and usually is the result of activation of peripheral high-threshold sensory receptors (i.e., nociceptors) that send electrical impulses from the periphery to the central nervous system (CNS; Fig. 49-1). Within the CNS the arriving neuronal signals are processed at various levels (within the spinal cord and lower and higher brain centers) before they eventually produce responses that serve to warn and protect the horse from impending tissue damage.
- Pain resulting from activation of nociceptors is commonly referred to as adaptive or physiologic pain because it minimizes tissue damage by activating reflex withdrawal mechanisms and increasing behavioral, autonomic, and neurohumoral responses that are aimed at maintaining body integrity, preventing further tissue damage, and promoting healing.
- Maladaptive pain, however, can be considered a disease (defined as a disorder with a specific cause and recognizable signs) and can be thought of as pain dissociated from the original noxious stimuli or the healing process.
    - It is expressed as abnormal sensory processing caused by damage to tissues (inflammatory pain) or the nervous system (neuropathic pain) or by abnormal function of the nervous system itself (functional pain).
    - It is pathologic and is accompanied by an exaggerated and prolonged response to noxious (hyperalgesia) and/or nonnoxious (allodynia) stimuli.
    - It often is responsible for persistent discomfort and stress of the horse, which can lead to abnormal behaviors; reduced quality of life; and if uncontrolled, distress and death.
- These latter aspects about maladaptive pain are particularly crucial in equine veterinary practice in which humane destruction of horses with uncontrollable or chronic pain is a common practice. Therefore, consider the following:
    - *Practice Tip: All surgical interventions should be considered as causing at least some degree of pain, which*

implies that analgesic therapy should begin before the pain-producing event whenever possible (preemptive analgesia).
- Patients often already suffer from pain caused by an underlying disease process or original tissue injury before any diagnostic or surgical procedure can take place. Nevertheless, pain therapy should be instituted as early as possible before further interventions are undertaken in an attempt to prevent worsening of the pain experience (preventive analgesia).
- Early recognition of pain as a significant component of injury or disease and a proactive approach to analgesic therapy with continued reevaluation of signs of nociception are mandatory if the risk of developing a chronic pain process is to be prevented.
- Left uncontrolled over extended periods, adaptive or physiologic pain may progress to maladaptive pain, which often fails to respond to conventional analgesic therapy.

Classification of Pain and Its Relevance to Pain Therapy

- Systems of pain classification have been widely used to direct analgesic therapy or to describe efficacy of therapeutic interventions. Most commonly pain is described in terms of:
    - Anatomic origin:
        - Superficial somatic (e.g., cutaneous) pain
        - Deep somatic (e.g., musculoskeletal) pain
        - Visceral (e.g., colic, urogenital) pain
    - Site of impulse generation:
        - Nociceptors (nociceptive pain)
        - Injured peripheral and central afferents (nonnociceptive or neuropathic pain)
    - Intensity:
        - Mild
        - Moderate
        - Severe
    - Duration:
        - Acute
        - Chronic
- *Note:* From a therapeutic standpoint these classifications are not particularly meaningful. The widespread convergence of nociceptive signals from cutaneous, musculoskeletal, and visceral tissues (often more than one visceral

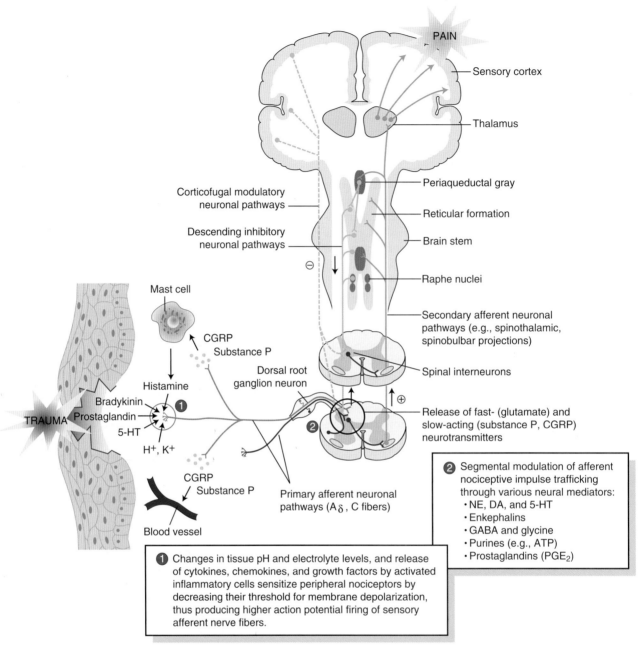

Figure 49-1 Ascending pathways of nociceptive impulses generated by peripheral sensory receptors (nociceptors) in response to noxious stimulation following tissue trauma. Once generated, impulses propagate along small-diameter (C and A_δ) ascending nerve fibers (primary afferent fibers) via the dorsal root ganglion cells to the dorsal horn of the spinal cord. Action potentials from activated peripheral nociceptors arriving at the spinal terminals of sensory afferent fibers in the dorsal horn of the spinal cord elicit the release of fast- and slow-acting neurotransmitters that chemically convey the nociceptive input to the spinal neurons (secondary afferent fibers) that conduct the information to the brain. In the brain, a complex integration of these signals occurs and, after their conduction through the thalamus as highest neuronal relay, the nociceptive input reaches the somatosensory cortex, where it is transformed into the sensation of pain. The inflammatory process associated with tissue injury causes pH and electrolyte changes in the close environment of peripheral nociceptors, production of inflammatory mediators, and the up-regulation of proinflammatory enzymes, all of which collectively sensitize nociceptors toward noxious and nonnoxious stimuli. Extensive processing of nociceptive signals involving inhibition and amplification takes place within the spinal cord. Simultaneously, descending neuronal pathways originating in the brain and terminating in the dorsal horn of the spinal cord, as well as spinal interneurons, modulate the conduction of nociceptive signals from the peripheral nerve fibers to ascending spinal neurons. *ATP,* Adenosine triphosphate; *CGRP,* calcitonin gene-related peptide; *DA,* dopamine; *GABA,* gamma-aminobutyric acid; *5-HT,* serotonin; *NE,* norepinephrine.

organ) or neuronal structures onto neurons in the CNS challenges the idea that the sensation of pain per se is qualitatively different. Furthermore, none of the analgesic agents available today have been shown to be exclusively effective toward pain of somatic, visceral, or nonnociceptive (neuropathic) origin. Likewise, separating acute from chronic pain is challenging.

- Although primary afferents transmitting signals from cutaneous, musculoskeletal, and visceral locations are mostly distinct both in type (primarily multimodal nociceptors in somatic versus primarily mechanoreceptors and some chemosensory receptors in visceral tissues) and numbers (somatic afferents > visceral afferents), these pathways converge at the dorsal horn so that the spinothalamic, spinoreticular, and spinomesencephalic tracts all contain neurons that respond to somatic and visceral, as well as nonnociceptor-generated stimuli, and convey information to various brain centers from where signal pathways are again bundled and project to the cerebral cortex.
  - As a result, a common neuronal network in the cerebral cortex subserves all three somatic and visceral nociceptive and nonnociceptor (neuropathic stimuli) input.
- According to the taxonomy of the IASP, chronic pain is defined by duration of more than *3 months*. Therefore, acute pain covers a long period of time during which many neurophysiologic and pathologic processes take place simultaneously that should be addressed therapeutically.
- As nociceptive input continues and becomes persistent, central sensitization goes through three increasingly longer-lasting, irreversible, and pathologic stages, namely:
  - Activation—transient, activity-dependent
  - Modulation—slower but still reversible functional changes
  - Modification—chronic structural and architectural alterations
- Activation is a rapidly reversible physiologic process involving use-dependent augmentation of transduction and transmission (e.g., wind-up).
- Modulation, a more slowly reversible process with early pathologic connotations, is mainly due to phosphorylation of neuronal receptors and ion channels (e.g., the *N*-methyl-D-aspartate (NMDA) receptor and associated calcium channel).
- Modification, generally considered the basis of chronic, pathologic pain, involves altered regulation and cell connectivity together with cell death. Typical changes include modified gene transcription combined with loss of inhibition, both functionally and via death of inhibitory neuron populations.
- A numeric classification of pain (types I, II, and III), adopted from a system originally described for human patients, has recently been proposed for use in equine practice. The classification scheme may provide the veterinarian with better direction in how to approach pain therapeutically because it signifies the underlying neurobiologic and neuropathologic mechanisms involved:

- *Type I* (adaptive or physiologic) pain:
  - Occurs in the state of normal responsiveness and is commonly caused by a wound, sprain, strain, burn, or a primarily inflammatory condition
  - Represents the result of physiologic processes of nociceptive signal generation, conduction, and CNS integration after tissue injury, whether somatic or visceral
  - Generally sharp, intense, and well localized if originating from somatic areas, and temporally well defined
  - Commonly accompanied by an inflammatory response and release of inflammatory mediators causing peripheral sensitization (primary hyperalgesia), characterized by locally heightened responsiveness to both noxious and nonnoxious stimuli
  - Usually disappears once tissue healing is complete and/or inflammation resolved
  - Its primary purpose is to aid in maintaining body integrity, preventing further tissue damage and promoting healing
- *Type II* pain (central sensitization):
  - Results from processes of central sensitization (secondary hyperalgesia)
  - Generated and conducted primarily by high-threshold, polymodal C fibers
  - Pain is diffuse, poorly localized, and persistent.
  - Develops when firing activity of secondary afferent neurons (primarily wide dynamic range neurons [WDR]) is enhanced in response to primary afferent nociceptive signaling through decreased inhibitory modulation, increased facilitatory activity or both, at the spinal level
  - Recognized when nonnoxious stimuli applied to intact peripheral areas surrounding site of tissue trauma elicit nociceptive responses and sensation
- *Type III* (maladaptive or pathologic) pain:
  - Represents a pathologic condition in and of itself and is the result of altered nerve firing and neuronal plasticity
  - Damage to peripheral nerve fibers and/or morphologic (plastic) remodeling within the neuronal circuitry of the dorsal horn of the spinal cord and supraspinal centers can lead to altered firing patterns in afferent pathways and abnormal conveyance and processing of sensory information.
  - Spontaneous discharge activity in ascending WDR pathways causes uncontrolled nociceptive signaling to supraspinal centers even in the absence of ongoing tissue compromise and painful responses to normally innocuous stimuli (allodynia).
  - Traditional pain therapeutic agents alone are often not effective or only minimally effective, requiring inclusion of nontraditional therapies to provide at least some pain relief and increase the comfort level of the horse to what is considered acceptable.

ANESTH

- **Note:** The above scheme must be applied in the context of the many dynamic processes that are initiated by nociceptive signaling. Therefore, transitions from one type of pain to another (especially from type I to II) may occur in many cases of tissue trauma, sometimes making a clear distinction between different types of pain difficult.
- *Primary hyperalgesia* is a normal and expected feature of any tissue insult, always accompanies type I pain, and should be considered when pain therapy is being prescribed.
- Type II pain and hence *secondary hyperalgesia* have physiologic and adaptive importance. Central sensitization results in persistent discomfort/pain from low-intensity activity, thereby serving to protect injured areas from further damage until tissue healing has sufficiently progressed. Nonetheless, persistent pain and central sensitization should be addressed early on by the pain therapist because they can lead to further loss of function and structural damage.
- Type III pain may persist even in the absence of any inflammation, detectable tissue injury, or after supposedly complete wound/tissue healing. In horses, it may arise from various conditions such as surgical or traumatic injury resulting in sensory nerve damage, equine fibromyalgia syndrome (EFMS), arthritis, spondylosis of the spine with dorsal root radiculopathy, tumor growth with progressive compression of adjacent sensory fibers, compartment syndromes, or chronic laminitis.
- Type III pain is certainly the most difficult pain to treat and often calls for nonconventional locoregional (e.g., continuous perineural administration of local anesthetics, local administration of capsaicin or resiniferatoxin) and systemic drug therapies (e.g., gabapentin, pregabalin) or even nonpharmacologic interventions such as high power shock wave therapy, acupuncture, or other similar methods.

Recognition of Pain

- To approach pain therapeutically it is important to apply a reliable method to measure its intensity and duration and to record the response to treatment.
- Pain in horses, especially when acute or severe, is commonly associated with changes in activity of autonomic nervous functions:
  - Tachycardia
  - Hypertension
  - Tachypnea
  - Diaphoresis (sweating)
  - Mydriasis
  - Increased plasma beta-endorphin, catecholamine, and corticosteroid levels
- **Practice Tip:** *Physiologic parameters such as heart and respiratory rates and blood pressure are nonspecific and the result of sympathetic nervous system activation and do not necessarily correlate well with intensity of perioperative pain*

because they are often also influenced by other perioperative factors such as anxiety, excitement, stress, hypovolemia, shock, sepsis, and endotoxemia.

- Studies in different species have demonstrated that evaluation of behavioral changes is generally the best way to assess pain in animals. In the horse, systematic studies of behavioral changes indicative of pain are still lacking. However, currently available data indicate that prolonged observation of behavioral activity promises to be a much more sensitive method of identifying pain-related behaviors in horses than intermittent (short-term) subjective evaluations.
- Several behavioral parameters were identified as most useful and quantifiable for pain scoring in horses:
  - Behaviors associated with superficial pain:
    - Immediate, forceful avoidance reaction in response to superficial pain stimulus
  - Behaviors associated with visceral pain:
    - Pawing, flank watching, rolling, sweating in response to abdominal pain
    - Consistent lowering of head to levels at or below the withers
    - Reduced or altered interest in food
    - Reduced exploratory behavior
    - Bruxism
    - Recumbency
    - Altered demeanor
  - Behaviors associated with musculoskeletal pain:
    - Abnormal exploratory behavior
    - Altered head and ear positioning
    - Altered gait
    - Altered hoof lifting on command
    - Reduced locomotion
    - Increased weight shifting
    - Pawing
    - Abnormal posture in box stall
    - Recumbency
    - Bruxism
    - Restlessness
    - Reduced or altered interest in food
    - Altered demeanor
- Independent of which behavioral factors are used to evaluate pain in horses, it is important to realize that familiarity with the breed and the individual horse's normal behavior is essential to any meaningful interpretation of observational parameters. Behaviors may be confounded by a number of other factors, such as the following:
  - Temperament (age-, breed-, sex-, stress-dependent)
  - Instinctive behavior as flight-response animal
  - Foraging and hunger-related activity
  - Mechanical (injury or bandage; cast-related) impairment of locomotor activity
  - Pharmacologic side effects or residual effects of analgesics, sedatives, and anesthetics previously administered
- **Important Note:** Pain is always subjective and is perceived by the horse as an aversive sensory and emotional

experience. Thus, it is best assessed by careful and repetitive observation and recording of changes in behavioral activity.

Anatomy and Physiology of Nociceptive Input Transmission and Processing

- To understand the pharmacologic mechanisms of action of available analgesics and to prescribe an effective pain management protocol, it is important to know which anatomic sites and physiologic/pathophysiologic processes are participating in the generation, conduction, and integration of nociceptive signals and which mechanisms are involved in the maintenance and exacerbation of the pain experience.
- In principle, four anatomic structures participate in the production of pain (see Fig. 49-1):
  - Nociceptors:
    - Mechanical
    - Thermal
    - Chemical
    - Polymodal
    - Primary afferent neuronal pathways (ascending nerve fibers)
    - Spinal cord
    - Brain
- Nociceptors are specialized neuronal structures that generate action potentials in response to noxious stimulation and thus transform the original mechanical, thermal, or chemical stimulus into electrical impulses.
- Certain nociceptors are specialized and respond to only one type of noxious stimulus, whereas others are polymodal; that is, they can be activated by a number of qualitatively different noxious stimuli.
- Nociceptive signaling is carried from the affected peripheral region to the dorsal horn of the spinal cord through *small myelinated (A$_\delta$)* and *nonmyelinated (C)* afferent nerve fibers (primary afferents) that are responsive only to high-threshold stimuli.
- The faster-conducting A$_\delta$ fibers carry information from nociceptors responsive to high-threshold thermal (hot or cold) or high-threshold mechanical stimuli.
- Slower conducting C fibers transmit signals from free nerve endings that are responsive to both high-threshold mechanical and thermal stimulation, as well as chemical stimuli (e.g., products of cellular damage, cytokines, autocoids, hydrogen ions, and various inflammatory mediators).
- From the dorsal horn of the spinal cord, the nociceptive input travels along multiple spinal ascending pathways called secondary afferent fibers, often referred to as spinothalamic, spinoreticular, and spinomesencephalic projections, to various areas of the brain.
- The ultimate destination of the nociceptive input is the somatosensory cerebral cortex.
- The complex integration of nociceptive signals within the CNS (especially at the level of the cerebral cortex)

transforms the nociceptive input into the unpleasant sensory and emotional experience that is described as pain and that evokes the multiple reflex withdrawal, behavioral, autonomic, and neurohumoral responses associated with pain.
- The observation in human beings that the experienced pain intensity often does not correlate well with the strength of the original noxious stimulus and varies from individual to individual indicates that extensive processing of nociceptive signals involving inhibition and amplification takes place once they are perceived by peripheral nociceptors.
- The spinal cord is the first relay station where significant modulation of the nociceptive input from the periphery occurs.
- Electrical impulses from activated peripheral nociceptors arriving at the spinal terminals of sensory afferent fibers elicit the release of fast-acting neurotransmitters (especially glutamate) and slower-acting neuropeptides (substance P, calcitonin gene-related peptide [CGRP], neurotensin, neurokinin), which are responsible for the electrochemical transmission of the nociceptive signals to secondary afferent fibers that convey the information to the brain.
- Simultaneously, descending neuronal pathways originating in the brain and terminating in the dorsal horn of the spinal cord, as well as spinal interneurons, modulate the conduction of peripheral signals by releasing inhibitory neurotransmitters or other neuroactive mediators (e.g., nitric oxide [NO], adenosine triphosphate [ATP], prostaglandins [PGE$_2$]) that elicit positive feedback, thus controlling as "gatekeepers" the flow of nociceptive signals to the brain.
- The spinal cord is also involved in activation of simple monosynaptic and polysynaptic spinal reflex responses (e.g., withdrawal reflexes and reflex muscle spasms) to noxious stimulation.
- ***Practice Tip:*** *The components of the peripheral nervous system and CNS that are involved in generation, transmission, and integration of nociceptive signals (peripheral nociceptors and ascending nerve fibers, spinal cord, and brain) are target sites for pharmacologic and nonpharmacologic modulation of the pain experience.*

Pathophysiology of Nociception

- As described earlier, normal pain (type I pain) is produced only by intense stimuli that are potentially or actually damaging to tissue. Thus, only high-threshold peripheral and central neurons are designed to respond to such noxious stimuli, and therefore nociceptive pain is essentially an early warning mechanism designed to make the horse aware of damage or threat to the integrity of its tissues.
- Type II pain and type III pain, by contrast, occur in response to tissue injury and inflammation, damage to the nervous system (neuropathic pain), and alterations in the normal functioning of the peripheral and central nervous

ANESTH

systems, and are associated with development of pain hypersensitivity that takes two forms:

- Responsiveness is increased, so that noxious stimuli produce an exaggerated and prolonged pain (hyperalgesia or *winding-up*).
- Thresholds are lowered so that stimuli that would normally not produce pain now begin to (allodynia).

- In type II pain, hypersensitivity is often an adaptive response after an injury because it helps healing by ensuring that contact with or use of the injured tissue/organ is minimized until repair is complete.

- However, in type III pain, hypersensitivity may persist long after an injury has healed or occur in the absence of any injury. In this case, pain provides no benefits and is the manifestation of a pathologic change in the functioning of the nervous system.

- Two mechanisms are primarily responsible for rendering neurons more sensitive to noxious stimuli or sensory inputs:
  - Peripheral sensitization or *primary hyperalgesia*
  - Central sensitization or *secondary hyperalgesia*

- Within minutes following an initial noxious stimulation caused by tissue injury, surgery, or infection, *peripheral sensitization* occurs and is noted as a reduction in stimulus threshold and an increase in responsiveness of the peripheral high-threshold nociceptors. Changes in the local chemical environment of the peripheral nociceptors are primarily responsible and include:
  - Changes in temperature, tissue pH, and local electrolyte (K^+) concentrations
  - The production and release of cytokines (tumor necrosis factor-α), adenosine triphosphate (ATP), chemokines (bradykinin), and growth factors by inflammatory cells
  - The products of up-regulation enzyme systems (cyclooxygenase, protease, phospholipase) collectively activate or sensitize expressed and silent nociceptors and sensitize them to noxious and non-noxious stimuli.
  - Mechanisms leading to peripheral sensitization include:
    ◦ Changes in key proteins
    ◦ Ion channels (known as transduction proteins) that determine the excitability of the nociceptor terminal
  - The transduction proteins are the means by which a noxious stimulus is converted into an electrical signal.

- After peripheral inflammation, the thresholds for heat, cold, and mechanical stimuli fall considerably. Two processes have been implicated in this increase in sensitivity:
  - Changes to existing nociceptor proteins (posttranslational processing)
  - Changes to the proteins being made by the nociceptor (altered gene expression)

- Posttranslational changes usually involve the phosphorylation of some of the nociceptor protein's amino acids by enzymes known as kinases. This phosphorylation can dramatically alter functions of the nociceptor; for example,

phosphorylation of a nociceptor's Na^+ channel can drastically lower the threshold at which the channel opens and makes the channel stay open for longer, so that any stimulus to the terminal evokes a greater response.

- Some inflammatory signals, however, are transported from the terminal along the axon or nerve fiber to the cell body of the sensory neurons in the dorsal root ganglion. Here they either change transcription (increase expression of particular genes) or increase translation (ensure more protein is produced from messenger RNA).

- The increased protein is then shipped back down to the terminal where it contributes to an increased responsiveness of the terminal to peripheral stimuli. One example is the TRPV1 protein, an ion channel that responds to heat stimuli.

- Activation of kinases takes minutes, changes in protein levels a day or so.

- Centrally mediated sensitization, or *secondary hyperalgesia,* is an increase in the excitability of neurons within the CNS, so that normal inputs begin to produce abnormal responses. It is a complex and still incompletely understood process at the level of the spinal cord that affects primarily the surrounding noninjured, noninflamed tissues and is initiated as early as primary hyperalgesia.

- The increased excitability is typically triggered by a burst of activity in nociceptors (such as that evoked by an injury), which alter the strength of synaptic connections between the nociceptor and the neurons of the spinal cord (so-called activity-dependent synaptic plasticity).

- Low-threshold sensory fibers activated by a very light touch of the skin, for example, begin to activate neurons in the spinal cord (for inputs from the body) or in the brainstem (for inputs from the head) that normally only respond to noxious stimuli. As a result, an input that would normally evoke an innocuous sensation now produces pain.

- In effect, the synaptic changes act like an amplifier mechanism. Thus, central sensitization is responsible for tactile allodynia (pain in response to, for example, a light brushing of the skin) and for the spread of pain hypersensitivity beyond an area of tissue damage so that adjacent nondamaged tissue is uncomfortable.

- Central sensitization also has two phases:
  - An immediate but relatively transient phase
  - A slower onset but longer-lasting phase

- As with peripheral hyperalgesia, the first phase depends on changes to existing proteins while the second phase relies on new gene expression. The early phase reflects changes in synaptic connections within the spinal cord, after a signal has been received from nociceptors.

- The central terminals of the nociceptor release a host of signal molecules, including the excitatory amino acid synaptic transmitter glutamate, neuropeptides (substance P and CGRP), and synaptic modulators including brain-derived neurotrophic factor (BDNF). These transmitters/modulators act on specific receptors on the spinal cord neurons, activating intracellular signaling pathways that lead to the phosphorylation of membrane receptors and channels, particularly the *N*-methyl-D-aspartate (NMDA) and the α-amino-3-hydroxy-5-methyl-4-isoxazolepropionic acid (AMPA) receptors for the excitatory neurotransmitter glutamate.

- These posttranslational changes lower the threshold and opening characteristics of these channels, thereby increasing the excitability of the neurons.
- A later transcription-dependent phase of central sensitization is mediated by increased levels of protein production.
- The net effect of these changes is that normally subliminal inputs begin to activate the neurons, and pain sensibility is drastically altered.
- Among the proteins mediating this effect are dynorphin, an endogenous opioid that increases neuronal excitability, and cyclooxygenase, the enzyme that produces prostaglandin E_2.
- As well as being involved in peripheral sensitization, prostaglandins also affect central neurons, contributing to central sensitization.
- As the neuronal network within the spinal cord is undergoing changes in response to continuous nociceptive input, a morphologic correlate of "pain memory" is developing. Morphologic changes may include alterations in the ratio of facilitatory and inhibitory interneurons and descending neuronal pathways, thereby altering the bidirectional control over dorsal horn nociceptive transmission neurons.
- Furthermore, physical rearrangement of the dorsal horn circuitry by abnormal sprouting of neurons and formation of new synaptic contacts among nerve cells can transform areas of the spinal cord normally involved in transmission of low-threshold mechanoreceptor signals (touch) into areas transmitting exclusively nociceptive input, thus producing the sensation of pain when low-threshold pressure (touch) receptors are activated.
- It appears that these structural changes at the spinal level contribute to the phenomenon that, with time, central hyperalgesia becomes increasingly less dependent or even independent of nociceptive input from the periphery, causing the development of chronic maladaptive pain.
- Peripheral and central sensitization processes have been demonstrated in the horse.
- ***Practice Tip:*** *Rapid development of primary and secondary hyperalgesia associated with moderate to severe noxious stimulation dictates that treatment of pain must commence as early as possible and shall include administration of drugs that target different mechanisms involved in the intra- and intercellular signaling cascades responsible for sensitization.*

Pain Management in the Horse
Concept of Multimodal Pain Therapy (Balanced Analgesia)
- Advancements in the understanding of the complex physiology and pathophysiology of pain have led to widespread

implementation of a strategy, often referred to as *multimodal* or *balanced* analgesia (Fig. 49-2) as opposed to the traditional *unimodal* pain therapy. This applies particularly to horses in which signs have progressed to type II or III pain.
- Given the multiple mechanisms and dynamic neuronal processes involved in generation and aggravation of the pain experience, it is unreasonable to assume in horses suffering from moderate to severe pain as a result of major tissue trauma, surgery, and/or inflammation that monotherapy (i.e., administration of a single analgesic drug with a single mechanism of action) produces adequate analgesia and long-term pain relief.
- *Multimodal or balanced analgesia* involves the combination of drugs with different pharmacologic mechanisms of action, and often both systemic drug administration and local or regional anesthesia/analgesia techniques, and may also include complementary modalities of pain treatment (Box 49-1; Fig. 49-2).
- The purpose of *multimodal or balanced analgesia* is to choose drugs and techniques that target different sites of the neural conduit conveying nociceptive signals from the

---

Box 49-1 Multimodal Approach to Analgesia or Balanced Analgesia

Anti-inflammatory Treatment
Nonsteroidal anti-inflammatory drugs
Steroids

Systemic Analgesia
Opioids
Alpha$_2$-agonists
Local anesthetics (lidocaine)
Nonconventional therapeutics:
- Butylscopolamine
- Ketamine
- Alpha$_2$delta ligands:
  - Gabapentin
  - Pregabalin

Local/Regional Anesthesia and Analgesia
Peripheral nerve blocks using topical, infiltrative, perineural, and intraarticular administration techniques:
- Local anesthetics
- Ketamine
- Morphine
- Alpha$_2$-agonists
Local intravenous administration (intravenous regional analgesia/anesthesia [IVRA]; Bier block):
- Lidocaine 1% to 2%
- Mepivacaine 1% to 2%
Epidural/spinal anesthesia/analgesia:
- Local anesthetics
- Opioids
- Alpha$_2$-agonists
Local capsaicin or resiniferatoxin application
Complementary therapies:
- Acupuncture/electroacupuncture
- Chiropractic treatment
- Mesotherapy
- High-power extracorporeal shock wave therapy

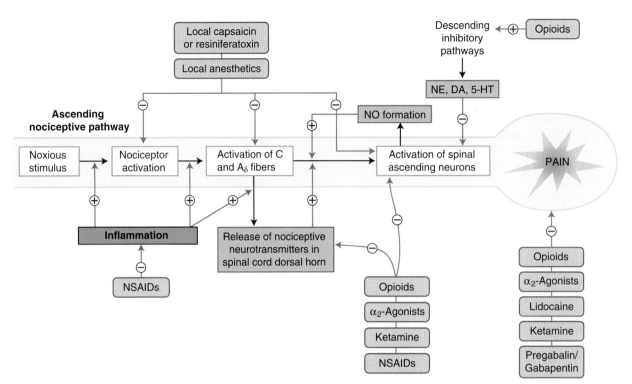

Figure 49-2 Indicated are target sites within the nociceptive conduit where different analgesics elicit their pharmacologic effects in a synergistic manner. The concept of multimodal or balanced analgesia is built on the idea that analgesics with different modes of action, when administered together, interfere with generation, conduction, and integration of nociceptive signals more effectively than when administered alone, and thus provide better analgesia. Furthermore, it must be a goal of multimodal or balanced analgesia to suppress or at least inhibit the development of primary and secondary hyperalgesia because those processes favor the transition of type I to type II and eventually type III pain. *DA, Dopamine, 5-HT,* serotonin; *NE,* norepinephrine; *NO,* nitric oxide; *NSAIDs,* nonsteroidal anti-inflammatory drugs.

periphery to the CNS and that act synergistically, thereby achieving five main goals:

- Blockade of nociceptive signal generation in primary afferent terminals
  ○ Tissue infiltration with local anesthetics
- Inhibition/decrease of nociceptive signal conduction from the periphery to CNS and suppression of primary hyperalgesia
  ○ Peripheral nerve blocks with local anesthetic agents
  ○ Systemic nonsteroidal anti-inflammatory drugs (NSAIDs)
  ○ Systemic and or local opioids
- Inhibition/decrease of spinal nociceptive signal transmission and suppression of secondary hyperalgesia
  ○ Peripheral nerve blocks without spinal/epidural administration of local anesthetic agents
  ○ Peripheral nerve or dorsal root ganglion blocks with local anesthetics or TRPV-1 agonists (e.g., capsaicin, resiniferatoxin)
  ○ Spinal or epidural administration of opioids
  ○ Spinal or epidural administration of alpha$_2$-agonists
  ○ Systemic NSAIDs (much less spinal than peripheral effect)
  ○ Systemic ketamine administration
  ○ Systemic gabapentin or pregabalin administration

- Inhibition/decrease of the pain experience by interfering with cerebral nociceptive signal processing
  ○ Systemic lidocaine
  ○ Systemic opioids
  ○ Systemic alpha$_2$-agonists
  ○ Systemic NSAIDs (much less central than peripheral effect)
  ○ Systemic ketamine
  ○ Systemic gabapentin or pregabalin administration
- Restoration of homeostasis and function
  ○ All treatment modalities
- In most instances, analgesic agents and techniques can be tailored to the specific situation of the individual horse with continuation for a minimum of 3 days following surgical procedures, trauma, and/or inflammation. ***Practice Tip:*** *Pain treatment should be continued as long as required based on repeated pain assessment.*
- ***Important Note:*** Whatever pharmacologic approach and technique are chosen in an individual *multimodal* or *balanced analgesia* protocol, the objective is to achieve optimum pain control for a particular situation while at the same time minimizing the risk for adverse responses to pain therapy. Thus, any analgesic protocol is tailored to an individual patient's situation.
- Multimodal approach to pain therapy is commonly used in equine practice. Horses undergoing surgery for elective

and emergency procedures are frequently being treated with systemic administration of a combination of drugs that target peripheral and central mechanisms of nociceptive signal generation, transmission, and integration (see Table 49-1 for a selection of drugs commonly used for pain management in the horse):

- An alpha$_2$-agonist and an opioid to provide preoperative and postoperative sedation and analgesia
- Ketamine, an NMDA-receptor antagonist for induction of anesthesia

- Systemic lidocaine, an opioid, or alpha$_2$-agonist intraoperatively as part of a balanced anesthesia protocol (partial intravenous anesthesia [PIVA])
- An NSAID given preoperatively and postoperatively
- Intermittent or continuous administration of opioids (e.g., butorphanol) postoperatively
- Continuous systemic infusion of analgesic drugs (Table 49-2) is often used as part of a balanced anesthetic (PIVA) protocol (i.e., a combination of one or more potent intravenous analgesic agents with a low-dose inhalant

Table 49-1 Drugs Commonly Used for Systemic Analgesia and Reported Doses

Drug	Dosage (mg/kg)	Route of Administration	Dosing Interval	Comments
Nonsteroidal Anti-inflammatory Drugs (NSAIDs)				
NSAIDs are effective analgesic adjuncts that primarily suppress inflammation as a cause of nociception and development of primary hyperalgesia. They are indicated in mild to moderate pain associated with acute (e.g., after surgery or trauma) or chronic inflammatory processes (e.g., osteoarthritis). NSAIDS are commonly combined with other analgesics in situations of more severe pain. All drugs of this class bear the risk of aggravating gastrointestinal ulceration, and causing renal and coagulation dysfunctions. An important advantage is that most can also be orally administered.				
Flunixin meglumine	0.2-1.1	IV, IM, PO	q8-12h	Most often used for acute abdominal pain and postoperatively; also exhibits anti-endotoxic activity
Phenylbutazone	2.2-4.4	IV, PO	q12-24h	Most often used in patients with musculoskeletal pain or before/after soft tissue and orthopedic surgery
Dipyrone (Metamizole)	10-20	IV, IM	q8-12h	Most often used for acute abdominal pain; also exhibits spasmolytic and strong antipyretic activity
Ketoprofen	2-2.5	IV, IM	q24h	
Carprofen	0.7-1.4	IV, PO	q12-24h	Not cyclooxygenase-2 (COX-2) selective in horses
Meloxicam	0.6 0.6 0.6	IV, PO PO PO	q12-24h q24h adults PO q12h foals	q24h for adults; q12 for foals Foals eliminate NSAIDs more rapidly than adults
Acetylsalicylic acid	5-20	PO	q24-48h	Also possesses antithrombotic activity
Naproxen	5 (10)	IV (PO)		Initially slow intravenous bolus followed by oral dose every 24 hours
Etodolac	10-20	IV, IM, PO	q12-24h	Developed as alternative to flunixin meglumine with fewer side effects in gastrointestinal tract
Eltenac	0.5-1	IV	q24h	Has significant anti-endotoxic activity
Vedaprofen	1-2	IV	q12-24h	Alternative to ketoprofen
Firocoxib	0.09 (0.1)	IV (PO)	q24h	Most COX-2 selective NSAID 0.2 to 0.3 mg/kg PO q24h; or 0.2 mg/kg IV q24h to reach steady state
Opioids				
Opioids are indicated in moderate to severe pain; however, evidence is less well defined for analgesic efficacy in horses compared with other species; opioids are commonly used in combination with sedatives (alpha$_2$-agonists, acepromazine) to control central excitatory effects; they carry an increased risk for ileus development upon repeated administration.				
Morphine	0.1-0.7	IV, IM	q4-6h	Ileus may be more likely than with other opioids
Methadone	0.1-0.2	IV, IM	q4-6h	
Meperidine	1-2	IM	q2-4h	Intravenous administration may cause hypotension because of histamine release.
Butorphanol	0.01-0.4	IV, IM	q2-4h	None or very short-lived analgesic effect at lower (<0.1 mg/kg) doses; excitatory responses at higher doses
Buprenorphine	0.005-0.02	IV, IM	q6-8h	Significant excitatory effects at doses of ≥0.01 mg/kg
Fentanyl	One 10-mg patch per 115 kg	Transdermal	q48-72h	Very variable uptake of fentanyl with plasma levels below analgesic (≤1 ng/mL) concentrations in up to one third of horses

Continued

| Table 49-1 | **Drugs Commonly Used for Systemic Analgesia and Reported Doses—cont'd** |

Drug	Dosage (mg/kg)	Route of Administration	Dosing Interval	Comments
Alpha₂-Agonists				
Alpha₂-agonists are potent analgesics indicated in moderate to severe pain; however, significant cardiovascular side effects (bradycardia, hypertension) and sedation accompany analgesia when given at higher doses; these are commonly used in combination with opioids to control acute pain and cause long-lasting reduction in gut motility (large intestines more than small intestines) upon repeated administration.				
Xylazine	0.2-1	IV, IM	q0.3-1h	Commonly used in colic patients for acute pain
Detomidine	0.005-0.02	IV, IM	q1-2h	Commonly used in colic patients for acute pain
Dexmedetomidine	0.003-0.007	IV, IM	q4h	Characterized by shortest plasma half-life (≈23 min) and highest alpha₂:alpha₁ receptor selectivity among all alpha₂-agonists
Romifidine	0.02-0.12	IV, IM	q4h	Longest lasting alpha₂-agonist with lowest alpha₂: alpha₁ receptor selectivity

Nonconventional Drugs Used in Pain Therapy

Drug	Dosage (mg/kg)	Route of Administration	Dosing Interval	Comments
In most situations of severe and chronic pain (e.g., laminitis, septic osteitis, and osteomyelitis) and in horses suffering from intestinal spasms, some adjunctive drugs have been reported to be efficacious when combined with conventional—e.g., opioid-, alpha₂-agonist–, and NSAID-based—analgesic drug regimens.				
Ketamine	0.2-0.5	IV, IM	q4-6h	Provides 30-60 min of analgesia; used when medication with alpha₂-agonists alone is ineffective
Gabapentin	20-40	PO	q6-8h	Effective for certain types of chronic pain syndromes (e.g., neuropathic pain) not amenable to conventional analgesic treatment; low oral bioavailability (~16%)
Pregabalin	2-4	PO	q8h	Effective for certain types of chronic pain (e.g., neuropathic pain); bioavailability nearly 100%; lower dose or increase treatment interval if the horse becomes overly depressed
Butylscopolamine	0.2-0.3	IV	One dose only	Primarily spasmolytic activity of short duration (~30 min)

| Table 49-2 | **Drugs Used for Systemic Analgesia via Continuous Rate Infusion** |

Drug	IV Bolus Dose (mg/kg)	IV CRI Rate (mg/kg per hour)	Comments
Opioids			
Morphine	0.05-0.3	0.1-0.4	Has been studied as adjunct to inhalant anesthesia
Butorphanol	0.02	0.013-0.024	Short-lived analgesic effect at lower doses; excitatory responses at higher doses (>0.02 mg/kg)
Fentanyl	0.00028-0.005 0.002	0.0004-0.008 0.0004	No unequivocal evidence for analgesic effects has been observed Predicted doses calculated based on published pharmacokinetic data in horses and a target plasma concentration of 1 ng/mL
Alpha₂-Agonists			
Xylazine	0.2-1.0	1.0-4.0	Significantly decrease requirement for anesthetic agents and thus often used in balanced anesthesia (PIVA) and total intravenous anesthesia (TIVA) protocols; provide effective analgesia for surgery in standing horses
Detomidine	0.006-0.04	0.007-0.036	
Medetomidine	0.003	0.0015-0.0036	
Dexmedetomidine	0.0015-0.0035	0.00075-0.0018	
Romifidine	0.01-0.04	0.1-0.4	
Local Anesthetics			
Lidocaine	1.3-2.5 (over 10-30 min)	1.8-3.0	Commonly used intraoperatively as part of a balanced anesthesia (PIVA) protocol and in the postoperative period after abdominal surgery and in horses with severe pain
Anesthetics			
Ketamine	None or 1.0-2.3 (over 30-40 min)	0.4-1.5	Administered at subanesthetic doses; most often used in horses with severe acute or chronic pain; no significant adverse excitatory effects observed
In combination with lidocaine CRI	None or 1.0 (over 30 min)	0.2	

CRI, Constant rate infusion.

anesthetic) or in total intravenous anesthesia (TIVA) to provide sufficient pain control during surgery.

- Intravenous infusion of a potent analgesic/sedative agent such as alpha$_2$-agonists alone or in conjunction with opioids is also indicated for surgical procedures in the standing, sedated horse.
  - In these situations, these drugs are usually used in conjunction with local or regional anesthesia to control short periods of acute pain.
  - Lidocaine infusions have been shown to be efficacious in controlling pain in the perioperative period, more for pain of soft tissue than musculoskeletal origin, and can be extended into the postoperative period.
- In patients with persistent moderate to severe pain of somatic or visceral origin, a combination of repetitive and continuous analgesic drug treatment is indicated and can entail one or all of the following agents:
  - NSAIDs administered at intervals of 8 to 24 hours
  - Opioids (e.g., butorphanol, morphine, or methadone) administered at intervals of 3 to 8 hours or as a continuous rate infusion
  - Low-dose alpha$_2$-agonists (preferentially dexmedetomidine because of its greater alpha$_2$-receptor selectivity and shorter plasma half-life compared with other alpha$_2$-agonists) via constant rate infusion
  - Ketamine administered as continuous rate infusion
  - Systemic lidocaine administered as a continuous rate infusion
  - Antiepileptic agents (e.g., gabapentin) given intermittently

Local/Regional Anesthesia and Analgesia

- The neuropathophysiologic processes leading to the development of central hyperalgesia, allodynia, and neuropathic pain are primarily triggered by barrages of firing activity in ascending sensory nerve fibers during the first 4 to 5 days following tissue trauma and associated peripheral nerve injuries.
- Local/regional anesthesia and analgesia should play a key role in the early management of most patients with moderate to severe and/or persistent pain.
- Clinical studies in human beings have demonstrated that the need for immediate postoperative and long-term pain medication is significantly reduced when local/regional anesthesia and analgesia techniques are applied preoperatively.
- Experimental evidence and clinical experiences in human medicine indicate that not only acute, but also persistent pain with development of central hyperalgesia, is obliterated by no other treatment modality more effectively than with locoregional anesthesia and analgesia.
- ***Practice Tip:*** *Techniques of locoregional anesthesia and analgesia may include wound infiltration or intraarticular injections with local anesthetics and opioids; topical local anesthetic application using 5% lidocaine patches (Lidoderm); single, repetitive or continuous peripheral nerve blocks; and epidural or intrathecal anesthesia and analgesia.*
- Box 49-1 lists the techniques and drugs used for local and regional anesthesia and analgesia in the equine with dosages for locoregional anesthesia given in Table 49-3

Table 49-3	Drugs Used for Local and Regional Anesthesia/Analgesia and Reported Concentrations and Dosages		
Drug	**Route of Administration**	**Onset of Action**	**Comments**
Local Anesthetics of Short Action (60-90 Minutes)			
Procaine 1%-2%	Topical	Slow	Has vasoconstrictive properties
Proparacaine 0.5%	Topical	Rapid	Used primarily for ophthalmologic procedures
Local Anesthetics of Intermediate Action (90-240 Minutes)			
Lidocaine 1%-2%	SQ, infiltration, epidural, spinal, perineural, IV, intraarticular	Fast	
Mepivacaine 1%-2%	SQ, infiltration, epidural, spinal, perineural, IV, intraarticular	Fast	Most commonly used for diagnostic blocks in lameness examinations and in trauma
Local Anesthetics of Long Action (180-360 Minutes)			
Bupivacaine 0.5%-0.75% or lower	SQ, IV, spinal, epidural, perineural, intraarticular	Intermediate	
Ropivacaine 0.2%-1.0% or lower	SQ, IV, spinal, epidural, perinerual, intraarticular	Fast	Vasoconstrictive action at lower concentrations; fewer motor blockade effects
Combinations of Local Anesthetics to Achieve Fast Onset and Long Action (>240 Minutes)			
Lidocaine 2% plus bupivacaine 0.5%-0.75%	SQ, infiltration, perineural		No evidence as to the benefit of this combination has been reported
Others			
Ketamine 1%-2%	Perineural		Very short action (5-15 min)

Table 49-4	Adjuvants Used for Local and Regional Anesthesia/Analgesia and Reported Concentrations and Dosages	
Drug	**Dose per Milliliter of Local Anesthetic (LA)**	**Comments**
Epinephrine 1 : 200,000	5 μg	Decreases local perfusion and delays absorption, thereby prolonging LA effect; when administered into epidural or subarachnoid space, epinephrine may enhance analgesia via alpha$_2$-agonistic action
NaHCO$_3^-$ 0.042%	5 μL NaHCO$_3^-$ 8.4%	Increases pH of LA solution, thereby increasing amount of un-ionized drug fraction available to diffuse across nerve membranes and thus accelerates onset of LA action
Buprenorphine 0.003%	30 μg	Reported in human beings to enhance and prolong regional analgesic effect of LAs
Dexmedetomidine	0.5 μg	Reported in human beings and small animals to enhance and prolong regional analgesic effect of LAs

and adjunctive agents that enhance their effect or duration in Table 49-4.

- Especially in the patient with severe and chronic pain, repeated or continuous administration of low doses of concentrated local anesthetic solutions alone or in conjunction with analgesics *(balanced regional analgesia)* in proximity to peripheral nerves (perineural nerve blocks, dental nerve blocks) or in the epidural space may offer significantly better pain relief with many fewer side effects than long-term systemic administration of analgesics.
- ***Practice Tip:*** *Local/regional anesthesia and analgesia should be considered an integral part of any balanced analgesia protocol for treatment of moderate to severe pain.* This is to inhibit the rapid development of primary and secondary hyperalgesia, which promotes the deterioration of adaptive or physiologic pain into maladaptive pain.

Caudal Epidural Catheterization

- Catheterization of the caudal epidural space is a relatively safe technique that is commonly employed in equine clinical practice and offers the advantage of long-term regional pain therapy beyond the immediate perioperative period by repeated or continued administration of local anesthetics and/or analgesic agents into the epidural space.

Technique of Caudal Epidural Catheter Placement

- Required materials and equipment:
  - Epidural catheter set (e.g., Perifix[1] epidural catheter or TheraCath[2] epidural catheter set, the latter providing exceptional long-term patency) with 18- or 17-gauge Tuohy Schliff epidural needle and 20- or 19-gauge epidural catheter labeled with markings indicating distance from tip, and catheter adaptor with injection port, respectively. Catheters may have open or closed tips. (Catheter lengths of >60 cm are suitable for use in adult horses.)
  - Sterile gloves
  - #11 blade

- Lidocaine 1% to 2% for skin desensitization
- 16-gauge, 1½-inch hypodermic needle
- Anatomy:
  - The spinal cord in the horse extends to the caudal half of the second sacral vertebra (S$_2$).
  - The epidural space is preferentially accessed via the intervertebral space between the first coccygeal vertebrae (Co$_1$-Co$_2$), although the sacrococcygeal (S-C) and second intercoccygeal (Co$_2$-Co$_3$) space can be used as alternative routes, without risk of entering the spinal canal.
  - Either access site can be easily palpated when moving the tail up and down with the other hand (Fig. 49-3, *A*).
- Procedure:
  - If performed in the awake horse, it is recommended to restrain the equine patient in stocks and to provide sedation with an alpha$_2$-agonist (i.e., xylazine, detomidine).
  - Clip and disinfect a rectangular, 2- to 2½-hand-wide area extending from the sacrum to the third coccygeal vertebra (Co$_3$; see Fig. 49-3, *A*) before catheter placement.
  - Observe strict aseptic technique when inserting the Tuohy needle and epidural catheter.
  - Infiltrate the skin and subcutaneous tissue at the preferred site of spinal needle insertion (Co$_1$-Co$_2$) with 1 to 3 mL of 1% to 2% lidocaine solution to avoid any pain response to needle and catheter placement (Fig. 49-3, *B*).
  - Tuohy needle insertion is greatly facilitated after making a 1- to 2-mm midline stab incision through the locally blocked skin and subcutaneous tissue.
  - Slowly advance the Tuohy needle with the bevel pointing cranially through the skin incision site at a 60- to 90-degree angle to the plane of the skin until a sudden loss of resistance is felt, indicating entrance into the epidural space following crossing the interarcuate ligament (Fig. 49-3, *C*).
  - Correct placement of the Tuohy needle must be confirmed before insertion of the catheter using any one of the following techniques:
    - *Hanging drop technique.* Soon after passing the skin and subcutaneous tissues, remove the stylet from the

---

[1]Perifix epidural catheter (B. Braun Medical, Inc., Bethlehem, Pennsylvania; product code CE-18T or alternatively, a spring-wire reinforced epidural catheter).

[2]TheraCath (Arrow International, Reading, Pennsylvania, USA).

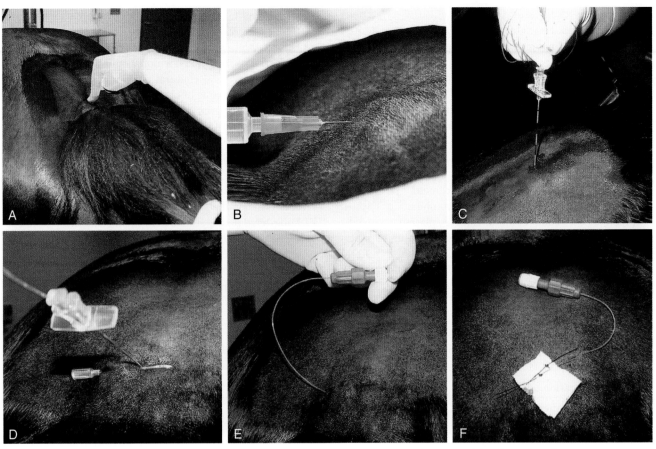

Figure 49-3   **A** to **F,** Step-by-step depiction of the placement of a 20-gauge radiopaque and closed tip polyamide epidural catheter into the first intercoccygeal space using an 18-gauge, 3½-inch (8.9-cm) Tuohy Schliff epidural needle for entrance into the epidural space (Perifix epidural catheter set). See text for detailed information.

Tuohy needle and place a drop of sterile saline solution into the hub of the needle; as soon as the epidural space has been entered, the saline drop is aspirated into the needle because of the negative pressure in the epidural space.

- *Loss of resistance techniques.* After sudden loss of resistance is noted following penetration of the interarcuate ligament, remove the stylet and attach a 5-mL syringe filled with air to the Tuohy needle: loss of resistance to air injection indicates correct positioning of the needle. Alternatively, a 5-mL syringe filled with saline and an air bubble may be attached to the Tuohy needle: loss of any deformation or compression of the air bubble in the syringe during saline injection indicates the correct position of the Tuohy needle.

- Once correct location of the Tuohy needle has been verified, the catheter can be advanced into the epidural space. Some resistance may be felt at the time the catheter tip is exiting the end of the needle, but thereafter the catheter can be pushed forward with little resistance. Any significant resistance at this point indicates that the catheter is *not* in the epidural space. The catheter should be advanced for a minimum of 10 cm in a cranial direction, that is, 2 cm beyond the end of the

Tuohy needle to avoid pulling out of the epidural space; it may also be advanced cranially for up to 30 to 35 cm.

- Once the catheter has been advanced to the desired length, carefully retract the Tuohy needle while one hand of the operator holds the catheter in place. To prevent the catheter from pulling out of the puncture site in the skin, the free end of the catheter should be tunneled subcutaneously using a 16-gauge hypodermic needle, forming a loop that can be fixed to the skin with a butterfly-shaped tape flap (Fig. 49-3, *D*). Simple polyamide catheters may be trimmed to a length of 10 to 20 cm extending from the skin before being capped with an adaptor with injection port (Fig. 49-3, *E*). Finally, cover the epidural site where the catheter exits the skin with a sterile dressing and secure the catheter loop using a butterfly-shaped tape or other suitable padding and suture or staple it to the skin (Fig. 49-3, *F*).

- Attachment of an epidural catheter to a lightweight, battery-powered mini-infusion pump[3] or a viscoelastic pump[4] that can be mounted on the equine patient allows continuous epidural drug infusion.

[3]Curlin 6000 CMS, B. Braun Medical, Inc., Bethlehem, Pennsylvania.
[4]ON-Q system (I-Flow Corp., Lake Forest, California).

- Continuous drug infusion reduces the risk of catheter contamination associated with intermittent drug administration and reduces the risk of early clotting of catheters.
- Epidural catheters have been kept in place for up to 28 days.
- Contraindications to caudal epidural catheter placement:
  - Skin infection at the site of catheter insertion
  - Spinal cord disease
  - Preexisting impairment of motor function (pelvic limb ataxia, reduced proprioception)

Indications for Epidural Catheter Placement

- Depending on the drug or drug combination selected (Table 49-5), caudal epidural catheter placement may be indicated in a wide variety of patients with various surgical and nonsurgical conditions associated with significant pain. Examples include problems involving the rectum, anus, perineum, tail, urethra, bladder, kidneys, uterus, vulva, vagina, pelvis, hind limbs, and potentially even forelimbs.
- Patients with persistent, moderate to severe pain in the hind part of their body, which would require repeated or continuous caudal epidural drug administration, benefit from this technique of pain management.
- When administered in volumes of 50 to 70 mL epidurally, opioids (e.g., morphine 0.05 to 0.3 mg/kg; methadone 0.1 mg/kg) diffuse far enough cranially to reach the thoracic and cervical segments of the spinal cord. Therefore, these opioids may also inhibit nociception originating from organs and tissues within the thoracic cavities, abdominal and chest walls, as well as the thoracic limbs.
- Long-term postoperative pain management is possible.
- Patients, in which the duration of a surgical procedure is likely to exceed the duration of action of a one-time local anesthetic or analgesic administration may require repeated epidural drug dosing.

Table 49-5   **Drug Regimens Used for Epidural Anesthesia/Analgesia and Reported Volumes and Dosages**

Drug (Concentration or Dosage)	Volume (mL)	Site of Injection	Onset / Duration of Effect (hours)	Comments
Caudal Epidural Anesthesia/Analgesia				
(a) Single drug				
Lidocaine 1%-2%	5-8	Co_1-Co_2	0.5 / 0.75-1.5	Repeated injections of 3 mL at 1-hr intervals
Lidocaine 1%	20	Co_1-Co_2	0.75 / 3.0	Causes moderate ataxia
Mepivacaine 2%	5-8	Co_1-Co_2	0.5 / 1.5-3.0	
Bupivacaine 0.2%-0.5%	5-8	Co_1-Co_2	0.5 / 3.0-8.0	
Ropivacaine 0.2%-0.5%	5-10	Co_1-Co_2	0.5 / 3.0-8.0	Fast onset of effect (10 min); less risk of ataxia
Xylazine, 0.17 mg/kg	10	Co_1-Co_2	0.5 / 1.0-1.5	May cause sedation/ataxia
Detomidine, 30 µg/kg	10	Co_1-Co_2	0.5 / 2-4	May cause sedation/ataxia
Dexmedetomidine, 1.0-2.5 µg/kg	10-30	Co_1-Co_2	0.5 / 4-6	May cause sedation/ataxia
Morphine, 0.05-0.2 mg/kg	10-30 (up to 50)	Co_1-Co_2	1-3 / 3-16	Also useful for CRI (0.5-2 mL/h) via epidural catheter
Methadone, 0.1 mg/kg	10-30 (up to 50)	Co_1-Co_2	0.5-1.0 / 5	
Ketamine, 0.5-2.0 mg/kg	10-30	Co_1-Co_2	0.5 / 0.5-1.25	
(b) Drug combinations("balanced regional analgesia")				
Lidocaine 2% + Xylazine, 0.17 mg/kg	5-8	Co_1-Co_2	0.5 / 4-6	
Lidocaine 2% + Morphine, 0.1-0.2 mg/kg	5-8	Co_1-Co_2	0.5 / 4-6	
Bupivacaine 0.125% + Morphine, 0.1-0.3 mg/kg	10-30	Co_1-Co_2/L-S	0.5-0.75 / 8 to >12	Also useful for CRI (0.5-2 mL/h) via epidural catheter
Xylazine, 0.17 mg/kg + Morphine, 0.1-0.3 mg/kg	10-30	Co_1-Co_2/L-S	0.5-1.0 / ≥12	
Detomidine, 30 µg/kg + Morphine, 0.1-0.3 mg/kg	10	Co_1-Co_2/L-S	0.5 / 24-48	For mild-to-moderate pain
Detomidine, 30 µg/kg + Morphine, 0.1-0.3 mg/kg	10	Co_1-Co_2/L-S	0.5 / 6-8	For severe pain
Lidocaine 1%-2% plus	5	Co_1-Co_2	0.5-1.0 / 0.75-1.5	Via Tuohy needle before epidural catheter placement
Morphine, 0.1-0.2 mg/kg + Bupivacaine 0.125%	together in 30	L-S	0.5-1.0 / 12 to >24	Via epidural catheter advanced ≥5 cm cranially

CRI, Constant rate infusion.

Risks, Side Effects, and Complications Associated with Repeated or Continuous Caudal Epidural Anesthesia and Analgesia

- Proprioceptive deficits caused by A_β-fiber blockade
  - May occur with all local anesthetics and xylazine
- Motor blockade evident as ataxia or sudden recumbency and caused by blockade of motor neurons
  - May occur with all local anesthetics
    - Less risk with ropivacaine than other local anesthetics
    - Increased risk when local anesthetics are administered in large volumes or via a catheter advanced further cranially into the lumbosacral epidural space
    - Significantly reduced risk when using long-acting local anesthetics at low concentrations (e.g., bupivacaine 0.125% or ropivacaine 0.125% to 0.180%)
  - Alpha$_2$-agonists at higher doses
- Blockade of sympathetic nerve fibers
  - May occur with local anesthetics only
- Systemic side effects caused by rapid systemic absorption:
  - Sedation (especially alpha$_2$-agonists [detomidine > xylazine])
  - Excitement (opioids; rare)
  - Mild to moderate cardiopulmonary and gastrointestinal effects (especially alpha$_2$-agonists)
    - Hypertension
    - Bradycardia and bradyarrhythmias
    - Hypotension
    - Respiratory depression
    - Decreased gut motility
- Pruritus
  - Opioids (more common)
  - Alpha$_2$-agonists (rare)

References

References can be found on the companion website at www.equine-emergencies.com.

ANESTH

CHAPTER 50

Medical Management of the Starved Horse

Dominic Dawson Soto

Etiology

- Underlying disease
- Owner negligence or abuse
- Insufficient resources for environmental conditions
- Herd dynamics
- Dental disease

Diagnosis and Initial Assessment

- Loss of body weight (body condition score (BCS) ≤3) or poor growth in young horses. See Table 50-1 for BCS calculations.
- Rough hair coat with poor shedding
- Depression
- Severity is cumulative and can be defined as:
  - Partial
  - Complete
- Can occur over weeks to months depending on etiology
- Question caretaker carefully on:
  - Feeding
  - Housing
  - Water access
  - Herd dynamics
  - Vaccination
  - Deworming
  - Dental care
  - Routine health maintenance
- Inspect premises for adequate water, forage, and/or concentrates (tactfully ask about feed receipts if necessary)
- Record BCSs on herd mates.
- Check for pregnancy in females
- If negligence or abuse is suspected, contact the local authorities immediately and carefully document, by written and photographic records:
  - Conditions of the patient
  - Housing, feed/water
  - Herd mates

- Perform a comprehensive physical examination; a heart murmur (i.e., aortic region systolic murmur) may be present with anemia secondary to chronic disease and/or malnutrition.
- Complete blood count and blood chemistry are needed to assess for underlying disease, dehydration, and secondary complications from starvation such as anemia. Special testing for glucose, triglycerides, and electrolytes (Na^+, K^+, PO_4^{3-}, and Mg^{2+}) may also be necessary. Use caution when interpreting electrolytes (i.e., Na^+, K^+, PO_4^{3-}, and Mg^{2+}) because serum measurements can be within reference intervals despite total body deficits, i.e., maintained at sufficient serum levels while depleted intracellularly.
- *Practice Tip: Routine laboratory findings supporting starvation:*
  - *Hypoproteinemia*
  - *Hyperbilirubinemia*
  - *Hypertriglyceridemia*
- *Note:* If fat stores are depleted, triglycerides may be normal.
- Muscle wasting indicates *severe* starvation.
- Horses that have lost up to or over 40% of their body weight may be recumbent.
- *Practice Tip: Decubitus ulcers may develop more quickly after recumbency in starved horses, often after only 48 hours of recumbency.*
- Observe for evidence of specific mineral deficiencies secondary to malnutrition:
  - White muscle disease—vitamin E and/or selenium deficiency
  - Rickets—vitamin D deficiency
- Necropsy findings if horse was recumbent:
  - Severe serous fat atrophy
  - Muscle wasting
  - Decubitus ulcers

Table 50-1	Characteristics of Individual Body Condition Scores					
Condition	**Neck**	**Withers**	**Loin**	**Tailhead**	**Ribs**	**Shoulder**
1 Poor	Bone structure easily noticeable; horse extremely emaciated; no fatty tissue can be felt	Bone structure easily noticeable	Spinous processes project prominently	Spinous processes project prominently	Tailhead (tuber ischii or tuber sacralae) and hook bones project prominently	Bone structure easily noticeable
2 Very Thin	Faintly discernible, horse emaciated	Faintly discernible	Slight fat covering over base of spinous processes, transverse processes of lumbar vertebrae feel rounded, spinous processes are prominent	Tailhead prominent	Slight fat cover over ribs; ribs easily discernible	Shoulder accentuated
3 Thin	Neck accentuated	Withers accentuated	Fat buildup halfway on spinous processes but easily discernible, transverse processes cannot be felt	Tailhead prominent but individual vertebrae cannot be visually identified, tuber coxae appear rounded but are still easily discernible, tuber ischii not distinguishable	Slight fat cover over ribs; ribs easily discernible	Shoulder accentuated
4 Moderately Thin	Neck not obviously thin	Withers not obviously thin	Negative crease along back	Prominence depends on conformation; fat can be felt, tuber coxae not discernible	Faint outline discernible	Shoulder not obviously thin
5 Moderate	Neck blends smoothly into body	Withers rounded over spinous processes	Back is level	Fat around tailhead beginning to feel spongy	Ribs cannot be visually distinguished but can be easily felt	Shoulder blends smoothly into body
6 Moderately Fleshy	Fat beginning to be deposited	Fat beginning to be deposited	May have slight positive crease down back	Fat around tailhead feels soft	Fat over ribs feels spongy	Fat beginning to be deposited
7 Fleshy	Fat deposited along neck	Fat deposited along neck	May have positive crease down back	Fat around tailhead is soft	Individual ribs can be felt, but noticeable filling between ribs with fat	Fat deposited behind shoulder
8 Fat	Noticeable thickening of neck, fat deposited along inner buttocks	Area along withers filled with fat	Positive crease down back	Tailhead fat, very soft	Difficult to feel ribs	Area behind shoulder filled in flush with body
9 Extremely Fat	Bulging fat, fat along inner buttocks may rub together, flanks filled in flush	Bulging fat	Obvious positive crease down back	Bulging fat around tailhead	Patchy fat appearing over ribs	Bulging fat

From Henneke et al: *Equine Vet J* 15(4):371-372, 1983.

NUTR

◉› WHAT TO DO

Starvation Cases That Are Not Experiencing Refeeding Syndrome

- If electrolytes are stable, feed high-quality, leafy alfalfa hay at 50% to 75% of DE of ideal body weight for first 5 days divided into small, frequent meals.
- Recognize patients at risk for developing RFS.
- Monitor vital signs (TRR) and electrolytes during first 5 to 7 days of refeeding.
- Document horse's BCS along with living and feeding conditions.
- If horse is tolerating refeeding with no signs of RFS, increase to 100% DE of ideal body weight over days 7-10.
- Fresh, clean water or water with electrolytes (Na or KCl) should be offered often.

BCS, Body condition score; *DE,* digestible energy; *RFS,* refeeding syndrome.

Refeeding Syndrome

- *Refeeding syndrome* (RFS) encompasses the metabolic, electrolyte, and organ dysfunction occurring as a result of reintroduction of feed nutrition, particularly carbohydrates, in the chronically malnourished patient. Derangements of the cardiovascular, respiratory, and neurologic systems can occur, and if RFS remains untreated, death may occur.
- Hallmarks of RFS include:
  - Severe hypophosphatemia—hypophosphatemia may occur following carbohydrate/glucose supplementation and is believed to be responsible for much of the progressive weakness seen in RFS.
  - Hypokalemia
  - Hypomagnesaemia
  - Potentially glucose derangements because of sudden glucose increases in a body adapted for fat metabolism
  - Hyponatremia or hypernatremia
  - Fluid overload
  - Vitamin (i.e., thiamine) and trace mineral deficiencies
  - Possible hypocalcemia
- *Practice Tip: The reintroduction of carbohydrates causes the release of insulin, leading to influx of glucose and other electrolytes into the cell, resulting in serum electrolyte deficiencies (e.g., phosphorus and potassium).*
- Initial clinical signs may include:
  - Cardiac arrhythmias and/or insufficiency
  - Peripheral edema
  - Respiratory failure due to diaphragmatic dysfunction
  - Rhabdomyolysis
  - Seizures
  - Weakness, coma, and/or death within the first 3 to 5 days after initiation of refeeding
- *Note: Hypophosphatemia* may occur even if phosphate levels are within reference intervals at the start of refeeding due to glucose/insulin-driven cellular uptake of phosphate allowing for:
  - Phosphorylation of glucose
  - Synthesis of adenosine triphosphate (ATP), proteins, and other essential compounds after glucose absorption

- *Anemia* may occur due to decreased PO_4 in RBCs. Anemia can lead to:
  - Hemolysis
  - Inadequate oxygen delivery to tissues
  - If left untreated, generalized ischemia and multiple organ failure
- *Fluid overload* can occur as a result of insulin-driven retention of Na^+.
- *Practice Tip: Parenteral feeding may have a higher risk for RFS and therefore enteral or oral feeding is recommended if possible; however, these are not without some risk.*
- Concentrations of *thiamine*, along with other vitamins, can decrease dramatically during starvation. Thiamine levels can decrease further as glucose metabolism begins at initial refeeding. Along with causing neurologic abnormalities such as ataxia and muscle tremors, thiamine deficiency inhibits aerobic metabolism, eventually leading to lactic acidosis.
- *Infections* may be more common because hyperglycemia inhibits appropriate neutrophil function.
- Alfalfa-based diets may improve Mg^{2+} levels.
- Oversupplementation with PO_4^{3-} may lead to:
  - Hypocalcemia
  - Hyperkalemia
  - Hypernatremia
- All electrolyte abnormalities should be corrected before refeeding, especially PO_4^{3-}, Mg^{2+}, and K^+ ($MgSO_4$, 50 to 100 mg/kg IV SID; PO_4^{3-}, 0.6 mg/kg/h and monitor q6h or 1200 to 1500 mg/day PO; K^+, 0.02 to 0.08 mEq/kg/L—*do not exceed* 0.5 mEq/kg/L). If phosphorus is less than 0.5 mg/dL, 2 to 5 mL of a sterile aqueous phosphate enema solution, which would supply approximately 170 mg P/mL, (do *not* use enema solutions with mineral oil) can be administered IV, at 0.6 mg/kg per hour or 50 mL can be given per rectum. If the patient is too weak to eat, enteral feeding can be started with electrolyte solutions containing Na^+, Cl^-, K^+, PO_4^-, Mg^{2+}, and dextrose (do not use dextrose solution, 5%).

◉› WHAT TO DO

Refeeding Syndrome

- Offer shelter if possible.
- If recumbent, assist to stand, and if severe, provide sling support (see Chapter 37, p. 634).
- Slow or discontinue nutritional support until patient's electrolytes and metabolic systems normalize. Dextrose in a balanced electrolyte solution can be started to prevent reflex hypoglycemia and hypophosphatemia. Once the patient is stable and symptoms of RFS have resolved, nutritional support can be restarted at ≤50% of previous rate when signs first developed.
- Rehydration should be incrementally performed. Starvation may cause hyponatremia or hypernatremia depending on concurrent water deprivation. Administer 2 to 4 L orally about 20 to 30 minutes apart until avid thirst has abated. If Na^+ derangements are present for >24 hours, adjustments in Na^+ administration should be no quicker than 0.5 mEq/L/h. Administer IV fluids if needed.
- Treat any fluid overload with diuretics (monitor K^+ closely if K^+-wasting diuretics are used, such as furosemide).
- Treat respiratory distress with oxygen supplementation.

- Monitor electrolytes during supplementation (PO_4^- as often as q4 to 6h; Mg^{2+} q12 to 24h) if severe derangements develop that require aggressive supplementation.
- Treat hypomagnesemia promptly ($MgSO_4$, 50 to 100 mg/kg IV q24h) because this can cause refractory hypocalcemia and hypokalemia.
- Provide phosphorus supplementation, PO and IV with severe hypophosphatemia (see previous page).
- Thiamine (10 mg/kg IM or IV diluted in fluids) should be given before and during any nutritional supplementation.
- Vitamin C can also be given (0.022 to 0.44 mg/kg PO q24h) during nutritional supplementation.
- If enteral or parenteral supplementation is used, begin at 25% of estimated goal needs for the first 24 hours and gradually increase up to 100% over 3 to 5 days, monitoring the patient closely for any signs of RFS.
- Provide trace minerals (especially selenium, zinc, and iron) if deficiencies are likely.
- Delayed gastric emptying and decreased absorptive capabilities of intestinal villi may develop after 72 hours of starvation. Therefore, simple nutrients that require minimal digestion may be warranted in the early stages.
- ***Practice Tip:*** *Horses able to eat forage should be given small and frequent meals and monitored for dysphagia and/or signs of choke because starved horses may ravenously consume food.* If electrolytes are stable, forage should be fed at 50% to 75% of the calculated daily digestible energy (DE) requirement (Mcal DE/day = 1.4 + 0.03 BW, where BW is their estimated ideal weight) divided into small, frequent meals for the first 5 days. After 5 days a gradual increase up to 100% of their DE, based on their ideal body weight, can be achieved over the next 1 to 2 days.
- Diagnose and treat, if possible, any underlying causes (e.g., infection, pituitary pars intermedia dysfunction, severe dental disease). Deworming and extensive diagnostics and/or procedures should be delayed if possible until the affected individual is clinically stable.
- Antibiotics may be indicated if primary or secondary infection is diagnosed.
- ***Caution:*** Highly protein-bound drugs (i.e., lidocaine, phenylbutazone) should be administered with caution if patient is hypoalbuminemic to minimize adverse events.

Monitoring
- Daily vital signs (temperature, pulse, and respiration [TPR]), mentation, and daily weight gain if possible
- Urine output
- Perform an electrocardiogram (ECG) during first 7 days if electrolyte abnormalities are present and/or with the use of supplementation
  Important Note: Hypokalemia can lead to atrial and ventricular arrhythmias.
- Monitor plasma glucose q4 to 6h if possible until stable
- Monitor electrolytes daily, especially Mg^{2+}, K^+, Na^+, PO_4^-, and Ca^{2+} until stabilized
- Elevated free fatty acid levels may drop within days of refeeding
- Anemia may take longer than 10 days to resolve
- Monitor for evidence of fluid overload:
  - Peripheral edema
  - Increased respiratory rate or effort
  - Increased jugular pulses
- ***Important Note:*** Even patients on hypocaloric formulations can develop RFS; therefore, careful monitoring is warranted.

Prognosis
- It may require 6 to 10 months to reach acceptable body condition score depending on severity of emaciation.
- Horses recumbent for >72 hours or a BCS of 1/9 have a grave prognosis.

◉〉 WHAT NOT TO DO

Refeeding Syndrome
- Do not feed concentrates or carbohydrate-dense feeds.
- Do not cause hyperglycemia.
- Do not utilize aggressive fluid therapy for rehydration.

References
References can be found on the companion website at www.equine-emergencies.com.

NUTR

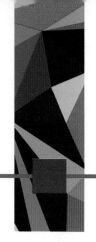

CHAPTER 51

Nutritional Guidelines for the Injured, Hospitalized, and Postsurgical Patient

Raymond J. Geor

- Assessment of nutritional status and the development of a feeding plan are important considerations in the overall management of injured, hospitalized, and postsurgical patients. In human medicine, both nutritional status at the time of injury or hospitalization and subsequent dietary management affect morbidity and mortality.
- Nutrient deprivation is associated with:
  - Immunosuppression
  - Alterations in gastrointestinal function, including:
    - Decreased motility
    - Villus atrophy
    - Decrease in gut barrier function due to an increase in intestinal permeability, particularly in patients with preexisting malnutrition
- Early nutritional intervention is known to improve health outcomes in human and animal studies.
- Although there are little data on the effects of different feeding practices on short- and long-term outcomes in sick, injured, or postsurgical horses, it is reasonable to assume that nutrition also impacts the recovery of equine patients.
- *Practice Tip: Healthy adult horses in good body condition can tolerate 2 to 3 days of feed withdrawal without ill effect.*
- Acute starvation invokes neuroendocrine responses that lower metabolic rate, conserve lean tissues (i.e., skeletal muscle), and promote use of fat stores to meet energy demands, which is a strategy to sustain bodily functions in the face of nutrient deprivation.
- The metabolic response to critical illness (e.g., sepsis, severe trauma, burn injury, or major surgical intervention) contrasts with that of simple starvation.
  - Increased sympathetic nervous system activity, inflammatory cytokines (e.g., interleukin [IL]-1β, IL-2, IL-6, tumor necrosis factor-α), and catabolic hormones (catecholamines, cortisol, and glucagon) combine to increase metabolic rate and induce a state of hypercatabolism.
  - Stimulation of proteolytic pathways in skeletal muscle provides amino acids for hepatic gluconeogenesis and synthesis of acute phase proteins. Amino acids (from catabolism of lean tissues) rather than fatty acids are the primary source of energy substrate. This hypercatabolic state can result in large nitrogen losses, severe muscle wasting, and compromise of immune function and tissue healing.

Assessment of Nutritional Status

- At presentation, or soon after initial assessment and institution of emergency treatment measures, an assessment of the horse's nutritional status should be performed. This guides the development of a nutritional plan including the need for assisted nutritional support or other form of special nutrition.
- The assessment should include:
  - Body condition score
  - Assessment of appetite
  - Identification of neurologic deficits or physical injury that may preclude or limit oral feed intake (e.g., fractured mandible or esophageal injury)
- *Practice Tips:*
  - *Horses in poor body condition (Henneke body condition score [BCS] <3; i.e., ribs easily seen, a concave neck, vertebral processes prominent in loin and tailhead area) may have impaired wound healing and be at increased risk of nosocomial infections.*
  - *Obese horses (BCS 8 to 9) are at greater risk for development of hypertriglyceridemia and potentially life-threatening hyperlipemia (mostly in ponies, donkeys, and Miniature horses) when inappetence or inanition (starvation) persists for more than 24 to 48 hours.*
- If possible, a dietary history should be obtained including the types and amounts of forages, feeds and other supplements provided, pasture access, and whether or not there has been a recent change in diet (e.g., an acute increase in the amount of grain fed or a change in type or batch of hay fed). This information may provide an indication as to the cause of the presenting problem (i.e., nutrition-associated laminitis, colic, or toxicities). Additionally, knowledge of the recent/current ration assists in the avoidance of an unintended major change in diet (type and amount of feed) that may cause additional problems during the period of hospitalization.
- If possible, serum triglyceride concentrations should be measured.
- *Practice Tip: Hypertriglyceridemia is a useful indicator of negative energy balance and the need for nutritional intervention, and serial measurements of serum triglycerides can be used to judge the efficacy of nutritional support.*
- Overweight and obese equids, especially ponies, donkeys and Miniature horses, are at risk to develop hypertriglyceridemia and hyperlipemia. Marked hypertriglyceridemia,

>500 mg/dL, has been described in horses with colic and/ or colitis that had clinical and/or laboratory evidence of systemic inflammation. The increase in circulating lipids likely reflects an increase in the mobilization of fat reserves (lipolysis) and a decrease in lipid clearance from blood. In affected horses, treatment with an intravenous dextrose solution or partial parenteral nutrition results in a decrease in serum triglyceride concentrations to reference limits and an improved appetite coincident with a decrease in circulating lipids.

Options for Nutritional Management

- Nutritional management of the injured, hospitalized, or postsurgical patient typically falls into one of the following categories:
  - No change in diet composition or amount or, at least, provision of forage and feed of the same type and quantity as provided before hospitalization
  - An increase in the variety of feedstuffs offered as a way to entice intake in horses with poor appetite
  - A change in amount, composition, and/or physical form of the ration based on medical or surgical condition (e.g., nutritionally associated laminitis, postcolic surgery, slurry diet for a horse with a fractured mandible). This includes a simple reduction in feed amount based on decreased caloric requirements in the face of stall confinement.
  - Assisted enteral feeding
  - Parenteral (intravenous) feeding
- Many sick or injured horses do *not* require special nutrition (e.g., severe lacerations or fractures, excluding mandibular fractures, in horses of good body condition with normal appetite). These horses should be provided a ration commensurate with physiologic status and activity level.
  - For mature (adult) horses, this typically comprises maintenance amounts (≈1.5% to 2.0% body weight [BW]/day) of good-quality forage (preferably the type fed before injury) with free access to water and salt.
  - Activity level is most often reduced because of stall confinement and, in general, mature horses do *not* require supplemental grain or feeds unless they are unable to maintain body weight and condition on the hay-only ration.
- *Practice Tips:*
  - *Growing horses (<2 years of age) and lactating mares should receive supplemental feed formulated for, respectively, growth and lactation, with the daily ration divided into 2 or 3 feedings.*
  - *Late pregnant mares (months 8 to 11) should be provided 0.5 to 1.0 kg/day of a "balancer" feed fortified with sources of protein/amino acids, vitamins, and minerals to ensure that the nutritional requirements of the mare and developing fetus are met.*
- The appetite of sick horses is often poor initially but gradually improves during convalescence; therefore, carefully monitor feed intake during the first few days of case management.

- Provide a variety of palatable feedstuffs (e.g., high-quality grass or legume hay, soaked hay cubes, small amounts [0.5 to 1.0 kg/meal] of commercial grain-based or fat-and-fiber–based feeds, the addition of molasses) to entice increased intake.
- Critically ill horses are often very selective about their food, and therefore it is important to remove any uneaten food and offer fresh food at each feeding interval.
- Fever, pain, and systemic inflammation all may reduce appetite, and thus the administration of nonsteroidal anti-inflammatory drugs also can help to improve feed intake.

●❯ WHAT TO DO

Supplemental Nutrition in the Critically Ill Horse

- Horses that have *not* eaten or consume <50% of daily nutrient needs for 48 to 72 hours are candidates for assisted nutritional support. Earlier implementation of nutritional support should be considered for horses with:
  - Increased metabolic demands in the face of poor appetite and feed intake (e.g., lactating mares, young growing horses)
  - Underlying endocrine and metabolic abnormalities that may worsen with a further period of little or no feed intake (e.g., obese horses with hypertriglyceridemia—triglycerides >500 mg/dL)
  - Ponies, donkeys, and Miniature horses
  - Metabolic syndrome or pituitary pars intermedia dysfunction
  - Severe illness that most likely results in increased metabolic demands and/or protein losses (e.g., sepsis, colitis, duodenitis-proximal jejunitis)

Estimating Nutrient and Feed Requirements

- The nutritional requirements of sick or severely injured horses have *not* been determined; therefore, recommendations are largely based on the requirements of healthy horses. Although severe illness or trauma, including surgery, may increase metabolic (energy) demands, overall energy requirement may be similar to that of healthy horses at maintenance because of decreased physical activity and reduced metabolic demands of digestion in the face of decreased feed intake.
- *Practice Tip 1: For most hospitalized or convalescing horses, the resting energy requirement (RER) is an appropriate target for initial nutritional management, where RER = [21 kcal × BW (kg)] + 975 kcal or approximately 23 kcal digestible energy (DE)/kg/day (≈11.5 Mcal/day for a 500-kg horse). The RER represents the energy requirements of horses kept in a stall with minimal to no activity ("stall maintenance").*
- *Practice Tip 2: With parenteral feeding, 80% of the RER (≈18 kcal/kg/day) is suggested as the initial caloric target because of a concern that overfeeding of calories may increase risk of complications such as hyperglycemia and hyperinsulinemia.*
- *Practice Tip 3: For easy reference, the true maintenance requirement for mature horses under normal living conditions is 30 to 35 kcal DE/kg/day (National Research Council [NRC], 2007); this level of DE intake may not be required until the horse returns to normal management after recovery from illness or injury.*

- Growing horses and late pregnant and lactating mares have higher energy requirements and this should be considered in the development of a nutritional plan (NRC, 2007).
- It is important to realize that individual horses have unique nutritional requirements; therefore, the calculated energy needs offered only represent a starting point.
- Regular measurement of bodyweight and assessment of BCS should be undertaken to judge the adequacy of energy provision and to provide a basis for adjustments in feeding.
- Protein requirements must be considered in light of caloric intake and underlying disease process.
  - ***Practice Tip:*** *When energy supply from carbohydrate and fat is limited, endogenous protein is used for energy, contributing to a loss of lean body mass. Therefore, develop a nutritional plan to first ensure that minimal energy needs are met, and then calculate protein requirements.*
  - For humans, suggested protein requirements range between 1.2 and 2.0 g protein/kg/day, with the higher end of this range recommended for patients undergoing major intestinal surgery.
- The crude protein (CP) requirement of healthy adult horses can be calculated from the equation:
  - CP (grams) = $40 \times$ DE (Mcal DE/day);
  - For a 500-kg horse at maintenance that is consuming ~16 Mcal DE per day, this equals 1.25 g CP/kg body weight.
  - Because the efficiency of digestion for most dietary proteins in horse feeds is about 70%, this level of CP provides approximately 0.9 g available protein/kg body weight.
  - There may be justification for higher levels of dietary protein (e.g., 2 g CP/kg/day), particularly for horses in poor body condition (BCS <3) or those with sepsis, hypoproteinemia, and/or hypoalbuminemia.
  - For parenteral feeding, a lower level of protein feeding is reasonable given the higher metabolic availability of amino acids administered by the intravenous route. In reports of parenteral feeding of horses, 0.6 to 0.8 g protein/kg/day (1 g/40 to 50 kcal) was administered as a balanced amino acid solution (Durham et al, 2004).
  - Some commercial feed supplements designed for use in sick horses (e.g., Well-Solve W/G[1]) are formulated to meet or exceed the maintenance protein requirement of healthy horses at a low feeding rate (0.3% BW/day or ≈1.5 kg/day for a 500-kg horse).

Nutritional Guidelines for Specific Conditions

Gastrointestinal Disease

Feeding After General Anesthesia and Upper Gastrointestinal Surgery

- *Nongastrointestinal surgery:* Feeding can be resumed when the horse has recovered from anesthesia and clinical

assessment indicates normal gastrointestinal function. In most circumstances, feeding can be initiated at 4 to 6 hours after the end of anesthesia, starting with small amounts of hay (≈1.0 kg/meal) and water with a gradual increase in the amount fed over the following 24 hours.

- *Dental surgery:* A change in diet is *not* normally required after routine dental procedures such as tooth extractions. A long-term modification of diet may be required, however, for horses with moderate or severe periodontal disease. The feeding of short-length fiber sources (hay chop <2 cm) or a complete feed is recommended to reduce the risk of feed impaction within periodontal pockets. During the early phases of management, pain associated with periodontal disease may necessitate the feeding of a slurry diet made from soaked hay cubes or pellets.
- *Esophageal surgery:* Voluntary consumption of feed and water is contraindicated for a minimum of 48 hours after surgical procedures involving repair of full-thickness esophageal injuries. Maintenance intravenous fluid therapy is recommended, as well as a 5% dextrose solution, to provide some calories during this period of feed withholding. Subsequently, a slurry diet of soaked forage cubes or pellets or "complete feed" is offered along with pasture, if available. Affected horses should *not* be offered dry forage until after complete healing of the esophageal surgery site. In cases where the esophageal injury or wound is left to heal by secondary intention, the equine patient is fed through a feeding tube that is placed via the nose, the esophageal wound, or an esophagostomy.
- *Esophageal choke:* Voluntary consumption of water is permitted after relieving an esophageal choke, but feed is withheld for a variable time depending on the duration of the choke and whether it is a recurrent problem. A wet mash or grass is introduced as the first feeding after choke. This type of feed is continued until the esophagus is physiologically normal (i.e., barium swallow or endoscopic evaluation of the "choke" site for more chronic or complicated cases). Recurrent episodes of choke should have an endoscopic examination before refeeding.

◗▸ WHAT TO DO

General Feeding Guidelines After Lower Gastrointestinal Surgery

- *Small-intestinal surgery:* There are a variety of opinions on when to feed horses after small-intestinal surgery.
  - Some clinicians prefer to wait 24 to 36 hours after surgery, especially in cases of strangulating obstruction that necessitate resection and anastomosis of the small intestine.
  - Others favor feeding as early as 6 to 8 hours after surgery, providing there is adequate gastrointestinal function.
  - Regardless, assessment of gut function by the monitoring of heart rate, borborygmi, and ultrasonographic evidence of small-intestinal motility provides the best guide as to the timing of the reintroduction of oral intake.
  - Water and feed should *not* be offered to horses with evidence of ileus, and feeding must be stopped if there is deterioration in intestinal function.

[1]Well-Solve W/G (Land O'Lakes Purina Feed, St. Louis, Missouri).

- Parenteral feeding is recommended if ileus persists for more than 48 hours.

Feeding After Small-Intestinal Surgery
- *Practice Tips:*
  - *Water is offered at 1-hour intervals to evaluate the effects of oral intake on gut function.*
  - *If no adverse effects are detected after 3 to 4 offerings of water, small amounts (1 to 2 handfuls) of very soft feed (preferably grass) is offered at 1-hour intervals.*
  - *Providing there are no complications, larger amounts of feed are offered every 2 to 3 hours starting as early as 12 hours after surgery (e.g., 0.5 kg of grass or alfalfa hay).*
  - *The amount of feed offered is gradually increased over the next 24 to 48 hours, with a concomitant decrease in the frequency of feeding.*
  - *Cereal grains or commercial grain-based feeds should not be fed for the first 10 to 14 days after surgery.*
  - *The feeding of a soft, low-bulk ration (e.g., a complete feed formulated for senior horses) for a few days is considered if there is concern about the impact of ingesta on the anastomosis site or in situations where the equine patient exhibits signs of colic after the reintroduction of feeding.*
  - *Fresh grass, hay cubes, and pellets that have been softened in water are suitable feedstuffs.*

Feeding After Large-Intestinal Surgery
- Diarrhea is a complication of all types of colic surgery, but the risk appears to be highest in horses undergoing celiotomy for large intestinal disorders.
  - Feeding hay appears to decrease risk of diarrhea after large intestinal surgery.
  - Water is offered as early as 4 to 6 hours after surgery, followed by small amounts of grass or soft grass hay (≈0.5 kg) at frequent intervals (every 2 to 3 hours) starting at 6 to 8 hours after surgery provided there is *no* evidence of gastric reflux or poor intestinal motility.
  - First cut hay is preferred because of higher dry matter digestibility compared with more mature forages. The equine patient is allowed to graze in-hand for 5 to 10 minutes, 3 to 4 times per day.
  - *No* grain or grain-based feed is fed until 10 to 14 days after surgery. A soft, low-bulk diet (as noted earlier) is recommended for feeding horses recovering from small colon surgery to limit stress on the colostomy or anastomosis site. Some clinicians also favor the nasogastric tube administration of mineral oil for the first 2 to 3 days to soften intestinal contents.

Feeding After Large Intestinal Impaction
- Horses with impaction of the large colon are fed soon after resolution of the obstruction.
- Fresh grass, alfalfa pellets, chopped alfalfa or grass hay, and other sources of highly digestible fiber are preferred. Pelleted feeds allow for increased rate of passage because of smaller particle size when compared with long-stem roughage.
- *Practice Tip: Careful dietary management is required of horses recovering from cecal impaction.*

- Affected horses are prone to reimpaction after resumption of feeding, perhaps reflecting a persistent decrease in cecal motility associated with marked distention of the cecum.
- Low-bulk pelleted feeds rather than long-stem hay are recommended during the first 10 to 14 days after cecal impaction. Careful clinical monitoring (e.g., repeat ultrasonographic examinations and palpations per rectum) is important during the first 48 to 72 hours when risk of reimpaction is highest.
- A thorough oral examination is recommended to determine whether poor mastication of feed is an underlying cause of the impaction.
- If sand accumulation is the cause of the impaction/colic, and there is risk of further sand ingestion, then administration of psyllium (0.5 to 1 g/kg BW daily) is indicated to enhance fecal sand output (see Chapter 18, p. 205).

Feeding a Horse with Diarrhea
- Systemic illness associated with acute colitis can result in inappetence or anorexia and parenteral feeding is often indicated.
- Grass hay is the primary component of the ration for affected horses that are willing to eat. In theory, colitis/diarrhea is associated with a decrease in intestinal transit time, raising the possibility of a more marked cecal delivery of feed ingredients normally digested in the small intestine (i.e., vegetable oils, nonstructural carbohydrate [NSC]).
- *Practice Tip: Dietary restriction of NSC (grains, grain-based feeds, access to rapidly growing pasture rich in fructans and other sugars and vegetable oils) is recommended until diarrhea has resolved.*
- Poor appetite is not uncommon and offering small amounts of different foods, even those that are not ideal, may stimulate their appetite.
- Initially, small (≈1.0 kg), frequent (6 to 8 times/day) meals of grass hay should be fed, with a steady return to the normal feeding pattern as the horse recovers.
- Other sources of highly digestible fibers such as sugar beet pulp (pre-soaked in clean water) may be offered.
- Abnormal serum concentrations of electrolytes (e.g., potassium, sodium, chloride, calcium, and magnesium) are commonly observed in horses with diarrhea. Oral electrolyte supplementation (e.g., NaCl, KCl, and/or $MgCl_2$,) is used as an adjunct to other fluid therapy.
- The administration of prebiotics (e.g., *Saccharomyces boulardi*) and other supplements purported to function as intestinal protectants or absorbents (e.g., di-tri-octahedral smectite; Bio-Sponge[2]) may be beneficial.

Laminitis
- Laminitis may develop under four major circumstances:
  - In association with sepsis/systemic inflammatory conditions (e.g., gastrointestinal disease, septic metritis, pneumonia)
  - Secondary to grain overload or pasture grazing
  - Horses with endocrine/metabolic diseases (equine metabolic syndrome and pituitary pars intermedia dysfunction)
  - Mechanical overload (supporting limb laminitis)

---

[2]Bio-Sponge (Platinum Performance, Buellton, California).

- Regardless of inciting cause, modification of the ration is usually required to avoid the potential for diet-associated exacerbation of the laminitis.
- Similar principles apply in the dietary management of horses and ponies that develop pasture-associated laminitis.
  - Affected horses must be removed from pasture, housed either in a dry lot (mild laminitis) or a box stall with deep bedding (more severe laminitis) and introduced to a low NSC, preserved forage-based ration with an appropriate forage balancer.
  - The duration of confinement and restricted diet, as well as decisions regarding a return to pasture grazing, depends on the severity and time course of the laminitis and the presence of underlying endocrine and metabolic problems.

●› WHAT TO DO

Feeding a Horse with Laminitis
- Removal of feeds that may have been involved in the development of laminitis and have the potential to exacerbate severity of current laminitis is essential.
- In horses that have consumed excessive grain but do *not* have clinical signs of grain overload, withhold feed for 24 hours followed by a gradual introduction to feeding of hay or alternate preserved forage over the next 24 to 48 hours (see Chapter 18, p. 184).
- Restriction of NSC intake (i.e., hay with NSC content <10% to 12% dry matter [DM]) is recommended to minimize postfeeding increases in circulating insulin that may increase risk for development of laminitis.
- For horses with clinical signs of grain overload, feed should be withheld until resolution of signs of colic, gastric/large intestinal distention, and gastric reflux.
- If laminitis does *not* develop, a gradual return to normal diet can be started 48 to 72 hours after grain engorgement.
- Conversely, a longer period of special dietary management is indicated for horses that develop laminitis; hay with low NSC content (<10% to 12% DM) should be fed at 1.5% to 2% of BW until resolution of laminitis.
- An appropriate "ration balancer" feed, 0.5 to 1.0 kg/day for a 400- to 600-kg horse, is added to the diet for amino acids, vitamins, and minerals lacking in the hay ration.
- Alternatively, a complete diet appropriately fortified and shown to produce a low glycemic/insulinemic response can be fed.
- In the unusual situation that the equine patient needs additional calories, they should be provided in the form of fat and not carbohydrates.

Renal Failure
- In horses with evidence of acute renal failure (or injury), or an acute exacerbation of chronic renal failure, nutritional support generally involves offering a variety of highly palatable feeds to encourage voluntary intake. Affected horses often have a poor appetite and assisted enteral or parenteral feeding is recommended when feed intake remains below requirements for >48 hours.
- Renal tubular dysfunction with a resultant "wasting" of sodium and chloride can persist for some time after

recovery from the acute renal insult. Loose salt (25 g twice daily for a 500-kg horse) and/or a hypotonic saline solution (0.45% NaCl) is offered to compensate for these ongoing urinary losses.
- ***Practice Tip:*** *Loss of body condition/muscle mass is a primary concern in horses with chronic renal disease.*

●› WHAT TO DO

Feeding a Horse with Renal Failure
- Good-quality grass hay should be the primary component of the diet with avoidance of legume hays (alfalfa, clover, and products) because of their high protein and calcium contents.
- Cereal grain (e.g., oats) or a commercial feed (preferably a feed with added vegetable oil) is usually indicated to increase daily energy intake and promote weight gain.
- The ration should contain an adequate but *not* excessive amount of dietary protein (1.0 to 1.5 g/kg BW/day).
- ***Practice Tip:*** *The adequacy of dietary protein intake can be indirectly assessed by monitoring the blood urea nitrogen to creatinine ratio: values >15 mg/dL suggest excessive protein intake, whereas values <10 mg/dL may indicate inadequate protein intake. A ration of grass hay plus a commercial feed or ration balancer provides at least 1.5 g protein/kg BW/day.*

Liver Failure
See Chapter 20, p. 268, for complete information on the topic.

●› WHAT TO DO

Feeding a Horse with Liver Failure
- The maintenance of blood glucose concentrations is a primary concern in acute hepatic insufficiency.
- Sweet feed or other similar grain-based feed should be provided as a supplement to forage, with the ration divided into 4 to 6 daily feedings to provide an almost continuous supply of exogenous glucose and thus reduce reliance on gluconeogenesis.
- This "trickle feeding" of the ration also may avoid disruption of the hindgut microflora, and thus reduce excessive ammonia production.
- Starch should *not* be fed at greater than 1 g/kg BW/meal (no more than 1 to 1.2 kg of sweet feed or oats per meal for a 500-kg horse).
- Avoiding large quantities of protein-rich dietary ingredients (e.g., alfalfa, soybean meal, linseed) is recommended because of a concern that a high-protein ration may precipitate or exacerbate signs of hepatoencephalopathy.
- The diet must provide adequate protein, and a commercial ration balancer product (0.5 to 1.0 kg/day) may be needed in the face of poorer quality forage.
- For horses with access to pasture, night-time turnout is recommended to avoid photodermatitis.

Refeeding the Starved Horse
- A conservative approach is indicated for the initial nutritional support of starved horses (see Chapter 50, p. 764).
- In malnourished human patients, aggressive refeeding can result in potentially fatal shifts in fluids and electrolytes

due to hormonal and metabolic responses to diet, whether enteral or parenteral, and is named *refeeding syndrome.*

- **Practice Tip:** *The hallmark biochemical feature of refeeding syndrome is hypophosphatemia, but other electrolyte abnormalities may occur, including hypokalemia and hypomagnesemia.*
- Cardiac dysfunction (e.g., arrhythmias, cardiac arrest, and neuromuscular complications) can develop as a result of these electrolyte abnormalities.
- Anecdotally, metabolic and electrolyte derangements similar to those observed in humans with refeeding syndrome have been observed in starved horses provided a diet rich in starches and sugars (i.e., high NSC).
- It is therefore recommended to restrict dietary NSC in the ration provided to chronically starved horses, specifically less than 20% NSC in the total diet.

●》 WHAT TO DO

Refeeding a Starved Horse
- In general, a predominantly forage-based diet (i.e., hay) is recommended during the rehabilitation of chronically starved horses (see Chapter 50, p. 766).
- Such horses should be fed grass or legume hay, or a mixture of the two.
- The NSC content of these forages is generally less than 15% DM. Alfalfa hay is a good choice for initial refeeding because it has a higher mineral content compared with grass hay.
- Grains (oats, corn, or barley) and sweet feeds are *not* recommended because of their high NSC content.
- It is recommended to supplement the hay ration with a vitamin-mineral supplement or ration balancer pellet.
- The energy density of the ration may be increased by the direct addition of vegetable oil (e.g., $\frac{1}{4}$ to 1 cup per day, starting at the low end of this range) or by providing a commercial fat-supplemented feed (8% to 12% fat) as fed with NSC <20%.
- **Practice Tip:** *The DE caloric requirement of starved horses should be calculated based on RER at the current BW (23 kcal/kg/day), and the true maintenance requirements at the ideal BW (30 to 35 kcal/kg/day).*
- Starved, emaciated horses may have lost 25% to 30% of BW; therefore, maintenance DE needs for ideal BW is based on 125% to 130% of BW measured at the time of first examination.
- A gradual increase in daily DE intake is recommended, starting at 25% to 50% of RER at current BW, building to 100% of resting requirements over 2 to 3 days, and followed by a gradual (over 7 to 10 days) transition to maintenance energy requirements for the ideal BW.
- Energy provision should *not* exceed 100% of resting requirements if assisted enteral feeding (AEF) is used for provision of the ration, with transition to true maintenance after the start of voluntary feed consumption.
- Regardless of feeding method (voluntary vs. AEF), the ration should be divided into 4 to 6 feedings per day during the first 10 to 14 days of rehabilitation.
- Thereafter the ration is divided into 2 to 3 meals per day.

Assisted Enteral Feeding
- Assisted enteral feeding (AEF) is accomplished by the infusion of a liquid diet through a nasogastric tube.

- Diet options include:
  - Equine and human enteral products
  - Commercial pelleted horse feeds
  - Homemade recipes
- Human formulations that have been administered to adult horses include Vital HN and Osmolyte HN.[3]
  - Both formulations are devoid of fiber, an advantage with respect to ease of administration through a small-diameter nasogastric tube but a possible cause for diarrhea when these products are fed to horses.
  - The mix of energy substrates in these fiber-free human enteral formulas differs from that in typical equine rations.
    - Osmolyte HN contains approximately 29% of calories from lipid and 54% of calories from hydrolyzable carbohydrate (mostly sugars).
    - Vital HN provides about 10% of calories from lipid and 74% from sugars.
    - The high lipid content of Osmolyte HN may contribute to digestive disturbances in horses *not* adapted to fat-supplemented rations, while use of a high carbohydrate diet such as Vital HN may be contraindicated for horses with insulin resistance.
    - Collectively, these considerations argue against the use of human enteral products in sick horses.
- Instead, enteral supplements or feeds formulated for use in horses should be used.
  - Several fiber-containing (10% to 15% crude fiber) enteral formulas for horses are commercially available in the United States (e.g., Critical Care Meals for Horses[4]; Well-Solve W/G[5]; Enteral Immunonutrition Formula[6]).
  - These products can be fed as an adjunct to other feeds (voluntary consumption) or as the sole component of the diet in AEF.
    - If using a commercially available enteral formula, follow the specific label instructions or calculate the amount to feed based on stall maintenance energy requirements.
    - A commercially available pelleted feed that contains a source of fiber, a so-called "complete feed," is a cost-effective alternative. However, a large-bore feeding tube is required for administration of these feeds.
- A suggested feeding protocol for a completed pelleted feed with supplemental vegetable oil is presented in Table 51-1. The feed in this example contains about 14% crude fiber and provides 2.6 Mcal DE/kg diet as fed. Therefore, 3.5 to 4.0 kg of diet is needed to meet the RER of a 500-kg horse.

---

[3]Vital HN and Osmolyte HN (Ross Laboratories, Columbus, Ohio).
[4]Critical Care Meals for Horses (MD's Choice, Louisville, Tennessee).
[5]Well-Solve W/G (Land O'Lakes-Purina Feed, St. Louis, Missouri).
[6]Enteral Immunonutrition Formula (Platinum Performance Vet, Buellton, California).

| Table 51-1 | **Enteral Formulation Based on a Complete Pelleted Ration with Supplemental Vegetable Oil and Recommended Feeding Schedule for a 500-kg Horse*** |

Ingredient	Day 1 (¼ ration)	Day 2 (½ ration)	Day 3 (¾ ration)	Day 4 (Full ration)
Complete pelleted horse feed (g)	885	1770	2650	3530
Vegetable oil (mL)	100	177	265	354
Water (L)	8	16	24	24
Digestible energy (Mcal)	3	6	9	12

*Energy requirements are at *stall maintenance* for a 500-kg horse (~12 Mcal DE/day). These allowances should be divided and administered into a minimum of 4 feedings daily.

- Vegetable oil (¼ to 1½ cup or 75 to 375 mL per day) is added to increase the caloric density of the diet. One standard cup (≈225 mL or 210 g) of oil provides about 1.7 Mcal of DE. Vitamin E (100 to 200 IU per 100 mL of oil) is added to the ration if supplemental vegetable oil is provided.
  - When providing supplemental fat to a sick horse (450- to 500-kg body weight), 75 to 125 mL per day (¼ to ½ cup) is given initially and then gradually increased if *no* adverse response is seen (e.g., diarrhea or steatorrhea).
  - ***Practice Tip:*** *Feeding vegetable oil may be contraindicated in horses and ponies with hypertriglyceridemia (triglyceride concentration >500 mg/dL) and/or hepatic lipidosis.*
- The rate of diet administration is gradually increased over a 3- to 5-day period. A suggested rate of introduction is:
  - One-quarter the final target volume of feed on day 1
  - One-half the total volume on day 2
  - Three-quarters the total volume on day 3
  - Total volume on day 4 or 5
- Clinical signs of intolerance to enteral feeding dictate a slower rate of introduction (see p. 775).
- ***Practice Tip:*** *In the hospital setting, the enteral diet is administered in a minimum of 4 and preferably 6 feedings per day with no more than 6 to 8 L per feeding for a 450- to 500-kg horse, including the volume of water used to flush the tube.* Administer the volume over a 10- to 15-minute period.
- In field settings, a more practical approach is to administer 2 treatments per day although it is *not* possible to meet stall maintenance nutritional requirements with this treatment regimen.

- Pelleted feeds are soaked in warm water to soften before mixing in a blender (ratio of 1 kg pelleted feed to 6 L of water). A fresh batch of diet is made before each feeding. A soft tube with a ½-inch (12-mm) inner diameter is suitable for most enteral diets that contain fiber. *The end of the tube should be open-ended, rather than fenestrated,* to prevent the tube from becoming clogged. Intermittent nasogastric intubation or preferably, placement of an indwelling nasogastric tube, is used to facilitate feeding.
- In hospitalized horses, feeding tubes are left in place for up to 7 to 8 days; however, some degree of nasopharyngeal irritation and mucoid nasal discharge are expected outcomes; when longer term AEF is anticipated, placement of the tube via cervical esophagostomy is recommended (see Chapter 18, p. 161).
- Softer silicon tubes:
  - Are less irritating compared with tubes made of polyvinyl chloride
  - Do *not* tend to harden when left in place
  - Are generally recommended for horses requiring AEF for several days or more
- Before placement of the indwelling tube, the clinician should confirm that the diet solution flows easily through the tube. It may be necessary to add more water or to mix the feed in a blender a second time.
- The tube should be positioned in the stomach rather than the distal esophagus to minimize risk of reflux of feed around the tube. The tube should be secured to the halter; between feedings, a muzzle may be needed to prevent the horse from dislodging the tube. A marine bilge pump is recommended for infusion of fiber-containing diets. After administration of the diet, the tube should be flushed with approximately 1 L of water followed by a small volume of air to ensure that *no* feed material remains in the tube. The end of the tube should be capped with a syringe case between feedings.
- ***Practice Tip:*** *Close clinical monitoring, particularly of gastrointestinal function, is imperative for horses receiving AEF. Repeated ultrasonographic examinations can be useful for evaluation of gastric distention and intestinal motility.*
- The presence of residual gastric fluid should be assessed (i.e., by siphoning before each feeding). Substantial gastric reflux (>1 to 2 L) is an indication to withhold enteral feeding for at least 1 to 2 hours with reevaluation before recommencement of feeding.
- Persistent gastric reflux indicates intolerance to enteral feeding and the need for parenteral nutrition support. Similarly, signs of colic, ileus, abdominal distention, and/or increased digital pulses suggest intolerance to enteral feeding and are an indication to discontinue treatment or decrease the volume and frequency of feedings.
- ***Practice Tip:*** *The passage of loose feces is not uncommon in horses receiving AEF and of minimal concern if not accompanied by clinical signs of depression, dehydration, ileus, and/or colic.*
- It is important to measure the total volume of water administered via the nasogastric tube. Daily water

requirements (approximately 50 mL/kg/day) are generally met during AEF if the horse is fed 4 to 5 times per day.

- Serial measurements of hematocrit and plasma total protein concentration are recommended but *not* useful for monitoring hydration status and the adequacy of water administration in horses that do *not* have excessive fluid loss.
- Horses should be monitored for development of complications associated with repeated or indwelling nasogastric intubation, including rhinitis, pharyngitis, and esophageal ulceration.
- Body weight is measured daily to assess the adequacy of nutritional support, although changes in BW may reflect alterations in fluid balance rather than the effect of feeding.

Parenteral Nutritional Support

- Intravenous nutritional support is considered for horses that remain anorectic for more than 48 to 72 hours and where AEF is *not* a viable option.
- Specific indications for parenteral nutrition (PN) include:
  - Dysphagia
  - Esophageal obstruction
  - Duodenitis–proximal jejunitis
  - Other gastrointestinal tract disorders that result in ileus and/or persistent gastric reflux
  - Any neonatal foal unable to tolerate, digest, or absorb sufficient nutrients to prevent weight loss
- There are three primary options for PN:
  - *Dextrose supplementation:* The administration of dextrose alone is a relatively inexpensive means to provide supplemental calories in situations where only short-term nutritional support is required (<72 hours).
    - Intravenous dextrose administration also can be used as an adjunct to oral feed intake. The infusion of a 5% dextrose solution (50 g dextrose/L crystalloid solution; 170 kcal/L) is recommended.
    - Dextrose administration rates of between 0.5 and 2.0 mg/kg/min are suggested; the risk of hyperglycemia is greater at the higher end of the range.
    - The infusion of 5% dextrose solution at 1.7 mg/kg/min (1 L/h for a 500-kg horse) provides about 4080 kcal/day for a 500-kg horse, or about 35% of RER.
  - *Glucose–amino acid solution:* This combination is suitable for PN support of <7 to 10 days; fatty acid deficiency may develop with longer-term use and lipid-containing PN is used for long-term parenteral feeding.
    - A 50:50 mixture of 50% dextrose and 8.5% amino acid solutions (e.g., Travasol 8.5%[7]) results in a solution containing 1.02 kcal/mL (50% dextrose = 1.7 kcal/mL; 8.5% amino acid solution = 0.34 kcal/mL).

Table 51-2 Formulation of Parenteral Nutrition Solutions and Calculation of Administration Rate for a 500-kg Horse

Formulation	Composition	Caloric Density (Kcal/mL)
Formula 1	1500 mL 50% dextrose, 1500 mL 8.5% amino acids	1.02
Formula 2	1000 mL 50% dextrose, 500 mL 20% lipids, 1500 mL 8.5% amino acids	1.07

The resting energy requirements (RER) for a 500-kg horse = 500 kg × 0.021 kcal/kg BW/day + 0.975 = 11,500 kcal/day
To provide this energy requirement with:
Formula 1: PN rate: 11,500 kcal/day ÷ 1.02 kcal/mL = 11,275 mL/day or 470 mL/h
Formula 2: PN rate: 11,500 kcal/day ÷ 1.07 kcal/mL = 10,748 mL/day or 448 mL/h
Both formulas provide 0.9 g protein/kg BW/day. Formula 1 is diluted by administering 150 mL sterile water/h as a piggyback to the PN solution.

- Accordingly, approximately 11.2 L of this mixture is required to meet the daily RER of a 500-kg horse, or ≈9.1 L if 80% of RER is the initial caloric target. Table 51-2 outlines recommended rates of administration.
- The osmolarity of this solution is ≈1700 mOsm/L and dilution with sterile water is recommended (3:1 ratio of PN:water) to reduce the irritating effects of a hyperosmolar solution (e.g., a piggyback infusion of sterile water).
- *Glucose-lipid–amino acid PN solution:* A typical formulation is 50% dextrose, 8.5% amino acids, and 20% lipid (Intralipid 20%[8]) at a ratio of 1 to 1.5 to 0.5 (see Table 51-2). Each milliliter of this mixture provides 1.07 kcal/mL and has an osmolarity of 1317 mOsm/L.
- Electrolyte needs are met via maintenance crystalloid fluid therapy. Water-soluble vitamins should be added to the PN solution; commercially available human products can be used for this purpose.
- *Practice Tip: Fat-soluble vitamins and trace minerals are stored in the body and it is only necessary to add these nutrients to the PN solution with long-term (>7 to 10 days) parenteral feeding.*
- PN is most commonly administered through an intravenous catheter inserted into a jugular vein although a cephalic vein is a viable alternative (see Chapter 1, p. 3). Polyurethane double- or triple-lumen catheters are good choices, allowing one port to be dedicated for PN administration and the other port(s) for delivery of crystalloid fluids and other medications, thereby avoiding the need to inject other medications into the PN line (see Chapter 3, p. 10).
- The fluid lines used for delivery of the PN solution need to be changed every 24 hours. An infusion pump is required to ensure accurate delivery of the PN solution.

[7]Travasol 8.5% (Baxter Healthcare Corp.).

[8]Intralipid 20% (Baxter Healthcare Corp.).

The PN solution bag(s) ideally are covered with a brown bag during administration if the solution is exposed to strong light, which can degrade the amino acids (and any B vitamins) in the solution.

- ***Practice Tip:*** *The initial rate of PN solution administration is approximately 25% of target calorie provision and 80% of RER. The rate of infusion can be increased every 4 to 6 hours until the target rate is reached, typically at 24 hours after the start of parenteral feeding.*
- Close monitoring for potential complications is essential and includes:
  - Serial measurement of blood and urine glucose
  - Serum blood urea nitrogen (BUN), electrolyte, and triglyceride concentrations
  - Evaluation of the catheter site for evidence of phlebitis
- Body weight is also measured daily along with periodic assessment of hydration status, including packed cell volume and total plasma protein concentrations.
- ***Practice Tip:*** *Hyperglycemia and hyperlipemia are the most common complications of postoperative PN in horses after intestinal surgery.*
- Hyperglycemia was observed in 52 of 79 horses receiving PN in one report, believed due to insulin resistance and/or an excessive rate of administration.
- Blood glucose concentrations are measured every 4 to 8 hours in horses receiving PN, and the rate of dextrose administration is decreased if glucose concentrations exceed the renal threshold (approximately 180 to 200 mg/dL).
- A constant-rate insulin infusion (e.g., regular insulin at a starting dose of 0.05 to 0.1 IU/kg/h) can be instituted if the reduction in dextrose administration rate fails to correct the hyperglycemia.
  - Blood glucose concentrations must be closely monitored (e.g., every 2 to 6 hours). Adjustments in insulin dose may be needed to achieve glycemic control.

Transition to Voluntary Feeding

- A decrease in AEF or PN is indicated when appetite returns or when voluntary oral feeding is *no* longer contraindicated.
- Initially, small amounts of palatable feed (e.g., fresh grass or leafy hay) should be offered. If these feedings are tolerated, the level of tube or parenteral feeding is gradually reduced as the provision of feed for voluntary consumption is increased.
- Nutritional support can be withdrawn when voluntary feed intake provides at least 75% of stall maintenance DE and protein requirements.
- ***Practice Tip:*** *All changes in diet should be gradual, as recommended for any feeding program.*

References

References can be found on the companion website at www.equine-emergencies.com.

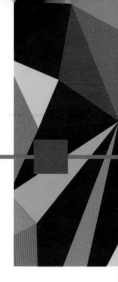

SECTION IV Biosecurity

CHAPTER 52

Contagious and Zoonotic Diseases

Helen Aceto and Barbara Dallap Schaer

- Before evaluating an equine emergency patient, one must consider the following as possible differential diagnoses:
  - Contagious diseases
  - Zoonotic diseases
- The period during which the patient is initially stabilized and preliminary diagnostics are performed can present significant potential risks to patients already in hospital, any individuals in contact with the presenting patient, and the environs of the hospital itself. This is particularly true when the patient is critical and all efforts are focused on ensuring the patient's survival such that infection control measures get overlooked. Moreover, in emerging situations, the need for infection control may not be readily apparent.
- No matter what the circumstance, it is always better to err on the conservative side when it comes to infection control and to at least have some minimal level of containment in place at all times.
- Having written protocols that are relayed to and understood by all staff for how specific categories of patients should be handled (vigilant preparation before admission, followed by implementation of rigorous infection control protocols during hospitalization) can all assist the clinician in providing the highest level of care while protecting the hospital and personnel.
- The information in this chapter helps the clinician identify the likelihood of contagious or zoonotic disease in the critically ill equine patient and provides strategies for the protection of owners, personnel, patients, and the hospital.

Useful Definitions

- *Infectious diseases* are those caused by an agent or organism capable of producing an infection or illness. The method of transmission or location of reservoir is not specifically defined, and the risks for potential spread from horse-to-horse or between vertebrate animal and human beings are not characterized. It is important to realize that infectious agents are always changing, requiring constant vigilance and attention to infection control procedures.
- *Contagious diseases* are those transmitted from horse-to-horse through direct or indirect contact. Literally

translated, "contagious" means communicable by contact. As stated, transmission may be by direct animal contact or by means of vector transmission or environmental contamination or through various kinds of fomites.
- *Zoonotic diseases* are those that are transmissible between human beings and animal species, or more precisely, from vertebrate animals to human beings. The reservoir for zoonotic diseases is the vertebrate animal population, and transmission may be by direct or indirect routes, through contact or vector mediation.
  - *Direct transmission* is defined as spread by intimate contact with the infected reservoir horse, through mechanisms such as contact with infected bodily fluids (respiratory secretions, urine, reproductive fluids) or via bite or scratch wound.
  - *Indirect transmission* is defined as spread by contact with an arthropod vector, airborne spread, or via an inanimate object (fomite) that permits survival of the infectious organism on it for long enough to reach a susceptible animal or human host (e.g., barn floor, feed trough, clothing, hands, and feet).

Key Points

- The recognition of contagious and zoonotic diseases has been a relatively recent historical development, mostly occurring in the late 1700s and 1800s, following the discovery of the microscope. Historically, animal products consumed as food have represented the greatest zoonotic risk. As human beings continue to encroach on the natural habitat of vertebrate animals and international travel and globalization expand, new zoonotic diseases are likely to emerge. Moreover, climatic change may cause shifts in the distribution of competent insect vectors that may in turn change the geographic distribution of equine diseases.
- There is no doubt that veterinary personnel are at greater risk of exposure to, and potentially infection by, zoonotic agents than are the public at large. Because of this, all veterinary clinics should take steps to educate staff about these agents and reduce risk wherever possible.
- Table 52-1 lists the most important zoonotic diseases that affect the horse, and Table 52-2 lists those important

Text continued on p. 790

Table 52-1 Equine Diseases of Zoonotic Importance*

Disease	Agent and Incubation Period	Mode of Transmission	Clinical Signs in Animal	Clinical Signs in Humans	Diagnostic Testing	Disinfection	Biosecurity and Precautions for Personnel
Acariasis (mange), zoonotic scabies[†]	Sarcoptes, psoroptes, chorioptes, demodex (rare in horses) and other mites 1-2 weeks after infestation.	Highly contagious by direct contact with infected animal. Also transmitted on fomites.	Intense pruritis, alopecia, crusting may be lichenification of skin. Location depends on mite involved.	Transient infestation possible primarily with sarcoptic mites. Intensely pruritic, resolves spontaneously, not transmitted between humans.	Direct exam. Microscopic examination of skin scrapings or skin biopsy.	Most effectively controlled by treating affected animal with acaricides.	Gloves, boots and protective clothing. Do not share equipment. Discard or disinfect equipment used on infected animal.
Anthrax (H,A)[†]	Bacillus anthracis. Gram-positive spore-forming anaerobic bacterium. 1 to 7 days.	Direct contact (cutaneous), aerosol (pulmonary), possibly vector (e.g., horseflies [cutaneous], ingestion of under-cooked contaminated meat [GI]).	Horses very susceptible, can present as acute enteritis with signs of colic, usually very rapid progression; septicemia, fever, hemorrhagic enteritis, depression, death.	Cutaneous (most common), pruritic macule leading to black eschar. Pulmonary, febrile respiratory disease rapidly fatal. Intestinal, febrile GI disease.	High level of bacteremia on smears of blood or aspirated edema fluid. Culture and ID possible but fluorescent antibody testing of smears of froth, blood or splenic aspirate safer for personnel.	Anthrax spores resistant to heat, drying and many disinfectants. Spores killed by 2% glutaraldehyde or 5% formalin.	Complete protection (gloves, boots, protective coveralls respiratory and eye protection) required when handling suspects. Avoid necropsy of infected or suspect cases beyond blood collection. Unopened carcass decomposes rapidly and spores are destroyed. Burn or deep bury carcass.
Brucellosis (H,A)	Brucella abortus, B. suis (both rare but B. abortus most common) 5 days to several months, usually 2-4 weeks.	Direct contact with infected tissues (e.g. aborted fetus) or fluids (including placental, urine), also shed in feces. Aerosol, ingestion, indirectly on fomites all possible routes. Horses most often infected by contact with cattle.	Suppurative bursitis (fistulous withers, poll evil, occasionally other bursal infections), rarely abortion.	Horses unlikely source for human infection. Gradual onset undulant fevers, myalgia, fatigue. Arthritis seen with long term infection. Long convalescence.	Culture of acute blood, lesions or other tissues and fluids (e.g., placenta, fetus, semen). Can be difficult to culture in bursitis due to presence of other bacteria. Concomitant paired sera tested by agglutination or complement fixation is useful.	Can survive for months in the environment. Destroyed by heat. Susceptible to bleach, 70% ethanol, iodine/alcohol, glutaraldehyde, formaldehyde, direct sunlight.	Protective clothing (boots, barrier gown, gloves, eyewear, face mask) with infected cases or when handling reproductive tissues. Good general hygiene strict hand hygiene. Proper disposal of aborted fetuses, placenta.

Disease	Etiology / Incubation	Transmission	Clinical Signs (Animals)	Clinical Signs (Humans)	Diagnosis	Survival / Disinfection	Prevention / Control
Clostridial enteritis†	Gram-positive spore-forming anaerobic bacterium. *Clostridium difficile* neonatal foals, adults primarily during or immediately after antimicrobial therapy and *Clostridium perfringens* neonatal foals. *C. difficile* most important nosocomially. Foals 8-24 hours. Adult incubation period unknown as present in feces of clinically normal horses in low numbers. Antibiotic-induced clostridial diarrhea highly variable but usually within one week of first dose.	Fecal-oral spread by direct contact, environmental contamination, on fomites, via humans on hands, etc. Public health risk of equine clostridial infections uncertain.	Acute colitis, abdominal pain, diarrhea of varying severity, may be accompanied by dehydration, fever, toxemia and leukopenia.	Sudden onset abdominal discomfort, diarrhea, nausea; vomiting and fever usually absent. Generally self-limiting, short duration but may be more severe disease; necrotizing enteritis, sepsis. *C. difficile* common cause of antimicrobial-associated and nosocomial diarrhea. *C. perfringens* more frequently foodborne.	Culture *and* toxin detection in fecal samples, blood culture.	Vegetative form killed by exposure to air, spores resistant to many disinfectants but can be reduced by thorough cleaning with a detergent followed by disinfection with diluted (1:10) bleach solution.	Isolation of confirmed cases with protective clothing (boots, barrier gown, gloves). Strict hand hygiene. Minimize stress especially dietary. Judicious use of antimicrobials. Consider routine examination for *C. difficile* and toxins A and B in foals and with antimicrobial-associated diarrhea.
Cryptosporidiosis (H)	*Cryptosporidium parvum* (primarily genotypes *bovis* and *hominis*) Apicomplexan protozoal parasite. 3-7 days.	Fecal-oral transmission through direct or indirect (fomites) contact with infected animals and their environment. Infection can also occur via droplet exposure during cleaning. Ingestion of contaminated water or food.	Uncommon in horses except SCID foals, most commonly young ruminants. Affected young animals often have diarrhea, lethargy, poor appetite, weight loss. Usually mild but can be serious in already debilitated animals. Inapparent carriage in horses appears rare.	GI disease including abdominal pain, nausea, anorexia, profuse watery diarrhea. Usually self-limiting but can cause severe life-threatening disease in immunocompromised individuals. Rarely a pulmonary form of infection occurs. Important zoonosis among veterinary personnel.	Fecal examination for thick-walled infective oocysts. Usually requires special stains (acid-fast).	Resistant to most disinfectants. Dessication and prolonged exposure to sunlight are effective. Moist heat >130°F effective. !8 h exposure to 10% ammonia or 10% formalin also kills oocysts.	Strict hand hygiene. Avoid eating and drinking near animals and their environments. Wear protective clothing including respiratory protection when working with infected animals or cleaning areas inhabited by infected animals.

Continued

BIOS

Table 52-1   Equine Diseases of Zoonotic Importance—cont'd

Disease	Agent and Incubation Period	Mode of Transmission	Clinical Signs in Animal	Clinical Signs in Humans	Diagnostic Testing	Disinfection	Biosecurity and Precautions for Personnel
Dermatophilosis (rain rot)[†]	*Dermatophilus congolensis.* Gram-negative actinomycete bacterium. Less than 7 days.	Direct contact. Trauma and biting insects may aid in spread.	Exudative crusted skin lesions, hair in "paint-brush" clumps.	Rare zoonosis. Afebrile, acute to chronic pustular to exudative dermatitis. May be pruritic or painful.	Cytology—gram stain of crust, histology, culture.	Diluted (1:10) bleach (sodium hypochlorite) solution.	Gloves, strict hygiene, disposal or disinfection of grooming and other equipment. Minimize exposure to excessive moisture, employ insect control/repellents.
Dermatomycosis (ringworm)[†]	Many fungi of *Trichophyton* and *Microsporum* spp. In horses *Trichophyton equinum* most common; also *T. mentagrophytes Microsporum equinum* (*M. canis* and *M. gypseum*). 4-14 days.	Direct contact or indirect contact with fomites— saddle blankets, grooming equipment, etc. Some ringworm fungi can be found in soil and may cause infections under the right conditions.	Round, hairless, scaly skin lesions.	Circular or annular lesions with scaling, occasionally erythema, itching.	Direct exam of hair, culture, histology of biopsy. Wood's lamp unreliable for equine dermatomycosis.	Diluted (1:10) bleach solution.	Gloves, strict hand hygiene, disposal or disinfection of grooming and other equipment.
Equine Encephalitides caused by Alphaviruses (WEE, VEE, EEE) (H,A)	Alphaviruses of the family Togaviridae. EEE 7-10 days humans, 18-24 hours horses VEE 1-6 days humans, 1-3 days horses WEE 5-10 days humans, 1-3 weeks horses	Mosquito vector. Natural reservoirs birds or rodents, horse is major amplifier for VEE but dead-end host and low viremia for WEE and EEE, probably no horse to human transmission of WEE or EEE.	Fever, depression, drowsiness. Paralysis, circling, dysphagia, stupor. Mortality rates WEE 20-40%, EEE 50-90%, VEE 50-80%	VEE ranges from non-specific fever with flu-like signs to encephalitis but most commonly mild to severe respiratory infection case fatality rate 0.2-1% cf 65-80% for EEE, more severe neurologic disease.	No reliable antemortem test to detect virus in clinically affected horses. Serology principal means of presumptive ante-mortem diagnosis. Detection of IgM in blood or CSF, paired sera less reliable.	Readily inactivated by most common disinfectants. Peroxygen-based disinfectants, 2% glutaraldehyde.	Protective clothing and insect repellents, vector control, vaccination. Handle blood and tissue from VEE infected horses as infectious biohazards. Wear full protection during post-mortem examination, (see Flaviviruses below).

Encephalitides caused by Flaviviruses (Japanese, West Nile, and St. Louis encephalitis viruses) (H,A)	Japanese encephalitis virus group of the family Flaviviridae. 5-15 days humans, 7-10 days horses.	Mosquito vector. Mammalian or avian reservoirs. Horses and humans dead-end hosts, viremia too low to infect mosquitoes. Transmission via oral ingestion demonstrated in both mammals and birds. Blood and organ donation from viremic donors.	Many infections subclinical. Clinical signs highly variable in duration, severity, and combination. Fever, anorexia depression most common initially. May be signs of colic. Muscle fasciculations. Onset of neurologic signs sudden and progressive. Gait and behavioral changes. Ataxia, paresis, cranial nerve abnormalities. Fatal JEV infection usually blindness, coma, and death, not seen with WNV. May be recrudescence after apparent recovery.	The elderly most vulnerable (same appears true in horses). Most infections asymptomatic. Mild—fever, headaches, aseptic meningitis. Severe—usually acute onset, headache, high fever, meningeal signs, stupor, disorientation, coma, tremors. Occasional convulsions (infants) and paralysis (usually spastic).	WNV serology, IgM capture ELISA (MAC-ELSA) preferred. Paired sera in non-vaccinated horses. Postmortem, PCR for detection of WNV in tissues. JEV serology, but can be difficult to interpret in areas where other flaviviruses endemic. Potsmortem virus isolation, PCR, and IHC from CNS.	Readily inactivated by most common disinfectants. Peroxygen-based disinfectants, 2% glutaraldehyde.	Insect repellents, vector control, vaccination. Little risk of human infection by direct contact except at necropsy. During post-mortem examination protective clothing, gloves, face shield, and mask rated for biohazards (N95 or better).
Equine influenza (A)†	Orthomyxovirus A. Enveloped, single-stranded RNA virus. Usually 1-3 days, range 18 hours to 5, or rarely 7, days. Most frequently diagnosed and economically important viral respiratory disease of the horse.	Respiratory route; aerosol, direct contact with infected secretions. Survives and may spread on fomites for several hours. Highly contagious, despite careful hygiene horses sharing same air space likely to become infected.	Acute, febrile, respiratory disease. High fevers, coughing, nasal discharge common; as are depression, anorexia, weakness. Occasionally pneumonia or other complications.	Although influenza A viruses can infect humans, equine-lineage viruses have very limited zoonotic risk. Recently, however, transmission of equine-lineage H3N8 virus has caused influenza in dogs in the United States.	PCR and/or virus isolation from nasopharyngeal swab collected as soon as possible after onset of illness, or paired serology. Directigen Flu-A test can be used "stall-side."	Easily killed by many disinfectants including 1% bleach, 70% ethanol, iodine-based disinfectants, quaternary ammonium disinfectants, peroxygen disinfectants, accelerated hydrogen peroxide disinfectants, phenolics, etc.	Isolation. Avoid sharing equipment. Strict hand hygiene. Maintain isolation until no symptoms and body temperature normal for ≥ 5 days. Consider vaccination of contact animals to control an outbreak.

Continued

BIOS

BIOS

Table 52-1	Equine Diseases of Zoonotic Importance—cont'd				
Disease	**Agent and Incubation Period**	**Mode of Transmission**	**Clinical Signs in Animal**	**Clinical Signs in Humans**	**Diagnostic Testing**	**Disinfection**	**Biosecurity and Precautions for Personnel**
Giardiasis (H)	Multiple species but *Giardia intestinalis* (*lamblia*) almost exclusive cause of disease in humans. Flagellated protozoan parasite. Within 7 days.	Fecal-oral transmission through direct or indirect (fomites) contact with infected animals and their environment. Ingestion of contaminated water or food.	Infrequent infection in horses, subclinical shedding in foals may be more common. Primarily ruminants. Most infected animals show no signs of disease. Diarrhea most common in young animals feces pale, may contain mucus. Intestinal gas and bloating, poor hair coat, failure to thrive.	GI disease, including diarrhea, intestinal gas, cramps, and nausea. Usually self-limiting in 1-2 weeks but can be a chronic infection lasting months to years.	Fecal examination for cysts or trophozoites. Usually requires special stains.	Resistant to most disinfectants. Dessication, boiling and freeze thaw cycles effective.	Strict hand hygiene. Avoid eating and drinking near animals and their environments. Protective clothing (gowns, gloves) when working with infected animals.
Leptospirosis (A)	*Leptospira* spp. Spirochete bacterium. 2-30 days, usually 7-12 days.	Contact particularly with urine or infected tissues, may also be aerosol. Enters via ingestion or mucous membranes, or by contact with abraded skin.	Usually inapparent, may cause fever and abortion in mares, septicemia foals, may be icteric. Recurrent uveitis is possible sequellum.	Inapparent to severe disease. Onset abrupt, non-specific fever, chills, headache, severe myalgia. May be multi-organ failure, liver, kidney, CNS.	Culture of blood, urine, or kidney. Dark field examination of a urine sample for leptospires only diagnostic if organisms are observed. Paired sera with microscopic or plate agglutination usually unrewarding.	1% bleach, 70% ethanol, detergents, most disinfectants	Proper hygiene, gloves, frequent hand washing. Isolate infected or suspect animals. Boots, protective clothing, eyewear and/or face shield with suspect or known cases. Uveitis occurs long after initial infection, no evidence that these animals represent an infection risk, special precautions not required.

Rabies (H,A)	Rhabdovirus of genus Lyssavirus. Enveloped, single-stranded RNA virus. Few days to several years, most cases apparent after 1-3 months.	Contact (saliva, CSF, neural tissue). Mucous membranes or compromised skin, cuts, etc.	Wide range of possible clinical signs. Progression of encephalitic signs may be aggression (furious form, more common), or depression (paralytic, dumb form). Average survival from onset of clinical signs 5 days, maximum 10 days.	Early signs malaise, fever, headache, pruritis at site of virus entry. Progressive anxiety, confusion, abnormal behavior. Encephalitic or paralytic form can occur. Death usually in 2-10 days.	No definitive antemortem test. Brain from suspect animal must be submitted to an approved laboratory for rabies testing.	Lipid solvents (soap solutions, acetone), 1% bleach, 2% glutaraldehyde, 45-75% ethanol, iodine-based disinfectants, quaternary ammonium disinfectants. Inactivated by sunlight, limited environmental survival.	Clearly label as rabies suspect. Strictly limit number of personnel involved in managing suspect animal. Record all in-contact personnel. Clearly label any laboratory specimens as rabies suspect. Full barrier precautions including gloves, boots, protective clothing, protective eyewear and face shield, N95-type mask should also be considered. Promptly submit necropsy samples using approved methods. Full protective clothing required during postmortem examination (see Flaviviruses).
Rhodococcus equi infection[†]	*Rhodococcus equi* likely 1-3 months for respiratory disease. Gram-positive, facultative intracellular bacterium Incubation period uncertain, in foals earliest isolation from feces at 1-2 weeks, most foals positive by 4 weeks of age. Often insidious onset, median age at time of diagnosis of pneumonia on endemic farms reported as 37-49 days.	Environmental exposure (soil), aerosol, contact, rarely via wound contamination.	Most often respiratory but other body systems can be involved. Most commonly fever, coughing, increased respiratory rate and effort, muco-purulent nasal discharge, pyogranulomatous pneumonia. Primarily foals 1-6 months old.	Rare human infection, only in the severely immunocompromized, appears to be *via* environmental exposure. Slowly progressive granulomatous pneumonia.	Culture of tracheobronchial aspirate or other samples. PCR can be valuable but best used in conjunction with culture. Radiographs useful.	70% ethanol, 2% glutaraldehyde, phenolics, and formaldehyde.	Bacteria shed in feces and respirate secretions/aerosol, prompt removal of manure and good hygiene limits accumulation. Frequent hand washing. Uncertain infection risk but consider barrier precautions on affected foals (at least up to 72 hrs after starting antimicrobial therapy) if susceptible foals housed in same area.

Continued

BIOS

BIOS

Table 52-1	Equine Diseases of Zoonotic Importance—cont'd					
Disease	**Agent and Incubation Period**	**Mode of Transmission**	**Clinical Signs in Animal**	**Clinical Signs in Humans**	**Diagnostic Testing**	**Disinfection**	**Biosecurity and Precautions for Personnel**
Salmonellosis (H)†	Various *Salmonella enterica*. Gram-negative bacterium. 12-72 hours in humans, possibly similar in debilitated horses, incubation in the healthy exposed animal variable and uncertain.	Contact with feces from an infected animal, most commonly ingestion, possibly via inhalation. Readily spread on fomites, in feed, water or via vermin, birds, insects. Good environmental survival but tends to be serotype dependent, can be very difficult to control.	Inapparent, to fever, leukopenia, severe diarrhea, to septicemia. Anorexia and depression common.	Inapparent, to self-limiting but often severe gastroenteritis (diarrhea generally much more prominent than vomiting), fever, myalgia, can be invasive leading to septicemia.	Fecal culture (sensitivity for MDR), gastrointestinal reflux may also be cultured. Consider additional molecular ID if a nosocomial problem is suspected. Where PCR is available, faster return of results can be a great aid to control but PCR positives should be subject to follow-up culture.	2% bleach, 70% ethanol, 2% glutaraldehyde, iodine-based disinfectants, phenolics, peroxygen or accelerated hydrogen peroxide disinfectants and formaldehyde.	Isolate confirmed cases. Strict hygiene. Prompt cleaning of all areas contaminated with feces. Gloves, frequent hand washing, protective clothing, boots or footwear that can be easily cleaned, face mask/shield with pipe-stream diarrhea.
Sporotrichosis (rose thorn disease)	*Sporothrix schenckii* Dimorphic fungus 7 days to 6 months	Direct contact with infected animal or material e.g. pus, organism can invade intact skin. In humans more commonly gardeners, horticulturalists. Has been associated with moss, timbers, soil, baled hay. Zoonotic infections most commonly from cats.	Skin nodules, may ulcerate, firm cord-like lymph nodes. Rarely, disseminated disease—arthritis, meningitis, other visceral infections.	Hard painless nodule at site of skin injury, may be multiple nodules extending along lymphatics. Nodules ulcerate. Occasional disseminated disease. Rarely pulmonary disease through inhalation of conidia.	Culture of biopsy, pus or exudates.	Organic iodine	Immunocompromised at greatest risk. Gloves, strict hand hygiene, eye protection (eye infections have been reported) careful general hygiene.

Disease	Etiology / Incubation	Transmission	Clinical signs (animal)	Clinical signs / forms	Diagnosis	Disinfection	Precautions
Staphylococcosis (H MRSA)†	Staphylococcus spp. Gram-positive bacterium. Methicillin (oxacillin) resistant S. aureus of special concern. Suppuration 4-10 days, gastroenteritis 0.5-7 h.	Direct contact most important, particularly hand-to-nose transfer. Purulent discharge from infected sites very infectious. Aerosol less important but can occur with coughing or snorting.	Inapparent nasal carriage (including of MRSA), to thrombophlebitis, other suppurative draining or nondraining lesions.	Subclinical, can become nasal carriers of MRSA and spread to other animals or people. Clinical may be suppurative lesions, usually skin (impetigo, boils) or gastroenteritis associated with toxin ingestion - sudden onset nausea, cramps, vomiting.	Standard culture with speciation to identify S. aureus because MRSA strains in horses can be very weakly coagulase positive and may be misidentified. Sensitivity; oxacillin resistant = MRSA.	Chlorohexadine, 1% bleach, 70% ethanol, 2% glutaraldehyde, quaternary ammonium disinfectants phenolics, peroxygen, accelerated hydrogen peroxide disinfectants.	Gown, gloves, boots strict hand hygiene. Surgeon-type face mask may help limit hand-to-nose transfer in personnel. Consider isolation with full barrier precautions for MRSA positive animals, particularly where active drainage from infection site.
Tularemia (H,A)	Francisella tularensis Gram-negative bacterium. 3-15 days.	Vector (ticks and biting flies), contact (through skin and mucous membranes), aerosols highly infectious.	Sudden onset high fever, lethargy, anorexia, stiffness, signs of septicemia.	Six different forms depending on inoculation site. Most forms first manifest as sudden onset of flulike symptoms.	Paired sera, ELISA-based most specific. Culture, PCR or FA of ulcer exudates, lymph node aspirates (risk of bacteremia with the latter).	Easily killed by many disinfectants including 1% bleach, 70% ethanol.	Vector control, gloves, protective clothing including eye protection and face mask, strict hand hygiene.
Vesicular stomatitis (A)†	Rhabdovirus, Rhabdovirus of genus Vesiculovirus. Enveloped, single-stranded RNA virus. 3-7 days.	Direct contact or aerosol, insect vectors (sand flies, black flies). In endemic areas, oral examination prior to admission may prevent introduction during outbreaks.	Horses, donkeys, mules, can be affected. Excess salivation, fever, vesicles on mucous membranes of mouth, epithelium of tongue, coronary band or on teats. Can lead to lameness, weight loss.	Infection rates in exposed humans low. Fever, headache, myalgia, rarely oral blisters. Recovery usually in 4-7days.	Standard test for VSV antibodies is virus neutralization, complement fixation or ELISA can also be used.	2% sodium carbonate, 4% sodium hydroxide, 2% iodophor disinfectants, chlorine dioxide.	Vector control, gloves, protective clothing including face mask, strict hand hygiene.

*Diseases that are nationally reportable for humans (H) or animals (A) in the United States are indicated in the first column. Cases may also be notifiable at the state level. Check with your state veterinarian or state public health veterinarian for a current listing of reportable diseases in your area.

†Agents that have been linked to nosocomial outbreaks of disease.

BIOS

Table 52-2 Equine Contagious Diseases of Nosocomial Importance*

Disease	Agent and Incubation Period	Mode of Transmission	Clinical Signs in Animal	Clinical Signs in Humans	Diagnostic Testing	Disinfection	Biosecurity and Precautions for Personnel
Equine herpesvirus infection (equine rhinopneumonitis—EHV1 and EHV4; equine myeloencephalopathy EHM - EHV1; abortion EHV1, occasionally EHV4; coital exanthema EHV3.[†]	Nine different types, EHV-1, EHV-3, and EHV-4 of major concern in domestic horses. Enveloped, double-stranded linear DNA virus. Incubation 2 to 10 days. Abortions occur 2-12 weeks after infection, usually between 8 and 11 months of gestation. EHV3, lesions appear within 1 week	Direct contact, aerosol (up to 35 feet), fomites.	EHV-1 inapparent to mild respiratory disease with fever, to abortion in mares, to rapidly progressing, often fatal, neurological disease, EHM (ascending paralysis, urinary incontinence). EHV-4 rhinopneumonitis primarily horses ≤ 3 years of age. EHV3 uncommon, nodules progressing to painful ulcerative lesions on the genitalia.	Nonzoonotic.	PCR or virus isolation from nasopharyngeal secretions and/or white blood cells (buffy coat).	Easily killed by many disinfectants including 1% bleach, 70% ethanol, iodine-based disinfectants, quaternary ammonium disinfectants, peroxygen disinfectants, accelerated hydrogen peroxide disinfectants, phenolics, etc.	Isolation for EHV-1 infection, monitor temperature of surrounding animals, submit samples for testing if fever (≥ 101.5 °F) develops. Proper disposal of aborted fetuses and related material. EHV-4 barrier precautions, no sharing of equipment. Avoid breeding of animals with clinical signs of coital exanthema.
Equine infectious anemia (EIA, swamp fever) A[†]	Retrovirus of the genus lentivirus, related to other important lentiviruses including HIV but not zoonotic. Enveloped single-stranded (2 copies) RNA virus. 1-3 weeks but may be as long as 3 months.	Primarily via transfer of contaminated blood by biting insects (most often tabanids) or fomites contaminated with blood.	Intermittent fever, depression, inappetance, weight loss, edema, thrombocytopenia, transitory or pro-gressive anemia. No therapy.	Nonzoonotic.	AGID (Coggins test); for animals testing positive a second con-firmatory test recommended. Other ELISA tests available.	Diluted (1:10) bleach solution, 70% ethanol, 2% glutaraldehyde peroxygen disinfectants, accelerated hydrogen peroxide disinfectants, phenolics.	Proper handling and disposal of biohazard material. Strict insect-proof isolation until testing confirmed. Due to life-long infection risk, consider euthanasia for positive animals.

Disease	Agent	Transmission	Clinical signs	Zoonotic	Diagnosis	Treatment/Disinfection	Control
Equine piroplasmosis A‡	Hemoprotozoan apicomplexan parasites of the order *Piroplasmidae*. *Theileria equi* (formerly *Babesia Equi*) and *Babesia caballi*. 12-19 days *T. equi*, 10-30 days *B. caballi*.	Tick vectors in *Dermacentor*, *Hyalomma*, and *Rhipicephalus* genera. Also *Boophilus* for *T. equi*. Contaminated blood by transfusion, contaminated needles, surgical instruments or other equipment contaminated with infected blood. Transplacental, possibly semen if blood contaminated.	Vast majority seropositive horses inapparent carriers. Clinically *B. caballi* milder than *T. equi*. Peracute, acute, subacute and chronic forms. Mild—weak, inappetence. More serious acute signs fever, anemia, jaundice, swollen abdomen, labored breathing. May also see CNS disturbances, rough hair coat, colic, hemoglobinuria.	*T. equi* implicated in rare human cases but *B. equi* and *B. caballi* generally regarded as non-zoonotic. Human infection described with bovine, canine white-footed mouse, and white-tailed deer pathogens.	Authorities must be notified prior to submission of samples. Giemsa stained blood or organ smears. CF, IFA, ELISA, and PCR also available.	Treat affected animals with acaricides. Eliminating contact with ticks and preventing transfer of blood between animals vital in preventing spread. Disinfectants and sanitation not generally considered effective against spread but scrupulous hygiene should be observed with hospitalized animals.	Isolate infected animals. Vector control, disinfection and proper sanitation crucial to prevent spread. Single use or complete cleaning and disinfection of equipment that may be blood contaminated. *T. equi* appears to be life-long carriage, *B. caballi* up to 4 years but may be possible to clear infection. Due to prolonged carriage and difficulty in controlling spread, euthansia should be considered.
Equine viral arteritis (EVA) A†	Arterivirus, equine arteritis virus. Enveloped, single-stranded RNA virus. Average 7 days, range 2 to 13 days.	Respiratory from acutely infected horse, direct contact or via relatively close contact (e.g., adjacent stall, limited spread on fomites). Venereal from acute or chronically infected stallion.	May be subclinical or only transient edema, or acute fever, depression, dependent edema especially limbs, scrotum and prepuce in stallions, conjunctivitis, nasal discharge, abortion.	Nonzoonotic.	Virus isolation or PCR from nasal secretions, conjunctival swabs or buffy coat. Paired serology. Virus isolation from semen of infected stallions.	Easily killed by many disinfectants—see EHV above.	Isolation of cases. Quarantine close contacts for at least 21 days after last clinical case, 30 days used in some previous outbreaks.

Continued

BIOS

Table 52-2   Equine Contagious Diseases of Nosocomial Importance—cont'd

Disease	Agent and Incubation Period	Mode of Transmission	Clinical Signs in Animal	Clinical Signs in Humans	Diagnostic Testing	Disinfection	Biosecurity and Precautions for Personnel
Multidrug-resistant bacterial infections or infections caused by organisms with antimicrobial resistance of concern. (H,A organism dependent) [†]	Various including *Salmonella*, MRSA, *E. coli*, *Klebsiella*, *Enterobacter*, *Enterococcus* (VRE and non-VRE), *Pseudomonas*, *Acinetobacter*, organisms resistant to extended spectrum beta lactams, etc. Incubation period varies by organism, may be hours to several days.	Multiple including fecal-oral, by direct contact with infected animals, *via* humans, or on fomites, in some cases aerosol. For some organisms (e.g., MRSA), *Salmonella* animals and/or humans can be inapparent carriers.	Depending on organism, many different clinical presentations e.g., GI, respiratory, catheter-related, or surgical site infections, septicemia (especially in foals), etc. Nosocomial cases may occur as low level endemic infections or in epidemic outbreaks of varying severity.	Many have zoonotic potential. Clinical signs depend on organism involved.	Culture and sensitivity. Regular monitoring required to assess incidence and detect changes that may require investigation or intervention. Additional molecular ID may be necessary if a nosocomial problem is suspected.	Often susceptible to many disinfectants. Regular cleaning and disinfection controls environmental load. If nosocomial problem identified additional cleaning and disinfection of specific areas may be required. Conduct of disinfectant kill-curves to ensure choice is efficacious may aid in control.	Judicious use of antimicrobials. Barrier precautions or possibly isolation for confirmed cases (organism dependent). Strict hand hygiene. Maintenance of good, regular hygienic practices for equipment and environment.
Pediculosis [†]	Biting or chewing lice *Werneckiella (Damalinia) equi* or sucking lice *Hematopinus asini*. Obligate parasite, all stages on horse, egg to egg development time 4-5 weeks.	Direct contact but can possibly spread on blankets and other equipment.	Itching and skin irritation leading to scratching, rubbing, and biting. Most common locations affected are head, mane and ventral neck area.	Nonzoonotic.	Physical examination.	As above, treat with insecticides such as pyrethrins.	Separate grooming equipment, blankets etc. Lice can live 2-3 weeks off host, but a few days more typical. Eggs may continue to hatch over 2-3 weeks in warm weather. Rigorously clean and disinfect areas that housed infested animals.

Rotavirus infection[†]	Rotavirus Group A, of the family Reoviridae. Non-enveloped, double-stranded RNA virus. 12-24 hours.	Fecal-oral, highly contagious, spreads readily on fomites or other contaminated material.	Variable severity of diarrhea in foals from mild to life threatening.	Nonzoonotic, but precautions such as strict hand hygiene should always be exercised with any equine diarrheal disease.	Shed in feces of foals for several weeks after diarrhea ceases. Where introduction a concern, test fecal swab using fecal antigen test (e.g., Virogen Rotatest, Rotazyme).	Phenolics are virucidal even in presence of organic material.	Isolate. Full barrier precautions. Proper sanitation and disinfection of contaminated material and equipment. In general, without other explanation e.g., typical foal heat, diarrheic foals should be considered infectious and possibly contagious until proven otherwise. Good hygiene critical.
Strangles[†]	Streptococcus equi equi. Gram-positive bacterium. 3 to 15 days.	Direct contact, also spread on fomites contaminated with infected secretions. Survival is few days in dry, sunlight.	Abrupt onset fever, mucopurulent nasal discharge, acute swelling and subsequent abscessation of submandibular, retropharyngeal lymph nodes. May be metastatic spread, purpura hemorrhagica or other complications.	Nonzoonotic.	PCR and aerobic culture of nasal/pharyngeal wash or swab, pus from abscesses ± guttural pouch/upper airway endoscopy especially in suspected carriers.	Quaternary ammonium disinfectants, 1% bleach, 70% ethanol, iodine-based disinfectants, phenolics.	Isolation. Fever occurs 2-3 days before nasal shedding; promptly isolate febrile horses in an outbreak. Good hygiene and sanitation, careful cleaning or disposal of contaminated equipment or other material, especially watering and feeding containers.

*Acariasis (mange), anthrax, dermatomycoses, salmonellosis, and leptospirosis are of nosocomial importance but are also zoonotic diseases and are covered in Table 53-1. Diseases that are nationally reportable for humans (H) or animals (A) in the United States are indicated in the first column. Cases may also be notifiable at the state level. Check with your state veterinarian or state public health veterinarian for a current listing of reportable diseases in your area.

[†]Agents that have been linked to nosocomial outbreaks of disease.

[‡]Although still considered exotic to the United States recent outbreaks of piroplasmosis indicate competent tick vectors exist at least in the southern US so given the potential importance of this disease it is included here.

BIOS

nonzoonotic contagious diseases that are not included in Table 52-1. Disease description, clinical signs, mode of transmission, and suggested protective measures (barrier precautions, housing recommendations) are described.

●〉 WHAT TO DO

Contagious and Zoonotic Diseases

- In many instances, known positive horses should be isolated, which implies full barrier precautions (foot baths, boots, gloves, and gowns: coveralls or other protective clothing; scrupulous hand hygiene; no shared equipment) in a dedicated isolation facility or segregated section of a larger facility with strictly controlled human and equine traffic. In the case of some zoonotic diseases, additional personal protective equipment such as eyewear or face shields and face masks effective against aerosols (e.g., N-95 type[1]) is required.
- Although a major expense, consideration must be given to the use of disposable protective items such as gowns or disposable coveralls in addition to gloves and plastic boots. Items hung on stall doors to be reused can be contaminated inside and out during use or while hanging. This is a particularly important decision in the case of foals, where handling generally involves more intimate physical contact.
- Tables 52-1 and 52-2 list some disinfectant choices, but before application of disinfectants, it is often necessary to wash (scrub) surfaces with an appropriate detergent (most often anionic) and rinse in order to achieve maximum disinfectant effect. This and other general biosecurity and infection control practices are discussed in Chapter 53, p. 791.
- *Practice Tip:* Frequent hand washing is very important in controlling the spread of contagious and zoonotic disease. The need for proper hand washing or the correct use of alcohol-based hand sanitizers should be repeatedly emphasized to all personnel and clients. Hand washing is necessary even when gloves are required in patient handling. To promote proper hand hygiene, ready access to hand-washing facilities or hand sanitizers should be available at all times.
- Because many zoonotic organisms—including *Salmonella,* which is the most common equine zoonosis and also one of the most important nosocomial infections capable of causing serious disease outbreaks in equine hospitals—can be spread by the oral route, individuals should not be permitted to eat or drink in equine housing or clinical areas.
- Education and awareness of zoonotic and contagious diseases of importance and the routes of transmission by which causative organisms spread from horse-to-horse, horse-to-human being, or human being-to-horse are key to reducing the risks of infection and preventing outbreaks of disease.
- Based on routes of transmission, all means of spread must be considered. For example, in the case of fecal-oral spread, in addition to general cleanliness, hand hygiene, and preventing contamination of feed and water sources, one must consider rodent control, bird control, and even insect control.
- There is ample evidence to indicate that airborne particulates such as dust can provide vehicles for the transport of contagious organisms. Care should be taken to control dust levels and potential

means by which particulates can be dispersed, such as forced air fans for either heating or cooling, particularly in sensitive areas such as isolation.
- Equine bites can transmit pasteurellosis to human beings; therefore, scrupulous cleansing should occur in the case of bites, and the attention of a physician should be sought if necessary.
- For zoonotic diseases, the *Compendium of Veterinary Standard Precautions* available at http://nasphv.org/Documents/Veterinary Precautions.pdf provides details on the prevention of zoonotic disease in veterinary personnel. The document includes a model infection control plan for veterinary practices, a modifiable electronic template that is available for download in MS Word format at http://nasphv.org/documentsCompendia.html. It should be standard practice for all veterinary facilities to develop a model infection control plan.
- *Practice Tip:* As with all zoonoses, if personnel suspect they have been exposed to a zoonotic disease, they should consult their health care provider as soon as possible.

Zoonotic and Contagious Diseases Restricted to Other Parts of the World

- See Chapter 40, p. 656.
  - Glanders (zoonotic: Asia, eastern Mediterranean)
  - Melioidosis (zoonotic: Southeast Asia, Africa, and northern Australia)
  - Equine morbillivirus pneumonia/Hendra virus (zoonotic: Australia)
  - Epizootic lymphangitis/Farcy (zoonotic: northeast Africa, Middle East, India, Far East)
  - African horse sickness (Africa)
  - Contagious equine metritis/CEM (Europe, Japan, Morocco)
  - Dourine (Asia, southeastern Europe, South America, North and South Africa)
- Although these conditions are considered exotic to North America, persons involved in infection control should be aware of these diseases and should remain vigilant for emergent zoonotic and contagious disease threats and for those that may be regularly reintroduced to North America via imported animals, such as CEM.
- As part of their duties, the individual(s) responsible for infection control should be aware of trends in disease threats and infection control practices. Today, with rapid global dissemination of information, this can be readily achieved by subscribing to appropriate listserves, Internet-based reporting systems such as ProMED-mail, and health emergency notification systems.

References

References can be found on the companion website at www.equine-emergencies.com.

---

[1]Particulate filtering face piece respirators certified by the CDC/National Institute for Occupational Safety and Health (NIOSH) are sometimes referred to as disposable respirators because the entire respirator is discarded when it becomes unsuitable for further use because of considerations of hygiene, excessive resistance, or physical damage. These are also commonly referred to as "N-95s."

CHAPTER 53

Standard Precautions and Infectious Disease Management

Helen Aceto and Barbara Dallap Schaer

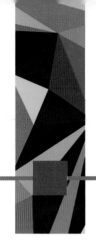

Thinking Critically About Biosecurity

- According to the U.S. Centers for Disease Control and Prevention, approximately 1.8 million (about 1 in 20) patients contract hospital-associated infections (HAI) each year. Of those, about 99,000 die, making HAI the fourth leading cause of death in the United States. The annual estimate of excess health care costs due to HAI is $40 USD billion.
- As a result, HAI are gaining increasing attention from investigative groups, insurance companies and the news media, and human health care facilities all have programs in place to limit HAI.
- HAI, which may represent both a nosocomial problem as well as infections associated with invasive procedures commonly performed in the critically ill/emergency patient, figure prominently in human intensive-care facilities.
- As large referral hospitals become more common and medical advances allow us to treat more critical and emergency cases in veterinary medicine, the potential vulnerability of our patient population increases.
- Although veterinary hospitals have been slower to adopt rigorous infection control practices than their human counterparts, HAI are undoubtedly going to become increasingly important in veterinary hospitals, and veterinarians must take an active role in developing infection control strategies that protect the hospitalized patient, the personnel who take care of them, and the entire veterinary facility.
- Veterinary facilities in the position of providing advanced care to critically ill horses must be particularly aggressive in developing and implementing an integrated infection control program (ICP).
- Appropriate ICPs facilitate:
  - Providing the best patient care
  - Ensuring a safe working environment for employees, students (in teaching institutions), and clients
  - Protecting the hospital from financial loss and possible litigation
- Today, the mobility of many horses (particularly those involved in athletic activities) and the number of contacts that they make as a result, means their risk of

contracting contagious disease–causing agents is probably only exceeded by humans.
- Consequently, directly transmitted infections can spread through equine populations with relative ease and rapidity. Active infection control and biosecurity efforts are integral to reducing the risk of infection and controlling the spread of infectious disease.
- The information presented here focuses on biosecurity and infection control in the setting of a veterinary hospital; the general principles described are relevant to all equine facilities.

Hospital-Associated Infections (HAI)

- There are generally two broad groups of infections that are hospital-associated and cause for concern in our equine patients:
  - Those commonly reported infections associated with the hospitalization and treatment of patients
  - Systemic infectious diseases, which may be transmitted nosocomially
  - Either type could also represent a zoonotic risk!
- Traditionally, frequently reported HAIs in human hospitals are:
  - Urinary tract infections
  - Surgical site infections
  - Catheter-related infections
  - Pneumonia
  - Bloodstream infections
- Although there is little information on similar endemic infections that commonly occur at low levels in equine hospitals, there is ample evidence that nosocomial outbreaks of disease are *not* uncommon.
- In a recent survey of biosecurity experts at 38 veterinary teaching hospitals located in North America, Europe, Australia, and New Zealand, 31 of 38 (82%) reported the occurrence of at least one nosocomial outbreak in the previous 5 years.
- In the same survey, when asked to rank which species was of most concern to them for introducing contagious agents into the hospital environment, more respondents reported that equine patients represented a greater risk than any other species.

- **Important:** Reports of nosocomial outbreaks of infectious disease in equine veterinary hospitals (particularly referral facilities) are abundant in the literature and include:
  - Salmonellosis, the most common
  - Methicillin-resistant *Staphylococcus aureus* (MRSA) associated infections
  - Clostridial enterocolitis
  - Strangles caused by *Streptococcus equi*
  - Herpesvirus myeloencephalitis
  - Equine influenza
  - Equine viral arteritis
  - Equine infectious anemia
  - Possible outbreak of infections caused by *Serratia spp.*
  - In addition to these reported nosocomial infections, other important pathogens include:
    - Rotavirus
    - Coronavirus
    - Cryptosporidia
    - Multidrug-resistant enterococci
- Temporary suspension of specific services or even hospital closures are *not* infrequent. In the survey mentioned above, 71% of hospitals that had reported a nosocomial outbreak had restricted patient admissions, and 38% closed part or all of the facility.
- **Practice Tip:** Salmonella *is most commonly (77%) cited as the reason for restricting patients' admissions.*
- Medical and economic consequences of HAI include:
  - Increased length of hospital stay
  - Increased treatment costs
  - Possible indemnification and legal costs
  - Loss of future business
- In the case of an outbreak, particularly one leading to hospital closure, the expense associated with the decontamination and remediation efforts often necessary in such circumstances, combined with any accompanying decrease in revenue, can pose a very serious financial burden to the affected facility. Deleterious influence on client confidence can have long-term effects on the business and financial health of any hospital or other facility that has suffered an outbreak of infectious disease.
- Definitions for nosocomial infection have been the subject of much debate and a number of different definitions exist in human medicine:
  - Human intensive care unit (ICU) HAI is defined as an infection that occurs after admission to the facility or within 48 hours following transfer from the ICU.
  - A general HAI has been defined as one that first appears 3 days after a patient is admitted to a health care facility.
- Such definitions are *not* always appropriate for equine patients. For example, there is evidence to indicate that at least one major nosocomial threat *(Salmonella)* could manifest in as little as 12 hours after admission and still be hospital associated, or *not* be apparent until after 3 days of hospitalization and still be community associated.
- **Practice Tip:** *The best strategy is to have an ICP in place that limits the risk of HAI in the first place. Part of the ICP*

should include when and how to initiate a more in-depth epidemiologic investigation designed to determine whether particular infections are more likely community associated or nosocomial in origin.

The Hospitalized Horse

- Hospitalized patients are *not* the same as the general population. In hospital, horses are more likely to shed or acquire an infectious agent than those in the general population because they:
  - Are more likely to be under stress
  - May be less able to respond immunologically to infectious agents
  - Have altered nutrition
  - Have disturbances to their normal flora
  - May be receiving antimicrobials
  - May undergo procedures that are known risk factors for various types of infection
  - Are concentrated in close proximity with other animals that have similar risk factors
  - Moreover, the horses in a hospital come from different herds so every patient admission is essentially admixing horses from separate populations, thereby providing an opportunity to introduce infectious organisms to potentially naïve individuals.
- Therefore, veterinary facilities that provide care to hospitalized horses are without doubt places where introduction and reintroduction of infectious agents occur because such facilities are where:
  - Contagious disease-causing organisms reside
  - A greater proportion of infectious agents are multidrug resistant (MDR) than in the general community
  - Infectious agents are present in high numbers and able to contact susceptible patients
- As with hospitalized humans, nosocomial infections in equine patients are an inherent risk of hospitalization, and it is essential that these potential risks are properly conveyed to clients when their horses are admitted to the hospital. Although the period immediately after admission, during which the patient is initially stabilized and preliminary diagnostics are performed, can be multilayered and communications with the client delayed, a discussion on prognosis should take place as soon as possible. As with any discussion of prognosis, the case clinician should inform the client of the possible favorable and unfavorable outcomes, noting HAI as one of the unfavorable outcomes.

Developing a Biosecurity Program

- A successful biosecurity program addresses areas of:
  - Hygiene
  - Patient surveillance
  - Patient contact
  - Education of faculty, staff, referring veterinarians, and clients; as well as house officers and students in the case of teaching institutions

- Although there is no "one-size-fits-all" program that can be used interchangeably for all veterinary facilities, *everyone* should understand their responsibilities in maintaining high standards of hygiene, with particular emphasis on strict hand hygiene, rigorous routine cleaning and disinfection, and reducing risk whenever possible.
- Additionally, it should be recognized that personnel working with hospitalized horses are likely to be exposed to a variety of infectious agents, including those with zoonotic potential, and all ICPs should be designed to limit the risk of human exposure.
- The extent to which an individual veterinary facility implements biosecurity practices is contingent on a number of factors:
  - Size and type of caseload
  - Facility size and design
  - Personnel
  - Economic issues
  - Level of risk aversion
- This chapter provides a general outline of the components of an ICP with details pertaining to specific standard precautions. Excellent resources are available in the literature, online, and in the bibliography to this chapter if more detail is needed.

Biosecurity Personnel

- It is best to have a designated Biosecurity Officer with specialized training in epidemiology or infectious disease to oversee the program. The training of the individual and associated staff may vary depending on the size and scope of the hospital; an individual capable of reviewing and manipulating surveillance data and monitoring infection control activities on a *daily* basis, who then reports to a veterinarian responsible for making biosecurity policy may be a reasonable alternative.
- It should be the responsibility of the individual(s) tasked with overseeing the program to adjust the focus of surveillance and any associated testing based on developments in the hospital, literature, and knowledge of active outbreaks in the hospital referral area.
- Subscription to selected listserves and Internet-based reporting systems such as ProMED mail (www.promedmail.org) can provide rapid notification of infectious disease outbreaks. An awareness of articles about infectious diseases that are published in the lay literature and directed at horse owners can be very useful in client and staff education.

Identification of Patients at Risk: Patient Surveillance

- ***Practice Tip:*** *Patient surveillance is a cornerstone of infection control!*
- Patient monitoring can include:
  - Collection and collation of data with respect to HAI, such as:
    - Unexplained fevers
    - Catheter-associated thrombophlebitis
    - Anesthetic or ventilator-associated pneumonia
    - Surgical-site infections
- Report any methicillin-resistant *Staphylococcus aureus* (MRSA) or vancomycin-resistant *Enterococcus* infections. In a large equine referral hospital setting, monitoring and evaluation of MDR infections and trends in microbial resistance in isolates obtained from clinical submissions should also be part of the biosecurity effort.
- It is essential to ensure a good working relationship among those individuals involved in biosecurity and the diagnostic laboratory.
- Use software developed for the management of microbiology laboratory data and the analysis of antimicrobial susceptibility test results to help provide close to real-time trend analysis and enhance the use of laboratory data for the complex question of guiding therapy, assisting with infection control, and characterizing resistance epidemiology.
- ***Practice Tip:*** *There are many examples of such software, but the World Health Organization's WHONET software has a veterinary module and is available for free download at www.who.int/drugresistance/whonetsoftware/en.*
- It can be particularly useful in an emergency setting to have knowledge of the most common organisms from specific clinical sample types and the resistance patterns those organisms typically exhibit, thus guiding rational empirical therapy in advance of culture results.
- Surveillance for *Salmonella* shedding by patients and subsequent environmental contamination can be a good indicator of the efficacy of the ICP.
- ***Practice Tip:*** Salmonella *serves as the primary model for organizing an ICP in a large equine hospital.*
- Fecal cultures or a combination of polymerase chain reaction (PCR) and culture for detection of *Salmonella* can be used on a patient population to determine the overall incidence of shedding and identify groups of patients that are at high risk for shedding *Salmonella*.
- Identification of patients as "high-risk" directs biosecurity and any related testing efforts (both of which can be costly) toward the proper sector of the patient population.
- The correlation of shedding with particular clinical signs triggers additional culturing and/or increasingly stringent isolation procedures for the patient once specific thresholds have been reached. For example, typical measures associated with *Salmonella* surveillance include:
  - Decreased white blood cell count
  - Increased rectal temperature
  - Diarrhea
  - Inappetence
  - Lethargy
- Systems for implementation of additional barrier precautions or movement of patients to isolation facilities are an important part of both patient handling and protecting the hospital environment.
- With respect to patient surveillance, horses should be monitored for the duration of their stay if they represent

a high-risk patient population. If surveillance relies only on information gathered at admission or during early hospitalization, the risk of the patient to the environment or hospital may be underestimated.

- In the case of *Salmonella,* monitoring could be by way of clinical monitoring and/or fecal culture (or PCR if available).
- Surveillance data from the University of Pennsylvania's George D. Widener Hospital serves to illustrate how the information obtained is used to adjust protocols to optimize the benefit-to-risk-ratio and control costs.
  - Samples are collected at admission and during hospitalization at the following times:
    - Twice weekly for high-risk colic, ICU/NICU (neonatal ICU), isolation, and bovine patients
    - Once weekly for all other patients
  - The data revealed that among horses:
    - Of elective and nongastrointestinal emergency patients, 1.2% were positive for *Salmonella*
    - In equine colic patients and those admitted with either fever and/or diarrhea as their presenting complaint (i.e., essentially all equine gastrointestinal [GI] emergency admissions), positive rates were 13.0% and 21.1%, respectively.
  - The data obtained indicated that surveillance in low- to medium-risk groups could be eliminated; high-risk patients are still subject to active surveillance.
- It is useful to perform pulsed-field gel electrophoresis "fingerprinting" on isolates, especially when monitoring an epidemic or endemic problem, to determine:
  - An index source of infection
  - Maintenance source of infection
  - Separate or new sources of infection

Patient Handling

- Patient handling to optimize patient care and infection control involves:
  - Patient segregation
  - Personnel segregation
  - Proper implementation of barrier precautions in high-risk patient populations
- Wherever possible, patients in the hospital should be segregated by risk category. Risk may be represented as either:
  - Risk to the hospital from the patient
  - Risk to the patient of hospitalization
- Patients in the ICU/NICU are considered at a higher risk for contracting infectious diseases, and may be more susceptible to all types of HAI, so rigorous barrier precautions and personnel segregation are required in these areas.
- Patients admitted for colic and without fever should preferably be segregated in one facility/area, while those with diarrhea, colic, and fever or suspected enterocolitis should be admitted directly to isolation. Because these patients both have increased rates for shedding *Salmonella,* having dedicated personnel to take care of these two populations as a group is ideal.

- Barrier precautions in these areas could include:
  - Disposable gowns or coveralls
  - Gloves
  - Face masks
  - Hair covers
  - Dedicated footwear
  - Footbaths
- Additional footbaths or mats may be placed at areas that function as "choke-points" or have the effect of concentrating foot traffic. Proper maintenance of footbaths and mats is critical to their efficacy and includes:
  - Monitoring disinfectant levels
  - Timely changing of disinfectant
  - Minimizing organic contamination and exposure to the elements such as sunlight and rain
- ***Practice Tip:*** *Even with proper maintenance, the efficacy of footbaths is questionable. Other considerations with footbaths include:*
  - The expense and difficulty of maintaining them
  - The damage to surfaces caused by constant exposure to disinfectant residues from foot traffic
  - Safety issues where disinfectants on some surfaces can cause a slip hazard
- In terms of personal protective equipment (PPE) for personnel working with isolated patients, disposable coveralls offer the best protection. Reusing any type of garment is a contamination risk and gowns *do not* sufficiently protect the lower legs, even when over-boots are worn. A waterproof coverall (e.g., Tyvek[1]) is recommended if there is any risk of getting wet, such as:
  - Kneeling in a stall to work with a foal
  - Close-contact restraint of a foal with diarrhea
  - Working with an adult that has pipe-stream diarrhea
- No matter what type of PPE is required, it is important that everyone understands the rationale behind its use and, most importantly, the distinction between *"clean"* vs. *"dirty"* so that PPE is properly applied and removed in the correct area and that all individuals move about the facility in an appropriate manner.
- Barrier precautions in low- or medium-risk patient populations may be minimal and should be based on incidence of infectious disease in this population.
  - If possible, low-risk patients should be housed separately from those at higher risk of developing HAI secondary to hospitalization, and, when practical, personnel segregation should also be implemented.
  - Ideally, elective cases are housed separately from those patients on antimicrobials for more than 72 hours and non-GI emergencies.

---

[1]Tyvek is a brand of flashspun high-density polyethylene fibers; the name is a registered trademark of DuPont. Tyvek is a strong waterproof material; water vapor can pass through it (highly breathable), but not liquid water. Because they are expensive, Tyvek coveralls should be reserved for uses where it is more likely personnel will get wet. Less expensive polypropylene, nonwaterproof coveralls can be used in all other situations when getting wet is not a concern.

- Ready access to hand-washing facilities or alcohol-based hand sanitizers is a must for patients of all risk categories. Hand sanitizers have been shown to work effectively even when hands are slightly dirty and should be readily accessible in all areas including animal housing, examination, and diagnostic spaces. If hands are grossly dirty they must be washed properly with soap and water! Hand washing/sanitizing is necessary even when gloves are worn for patient handling.
- The presenting complaint and a good history should guide handling of emergency patients, even in the absence of obvious clinical signs, especially where there is a known or suspected outbreak of a contagious disease.
- Tests and clinical monitoring may be something as simple as increased frequency of measuring rectal temperature. For example, with equine herpesvirus, which may spread by aerosol or fomites, it is important to increase clinical monitoring of other horses housed in the same area.
- Clinical signs such as diarrhea, retropharyngeal lymph node swelling or abscesses, accompanied by an appropriate or uncertain history in any horse, should mandate isolation.
- It is important to know the vaccine status of admitted patients for neurologic emergency admissions in rabies-endemic areas.
- *Practice Tip: In terms of infection threat to the hospital, the most difficult patient to handle is the unknown threat or unrecognized case (i.e., the patient that is incubating a contagious disease but has* no *suspect history and* no *clinically apparent disease at presentation).*
  - *Important:* There may be no way to identify this horse on admission, but a proactive infection control program including daily updates on patient clinical status and a heightened awareness of infection risks can rapidly identify potential infection problems and limit spread.

Monitoring of the Environment

- Monitoring the hospital environment is critical for a successful biosecurity program. This includes close monitoring of areas to ensure proper cleaning practices and minimizing clutter that impedes proper cleaning, but does not always imply microbiologic testing of the environment.
- The focus of environmental monitoring should be:
  - High traffic areas
  - Treatment areas
  - Facilities that house high-risk patients
- *Practice Tip: Overall, in a large equine hospital, environmental monitoring based on culturing for* Salmonella *is an effective way of evaluating an ICP.* Careful analysis of environmental cultures plays an important role in modifying biosecurity practices, including:
  - Directing disinfection protocols
  - Determining patient segregation and traffic
  - Optimizing personnel traffic and utilization
- Using *Salmonella* as a general "biosensor" does *not* preclude initiating investigation of other organisms, and part of a proactive biosecurity program should determine trigger points for the initiation (and cessation) of testing for other/additional organisms.
- Investigating specific problems is a legitimate use of environmental monitoring, but randomly testing "this and that" is *not* an effective surveillance strategy.
- Sites chosen for routine sampling should be those most likely to reflect changes in environmental pathogen load. High traffic "choke-points" where there may be crossover between risk groups are good choices, and it is just as important to consider hand surfaces as well as floors.

Microbiologic and Other Test Techniques

- Surveillance tests and strategies should be under constant review. Critical evaluation of the microbiologic techniques used for patient and environmental surveillance must be performed periodically.
- *Important:* If the "hospital's clinical presentation" does *not* match culture information, or if the surveillance protocols in place *do not* adequately address changing infection threats, further investigation and/or implementation of new procedures is warranted.
- Care should be exercised to ensure that any new tests are properly validated and that information is available on the test's characteristics and performance (e.g., sensitivity and specificity) before it is used in any surveillance protocol.

Disinfection Protocols

- Disinfection protocols should be frequently reviewed and changed based on evidence gathered through patient and environmental surveillance.
- Bacterial resistance is a constant worry, and disinfectant kill-curves directed toward organisms of concern may be periodically warranted.
- Consideration should also be given to the effect of the disinfectants on equipment, personnel, and the environment. If prolonged use of a disinfectant damages surfaces, an alternative should be found because loss of surface integrity defeats the goal of maintaining sealed, cleanable surfaces in potentially critical areas.
- At a minimum, cleaning and disinfection protocols should include four steps:
  - Detergent step
  - Rinsing
  - Drying
  - Application of a disinfectant, with further rinsing and drying
- In areas of high risk, multiple disinfectant steps may be useful (Box 53-1). Check to ensure that the properties of the detergent and disinfectant are compatible. Application of a disinfectant in an area that is water-logged may result in dilution to the point of inefficacy.
- *Practice Tip: Remember a surface* cannot *be properly disinfected if it's* not *clean!*
- Intensive care units with specialized equipment and environmental control can be particularly challenging to effectively disinfect. Disinfectant wipes, notably glutaraldehyde

---

| Box 53-1 | Protocol for Effective, Broad Application of Cleaning and Disinfection |

1. Have all material safety data sheets (MSDS) for cleaning and disinfection materials available and follow instructions for proper mixing, disposal, and personal protective equipment (e.g., gloves, eye protection, etc.).
2. Remove all visible organic material (e.g., bedding and manure) before cleaning.
3. Clean surfaces with an anionic detergent (2 oz per gallon of water). Mechanical disruption (scrubbing) of surfaces is often necessary to remove biofilms and stubborn organic debris, especially in horse housing areas.
4. Rinse with clean water.
5. Allow to dry or at least ensure that the bulk of surface water is removed. If excess water remains disinfectants may be diluted to the point of inefficacy.
6. Apply disinfectant solution and allow the appropriate contact time. A dilute solution of bleach (2% to 4%) with at least 15 minutes contact time is inexpensive but may *not* be the most effective choice. There are many other options available. Alternatives include quaternary ammonium disinfectants (e.g., Roccal D), those containing quaternary ammonium and glutaraldehyde (e.g., Synergize), phenolics (e.g., 1-Stroke Environ), accelerated hydrogen peroxide (e.g., Accel TB), or peroxygen-based disinfectants (e.g., Virkon-S). Dilution rates and recommended contact times vary by product.
7. Rinse thoroughly with clean water and allow the treated area to dry as much as possible.
8. In known contaminated or high-risk areas, a second application of disinfectant with an accelerated hydrogen peroxide product should be considered as a final decontamination step. Allow at least 10 minutes' contact time.
9. Rinse with clean water.
10. Drying is important in achieving maximum effect so allow the area to dry as much as possible before rebedding or reintroducing horses. If postcleaning environmental samples are being collected, the area must be completely dry.

or accelerated hydrogen peroxide–based wipes, as opposed to those containing quaternary ammonium disinfectant, can be particularly useful in these settings where delicate equipment needs special attention. Diligence with respect to infection control is probably most important in these areas.

Facility Evaluation
- All aspects of the hospital must be evaluated with biosecurity in mind.
- In a large equine hospital setting, this refers to everything from manure handling to flooring choices to the development of appropriate isolation facilities.
- The goal should be to have as many cleanable, nonporous surfaces as possible. Critically evaluate the environment. Noncleanable surfaces in high-risk patient areas provide a threat to the care of all horses, especially the critically ill.

- Isolation and other facilities for housing high-risk patients must have the ability to:
  - Care for the critically ill equine patient
  - Ventilate a patient
  - Provide intranasal oxygen
  - Provide climate control
  - Make a sling/hoist system available

"Clinical Impression" vs. "Evidence-Based Decision-Making"
- The needs of the hospital as a "patient" are best met by making evidence-based decisions.
- Biosecurity efforts are most effectively directed by collection and critical evaluation of *data*.
- Efforts and resources can be wasted by making decisions based solely on clinical impression.
- The implementation of an effective biosecurity program must be focused on the principles of:
  - Hygiene
  - Patient contact
  - Education and awareness
  - Surveillance
- In the wake of an outbreak, the level of risk aversion is *high*. It is important to appreciate that just as disease-causing organisms evolve and change, evidence-based evolution of biosecurity protocols is inevitable and indeed crucial to ongoing program success.
- The data gathered from monitoring and surveillance are used to:
  - Make evidence-based decisions on the effectiveness of the biosecurity protocols
  - Define the level of risk that different types of cases represent
  - Keep pace with infection threats
  - Optimize the benefit-to-risk ratio of the program
- The appearance of increasingly resistant organisms in both community and hospital settings and the mobility of our equine populations increase the risk of disease outbreaks caused by infectious agents and make HAI increasingly difficult to treat. A demonstrably effective ICP improves the quality of the facility by:
  - Optimizing patient care
  - Reducing HAI
  - Protecting personnel and clients from zoonotic agents
  - Providing educational opportunities
  - Limiting financial losses and liability
  - Instilling confidence in staff and clients
- ***Practice Tip:*** *Written plans, careful data management, attention to detail, good communications, and a persistent message are imperative to success.*

References
References can be found on the companion website at www.equine-emergencies.com.

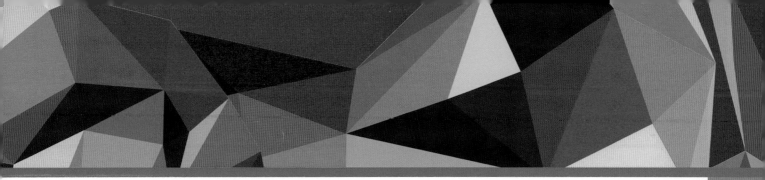

Appendices

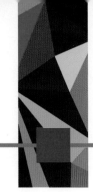

APPENDIX 1

Reference Values

Reference Values for *Selected** Blood Chemistries in Adults[†]

Assay	Reference Values	Assay	Reference Values
Acetylcholinesterase	450-790 IU/L	Lactate	1.11-1.78 mmol/L 10-16 mg/dL
Ammonia/plasma (on ice)	7.63-63.4 μmol/L (mean 35.8 ± 17.0) 13-108 μg/dL	Leptin	1-4 mg/mL
Amylase	75-150 IU/L	Triglycerides	12-67 mg/dL or 0.13-0.76 mmol/L May be higher in ponies—(adults and foals)
Bile acids (total)	5-15 μmol/L; ± 20 μmol/L in anorexia	Serum amyloid (SAA)[‡]	0-20 mg/L[‡]
Cardiac troponin I	0.00-0.06 ng/mL	Serum haptoglobin[‡]	0.2-2.3 mg/mL[‡]

*Laboratory assays that may not have normal ranges reported on commercial test results.
[†]A complete listing of all "Adult Assays" can be found at www.equine-emergencies.com, Web Appendix 3.
[‡]Can be performed at the University of Miami, Miller School of Medicine on either serum or plasma. www.cpl.med.miami.edu.

Age-Related Changes in Serum Electrolyte Concentrations in Foals (Mean ± 2 SD)

Age	Na^+ (mEq/L)	K^+ (mEq/L)	Cl^- (mEq/L)	CO_2 (mEq/L)	HPO_4^+ (mg/dL)	Ca^{2+} (mg/dL)*	Mg^{2+} (mg/dL)	Anion Gap (mEq/L)
Hours								
<12	148 ± 15	4.4 ± 1	105 ± 12	25 ± 5	4.7 ± 1.6	12.8 ± 2	1.5 ± 0.8	21 ± 12
Days								
1	141 ± 18	4.6 ± 1	102 ± 12	27 ± 6	5.6 ± 1.8	11.7 ± 2	2.4 ± 1.8	16 ± 8

*Ionized calcium conversion factor from mg/dL to mmol/L is division by 4.

Age-Related Changes in Serum Iron and Related Parameters in Foals

Age	Iron (μg/dL)	UIBC (μg/dL)	TIBC (μg/dL)	Iron Saturation (%)	Ferritin (ng/mL)
Hours					
<1	345-592	4-156	386-663	73-99	34-161
<12	262-488	10-133	339-535	69-98	
Days					
1	78-348	28-416	208-620	22-90	79-263
3	29-191	47-494	175-552	6-66	52-200
5	21-258	129-460	250-581	7-59	54-170
Weeks					
1	30-273	35-503	222-619	10-72	57-173
2	22-215	168-643	337-706	4-52	21-136
3	46-241	228-669	408-745	7-46	27-117

Age	Iron (μg/dL)	UIBC (μg/dL)	TIBC (μg/dL)	Iron Saturation (%)	Ferritin (ng/mL)
Months					
1	49-288	250-668	437-777	9-50	33-140
2	43-340	201-529	397-716	19-57	32-144
Adult	74-209	177-379	305-542	21-48	58-365

From Koterba AM, Drummond WH, Koseh PC: *Equine clinical neonatology,* Philadelphia, 1990, Lea & Febiger.
TIBC, Total iron-binding capacity; *UIBC,* unbound iron-binding capacity.
Low iron with normal or high TIBC could indicate iron deficiency, which may occur rarely in young foals.

Age-Related Changes in Erythrocyte Values in Foals

Age	PCV	Hb (g/dL)	RBC(×10⁶/μL)	MCV (ff)	MCHC (g/dL)
Hours					
<1*	40-52	13.4-19.9	9.3-12.9	37-45	33-39
<12†	37-49	12.6-17.4	9-12	36-45	32-40
Days					
1	32-46	12-16.6	8.2-11.0	36-46	32-40
3	30-46	11.5-16.7	7.8-11.4	35-44	34-40
5	30-44	11-16.6	7.2-11.6	35-45	34-40
Weeks					
1	28-43	10.7-15.8	7.4-10.6	35-44	35-40
2	28-41	10.1-15.3	7.2-10.8	35-41	34-40
3	29-40	10.5-14.8	7.8-10.6	34-41	34-40
Months					
1	29-41	10.9-15.3	7.9-11.1	33-40	34-40
Years					
>4	31-47	11-18	5.9-9.9	41-51	33-41

From Koterba AM, Drummond WH, Koseh PC: *Equine clinical neonatology,* Philadelphia, 1990, Lea & Febiger.
ff, Free fraction; *Hb,* hemoglobin; *MCHC,* mean corpuscular hemoglobin concentration; *MCV,* mean corpuscular volume; *PCV,* packed cell volume; *RBC,* red blood cells.
*Before nursing.
†After nursing.

Age-Related Changes in Normal Hematologic Values in Foals

Age	Total Plasma Protein (g/dL)	Fibrinogen (mg/dL)*	Haptoglobin (mg/dL)	Icterus Index (units)	Platelets (×10³/μL)
Hours					
<1	4.4-5.9	100-500		20-100	
<12	5.1-7.6	100-350	8-120	15-50	105-446
Days					
1	5.2-8.0	100-400	0-136	10-75	129-409
3	5.3-7.9	150-500	8-162	10-50	105-353
5	5.4-7.6	100-500		15-50	
Weeks					
1	5.2-7.5	150-450	0-143	5-25	111-387
2	5.2-7.2	150-600	0-202	5-25	133-457
3	5.2-6.8	150-600	11-184	5-20	134-442
Adults	6.2-8	100-600	19-177	5-20	100-350

From Koterba AM, Drummond WH, Koseh PC: *Equine clinical neonatology,* Philadelphia, 1990, Lea & Febiger.
*Values vary considerably between laboratories.

Age-Related Changes in Serum Enzyme Activities in Foals

Age	ALP	GGT	SDH	AST*	ALT	CK*
			(Range, IU/L)			
Hours						
<12	152-2835	13-39	0.2-4.8	97-315	0-47	65-380
Days						
1	861-2671	18-43	0.6-4.6	146-340	0-49	40-909
3	283-1462	11-50	0.6-3.7	80-580	0-52	21-97
5	156-1294	8-89	0.8-5.3			29-208
7	137-1169	16-98	0.8-8.2	237-620	4-50	52-143
14	182-859	13-59	0.6-4.3	240-540	1-9	46-208
21	146-752	16-64	1-8.4	226-540	0-45	44-210
28	210-866	17-44	1.2-5.9	252-440	5-47	81-585
Months						
2	201-747	8-38	1.1-4.6	282-484	7-57	50-170

From Koterba AM, Drummond WH, Koseh PC: *Equine clinical neonatology*, Philadelphia, 1990, Lea & Febiger; and Barton MH, LeRoy BE: Serum bile acids concentrations in healthy and clinically ill neonatal foals, *J Vet Intern Med* 21(3):508-513, 2007.

ALP, Alkaline phosphatase; *ALT*, alanine transaminase; *AST*, aspartate aminotransferase; *CK*, creatine kinase; *GGT*, gamma-glutamyltransferase; *SDH*, sorbitol dehydrogenase.

*Upper range may be considered abnormal.

Age-Related Changes in Leukocyte Counts in Foals

Age	Total Leukocytes (×10³/μL)	Neutrophils (×10³/μL)	Lymphocytes (×10³/μL)	Monocytes (×10³/μL)	Eosinophils (×10³/μL)	Basophils (×10³/μL)
Hours						
<12	6.9-14.4	5.55-12.38	0.46-1.43	0.04-0.43	0	0-0.02
Days						
1	4.9-11.7	3.36-9.57	0.67-2.12	0.07-0.39	0-0.02	0-0.03
3	5.1-10.1	3.21-8.58	0.73-2.17	0.08-0.58	0-0.22	0-0.12
Weeks						
1	6.3-13.6	4.35-10.55	1.43-2.28	0.03-0.54	0-0.09	0-0.18
2	5.2-11.9	3.99-9.08	1.32-3.12	0.07-0.58	0-0.10	0-0.1
3	5.4-12.4	3.16-8.94	1.47-3.26	0.06-0.69	0-0.16	0-0.09
Months						
1	5.3-12.2	2.76-9.27	1.73-4.85	0.05-0.63	0-0.12	0-0.08
Adults	5.4-14.3	2.26-8.58	1.5-7.7	0-1	0-1	0-0.4

From Koterba AM, Drummond WH, Koseh PC: *Equine clinical neonatology*, Philadelphia, 1990, Lea & Febiger.

Premature foals commonly have lower neutrophil counts at birth. Premature foals with normal or high neutrophil count indicates in utero stress and may suggest expedited development and improved prognosis.

Age-Related Changes in Serum Protein Values in Foals

Age	Total Protein* (g/dL)	Albumin (g/dL)	Total Globulin (g/dL)	Clotting Times†
Hours				
<12	4-7.9	2.7-3.9	1.1-4.8 Range includes before and after nursing	PT = 10-11 sec APTT = 52-63 sec
Days				
1	4.3-8.1	2.5-3.6	1.5-4.6	
3	4.4-7.6	2.8-3.7	1.6-4.5	
5				
7	4.4-6.8	2.7-3.4	2.7-3.4	PT = 9-10 sec APTT = 36-44 sec
14	4.8-6.7	2.6-3.3	2.6-3.3	
21	4.7-6.5	2.6-3.2	2.6-3.2	
28	5-6.7	2.7-3.4	2.7-3.4	
Months				
2	5.2-6.5	2.7-3.5	1.9-3.8	PT = 9-10 sec APTT = 35-47 sec
Adults	5.5-7.9	2.8-4.8	1.9-3.8	PT = 9-10 sec APTT = 33-51 sec

From Koterba AM, Drummond WH, Koseh PC: *Equine clinical neonatology,* Philadelphia, 1990, Lea & Febiger.
APTT, Activated partial thromboplastin time; *PT,* prothrombin time.
*Some values within these reported ranges may be considered abnormal.
†Values from Barton MH et al: Hemostatic indices in healthy foals, from birth to one month of age, *J Vet Diag Lab Invest* 7(3):380-385, 1995. Note: Fibrin degradation products and D-dimers may be higher in normal foals some of which may be related to fibrinolysis of normally clotted umbilical vessels. Antithrombin III activity is reported to be lower in healthy newborn foals but protein C antigen is increased. Normal antithrombin III activity in adult horses is 90% to 113%.
Thromboelastography studies "suggest" that time to clot formation may be prolonged in normal foals compared with normal horses, and clot strength is less in septic foals than healthy foals. There is also a decrease in antithrombin III and protein C.

Age-Related Changes in Serum Basal Cortisol and Serum Basal ACTH in Foals

Age	Cortisol (µg/dL)	ACTH (pg/mL)	ACTH:Cortisol Ratio
Birth	8.9-11.6	199.6-371.4	13.3-41.5
Hours			
12-24	2.6-4.6	17.9-21.3	5.0-7.4
36-48	2.0-3.2	16.3-49.1	9.4-18.4
Days			
5-7	1.5-2.5	20.2-47.4	12.8-19.0

From Hart KA, Heusner GL, Norton NA et al: Hypothalamic-pituitary-adrenal axis assessment in healthy term neonatal foals utilizing a paired low dose/high dose ACTH stimulation test, *J Vet Intern Med* 23(2):344-351, 2009. Results reflect 95% confidence interval.
ACTH, Adrenocorticotropic hormone.

Age-Related Changes in Serum Chemistry Concentrations: Small Organic Molecules in Foals

	Glucose	BUN	Creatinine	TBR	CJBR	UNCJBR	Bile Acids*	Triglycerides
Age				**(Range, mg/dL)**				
Hours								
<12	108-190	12-27	1.7-4.2	0.9-2.8	0.1-0.4	0.8-2.5	24-38	11-33
Days								
1	121-233	9-40	1.2-4.3	1.3-4.5	0.1-0.4	1-3.8	7-38	4-154
3	101-226	2-29	0.4-2.1	0.5-1.2	0.1-0.4	0.2-3.3		63-342
5				1.2-3.6	0.1-0.4	0.8-2.8		52-340
7	121-192	4-20	1-1.7	0.8-3	0.1-0.4	0.5-2.3	4-15	35-200
14	137-205	6-13	0.9-1.8	0.7-2.2	0.1-0.3	0.5-1.6	6-9	28-91
21	130-240	6-14	0.6-2	0.5-1.6	0.1-0.3	0.2-1.1	6-7	34-124
28	130-216	6-21	1.1-1.8	0.5-1.7	0.1-0.3	0.4-1.2	4-6	45-155
Months								
2	119-204[†]	6-11	1.1-1.2	0.5-2	0.1-0.3	0.3-1.5	5-11	10-148
Adults	57-96	12-24	0.9-2	0.5-1.8	0.1-0.3[‡]	0.3-1	58-109	6-44

From Koterba AM, Drummond WH, Koseh PC: *Equine clinical neonatology,* Philadelphia, 1990, Lea & Febiger; and Barton MH, LeRoy BE: Serum bile acids concentrations in healthy and clinically ill neonatal foals, *J Vet Intern Med* 21(3):508-513, 2007.
BUN, Blood urea nitrogen; *CJBR,* conjugated bilirubin; *TBR,* total bilirubin; *UNCJBR,* unconjugated bilirubin.
*Radioimmunoassay (RIA) values; enzymatic assays may be double RIA values.
[†]Higher than normal horse values may be somewhat explained by stress of blood collection.
[‡]Some laboratories have normal ranges up to 0.6.

Summary of Important Age-Related Changes in Complete Blood Cell Count and Chemistries

	Neonatal TB 24-48 Hours	TB 3 Weeks	TB Yearling	TB 2 Years	TB Adult	Non-TB Adult
PCV	30-44	30-38	30-41	34-45	35-47	31-43
WBC (×10³)	6.2-12.4	6.9-15.2	6.0-15.0	7.3-12.7	4.1-10.1	6-10
Segments (×10³)	4.1-9.5	4.1-9.1	3.7-5.4	4.0-6.0	1.4-5.8	3.4-5.4
Lymphocytes (×10³)	1.0-3.1	0.9-5.9	3.5-4.9	2.7-4.4	1.4-4.7	2.0-3.2
TP (g/dL)	4.1-6.6	4.2-6.6	5.0-7.0	5.9-6.6	6.5-7.5	5.3-7.3
AST (IU/L)	111-206	329-337	329-441	308-520	256-369	102-350
CK (IU/L)	165-761	204-263	190-370	165-472	157-270	110-250
GGT (IU/L)	10-32	13-30	10-30	12-40	14-28	1-40
BUN (mg/dL)	9-40	6-14	15-24	15-24	12-24	12-24
Creatinine (mg/dL)	1.7-4.3	0.6-2.0	1.3-2.1	1.3-2.1	0.9-1.8	0.9-2.2
Bile acids (µmol/L)	11-30*	11-22*	6-12	6-12	6-12	6-12
Glucose (mg/dL)	101-233[†]	130-240[†]	105-165	90-104	84-104	84-104
Triglycerides (mg/dL)	30-340	34-124	38-86	20-56	20-56	20-56
Thyroxine	21.5-35.7 µg/dL Declines in first weeks of life		Adult values 0.85-2.4 µg/dL fT₄, 1.2-1.8 ng/dL			
Triiodothyronine	7-12× adult values Declines in first weeks of life		Adult values 0.3-0.8 ng/mL			

Information gathered from several books, particularly Ricketts S et al: *Guide to equine clinical pathology,* Newmarket, UK, 2006, Rossdale and Partners.
TB, Thoroughbred; *PCV,* packed cell volume; *WBC,* white blood cell; *TP,* total protein; *AST,* aspartate transaminase; *CK,* creatine kinase; *fT₄,* free thyroxine test; *GGT,* gamma-glutamyltransferase; *BUN,* blood urea nitrogen.
*May be even higher in some normal foals if enzymatic assay used.
[†]Significantly high normals may be caused by stress of restraint and blood collection.

Arterial Blood Gas Parameters in Young and Old Horses

Age	PaO$_2$ (mmHg)	PaCO$_2$ (mmHg)	pH	HCO$_3$ (mEq/L)
Young horses (3-8 years)	98.6-104.8	41.6-44.4	7.394-7.414	25.6-27.2
Old horses (>20 years)	85.9-94.5	39.5-43.5	7.414-7.442	25.0-28.6

From Aquilera-Tejero E, Estepa JC, Lopez I, et al: Arterial blood gases and acid-base balance in healthy young and aged horses, *Equine Vet J* 30(4):352-354, 1998. Results reflect 95% confidence interval.

Arterial Blood Gas Parameters in Foals at Sea Level and 1500-Meter Altitude

Age	PaO$_2$ (mm Hg) Sea Level *(1500-m Altitude)*	PaCO$_2$ (mm Hg) Sea Level *(1500-m Altitude)*	pH Sea Level *(1500-m Altitude)*	HCO$_3$ (mEq/L) Sea Level *(1500-m Altitude)*
Birth	51.2-61.6 *(47.1-58.9)*	49.6-58.8 *(42.0-46.2)*	7.276-7.348 *(7.370-7.418)*	21.3-26.7 *(24.7-28.3)*
Hours				
3	61.1-71.9 *(55.0-63.4)*	43.7-51.7 *(40.6-44.1)*	7.334-7.390 *(7.381-7.424)*	22.9-27.1 *(25.0-28.0)*
6	64.6-86.8 *(59.3-74.2)*	40.7-49.3 *(39.8-44.3)*	7.317-7.393 *(7.381-7.424)*	21.1-26.1 *(24.5-27.0)*
12	66.7-80.3 *(53.6-64.9)*	41.6-47.0 *(40.8-44.9)*	7.303-7.411 *(7.377-7.415)*	20.3-26.1 *(24.5-27.0)*
24	57.5-77.7 *(55.4-64.5)*	42.0-49.0 *(39.6-43.5)*	7.365-7.421 *(7.380-7.413)*	23.7-28.7 *(23.7-26.2)*
48	67.1-82.7 *(64.0-71.1)*	43.5-48.7 *(35.9-40.6)*	7.377-7.415 *(7.369-7.399)*	24.5-26.9 *(20.6-23.7)*

From Stewart JH, Rose RJ, Barko AM: Respiratory studies in foals from birth to seven days old, *Equine Vet J* 16:323-328, 1984; and Hackett ES, Traub-Dargatz JL, Knowles JE et al: Arterial blood gas parameters of normal foals born at 1500 meters elevation, *Equine Vet J* 42:59-62, 2010. Results reflect 95% confidence interval.

Normal foals should have a PaO$_2$-Fio$_2$ ratio (mm Hg) of 250 or more at birth and 350 within 48 hours.

All values above and ratio value are from sampling in lateral recumbency, which on average causes a 14-mm Hg lower measurement than when standing!

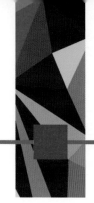

Calculations in Emergency Care

Eileen Sullivan Hackett

A-a Gradient

$$P_{(A-a)}O_2 = P_AO_2 - P_aO_2$$

Alveolar-arterial oxygen difference

$$P_AO_2 = P_IO_2 - (1.25 \times PaCO_2)$$

P_AO_2 = Alveolar oxygen tension
P_IO_2 = Inspired oxygen tension
$PaCO_2$ = Arterial carbon dioxide tension

$$P_IO_2 = (\text{Barometric pressure} - 47) \times F_IO_2$$

F_IO_2 = Inspired oxygen concentration

$$A - a: (P_{BAR} - 47)0.21 - \frac{PaCO_2}{0.8} - PaO_2$$

P_{BAR} = Barometric pressure

Albumin Deficit

$$AD = 10 \times (\text{desired [alb]} - \text{patient [alb]}) \times \text{body weight (kg)} \times 0.3$$

AD = Albumin deficit
[alb] = Albumin concentration

Anion Gap

$$AG = [Na^+ + K^+] - [Cl^- + HCO_3^-]$$

Base Deficit

HCO_3^- needed for correction (mEq) = mEq base deficit × Body mass (kg) × 0.50*
mEq base deficit = Normal HCO_3^- − Measured HCO_3^-
HCO_3^- = Serum bicarbonate

Blood Transfusion

$$\text{Transfusion volume (L)} = \frac{PCV_{desired} - PCV_{recipient}}{PCV_{donor}} \times 0.08 \text{ (BW)}$$

PCV = Packed cell volume
BW = Body weight in kg
Administration rate of 10 to 20 mL/kg/h

Body Weight

$$\text{Pony: Weight in kilograms} = \frac{\text{Chest girth (cm)}^2 \times \text{Length (cm)}}{11,877}$$

$$\text{Horse: Weight in kilograms} = \frac{\text{Umbilical girth (cm)}^{1.78} \times \text{Length (cm)}^{1.05}}{3011}$$

*0.50 for neonates and 0.30 for adults.

Carbonic Anhydrase Equation

$$CO_2 + H_2O \xrightarrow[CA]{} H_2CO_3 \leftrightarrow H^+ + HCO_3$$

Carbonic anhydrase enzyme facilitates first reaction; second reaction occurs spontaneously.

Cardiac Output

$$CO \text{ (L/min)} = SV \times HR$$

or

$$CO = CI \times BSA$$

CO = Cardiac output
SV = Stroke volume
HR = Heart rate
CI = Cardiac index
BSA = Body surface area (m^2)

Cardioversion

1 to 4 J/kg, increasing energy by 50% at each defibrillation attempt
50 to 200 J for a 50-kg foal

Cerebral Perfusion Pressure

$$CPP = MAP - ICP$$

MAP = mean arterial blood pressure
ICP = intracranial pressure

Colloid Osmotic Pressure

Foals (Landis-Pappenheimer equation)

$$COP = 2.1 TP + (0.16 TP^2) + (0.009 TP^3)$$

TP = total protein
Adults

$$COP = 0.986 + 2.029 A + 0.175 A^2$$

A = Albumin

$$COP = -0.059 + 0.618 G + 0.028 G^2$$

G = Globulin

$$COP = 0.028 + 1.542 P + 0.219 P^2$$

P = Protein

$$COP = -1.989 + 1.068 TS + 0.176 (TS)^2$$

$$\text{Simplified: } COP = 3.02 \times TS + 0.65$$

TS = Refractometer total solids

$$COP = -4.384 + 5.501A + 2.475G$$

Continuous Rate Infusion

Step 1: Calculate amount of drug (mcg or mg) for 1 unit of infusion time (minute or hour): dosage (mcg/kg or mg/kg) × body weight (kg) = X amount drug.

Step 2: Calculate volume of drug needed for 1 unit infusion time: divide X (amount of drug, mcg or mg) by drug's concentration (mcg/mL or mg/mL): X ÷ concentration = Y volume of drug (mL).

Step 3: Calculate volume of drug for duration of infusion: Y mL × anticipated infusion time.

Step 4: Calculate infusion volume by summing the volume of drug (Y) and crystalloid volume infused over anticipated infusion time.

Step 5: Calculate infusion rate by dividing total volume by infusion time.

Example: 500-kg horse to receive a 1-hour lidocaine CRI at 0.05 mg/kg/min prepared with lidocaine 2% (20 mg/mL) solution added to 1 L of crystalloid fluid

Step 1: 0.05 mg/kg × 500 kg = 25 mg lidocaine

Step 2: 25 mg ÷ 20 mg/mL = 1.25 mL lidocaine per minute

Step 3: 1.25 mL/min × 60 min = 75 mL of 2% lidocaine

Step 4: 75 mL lidocaine + 1000 mL crystalloid = 1075 mL total infusion volume

Step 5: 1075 mL ÷ 60 min = 17.9 mL, or 18 mL per minute infusion rate

Crystalloid Fluid Rate Calculation

Shock dose = 50 to 80 mL/kg; give in 25% increments and reassess

Adult maintenance fluid rate = 60 mL/kg/day

Foal calculation based on body surface area:

$$\text{Daily fluid need (mL)} = [100\,\text{mL} \times \text{First 10 kg}] + [50\,\text{mL} \times \text{Second 10 kg}] + [25\,\text{mL} \times \text{Remaining body mass}]$$

Electrolyte supplementation:

$$\text{Body weight (kg)} \times 0.3\,\text{ECF} \times (\text{Normal} - \text{Measured in mEq}) = \text{Deficit in mEq/L}$$

ECF = Extracellular fluid

$$\text{Rate} = \text{drops/min} = [\text{mL/min} \times \text{drops/mL}]$$

Dead Space Ventilation Fraction

$$\frac{Vd}{Vt} = \frac{(Paco_2 - PEco_2)}{Paco_2}$$

Vd = Dead space volume
Vt = Tidal volume
$Paco_2$ = Arterial carbon dioxide tension
$PEco_2$ = End-tidal carbon dioxide tension

Dehydration Correction

Estimate of dehydration (%) × Body mass (kg) = Liter volume to correct dehydration

Extracellular Fluid Volume

$$ECF\,(L) = 0.25^* \times BW\,(kg)$$

ECF = Extracellular fluid volume
BW = Body weight
*Higher for neonates: 35%-50% (0.35-0.5)

Fick Equation

$$V = Q\,(C_A - C_V)$$

or

$$Q = \frac{V}{(C_A - C_V)}$$

C_A = Arterial concentration
C_V = Venous concentration
V = Amount of substance removed by an organ or circuit
Q = Blood flow to the organ or circuit

Fractional Excretion of Quantity "X"

$$FEx = \frac{[\text{serum creatinine}]}{[\text{urine creatinine}]} \times \frac{[\text{urine x}]}{[\text{serum x}]}$$

Global Oxygen Delivery

$$DO_2 = Q \times CaO_2$$

Q = Cardiac output (L/min)
CaO_2 = Arterial oxygen content

Henderson-Hasselbalch Equation

$$pH = pKa + \frac{\log[HCO_3]}{\text{Total } CO_2}$$

Intracellular Fluid Volume

$$ICF\,(L) = 0.40 \times BW\,(kg)$$

ICF = Intracellular fluid volume
BW = Body weight

K⁺ Max

Maximum potassium infusion = 0.5 mEq/kg/h

Mean Arterial Pressure

$$MAP = DAP + \frac{(SAP - DAP)}{3}$$

MAP = Mean arterial pressure
DAP = Diastolic arterial pressure
SAP = Systolic arterial pressure

Milliequivalents

$$mEq = \frac{\text{Milligram} \times \text{Valence}}{\text{Molecular weight}}$$

or

$$mEq = \text{mmol/L} \times \text{Valence}$$

Comment: if the substance is a +1 and −1 charge (i.e., NaCl) then 1 mEq = 2 mmol

Molality

$$\text{Molality (mOsm/kg)} = \frac{\text{Grams/Molecular weight}}{\text{Liter}}$$

Molarity

$$M = \frac{\text{Grams/Molecular weight}}{\text{Liter}}$$

Oxygen Consumption

See Tissue Oxygen Consumption.

Oxygen Content (Arterial)

$$CaO_2 = (1.34 \times Hb \times SaO_2) + (0.003 \times PaO_2)$$

Hb = hemoglobin content (g/dL)
SaO_2 = Arterial oxygen saturation
PaO_2 = Arterial oxygen tension (mm Hg)

Oxygen Extraction Ratio

$$OER = VO_2/DO_2 = \frac{SaO_2 - SvO_2}{SaO_2}$$

Ratio of O_2 uptake to O_2 delivery (fraction of O_2 delivered to tissues)
VO_2 = Tissue oxygen uptake
DO_2 = Global oxygen delivery

Oxygen Index (Arterial)

$$\text{Oxygen index} = \frac{P_aO_2}{F_IO_2} \times 100$$

Percent Solution

$$xL\% = \frac{x \text{ Grams}}{100 \text{ mL}}$$

Plasma Osmolality

$$\text{Osmolality (mOsm/kg)} = 1.86\,(Na + K) + BUN/2.8 + \text{Glucose}/18 + 9$$

or

$$\text{Osmolality} = (Na \times 2) + BUN/2.8 + \text{Glucose}/18$$

or

$$\text{Osmolality} = 2.1\,(Na)$$

BUN = Blood urea nitrogen
Osmolality and *osmolarity* are measurements that are "technically" different, but "functionally" the same for normal use. Osmolality is a measure of the *osmoles* (Osm) of a solute per *kilogram* of *solvent* (osmol/kg or Osm/kg); osmolarity is defined as the number of osmoles of a solute per *liter* (L) of *solution* (osmol/L or Osm/L).

Plasma Volume

$$\text{Plasma volume} = \text{blood volume} \times (1 - PCV)$$

PCV = Packed cell volume

Poiseuille's Law of Flow

$$Q = \Delta P/R$$

Blood flow (Q) is equal to perfusion pressure (ΔP) over resistance to flow (R).

$$R = 8\eta L/\pi r^4$$

Resistance to flow is proportional to viscosity (η) and length (L) and inversely proportional to radius (r).

$$Q = \frac{\Delta P r^4 \pi}{\eta L 8}$$

Resting Energy Requirement

Foal: DE = 30 to 50 kcal/kg per day
Adult: DE = $(0.03 \times kg) + 1.4$ kcal/d when body mass < 600 kg
    DE = $1.82 + (0.0383 \times kg) - (0.000015 \times kg^2)$ kcal/d when body mass > 600 kg
    DE = Digestible energy

Shunt Fraction

$$Qs/Q = ScO_2 - SaO_2/ScO_2 - SvO_2$$

Qs = Shunt fraction
Q = Total flow
SaO_2 = Arterial oxygen saturation
ScO_2 = Capillary oxygen saturation
SvO_2 = Mixed venous oxygen saturation
Assume ScO_2 is 100 if breathing 100% oxygen

Sodium Correction Rate

0.5 mEq/h

Starling Equation

$$J = K_f[(P_c - P_t) - s(p_p - p_t)]$$

J = Volume of flow across capillary wall
K_f = Filtration coefficient of capillary wall
P_c = Capillary hydrostatic pressure
P_t = Interstitial fluid hydrostatic pressure
s = Osmotic reflection coefficient
p_p = Colloid osmotic (oncotic) pressure of plasma
p_t = Colloid osmotic (oncotic) pressure of interstitial fluid

Strong Ion Difference—Stewart

$$SID = (\text{Plasma }[Na] + \text{Plasma }[K]) - (\text{Plasma }[Cl] + \text{Plasma }[\text{Lactate}])$$

Simplified version of SID = (Plasma [Na] + Plasma [K]) − (Plasma [Cl])

Systemic Vascular Resistance

$$SVR(\text{dynes} \cdot s \cdot cm^{-5}) = \frac{(MAP - CVP) \times 80}{\text{Cardiac output}}$$

MAP = mean arterial pressure
CVP = central venous pressure

Tissue Oxygen Consumption

$$VO_2 \ (mL \ O_2/min) = Q \times (CaO_2 - CvO_2)$$

Product of cardiac output and difference in arterial and venous oxygen content

$$VO_2 = Q \times 13.4 \times Hb \times (SaO_2 - SvO_2)$$

(Multiply by 10 to correct unit differences)
Q = Cardiac output
Hb = Hemoglobin content (g/dL)
Sa_{O_2} = Arterial oxygen saturation
Sv_{O_2} = Venous oxygen saturation

Total Body Water

$$TBW = 0.6 \times BW \ (kg)$$

TBW = Total body water
BW = Body weight

Water Deficit*

$$Water \ deficit \ (L) = 1 - Na^+_{Normal}/Na^+_{Measured} \times TBW_{Normal}$$

TBW = 0.6 × body weight in kg

---

*Calculation for water deficit only with no abnormal sodium loss.

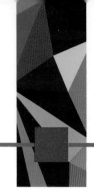

Equivalents

Needle and Catheter Reference Chart

Gauge	Regular ID	Thin ID	Inches OD	French Size	Inches OD
36	0.002	0.003	0.004		0.109
35	0.002	0.003	0.005		0.118
34	0.003	0.004	0.007		0.12
33	0.004	0.005	0.008		0.131
32	0.004	0.005	0.009		0.134
31	0.005	0.006	0.01		0.144
30	0.006	0.007	0.012		0.148
29	0.007	0.008	0.013	1	0.158
28	0.007	0.008	0.014		0.165
27	0.008	0.01	0.016		0.17
26	0.01	0.012	0.018		0.18
25	0.01	0.012	0.02		0.184
24	0.012	0.014	0.022		0.197
23	0.013	0.015	0.025		0.203
22	0.016	0.018	0.026	2	0.21
21	0.02	0.022	0.028		0.223
20	0.023	0.025	0.032		0.236
19	0.027	0.031	0.035		0.249
18	0.033	0.042	0.039	3	0.263
17	0.041	0.046	0.042		0.276
16	0.047	0.052	0.05		0.288
15	0.054	0.059	0.053	4	0.302
14	0.063	0.071	0.059		0.315
13	0.071	0.077	0.065		0.328
12	0.085	0.091	0.066	5	0.341
11	0.094	0.1	0.072		0.354
10	0.106	0.114	0.079	6	0.367
9	0.118	0.126	0.083		0.38
8	0.135	0.143	0.092	7	0.393
7	0.15	0.158	0.095		0.407
6	0.173	0.181	0.105	8	0.42
					0.433
					0.446

ID, Inner diameter; *OD,* outer diameter.

Physical Equivalents
Weight Equivalents

1 lb	453.6 g = 0.4536 kg = 16 oz
1 oz	28.35 g
1 kg	1000 g = 2.2046 lb
1 g	1000 mg = 0.0353 oz
1 mg	1000 µg = 0.001 g
1 µg	0.001 mg = 0.000001 g

1 µg/g or 1 mg/kg is the same as
1 ppm.

Volume Equivalents

1 drop (gt)	0.06 mL
15 drops (gtt)	1 mL (1 cc)
1 teaspoon (tsp)	5 mL
1 tablespoon (tbs)	15 mL
2 tbs	30 mL
1 teacup	180 mL (6.0 oz)
1 glass	240 mL (8.0 oz)
1 measuring cup	240 mL ($\frac{1}{2}$ pt)
2 measuring cups	480 mL (1 pt)
1 fl oz	29.57 mL
1 pt	0.473 L
1 pt	16 fl oz
1 gal	3.785 L
1 gal (US)	0.833 gal (imperial)
1 mL	0.03382 fl oz
1 L	2.1134 pt
1 L	0.26417 gal

Pressure Equivalents

1 centimeter water (cm H_2O) = 0.736 mm Hg = 0.098 kPa
1 millimeter mercury (mm Hg; torr) = 1.36 cm H_2O = 0.133 kPa
1 kilopascal (kPa) = 7.5 mm Hg = 10.2 cm H_2O
1 atmosphere (atm) = 760 mm Hg = 1033.6 mm H_2O

Temperature Conversion

Degrees Celsius to degrees Fahrenheit: (C)(9/5) + 32
Degrees Fahrenheit to degrees Celsius: (F − 32)(5/9)

Weight-Unit Conversion Factors

Unit Given	Unit Wanted	For Conversion Multiply By
lb	g	453.6
lb	kg	0.4536
oz	g	28.35
kg	lb	2.2046
kg	mg	1,000,000
kg	g	1000
g	mg	1000
g	µg	1,000,000
mg	µg	1000
mg/g	mg/lb	453.6
mg/kg	mg/lb	0.4536
µg/kg	µg/lb	0.4536
Mcal	kcal	1000
kcal/kg	kcal/lb	0.4536
kcal/lb	kcal/kg	2.2046
ppm	µg/g	1
ppm	mg/kg	1
ppm	mg/lb	0.4536
mg/kg	%	0.0001
ppm	%	0.0001
mg/g	%	0.1
g/kg	%	0.1

Conversion Factors

1 mg	$\frac{1}{65}$ grain ($\frac{1}{60}$)
1 g	$\frac{15}{43}$ grains (15)
1 kg	2.20 lb (avoirdupois) 2.65 lb (troy)
1 mL	16.23 minims (15)
1 L	1.06 quarts (1+) 33.80 fl oz (34)
1 grain	0.065 g (60 mg)
1 dram	3.9 g (4)
1 oz	31.1 g (30+)
1 minim	0.062 mL (0.06)
1 fluid dram	3.7 mL (4)
1 fl oz	29.57 mL (30)
1 pt	473.2 mL (500−)
1 qt	946.4 mL (1000−)

EQUIV

Length-Unit Conversion Factors

cm	inches	cm	inches	mm	inches	inches	cm
1	0.394	41	16.142	0.125	0.0049	$\frac{1}{8}$	0.32
2	0.787	42	16.535	0.25	0.0098	$\frac{1}{4}$	0.64
3	1.181	43	16.929	0.5	0.0197	$\frac{1}{2}$	1.27
4	1.575	44	17.323	0.75	0.0295	$\frac{3}{4}$	1.91
5	1.969	45	17.717	1	0.0394	1	2.54
6	2.362	46	19.11	2	0.0787	2	5.08
7	2.756	47	18.504	3	0.1181	3	7.62
8	3.15	48	18.898	4	0.1585	4	10.16
9	3.543	49	19.291	5	0.1968	5	12.7
10	3.937	50	19.685	6	0.2362	6	15.24
11	4.331	51	20.1	7	0.2756	7	17.78
12	4.724	52	20.5	8	0.315	8	20.32
13	5.118	53	20.9	9	0.3543	9	22.86
14	5.512	54	21.2	10	0.3937	10	35.4
15	5.906	55	21.6	11	0.4331	11	27.94
16	6.299	56	22	12	0.4724	12	30.48
17	6.693	57	22.4	13	0.5118	13	33.02
18	7.087	58	22.8	14	0.5512	14	35.56
19	7.48	59	23.2	15	0.5905	15	38.1
20	7.874	60	23.6	16	0.6299	16	40.64
21	8.268	61	24	17	0.6693	17	43.18
22	8.661	62	24.4	18	0.7087	18	45.72
23	9.055	63	24.8	19	0.748	19	48.26
24	9.449	64	25.2	20	0.7874	20	50.8
25	9.843	65	25.6	21	0.8268	21	53.34
26	10.236	66	26	22	0.8661	22	55.88
27	10.63	67	26.4	23	0.9055	23	58.42
28	11.024	68	26.8	24	0.9449	24	60.96
29	11.417	69	27.1	25	0.9842	25	63.5
30	11.811	70	27.6	26	1.0236	26	66.04
31	12.205	71	28	27	1.063	27	68.58
32	12.598	72	28.3	28	1.1024	28	71.12
33	12.992	73	28.7	29	1.1417	29	73.66
34	13.386	74	29.1	30	1.1811	30	76.2
35	13.78	75	29.5	31	1.2205	31	78.74
36	14.173	76	29.9	32	1.2598	32	81.28
37	14.567	77	30.3	33	1.2992	33	83.82
38	14.961	78	30.7	34	1.3386	34	86.36
39	15.354	79	31.1	35	1.3779	35	88.9
40	15.748	80	31.5	36	1.4173	36	91.44
				37	1.4567	37	93.98
				38	1.4961	38	96.52
				39	1.5354	39	99.06
				40	1.5748	40	101.6

Conversion of Grams to Milliequivalents of Common Substances*

1 g $NaHCO_3$	12 mEq Na or HCO_3*	1 g Calcium gluconate	4.5 mEq Ca
1 g NaCl	17 mEq Na or Cl	1 g Calcium borogluconate	4.1 mEq Ca
1 g KCl	13.4 mEq K or Cl	1 g $MgSO_4$	8.1 mEq Mg
1 g $CaCl_2$	18 mEq Ca or Cl	1 g $MgCl_4$	9.1 mEq Mg or Cl

*Conversion to mmoles is easy for substances that are +1 and −1. For example, 1 g $Na^{+1}HCO_3^{-1}$ = 12 mEq $NaHCO_3$ = 24 mmoles.

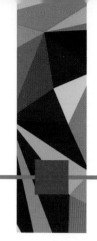

APPENDIX 4

Adverse Drug Reactions, Air Emboli, and Lightning Strike

Thomas J. Divers

Important Adverse Drug Reference Information

Adverse event reporting

FDA Center for Veterinary Medicine

Adverse event reporting: 888-332-8387; 240-276-9300; 888-463-6332 (FDA)

http://fdable.com or www.fda.gov/AnimalVeterinary/default.htm

U.S. Department of Agriculture

Veterinary Biologics and Diagnostics Hotline

1-800-752-6255 weekdays 8 AM to 4:30 PM Central Time (message service after hours)

www.aphis.usda.gov/animal_health/vet_biologics/vb_adverse_event.shtml

National Animal Poison Control Center Hotline

1-888-426-4435

Veterinary Practitioners' Reporting Program (for adverse reactions; reports to the FDA/USDA drug manufacturer and the AVMA)

1-800-487-7776

www.usp.org

EPA—pesticide information

http://www.epa.gov/pesticides

http://pesticides.supportportal.com/ics/support/default.asp?deptID=23008

U.S. Equestrian Federation, Drug and Medication Guidelines

www.usef.org/issuu/flipbook.ashx?docname=drugsmedsguidelines2012&pdfurl=

www.usef.org/_IFrames/Drugs/Default.aspx

Intracarotid Injections

Many of the immediate adverse reactions to parenterally administered xylazine, detomidine, phenylbutazone, and trimethoprim-sulfadiazine (where available) are probably the result of inadvertent intracarotid injections.

Water-Soluble Drugs—Intracarotid Administration

Water-soluble intracarotid drugs include acepromazine, detomidine, some barbiturates, and xylazine.

Clinical Signs
- Immediate hyperexcitability occurs and possibly collapse.
- Seizure or coma may follow.

● WHAT TO DO

Water-Soluble Drugs—Intracarotid Administration
- Reaction usually can be successfully managed by sedation with pentobarbital or phenobarbital, 5 to 12 mg/kg IV (or to effect) q12h or as needed.
- Alternatively, administer diazepam intravenously to effect as a relatively safe sedative.
- Administer anti-inflammatory, edema-reducing drugs (e.g., dimethyl sulfoxide [DMSO]), 1 g/kg, or dexamethasone, 0.5 mg/kg.
- Some patients may remain recumbent for several hours or days before standing.
- Manage wounds and corneal trauma that may occur as a result of the seizure.
- Cortical blindness occurs in some cases.
- Include anti-edema therapy:
  - DMSO, 1 mg/kg IV diluted in polyionic crystalloid fluid
  - Dexamethasone, 0.2 mg/kg IV
  - Mannitol (20%), 0.25 to 2.0 g/kg slowly IV

Oil-Based, High pH Drugs—Intracarotid Administration

Oil-based intracarotid drugs include:
- Propylene glycol
- Trimethoprim-sulfadiazine
- Diazepam
- Penicillin procaine
- Phenylbutazone

Clinical Signs
- Signs are seizure, collapse, and sometimes rapid death.
- Contralateral cortical blindness is a frequent finding among patients that survive.
- Cerebral hemorrhage often is present.

● WHAT TO DO

Oil-Based Drugs—Intracarotid Administration
- If the patient does *not* die immediately, administer treatment as for water-soluble drugs.

Flunixin Meglumine

Intracarotid injection does *not* produce signs as severe as those of some of the drugs listed as oil-based drugs. Flunixin meglumine may produce neurologic signs such as ataxia and hysteria, hyperventilation, and muscle weakness. These signs are transient, according to the package insert, and require *no* antidote.

Practice Tip: When a 20-gauge needle is used to penetrate the carotid artery, blood may not spurt from needle hub.

Intravenous or Intraarterial Administration of Penicillin Procaine

Administration of penicillin procaine is one of the most common causes of serious and immediate adverse drug reaction in equine practice. Penicillin procaine can cause procaine reactions when the drug is inadvertently injected into a small vessel, most likely arterial. This is more common among individuals receiving injections long-term in the same muscle mass, presumably because of increased vascularity of the area. Clinical signs and frequently death may also occur when penicillin procaine is mistakenly given intravenously.

Practice Tip: A general rule of practice is: "If the medication to be administered is white, do not administer intravenously."*

Horses experiencing a procaine reaction have a sudden (often by time the intramuscular injection is completed) onset of terror (overly alert, snorting, unusually erect appearance) followed immediately by uncontrollable circling, collapse, seizure, and sometimes death.

●〉 WHAT TO DO

Penicillin Procaine Reaction
- The first response of the attending veterinarian is to evacuate all personnel from the stall.
- If the horse does *not* collapse and can be safely approached or after collapse, one may enter the stall to administer diazepam or pentobarbital intravenously as needed to calm the horse and control any seizures.
- Horses that do *not* die within the first 15 minutes have a good chance of survival, often with *no* permanent neurologic signs.

●〉 WHAT NOT TO DO

Penicillin Procaine Reaction
Do *not* administer epinephrine unless there is a strong suspicion that clinical signs are due to rarely observed "penicillin allergy."

Intravenous Trimethoprim-Sulfadiazine Reaction

Injectable trimethoprim-sulfadiazine (available in Europe) can cause fatal reactions when detomidine is administered intravenously along with intravenous administration of trimethoprim-sulfadiazine (see Appendix 5, p. 822).

●〉 WHAT TO DO

Trimethoprim-Sulfadiazine Reaction
- See What to Do: Penicillin Procaine Reaction!

Air Emboli

Catheters become disconnected frequently in equine practice, and in the majority of cases there are no problems with

*Exceptions are propofol and TMP-5.

air emboli. If the horse holds its head high, there is more risk for air aspiration than when the head is lowered and retrograde bleeding from a disconnected intravenous catheter is increased. If the air remains on the venous side (the usual case), clinical signs are either nonexistent or those of poor perfusion and hypoxemia, elevated heart and respiratory rates, discolored mucous membranes, trembling, weakness, and disorientation. The air that accumulates in the right atrium could interfere with venous return (air lock) resulting in decreased cardiac output. A bubbling or swishing sound may be heard at cardiac auscultation, and an ultrasound examination reveals air in the right side of the heart. Microbubbles of air in the pulmonary artery usually escape into the capillaries and then into the alveolus to be exhaled; however, larger volumes of air in the pulmonary circulation may induce pulmonary constriction and endothelial damage and lead to pulmonary edema.

●〉 WHAT TO DO

Air Emboli
Venous air emboli include:
- Intranasal oxygen administration at the highest flow rate to maintain oxygenation of blood and tissues and force nitrogen from the air bubbles.
- Intravenous fluids to support cardiac output.
- Flunixin meglumine to reduce prostanoid-associated inflammation.
- If the air emboli appears serious and a large volume of air is seen in the right heart on ultrasound evaluation, insert a long catheter via the jugular vein into the right atrium and aspirate the air.
- If the problem is severe enough to cause cardiac arrest, perform cardiac massage.
- In the rare instance where air passes to the arterial side, neurologic signs predominate (e.g., seizure). This is more likely to occur if the horse is recovering from anesthesia and has atelectasis or preexisting pulmonary disease, which may allow right-to-left shunting of the air!
Treatment for arterial air emboli includes:
- Seizure management:
  - Pentobarbital: 5 to 12 mg/kg IV
  - High-flow oxygen
  - Mannitol
  - Fluids to decrease viscosity
  - Plavix and pentoxifylline
- Hyperbaric oxygen is effective in the early treatment of venous and arterial air emboli.
- The hyperoxia, a result of hyperbaric treatment, ensures that oxygen is available for tissue and creates a strong diffusion gradient for nitrogen reabsorption.
- **Practice Tips:** *Air emboli may occur:*
  - *With prolonged cystoscopy and repeated injection of air into the bladder with the belief that air is absorbed into the venous or arterial circulation.*
  - *During arthroscopy if nitrous oxide is used; nitrous oxide is more diffusible than oxygen and causes large bubbles in the circulation.*
  - *With death in young foals receiving rapid fluid boluses when air is pumped into the fluids to speed delivery; this practice is discouraged!*

Lightning Strike

- Horses pastured at the time of electrical storms and congregating near metal fences and under trees are at increased risk of lightning strike.
- Acute death due to cardiopulmonary arrest is common if there is a direct strike.
- Because of the distance between the horse's limbs, they are susceptible to a "*stride potential*" (current flows from one limb to another) if the strike occurs on the ground near the horse. This may cause thermal injury to:
  - Skin
  - Musculoskeletal system
  - Pulmonary edema
  - Neurologic signs, including vestibular signs

●› WHAT TO DO

Lightning Strike

- Treat the affected organ system.
- For treatment of pulmonary edema, see Chapter 25, p. 473.
- If the electrical current quickly flashes over the horse, then ocular damage (cornea, lens, and retina) and dermal injury may occur and are treated with anti-inflammatory and anti-edema medications.
- Horses suspected of sustaining a lightning strike injury should be examined by an ophthalmologist.

Acute Drug-Induced Anaphylaxis

Anaphylactic reactions are most frequent with intravenous administration of vaccines, occasionally penicillin or other antibiotics, selenium, plasma, whole blood, phytonadione (vitamin K), and other vitamins and minerals. In most cases, this is *not* a result of previous sensitization and antigen-antibody reaction but is an immediate "triggering" of the complement-kinin system caused by some part of the drug.

●› WHAT TO DO

Mild Forms

- Mild forms of anaphylaxis cause urticaria and minor increases in respiratory rate. These may be simply treated with any of the following antihistamines:
  - Diphenhydramine: 0.5 to 1.0 mg/kg IM or *slowly* IV
  - Doxylamine succinate: 0.5 mg/kg *slowly* IV, IM, or SQ q8 to 12h
  - Pyrilamine maleate: 1.0 mg/kg *slowly* IV, IM, or SQ
  - Tripelennamine: 1.1 mg/kg IM or SQ

  Practice Tip 1: *Administer all antihistamines slowly if given intravenously because excitement and hypotension are occasional adverse effects. These adverse effects are rarely seen when antihistamines are administered intramuscularly or subcutaneously.*

  Practice Tip 2: *Alternatively, **but not simultaneously**, administer epinephrine (1:1000) intramuscularly, 5 to 8 mL/450-kg adult, because when antihistamines and epinephrine are used together, antihistamines potentiate the effect of epinephrine on vascular resistance.*

●› WHAT TO DO

Severe Forms

- See pulmonary edema Chapter 25, p. 473.
- Administer epinephrine, 3 to 7 mL (1:1000 undiluted) slowly IV to a 450-kg adult. Epinephrine may be administered intramuscularly

in less severe cases at the same dosage or 2 times this dosage intramuscularly for severe anaphylaxis.

- **Practice Tip:** *Epinephrine by the intratracheal route, 5× IV dosage, may be used when intravenous access is* not *possible or limited.*
- Provide patent airway if needed by intubation. This is important when laryngeal edema is severe. Intubation is also of some benefit in managing pulmonary edema when the upper airway is edematous and compromised. **Practice Tip:** *Stridor may* not *appear until 80% or more of the upper airway is obstructed.*
- Administer furosemide: 1 mg/kg IV.
- Use plasma or hetastarch as an oncotic volume expander if pulmonary edema is believed to be progressive. If other fluids are needed for hypotension, administer hypertonic saline solution, 4 mL/kg.
- Corticosteroids: Although of *no* demonstrated clinical benefit, dexamethasone, 0.2 to 0.5 mg/kg, frequently is administered to prevent delayed edema formation in the lungs, pharynx, etc.
- Administer oxygen intranasally.

Special Considerations
Perivascular Injections

- Perivascular injections with irritating drugs are common.
- The most irritating drugs are those with high or low pH.

Clinical signs include pain, swelling, cellulitis, and vessel necrosis; if the injection is perivascular to the jugular vein signs of Horner syndrome may occur. Vessel necrosis may rarely occur several days after the perivascular injection and can be fatal.

●› WHAT TO DO

Perivascular Injections

- Stop the infusion.
- Infiltrate the area with 10 mL saline solution (can be mixed with ¼ mL penicillin procaine if infection is a concern).
- Apply heat to the area.
- Apply topical diclofenac at the site.
- If a large volume of irritating drug is administered, ventral drainage and flushing/lavage may be indicated.

●› WHAT TO DO

Drug Overdose

If an overdose of a drug occurs:

- Keep records and provide proper communication.
- Review clinical and physiologic effects of the overdose.
- **Practice Tip:** *Drugs that are highly protein bound may affect the protein binding of a toxic drug; therefore, check the percentage of protein binding of drugs being administered. Use lower percentage protein-bound drugs if possible.*
- Provide specific treatment if indicated.
- General treatment for most overdoses includes the following:
  - Intravenous fluid administration
  - Activated charcoal: 0.5 kg/450-kg adult PO, repeated doses may be needed for drugs that undergo enterohepatic recirculation or for ivermectin, which may return to the gut lumen after initial absorption.

- ***Practice Tip:*** *Even when the overdose has been administered parenterally, oral charcoal administration may act as a "sink" and "pull" some of the drug into the gastrointestinal tract for excretion.*
- If overdose is administered orally, give MgSO₄, 0.5 kg/450-kg adult PO, in addition to fluids and charcoal.

⬤〉 WHAT NOT TO DO

Drug Overdosage
- Do *not* administer drugs that decrease or compete for protein binding of the toxic drug.

Broken Jugular Catheters

Although alarming, a broken jugular catheter in an adult is *not* a life-threatening occurrence. The catheter usually passes through the right side of the heart and lodges in the pulmonary circulation, where it is walled-off and generally causes *no* clinical problems.

⬤〉 WHAT TO DO

Broken Jugular Catheters
- Perform an ultrasound examination to confirm passage of the catheter into the lungs.
- Chest radiographs may *not* allow visualization of the catheter in the lung of large horses.
- *In foals, the catheter often is too large to pass from the right side of the heart and must be removed or the sequela over a prolonged period is a heart wall defect and fatal hemorrhage.*
- For a foal or the rare adult in which the catheter or J wire is lodged in the heart, consult a vascular human surgeon regarding the current techniques for retrieval of catheters.
- Location of the broken end is important because some catheters or J wires lodge at the thoracic inlet and can be removed surgically.

Acute Drug Reactions

See Appendix 5, p. 817, Specific Acute Drug Reactions and Recommended Treatments.

Considerations for Drug Therapy in the Neonatal Foal

- Renal excretion of most drugs is approximately equal to that of adults.
- Premature foals may need prolonged treatment intervals if drug is excreted predominantly by the kidneys, particularly drugs with potential toxicity (e.g., aminoglycosides).
  - Peak (30- to 60-minute) and trough concentrations ideally should be determined.
    - For concentration-dependent antimicrobials (e.g., aminoglycosides) high peaks are best correlated with efficacy and trough levels should be low for potentially toxic drugs.
    - For time-dependent antimicrobials (β-lactams) serum concentrations should be 2-4× above the

minimum inhibitory concentration (MIC) for the targeted pathogen during the entire treatment period. It may not be necessary to have drug levels, at the site of the infection, much above the MIC.
  - Generally lipid-soluble drugs have tissue concentrations similar to or higher than serum concentrations while antibiotics with low tissue distribution may need to be 4 to 10 times the serum concentration to be clinically efficacious.
- Hepatic metabolism is slower in foals than in adults. The time of delayed metabolism varies because of drug-induced enhanced activity.
- ***Practice Tip:*** *Sulfonamides, phenobarbital, trimethoprim, nonsteroidal anti-inflammatory drugs (NSAIDs), diazepam, metronidazole, and theophylline may require extended dosing intervals, and in the case of inhalant anesthesia, lower concentrations. This has* not *been documented to be a clinically important concern.*
- The albumin concentration in young foals is approximately that of adults. Protein binding is *not* very different between age groups. If hypoalbuminemia, as from enteritis, is present, highly protein-bound drugs such as diazepam, sulfas, and NSAIDs may have an enhanced effect. This effect may be partially offset by more rapid elimination.
- Extracellular fluid volume in neonatal foals is nearly double that of adults. The results are decreased blood concentration and prolonged excretion of many drugs.
- ***Practice Tip:*** *In the management of life-threatening infection, it is recommended to administer a larger loading dosage (approximately 30% larger than an adult dose) of an antibiotic to help ensure therapeutic levels in the plasma during treatment.*
  - This applies to both time-dependent (e.g., β-lactams, to ensure drug concentration above the MIC for the whole treatment period) and concentration-dependent antimicrobials (e.g., aminoglycosides), which have increased efficacy and more prolonged postantibiotic effect with increasing plasma concentrations.
- Oral absorption of many drugs may be more variable (usually increased absorption) in foals than in weanlings, yearlings, or adults.

⬤〉 WHAT TO DO

Drug Dosing Adjustments in Renal Failure
- Discontinue all nephrotoxic drugs if possible.
- If it is necessary to administer potentially nephrotoxic drugs during renal failure, the interval of the treatments should be prolonged in accordance with the estimated decline in glomerular filtration rate (GFR). For example, occasionally it is necessary to continue administration of aminoglycosides, tetracycline, polymyxin B, sulfonamides, or NSAIDs despite an abnormally low GFR.
- ***Practice Tip:*** *Example: A Thoroughbred mare with a creatinine concentration of 2.2 to 2.4 mg/dL conceivably has only 50% normal GFR. Therefore, if any of the aforementioned treatments are required, the treatment interval should be doubled. Intravenously administered fluids also should be provided.*

- There are more elaborate methods of estimating GFR (e.g., radionuclide studies), but serum creatinine concentration generally provides a reasonable estimate in a euvolemic (normal water content) patient. Most light-breed horses and foals have serum creatinine concentrations between 0.9 and 1.4 mg/dL. Quarter Horses may have a normal value as high as 2.1 mg/dL. The value in some foals born of mares with placentitis may be very high for the first 3 days of life without any abnormality in GFR.
- Increasing the interval of administration generally is preferred to decreasing dosage although either method may be used.
- Measurement of peak and trough levels is ideal, if assays are available.
- For drugs that are *not* nephrotoxic but are eliminated exclusively by the kidney (e.g., digoxin) similar adjustments should be made if there is concern about toxic effects. Many drugs (e.g., penicillins, doxycycline, cephalosporins, lidocaine, and barbiturates) do *not* require interval or dosage adjustments.

●› WHAT TO DO

Drug Dosing Adjustment in Liver Failure
- Prolongation of interval of treatment should be considered for potentially toxic drugs excreted predominantly by the liver (e.g., lidocaine and metronidazole).
- Foals younger than 2 weeks of age may also have decreased hepatic clearance of these and other drugs, such as diazepam, barbiturates, and aminophylline.

References

References can be found on the companion website at www.equine-emergencies.com.

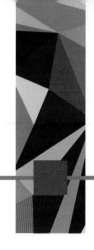

APPENDIX 5

Specific Acute Drug Reactions and Recommended Treatments

Thomas J. Divers

Drug	Clinical Signs and Overdose Information	Treatment
Acepromazine	Weakness, sweating, pale membranes, death, low PCV (chronic), penile paralysis	4 mL/kg hypertonic saline solution IV for hypotension (for paraphimosis, see Chapter 24, p. 428)
Albuterol	Tremors, tachycardia, CNS excitement, some of which may be caused by hypokalemia, poorly absorbed in horses	Usually requires no treatment; however, check serum K$^+$; if hypokalemia present, administer supplemental K$^+$
Altrenogest, oral	Colic, sweating rarely reported. Avoid human skin exposure	Symptomatic
Aminocaproic acid	Trembling if given too fast and potential for hyperkalemia	Slow infusion
Aminoglycoside antibiotics	A single dose even 10× normal dosage is unlikely to cause clinical problems in a horse with normal renal function. Treatment of a dehydrated patient with aminoglycosides is the most common predisposing factor for aminoglycoside toxicity. Weakness caused by neuromuscular blockade occurs rarely, unless other neuromuscular blocking drugs are administered or a neuromuscular disease (e.g., botulism) is present	IV fluid therapy (see Chapter 32, p. 567); monitoring of serum creatinine values and urine production is advisable for prevention For renal failure, see Chapter 26, p. 487 If toxicity occurs, neuromuscular blockage can be reversed with neostigmine, 0.01 mg/kg SQ, or slowly administered calcium IV mixed in polyionic fluids
Aminophylline (theophylline)	Seizures, tachydysrhythmia	If possible, discontinue drugs that reduce clearance: H$_2$ blockers, enrofloxacin, erythromycin. Administer phenobarbital to control seizures and enhance clearance. Keep serum concentration <15 mg/mL
Amitraz	Accidental exposure	See Chapter 34, p. 582
Amphotericin B	Rarely recommended in treatment of horses, but can cause renal failure unless sodium diuresis is administered during treatment	Fluid diuresis
Anthelmintics	Colic, diarrhea Ascarid impactions in foals within 24 hours of administration	Supportive Surgery for ascarid impactions Ascarid impactions may be less common with fenbendazole than many other anthelmintics
Antihistamines	When given IV, antihistamines may cause head tremors, agitation, and excitement	Valium: 0.1 mg/kg IV Do not use epinephrine
Arginine vasopressin	Colic, hyponatremia, bradycardia	Diuresis; hypertonic saline or mannitol
Atropine	Colic, abdominal distention	Analgesics plus neostigmine, 0.01-0.02 mg/kg SQ q2-4h or cecal trocarization
Azithromycin and other macrolides	Diarrhea, colic, toxemia	Metronidazole, analgesics, fluids, intestinal protectants, prokinetics
Barbiturates	Respiratory depression, hypothermia; irritating when administered perivascularly	Assisted respiration
Bethanechol	Rarely produces adverse effects other than salivation	None

Continued

Drug	Clinical Signs and Overdose Information	Treatment
Buprenorphine Butorphanol	Head tremors, excitement, ataxia, death (rare); most often occurs when used without tranquilizers	Xylazine
Buscopan (N-butylscopolammonium bromide)	Transient mydriasis, tachycardia (when given IV) and ileus	None
Ceftiofur	As with any antibiotic, can cause colitis; excede may cause local reactions	Stop treatment (see p. 232) Limit volume/site to 7 mL and massage injection
Chorionic gonadotropin	Rare CNS or GI sign when given IV; may cause muscle swelling when administered IM	
Ciprofloxacin	Rare psychotic behavior. Because of poor bioavailability and colitis in adult horses, do *not* give orally	Diazepam; treat for anaphylaxis (Appendix 4, p. 814) if needed; may cause abortion in early pregnancy
Clenbuterol	(see Albuterol)—Do *not* use for more than 14 days consecutively	
Corticosteroids	Risk of laminitis is related mostly to individual horse predisposition (i.e., horses with metabolic syndrome) and degree of insulin resistance caused by the different corticosteroids; triamcinolone > dexamethasone > prednisolone; dose and duration are secondary risk factors; immunosuppression also occurs	Cryotherapy Bactericidal antibiotics if needed
Detomidine	Do *not* administer with IV trimethoprim-sulfamethoxazole or sulfadiazine; sweating, cardiovascular and respiratory depression, collapse; can be used in pregnant mares, although romifidine is considered safer; *tachypnea may occur when administered to febrile horses!* Some horses may become aggressive after administration!! Urticaria	For detomidine or medetomidine overdose, give antisedan at up to 3-4× the detomidine/medetomidine dose. Yohimbine: 0.07-0.1 mg/kg, or tolazoline: 0.5-1 mg/kg IV; may be used in place of antisedan. All of these reversal drugs can cause adverse cardiac effects when given rapidly IV. *Generally* no *treatment required*
Diazepam	Ataxia; coma with massive overdosage	None for ataxia; flumazenil: 0.01 mg/kg slowly, for coma
Dichlorvos	Colic or signs of organophosphate toxicity (salivation, miosis, diarrhea); rarely neuromuscular weakness	NSAIDs for colic; atropine only if certain organophosphate toxicity has occurred
Digoxin	See Chapter 17, p. 135	See Chapter 17, p. 149
Dimethyl sulfoxide	Hemolysis; do *not* use in concentrations greater than 10% dextrose	*No* treatment required unless severe; transfusion
Dinoprost tromethamine (prostaglandin F$_{2\alpha}$)	Colic, sweating	Usually none required
Dobutamine	Heart rate increases more than 30%-50%, arrhythmias	Usually none required; decrease rate of administration or stop infusion
Domperidone (adult dose to a foal)	Somnolence	Supportive, usually complete recovery
Dopamine	Tachycardia, very irritating if perivascular administration, decreased GI perfusion	Usually none required; decrease rate of administration
Doxapram HCl	Seizures	Pentobarbital to effect; intranasal oxygen
Doxycycline	Collapse, death, supraventricular tachycardia, hypertension when administered IV, rarely diarrhea after administration of 10 g or more, teratogenic	*Do* not *use IV* Do not use with Rifampicin—causes liver disease
Embutramide, mebezonium, tetracaine	CNS signs, hyperactivity	Sedation rarely needed
Enrofloxacin	Swollen joints and tendons in foals; erosions in mouth after oral administration of injectable product	Discontinue treatment, rinse mouth after administering Baytril 100
Epinephrine	Collapse	Usually none; monitor cardiac rhythm and blood pressure. A beta-blocker proponent should be used only if hypertension is demonstrated

Drug	Clinical Signs and Overdose Information	Treatment
Epogen (recombinant human erythropoietin)	Nonregenerative anemia (possibly life-threatening) may develop in horses receiving one or usually more injections of this product. Diagnosis is by history, presence of nonregenerative anemia, or low or absent levels of erythropoietin (EPO-Trac RIA, INCSTAR) 1 week or more after the last injection	Treatment is blood transfusion Steroids are used but of unknown efficacy. Recovery can occur in many cases
Fenbendazole (larvicidal dose) and other anthelmintics with efficacy against encysted small strongyles	Diarrhea after treatment of encysted small strongyles	Corticosteroids
Fentanyl	*No* adverse effects reported in horses, but could cause respiratory and CNS depression	Naloxone
Flunixin meglumine *Do not administer to dehydrated horses; use sparingly in foals Do not give IM unless there are no other reasonable options*	Injection site swelling including clostridial myositis most common; collapse if administered into carotid artery, right dorsal colitis, gastric ulcers, and renal disease	If swelling at injection site occurs, monitor closely for sepsis Monitor plasma protein to prevent right dorsal colitis—treatment is misoprostol
Fluphenazine decanoate (Prolixin), *a derivative that blocks phenothiazine dopamine receptors*	Bizarre behavior, restlessness (refractory to treatment with xylazine), recumbency, seizure	Benztropine mesylate: 0.002 mg/kg IV or phenobarbital: 12 mg/kg, administered in 1 L over 20 minutes rather than by bolus; antihistamines (e.g., diphenhydramine). Supportive therapy
Fluprostenol sodium	Sweating, colic	Treatment generally *not* needed
Glycopyrrolate	Tenesmus, small-colon impaction, possible cardiovascular effects	Analgesics, oral and IV fluid administration for impaction
Guaifenesin	Toxic at high dosage (3× normal) causes hypotension; perivascular injections irritating, rarely causes hemolysis	IV fluid administration See previous treatments for perivascular injections.
Halothane	Respiratory or cardiac depression, arrhythmia	Stop anesthesia; CPR if arrest occurs
Heparin (nonfractionated)	Anemia	Discontinue treatment; PCV should return to pretreatment values within 2-4 days
Hyaluronate sodium	Swollen joints and lameness. See Polysulfated Glycosaminoglycan.	NSAIDs, joint lavage, hydrotherapy, antibiotics—especially if swelling does *not* occur for several hours
Imidocarb	See Chapter 40, p. 685	
Imipramine	Tricyclic overdosage causes CNS signs and hypotension	Diazepam or phenobarbital for CNS signs; fluids with $NaHCO_3$ for hypotension
Insulin	*Overdosage can lead to hypoglycemia*	*Check glucose and potassium and administer 20%-50% dextrose with KCl if needed. Save blood sample if malicious intention suspected.*
Iohexol (myelography)	Do *not* use more than 60 mL of 240 mg iodine/mL in a 500 kg horse; seizures and blindness (unilateral or bilateral) are *not* uncommon; fever for 48 hours is also seen after myelography in some cases	Dexamethasone: 0.1 mg/kg IV; Valium: 0.1 mg/kg IV for seizures; phenobarbital to effect for refractory cases; thiamine: 2 mg/kg IV slowly; vitamin C: 30 mg/kg IV; flunixin meglumine: 1 mg/kg for fever
Iron	In newborn foals, produces acute hepatic failure and death when administered orally before colostrum. Can cause acute collapse followed by hepatic or renal disease in some patients when administered IV	Fluids, Desferrioxamine (see p. 841)
Isoflurane	Respiratory or cardiac depression	CPR if arrest occurs, O_2 therapy, stop anesthesia
Isoxsuprine	When administered IV, can cause hyperexcitability and hypotension	Diazepam and IV fluid administration

Continued

Drug	Clinical Signs and Overdose Information	Treatment
Ivermectin (oral) *Do not give injectable ivermectin to horses* *Do not give if horses ingesting solanum*	Rare severe systemic reaction, such as blindness and ataxia (more likely in newborn foals), diarrhea, colic, ventral abdominal swelling caused by death of *Onchocerca* microfilariae *not* unusual. Injection of ivermectin (SQ or IM) can result in severe local swelling	For *Onchocerca* reaction, symptomatic usually. For CNS signs, administer 20% intralipids: 1.5 mL/kg as an IV bolus. Supportive therapy Sarmazenil: 0.04 mg/kg IV may also be used if there is *no* response to the above.
Ketamine	Respiratory depression	Mechanical or physical ventilation
Ketoprofen	Injection site reactions; collapse and death with intracarotid administration	None
Levamisole	Salivation, ataxia, nervousness, GI signs	
Lidocaine *Do not use lidocaine with epinephrine IV*	CNS signs, hypotension, rarely arrhythmia; blood concentration may increase over time with 0.05 mg/kg/min. Highly protein-bound drugs (NSAIDs, ceftiofur) increase lidocaine activity	Diazepam, hypertonic saline solution for hypotension
Lincomycin	*Contraindicated* in horses; severe colitis	IV fluid administration; metronidazole: 25 mg/kg PO q12h
Magnesium toxicity	Rare, can produce weakness and respiratory distress when administered to oliguric patients	Slow IV fluid administration with calcium borogluconate
Mannitol	Electrolyte imbalances, pulmonary edema if patient is anuric	Stop treatment if urination is inadequate
Marbofloxacin	Diarrhea occasionally	Stop treatment and administer metronidazole, Biosponge, and transfaunation if possible.
Meperidine HCl	Overdosage may produce respiratory depression and hypotension. Excitement may occur when used without tranquilization	Naloxone: 0.01 mg/kg IV, repeated if necessary, and IV fluid administration
Methocarbamol	Sedation and ataxia	Supportive
Metoclopramide HCl	Bizarre behavior, head tremors, ataxia	Diphenhydramine and phenobarbital. *Do not use tranquilizers.* Chloral hydrate can be administered to effect as a sedative
Metronidazole	When given orally, horses may salivate and have decreased appetite, may cause CNS sign in neonatal foals; if CNS signs develop, stop treatment	Can be given per rectum at 30 mg/kg q8h
Misoprostol	High dosages can cause diarrhea and colic. Abortion in pregnant animals including human beings	Stop treatment or reduce dosage if diarrhea occurs, especially in foals Do *not* dispense for treatment of pregnant horses or if any chance of being handled by pregnant women!
Monensin (oral)	Increased heart rate, diarrhea, colic, recumbency, death	Supportive (see Chapter 17, p. 154; Chapter 34, p. 602)
Morphine sulfate, oxymorphone, and pentazocine	After IV administration, hyperexcitability; ataxia may occur when pretreatment with tranquilizers has *not* been administered. Large dosages may depress respiration	Naloxone: 0.01 mg/kg IV, repeated if necessary. Efficacy of naloxone in treating drugs (pentazocine, butorphanol) with opiate agonist and antagonist properties is unknown; therefore, use with caution
Moxidectin	A leading cause of serious adverse reaction in foals <4 months of age. Coma, death, hypothermia, bradycardia, blindness. Identical signs reported in a premature foal treated with ivermectin	Sarmazenil: 0.04 mg/kg IV q2h Administer 20% intralipids: 1.5 mL/kg as an IV bolus With supportive treatment, some recover
Neostigmine	Colic	Analgesics and fluids
Nitazoxanide	Colic, diarrhea, laminitis	Metronidazole, gastroprotectants
Nitric oxide (inhaled)	Has little effect on systemic blood pressure. High levels (>40 ppm) can cause methemoglobinemia	Methylene blue for confirmed methemoglobinemia
Nitroglycerin ointment	If used for laminitis in a hypotensive patient, hypotension can worsen	IV fluid administration; remove ointment. *Avoid human contact*

Drug	Clinical Signs and Overdose Information	Treatment
Organophosphate anthelmintics, such as trichlorfon	Rarely causes signs; loose feces, diarrhea, increased salivation, sweating, colic, ataxia, death	Supportive treatment, fluids, and analgesics. If classic signs (salivation, miosis) of organophosphate poisoning are present and overdosing is known to have occurred, administer atropine, 0.22 mg/kg. *Do not use atropine unless certain of organophosphate toxicity*
Oxytetracycline	Rapid IV infusion can cause collapse and hemolysis Large dosages (3 g) administered to foals only to treat contracted/deformed tendons rarely results in renal failure. Do *not* use >15 mg/kg per day for prolonged periods	Treatment usually *not* required IV fluid diuresis
Oxytocin	Colic	Treatment usually *not* required
Penicillin	Penicillin procaine reactions are more common in patients receiving long-term injections in the same muscle mass

Heating penicillin procaine increases procaine toxicity.

Rarely, immune-mediated anaphylaxis or hemolytic anemia.
IV penicillin salts administration may cause salivation, "smacking" of lips, head movement (*no* treatment required).
Immediate passage of loose stool upon each IV administration | Prevent injury to the individual by removing dangerous objects from the area. Human beings should leave the stall to prevent bodily harm unless the patient is persistently circling, in which case an experienced person may walk *carefully* with the horse. Diazepam has *no* effect after excitability has occurred
For anaphylaxis, see Appendix 4, p. 814
For hemolytic anemia, see Chapter 20, p. 277
Generally do *not* need to discontinue treatment but in some cases diarrhea may become more persistent |
| Pergolide | Gross overdosage can cause CNS signs similar to those of metoclopramide | Sedation (barbiturates) and fluid therapy |
| Phenobarbital | Sedation, ataxia, coma, respiratory depression | Activated charcoal orally decreases serum levels, fluids |
| Phenoxybenzamine | May cause hypotension when administered IV (little or *no* indication for IV use in horse) | Hypertonic saline solution IV; if sodium fluid loading *not* indicated, administer phenylephrine
Epinephrine contraindicated with any alpha-adrenergic blocking agent—adverse reaction |
Phenylbutazone	Gross overdosing can cause GI ulceration, colic, diarrhea, hemorrhage, and ARF with hematuria. Perivascular injection can cause necrosis	Misoprostol, omeprazole, sucralfate, and fluids
Phenylpropanolamine	Relatively safe in horses; gross overdosing can cause CNS signs and cardiovascular collapse	IV fluids and oral charcoal and MgSO$_4$ if treatment within last hour
Phenytoin	Ataxia, depression, weakness, recumbency	Treatment usually *not* required; however, may administer IV fluids
Phytonadione (vitamin K)	Immediate death when given IV; anaphylaxis?	Do *not* administer IV
Piperazine	Gross overdosing has occurred in horses and has caused paralysis, salivation, and CNS signs. As with any anthelmintic effective against *Parascaris equorum,* it can cause colic if large numbers of the worms are killed.	IV fluids and oral charcoal and MgSO$_4$ for overdosage
Plasma, whole blood	Tremors, pyrexia, agitation, tachypnea, tachycardia, piloerection, hepatitis	If hemolysis occurs, stop the transfusion Slow plasma, blood infusion and administer antihistamine if other reactions
Polysulfated glycosaminoglycan	When administered intraarticularly, may cause subacute (within hours) swelling and pain. This usually is a nonseptic inflammatory response. Sepsis is always a concern and should be ruled out with arthrocentesis and cytologic examination if pain or lameness does *not* occur for 12-24 hours or more.	Phenylbutazone systemically and cold hydrotherapy. Joint lavage if swelling is severe or sepsis is suspected. If sepsis is suspected, therapy should be directed against the most common organism, *Staphylococcus aureus.*

Continued

Drug	Clinical Signs and Overdose Information	Treatment
Procainamide	Rarely used in horses; however, when used can cause hypotension, sweating.	IV hypertonic saline solution
Promazine	See Acepromazine	Fluids or pressor drugs for hypotension
Propantheline bromide	GI ileus, colic	Dipyrone or low-dose flunixin meglumine: 0.3 mg/kg IV; cecal trocarization if needed; neostigmine: 0.01-0.02 mg/kg SQ; IV fluids
Propranolol	Rarely used in horses; however, can cause severe bradycardia and collapse.	Atropine: 0.07 mg/kg IV; fluids
Propylene glycol	CNS depression, colic, diarrhea, respiratory distress	IV fluids and sodium bicarbonate to combat the D-lactic acidosis
Pyrantel	Colic, diarrhea	Supportive
Quinidine	Tachycardia, sweating, colic (ileus), collapse, hypotension, ataxia (usually mild), mild nasal stridor, ileus, and colic	Digoxin: 1 mg/450-kg IV for super ventricular tachycardia, fluids for hypotension, $NaHCO_3$ IV to increase excretion, and KCl (see p. 132) Flunixin meglumine for colic
Rifampin	Hepatotoxic when used with doxycycline	Stop treatment as support IV core (see pp. 275 and 277)
Selenium	Collapse occurs occasionally with IV injections, death, colic, ataxia	Supportive; do *not* administer IV
Sodium bicarbonate	Gross overdosage IV or orally can cause alkalosis and synchronous diaphragmatic flutter	0.9% NaCl with KCl and calcium borogluconate
Succinylcholine chloride	Respiratory paralysis	Mechanical ventilation
Terbutaline	Excitement, tachycardia, sweating, tremors	IV fluids containing potassium
Tetracycline	ARF, in dehydrated or hypotensive individuals. Rarely causes ARF in foals. Occasional collapse or hemolysis when administered undiluted	Fluids for ARF
Tiludronic acid	Occasionally colic, acute renal failure	Colic treatment supportive Renal failure treatment, see p. 487
Tolazoline	Cardiovascular collapse when administered in high dosages to some horses	Use with caution, lowest dosage possible; administer slowly
Trimethoprim-sulfamethoxazole or trimethoprim-sulfadiazine	Oral, rarely diarrhea; IV, rarely collapse	Diarrhea (see Chapter 18, p. 232). Do *not* administer with detomidine. Fatal if administered by intracarotid route
Vasopressin	If administered IV, can cause CNS signs	Treatment usually *not* required
Vincristine	Rarely causes acute neutropenia, thrombophlebitis	Bactericidal antibiotics, hot pack to area
Warfarin	See Chapter 16, p. 122, and Chapter 34, p. 605	Charcoal and $MgSO_4$ PO, vitamin K, plasma
Xylazine	Hyperventilation (especially in febrile horses), death from pulmonary edema on rare occasions (when preexisting respiratory disease is present)	Usually *no* treatment required for hyperventilation. Do *not* use with upper respiratory obstruction. Treat with yohimbine: 0.075 mg/kg IV, or preferably tolazoline: 2.2 mg/kg slowly IV. Use diazepam rather than xylazine, when possible, in foals <1 week of age
	Intracarotid administration.	Supportive, most recover
	Some horses (e.g., Draft breeds, Warmbloods, foals) can become recumbent with recommended dosage	Treatment usually *not* required; however, if patient is severely hypotensive, administer IV fluids

Note: For any adverse drug reaction, read the package insert.
ARF, Acute renal failure; *CNS,* central nervous system; *CPR,* cardiopulmonary resuscitation; *GI,* gastrointestinal; *IM,* intramuscularly; *IV,* intravenous(ly); *NSAID,* nonsteroidal anti-inflammatory drug; *PO,* per os; *PCV,* packed cell volume; *SQ,* subcutaneously.
Results of reported adverse drug experiences can be found at www.fda.gov/cvm/ade_cum.htm.

Quick Reference Protocols for Emergency and Clinical Conditions

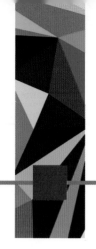

Eileen S. Hackett

Cardiac Protocols

- Antiarrhythmic Therapy: See Chapter 17, p. 135
- Adverse Effects of Antiarrhythmic Drugs: See Chapter 17, p. 135
- Drug Therapy for Myocardial, Valvular Disease and Congestive Heart Failure: See Chapter 17, pp. 148-149

Colitis

Name, Formulation Concentration	Dosage	1000-lb (450-kg) Dose	Considerations
Bismuth subsalicylate (1.75%) 525 mg/30 mL	4.5 mL/kg PO q 4-12h	2000 mL	
Charcoal, activated	0.5-1 g/kg	225-450 g	
Di-tri-octahedral smectite (BioSponge) powder	PO q12-24h	0.5-3 lb	
Flunixin meglumine 50 mg/mL	0.25-1.1 mg/kg IV or IM q8-12h	2.3-9.9 mL	IM injections associated with clostridial myositis, inhibits intestinal repair
Hetastarch (6%) or VetStarch (6%)	Up to 10 mL/kg IV q24-48h	Up to 4500 mL	Higher doses of Hetastarch may inhibit coagulation
Hypertonic saline (7.2%)	4-5 mL/kg IV	1800-2250 mL	
Lidocaine (2%) 20 mg/mL	1.3 mg/kg IV slowly followed by 0.05 mg/kg/min	30-mL bolus 1.1 mL/min	Analgesia and inflammation
Mannan oligosaccharide	100-200 mg/kg PO q8-24h		
Polymyxin B	1000-6000 units/kg IV q8-12h	0.45-2.7 million units	Dilute and administer slowly IV

Epidural Analgesia

Name	Method	1000-lb (450-kg) Dose	Considerations
Detomidine 10 mg/mL	Detomidine 0.03-0.05 mg/kg	1.4-2.3 mL Smaller amounts are frequently used	Peak sedative actions between 5-20 minutes after injection; provides analgesia for 2-4 hours
Hydromorphone (H) 2 mg/mL or Morphine (M) 15 mg/mL *with* Xylazine (X) 100 mg/mL	Hydromorphone: 0.01-0.04 mg/kg Morphine: 0.1 mg/kg Xylazine: 0.17 mg/kg	H: 2.3-9 mL M: 3 mL X: 0.76 mL	Rapid onset; provides analgesia for approximately 12 hours Morphine also available in 10-mg/mL concentration
Ketamine 100 mg/mL	Ketamine: 0.5-2 mg/kg	2.3-9 mL	Provides analgesia for 30-75 minutes

Continued

Name	Method	1000-lb (450-kg) Dose	Considerations
Lidocaine 20 mg/mL (2%)	Lidocaine: 0.2-0.25 mg/kg	4.5-5.6 mL	Rapid onset of <6-10 minutes; provides analgesia for 45-60 minutes
Lidocaine (2%) (L) 20 mg/mL and Xylazine (X) 100 mg/mL	Lidocaine: 0.22 mg/kg Xylazine: 0.17 mg/kg	L: 5 mL X: 0.75 mL (0.77)	Combination prolongs duration of action
Mepivacaine (2%) 20 mg/mL	0.2-0.25 m/mg/kg	4.5-5.6 mL	Rapid onset of 10 minutes; provides analgesia for 45-60 minutes
Methadone 10 mg/mL	Methadone: 0.1 mg/kg	4.5 mL	Analgesia onset 15 minutes, lasting approximately 5 hours
Morphine 25 mg/mL preservative free if available	Morphine: 0.1 mg/kg	1.8 mL	Analgesia onset 1-8 hours, lasting up to 18 hours; does not result in altered motor function
Morphine (M) 15 mg/mL and Detomidine (D) 10 mg/mL	Morphine: 0.1 mg/kg Detomidine: 0.01-0.03 mg/kg	M: 3 mL D: 0.45-1.4 mL	
Morphine (M) 15 mg/mL and Xylazine (X) 100 mg/mL	Morphine: 0.1 mg/kg Xylazine: 0.17 mg/kg	M: 3 mL X: 0.75 mL (0.77)	Analgesia for 2-4 hours Morphine also available in 10 mg/mL concentration

General Anesthesia: Induction with Injectable Drugs

Name	Method	1000-lb (450-kg) Dose	Considerations
Xylazine (X) 100 mg/mL Diazepam (D) 5 mg/mL Ketamine (K) 100 mg/mL	Xylazine sedation: 1.1 mg/kg D/K induction: D: 0.05-0.1 mg/kg K: 2.2 mg/kg	Xylazine: 5 mL Diazepam: 4.5-9 mL Ketamine: 10 mL	Diazepam extends short-acting anesthesia from 20 to 25 minutes over ketamine alone
Xylazine (X) 100 mg/mL Propofol (1%) (P) 10 mg/mL Ketamine (K) 100 mg/mL	Xylazine sedation: 1.1 mg/kg P/K induction: P: 0.5 mg/kg K: 1.5-1.7 mg/kg	Xylazine: 5 mL Propofol: 22.5 mL Ketamine: 7-8 mL	Propofol inductions may be violent or associated with limb paddling
Telazol 100 mg/mL	Xylazine sedation: 1.1 mg/kg Telazol induction: 1.1 mg/kg	Xylazine: 5 mL Telazol: 5 mL	May result in respiratory depression
Xylazine 100 mg/mL Ketamine 100 mg/mL	Xylazine sedation: 1.1 mg/kg Ketamine induction: 2.2 mg/kg	Xylazine: 5 mL Ketamine: 9.9 mL	

General Anesthesia: Maintenance with Injectable Drugs

Name	Method	1000-lb (450-kg) Dose	Considerations
Guaifenesin/Ketamine/ Detomidine (GKD) Guaifenesin Ketamine 100 mg/mL Detomidine 10 mg/mL	Combine guaifenesin 100 mg/mL, ketamine 4 mg/mL, and detomidine 0.04 mg/mL and administer at 0.6-1.0 mL/kg/h	270-450 mL/h	Limit anesthesia to 60 minutes 2 mg/kg ketamine is preferred by some practitioners
GKX (see Triple Drip)	See p. 847 and below		
Propofol 10 mg/mL	Administer propofol 0.14-0.22 mg/kg/min	6.3-9.9 mL/min	Profound respiratory depression may necessitate assisted ventilation; limit anesthesia to 60 minutes and may not keep horse immobile
Triple Drip—GKX Guaifenesin Ketamine 100 mg/mL Xylazine 100 mg/mL	Combine guaifenesin 50 mg/mL, ketamine 1-2 mg/mL, and xylazine 0.5 mg/mL and administer at 1.5-2.2 mL/kg/h	675-990 mL/h	Higher concentration of ketamine used for more painful procedures; limit anesthesia to 60 minutes
Xylazine 100 mg/mL Ketamine 100 mg/mL	Administer xylazine 2.1 mg/kg/h and ketamine 7.2 mg/kg/h	945 mg/h xylazine 3240 mg/h ketamine Remove 42 mL from 250 mL bag IV fluid, add 9.5 mL X, 32.5 mL K, administer 1 drop/sec with 15 drop/mL set	Limit anesthesia to 60 minutes

Head Trauma

Name	Dosage	1000-lb (450-kg) Dose	Considerations
Hypertonic saline (7.2%)	4-5 mL/kg IV	1800-2250 mL	Initial bolus dose should be followed with CRI to maintain serum sodium of approximately 160 mEq/L
Mannitol (20%)	0.25-2 g/kg q6-24h	560-4500 mL	Administer over 20-30 minutes IV, effect lasts for 4-6 hours.

Hemorrhage

Name	Dosage	1000-lb (450-kg) Dose	Considerations
Acepromazine 10 mg/mL	0.01-0.02 mg/kg IV or IM q6-8h	0.45-0.9 mL	"Permissive hypotension" (e.g., uterine bleed) Results in hypotension
Aminocaproic acid 250 mg/mL	10-40 mg/kg IV q6h per 40 mg/kg loading dose	18-72 mL	Administer slowly IV; see p. 836
Naloxone 0.4 mg/mL	0.01-0.03 mg/kg IV	11.25-33.75 mL	Active hemorrhage
Tranexamic acid 100-mg/mL injection, or 650-mg tablets	10 mg/kg IV q8-12h or 20 mg/kg q6h PO	45 mL 14 tabs	

Neonatology Protocols

- Hypoglycemia: See Chapter 31, p. 530
- Seizures: See Chapter 31, p. 538
- Emergency Stabilization: See Chapter 31, p. 541
- Septicemia: See Chapter 31, p. 554
- Colic: See Chapter 31, p. 559
- Persistent Pulmonary Hypertension: See Chapter 31, p. 549
- Respiratory Compromise: See Chapter 31, p. 550
- Prematurity/Dysmaturity: See Chapter 31, p. 551
- Uroperitoneum: See Chapter 31, p. 553
- Meconium Impaction: See Chapter 31, p. 560
- Diarrhea: See Chapter 31, p. 563

REF VALS

Laminitis Treatment

Name	Dosage	1000-lb (450-kg) Dose	Considerations
Acepromazine 10 mg/mL	0.04 mg/kg IM q6h	2 mL (1.8)	Not recommended for use concurrently with cryotherapy
Analgesic CRI Acepromazine 10 mg/mL, Ketamine 100 mg/mL, Lidocaine (2%) 20 mg/mL Morphine 15 mg/mL	Acepromazine: 0.166 mg/kg/h Ketamine: 0.6 mg/kg/h Lidocaine: 3 mg/kg/h Morphine: 0.0093 mg/kg/h	A: 0.75 mL/h K: 2.7 mL/h L: 67.5 mL/h M: 0.28 mL/h Can be added to crystalloid fluids and rate regulated by infusion pump	Detomidine is often added, administered at 0.00155 mg/h
Aspirin 15.4 g	10-20 mg/kg PO q48h	$\frac{1}{4}$-$\frac{1}{2}$ bolus	
Fentanyl patch	Dermal	2-3 × 100 µg/h patches	
Firocoxib paste or 20 mg/mL injection	0.1 mg/kg PO q24h after 0.2 mg/kg loading dose 0.09 mg/kg IV q24h	0.8 tube (45.5 mg) 2 mL	
Flunixin meglumine 50 mg/mL	1.1 mg/kg IV q12h	9.9 mL	Limit use if laminitis is associated with NSAID toxicity
Gabapentin 300-mg, 400-mg capsules 600-mg, 800-mg tablets	20 mg/kg PO q8-12h	300 mg × 30 capsules or 600-mg tabs × 15	
Heparin 1000 units/mL	40-80 IU/kg IV or SQ q8h	18-36 mL	
Isoxsuprine 20-mg tablets	0.6 mg/kg PO q12h	13.5 tabs	Bioavailability unknown
Lidocaine (2%) 20 mg/mL	1.3 mg/kg loading 0.05 mg/kg/min CRI	30-mL bolus 1.1 mL/min	
Morphine 15 mg/mL	0.05-0.1 mg/kg IM q24h	1.5-3 mL	
Pentoxifylline 400-mg tablets	8.5 mg/kg PO q12h	9.5 tabs	
Phenylbutazone 200-mg/mL injection or 1-g tablets	2.2-4.4 mg/kg IV or PO q12-24h	5-10 mL 1-2 tabs	
Pregabalin 50-, 75-, 100-, 150-, 200-, 225-, and 300-mg capsules	4 mg/kg PO q8-12h	300-mg capsules ×6	If horse becomes noticeably depressed or ataxic, reduce dose to 2 mg/kg.

CRI, Continuous rate infusion; *NSAIDs,* nonsteroidal anti-inflammatrory drugs.

Physical and Chemical Restraint

Name	Dosage	1000-lb (450-kg) Dose	Considerations
Acepromazine 10 mg/mL	0.02-0.05 mg/kg IV or IM	0.9-2.25 mL	
Buprenorphine 0.3 mg/mL	0.001-0.006 mg/kg IV or IM	1.5-9 mL	Combine with α_2-agonists
Butorphanol 10 mg/mL	0.01-0.1 mg/kg IV or IM 13-22 µg/kg/h IV CRI	0.45-4.5 mL 5.9-9.9 mg/h	Combine with α_2-agonists
Detomidine 10 mg/mL	5-40 µg/kg IV or IM sedation 6.7-11.1 µg/kg/h IV CRI	0.23-1.8 mL; 0.3-0.5 mL/h	
Morphine 15 mg/mL	0.3-0.5 mg/kg IV	9-15 mL	Combine with α_2-agonists; reversible with naloxone
Romifidine 10 mg/mL	0.04-0.12 mg/kg IV or IM	1.8-5.4 mL	
Xylazine 100 mg/mL	0.2-1.1 mg/kg IV or IM	1-5 mL	

Prokinetics

Name	Dosage	1000-lb (450-kg) Dose	Considerations
Cisapride compounded	mg/kg IM q8h 0.1-1.0 mg/kg PO q4-8h 10 mg/tab	4.5-45 tabs	Must be reformulated before IM administration; not available in the United States
Erythromycin 100 mg/mL	1-2.5 mg/kg as 1-hour infusion IV q6h	4.5-11 mL	
Lidocaine (2%) 20 mg/mL	1.3 mg/kg IV slowly, followed by 0.05 mg/kg/min IV	30-mL bolus 1.1 mL/min	
Metoclopramide 5 mg/mL	0.1-0.5 mg/kg IV slowly q4-8h; 0.04 mg/kg/h IV	9-45 mL	May produce CNS excitement
Neostigmine 0.5 mg/mL or 1 mg/mL	0.005-0.02 mg/kg SQ or IM q4-6h	2.3-4.5 mL of 1 mg/mL (9 mL)	

CNS, Central nervous system.

Seizure Control

Name	Dosage	1000-lb (450-kg) Dose	Considerations
Diazepam 5 mg/mL	Adult: 0.05-0.44 mg/kg IV Foal: 0.1-0.2 mg/kg IV	Adult: 4.5-39.6 mL Foal: 1-2 mL	
Midazolam 1 mg/mL and 5 mg/mL	Adult: 0.05-0.1 mg/kg Foal: 0.1-0.2 mg/kg IV or CRI 0.06-0.12 mg/kg/h	Adult: 4.5-9 mL using 5 mg/mL Foal: 1-2 mL using 5 mg/mL or 0.6-1.2 mL/h	
Phenobarbital 15-mg, 30-mg, 60-mg, and 100-mg tablets 130-mg/mL injection	2-10 mg/kg PO q8-12h; 5-15 mg/kg IV slowly	100-mg tabs ×9— 45 tabs 17-52 mL	Monitor seizure control and therapeutic drug levels
Potassium bromide Compounded 250 mg/mL KBr solution for oral use, or 250 mg/mL NaBr for injection	60-90 mg/kg PO KBr Or IV q24h NaBr	108-162 mL	Monitor seizure control and therapeutic drug levels Higher doses than 60-90 mg/mL PO have also been recommended

Drug Trade Name Index

Drug trade names (bold) and common names are listed in alphabetical order and followed by the ingredient names (italics), as listed in the equine emergency drug index. Other generic products are often available.

A

Accupril—*quinapril*
ADH—*vasopressin, arginine*
Adrenalin—*epinephrine*
Adriamycin—*doxorubicin*
Amicar—*aminocaproic acid*
Amiglyde-V—*amikacin*
Amp-Equine—*ampicillin sodium*
Amphocin—*amphotericin B*
Anafranil—*clomipramine*
Ancef—*cefazolin*
Antagonil—*yohimbine*
Anthelcide—*oxibendazole*
Antisedan—*atipamezol*
Antizol-Vet—*fomepizole*
Apresoline—*hydralazine*
Aquasol E—*vitamin D, vitamin E*
Arquel—*meclofenamic acid*
Ascorbic acid—*vitamin C*
Atarax—*hydroxyzine hydrochloride*
Atrovent—*ipratropium bromide*
Azium—*dexamethasone*

B

Banamine—*flunixin meglumine*
Baycox—*toltrazuril*
Baytril—*enrofloxacin*
Beclovent—*beclomethasone*
Benadryl—*diphenhydramine hydrochloride*
Benzelmin—*oxfendazole*
Betapace—*sotalol*
Beuthanasia—*pentobarbital*
Biaxin—*clarithromycin*
Bio-Mos—*mannan oligosaccharide*
Biosol—*neomycin*
Bio-Sponge—*di-tri-octahedral smectite*
Brethine—*terbutaline*
Bumex—*bumetanide*
Buprenex—*buprenorphine*
Burinex—*bumetanide*
Buscopan—*butylscopolammonium bromide*

Buspar—*buspirone*
Butazolidin—*phenylbutazone*

C

Carafate—*sucralfate*
Cefadyl—*cephapirin*
Cefa-Lak—*cephapirin sodium*
Cefobid—*cefoperazone*
Chloral hydrate—*chloropent*
Chloromycetin—*chloramphenicol*
Chorisol—*chorionic gonadotropin*
Chronulac—*lactulose*
Claforan—*cefotaxime*
Clavamox—*amoxicillin—clavulanic acid*
Clinacox—*diclazuril*
Clomicalm—*clomipramine*
Cobactan—*cefquinome*
Cogentin—*benztropine mesylate*
Cordarone—*amiodarone*
Corlopam—*fenoldopam*
Corophyllin—*aminophylline*
Cortrosyn—*cosyntropin*
Cytotec—*misoprostol*
Cytovene—*ganciclovir*
Cytoxan—*cyclophosphamide*

D

Dantrium—*dantrolene*
Daraprim—*pyrimethamine*
Delta Cortef—*prednisolone*
Demerol—*meperidine hydrochloride*
Denosyl—*S-adenosylmethionine*
Dexdomitor—*dexmedetomidine*
Diamox—*acetazolamide*
Dibenzyline—*phenoxybenzamine*
Diflucan—*fluconazole*
Di-Gel—*antacid*
Dilantin—*phenytoin*
Dioctynate—*dioctyl sodium sulfosuccinate*
Diprivan—*propofol*
DMSO—*dimethyl sulfoxide*
Dobutrex—*dobutamine*
Domitor—*medetomidine*
Domoso—*dimethyl sulfoxide*
Dopram V—*doxapram*

Dormosedan—*detomidine hydrochloride*
Duragesic—*fentanyl*

E
Enacard—*enalapril*
Epogen—*epoetin alfa*
Epsom salts—*magnesium sulfate*
Equidone—*domperidone*
Equimate—*fluprostenol sodium*
Equioxx—*firocoxib*
Eqvalan—*ivermectin*
Ergamisol—*levamisole*
Erythropoietin—*epoetin alfa*
E Se—*selenium vitamin E*
Eskazole—*albendazole*
EtoGesic—*etodolac*
Excede—*ceftiofur*

F
Feldene—*piroxicam*
Flagyl—*metronidazole*
Flovent—*fluticasone*
Flumadine—*rimantadine*
Fluorescite—*fluorescein sodium*
Follutein—*chorionic gonadotropin*
Fomepizole—*4-methylpyrazole*
Fortamet—*metformin*
Fortaz—*ceftazidime*
Fragmin—*heparin, low molecular weight (dalteparin)*
Fulvicin—*griseofulvin*
Fungizone—*amphotericin B*

G
GastroCote—*bismuth subsalicylate*
Gastrogard—*omeprazole*
Gecolate—*guaifenesin*
Gentocin—*gentamicin*
Gentran—*dextran 70*
GG—*guaifenesin*
Glucophage—*metformin*

H
HCG—*chorionic gonadotropin*
Hespan—*hetastarch*
Hextend—*hetastarch*
Histavet P—*pyrilamine maleate*
Humatin—*paromomycin*
Humulin—*insulin, regular*
Hydrozide—*hydrochlorothiazide*

I
Imizol—*imidocarb*
Imodium—*loperamide*
Imuran—*azathioprine*
Inderal—*propranolol*
Indocin—*indomethacin*
Intropin—*dopamine*
Isuprel—*isoproterenol*

K
Keflex—*cephalexin*
Keflin—*cephalothin*
Ketaset—*ketamine*
Ketaved—*ketamine*
Ketex—*telithromycin*
Ketofen—*ketoprofen*

L
LA 200—*oxytetracycline*
Lanoxin—*digoxin*
Lasix—*furosemide*
Leucovorin—*folinic acid*
Lodine—*etodolac*
Losec—*omeprazole*
Lotensin—*benazepril*
Lovenox—*heparin, low molecular weight (enoxaparin)*
Lutalyse—*dinoprost tromethamine*
Lyrica—*pregabalin*

M
Maalox—*antacid*
Marquis—*ponazuril*
Maxipime—*cefepime*
Mefoxin—*cefoxitin*
Metacam—*meloxicam*
Meta-Dote—*Ca-EDTA*
Metamizole—*dipyrone*
Metamucil—*psyllium hydrophilic mucilloid*
Methylpyrazole—*fomepizole*
Mucomyst—*acetylcysteine*

N
Naprosyn—*naproxen*
Naquasone—*dexamethasone trichlormethiazide*
Narcan—*naloxone*
Nasalcrom—*cromolyn sodium*
Naxcel—*ceftiofur*
Neoprontosil—*azosulfamide*
Neo-Synephrine—*phenylephrine hydrochloride*
Neupogen—*colony-stimulation factor*
Neurontin—*gabapentin*
Nitro Bid—*nitroglycerin cream*
Nizoral—*ketoconazole*
NoDoz—*caffeine*
Novin—*dipyrone*
NuFlor—*florfenicol*
Numorphan—*oxymorphone*

O
Oncovin—*vincristine*
Osmitrol—*mannitol*

P
Palaron—*aminophylline*
2-PAM—*pralidoxime*
Panacur—*fenbendazole*

Pepcid AC—*famotidine*
Pepto-Bismol—*bismuth subsalicylate*
Periactin—*cyproheptadine*
Phytonadione—*vitamin K₁*
Plavix—*clopidogrel*
Poly-Flex—*ampicillin trihydrate*
Prascend—*pergolide*
Predef 2x—*isoflupredone acetate*
Premarin—*estrogen conjugates*
Primacor—*milrinone*
Primaxin IV—*imipenem*
Prion—*phenylpropanolamine*
Procrit—*epoetin alfa*
Program—*lufenuron*
Prolixin—*fluphenazine decanoate*
Promace—*acepromazine*
Pronestyl—*procainamide*
Propulsid—*cisapride*
Prostigmin—*neostigmine*
Prostin F2 Alpha—*dinoprost tromethamine*
Protozil—*diclazuril*
Proventil—*albuterol*
ProZinc—*insulin, protamine zinc*
Pyridium—*phenazopyridine*

Q
Quest—*moxidectin*
Quinidex—*quinidine sulfate*

R
Rapinovet—*propofol*
Re-Covr—*tripelennamine HCl*
Reglan—*metoclopramide*
Regu-Mate—*altrenogest*
Rifadin—*rifampin*
Rimadyl—*carprofen*
Robaxin—*methocarbamol*
Robinul V—*glycopyrrolate*
Rocephin—*ceftriaxone*
Romazicon—*flumazenil*
Rompun—*xylazine hydrochloride*
Rythmol—*propafenone*

S
Salix—*furosemide*
SAMe—*S-adenosylmethionine*
Sandostatin—*octreotide acetate*
Sedazine—*xylazine hydrochloride*
Sedivet—*romifidine*
Sepracoat—*sodium hyaluronate solution*
Serevent—*salmeterol*
Siliphos—*milk thistle phospholipid*
Solu-Delta Cortef—*prednisolone sodium succinate*
Solu-Medrol—*methylprednisolone sodium succinate*
Sporanox—*itraconazole*
Surpass—*diclofenac sodium*
Symmetrel—*amantadine*

T
Tagamet—*cimetidine*
Talwin—*pentazocine*
Tegretol—*carbamazepine*
Telazol—*tiletamine and zolazepam*
Tensilon—*edrophonium*
Thyro-L—*levothyroxine*
Ticar—*ticarcillin*
Tildren—*tiludronate*
Timentin—*clavulanic acid-ticarcillin*
Tofranil—*imipramine*
Tolazine—*tolazoline*
Torbugesic—*butorphanol tartrate*
Tosylate—*bretylium*
ToxiBan—*activated charcoal*
Tracurium—*atracurium*
Trental—*pentoxifylline*
Tribrissen—*trimethoprim sulfadiazine*
Trienamine—*tripelennamine HCl*
Trilafon—*perphenazine*

U
Ulcergard—*omeprazole*
Ultram—*tramadol*
Uniprim—*trimethoprim-sulfadiazine*
Urecholine—*bethanechol*

V
Valbazen—*albendazole*
Valium—*diazepam*
Valtrex—*valacyclovir*
Vanceril—*beclomethasone*
Vantin—*cefpodoxime proxetil*
Vasotec—*enalapril*
Veda K1—*vitamin K₁*
Ventipulmin—*clenbuterol*
Vermox—*mebendazole*
Versed—*midazolam*
Vetalar—*ketamine*
Vfend—*voriconazole*
Viagra—*sildenafil citrate*
Vibramycin—*doxycycline*
Vistaril—*hydroxyzine hydrochloride*
Vivarin—*caffeine*

X
Xylocaine—*lidocaine*

Y
Yocon—*yohimbine*

Z
Zantac—*ranitidine*
Zeniquin—*marbofloxacin*
Zithromax—*azithromycin*
Zovirax—*acyclovir*

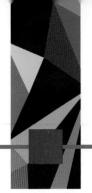

APPENDIX 8

Drug Category Index

Drugs are listed by ingredient/generic name (bold print) and trade name (regular print). Dosage information is located within Appendix 9, Equine Emergency Drugs, under ingredient name.

Analgesics

Buprenorphine, Buprenex
Butorphanol tartrate, Torbugesic
Fentanyl, Duragesic
Gabapentin, Neurontin
Hydromorphone
Meperidine hydrochloride, Demerol
Methadone
Morphine sulfate
Nalbuphine
Oxymorphone, Numorphan
Pentazocine, Talwin
Pregabalin, Lyrica
Tramadol, Ultram

Anesthetics

Diazepam, Valium
Guaifenesin, GG, Gecolate
Ketamine, Ketaset, Ketaved, Ketavet, Vetalar
Lidocaine, Xylocaine
Midazolam, Versed
Propofol, Diprivan, Rapinovet
Ropivacaine
Thiopental sodium*
Tiletamine and zolazepam, Telazol

Antifungals

Amphotericin B, Fungizone, Amphocin
Fluconazole, Diflucan
Griseofulvin, Fulvicin
Iodide potassium
Itraconazole, Sporanox
Ketoconazole, Nizoral
Lufenuron, Program
Sodium Iodide
Voriconazole, Vfend

Antihistamines

Diphenhydramine hydrochloride, Benadryl
Doxylamine succinate

Hydroxyzine hydrochloride, Vistaril, Atarax
Pyrilamine maleate, Histavet-P
Tripelennamine HCl, Trienamine, Re-Covr

Anti-inflammatories

Nonsteroidal Anti-inflammatory Drugs

Acetylsalicylic acid, Aspirin
Carprofen, Rimadyl
Diclofenac sodium, Surpass
Eltenac
Etodolac, EtoGesic, Lodine
Firocoxib, Equioxx
Flunixin meglumine, Banamine
Ketoprofen, Ketofen
Meclofenamic acid, Arquel
Meloxicam, Metacam
Naproxen, Naprosyn
Phenylbutazone, Butazolidin
Piroxicam, Feldene
Vedaprofen

Steroids

Beclomethasone, Beclovent, Vanceril
Dexamethasone, Azium
Dexamethasone trichlormethiazide, Naquasone
Fluticasone, Flovent
Isoflupredone acetate, Predef 2x
Methylprednisolone sodium succinate, Solu-Medrol
Prednisolone, Delta-Cortef
Prednisolone sodium succinate, Solu-Delta Cortef

Other

Dimethyl sulfoxide (DMSO), Domoso
Dipyrone, Novin, Metamizole

Antimicrobials

Amikacin, Amiglyde
Amoxicillin Clavulanic Acid, Clavamox
Ampicillin sodium, Amp-Equine
Ampicillin trihydrate, Poly-Flex
Azithromycin, Zithromax
Cefazolin, Ancef
Cefepime, Maxipime
Cefixime, Suprax
Cefoperazone, Cefobid
Cefotaxime, Claforan
Cefoxitin, Mefoxin

---

*Limited availability in many countries

Cefpodoxime proxetil, Vantin
Cefquinone, Cobactam
Ceftazidime, Fortaz
Ceftiofur, Naxcel, Excede
Ceftriaxone, Rocephin
Cephalexin, Keflex
Cephalothin, Keflin
Cephapirin, Cefa-Lak
Cefixime, Suprax
Chloramphenicol, Chloromycetin
Clarithromycin, Biaxin
Clavulanic acid—ticarcillin, Timentin
Dapsone
Doxycycline, Vibramycin
Enrofloxacin, Baytril
Erythromycin
Florfenicol, NuFlor
Gentamicin, Gentocin
Imipenem, Primaxin IV
Marbofloxacin, Zeniquin
Metronidazole, Flagyl
Neomycin, Biosol
Oxytetracycline, LA 200
Penicillin, Na$^+$ or K$^+$
Penicillin, procaine
Polymyxin B
Rifampin, Rifadin
Telithromycin, Ketex
Ticarcillin-clavulanate, Timentin
Trimethoprim-sulfadiazine, Uniprim, Tribrissen
Vancomycin

Antiprotozoals

Diclazuril, Protozil
Imidocarb, Imizol
Metronidazole, Flagyl
Nitazoxanide
Paromomycin, Humatin
Ponazuril, Marquis
Pyrimethamine, Daraprim
Toltrazuril, Baycox

Antivirals

Acyclovir, Zovirax
Amantadine, Symmetrel
Ganciclovir, Cytovene
Rimantadine, Flumadine
Valacyclovir, Valtrex

Autonomics

Atropine
Benztropine mesylate, Cogentin
Butylscopolammonium bromide, Buscopan

Behavior Modification

Buspirone, Buspar
Clomipramine, Clomicalm, Anafranil

Cardiovascular

Amiodarone, Cordarone
Benazepril, Sotalol
Bretylium, Tosylate
Calcium chloride
Digoxin, Lanoxin
Diltiazem
Dobutamine, Dobutrex
Dopamine, Inotropin
Edrophonium, Tensilon
Enalapril, Vasotec, Enacard
Ephedrine
Epinephrine, Adrenalin
Glycopyrrolate, Robinul-V
Hydralazine, Apresoline
Isoproterenol, Isuprel
Isoxsuprine
Lidocaine, Xylocaine
Magnesium oxide
Magnesium sulfate
Milrinone, Primacor
Nitroglycerin cream, Nitro-Bid
Norepinephrine
Phenylephrine hydrochloride, Neo-Synephrine
Phenytoin, Dilantin
Procainamide, Pronestyl
Propafenone, Rythmol
Propranolol, Inderal
Quinidine gluconate
Quinidine sulfate, Quinidex
Vasopressin arginine, ADH
Verapamil

Chemotherapeutic

Cyclophosphamide, Cytoxan
Doxorubicin, Adriamycin
Piroxicam, Feldene
Vincristine, Oncovin

Coagulation

Aminocaproic acid, Amicar
Clopidogrel, Plavix
Heparin, unfractionated
Heparin, low molecular weight, Dalteparin, Fragmin, Enoxaparin, Lovenox

Diuretics

Acetazolamide, Diamox
Bumetanide, Bumex, Burinex
Furosemide, Salix, Lasix
Hydrochlorothiazide, Hydrozide
Mannitol, Osmitrol

Fluids

Albumin
Calcium borogluconate

Dextran 70, Gentran
Dextrose
Equine plasma
Hetastarch, Hespan, Hextend
Hyperimmune plasma
Pentastarch
Potassium chloride
Saline solution hypertonic
Sodium bicarbonate

Gastrointestinal

Antacids, Maalox, Di-Gel
Bismuth subsalicylate, Pepto-Bismol, Gastrocote
Carboxymethylcellulose sodium
Charcoal (activated), ToxiBan
Cimetidine, Tagamet
Cisapride, Propulsid
Dioctyl sodium sulfosuccinate, Dioctynate
Di-tri-octahedral smectite, Bio-Sponge
Famotidine, Pepcid AC
Fluorescein sodium, Fluorescite
Kaolin/Pectin
Lidocaine, Xylocaine
Loperamide, Imodium
Magnesium sulfate, Epsom salts
Mannan oligosaccharide, Bio-Mos
Metoclopramide, Reglan
Milk of magnesia
Mineral oil
Misoprostol, Cytotec
Neostigmine, Prostigmin
Omeprazole, Gastrogard, Ulcergard, Losec
Pectin-kaolin
Pentoxifylline, Trental
Phenoxybenzamine, Dibenzyline
Phenylephrine hydrochloride, Neo-Synephrine
Polymyxin B
Propantheline bromide
Psyllium hydrophilic mucilloid, Metamucil
Ranitidine, Zantac
Sodium hyaluronate solution, Sepracoat
Sucralfate, Carafate

Hormones

Altrenogest, Regu-Mate
Chorionic gonadotropin, Chorisol, Follutein, HCG
Cosyntropin, Cortrosyn
Dinoprost tromethamine, Lutalyse, Prostin F2 Alpha
Estrogen conjugates, Premarin
Fluprostenol sodium, Equimate
Levothyroxine, Thyro-L
Octreotide acetate, Sandostatin
Oxytocin
Progesterone

Immune

Azathioprine, Imuran
Cyclophosphamide, Cytoxan
Levamisole, Ergamisol

Liver

Colchicine
Lactulose, Chronulac
Milk thistle phospholipid, Siliphos
Neomycin, Biosol
Pentoxifylline, Trental
***S*-adenosylmethionine,** SAM-e, Denosyl
Ursodiol, Actigall

Metabolic Disease

Cyproheptadine, Periactin
Metformin, Fortamet, Glucophage
Pergolide, Prascend
Trilostane

Muscle

Atracurium, Tracurium
Dantrolene, Dantrium
Guaifenesin, GG, Gecolate
Methocarbamol, Robaxin
Propantheline bromide
Selenium-vitamin E, E-Se
Succinylcholine

Neurologic

Carbamazepine, Tegretol
Gabapentin, Neurotin
Imipramine, Tofranil
Mannitol, Osmitrol
Phenobarbital
Potassium bromide
Pregabalin, Lyrica
Thiamine
Thyrotropin-releasing hormone
Vitamin D, Vitamin E, Aquasol E, Vital E-300

Paraciticides

Albendazole, Eskazole
Febantel
Febendazole, Panacur
Ivermectin, Eqvalan
Levamisole, Ergamisol
Mebendazole, Vermox
Moxidectin, Quest
Oxfendazole, Benzelmin
Oxibendazole, Anthelcide
Piperazine
Praziquantel
Pyrantel pamoate
Thiabendazole

Respiratory Drugs

Acetylcysteine, Mucomyst
Albuterol, Proventil
Aminophylline, Corophyllin, Palaron
Beclomethasone, Beclovent, Vanceril
Caffeine, No-Doz, Vivarin
Clenbuterol, Ventipulmin
Cromolyn sodium, Intal, Nasalcrom
Doxapram, Dopram-V
Fluticasone, Flovent
Glycopyrrolate, Robinul-V
Ipratropium bromide, Atrovent
Isoflupredone acetate, Predef 2x
Isoproterenol, Isuprel
Nitric oxide
Salmeterol, Serevent
Sildenafil citrate, Viagra
Terbutaline, Brethine
Thyrotropin-releasing hormone
Xylazine hydrochloride, Rompun, Sedazine

Reversal Agents

Atipamezol, Antisedan
Edrophonium, Tensilon
Flumazenil, Romazicon
Naloxone, Narcan
Tolazoline, Tolazine
Yohimbine, Antagonil, Yocon

Sedative/Tranquilizers

Acepromazine, Promace
Chloral hydrate, Chloropent
Detomidine hydrochloride, Dormosedan
Dexmedetomidine, Dexdomitor

Diazepam, Valium
Fluphenazine decanoate, Prolixin
Haloperidol decanoate
Medetomidine, Domitor
Meperidine hydrochloride, Demerol
Midazolam, Versed
Romifidine, Sedivet

Toxicity Therapies

CaEDTA, Meta-Dote
Charcoal (activated), ToxiBan
Desferrioxamine
Di-tri-octahedral smectite, Biosponge
Dimercaprol
Fomepizole, Antizol-Vet, 4-methylpyrazole, Methylpyrazole
Methylene blue
Penicillamine
Perphenazine, Trilafon
Phenytoin, Dilantin
Physostigmine
Pralidoxime, 2-PAM
Sarmazenil
Sodium nitrate
Sodium thiosulfate
Thiamine
Vitamin K_1, phytonadione, Veda-K1

Urinary

Ammonium chloride
Azosulfamide, Neoprontosil
Bethanechol, Urecholine
Fenoldopam, Corlopam
Phenazopyridine, Pyridium
Phenoxybenzamine, Dibenzyline
Phenylpropanolamine, Prion

PHM

APPENDIX 9

Equine Emergency Drugs: Approximate Dosages and Adverse Drug Reactions*

Eileen S. Hackett, Thomas J. Divers, and James A. Orsini

Equine Emergency Drugs: Approximate Dosages*

Drug Name, Trade Name,* Conversion Factor	Indication	Dosage	Route	Estimated Dose Per 1000 lb (450 kg)	Precautions and Comments
Acepromazine, *Promace,* 10 mg/mL	Restraint, tranquilizer, preanesthetic, peripheral vasodilator	0.02-0.05 mg/kg q6-8h	IV, IM	0.9-2.25 mL	May result in hypotension; may cause paraphimosis when used in stallions or debilitated males
Acetaminophen, Tylenol, 500 mg/tab	COX-3 inhibitor, analgesia, laminitis	20-25 mg/kg q12h	PO	18 tabs	Clinical response seems variable
Acetazolamide, *Diamox,* 250 mg/tab[†]	Diuretic, glaucoma, HYPP prophylaxis, hyperkalemia	2-4 mg/kg q6-12h	PO	3.6-7.2 tabs	
Acetylcysteine, *Mucomyst,* 10% or 20% solution	Mucolytic, anticollagenase	50-140 mg/kg	PO or slowly IV	225-630 mL (10%)	ARDS, oxidative disorders, acute liver failure
		0.25-1 g q6-8h	Nebulization, IT	5 mL (10%)	ARDS or tenacious exudate in airways
N-Acetyl-L-cysteine (powdered)	Meconium impaction	Add 8 g powder and 1.5 tbsp (22.5 g) sodium bicarbonate (baking soda) to 200 mL water (4% solution); infuse solution	Per rectum	120-180 mL	Use Foley catheter and clamp for 20 minutes. Sedation with valium usually required. *DO NOT* use bicarbonate if serum sodium is elevated
Acetylsalicylic acid, aspirin, 240-gr. boluses,[†] 325-mg tablet	Antithrombotic	15-20 mg/kg q48h	PO	½ bolus	Decreases platelet aggregation in many normal horses (minimal effect in horses with SIRS); rectal administration results in higher blood levels than PO administration

Continued

---

*Dosage recommendations and routes of administration may change or vary from those listed in the book chapters depending on the intended use and clinician preference.

Equine Emergency Drugs: Approximate Dosages—cont'd

Drug Name, Trade Name,* Conversion Factor	Indication	Dosage	Route	Estimated Dose Per 1000 lb (450 kg)	Precautions and Comments
Albendazole, *Eskazole, Valbazen,* 600-mg tab, 114-mg/mL suspension	Benzimidazole	25-50 mg/kg q12-24h	PO	19-38 tabs 99-197 mL	
Albumin (human), 250 mg/mL)	Oncotic	250-750 mg/kg/h Smaller doses may be used	IV	450-1350 mL/h	Infrequent anaphylactoid reaction may occur
Albuterol, *Proventil,* 90 μg/puff, 0.5% for nebulization	Bronchospasm, bronchodilation	720 μg q4-6h for adult	Inhaler	5-8 puffs	**DO NOT** use in hypokalemic patients
			Nebulization	2-5 mL	Dilute with 0.9% saline
Allopurinol *Zyloprim (tablets), Aloprim (IV formulation),* 500 mg/30 mL vial	Antioxidant	5 mg/kg q4-6h for 1 day	IV, PO	~135 mL	Treat for 1-2 days
Altrenogest, *Altresyn, Regumate,* 2.2 mg/mL	Pregnancy maintenance, estrus suppression	0.044-0.088 mg/kg q24h	PO	9-18 mL	For pregnant mares experiencing toxemia, placentitis, or indications of premature delivery
Amantadine, *Symmetrel,* 100-mg cap	Antiviral	2.2-2.4 mg/kg q12-24h	PO	10-11 caps	Neurologic side effects at high doses (15 mg/kg)
Amikacin, *Amiglyde-V,* 250 mg/mL	Aminoglycoside antibiotic	15-25 mg/kg q24h 10-15 mg/kg q24h in adult 125-1000 mg	IV, IM IVRP	27-45 mL 18-27 mL 0.5-4 mL	Preferred over gentamicin in foals; nephrotoxic; use *only* if well hydrated
Aminocaproic acid, *Amicar,* 250 mg/mL	Hemorrhage, antifibrinolytic, plasminogen blocker	10-40 mg/kg q6h after 40 mg/kg loading dose	IV slowly (30-60 min) in 0.9% saline	18-72 mL	Used for uncontrolled bleeding when ligation is *not* an option
		70 mg/kg	IV over 20 min followed by CRI	126 mL	Maintains therapeutic levels for 60 min or more
		10-15 mg/kg/h	IV CRI	18-27 mL/h	For prolonged therapy
Aminophylline, *Corophyllin, Palaron,* 200 mg/tab,† 25 mg/mL	Bronchodilator, diminishes diaphragmatic fatigue, muscle fatigue, respiratory stimulant, anti-inflammatory, pulmonary edema diuretic, acute renal failure	4-10 mg/kg q8-12h 2-5 mg/kg q8-12h	PO IV (diluted slowly)	9-22 tabs 36-90 mL	May improve glomerular filtration rate; rarely recommended as a bronchodilator
Amiodarone, *Cordarone,* 50 mg/mL	Ventricular tachycardia, atrial fibrillation	5-7 mg/kg	IV	50 mL (45-63 mL)	Potassium channel blocker
		5 mg/kg/h 1st hour, 0.83 mg/kg/h up to 48 hours	IV CRI	45 mL 1st hour, 7.5 mL/h up to 48 hours	
Ammonium chloride, 5, 25, 100 g in poly bottle	Urinary acidifier	90-330 mg/kg	PO	40.5-148.5 g	Contraindicated in renal failure, poor palatability

Equine Emergency Drugs: Approximate Dosages—cont'd

Drug Name, Trade Name,* Conversion Factor	Indication	Dosage	Route	Estimated Dose Per 1000 lb (450 kg)	Precautions and Comments
Amoxicillin Clavulanic Acid, *Clavamox,* 250-mg tab†	Antibiotic	10-30 mg/kg q6-8h	PO	2 tabs/**50 kg**	Foals only
Amphotericin B, *Fungizone, Amphocin,* 5 mg/mL	Antifungal	0.3-1.0 mg/kg q24-48h	IV slowly	27-90 mL	Dilute in 1 liter D_5W
Ampicillin sodium, 1 and 3 g/vial (40 mg/mL)†	Antibiotic	15-50 mg/kg q8-12h	IV, IM	168-562 mL	More concentrated solutions may be used
Ampicillin trihydrate, *Poly-Flex,* 10 and 25 g/vial (40 mg/mL)	Antibiotic	11-22 mg/kg q8-12h	IM	123-247 mL	Volume required limits use
Antacids, *Maalox, Di-Gel*	Esophagitis, gastric hyperacidity, peptic ulcer, gastritis	0.6-2 mL/kg q3-4h	PO	30-100 mL/50 kg	Contain aluminum hydroxide and magnesium hydroxide that buffer acid for a brief period
Antivenin, 10-mL vial	Viperene snake envenomation	1-5 vials	IV slowly	10-50 mL	(4.5-18 mL) Dilute
Atipamezole, *Antisedan,* 5 mg/mL	α_2-Antagonist Especially detomidine or medetomidine	0.05-0.2 mg/kg	IV slowly IM	4-5 mL	Can produce excitement or have adverse cardiac effect when administered IV
Atracurium, *Tracurium,* 10 mg/mL	Neuromuscular blocker	0.1-0.2 mg/kg	IV	4.5-9.0 mL	Paralytic agent
Atropine, 15 mg/mL, 0.54 mg/mL	Bradyarrhythmias	0.005-0.01 mg/kg for sinus bradycardia	IV	0.15-0.3 mL (15 mg/mL) 4.5-9 mL (0.54 mg/mL)	Tachycardia, arrhythmia, ileus, mydriasis may occur; **DO NOT** use with inotropes
	Bronchodilator	0.014-0.02 mg/kg for bronchodilation	IV, IM	0.6 mL (15 mg/mL)	Repeat in 5 min if indicated
	Organophosphate toxicity	0.15 mg/kg or more	IV, IM, SQ	4.5 mL (15 mg/mL)	Administer for *confirmed* organophosphate toxicity and observe for signs of ileus
Azathioprine, *Imuran,* 50-mg tab	Immune-mediated thrombocytopenia, vasculitis, polyneuritis	2-3 mg/kg q12-24h; taper dose after 1 wk	PO	18-27 tabs	Monitor leukogram
Azithromycin, *Zithromax,* 100-mg/tab, 250-mg/tab	Antibiotic	10 mg/kg q24h for 5 days, then every other day	PO	18 tabs (250 mg)	*R. equi* pneumonia may cause hyperthermia. Dosing with rifampin should be separated by 2 hours
Azosulfamide, *Neoprontosil*	Urine dye for ectopic ureter detection	1.9 mg/kg	IV, IM		

Continued

Equine Emergency Drugs: Approximate Dosages—cont'd

Drug Name, Trade Name,* Conversion Factor	Indication	Dosage	Route	Estimated Dose Per 1000 lb (450 kg)	Precautions and Comments
Beclomethasone, *QVAR (Teva),* 40- and 80-µg/puff	Anti-inflammatory	3-8 µg/kg q12-24h	Inhaler	17-45 puffs (using 80 µg/ puff MDI)	
Benazepril *Lotensin,* also generic 40 mg/tab	Angiotension-converting enzyme inhibitor	0.5 mg/kg q24h	PO	5-6 tabs	
Benztropine mesylate, *Cogentin,* 1 mg/tab, 1 mg/mL	Anticholinergic	8-16 mg/450 kg 17 mg/450 kg	IV PO	8 mL 8 tabs	Use for priapism or fluphenazine toxicity
Bethanechol, *Urecholine,* 5 mg/mL 5 mg/tab†	Bladder atony, urinary retention, delayed gastric emptying	0.03-0.04 mg/kg q6-8h 0.22-0.45 mg/kg q6-8h	SQ, IV PO	3-4 mL 17 tabs (20-40 tabs)	Can be formulated for IV or SQ use Poorly absorbed
Beuthanasia solution, 290 mg/mL pentobarbital	Euthanasia	10-15 mL/100 lb (45 kg)	IV	100-150 mL	Has been approved for **euthanasia only;** some pentobarbital-based solutions have been used for seizure control when no other viable option: 5-20 mL/500 kg Use **ONLY** if no substitute available
Bismuth subsalicylate, *Pepto-Bismol, Gastrocote,* 262 mg/15 mL	Antidiarrheal	1-4.5 mL/kg q4-12 h	PO	500-2000 mL adult 50 mL foal	
Boldenone undecylenate, *Equipoise,* 10 mL vials	Anabolic steroid, 50 mg/mL	1.1 mg/kg	IM	9.5 mL	Treating debilitated horses with good appetite
Bretylium, *Tosylate,* 50 mg/mL	Ventricular fibrillation	5-10 mg/kg (every 10 min)	IV	45-90 mL	**DO NOT** exceed 30-35 mg/kg total dose (CPCR or Vtach) or 10 mg/kg adults
Bumetanide, *Bumex, Burinex,* 0.25 mg/mL	Congestive heart failure, loop diuretic	15 µg/kg	IV, IM	27 mL	
Buprenorphine, *Buprenex,* 0.3 mg/mL	Opioid partial agonist, analgesia	0.001-0.01 mg/kg 0.004-0.006 mg/kg	IV, Sublingual IM	1.5-15 mL 6-9 mL	*Note:* Controlled substance— schedule III; may cause excitement, decreased gut motility
Buspirone, *Buspar,* 30-mg tab	Compulsive behaviors	0.5 mg/kg q8-12h	PO	7.5 tabs	
Butorphanol tartrate, *Torbugesic,* 10 mg/mL	Analgesic, sedation, preanesthetic, antitussive	0.01-0.1 mg/kg 13-22 µg/kg/h	IV, IM IV CRI	0.45-4.5 mL 0.6-1 mL/h	Ataxia and head tremors when used without tranquilization. *Note:* Controlled substance— schedule IV

Equine Emergency Drugs: Approximate Dosages—cont'd

Drug Name, Trade Name,* Conversion Factor	Indication	Dosage	Route	Estimated Dose Per 1000 lb (450 kg)	Precautions and Comments
Butylscopolammonium bromide, *Buscopan,* 20 mg/mL	Colic pain, antispasmodic, anticholinergic (used for colic, choke, meconium impactions, cervical relaxation)	0.3 mg/kg	IV, IM, or SQ	6.8 mL 1 mL in enema for meconium impaction; 1-3 mL topical application to relax cervix	Should not be used in horses with glaucoma; IV use results in elevated heart rate. ***DO NOT*** use in exhausted horses
Ca-EDTA, *Meta-Dote,* 50 mg/mL	Lead toxicity, chelator	75 mg/kg per day divided q12h	IV slowly	675 mL	Monitor serum lead levels
Caffeine, *NoDoz,*[†] *Vivarin,* 200-mg/tab	Respiratory stimulant (appears effective clinically but *no* evidence-based studies)	10 mg/kg loading dose, then 2.5-3 mg/kg, q12-24h maintenance dose	PO or per rectum	2.5 tabs/50 kg	Toxic level >40 µg/L Foals become hyperexcitable
Calcium borogluconate (23%), 230 mg/mL (20.7 mg Ca, 1.08 mEq/mL)	Hypocalcemia, hyperkalemia	150-250 mg/kg	IV slowly	300-450 mL	Can be mixed with most crystalloids; monitor cardiac rate and rhythm
Calcium chloride, 100 mg/mL	Cardiac resuscitation	5-7 mg/kg	IV slowly	22.5-31.5 mL slowly	
Carbamazepine, *Tegretol,* 200-mg tab	Anticonvulsant, head shakers	2-8 mg/kg q6-8h	PO	4.5-18 tabs	
Carboxymethylcellulose, sodium, 10 mg/mL	Adhesion preventative	7 mL/kg	Intraperitoneal	3 liters	
Carbaryl	Insecticide	10 gm of 50% pwdr mixed in 1 L of water	Topical	4.5 L 4.5%	No more than 1-2x/wk
Carprofen, *Rimadyl,* 100-mg/tab,[†] 50 mg/mL	Analgesic, anti-inflammatory	1.4 mg/kg q24h	IV, PO	6.3 tabs 12.5 mL	Commonly used in treatment of "joint ill"
Cefazolin *Ancef,* 1 g/vial 20g/vial	Antibiotic	11-22 mg/kg q6-8h 200 mg 0.2 mL of 50 mg/mL	IV Subconjunctivally Subpalpebral catheter	0.25-0.5 vial (20 g/vial) 0.2 mL of 50 mg/mL	First-generation cephalosporin
Cefepime, *Maxipime,* 500 mg, 1-g, and 2-g vials	Antibiotic	2.2 mg/kg q8h adults 11 mg/kg q8h foals	IV, IM IV, IM	990 mg (1-g vial) 550 mg/50 kg (500 mg vial)	Fourth-generation cephalosporin
Cefoperazone, *Cefobid,* 1 g/vial (40 mg/mL)[†]	Antibiotic	30 mg/kg q8h	IV	37 mL/50 kg	Third-generation cephalosporin
Cefotaxime, *Claforan,* 500 mg (20 mg/mL)[†]	Antibiotic	40-50 mg/kg q6-8h	IV	**100-125 mL/ 50 kg**	Third-generation cephalosporin
Cefoxitin, *Mefoxin,* 1 g/ vial	Antibiotic	20 mg/kg q6h	IV, IM	9/1g vials	Second-generation cephalosporin
Cefpodoxime proxetil, *Vantin,* 200-mg tab	Antibiotic	10 mg/kg q6-12h	PO	2.5 tabs/50 kg	Third-generation cephalosporin
Cefquinome, *Cobactam*	Antibiotic	1-2.5 mg/kg q6-12h	IV, IM		Fourth-generation cephalosporin
Ceftazidime, *Fortaz,* 1 g/ vial (40 mg/mL)	Antibiotic	20-50 mg/kg q6-12h	IV, IM	**38 mL/50 kg (25-63 mL/ 50 kg)**	Third-generation cephalosporin

Continued

Equine Emergency Drugs: Approximate Dosages—cont'd

Drug Name, Trade Name,* Conversion Factor	Indication	Dosage	Route	Estimated Dose Per 1000 lb (450 kg)	Precautions and Comments
Ceftiofur, *Naxcel,* 50 mg/mL, 4 g/vial†	Antibiotic	1-5 mg/kg q6-12h 200 mg	IV, IM IVRP	9-45 mL	Dose varies with severity of disease; third-generation cephalosporin
Ceftiofur, *Excede,* 200 mg/mL	Antibiotic	6.6 mg/kg q4 days	IM SQ (foal) ***DO NOT*** give IV	15 mL	Inject a maximum of 7 mL per site (massage area after injection); requires 12-24 hours to reach peak blood levels
Ceftriaxone, *Rocephin,* 1-, 2-, 10-g vials, 100 mg/mL	Antibiotic	25-50 mg/kg q12h	IV, IM	112.5-250 ml (adult) if reconstituting to 100 mg/mL	Third-generation cephalosporin
Cephalexin, *Keflex,* 500-mg tab	Antibiotic	25 mg/kg q6h	PO	2.5 tabs/50 kg	First-generation cephalosporin
Cephalothin, *Keflin*	Antibiotic	20 mg/kg q6h	IV, IM		First-generation cephalosporin
Cephapirin, *Cefadyl, Cefa-Lak,* 500 mg (20 mg/mL)†	Antibiotic	20-30 mg/kg q4-8h	IV, IM	**62 mL/50 kg (50-75 mL/ 50 kg)**	Reports of diarrhea, anaphylaxis; first-generation cephalosporin
	Intramammary antibiotic preparation		Topical Intramammary		First-generation cephalosporin
Cetirizine, *Zyrtec* 10 mg/tab	Antihistamine	0.2-0.4 mg/kg q12h	PO	9-18 tabs	Metabolite of hydroxyzine
Charcoal, activated *ToxiBan*† 200 mg/mL or chemical grade	Gastrointestinal adsorbent	0.5-1 g/kg	PO via NG intubation	1.1-2.3 liters	
Chloral hydrate, *Chloropent,* 120 mg/mL	Restraint, sedation, preanesthetic	22 mg/kg (moderate sedation) 30-60 mg/kg (profound sedation)	IV 12% solution by slow infusion	82.5 mL 112.5-225 mL	Perivascular administration may result in phlebitis, does *not* provide analgesia
Chloramphenicol, *Chloromycetin,* 500-mg tabs† Sodium succinate, 20-200 mg/mL	Antibiotic	40-60 mg/kg q6-8h 25 mg/kg q4-6h	PO IV IV	36-54 tabs ~550 mL/20 mg/ mL conc– 55 mL/200 mg/ mL conc	Compounded paste may decrease human contact during treatment; *illegal* in some countries.
Chorionic gonadotropin, *Chorisol, Follutein,* HCG, 1000 U/mL	Induce ovulation, cystic ovaries	2.2-6.7 U/kg 22.2 U/kg	IM IM	1000-3000 U 10,000 U	Luteinizing hormone schedule III
	Cryptorchid classification stimulation test	13-27 U/kg	IV	6000-12,000 U	If cryptorchid, expect testosterone >100 pg/mL 30-120 min after injection
Cimetidine, *Tagamet,* 150 mg/mL, 800 mg/tab	Gastroduodenal ulceration Melanoma	6.6 mg/kg q6-8h 16-25 mg/kg q6-8h 2.5 mg/kg q8-12h	IV PO PO	20 mL 9-14 tabs 1.4 tabs	H_2-receptor antagonist

Equine Emergency Drugs: Approximate Dosages—cont'd

Drug Name, Trade Name,* Conversion Factor	Indication	Dosage	Route	Estimated Dose Per 1000 lb (450 kg)	Precautions and Comments
Cisapride, *Propulsid* 10 mg/tab	Ileus	0.1 mg/kg q8h 0.1-1.0 mg/kg q4-8h	IM PO	 4.5-45 tabs	Must be reformulated before IM administration; cardiac arrhythmia possible with IV administration; negligible rectal absorption
Clarithromycin, *Biaxin,* 500-mg tab	*Rhodococcus equi* infections, used in conjunction with rifampin	7.5 mg/kg q12h	PO	0.75 tab/50 kg	Not for use in adult horses because of risk of severe colitis; best to separate by 2 hours when administered concurrently with rifampin
Clavulanic acid– ticarcillin, *Timentin,* 3.1- and 31-g vial	Antibiotic	100 mg/kg loading dose, then 50 mg/kg q6h	IV	Loading dose: 1.5 vials (31-g vial), maintenance: 0.75 vial (31-g vial)	
Clenbuterol, *Ventipulmin,* 72.5 µg/mL	Bronchodilator, tocolytic	0.8-3.2 µg/kg q12h	IV, PO	5-20 mL	Tachycardia and restlessness may occur at higher doses; ***DO NOT*** use for more than 14 days concurrently with inhaler
Inhaler†		0.5 µg/kg q8h	Nebulization		***DO NOT*** use concurrent with oral or IV
Clomipramine, *Clomicalm, Anafranil,* 80-mg tab	Compulsive behaviors Chemical ejaculation	1-2 mg/kg q24h 2.2 mg/kg	PO IV	5.6-11.3 tabs	Used in conjunction with alpha-adrenergic agonists
Clopidogrel, *Plavix,* 75-mg tab	Antiplatelet agent	2 mg/kg q24h 4 mg/kg loading dose	PO	12 tabs 24 tabs	Generally inhibits platelet aggregation in most healthy and ill horses; +/− bleeding
Cloprostenol sodium, *Estrumate or estroPLAN,* 250 mcg/mL, 20 mL vials	Induce abortion	0.5 µg/kg	IM	250 µg/450-kg horse	Must be >80d pregnant
Colchicine, 0.6-mg tabs	Hepatic fibrosis	0.03 mg/kg q12-24h	PO	22 tabs	
Colony-stimulating factor, *Neupogen,* 300 µg/mL	Life-threatening leukopenia	5 µg/kg q24h	IV slowly over 30 min	1 mL/50 kg	Failure to respond negative prognostic indicator
Cosyntropin, *Cortrosyn,* 0.25 mg/mL	ACTH stimulation test High-dose stimulation test Low-dose stimulation test	0.1-0.5 µg/kg 2 µg/kg 0.2 µg/kg	IV IV IV	0.18-0.9 mL 0.4 mL/50 kg 0.04 mL/50 kg	Stable for 4 months following saline dilution, if frozen

Continued

Equine Emergency Drugs: Approximate Dosages—cont'd

Drug Name, Trade Name,* Conversion Factor	Indication	Dosage	Route	Estimated Dose Per 1000 lb (450 kg)	Precautions and Comments
Cromolyn sodium, *Intal, Nasalcrom,* 40 mg/mL	Chronic obstructive pulmonary disease	0.2-0.5 mg/kg	Nebulization	2.25-5.6 mL	Availability unpredictable
Cyclophosphamide, *Cytoxan,* 20 mg/mL	Immune-mediated disease Chemotherapy	1.1 mg/kg q24h 2.2 mg/kg q 2 weeks	IM IV slowly following saline dilution	24.8 mL 49.5 mL	Immunosuppressive
Cyproheptadine, *Periactin,* 4 mg/tab	Pituitary hyperplasia, head shaking	0.25-0.6 mg/kg q12-24h	PO	28-67.5 tabs	Efficacy unproven
Dantrolene, *Dantrium,* 100-mg capsules, 20-mg vial	Rhabdomyolysis, muscle relaxation, malignant hypothermia	2.5-5 mg/kg q8-24h 10-mg/kg loading dose 2-4 mg/kg q1-2h	PO PO IV	11-22 capsules 45 capsules 67 vials slowly; mixed in saline	May cause sedation at higher doses
Dapsone, 100-mg tab	Antibacterial drug useful in treatment of *Pneumocystis carinii* pneumonia	3 mg/kg q24h	PO	13.5 tabs	
Decoquinate	Antiprotozoal	0.5 mg/kg q24h	PO		Paste being evaluated for EPM; often combined with levamisole
Deracoxib, *Deramaxx,* 12-mg, 25-mg, 75-mg, or 100-mg chewable tabs in U.S.	NSAID COX-2 selective 1:25 in dogs	2 mg/kg q12-24h	PO	9 tabs/100-mg tab	Not approved for use in horses
Desferrioxamine, 500 mg, 2 g vials available (200 mg/mL)	Iron toxicity	10 mg/kg	IM, IV slowly	22.5 mL adult 2.5 mL foal	
Detomidine hydrochloride, *Dormosedan,* 10 mg/mL	Sedation, analgesia Epidural Standing surgical procedures, IV bolus followed by maintenance CRI	5-40 µg/kg 30-50 µg/kg or less 8.4 µg/kg, 0.5 µg/kg/min	IV, IM Epidural IV bolus follows by CRI	0.23-1.8 mL Dilute to 10 mL (saline)	Higher dosage for IM only. ***Caution:*** May cause unexpected aggression See Chapter 47, p. 738.
Detomidine gel, *Dormosedan,* 7.6 mg/mL		40-80 µg/kg or more in excited horses	PO	2.3-4.7 mL	4-8 × the IV dose. ***DO NOT*** get in administrator's eyes or mouth!
Dexamethasone, *Azium,*† 2 mg/mL	Anti-inflammatory	0.02-0.1 mg/kg q24h	IV, IM	4.5-22.5 mL	Prolonged treatment may cause laminitis; prolonged high dose may cause abortion
		0.04-0.067 mg/kg	PO	20-30 mL	Injectable preparation given PO has variable bioavailability of 30%-60%
Azium SP, 4 mg/mL (equivalent to 3 mg dexamethasone)	Anti-edema	0.1-0.5 mg/kg q6-24h	IV	11-56 mL	
Dexamethasone-trichlormethiazide, *Naquasone*	Inflammatory edema	5 mg/200 mg boluses q24h	PO		

Equine Emergency Drugs: Approximate Dosages—cont'd

Drug Name, Trade Name,* Conversion Factor	Indication	Dosage	Route	Estimated Dose Per 1000 lb (450 kg)	Precautions and Comments
Dexmedetomidine, *Dexdomitor,* 0.5 mg/mL	Sedation, analgesia	0.0025-0.01 mg/kg	IV, IM	2.25-9 mL	
Dextran 70, *Gentran*	Plasma volume expansion	4-10 mL/kg	IV slowly	1.8 liters	Watch for anaphylaxis
Dextrose	Hypoglycemia, hyperkalemia	5% or 10% solution at 4-8 mg/kg per minute; 0.5 mL/kg bolus	IV	225 mL	May cause rebound hypoglycemia or hypokalemia
Diazepam, *Valium,* 5 mg/mL	Tranquilizer, anticonvulsant, preanesthetic, anxiolytic	0.05-0.44 mg/kg for adult; 0.1-0.2 mg/kg for foal	IV	4.5-39.6 mL; 1-2 mL foal	Respiratory depression may occur at higher doses; may precipitate in PVC lines. **Note:** Controlled substance—schedule IV
	Appetite stimulant	0.02 mg/kg	IV	2 mL	
Diclazuril, *Protozil,* 1.56% oral pellets	Protozoal myelitis	1 mg/kg q24h	PO		28-day course of treatment recommended
Diclofenac sodium, *Surpass,* 10 mg/mL	Joint pain and inflammation associated with osteoarthritis	q12h	Topical	5-inch ribbon over affected area	Wear gloves during application
Digoxin, *Lanoxin,* 0.1 mg/mL	Cardiac failure, supraventricular arrhythmias, poor systolic function	0.0022-0.0075 mg/kg q12h	IV	10-33 mL	Depression, anorexia, colic may occur; lower dose most commonly used
0.5-mg tab		0.011-0.0175 mg/kg q12h	PO	10-15 tabs	For longer-term use, monitor serum levels
Di-tri-octahedral smectite, *Bio-Sponge,* powder	Gastrointestinal adsorbent, enterocolitis	q12-24h	PO or per NG intubation	0.5-3 lb	Does **NOT** interfere with metronidazole absorption
Diltiazem, 5 mg/mL	Calcium channel blocker	0.125 mg/kg	IV over 2 min	11.25 mL	May repeat, **not** to exceed 1.0 mg/kg
Dimercaprol, 100 mg/mL	Arsenic, lead toxicity	2.5-5 mg/kg	IM	11.25-22.5 mL	
Dimethyl sulfoxide (DMSO), *Domoso,* 900 mg/mL	Anti-edema	10%-20% solution at 0.5-1.0 g/kg q12-24h	IV in 0.9% saline or D_5W	500 mL	May cause hemolysis when given IV
	Anti-inflammatory	10%-20% solution at 20-100 mg/kg q8-12h	IV in 0.9% saline or D_5W	10-50 mL	Postoperative treatment, reperfusion injury
Diminazene aceturate (1.05 g), *Tryponil* *(1.31 g)*	Trypanosomiasis	3.5-5 mg/kg as single dose, repeat in 5 weeks	SC, IM		Administer antihistamine before treatment. General: 1 mL per 20 kg body weight (2.36 gram per 300 kg body weight). Dissolve 2.36 gram powder in 15 mL sterile water before use (=157.3 mg/mL).

Continued

Equine Emergency Drugs: Approximate Dosages—cont'd

Drug Name, Trade Name,* Conversion Factor	Indication	Dosage	Route	Estimated Dose Per 1000 lb (450 kg)	Precautions and Comments
Dinoprost tromethamine, *Lutalyse, Prostin F2 Alpha,* 5 mg/mL	Abortion	0.011-0.022 mg/kg	IM	0.9-1.98 mL (1-2 mL)	Early and midgestation; abortifacient
Dioctyl sodium sulfosuccinate, *Dioctynate,* 50 mg/mL	Laxative	10-20 mg/kg; up to 2 doses, 48 hours apart	PO	90-180 mL	GI irritant
Diphenhydramine hydrochloride, *Benadryl,* 50 mg/mL	Antihistamine, antipyretic, analgesic, anaphylaxis	0.5-2 mg/kg	IV, IM	IV slowly, 4.5-18 mL	May enhance or inhibit the effects of epinephrine
Dipyrone, *Novin, Metamizole*	Anti-inflammatory, analgesic, antipyretic	10-22 mg/kg	IV, IM		Compounded only in United States
Dobutamine, *Dobutrex,* 12.5 mg/mL	Cardiac failure, hypotension, AV block, inotrope, beta$_1$-adrenergic agent	1-15 µg/kg/min	IV CRI after dilution in D$_5$W or 0.9% saline to 500 µg/mL		***DO NOT*** use with magnesium, lidocaine, furosemide, or calcium bicarbonate
Domperidone, *Equidone,* 110 mg/mL	Agalactia, fescue toxicity	1.1 mg/kg q12h	PO	4.5 mL	May enhance GI motility; foal accidentally receiving mare dose may have transient CNS signs
Dopamine, *Intropin,* 40 mg/mL	Lower dose: Oliguric renal failure, cardiac failure, AV block, renal perfusion Higher dose: beta$_1$-adrenergic agent	1-20 µg/kg/min	IV CRI		Dilute with D$_5$W
Doxapram, *Dopram-V,* 20 mg/mL	Respiratory stimulant	0.2-0.5 mg/kg loading dose followed by 0.03-0.08 mg/kg/min for 20 min	IV	0.5-1.25 mL/50 kg	Use if mechanical means of ventilation not possible. ***DO NOT*** mix with sodium bicarbonate
Doxorubicin, *Adriamycin,* 2 mg/mL	Chemotherapeutic	0.3 mg/kg	IV slowly following saline dilution	67.5 mL	Cardiotoxic; monitor cardiac troponin levels
Doxycycline, *Vibramycin,* 100 mg/tab[†]	Antibiotic	5-10 mg/kg q12h	PO	22-45 tabs	Poorly absorbed orally
Doxylamine succinate, 11.36 mg/mL	Antihistamine	0.5 mg/kg q6-12h	IV slowly, IM, SQ	20 mL	May enhance or inhibit the effects of epinephrine
Edrophonium, *Tensilon,* 10 mg/mL	Supraventricular arrhythmia, reversal of atracurium	0.5-1 mg/kg	IV	22-45 mL	Antagonist for atracurium
Eltenac	NSAID	0.5 mg/kg q24h	IV		Not available in U.S.
Enalapril, *Vasotec, Enacard,* 20 mg/tab[†]	Vasodilator, ACE inhibitor, congestive heart failure	1.0 mg/kg q12-24h	PO	22.5 tabs	Bioavailability reportedly very low in horses!

Equine Emergency Drugs: Approximate Dosages—cont'd

Drug Name, Trade Name,* Conversion Factor	Indication	Dosage	Route	Estimated Dose Per 1000 lb (450 kg)	Precautions and Comments
Enrofloxacin, *Baytril,* 68 mg/tab	Fluoroquinolone antibiotic	5-7.5 mg/kg q24h	IV PO	23-34 mL 33-50 tabs	May cause arthropathy in foals; IV preparation may be used orally; oral erosions a potential sequela
100 mg/mL		7.5 mg/kg q24h	IV	34 mL	For oral use
Ephedrine, 50 mg/mL	Vasopressor, splenic contracture	0.02-0.1 mg/kg	IV	0.2-0.9 mL	
Epinephrine, *Adrenalin,* 1:1000 (1 mg/mL)	Anaphylaxis, asystole, glaucoma, bradycardia, cardiac resuscitation, vasopressor	0.01-0.02 mg/kg anaphylaxis	IV, IM	4.5-9 mL	Continuous infusion of drug may be arrhythmogenic; *DO NOT* use with anithistamines
		0.1-0.2 mg/kg anaphylaxis	IT	45-90 mL	
		0.03-0.05 mg/kg for asystole	IV	13.5-22.5 mL	
		0.3-0.5 mg/kg for asystole	IT	135-225 mL	
Epoetin alfa, *Epogen, Erythropoietin Procrit,* 4000 U/mL	Stimulate RBC production, renal anemia	50 U/kg once weekly	SQ	5.6 mL	May cause aplastic anemia
Equine plasma	Sepsis, shock, hypogammaglobulinemia, hemorrhage, decreased oncotic pressure, specific antibodies	1 or more liters	IV		Can generally be administered rapidly; rarely causes anaphylaxis and very rarely associated with Theiler's disease
Erythromycin,† 100 mg/mL, 250 mg/tab	Macrolide antibiotic	25-30 mg/kg q6-12h	PO	45-54 tabs	May induce diarrhea, hyperthermia
		1 gram regional perfusion q8h for foals with *R. equi* physitis	RP		
	Ileus	1-2.5 mg/kg as 1-hour infusion q6h	IV	4.5-11 mL	To improve intestinal motility; observe for colic, diarrhea, intussusception
Estrogen, conjugates *Premarin,* 25-mg vial	Hemorrhage	0.05-0.1 mg/kg	IV	1-2 vials	For uncontrolled uterine hemorrhage
Etodolac, *EtoGesic, Lodine,* 500-mg tab	Inflammation	20 mg/kg q12-24h	PO	18 tabs	
Famotidine, *Pepcid AC,* 10 mg/mL	GI ulceration	0.23-0.5 mg/kg q8-12h	IV	10.5-22.5 mL/450 kg **1.2-2.5 mL/50 kg**	Minimal pharmacokinetic data
20 mg/tab	H₂-receptor antagonist	2.8-4 mg/kg q8-12h	PO	10 tabs (foal)	
Febantel (FBT), 93 mg/mL	Anthelmintic	6 mg/kg	PO	29 mL	
Fenbendazole (FBZ), *Panacur,* 100 mg/mL	Anthelmintic	5-10 mg/kg	PO	22.5-45 mL	Relatively safe for foals with ascarids

Continued

Equine Emergency Drugs: Approximate Dosages—cont'd

Drug Name, Trade Name,* Conversion Factor	Indication	Dosage	Route	Estimated Dose Per 1000 lb (450 kg)	Precautions and Comments
Fenoldopam, *Corlopam*, 10 mg/mL	Dopamine-1 antagonist, renal failure	0.04-0.1 µg/kg/min	IV	0.18-0.27 mL/h	Dilute in 0.9% saline or D₅W
Fentanyl, *Duragesic*, 25-, 50-, and 100-µg/h transdermal patches	Narcotic analgesia	Modify dosage with concurrent analgesia	Dermal	2-3 × 100 µg/h patches for adult	Change every third day; *DO NOT* use with butorphanol, decreases intestinal motility; *Note:* Controlled substance—schedule II
0.05 mg/mL	Monitoring of plasma concentration during administration suggested	3-6 µg/kg/h	CRI	27-54 mL/h	Agitation and tachycardia may be observed at higher doses
Firocoxib, *Equioxx*, 6.93 g/tube (56.8 mg of firocoxib), 20 mg/mL	Analgesia, NSAID, osteoarthritis, COX-2 selective	0.1 mg/kg q24h (0.2 mg/kg loading dose) 0.09 mg/kg q24h	PO IV	0.8 paste syringe (45.5 mg) or 1 paste syringe/ 1250 lb 2 mL	Stop treatment if signs of inappetence, colic, abnormal feces, or lethargy are observed
Florfenicol, *NuFlor*, 300 mg/mL	Antibiotic	20 mg/kg q24-48h	IM	3.3 mL/50 kg	For use in foals between 2 weeks and 4 months
Fluconazole, *Diflucan*, 200 mg/tab	Antifungal	8-14 mg/kg loading dose; 4-5 mg/kg maintenance q12-24h	PO	18-31 tabs loading; 9-11 tabs maintenance	Provides higher tissue levels than most other antifungal drugs
Flumazenil, *Romazicon*, 0.1 mg/mL	Benzodiazepine (Valium) antagonist, uncontrolled hepatic coma	0.011-0.022 mg/kg	IV slowly	50-100 mL	Expensive treatment with questionable benefit for hepatic encephalopathy
Flunixin meglumine, *Banamine*, 50 mg/mL, 1500 mg/30-g oral paste syringe	Endotoxemia	0.25 mg/kg q8h	IV	2.3 mL	IM injections infrequently associated with clostridial myositis
	Analgesia, anti-inflammatory, antipyretic	0.25-1.1 mg/kg q8-12h	PO IV, IM	2.3-9.9 mL	1000-lb oral dose equivalent to 500 mg flunixin
Fluorescein sodium, *Fluorescite*, 100 mg/mL	Assess intestinal viability	6.6-15 mg/kg	IV	30-67.5 mL	Extravasation during injection may result in severe local tissue damage
Fluphenazine decanoate *Prolixin*, 25 mg/mL	Long-term tranquilization	0.06 mg/kg	IM once	1.1 mL	Adverse CNS signs possible
Fluprostenol sodium, *Equimate*, 50 µg/mL	Abortion	2.2 µg/kg	IM	20 mL	Induce parturition
Fluticasone, *Flovent*, 220 µg/puff	Heaves	2.2-4.4 mg/450 kg q12-24h	Inhaler	10-20 puffs	Lower range most commonly used
Folinic acid, *Leucovorin*, 10 mg/mL	Bone marrow suppression	0.09-0.22 mg/kg	IM	4-10 mL	

Equine Emergency Drugs: Approximate Dosages—cont'd

Drug Name, Trade Name,* Conversion Factor	Indication	Dosage	Route	Estimated Dose Per 1000 lb (450 kg)	Precautions and Comments
Fomepizole, *Antizol-vet, 4-methylpyrazole, Methylpyrazole,* 50 mg/mL	Ethylene glycol toxicity	20 mg/kg initial dose, then 17 hours later 15 mg/kg, then 25 hours after initial 5 mg/kg, then 36 hours after initial 5 mg/kg	IV	180 mL 135 mL 45 mL	Dilute before administration to avoid phlebitis
Furosemide, *Salix, Lasix,* 50 mg/mL	Diuretic, pulmonary edema	1-2 mg/kg bolus	SQ, IM, IV	9-18 mL	Protect solution from light; may result in acidosis and electrolyte imbalance, PO administration has very poor bioavailability
		0.12 mg/kg/hr	IV CRI	1.1 mL/h following IV bolus	CRI decreases fluctuations in plasma volume compared with intermittent administration
	EIPH	0.3-0.6 mg/kg	IV	2.7-5.5 mL	State regulated by racing commission
Gabapentin, *Neurontin,* 300-mg tab	Neuropathic pain	5-19 mg/kg q12-24h	PO	7.5-28.5 tabs	Low oral bioavailability
Gamithromycin, *Zactran,* 150 mg/mL	Macrolide antibiotic	6 mg/kg every 5-7 days	IM	18 mL	For macrolide sensitive *R. equi* pulmonary infections or *Streptococcus zooepidemicus* pneumonia in foals
Ganciclovir, *Cytovene,* 50 mg/mL	Antiviral	2.5 mg/kg q8h day 1, followed by q12h following days	IV	22.5 mL	
Gentamicin, *Gentocin,* 100 mg/mL	Aminoglycoside antibiotic	6.6 mg/kg q24h	IV, IM	30 mL	Nephrotoxic; use *cautiously* and only in well-hydrated foals and adults
Glycopyrrolate, *Robinul-V,* 0.2 mg/mL	Vagally induced bradyarrhythmias	0.002-0.01 mg/kg	IV	4.5-22.5 mL	Tachycardia, arrhythmia, ileus, mydriasis
	Bronchodilator	0.005 mg/kg q8-12h	IV, IM, SQ	11 mL	
Griseofulvin, *Fulvicin,* 2.5-g packets	Dermatophytic infection	10 mg/kg q24h	PO	2 packets	***DO NOT*** use in pregnant horses
Guaifenesin (GG), *Gecolate,*† 50 mg/mL	Central-acting muscle relaxant, preanesthetic, expectorant	60-90 mg/kg	IV as 5% solution	540-810 mL to effect	Should be administered by IV catheter to avoid perivascular reaction, overdose may result in apnea
Triple Drip: 1 L 5% GG 1-2 g ketamine 500 mg xylazine		1-3 mL/kg/hr	IV		

Continued

Equine Emergency Drugs: Approximate Dosages—cont'd

Drug Name, Trade Name,* Conversion Factor	Indication	Dosage	Route	Estimated Dose Per 1000 lb (450 kg)	Precautions and Comments
Haloperidol decanoate, 50 mg/mL	Long-acting tranquilizer	0.01 mg/kg 0.3 mg/kg	IM PO	0.1 mL 2.7 mL	Adverse effects occur; may cause sedation for 5-7 days; **DO NOT** give IV
Heparin, unfractionated, 1000 IU/mL[†]	Anticoagulant, hyperlipidemia, prevention of abdominal adhesions	40-100 IU/kg q6h	IV, SQ	18-45 mL	Monitor for RBC agglutination and decreasing hematocrit
Heparin, low molecular weight	Antithrombotic, anti-inflammatory				100 U/kg needed to inhibit factor Xa activity in foals
Dalteparin, *Fragmin*, 25,000 U/mL		50-100 U/kg q24h	SQ	1-2 mL	
Enoxaparin, *Lovenox*, 100 mg/mL		0.4-0.8 mg/kg q24h	SQ	2.25-4.5 mL (100 mg/mL)	
Hetastarch, *Hespan*, 60 mg/mL in saline *Hextend*, 60 mg/mL in Lactated Ringer solution or VetStarch 6%	Shock, low colloid osmotic pressure, plasma volume expansion	Up to 10 mL/kg q24-48h	IV	4500 mL	Alters refractometer plasma and urine protein measurement; high dosage may inhibit coagulation
Hydralazine, *Apresoline*, 50 mg/tab[†] 10 mg/2 mL ampule (10 mg/mL)	Congestive heart failure, vasodilator	0.5-1.5 mg/kg q12h 0.5 mg/kg	PO IV	4.5-13.5 tabs 22.5 mL	Arterial dilation Bioavailability per os is variable
Hydrochlorothiazide, *Hydrozide*, 25 mg/mL	Diuretic	0.56 mg/kg q24h	PO	10 mL	
Hydrocortisone, sodium succinate, *Solu-Cortef*, 100 mg/2 mL (50 mg/mL)		0.2-0.4 mg/kg q4h	IV	**0.2-0.4 mL/50 kg**	For adrenal gland exhaustion in septic foals
Hydromorphone, 2 mg/mL	Analgesia	0.01-0.04 mg/kg	Epidural	2-9 mL	
Hydroxyzine hydrochloride, *Vistaril*, *Atarax*, 100-mg tabs,[†] 25 mg/mL	Antihistamine, pruritus, urticaria	1-1.5 mg/kg q8-12h 0.5-1 mg/kg q12h	PO IM	5 tabs (4.5-6.75 tabs) 9-18 mL	May have unpredictable results when used with epinephrine
Hyperimmune plasma	Endotoxemia, *C. difficile*, *R. equi*, botulism, etc.	2-4 L/450 kg	IV	2-4 liters	
Hypertonic saline 7.5%	Hypotension, acute dehydration	3-5 mL/kg	IV	1-2 liters	**DO NOT** use for chronic dehydration
Imidocarb, *Imizol*, 120 mg/mL	Babesiosis	2.2-4 mg/kg q24h × 3 days, if needed	IM, SQ	8-15 mL	
Imipenem, *Primaxin IV*, 250 mg (10 mg/mL)	Antibiotic	10-15 mg/kg q6-8h	IV in fluids	50-75 mL/50 kg	
Imipramine, *Tofranil*, 50-mg tabs	Narcolepsy, cataplexy	1-2 mg/kg q8-12h	PO	9-18 tabs	IV preparation also available
Insulin, porcine Zn, *Vetsulin*, 40 IU/mL	Hyperglycemia	0.4 IU/kg q24h	SQ	4.5 mL	

Equine Emergency Drugs: Approximate Dosages—cont'd

Drug Name, Trade Name,* Conversion Factor	Indication	Dosage	Route	Estimated Dose Per 1000 lb (450 kg)	Precautions and Comments
Insulin, regular, *Humulin,* 100 IU/mL	Hyperglycemia Hyperkalemia	0.1 IU/kg PRN 0.1-1 IU/kg/hr	IM, IV IM, IV, or CRI	0.45 mL 0.45-4.5 mL	Most often used q8h IM Should be used as a last resort for hyperkalemia Flush catheter well before and after administration
Iodide potassium	Fungal disease	22-67 mg/kg q24h	PO, IV		Discontinue use when signs of iodism are encountered
Ipratropium bromide, *Atrovent,* 18 µg/puff	Bronchodilator	0.2-0.5 µg/kg q8h	Nebulization, inhaler	5-12 puffs	Can be used in addition to β$_2$-agonist
Isoflupredone acetate, *Predef 2x,* 2 mg/mL	Heaves	0.02 mg/kg q24h	IM	4.5 mL	Decrease dose and prolong interval after 3-5 days; hypokalemia **NOT** reported in horses
Isoproterenol, *Isuprel,* 0.2 mg/mL	Bronchodilator, resuscitation, beta-adrenergic	0.05-0.2 µg/kg/min	IV CRI	6.75-27 mL/h	Rarely used
Isoxsuprine, 20 mg/tab	Vasodilation	0.6-1.32 mg/kg q12h 0.4-1.2 mg/kg q24h	PO IM	13.5-30 tabs	Give on empty stomach; poor bioavailability IM product available in some countries
Itraconazole, *Sporanox,* 100 mg/tab	Antifungal	5 mg/kg q24h	PO	22 caps	Solution has better absorption than capsules
Ivermectin, *Eqvalan,* 10 mg/mL	Anthelmintic	200 µg/kg	PO	9 mL	Lethal to large and small strongyles, large strongyle larvae, ascarids, and bots
Kaolin/Pectin, 4-8 mL/kg	Gastrointestinal adsorbent	4-8 mL/kg q12h	PO	1800-3600 mL	
Ketamine, *Ketaset, Ketaved, Vetalar,* 100 mg/mL	Anesthesia	1-2 mg/kg for adult; 1 mg/kg for foal	IV	4.5-9 mL **5 mL/50 kg**	Sympathomimetic, may increase blood pressure. *Note:* Controlled substance—schedule III
	Analgesia	0.2 mg/kg q2h 0.01-0.04 mg/kg/min	IV, IM IV CRI	0.9 mL 2.7-10.8 mL/h	May induce muscle tremors and spasticity
		0.8-2.0 mg/kg q1-2h	Epidural	3.6-9 mL	Dilute to 5-10 mL with 0.9% saline
Ketoprofen, *Ketofen,* 100 mg/mL	Analgesia, anti-inflammatory, antipyretic	1.1-2.2 mg/kg q12-24h	IV	5-10 mL	
Lactulose, *Chronulac,* 666 mg/mL	Liver failure, hyperammonemia	0.2 mL/kg q6-12h	PO	60-120 mL (90)	May cause diarrhea, rectal administration may be used

Continued

Equine Emergency Drugs: Approximate Dosages—cont'd

Drug Name, Trade Name,* Conversion Factor	Indication	Dosage	Route	Estimated Dose Per 1000 lb (450 kg)	Precautions and Comments
L-asparaginase	Rescue drug for severe lymphona	200-400 U/kg	IM		Benefits would be short-term No equine data, anaphalaxis may occur
Levamisole, *Ergamisol,* 50 mg	Immunomodulator	2-10 mg/kg q24h	PO	18-90 tabs	Imidazothiazole
Levothyroxine, *Thyro-L,* 12 mg per teaspoon powder	Insulin resistance—related obesity	0.01-0.1 mg/kg q24h	PO	0.5-4 teaspoons	
Lidocaine, *Xylocaine,* 20 mg/mL	Ventricular tachyarrhythmias	0.25-1.0 mg/kg (bolus)	IV slowly	5.6-22.5 mL	For ventricular arrhythmias Excitement, seizures, ataxia may occur if drug is delivered too fast; **DO NOT** exceed 3 mg/kg total dose; NSAIDs may decrease protein binding and increase toxicity. If time interval between discontinuing (DC) lidocaine CRI and starting new CRI >4h, bolus administration of lidocaine recommended
	Systemic analgesia, anti-inflammatory, gastrointestinal ileus	1.3 mg/kg, followed by 0.05 mg/kg per minute	IV slowly IV CRI	30-mL bolus 1.1 mL/min	
	Perineal analgesia	0.2-0.25 mg/kg q1h	Epidural	4-6 mL; overdose may cause paresis of rear legs	
Loperamide, *Imodium,* 2 mg/tab	Antidiarrheal	4-16 mg/foal; then increase by 2-mg increments every 2-3 doses q6h	PO	2-8 tabs	Enhances toxin absorption in cases of acute, infectious enteritis
Lufenuron, *Program*	Fungal infection	5-20 mg/kg q24h	PO		
Magnesium oxide	Hypertension	3-5 g/500 kg	PO		
Magnesium sulfate 50%,† 500 mg/mL, 4 mEq/mL	Ventricular tachyarrhythmia	2.2-5.6 mg/kg/min for 10 min	IV CRI	20-50 mL over 10 min	**DO NOT** exceed 25 g IV total dose May be effective for quinidine-induced tachyarrhythmias
	Hypomagnesemia, reperfusion injury	50-100 mg/kg q24h	IV slowly	50 g	
	Malignant hyperthermia	6 mg/kg	IV	5.6 mL	
	Neonatal maladjustment	20-50 mg/kg over 1 hour followed by 10-25 mg/kg/h CRI	IV CRI	18-45 mL 9-22.5 mL/h	
Magnesium sulfate, Epsom salts	Osmotic cathartic laxative	0.2-1 g/kg diluted in warm water q24h	PO	450 g	**DO NOT** use longer than 3 days to avoid enteritis and magnesium toxicity
Mannan oligosaccharide, *Bio-Mos*	Antidiarrheal	100-200 mg/kg q8-24h	PO		

Equine Emergency Drugs: Approximate Dosages—cont'd

Drug Name, Trade Name,* Conversion Factor	Indication	Dosage	Route	Estimated Dose Per 1000 lb (450 kg)	Precautions and Comments
Mannitol, *Osmitrol,* 200 mg/mL	Cerebral edema, diuresis	0.25-2 g/kg q6-24h	IV slowly over 15-40 min	560-4500 mL	May exacerbate cerebral hemorrhage; examine closely for crystals
Marbofloxacin, *Zeniquin,* 100-mg tabs	Fluoroquinolone antibiotic	2-3 mg/kg 0.67 mg/kg	PO IV (in Europe)	9 tabs	Minimal risk of cartilage damage
Mebendazole (MBZ), *Vermox,* 100 mg/tab	Anthelmintic	8.8 mg/kg	PO	40 tabs	Large and small strongyles
Meclofenamic acid, *Arquel,* 5% dry weight granules	Anti-inflammatory	2.2 mg/kg q12-24h	PO		NSAID
Medetomidine, *Domitor,* 1 mg/mL	Analgesia	5-7 µg/kg q2-4h 3.5 µg/kg/h	IV IV CRI	2.25-3.15 mL 1.5 mL/h	
Meloxicam, *Metacam,* 5 mg/mL; *Mobic,* 15 mg/tab	NSAID (COX-2 selective)	0.6 mg/kg q12h 0.6 mg/kg q24 0.6 mg/kg q12	IV PO PO	54 mL Adult, 18 tabs Foals <7 weeks, 2 tabs	
Meperidine hydrochloride, *Demerol,* 50 mg/mL	Analgesia, sedation	0.55-2.2 mg/kg q4-8h	IV, IM	5-20 mL	IV administration may cause severe hypotension and excitement
Meropenem, *Merrem,* 1 g vials	Antibiotic	10-15 mg/kg q8h	IV	3/4 vial for 50 kg foal	
Metformin, *Fortamet, Glucophage,* 1000-mg tab	Equine metabolic syndrome	15-30 mg/kg q8-12h	PO	6.75-13.5 tabs	May result in hypoglycemia
Methadone, 10 mg/mL	Analgesia	0.1 mg/kg 0.1-0.22 mg/kg	Epidural IV, IM	4.5 mL 9.9 mL	*Note:* Controlled substance—schedule II
l-Methionine, 500-mg tabs	Laminitis	25 mg/kg	PO	22 tabs	
Methocarbamol, *Robaxin-V, Robaxin,* 500 mg/tab, 100 mg/mL	Muscle relaxant	40-60 mg/kg q12-24h 10-25 mg/kg q6h	PO IV	36-54 tabs 45-112 mL	
Methylene blue, 10 mg/mL	Nitrate/nitrite and cyanide toxicities	5-8.8 mg/kg	IV slowly	225-400 mL	
Methylprednisolone sodium succinate, *Solu-Medrol,* 125 mg/mL†	Anti-inflammatory	10-30 mg/kg over 15 min	IV	36-108	Glucocorticoid; for acute CNS injury
Metoclopramide, *Reglan,* 5 mg/mL 1 mg/mL oral solution	Ileus	0.1-0.5 mg/kg q4-8h 0.04 mg/kg/h 0.1-0.6 mg/kg q4-6h	IV slowly over 1 hr or SQ IV CRI PO	9-45 mL 3.6 mL/h 45-270 mL	May produce CNS excitement Start with low dose
Metronidazole, *Flagyl,* 500-mg tabs† 5 mg/mL	Antibiotic, antiprotozoal	15-25 mg/kg q6-8h 10-15 mg/kg q8-12 15-20 mg/kg q8-12h	PO, per rectum PO foals IV	13-22 tabs 1-1.5 tabs/50 kg 1350-1800 mL	Oral administration may result in anorexia Suppository bioavailability is 50% of orally administered drug
Midazolam, *Versed,* 5 mg/mL	Preanesthetic, anticonvulsant, tranquilizer, anxiolytic	0.1-0.2 mg/kg 0.04-0.12 mg/kg/h	IV IV CRI for foals	9-18 mL	*Note:* Controlled substance—schedule IV

Equine Emergency Drugs: Approximate Dosages—cont'd

Drug Name, Trade Name,* Conversion Factor	Indication	Dosage	Route	Estimated Dose Per 1000 lb (450 kg)	Precautions and Comments
Milk of magnesia	Laxative	6-8 L/500 kg	PO		
Milk thistle phospholipid, *Siliphos*	Liver disease	20 mg/kg q12h	PO	9 g	Equivalent to 6.5 mg/kg silibinin, phospholipid formulation increases bioavailability
Milrinone, *Primacor*, 1 mg/mL	Supports ventricular function PDE-3 inhibitor	10 µg/kg/min 0.5-1 mg/kg q12h	IV, short-term treatment	4.5 mL/min	Discontinue if ventricular arrhythmias occur
Mineral oil	Emollient cathartic laxative, liquid GI transit marker	4.5-9 mL/kg	PO via NG intubation	2-4 liters	
Misoprostol, *Cytotec*, 200 µg/tab†	Prevention of NSAID GI ulceration, mucosal protectant	2.5-5 µg/kg q12-24h	PO	5-11 tabs	*DO NOT* use in pregnant horses; *Caution: DO NOT allow pregnant women to handle*
Morphine sulfate, 15 mg/mL	Analgesic	0.05-0.1 mg/kg	IV	1.5-3 mL	Use with xylazine (0.66-1.1 mg/kg IV) or detomidine to avoid CNS excitement
Preservative-free morphine, 25 mg/mL	Epidural analgesic	0.1 mg/kg q24h	Epidural	1.8 mL, add sterile saline to 20 mL total volume	Use preservative-free solution for epidural (this can be compounded at a higher concentration per mL). *Note*: Controlled substance—schedule II
Moxidectin, *Quest*, 20 mg/mL	Anthelmintic	0.4-0.5 mg/kg	PO	9-11.25 mL	*DO NOT use in foals younger than 4 months* Large and small strongyles, large and small strongyle larvae, and ascarids
Nalbuphine, 10 mg/mL	Opioid agonist-antagonist	0.02-0.15 mg/kg	IV, SQ, IM	0.9-6.8 mL	
Naloxone, *Narcan*, 0.4 mg/mL	Opioid antagonist, hemorrhage	0.01-0.03 mg/kg	IV	11.25-33.75 mL	
Naproxen, *Naprosyn*, 100 mg/mL, 500-mg tab	Anti-inflammatory	5 mg/kg 10 mg/kg q12-24h	IV PO	22.5 mL 9 tabs	NSAID
Neomycin, *Biosol*, 50 mg/mL†	Antibiotic for decreasing enteric ammonia production	8-20 mg/kg q8-24h	PO	72-180 mL	Prolonged administration (3-4 doses) or higher doses may cause diarrhea
Neostigmine, *Prostigmin*, 2 mg/mL	Ileus	0.005-0.02 mg/kg q4-6h	SQ, IM	1-4.5 mL	Higher doses may cause increased abdominal pain
Nitazoxanide, *Alinia*, 500 mg/tab	Antiprotozoal	25-50 mg/kg	PO	2.5-5 tabs	For treatment of *Cryptosporidium* in foals

Equine Emergency Drugs: Approximate Dosages—cont'd

Drug Name, Trade Name,* Conversion Factor	Indication	Dosage	Route	Estimated Dose Per 1000 lb (450 kg)	Precautions and Comments
Nitric oxide	Pulmonary hypertension	20-80 ppm, 1:5 to 1:9 ratio with oxygen	Inhalation		
Norepinephrine, 1 mg/mL	Refractory hypotension and anuria	0.05-1 μg/kg/min Up to 5 μg/kg/min	IV CRI (Refractory cases)	1.35-2.7 mL/hr	*DO NOT* exceed 10 μg/kg/min
Octreotide acetate, *Sandostatin,* 200 μg/mL†	Somatostatin analogue	0.5-5.0 μg/kg q6h	SQ	1.1-11.3 mL	
Omeprazole, *Gastrogard, Ulcergard* *Losec,* 2.28 g/tube, 4 mg/1 mL	GI ulceration, proton pump inhibitor	1-4 mg/kg q24h increase gastric pH 0.5 mg/kg q24h	PO IV	0.2-0.8 tube 56 mL	May require 2-3 days to see clinical response *Losec* available in UK, Europe, New Zealand and Australia
Oxfendazole (OFZ), *Benzelmin,* 90.6 mg/mL†	Anthelmintic	10 mg/kg	PO	50 mL	Large and small strongyles, ascarids, and migrating large strongyle larvae
Oxibendazole (OBZ), *Anthelcide,* 100 mg/mL†	Anthelmintic	10-15 mg/kg	PO	45-67.5 mL	Large and small strongyles
Oxymorphone, *Opana,* 1 mg/mL	Narcotic analgesic	0.02-0.03 mg/kg	IV, IM, SQ	9-13.5 mL	*Note:* Controlled substance—schedule II
Oxytetracycline, *LA 200,* 200 mg/mL, 100 mg/mL	Antibiotic Contracted tendons in foals	6.6 mg/kg q12h 30-60 mg/kg 1-3 treatments EOD	IV slowly IV slowly	30 mL (100 mg/mL) 15 mL (200 mg/mL) 15-30 mL/50 kg (100 mg/mL)	Nephrotoxicity Ideally given in saline Monitor renal function during treatment
Oxytocin, 20 IU/mL	Milk letdown, retained fetal membranes Induction of parturition Choke	2.5-20 units/450 kg q4h 75 IU/450 kg 75 IU/450 kg 0.11-0.22 IU/kg	IV, IM, SQ IV over 1 hour OR IM divided into 5 doses IM 10 min apart IV	0.125-1 mL 3-4 mL 2.5-5 mL	Higher doses and IV produce more pain Questionable efficacy
Paromomycin, *Humatin,* 250 mg/tab	Antiprotozoal	100 mg/kg q24h ∞5 days	PO	20 tabs/50 kg	Efficacy unproven in foals; for *Cryptosporidium*
Pectin-kaolin, 4-8 mL/kg	GI adsorbent	4-8 mL/kg q12h	PO	1800-3600 mL	
Penicillamine	Heavy metal toxicosis	3 mg/kg q6h	PO	5.5 tabs	
Penicillin, Na+ or K+, 20,000 IU/mL†	Antibiotic	22,000-44,000 IU/kg q4-6h 4-11 IU/kg/h	IV, IM IV CRI		Higher dosages may be used for clostridial cellulitis; high and continuous dosage may lead to potassium overdose, especially in renal insufficiency

Continued

Equine Emergency Drugs: Approximate Dosages—cont'd

Drug Name, Trade Name,* Conversion Factor	Indication	Dosage	Route	Estimated Dose Per 1000 lb (450 kg)	Precautions and Comments
Penicillin, procaine, 300,000 IU/mL	Antibiotic	15,000-44,000 IU/kg q12h	IM	22.5-66 mL	
Pentastarch	Colloid	1-10 mL/kg	IV	450-4500 mL	
Pentazocine, *Talwin,* 30 mg/mL	Analgesia	0.3-0.6 mg/kg	PO, IV	4.5-9 mL	
Pentobarbital, *Beuthanasia-D,* 390 mg/mL See also Beuthanasia, p. 838	Anticonvulsant, anesthesia Euthanasia	3-10 mg/kg 85 mg/kg	IV IV	3.5-11.5 mL 98 mL	To effect for sedation/seizure control and humane destruction. *Note:* Controlled substance—schedule III
Pentoxifylline, *Trental,* 400 mg/tab	Endotoxemia, laminitis, vasodilator, rheologic agent, hepatitis, renal disease	7.5-10 mg/kg q8-12h	PO, IV	8-11 tabs	Can be prepared for IV use
Pergolide, *Prascend,* 1.0 mg/tab	Pituitary pars intermedia hyperplasia	0.0017-0.01 mg/kg q24h	PO	1 tab	
Perphenazine, *Trilafon,* 16 mg/tab	Fescue toxicity	0.3-0.5 mg/kg q8h	PO	3-14 tabs	
Phenazopyridine, *Pyridium,* 100, 200 mg/tab	Urinary irritation, urethritis	4-10 mg/kg q8-12h	PO	9 tabs (200 mg) 18 tabs (100 mg)	Expect urinary discoloration
Phenobarbital, 100-mg tablets, 130 mg/mL	Anticonvulsant, dopamine antagonist	2-10 mg/kg q8-12h Higher doses may be needed	PO	9-45 tabs	Respiratory depression, hypotension; monitor serum levels (10-40 µg/mL); clinical response may occur at 10 µg/mL
		5-15 mg/kg	IV slowly	17-52 mL	IV for seizure control; controlled substance—schedule IV
		2-3 mg/kg/foals	IV slowly over 15-20 min	0.4-0.8 mL/50 kg	
Phenoxybenzamine, *Dibenzyline,* 10 mg/cap	Laminitis, diarrhea, decrease urethral sphincter tone	0.4 mg/kg q6h	PO	18 caps	
Phenylbutazone, *Butazolidin,* etc., 1 g/tab, 200 mg/mL	Anti-inflammatory, analgesic, antipyretic	2.2-4.4 mg/kg q12h	PO, IV	5-10 mL 1-2 tabs	Perivascular injection may cause necrosis, use only if well hydrated
Phenylephrine hydrochloride, *Neo-Synephrine,* 10 mg/mL	Nephrosplenic colonic entrapment Hypotension Nasal, pharyngeal hemorrhage and edema Priapism	3 µg/kg/min for 15 min 0.2-1.0 µg/kg/min 10 mg diluted to 10 mL for nasal spray 5-20 mg into corpus cavernosum	IV IV CRI Intranasal	2 mL diluted in 1 L NaCl over 15 min 0.5-2 mL	Contracts spleen, increases vascular resistance, bradyarrhythmias and serious hemorrhage may result; perivascular injections may cause necrosis
Phenylpropanolamine, *Prion,* 25, 50, and 75 mg/tab†	Bladder atony, urethral sphincter hypotonus	0.5-2 mg/kg q8-12h	PO	4.5-18 tabs (50 mg)	

Equine Emergency Drugs: Approximate Dosages—cont'd

Drug Name, Trade Name,* Conversion Factor	Indication	Dosage	Route	Estimated Dose Per 1000 lb (450 kg)	Precautions and Comments
Phenytoin, *Dilantin,* 50 mg/mL†	Anticonvulsant, digoxin toxicity, supraventricular tachyarrhythmias	5-20 mg/kg (first 12 hours)	IV	4.5-180 mL slowly IV over 1+ hours	Sedation, drowsiness, lip and facial twitching, gait deficits
		20 mg/kg q12h × 3, followed by 10-15 mg/kg until conversion	PO	90 caps (load), 45-68 maintenance	
100-mg cap†	Stringhalt, chronic intermittent exertional rhabdomyolysis prophylaxis	2-7.5 mg/kg q12h	PO	9-33 caps	Erratic absorption may cause weakness; therapeutic levels 5 µg/mL; toxic 10 µg/mL
Physostigmine, 1 mg/mL	Atropine toxicity	0.6 mg/kg	IV	270 mL	Cholinesterase inhibitor
	Diagnostic induction of narcoleptic episode	0.06-0.08 mg/kg	IV	27-36 mL	Variable response as a diagnostic test
Pioglitazone, *Actos,* 15-, 20-, and 45-mg tablets	Equine metabolic syndrome	1 mg/kg q24h	PO	10 tablets/45-mg tablets	Plasma concentration lower and more variable to those considered therapeutic in humans
Piperazine (PPZ)	Anthelmintic	110 mg/kg	PO		
Piroxicam, *Feldene,* 10-mg cap	Carcinomas	80-100 mg q24h per adult horse	PO	8-10 caps	Larger capsules can be formulated
Polymyxin B, 500,000 U/ vial (10,000 U = 1 mg)	Antibiotic, endotoxemia	1000-6000 U/kg q8-12h	IV slowly diluted	2.7 million units or 5 vials	Check renal function
Ponazuril, *Marquis*	Antiprotozoal (for EPM)	5-10 mg/kg q24h 15 mg/kg loading dose	PO		28-day course of treatment recommended
Potassium bromide, 250 mg/mL	Anticonvulsant	25-90 mg/kg q24h	PO or IV	45-162 mL	
Potassium chloride, (KCl), 2 mEq/mL	Hypokalemia	1 mEq/kg	IC	225 mL	For ventricular fibrillation *only* if electrical defibrillation **NOT** available
		0.1-0.5 mEq/kg/h 0.1 g/kg	IV PO	22.5-112.5 mL 300 mL	***DO NOT*** exceed 0.5 mEq KCl/kg/h
Pralidoxime (2-PAM), 300 mg/mL†	Organophosphate toxicity	20 mg/kg q4-6h	IV	30 mL	Not effective for carbamate toxicity
Praziquantel, *Droncit,* 34 mg tabs	Pyrazino isoquinoline	1.5 mg/kg	PO	20 tabs (34 mg)	Lethal to tapeworm parasites
Prednisolone, *Delta- Cortef,* 20 mg/tab†	Anti-inflammatory	0.4-1.6 mg/kg q24h	PO	9-36 tabs	Anti-inflammatory
Prednisolone sodium succinate, *Solu-Delta Cortef,* 500 mg/vial (50 mg/mL), 100 mg/ vial (10 mg/mL)	Inflammatory shock Shock, cerebral edema	2-5 mg/kg 10 mg/kg q6h	IV IV	18-45 mL/ 50 mg/mL conc 90 mL/50 mg/ mL conc	
Pregabalin, 300 mg capsule	Neuropathic pain	2-4 mg/kg q8h	PO	3-6 capsules	Bioavailability near 100%

Continued

Equine Emergency Drugs: Approximate Dosages—cont'd

Drug Name, Trade Name,* Conversion Factor	Indication	Dosage	Route	Estimated Dose Per 1000 lb (450 kg)	Precautions and Comments
Procainamide, *Pronestyl,* 100 mg/mL	Supraventricular tachyarrhythmia	1 mg/kg/min	IV CRI	4.5 mL/min	***DO NOT*** exceed 20 mg/kg IV total dose, may induce hypotension
		25-35 mg/kg q8h	PO	22.5-31.5 tabs	GI, neurologic signs are similar to those of quinidine
Progesterone (in oil) compounded	Suppression of estrus, maintenance of pregnancy	0.8 mg/kg q24h	IM		For pregnant mares experiencing endotoxemia or premature separation of placenta; compounded product for injection
Propafenone, *Rythmol,* 300 mg caps	Supraventricular and ventricular tachyarrhythmias	0.5-1 mg/kg in 5% dextrose (slowly to effect over 5-8 min)	IV		GI, neurologic signs similar to those with quinidine; bronchospasm
		2 mg/kg q8h	PO	3 caps (300 mg)	
Propantheline bromide	Smooth muscle relaxant assist in rectal procedures	0.067 mg/kg	IV		
Propofol, *Diprivan, Rapinovet,* 10 mg/mL	Anesthesia	2-4 mg/kg	IV after tranquilization	90-180 mL 22.5 mL with ketamine and α-agonist	Respiratory depression may occur Can Rx with doxapram
Propranolol, *Inderal,* 1 mg/mL, 160 mg tabs	Ventricular tachycardia, beta-blocker	0.03-0.05 mg/kg 0.38-0.78 mg/kg q8h	IV PO	13.5-22.5 mL 1-2 tabs (160 mg)	Lethargy, worsening of COPD
Psyllium hydrophilic mucilloid, *Metamucil,* 400 g/kg†	Bulk laxative, sand colic	0.25-0.9 g/kg q6-12h	PO	113-405 g	Mix in cold water to prevent gel formation!
Pyrantel pamoate (PRT), 50 mg/mL	Anthelmintic	6.6-13.2 mg/kg	PO	60-120 mL	Large and small strongyles and tapeworm parasites
Pyrilamine maleate, *Histavet-P*	Hives, allergic dermatitis	1 mg/kg q12h 0.44 mg/kg foals	IV slowly, IM, SQ		IV administration may cause CNS signs
Pyrimethamine, *Daraprim,* 25 mg/tab	Antiprotozoal (for EPM)	1-2 mg/kg q24h	PO	18-36 tabs	
Quinapril, *Accupril,* 40-mg tab	Angiotensin-converting enzyme inhibitor	0.25-0.5 mg/kg q24h	PO	3-6 tabs	Low bioavailability; decreases ACE inhibition by 50%
Quinidine gluconate, 80 mg/mL	Atrial fibrillation, supraventricular and ventricular tachyarrhythmias	0.5-2.2 mg/kg (bolus every 10 min to effect)	IV	2.8-12.3 mL	***DO NOT*** exceed 12 mg/kg IV total dose; depression, paraphimosis, urticaria, wheals, nasal mucosal swelling, laminitis, neurologic, GI effects

Equine Emergency Drugs: Approximate Dosages—cont'd

Drug Name, Trade Name,* Conversion Factor	Indication	Dosage	Route	Estimated Dose Per 1000 lb (450 kg)	Precautions and Comments
Quinidine sulfate, *Quinidex,* 300 mg/tab†	Atrial fibrillation	20-22 mg/kg q2h until converted, toxic, or plasma quinidine concentration >4 µg/mL; often 3× q2h doses, then continue q6h until converted or toxic signs begin	NG tube	30-33 tabs	*DO NOT* exceed 6 doses q2h; depression, paraphimosis, urticaria, wheals, nasal mucosal swelling, laminitis, neurologic, GI effects
Ranitidine, *Zantac,* 300 mg/tab 25 mg/mL	Gastroduodenal ulceration H₂-receptor antagonist	6.6 mg/kg q6-8h 0.9-1.5 mg/kg q6-8h	PO IV, IM	10 tabs 16-27 mL	
Rifampin, *Rifadin,* 300 mg/tab	Antibiotic	5-10 mg/kg q12h	PO	7.5-15 tabs	Concurrent administration may interfere with macrolide bioavailability Hepatotoxic when used with doxycycline
Rimantadine, *Flumadine,* 100-mg tab	Antiviral	30 mg/kg q12h	PO	135 tabs	
Romifidine, *Sedivet,* 10 mg/mL	Analgesia, sedative Preanesthetic	0.04-0.12 mg/kg q2-4h 0.1 mg/kg	IV, IM IV	1.8-5.4 mL 4.5 mL	Duration of sedation is approximately 1 hour at lower end of dose range
Ropivacaine	Analgesia	0.8 mg/kg q3-4h	Epidural		
S-adenosylmethionine, SAM-e, *Denosyl,* 425-mg tab	Hepatic disease, cholestasis	10-20 mg/kg q24h	PO	10.5-21 tabs	
Salbutamol, 100 µg/puff	Bronchodilator, short acting	1-2 µg/kg q8-12h	Inhaler	5-10 puffs	
Saline solution, hypertonic, 5% or 7%	Shock, hypotension, cerebral trauma	4-5 mL/kg	IV	1800-2250 mL	Follow with isotonic fluid therapy
Salmeterol, *Serevent,* 50 µg/puff†	Bronchodilator, long acting	0.5 µg/kg q12h	Inhaler	4-5 puffs	Long-acting bronchodilator
Sarmazenil	Moxidectin toxicity	0.04 mg/kg	IV		Multiple treatments may be required
Selenium–vitamin E, *E-Se,* 2.5 mg Se and 68 U vitamin E per mL	Selenium and vitamin E deficiency	1 mL/100 lb (45 kg)	IM only	10 mL	*IV administration can cause death*
Sildenafil citrate, *Viagra,* 25-mg tab, 100-mg tab	Pulmonary hypertension	0.2-0.6 mg/kg q4-8h	PO	0.4-1.2 tabs (25 mg)/50 kg	Phosphodiesterase inhibitor; *DO NOT* use if patient has hypotension
Sodium bicarbonate, 1 mEq/mL 8.4%	Metabolic acidosis, hyperkalemia Quinidine toxicity	Variable according to base deficit (see Appendix 2, Calculations in Emergency Care) 0.5-1.0 mEq/kg	IV, PO IV		*DO NOT* use if patient has respiratory acidosis

Continued

Equine Emergency Drugs: Approximate Dosages—cont'd

Drug Name, Trade Name,* Conversion Factor	Indication	Dosage	Route	Estimated Dose Per 1000 lb (450 kg)	Precautions and Comments
Sodium hyaluronate solution 0.4%, *Sepracoat*	Adhesion preventative	2 mL/kg	Intraperitoneal	1 liter	
Sodium iodide, 200 mg/mL	Actinobacillosis	100 mg/kg q24h	IV	225-250 mL	
		20-40 mg/kg q24h	PO		
Sodium nitrate 1%, 10 mg/mL	Cyanide toxicity	16 mg/kg	IV	720 mL	
Sodium thiosulfate, 300 mg/mL	Cyanide and arsenic toxicity	30-500 mg/kg	IV slowly	45-750 mL	
Sotalol, *Betapace,* 160 mg/tab	To slow ventricular rate	2.5-4 mg/kg q24h	PO	7-11 tabs	Depresses atrial activity following atrial fib conversion
Succinylcholine, 20 mg/mL†	Neuromuscular blocker Muscle relaxation	0.1 mg/kg	IV	2.25 mL	Sometimes used with euthanasia solution to prevent "paddling"
Sucralfate, *Carafate,* 1 g/tab	GI ulceration	20-40 mg/kg q6-8h	PO	9-18 tabs 1-2 tabs for foals	*DO NOT* give within 1-2 hours of other oral medication
Telithromycin, *Ketex,* 400-mg tab	*Rhodococcus* infection	15 mg/kg q12-24h	PO	17 tabs	Reserve for resistant *R. equi*
Terbutaline, *Brethine,* 5 mg/tab	Bronchial, vascular dilator	0.04-0.13 mg/kg q8-12h	PO	3.5-11 tabs	
Thiabendazole (TBZ)	Benzimidazole	50-100 mg/kg	PO		
Thiamine, 200 mg/mL	Thiamine deficiency, lead poisoning, CNS injury, bracken intoxication	1-10 mg/kg q12-24h	IV, IM	2.25-22.5 mL	
Thiopental sodium, 20 mg/mL	General anesthesia, barbiturate	3-10 mg/kg	IV	67.5-225 mL	*Note:* Controlled substance—schedule III, not available in many countries
Thyrotropin-releasing hormone	CNS injury, dysmature lung, Cushing's testing	1 mg all ages	IV		
Ticarcillin, *Ticar*	Antibiotic	50 mg/kg q6h	IV, IM		
Ticarcillin-clavulanate, *Timentin* 3.1 and 31 g/vial	Antibiotic	50 mg/kg q6h	IV	Loading dose: 1.5 vials (31-g vial), maintenance: 0.75 vial (31-g vial)	High loading dose may be used in foals (100 mg/kg)
Tiletamine and zolazepam, *Telazol,* 100 mg/mL	Anesthesia	1.1-2.2 mg/kg	IV	5-10 mL	*Note:* Controlled substance—schedule III
Tiludronate, *Equidronate,* 5 mg/mL	Inhibits osteoclast-mediated bone resorption	0.1-1 mg/kg	IV slowly	9-90 mL	Dilute before administration May cause colic, acute renal failure
Tissue plasminogen activator (tPA), *Alteplase*	Thrombolytic	4-16 mg	Intrapleural/pericardial	Dilute in 1 liter saline	Also used for some hyphemas

Equine Emergency Drugs: Approximate Dosages—cont'd

Drug Name, Trade Name,* Conversion Factor	Indication	Dosage	Route	Estimated Dose Per 1000 lb (450 kg)	Precautions and Comments
Tolazoline, *Tolazine,* 100 mg/mL	α_2-Antagonist	0.5-2 mg/kg	IV slowly	2.25-9 mL	Occasional serious reactions; rapid administration of labeled dose may cause hypotension, cardiac arrhythmias, and death
Toltrazuril, *Baycox*		10 mg/kg q24h	PO		**NOT** approved for horses
Tramadol, *Ultram,* 50 mg/mL, 50-mg tab	Analgesia	1 mg/kg q6h 4 mg/kg 10 mg/kg	Epidural IV PO	9 mL 4 mL/50 kg 10 tabs/50 kg	Nonopiate μ-agonist Short T 1/2
Tranexamic acid, *Cyklokapron, Lysteda,* 100 mg/mL, 650-mg tab	Control of hemorrhage	10 mg/kg q8-12h 20 mg/kg q6h	IV slowly PO	45 mL 14 tabs	
Trilostane, *Vetoryl,* 120 mg cap	Equine metabolic syndrome	0.5-1 mg/kg q24h	PO	2-4 caps	
Trimethoprim-sulfadiazine,† *Uniprim, Tribrissen,* 960-mg (1:5) tabs,† 480 mg/mL (1:5)†	Antibiotic	20-30 mg/kg q12h	PO, IV	10-14 tabs 19-28 mL	**DO NOT** use if patient has ileus; **DO NOT** administer IV after detomidine
Tripelennamine HCl, *Trienamine, Re-Covr,*† 20 mg/mL	Antihistamine	1 mg/kg q6-12h	IM	22 mL	**DO NOT** give IV
Triple Drip: See Guaifenesin (GG), p. 847					
Tromethamine	Buffer	0.55 mmol/kg/h	IV CRI		
Ursodiol, 500 mg/tab	Cholestatic disease	15 mg/kg q24	PO SID	13.5 tabs	
Valacyclovir, *Valtrex,* 500-mg tabs	Antiviral (herpes)	22-30 mg/kg q8-12h for 2 days, then 18 mg/kg q12h	PO	20-27 tabs	Prodrug of acyclovir with improved bioavailability (30%)
Vancomycin, *Vancosin,* 50 mg/mL when reconstituted (then further diluted)	For amikacin-resistant MRSA, 7.5 mg/kg q8h 300 mg in 60 mL saline	IV IVRP	67.5 mL (50 mg/mL) then dilute further	**Reserve for amikacin-resistant MRSA**
Vasopressin, Arginine (ADH), 20 units/mL	Pressor, diabetes insipidus	0.05-0.8 IU/kg 0.0005-0.001 IU/kg/min	IV IV CRI	1.1-18 mL 0.7-1.35 mL/h	
Vedaprofen	NSAID	1 mg/kg q24h	IV		
Verapamil, 2.5 mg/mL	Supraventricular tachyarrhythmia	0.025-0.05 mg/kg every 30 min	IV	4.5-9 mL	**DO NOT** exceed 0.2 mg/kg IV total dose
Vincristine, *Oncovin,* 1 mg/mL	Immune thrombocytopenia, chemotherapeutic	0.005-0.02 mg/kg	IV	2.25-9 mL	*Give only* 2 treatments 3 days apart

Continued

Equine Emergency Drugs: Approximate Dosages—cont'd

Drug Name, Trade Name,* Conversion Factor	Indication	Dosage	Route	Estimated Dose Per 1000 lb (450 kg)	Precautions and Comments
Vitamin B complex, 100-mL vial	Nutrient	q24h	IV, IM	10-20 mL	
Vitamin C, Ascorbic acid 1 g/tab, 250 mg/mL	Antioxidant, urinary acidifier	0.2-1 g/kg q24h / 30 mg/kg q12-24h	PO / IV	90-450 tabs	Give slowly IV
Vitamin E, *Aquasol E,* 1000 U/cap†	Nutrient / Vitamin E deficiency, equine motor neuron disease, equine degenerative myeloencephalopathy prophylaxis and treatment	6.6 IU/kg / 10-20 IU/kg q24h	IM / PO	10 mL / 5-10 caps	Controls lipid peroxidation
Vital E-300, 300 U/mL	Acute neurologic injury	2000 IU/adult (once)	IM	7 mL	After initial treatment, switch to oral administration if possible
Vitamin K₁, phytonadione, *Veda-K1,* 10 mg/mL	Rodenticide (warfarin) toxicity	0.5-2 mg/kg	SQ, IM	22.5-90 mL	**DO NOT** administer IV
Voriconazole, *Vfend,* 200 mg caps	Antifungal	3-4 mg/kg q12-24h	PO	7-9 caps	Ophthalmic 0.5-1% q2-6h topical in eye
Xylazine hydrochloride, *Rompun, Sedazine,* 100 mg/mL	Restraint, sedation, preanesthetic, analgesia	0.2-1.1 mg/kg q8-12h	IV slowly, IM	1-5 mL	May cause tachypnea when given to febrile patients, may cause aggression
		0.17 mg/kg	Epidural	0.8 mL, dilute to 10 mL (saline)	Combined with morphine or lidocaine
Yohimbine, *Antagonil, Yocon,* 2 mg/mL	α₂-Antagonist	0.075-0.12 mg/kg	IV slowly	17-27 mL	Tachycardia
Yunnan baiyao, 250-mg capsule, powder	Hemostatic agent	10 mg/kg q8h	PO	18 capsules	Red pills, more concentrated = 16 capsules; 16 capsules per packet, containing 4 g total; Can apply topically to hemorrhage site

ACE, Angiotensin converting enzyme; *ACTH,* adrenocorticotropic hormone; *ARDS,* acute respiratory distress syndrome; *AV,* atrioventricular; *CNS,* central nervous system; *COPD,* chronic obstructive pulmonary disease; *COX,* cyclooxygenase; *CPCR,* cardiopulmonary cerebral resuscitation; *CRI,* constant rate infusion; *D₅W,* 5% dextrose solution; *EOD,* every other day; *EPM,* equine protozoal myelitis; *GI,* gastrointestinal; *HYPP,* hyperkalemic periodic paralysis; *IC,* intracardiac; *IM,* intramuscular; *IT,* intratracheal; *IV,* intravenous; *IVRP,* intravenous regional perfusion; *MRSA,* methicillin-resistant *Staphylococcus aureus*; *NG,* nasogastric; *NSAID,* nonsteroidal anti-inflammatory drug; *PDA,* patent ductus arteriosus; *PO,* by mouth; *PRN,* as necessary; *PVC,* polyvinyl chloride; *RBC,* red blood cell; *RP,* regional perfusion; *SIRS,* systemic inflammatory response syndrome; *SQ,* subcutaneous; *T 1/2,* drug half-time; *Vtach,* ventricular tachycardia.

*Italics indicate trade name.
†Other products and concentrations are available.

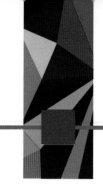

Index

Emergency Drug Charts*

Foal

Drug	Dosage per kg	Concentration	mL/kg	Dose mL/50 kg
Atropine[†]	0.02 mg	*0.54 mg/mL*	0.04	2.0
Beuthanasia solution	0.2-0.3 mL 58-87 mg	290 mg/mL	0.2-0.3	10-15 mL
Calcium[‡] borogluconate	150-250 mg	230 mg/mL	0.65-1.1	33-55
CaCl[‡]	20 mg	100 mg/mL (10%)	0.2	10
Defibrilation	2-4 jules (J)			100-200 J
Diazepan	0.1 mg	5 mg/mL	0.02	1.0
Doxapram	0.2-1.0 mg	20 mg/mL	0.01-0.05	0.5-2.5
Epinephrine *high* dose	0.1-0.2 mg	1 mg/mL	0.1-0.2	5-10
Epinephrine *low* dose	0.01-0.02 mg	1 mg/mL	0.01-0.02	0.5-1
Furosemide	1 mg	50 mg/mL	0.02	1.0
Glucose	50 mg[§]	10% 100 mg/mL	0.5 (initial bolus)	25
Glycopyrrolate	0.001-0.005 mg	0.2 mg/mL	0.005-0.025	0.25-1.25
Lidocaine	1.5 mg	2% 20 mg/mL	0.075	3.75
MgSO$_4$	25-50 mg	50% 500 mg/mL	0.05-0.1	2.5-5
NaHCO$_3$[‖]	0.5-1.0 mEq	1 mEq/mL	0.5-1.0	25-50
Norepinephrine	0.001-0.002 mg/kg	1 mg/mL	0.001-0.002	0.05-0.1
Vasopressin	0.4 U	20 U/ml	0.02	1.0

*Eileen Sullivan Hackett, DVM, PhD, Diplomate ACVS, and ACVECC.
[†]There are **two** concentrations of atropine sulfate for injection.
[‡]Slow administration over 10 minutes.
[§]50 mg/kg is followed by 4 to 8 mg/kg/min of a 10% solution.
[‖]Not routinely recommended; only when severe metabolic acidosis is suspected and adequate ventilation is established.

Adult

Drug	Dosage per kg	Concentration	mL/kg	Dose mL/450 kg
Atropine	0.01-0.02 mg	*15 mg/mL*	0.0006-0.001	0.3-0.45
Beuthanasia solution	0.2-0.3 mL 58-87 mg	290 mg/mL	0.2-0.3	~100-150
Calcium borogluconate	150-250 mg	230 mg/mL	0.65-1.1	293-495
CaCl[†]	20 mg	100 mg/mL (10%)	0.2	90
Digoxin	0.003-0.005	0.25 mg/mL	0.012-0.02	5.4-9.0
Epinephrine	0.02	1 mg/mL	0.02	9.0
Furosemide	1 mg	50 mg/mL	0.02	9.0
Glycopyrrolate	0.001-0.005 mg	0.2 mg/mL	0.005-0.025	2.25-11.25
Hyperonic saline	0.144-0.288 g NaCl	7.2%	2.0-4.0	1000-2000
Lidocaine	1.5 mg	20 (2%)	0.075	33.75
Mannitol	250-1000 mg	20% 200 mg/mL	1.3-4.7	~560-2250
MgSO$_4$	25-50 mg	50% 500 mg/mL	0.05-0.1	22.5-45
NaHCO$_3$*	0.5-1.0 mEq	1 mEq/mL (8.4%)	0.5-1.0	225-450

*Not routinely recommended; only when severe metabolic acidosis is suspected and adequate ventilation is established.
[†]Slow administration over 10 minutes.